Contemporary Fixed Prosthodontics

Contemporary Fixed Prosthodontics

Third Edition with 2800 illustrations

STEPHEN F. ROSENSTIEL, BDS, MSD
Professor and Chair
Section of Restorative Dentistry
Prosthodontics and Endodontics
The Ohio State University College of Dentistry
Columbus, Ohio

MARTIN F. LAND, DDS, MSD
Professor and Chair
Department of Restorative Dentistry
Southern Illinois University
School of Dental Medicine
Alton, Illinois

JUNHEI FUJIMOTO, DDS, MSD, DDSc
Part-Time Lecturer, Tokyo Medical and Dental University
Director of J.F. Occlusion and Prosthodontic
   Postgraduate Course
Private Practice, Tokyo, Japan

Artwork for Third Edition by
DONALD O'CONNOR
Medical Illustrator
St. Peters, Missouri

Artwork for Second Edition by
SANDRA CELLO-LANG
Bio-Medical Illustrator
Chicago, Illinois

SUE E. COTTRILL
Medical Illustrator
Chicago, Illinois

KERRIE MARZO
Medical Illustrator
Chicago Heights, Illinois

Artwork for First Edition by
KRYSTYNA SRODULSKI
Medical Illustrator
San Antonio, Texas

Photographic Services by
JAMES COCKERILL, RBP
Medical and Dental Photographer
Oak Park, Illinois

Editor-in-Chief: John Schrefer
Editor: Penny Rudolph
Developmental Editor: Kimberly Frare
Project Manager: Linda McKinley
Production Editor: Rich Barber
Designer: Kathi Gosche

THIRD EDITION

Permissions may be sought directly from Elsevier's Health Sciences Rights
Department in Philadelphia, PA, USA: phone: (+1) 215 239 3804, fax: (+1) 215 239 3805,
e-mail: healthpermissions@elsevier.com. You may also complete your request on-line
via the Elsevier homepage (http://www.elsevier.com), by selecting 'Customer Support'
and then 'Obtaining Permissions'.

Printed in the United States of America

Mosby, Inc.
An Affiliate of Elsevier
11830 Westline Industrial Drive
St. Louis, Missouri 63146

Library of Congress Cataloging in Publication Data

ISBN-13:978-0-8151-5559-1
ISBN-10:0-8151-5559-X

05 / 9 8 7 6 5

CONTRIBUTORS

ROBERT F. BAIMA, DDS
Associate Professor
Department of Periodontology and Dental Hygiene,
Restorative Dentistry
The University of Detroit Mercy
School of Dentistry
Detroit, Michigan

WILLIAM A. BRANTLEY, PhD
Professor and Director of the Graduate Program in Dental
Materials
Section of Restorative Dentistry, Prosthodontics
and Endodontics
The Ohio State University
College of Dentistry
Columbus, Ohio

ISABELLE L. DENRY, DDS, PhD
Associate Professor
Section of Restorative Dentistry, Prosthodontics
and Endodontics
The Ohio State University
College of Dentistry
Columbus, Ohio

ROBERT DUANE DOUGLAS, DMD, MS
Assistant Professor and Section Head Fixed Prosthodontics
Department of Restorative Dentistry
Southern Illinois University
School of Dental Medicine
Alton, Illinois

MARTIN A. FREILICH, DDS
Associate Professor
Department of Prosthodontics
University of Connecticut Health Center
Farmington, Connecticut

ANTHONY GEGAUFF
Associate Professor
Section of Restorative Dentistry, Prosthodontics and
Endodontics
The Ohio State University
College of Dentistry
Columbus, Ohio

A. JON GOLDBERG, PhD
Associate Department of Prosthodontics
Director Center for Biomaterials
University of Connecticut Health Center
Farmington, Connecticut

JULIE A. HOLLOWAY, DDS, MS
Associate Professor, Prosthodontics
Section of Restorative Dentistry, Prosthodontics
and Endodontics
The Ohio State University
College of Dentistry
Columbus, Ohio

WILLIAM M. JOHNSTON, PhD
Professor
Section of Restorative Dentistry, Prosthodontics
and Endodontics
The Ohio State University
College of Dentistry
Columbus, Ohio

PETER E. LARSEN, DDS
Professor and Chairman
Section of Oral and Maxillofacial Surgery
The Ohio State University
College of Dentistry
Columbus, Ohio

LEON W. LAUB, PhD
Manager of Engineering/Product Manager
Rocky Mountain Orthodontics, Inc.
Denver, Colorado

EDWIN A. McGLUMPHY, DDS, MS
Associate Professor
Section of Restorative Dentistry, Prosthodontics
and Endodontics
The Ohio State University
College of Dentistry
Columbus, Ohio

DONALD A. MILLER, DDS, MS
Private Practice Limited to Endodontics
Diplomate, American Board of Endodontics
Joliet, Illinois

JAMES L. SANDRIK, PhD
Assistant to Associate Executive Director,
Division of Science
American Dental Association
Chicago, Illinois

VAN THOMPSON, DDS, PhD
Professor of Prosthodontics and Biomaterials
Department of Prosthodontics and Biomaterials
University of Medicine and Dentistry of New Jersey
Newark, New Jersey

PREFACE

"The 'odd' editions, the first, the third, fifth and so on, are the toughest . . . by the time you get to a third edition, your specialty will have changed sufficiently that you will be forced to completely rethink the organization of your book" an experienced textbook author told us several years ago. He was absolutely right. Since 1988 and 1995, when the first and second editions of Contemporary Fixed Prosthodontics were published, our field has indeed evolved beyond previously predictable expectations. Many of the changes are driven by technological developments and newly available materials. Some, because the practice of dentistry has experienced changes in the demand for certain services. Throughout the process of formulating this new edition, we have sought to make the text more readable for the dental student while maintaining the core format previously so well received. Concurrently, every effort was made to maintain the in-depth comprehensive content for the established practitioner, graduate student, and researcher.

It remains a difficult task to achieve the best balance between comprehensive incorporation of current needs as driven by changes in the undergraduate dental curriculum, while continuing to provide the reader with comprehensive and clinically relevant information about as broad an array of topics and techniques. Some dental schools aim to de-emphasize student involvement in laboratory procedures, yet we firmly believe that, although few beginning dentists will achieve proficiency with the increasingly complicated laboratory steps, each graduate must have a thorough understanding of how dental prostheses are fabricated so he or she can exercise sound clinical judgment and decision making. Also, the dental profession must have ready access to a comprehensive reference that enables rapid retrieval of integrated and relevant information. Thus, one of our challenges was to maintain the comprehensive nature of the provided information, while subtly restructuring content so both novice and experienced practitioners can take full advantage with minimal digression to related but less than critical information.

ORGANIZATION

This edition retains the previous four-section format: Planning and Preparation; Clinical Procedures Part I; Laboratory Procedures, and Clinical Procedures Part II. Pertinent basic sciences continue to be presented throughout and are integrated with applicable content.

We are particularly grateful for the constructive comments and suggestions received from a large number of our colleagues who were kind enough to take the time to conduct an in-depth review of the text, and to comment and respond to a lengthy list of specific questions. Their recommendations to address specific issues, not adequately covered previously, helped considerably in formulating the initial template for this revision.

NEW TO THIS EDITION

Content and references were thoroughly updated throughout, and glossaries consistent with the most recent edition of *The Glossary of Prosthodontics Terms* were added to provide the reader with lists of terminology relevant to the chapter topics. Selected key words are listed at the beginning of the chapters, to facilitate rapid information retrieval. Also, essay format Study Questions were added to provide the student an opportunity to test his or her knowledge and comprehension after reading a chapter.

Section I. This section now consists of six chapters, the previous chapter on "History, Examination, Diagnosis and Prognosis" having been divided into two separate chapters: "History Taking and Clinical Examination" and "Diagnostic Casts and Related Procedures." The section now includes additional step-by-step sequences of photographs of commonly performed diagnostic procedures and new artwork to clarify hinge axis location and border movements.

Section II. The tooth preparation chapters in Section II were revised; new artwork was generated for inlays, onlays, and metal-ceramic preparations;

and content was thoroughly updated, in particular for all-ceramic restorations. The Implant chapter was comprehensively revised to be current with new developments in implant prosthodontics, as was the chapter on Provisional Restorations.

Section III. In an effort to emphasize the importance of the mutual collaboration between dentist and technician, Section III now begins with the chapter on Laboratory Communication. In addition to the many new illustrations throughout the section, for example those on occlusal waxing, the chapter on Pontic Design underwent an in-depth revision. It now includes emphasis on ridge shape and contour of the edentulous site, pontic classification, and various more contemporary techniques than the ones previously presented.

Similarly, the chapter on All-Ceramic Restoration Fabrication was again updated to incorporate the most recent developments and techniques. A section on esthetic considerations was added to the Color Science chapter, and a chapter on Fiber-Reinforced Composite Fixed Prostheses follows the comprehensively rewritten chapter on Resin-Retained Fixed Partial Dentures.

Section IV. This section now includes, among others, a more detailed discussion on luting agents, in an effort to make sense out of the myriad of choices confronting the practitioner when attempting to select the appropriate luting agents for various fixed prosthodontic procedures. The treatment presentations now include additional long-term follow up on simple and complex fixed prosthodontic treatments, emphasizing the goal of longevity when planning fixed prostheses.

GIVING CREDIT WHERE CREDIT IS DUE

After three editions, it is difficult, if not impossible, to be 100 percent accurate and complete in crediting all sources of information, ideas, illustrations, photographs, and concepts. Without the selfless help and support of so many others, we could not have managed this overwhelming task. Once again, whenever we approached colleagues, friends, and manufacturers, our requests for permission to include materials were invariably most kindly approved. Throughout, we have made every effort to correctly identify all sources and individuals who helped us bring this mammoth undertaking to a successful completion. We apologize for any omissions, which are certainly unintentional, and for which we are solely responsible.

ACKNOWLEDGMENTS

A special thank you to . . .

All those who contributed unselfishly to make this text better through donation of their time, energy, pictures, concepts for illustrations, or clinical photos.

Our reviewers who took time out of their busy schedules to provide input and suggestions to incorporate in this edition: Drs. Ralph DeLong, University of Minnesota; Ira Gulker, New York University; Ronald Gunderson, University of Maryland; David Koth, University of Alabama; Xavier Lepe, University of Washington; Terry Lindquist, University of Iowa; Mark Richards, West Virginia University; Terry Wilwerding, Creighton University; Gerald Woolsey, University of Missouri Kansas City.

James Cockerill, R.B.P., who one more time provided selected photographic support, building on his previous contributions to the first two editions.

Don O'Connor, who generated all new artwork for this edition emulating the styles used previously by Krystina Srodulski for edition one, and Sandra Cello for edition two.

Our contributors: Drs. Robert F. Baima, William Brantley, Isabelle Denry, Duane Douglas, Martin Freilich, Jon Goldberg, Julie Holloway, Peter Larsen, Donald Miller, Edwin McGlumphy, and Van Thompson.

Dr. Clifford W. VanBlarcom, Chairman of the Nomenclature Committee of the Academy of Prosthodontics, and Dr. Brien R. Lang, Chairman of the Editorial Council of The Journal of Prosthetic Dentistry, for generously supporting the integration of terms from *The Glossary of Prosthodontic Terms* into the various chapters. It is so important when teaching a discipline to use the correct word and as Mark Twain put it "The difference between the right word and the almost right word is the difference between lightning and a lightning bug."

Faculty and staff at Southern Illinois University, School of Dental Medicine, and The Ohio State University College of Dentistry for their help in making an already successful text even better: especially Tammy Duggan, Connie Mason, and Angela Evans for their tireless support and Pat Uhlemeyer for all the time spent word processing, and Drs. James A. Nelson, Gaylord J. James Jr., Kenneth Seckler, Cornell C. Thomas, and Robert Froemling for always being willing to take on another task.

The outstanding team at Mosby: especially Penny Rudolph, Kimberly Frare, Stacy Welsh, and Rich Barber for their patience and understanding in this endeavor. They are the professionals in this enterprise.

Enid, Karen, and Yoshiko have now 'survived' three editions. It takes special spouses to tolerate prosthodontists to begin with, but to support us throughout the completion of yet another edition shows how special they truly are.

A highly respected restorative dentist told us once: "It took me about 10 to 15 years after dental school, until I could routinely make excellent inlays and onlays." This illustrates but one small aspect of the lifetime challenge that fixed prosthodontics presents to student, practitioner, and scholar. We hope that this new edition may help those who are sufficiently motivated and interested to meet that challenge successfully.

Stephen F. Rosenstiel
Martin F. Land
Junhei Fujimoto

Contents

PLANNING AND PREPARATION

CHAPTER ONE

HISTORY TAKING AND CLINICAL EXAMINATION

KEY TERMS

chief complaint
click
communication
dental history
fixed prosthodontics
fremitus
medical history

palpation
percussion
periodontal evaluation
slide
systemic conditions
TMJ dysfunction

Fixed prosthodontic treatment involves the replacement and restoration of teeth by artificial substitutes that are not readily removable from the mouth. Its focus is to restore function, esthetics, and comfort.

Fixed prosthodontics can offer exceptional satisfaction for both patient and dentist. It can transform an unhealthy, unattractive dentition with poor function into a comfortable, healthy occlusion capable of years of further service while greatly enhancing esthetics (Fig. 1-1, *A, B*). Treatment can range from the fairly straightforward restoration of a single tooth with a cast crown (Fig. 1-1, *C*), replacement of one or more missing teeth with a fixed partial denture (Fig. 1-1, *D*), to a highly complex restoration involving all the teeth in an entire arch or dentition.

To achieve predictable success in this technically exacting and demanding field, there must be meticulous attention to every detail—from the initial patient

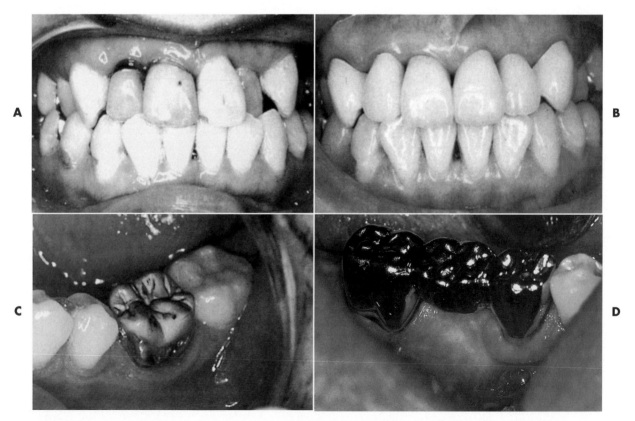

Fig. 1-1. A severely damaged maxillary dentition **(A)** restored with metal-ceramic fixed prostheses **(B)**. **C,** Complete cast crown restores mandibular molar. **D,** Three-unit fixed partial denture replacing missing mandibular molar.
(*C courtesy Dr. X Lepe.* *D courtesy Dr. J. Nelson*)

interview and diagnosis, through the active treatment phases, and to a planned schedule of follow-up care. Otherwise, the result is likely to be unsatisfactory and frustrating for both dentist and patient, resulting in disappointment and loss of confidence.

Problems encountered during or following treatment can often be traced to errors and omissions during history taking and initial examination. An inexperienced clinician may plunge into the treatment phase before collecting sufficient diagnostic information that will help predict likely pitfalls.

Making the correct diagnosis is prerequisite to formulating an appropriate treatment plan. This requires that all pertinent information be obtained. A complete history includes a comprehensive assessment of the patient's general and dental health, individual needs, preferences, and personal circumstances. This chapter reviews fundamentals of history taking and clinical examination, with special emphasis on obtaining the necessary information to make appropriate fixed prosthodontic treatment decisions.

HISTORY

A patient's history should include all pertinent information concerning the reasons for seeking treatment, along with any personal information, including relevant previous medical and dental experiences. The **chief complaint** should be recorded, preferably in the patient's own words. A screening questionnaire (Fig. 1-2) is useful for history taking; it should be reviewed in the patient's presence to correct any mistakes and to clarify inconclusive entries. If the patient is mentally impaired or a minor, the guardian or responsible parent must be present.

CHIEF COMPLAINT

The accuracy and significance of the patient's primary reason(s) for seeking treatment should be analyzed first. This may be just the tip of the iceberg, and careful examination will often reveal problems and disease of which the patient is unaware; nevertheless, the patient perceives the chief complaint as the major problem. Therefore, when a comprehensive treatment plan is proposed, special attention must be given to how it can be resolved. The inexperienced clinician trying to prescribe an "ideal" treatment plan can lose sight of the patient's wishes. The patient may then become frustrated because the dentist apparently does not understand or does not want to understand.

Chief complaints usually fall into one of the following four categories:
- Comfort (pain, sensitivity, swelling)
- Function (difficulty in mastication or speech)

- Social (bad taste or odor)
- Appearance (fractured or unattractive teeth or restorations, discoloration)

Comfort. If pain is present, its location, character, severity, and frequency should be noted, as well as the first time it occurred, what factors precipitate it (e.g., hot, cold, or sweet things), and any changes in its character. Is it localized or more diffuse in nature? It is often helpful to have the patient point at the area while paying close attention.

If swelling is present, the location, size, consistency, and color are noted as well as how long it has been felt and whether it is increasing or decreasing.

Function. Difficulties in chewing may result from a local problem such as a fractured cusp or missing teeth; it may also indicate a more generalized malocclusion or dysfunction.

Social. A bad taste or smell often indicates compromised oral hygiene and periodontal disease. Often social pressures prompt the individual to seek care.

Appearance. Compromised appearance is a strong motivating factor for patients to seek advice as to whether improvement is possible (Fig. 1-3). Such individuals may have missing or crowded teeth, or a tooth or restoration may be fractured. Their teeth may be unattractively shaped, malpositioned, or discolored, or there may be a developmental defect.

PERSONAL DETAILS

The patient's name, address, phone number, sex, occupation, work schedule, and marital and financial status are noted. Much can be learned in a 5-minute, casual conversation during the initial visit. In addition to establishing rapport and developing a basis for the patient to trust the dentist, small and seemingly unimportant personal details often have considerable impact on establishing a correct diagnosis, prognosis, and treatment plan.

MEDICAL HISTORY

An accurate and current general **medical history** should include any medication the patient is taking as well as all relevant medical conditions. If necessary, the patient's physician(s) can be contacted for clarification. The following classification may be helpful:
1. Conditions affecting the treatment methodology (e.g., any disorders that necessitate the use of antibiotic premedication, any use of steroids or anticoagulants, and any previous allergic

REG. NO. _____

Name _____ Date _____ Age _____

Write Yes or No.

1. Have you been hospitalized or under the care of a physician within the last 2 years? _____

2. Has there been a change in your general health within the past 2 years? _____

3. Are you allergic to penicillin or any other drugs? _____

4. Indicate **Yes** or **No** to any of the conditions below for which you are being treated or you have had:

Y / N	Heart attack	Y / N	Hives, skin rash	Y / N	Substance abuse
Y / N	Heart trouble	Y / N	Cancer treatment	Y / N	AIDS
Y / N	Heart surgery	Y / N	Radiation therapy	Y / N	HIV infection
Y / N	Angina (chest pain)	Y / N	Ulcers	Y / N	Diabetes
Y / N	High blood pressure	Y / N	Gastritis	Y / N	Hepatitis
Y / N	Prolapsed mitral valve	Y / N	Hiatus hernia	Y / N	Kidney trouble
Y / N	Heart murmur	Y / N	Easy bruising	Y / N	Psychiatric treatment
Y / N	Artificial heart valves	Y / N	Excessive bleeding	Y / N	Fainting spells
Y / N	Congenital heart lesions	Y / N	Artificial joint	Y / N	Seizures
Y / N	Cardiac pacemaker	Y / N	Arthritis	Y / N	Epilepsy
Y / N	Rheumatic fever	Y / N	Asthma	Y / N	Anemia
Y / N	Stroke	Y / N	Persistent cough		
Y / N	Allergies	Y / N	Emphysema		**Women Only**

Women Only:
Y / N Currently pregnant
Y / N Nursing
Y / N Female problems

Do you use tobacco? Y / N Type _____ How much? _____

Do you drink alcohol? Y / N Type _____ How much? _____

5. Have you had any serious illness, disease, or condition not listed above? _____

   If so, explain _____
   _____

6. Indicate date of your last physical examination _____

7. Name and address of your personal physician _____
   _____

8. List any medications you are currently taking _____
   _____

9. Have you had any problems or anxiety associated with previous dental care? _____

   If so, explain _____
   _____

DENTAL QUESTIONNAIRE

Indicate Yes or No to the Following:

Y / N 10. Does it hurt when you chew?
Y / N 11. Is a tooth sensitive or tender?
Y / N 12. Do you have frequent toothaches or gum pain?
Y / N 13. Do your gums bleed a lot when you brush your teeth?
Y / N 14. Do you have occasional dryness or burning in your mouth?
Y / N 15. Do you have occasional pain in the jaws, neck, or temples?
Y / N 16. Does it hurt when you open wide or take a big bite?
Y / N 17. Does your jaw make "clicking or popping" sounds when you chew or move your jaw?
Y / N 18. Do you suffer from headaches?
Y / N 19. Do you have occasional ear pain or pain in front of the ears?
Y / N 20. Does your jaw "feel tired" after a meal?
Y / N 21. Do you ever have to search for a place to close your teeth?
Y / N 22. Does a tooth ever get in the way?
23.   Is there anything you wish to tell us that has not been asked?

24.   Were there any items you did not understand?

I will inform the Clinic of any changes in the above
        Person completing form sign here: _____
                                    self   parent   guardian
                            Circle Relationship
                    If Minor: Parent or Legal Guardian Signature
        Date Signed: _____

Fig. 1-2. Screening questionnaire.

responses to medication or dental materials). Once these are identified, treatment usually can be modified as part of the comprehensive treatment plan, although some factors may severely limit available options.

2. Conditions affecting the treatment plan (e.g., previous radiation therapy, hemorrhagic disorders, extremes of age, and terminal illness). These can be expected to modify the patient's response to dental treatment and may affect the prognosis. For instance, patients who have previously received radiation treatment in the area of a planned extraction require special measures (hyperbaric oxygen) to prevent serious complications.

3. **Systemic conditions** with oral manifestations. For example, periodontitis may be modified by diabetes, menopause, pregnancy, or the use of anticonvulsant drugs (Fig. 1-4); in cases of hiatal hernia, bulimia, or anorexia nervosa, teeth may be eroded by regurgitated stomach acid[1,2] (Fig. 1-5); certain drugs may generate side

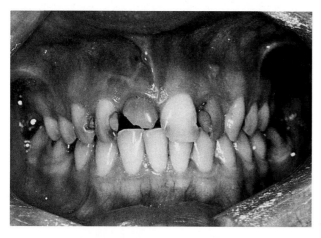

Fig. 1-3. Poor appearance is a common reason for seeking restorative dental treatment.

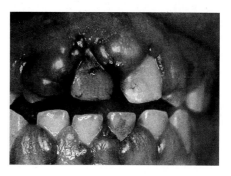

Fig. 1-4. Severe gingival hyperplasia associated with anticonvulsant drug use.
(Courtesy Dr. P.B. Robinson.)

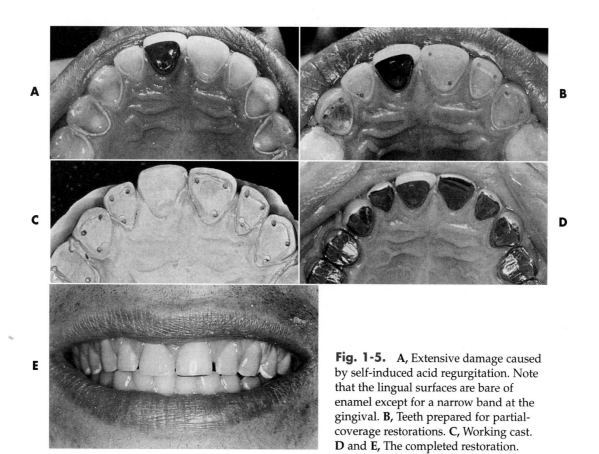

A

B

C

D

E

Fig. 1-5. **A,** Extensive damage caused by self-induced acid regurgitation. Note that the lingual surfaces are bare of enamel except for a narrow band at the gingival. **B,** Teeth prepared for partial-coverage restorations. **C,** Working cast. **D** and **E,** The completed restoration.

effects that mimic temporomandibular disorders (TMDs)[3] or reduce salivary flow.[4,5]

4. Possible risk factors to the dentist and auxiliary personnel (e.g., patients who are suspected or confirmed carriers of hepatitis B, acquired immunodeficiency syndrome, or syphilis).

Dental offices practice "universal precautions" to ensure appropriate infection control. This means that full infection control is taken for every patient; no additional measures are needed when treating known carriers.[6]

DENTAL HISTORY

Clinicians should be cautious when commenting before a thorough examination is completed. With adequate experience, a clinician can often assess preliminary treatment needs during the initial appointment. However, fairly assessing the quality of a previously rendered treatment can be difficult, because the circumstances under which the treatment was rendered are seldom known. When such an assessment is requested for legal proceedings, the patient should be referred to a specialist familiar with the "usual and customary" standard of care.

Periodontal History. The patient's oral hygiene is assessed, and current plaque-control measures are discussed, as are previously received oral hygiene instructions. The frequency of any previous debridements should be recorded, and the dates and nature of any previous periodontal surgery should be noted.

Restorative History. The patient's restorative history may include only simple composite resin or dental amalgam fillings, or it may involve crowns and extensive fixed partial dentures. The age of existing restorations can help establish the prognosis and probable longevity of any future fixed prostheses.

Endodontic History. Patients often forget which teeth have been endodontically treated. These can be readily identified with radiographs. The findings should be reviewed periodically so that periapical health can be monitored and any recurring lesions promptly detected (Fig. 1-6).

Orthodontic History. Occlusal analysis should be an integral part of the assessment of a postorthodontic dentition. If restorative treatment needs are anticipated, they should be undertaken by the restorative dentist. Occlusal adjustment (reshaping of the occlusal surfaces of the teeth) may be needed to promote long-term positional stability of the teeth and reduce or eliminate parafunctional activ-

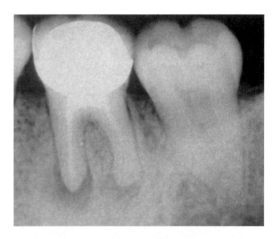

Fig. 1-6. Defective endodontics has led to recurrence of a periapical lesion. Retreatment will be required.

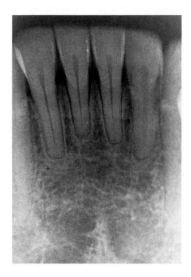

Fig. 1-7. Apical root resorption subsequent to orthodontic treatment.

ity. On occasion, root resorption (detected on radiographs) (Fig. 1-7) may be attributable to previous orthodontic treatment. As the crown/root ratio is affected, future prosthodontic treatment and its prognosis may also be affected. Restorative treatment can often be simplified by minor tooth movement. When a patient is contemplating orthodontic treatment, considerable time can be saved if minor tooth movement (for restorative reasons) is incorporated from the start. Thus good **communication** between the restorative dentist and the orthodontist may prove very helpful.

Removable Prosthodontic History. The patient's experiences with removable prostheses must be carefully evaluated. For example, a removable partial denture may not have been worn for a variety of reasons, and the patient may not even have mentioned its existence. Careful questioning and examination will usually elicit discussion concerning any such devices. Listening to the patient's comments about previously unsuccessful removable prostheses can be very helpful in assessing whether future treatment will be more successful.

Oral Surgical History. Information about missing teeth and any complications that may have occurred during tooth removal is obtained. Special evaluation and data collection procedures are necessary for patients who require prosthodontic care subsequent to orthognathic surgery. Before any treatment is undertaken, the prosthodontic component of the proposed treatment should be fully coordinated with the surgical component.

Radiographic History. Previous radiographs may prove helpful in judging the progress of dental disease. They should be obtained if possible, because it is generally better to avoid exposing the patient to unnecessary ionizing radiation. Dental practices will usually forward radiographs or acceptable duplicates promptly upon request. In most instances, however, a current diagnostic radiographic series is essential and should be obtained as part of the examination.

TMJ Dysfunction History. A history of pain or clicking in the temporomandibular joints or neuromuscular symptoms, such as tenderness to **palpation,** may be due to **TMJ dysfunction,** which should normally be treated and resolved before fixed prosthodontic treatment begins. A screening questionnaire will efficiently identify these problems. The patient should be questioned regarding any previous treatment for joint dysfunction (e.g., occlusal devices, medications, biofeedback, or physical therapy exercises).

EXAMINATION

An examination consists of the clinician's use of sight, touch, and hearing to detect conditions outside the normal range. To avoid mistakes, it is critical to record what is actually observed rather than to make diagnostic comments about the condition. For example, "swelling," "redness," and "bleeding on probing of gingival tissue" should be recorded rather than "gingival inflammation" (which implies a diagnosis).

Thorough examination and data collection are needed for the prospective fixed prosthodontic patient, and the protocol for this effort can be obtained from various textbooks of oral diagnosis.[7,8]

GENERAL EXAMINATION

The patient's general appearance, gait, and weight are assessed. Skin color is noted for signs of anemia or jaundice. Vital signs, such as respiration, pulse, temperature, and blood pressure, are measured and recorded. Fixed prosthodontic treatment is often indicated in middle-aged or older patients, who can be at higher risk for cardiovascular disease. Relatively inexpensive cardiac monitoring units are available for in-office use (Fig. 1-8). Patients with vital signs outside normal ranges should be referred for a comprehensive medical evaluation before definitive treatment is initiated.

EXTRAORAL EXAMINATION

Special attention is given to facial asymmetry because small deviations from normal may hint at serious underlying conditions. Cervical lymph nodes are palpated, as are the TMJs and the muscles of mastication.

Temporomandibular Joints. The clinician locates the TMJs by palpating bilaterally just anterior to the auricular tragi while having the patient open and close. This permits a comparison between the relative timing of left and right condylar movements during the opening stroke. Asynchronous movement may indicate an anterior disk displacement that prevents one of the condyles from making a normal translatory movement (see Chapter 4). Auricular palpation (Fig. 1-9) with light anterior pressure helps identify potential disorders in the posterior attachment of the disk. Tenderness, or pain on movement, is noted and can be indicative of inflammatory changes in the retrodiscal tissues, which are highly vascular and innervated. Clicking in the TMJ is often noticeable through auricular palpation but may be difficult to detect when palpating directly over the lateral pole of the condylar process, because the overlying tissues can "muffle" the **click.** Placement of the fingertips on the angles of the mandible will help identify even a minimal click, because very little soft tissue lies between the fingertips and the mandibular bone.

A maximum mandibular opening resulting in less than 35 mm of interincisal movement is considered to be restricted, because the average opening is greater than 50 mm.[9,10] Such restricted movement on opening can be indicative of intracapsular changes in the joints. Similarly, any midline deviation on opening and/or closing is recorded. The maximum lateral movements of the patient can be measured (normal is about 12 mm) (Fig. 1-10).

Muscles of Mastication. Next, the masseter and temporal muscles, as well as other relevant

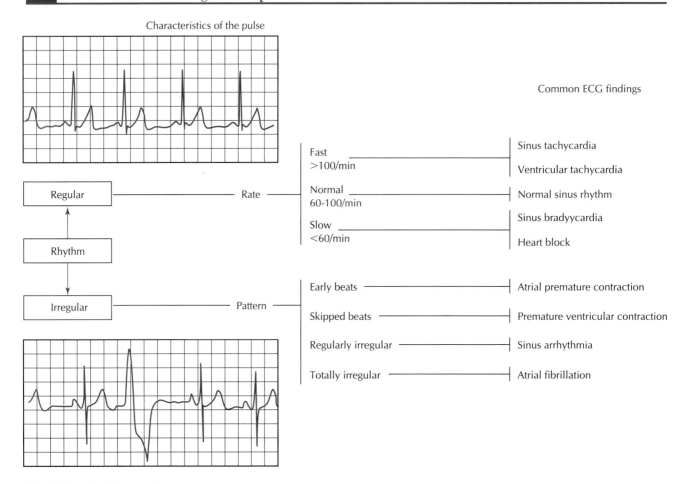

Characteristics of the pulse

Common ECG findings

Fast >100/min	—	Sinus tachycardia
		Ventricular tachycardia
Normal 60-100/min	—	Normal sinus rhythm
Slow <60/min	—	Sinus bradyycardia
		Heart block
Early beats	—	Atrial premature contraction
Skipped beats	—	Premature ventricular contraction
Regularly irregular	—	Sinus arrhythmia
Totally irregular	—	Atrial fibrillation

Fig. 1-8. Cardiac monitoring printout. *(Courtesy Dr. T. Quilitz.)*

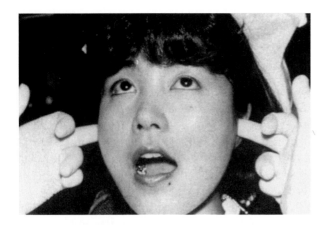

Fig. 1-9. Auricular palpation of the posterior aspects of the temporomandibular joints.

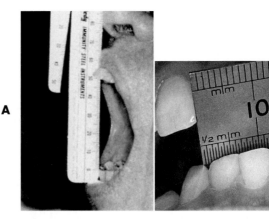

Fig. 1-10. Maximum opening of more than 50 mm **(A)** and lateral movement of about 12 mm **(B)** are normal.

postural muscles, are palpated for signs of tenderness (Fig. 1-11). Palpation is best accomplished bilaterally and simultaneously. This allows the patient to compare and report any differences between the left and right sides. Light pressure should be used (the amount of pressure one can tolerate when gently pushing on one's closed eyelid without feeling discomfort is a good comparative measure), and if any difference is reported between the left and right sides, the patient is asked to classify the discomfort as mild, moderate, or severe. If there is evidence of significant asynchronous movement or TMJ dysfunction, a systematic sequence for comprehensive muscle palpation should be followed as described by Solberg[9] and Krogh-Poulsen and Olsson.[11] Each palpation site is given a numerical score based on

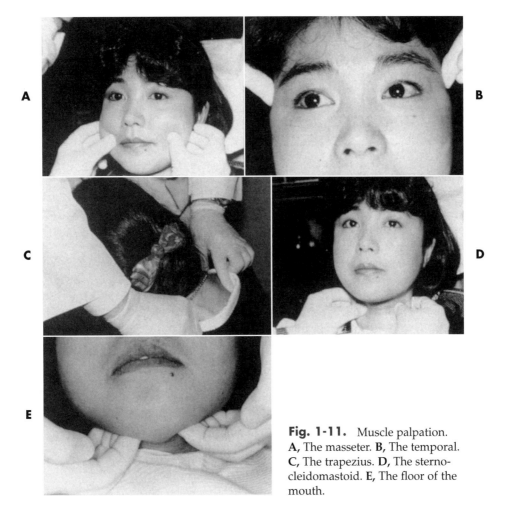

Fig. 1-11. Muscle palpation.
A, The masseter. **B,** The temporal.
C, The trapezius. **D,** The sternocleidomastoid. **E,** The floor of the
mouth.

the patient's response. If neuromuscular or TMJ treatment is initiated, the examiner can then repalpate the same sites periodically to assess the response to treatment (Fig. 1-12).

Lips. The patient is observed for tooth visibility during normal and exaggerated smiling. This can be critical in fixed prosthodontic treatment planning,[12] especially for margin placement of certain metal-ceramic crowns. Some patients show only their maxillary teeth during smiling. More than 25% do not show the gingival third of the maxillary central incisors during an exaggerated smile[13] (Fig. 1-13). The extent of the smile will depend on the length and mobility of the upper lip and the length of the alveolar process. When the patient laughs, the jaws open slightly and a dark space is often visible between the maxillary and mandibular teeth (Fig. 1-14). This has been called the *negative space*.[14] Missing teeth, diastemas, and fractured or poorly restored teeth will disrupt the harmony of the negative space and often require correction.[15]

INTRAORAL EXAMINATION
The intraoral examination can reveal considerable information concerning the condition of the soft tis-

sues, teeth, and supporting structures. The tongue, floor of the mouth, vestibule, cheeks, and hard and soft palates are examined, and any abnormalities are noted. This information can be properly evaluated during treatment planning only if objective indices, rather than vague assessments, are used.

Periodontal Examination

Robert F. Baima
A periodontal examination should provide information regarding the status of bacterial accumulation, the response of the host tissues, and the degree of irreversible damage. Because long-term periodontal health is essential to successful fixed prosthodontics (see Chapter 5), existing periodontal disease must be corrected before any definitive prosthodontic treatment is undertaken.

Gingiva. The gingiva should be lightly dried before examination so that moisture does not obscure subtle changes or detail. Color, texture, size, contour, consistency, and position are noted and recorded. The gingiva is then carefully palpated to express any exudate or pus that may be present in the sulcular area.

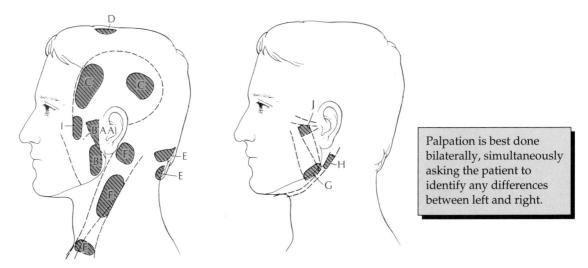

Fig. 1-12. Palpation sites for assessing muscle tenderness. *A*, TMJ capsule: lateral and dorsal. *B*, Masseter: deep and superficial. *C*, Temporal: anterior and posterior. *D*, Vertex. *E*, Neck: nape and base. *F*, Sternocleidomastoid: insertion, body, and origin. *G*, Medial pterygoid. *H*, Posterior digastric. *I*, Temporal tendon. *J*, Lateral pterygoid.
(From Krogh-Poulsen WG, Olsson A: Dent Clin North Am *10:627, 1966.)*

> Palpation is best done bilaterally, simultaneously asking the patient to identify any differences between left and right.

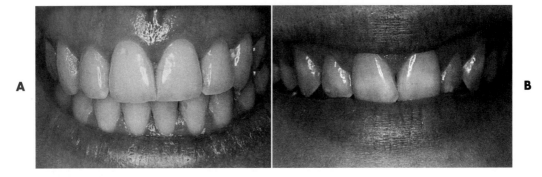

Fig. 1-13. Smile analysis is an important part of the examination, particularly when anterior crowns or FPDs are being considered. **A,** Some individuals show considerable gingival tissue during an exaggerated smile. **B,** Others may not show the gingival margins of even the central incisors.

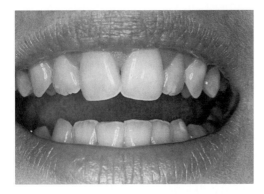

Fig. 1-14. The "negative" space between the maxillary and mandibular teeth is assessed during the examination.

Healthy gingiva (Fig. 1-15, *A*) is pink, stippled, and firmly bound to the underlying connective tissue. The gingival margin is knife-edged, and sharply pointed papillae fill the interproximal spaces. Any deviation from these findings should be noted. With the development of chronic marginal gingivitis (Fig. 1-15, *B*), the gingiva becomes enlarged and bulbous, loss of stippling occurs, the margins and papillae are blunted, and bleeding and exudate are observed.

The width of the band of attached keratinized gingiva around each tooth may be assessed by measuring the surface band of keratinized tissue in an apicocoronal dimension with a periodontal probe and subtracting the measurement of the sulcus depth. Another method to obtain this measurement by visual examination is to gently depress the marginal gingiva with the side of a periodontal probe or explorer. At the mucogingival junction (MGJ), the effect of the instrument will be seen to end abruptly, indicating the transition from tightly bound gingiva to more flexible mucosa. Injecting anesthetic solu-

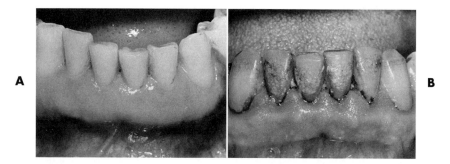

Fig. 1-15. **A,** Healthy gingivae—pink, knife-edged, and firmly attached. **B,** Gingivitis—plaque and calculus have caused marginal inflammation, with changes in color, contour, and consistency of the free gingival margin. Inflammation extends into the keratinized attached gingiva.

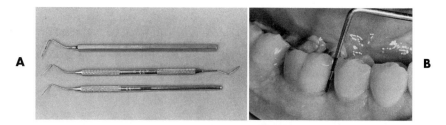

Fig. 1-16. **A,** Three types of sulcus/pocket-measuring probes. **B,** Correct position of a periodontal probe in the interproximal sulcular area, parallel to the root surface and in a vertical direction as far interproximally as possible.

tion into the nonkeratinized mucosa close to the MGJ to make the mucosa balloon slightly is a third method of visualizing the MGJ. However, this is done only if the other methods do not provide the desired information.

Periodontium. The periodontal probe (Fig. 1-16, *A*) is one of the most reliable and useful diagnostic tools available for examining the periodontium. It provides a measurement (in millimeters) of the depth of periodontal pockets and healthy gingival sulci on all surfaces of each tooth. In this examination the probe is inserted essentially parallel to the tooth and is "walked" circumferentially through the sulcus in firm but gentle steps, determining the measurement when the probe is in contact with the apical portion of the sulcus (Fig. 1-16, *B*). Thus any sudden change in the attachment level can be detected. The probe may also be angled slightly (5 to 10 degrees) in the interproximal areas to reveal the topography of an existing lesion. Probing depths (usually six per tooth) are recorded on a periodontal chart (Fig. 1-17), which also contains other data pertinent to the periodontal examination (e.g., tooth mobility or malposition, open or deficient contact areas, inconsistent marginal ridge heights, missing or impacted teeth, areas of inadequate attached keratinized gingiva, gingival reces-

sion, furcation involvements, and malpositioned frenum attachments).

CLINICAL ATTACHMENT LEVEL

Documenting the level of attachment helps the clinician determine the amount of periodontal destruction that has occurred and is essential when rendering a diagnosis of periodontitis (loss of connective tissue attachment).[16,17] This measurement also provides the clinician with more detailed and accurate information regarding the prognosis of an individual tooth. The clinical attachment level (CAL or AL) is determined by measuring the distance between the apical extent of the probing depth and a fixed reference point on the tooth, most commonly either the apical extent of a restoration and/or the cementoenamel junction (CEJ). This measurement can be documented on modified periodontal charts (Fig. 1-18) and incorporated with the standard periodontal documentation (see Fig. 1-17) to complete the clinical periodontal examination. When the free margin of the gingiva is located on the clinical crown and the level of the epithelial attachment is at the CEJ, there is no loss of attachment, and recession is noted as a negative number. When the level of the epithelial attachment is on root structure and the free margin of the gingiva is at the CEJ, the attachment loss equals the probing depth, and the

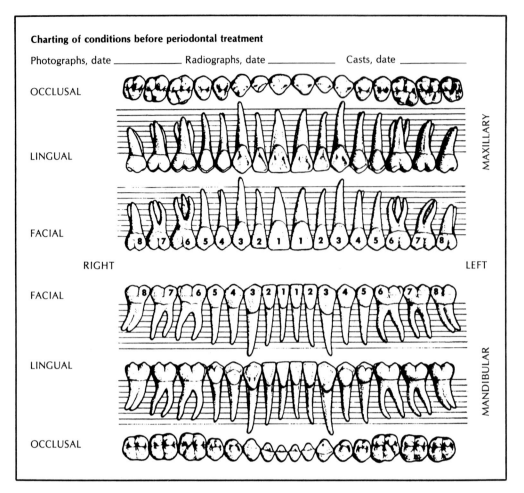

Charting of conditions before periodontal treatment

Photographs, date _____ Radiographs, date _____ Casts, date _____

Fig. 1-17. Chart for recording pocket depths. The parallel lines are approximately 2 mm apart. Following are the notations involved in using the chart:
1. Block out any missing teeth.
2. Draw a red *X* through the crown of any tooth that is to be extracted.
3. Record the gingival level with a continuous blue line.
4. Record pocket depths with a red line interrupted at the proximal surfaces of each tooth.
5. Shade the pocket form on each tooth with a red pencil (between the red and blue lines).
6. Indicate bifurcation or trifurcation involvements with a small red *X* at the involved area.
7. Record open contacts with vertical parallel lines (‖) through the area.
8. Record improper contacts with a wavy red line ($\sum$) through the area.
9. Record gingival overhang(s) with a red spur (∧) through the area.
10. Outline cavities and faulty restorations of periodontal significance in red.
11. Indicate rotated teeth by outlining in blue to show their actual position.
(Modified slightly from Goldman HM, Cohen DW: Periodontal therapy, ed 5, St Louis, 1973, Mosby.)

recession is *0*. In a situation in which there is increased periodontal destruction and recession, the loss of attachment measurement equals the probing depth plus the measurement of recession[18] (see Fig. 1-18, *B, C*). Clinical attachment loss is a measure of periodontal destruction at a site, rather than current disease activity, and it may be considered the diagnostic "gold standard" for periodontitis.[19] It should be documented in the initial periodontal examination.[20] It is an important consideration in the development of the overall diagnosis, treatment plan,

and prognosis of the dentition and can be an effective research tool.

• • •

Dental Charting

An accurate charting of the state of the dentition will reveal important information about the condition of the teeth and will facilitate treatment planning. Adequate charting (Fig. 1-19), in addition to all periodontal information, must show the pres-

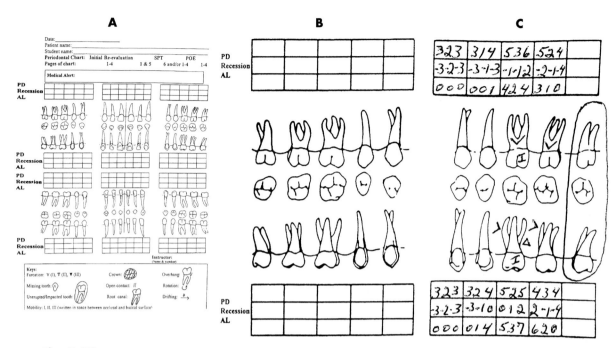

Fig. 1-18. **A,** Modified periodontal chart **B,** Maxillary right sextant of modified periodontal chart with areas to record probing depths *(PD),* recession, and attachment loss *(AL).* **C,** Maxillary left sextant of modified periodontal chart exhibiting clinical documentation.
(Courtesy University of Detroit Mercy School of Dentistry, Department of Periodontology and Dental Hygiene).

ence or absence of teeth, dental caries, restorations, wear faceting and abrasions, fractures, malformations, and erosions. Missing teeth will often have an impact on the position of adjacent teeth (see also the section on arch integrity in Chapter 3). Similarly, the presence of dental caries on one interproximal surface should alert the examiner to carefully inspect the adjacent proximal wall, even if caries is not apparent radiographically. The degree and extent of caries development over time can have a considerable impact on the eventual prognosis of fixed prosthodontic treatment. The condition and type of the existing restorations are noted (e.g., amalgam, cast gold, composite resin, all-ceramic). Open contacts and areas where food impaction occurs must also be identified. The presence of wear facets is indicative of sliding contact sustained over time and thus may indicate parafunctional activity (see Chapter 4). Wear facets are often easier to see on diagnostic casts, however (see Chapter 2); during the clinical examination, the location of any observed facets is recorded. Fracture lines in teeth may require fixed prosthodontic intervention, although minor hairline cracks in walls that are not subject to excessive loading can often go untreated and simply be observed at recall appointments (see Chapter 32). The location of fractures should be indicated on the chart, as should any other abnormalities.

Occlusal Examination. The initial clinical examination starts with the clinician asking the patient to make a few simple opening and closing movements while carefully observing the opening and closing strokes. The objective is to determine to what extent the patient's occlusion differs from the ideal (see Chapter 4) and how well the patient has adapted to this difference. Special attention is given to initial contact, tooth alignment, eccentric contacts, and jaw maneuverability.

Initial Tooth Contact. The relationship of teeth in both centric relation (see Chapter 4) and the intercuspal position should be assessed. If all teeth come together simultaneously at the end of terminal hinge closure, the centric relation position (CR) of the patient is said to coincide with the maximum intercuspation (MI) (see Chapters 2 and 4). The patient is guided into a terminal hinge closure to detect where initial tooth contact occurs (see the sections on bimanual manipulation and terminal hinge closure in Chapters 2 and 4). The clinician should ask the patient to "close featherlight" until any of the teeth touch and to have the patient help identify where that initial contact occurs by asking him or her to point at the location. If initial contact occurs between two posterior teeth (usually molars), the subsequent

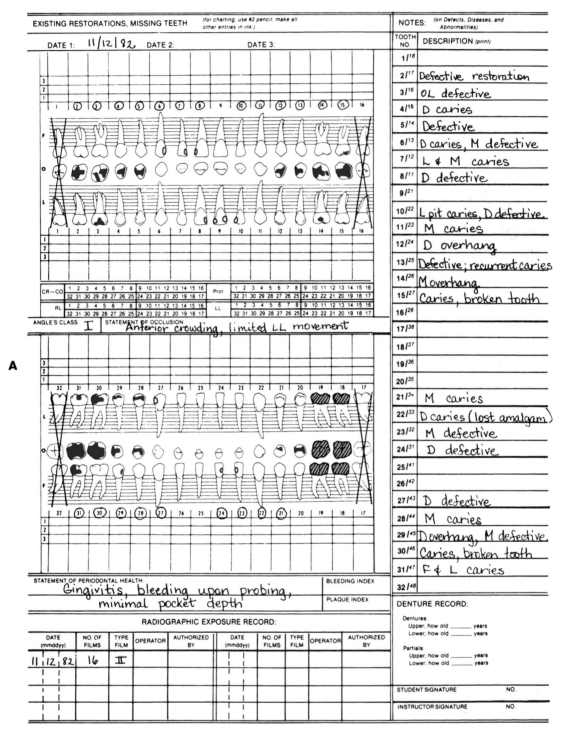

Fig. 1-19.   **A,** An appropriate charting system will designate the location, type, and extent of existing restorations and the presence of any disease condition, all of which become part of the permanent patient record.

Continued

movement from the initial contact to the MI position is carefully observed and its direction noted. This is referred to as a *slide from CR to MI.* The presence, direction, and estimated magnitude of the slide are recorded, and the teeth on which initial contact occurs are identified. Any such discrepancy between CR and MI should be evaluated in the context of other signs and symptoms

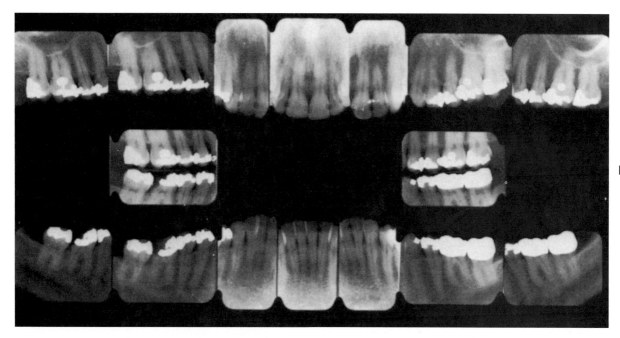

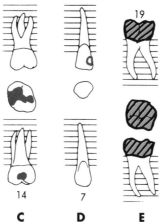

Fig. 1-19, cont'd. **B,** Radiographic findings obtained from a full-mouth series are correlated with the clinical findings and noted in the record. **C to E,** Charting is performed to provide a quick reference to conditions in the mouth. The following may be useful:

1. Amalgam restorations **(C)** are depicted by an outline drawing blocked in solidly to show the size, shape, and location of the restoration.
2. Tooth-colored restorations **(D)** are depicted by an outline drawing of the size, shape, and location of the restoration.
3. Gold restorations **(E)** are depicted by an outline drawing inscribed with diagonal lines to show the size, shape, and location of the restoration.
4. Missing teeth are denoted by a large *X* on the facial, lingual, and occlusal diagrams of each tooth that is not visible clinically or on radiographs.
5. Caries is recorded by circling the tooth number located at the apex of the involved tooth and noting the presence and location of the cavity in the description column corresponding to the tooth number on the right.
6. Defective restorations are recorded by circling the tooth number and noting the defect in the description column.

(Modified slightly from Sturdevant CM et al: The art and science of operative dentistry, ed 3, St Louis, 1994, Mosby.)

that may be present (e.g., elevated muscle tone previously observed during the extraoral examination, mobility on the teeth where initial contact occurs, wear facets on the teeth involved in the slide).

General Alignment (Fig. 1-20). The teeth are evaluated for crowding, rotation, supra-eruption, spacing, malocclusion, and vertical and horizontal overlap. Teeth adjacent to edentulous spaces often have shifted position slightly. Small amounts of

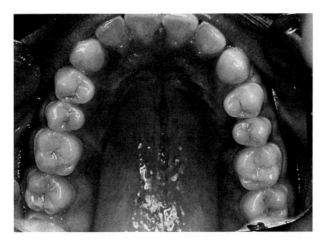

Fig. 1-20. Alignment of the dentition can be assessed intraorally, although diagnostic casts allow a more detailed assessment. This patient has caries-free teeth in good alignment.

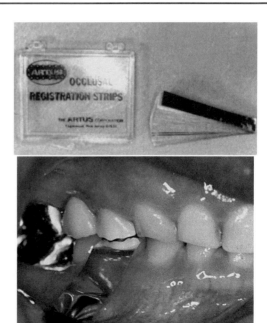

Fig. 1-21. Eccentric tooth contact can be tested with thin Mylar shim stock.

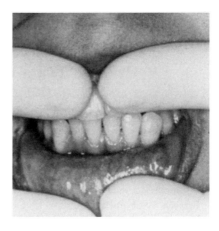

Fig. 1-22. Fremitus (movement on palpation) indicates tooth contact during lateral excursions.

tooth movement can significantly affect fixed prosthodontic treatment. Tipped teeth will affect tooth preparation design or in severe cases, may result in a need for minor tooth movement before restorative treatment. Supra-erupted teeth are often overlooked clinically but will often complicate fixed partial denture design and fabrication.

The relative relationship of adjacent teeth to teeth requiring fixed prosthodontic treatment is important. A tooth may have drifted into the space previously occupied by the tooth in need of treatment because a large filling was previously lost. Such changes in alignment can seriously complicate or preclude fabrication of a cast restoration for the damaged tooth and may even necessitate its extraction.

Lateral and Protrusive Contacts. Excursive contacts on posterior teeth may be undesirable under certain circumstances (see Chapter 4).

The degree of vertical and horizontal overlap of the teeth is noted. When asked, most patients are capable of making an unguided protrusive movement. During this movement, the degree of posterior disclusion that results from the overlaps of the anterior teeth is observed.

The patient is then guided into lateral excursive movements, and the presence or absence of contacts on the nonworking side and then the working side is noted. Such tooth contact in eccentric movements can be verified with a thin Mylar strip (shim stock). Any posterior cusps that hold the shim stock will be evident (Fig. 1-21). Teeth that are subject to excessive loading may develop varying degrees of mobility. Tooth movement (**fremitus**) should be identified by palpation (Fig. 1-22). If a heavy contact is suspected, a finger placed against the buccal or

labial surface while the patient lightly taps the teeth together will locate fremitus in MI.

Jaw Maneuverability. The ease with which the patient moves the jaw and the way it can be guided through hinge closure and excursive movements should be assessed, since these factors are a good guide to neuromuscular and masticatory function. If the patient has developed a pattern of protective reflexes, manipulating the jaw will be difficult. The patient's restricted maneuverability is recorded.

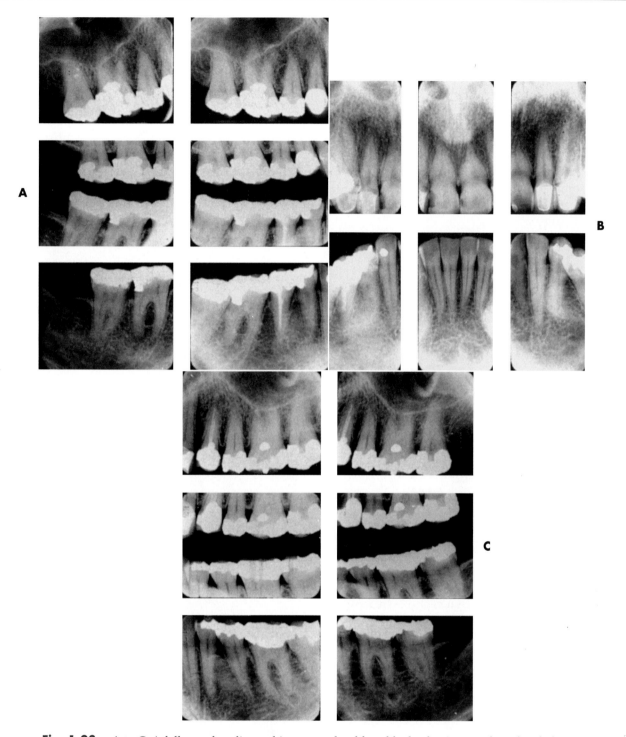

Fig. 1-23. **A** to **C,** A full-mouth radiographic survey should enable the dentist to make a detailed assessment of the morphology of each tooth and its bone support.

RADIOGRAPHIC EXAMINATION

Radiographs provide essential information to supplement the clinical examination. Detailed knowledge of the extent of bone support and the root morphology of each standing tooth is essential to establishing a comprehensive fixed prosthodontic treatment plan. Although radiation exposure guidelines recommend limiting the number of radiographs to only those that will result in potential changes in treatment decisions, a full periapical series (Fig. 1-23) is normally required for new patients so that a comprehensive fixed prosthodontic treatment plan can be developed. Patient exposure can be minimized by using a technique that provides the most information with a minimal need for repeat films and by using appropriate protection. The use of digital radiography can further help reduce radiation exposure.

Panoramic films (Fig. 1-24) provide useful information about the presence or absence of teeth. They are especially helpful in assessing third molars and impactions, evaluating the bone before implant placement (see Chapter 13), and screening edentulous arches for buried root tips. However, they do not provide a sufficiently detailed view for assessing bone support, root morphology, caries, or periapical pathology.

Special radiographs may be needed for the assessment of TMJ disorders. A transcranial exposure (Fig. 1-25), with the help of a positioning device, will reveal the lateral third of the mandibular condyle and can be used to detect structural and positional changes. However, interpretation may be difficult.[21] More information can be obtained from serial tomography, arthrography,[22] CT scanning,[23] magnetic resonance imaging[24-26] (Fig. 1-26), or digital subtraction radiography[27] of the joints.

VITALITY TESTING

Before any restorative treatment, pulpal health must be assessed, usually by measuring the response to **percussion** and thermal or electrical stimulation. A diagnosis of nonvitality can be confirmed by preparing a test cavity without the administration of local anesthetic. Vitality tests, however, assess only the afferent nerve supply. Misdiagnosis can occur if the nerve supply is damaged but the blood supply is intact. Careful inspection of radiographs is

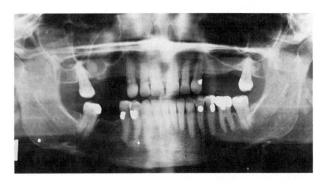

Fig. 1-24. A panoramic film cannot be substituted for a full-mouth series because the image is distorted. Nevertheless, it is very useful for assessing unerupted teeth, screening edentulous areas for buried root tips, and evaluating the bone before implant placement.

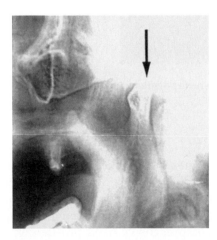

Fig. 1-25. A transcranial radiograph shows the lateral pole of the mandibular condyle (arrow).

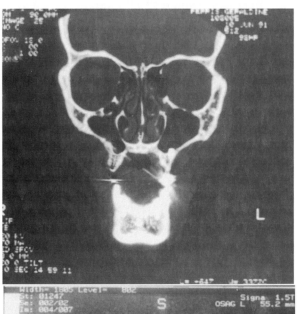

A

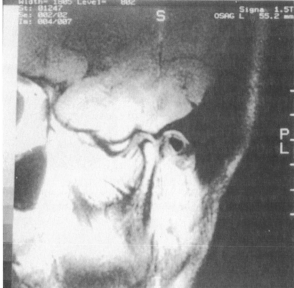

B

Fig. 1-26. More sophisticated techniques permit the generation of computer-assisted images of clinician-determined cross-sections. **A,** A CT scan. **B,** An MRI showing the soft tissue in greater detail.
(Courtesy Dr. J. Petrie.)

therefore an essential aid in the examination of such teeth.

DIAGNOSIS AND PROGNOSIS

Not all patients seeking fixed prosthodontic treatment will present diagnostic problems. Nevertheless, diagnostic errors are possible, especially when a patient complains of pain or symptoms of occlusal dysfunction. Treatment may be needed to eliminate obvious dental caries, to restore a fractured prosthesis, or to replace a missing tooth. A logical and systematic approach to diagnosis will help avoid mistakes.

DIFFERENTIAL DIAGNOSIS

When the history and examination are completed, a differential diagnosis is made. The practitioner should determine the most likely causes of the observed condition(s) and record them in order of probability. A definitive diagnosis can usually be developed after such supporting evidence has been assembled.

A typical diagnosis will condense the information obtained during the clinical history taking and examination. For instance, a diagnosis could read as follows: 28-year-old male, no significant medical history; vital signs normal. Chief complaint: Mesiolingual cusp fracture on tooth # 30. Teeth # 1, # 16, # 17, # 19, and # 32 missing. Patient reports significant postoperative discomfort after previous molar extraction. High smile line. Caries: # 6, mesial; # 12, distal; # 20, mesio-occlusal; and # 30, mesio-occlusal-distal. Tooth # 8 has received previous endodontic treatment. Generalized gingivitis four posterior quadrants, with recession noted on teeth # 23, # 24, and # 25. 5-mm pockets on teeth # 18, # 30, and # 31. Radiographic evidence of periapical pathology tooth # 30. Tooth # 30 tests nonvital.

This hypothetical scenario summarizes the patient's problems, allowing subsequent prioritization as a treatment plan is developed (see Chapter 3). In this case, the patient's chief complaint likely has a longer-term history that has only recently led to symptoms the patient could identify, causing him to seek care.

PROGNOSIS

The prognosis is an estimation of the likely course of a disease. It can be difficult to make, but its importance to patient understanding and successful treatment planning must nevertheless be recognized. The prognosis of dental disorders is influenced by general factors (age of the patient, lowered resistance of the oral environment) and local factors (forces applied to a given tooth, access for oral hy-giene measures). For example, a young person with periodontal disease will have a more guarded prognosis than an older person with the same disease experience. In the younger person, the disease has followed a more virulent course because of the generally less-developed systemic resistance; these facts should be reflected in treatment planning.

Fixed prostheses function in a hostile environment: the moist oral environment is subject to constant changes in temperature and acidity and considerable load fluctuation. A comprehensive clinical examination helps identify the likely prognosis. All facts and observations are first considered individually and then correlated appropriately.

General Factors. The overall caries rate of the patient's dentition indicates future risk to the patient if the condition is left untreated. Important variables include the patient's understanding and comprehension of plaque-control measures as well as the physical ability to perform those tasks. Systemic problems analyzed in the context of the patient's age and overall health provide important information. Diabetics are prone to a higher incidence of periodontal pathology, and special precautionary measures may be indicated before treatment begins. Such conditions also affect the overall prognosis.

Some patients are capable of an extremely high bite force, whereas others are not. If an elevated muscle tone of hypertrophied elevator muscles is identified during the extraoral examination and multiple intraoral wear facets are observed, loading of the teeth will be considerably higher than in the dentition of a frail 90-year-old who tires easily when asked to close. Other important factors in determining overall prognosis are the history and success of previous dental treatments. If a patient's previous dental care has been successful over a period of many years, a better prognosis can be anticipated than when apparently properly fabricated prostheses fail or become dislodged within a few years of initial placement.

Local Factors. The observed vertical overlap of the anterior teeth has a direct impact on the load distribution in the dentition and thus can have an impact on the prognosis. In the presence of favorable loading, minor tooth mobility is less of a concern than in the presence of unfavorable directed or high load. Impactions adjacent to a molar that will be crowned may pose a serious threat in a younger individual in whom additional growth can be anticipated, but it may be of lesser concern in an older individual.

Individual tooth mobility, root angulation, root morphology, crown-to-root ratios, and many other variables all have an impact on the overall fixed prosthodontic prognosis. They will be addressed later in this book.

SUMMARY

The history and clinical examination must provide sufficient data for the practitioner to formulate a successful treatment plan. If they are too hastily accomplished, details may be missed that can cause significant problems during treatment, when it may be difficult or impossible to make corrections. Also, the overall outcome and prognosis may be adversely affected. In particular, it is critical to develop a thorough understanding of special patient concerns relating to previous care and expectations about future treatment. Many problems encountered during fixed prosthodontic treatment are directly traceable to factors overlooked during the initial examination and data collection. A diagnosis is a summation of the observed problems and their underlying etiologies. The patient's overall prognosis is influenced by general and local factors.

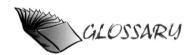 GLOSSARY

anterior guidance: *1:* the influence of the contacting surfaces of anterior teeth on tooth-limiting mandibular movements. *2:* the influence of the contacting surfaces of the guide pin and anterior guide table on articular movements. *3:* the fabrication of a relationship of the anterior teeth preventing posterior tooth contact in all eccentric mandibular movements.

anterior programming device: an individually fabricated anterior guide table that allows mandibular motion without the influence of tooth contacts and facilitates the recording of maxillomandibular relationships; also used for deprogramming.

apex: *n, pl* **apexes:** or **apices:** (1601) *1:* the uppermost point; the vertex. *2:* in dentistry, the anatomic end of a tooth root.

arthrography: *n 1:* roentgenography of a joint after injection of an opaque contrast material. *2:* in dentistry, a diagnostic technique that entails filling the lower, upper, or both joint spaces of the temporomandibular joint with a contrast agent to enable radiographic evaluation of the joint and surrounding structures; used to diagnose or confirm disk displacements and perforations.

articulate: *vb* (1691) *1:* to join together as a joint. *2:* the relation of contacting surfaces of the teeth or their artificial replicas in the maxillae to those in the mandible.

articulate: *adj* (1586) in speech, to enunciate clearly or be clearly spoken.

auscultation: *n* (ca, 1828) the process of determining the condition of various parts of the body by listening to the sounds they emit.

buccolingual relationship: any position of reference relative to the tongue and cheeks.

centric relation record: a registration of the relationship of the maxilla to the mandible when the mandible is in centric relation. The registration may be obtained either intraorally or extraorally.

centric slide: *obs* the movement of the mandible while in centric relation from the initial occlusal contact into maximum intercuspation (GPT-4).

chronic pain: pain marked by long duration or frequent recurrence.

Study Questions

1. Discuss the importance of the chief complaint and its management during examination and treatment plan presentation.
2. What is the classification of conditions observed as part of the medical history?
3. Describe the various areas included when taking a comprehensive dental history.
4. What systemic conditions may exhibit oral manifestations that can affect a fixed prosthodontic treatment plan?
5. What is included in a comprehensively conducted extraoral examination? Specify all structures included in palpation.
6. Discuss three critical observations that are part of a comprehensive periodontal evaluation. Why are they important for fixed prosthodontic evaluation?
7. What would be recorded as part of an intraoral charting?
8. Discuss the various types of radiographs available for diagnostic purposes. What are the advantages and limitations of each technique?
9. Give examples of general and local factors that may influence the patient's prognosis.

click: *n* (1611) a brief sharp sound; with reference to the temporomandibular joint, any bright or sharp sound emanating from the joint.

condylar axis: a hypothetical line through the mandibular condyles around which the mandible may rotate.

condylar hinge position: *obs* the position of the condyles of the mandible in the glenoid fossae at which hinge axis movement is possible (GPT-4).

crepitation: *n* a crackling or grating noise in a joint during movement, likened to the throwing of fine salt into a fire or rubbing hair between the fingers; the noise made by rubbing together the ends of a fracture bone.

deflection: *n* (1605) *1:* a turning aside or off course. *2:* a continuing eccentric displacement of the mandibular midline incisal path symptomatic of restriction in movement.

demineralization: *n* (ca. 1903) *1:* loss of minerals (as salts of calcium) from the body. *2:* in dentistry, decalcification.

dental cast: a positive life-size reproduction of a part or parts of the oral cavity.

deprogrammer: *n* various types of devices or materials used to alter the proprioceptive mechanism during mandibular closure.

deviation: *n* (15c) with respect to movement of the mandible, a discursive movement that ends in the centered position and is indicative of interference during movement.

disk derangement: an abnormal relationship of the articular disk to the condyle, fossa, and/or eminence.

diagnostic cast: a life-size reproduction of a part or parts of the oral cavity and/or facial structures for the purpose of study and treatment planning.

erosion: *n* (1541) *1:* an eating away; a type of ulceration. *2:* in dentistry, the progressive loss of tooth substance by chemical processes that do not involve bacterial action-producing defects that are sharply defined, wedge-shaped depressions often in facial and cervical areas.

etiologic factors: the elements or influences that can be defined as the cause or reason for a disease or lesion.

facet: *n* (1625) a small, planar surface on any hard body. Usage: the French spelling of facet, *facette,* has continued to confuse the profession regarding pronunciation.

fixed prosthodontics: the branch of prosthodontics concerned with the replacement and/or restoration of teeth by artificial substitutes that are not readily removed from the mouth.

forces of mastication: *obs* the motive force created by the dynamic action of the muscles during the physiologic act of mastication (GPT-4).

fremitus: *n* (1879) a vibration perceptible on palpation; in dentistry, a vibration palpable when the teeth come into contact.

high lip line: the greatest height to which the inferior border of the upper lip is capable of being raised by muscle function.

horizontal overlap: the projection of teeth beyond their antagonists in the horizontal plane.

incisal guidance: *1:* the influence of the contacting surfaces of the mandibular and maxillary anterior teeth on mandibular movements. *2:* the influence of the contacting surfaces of the guide pin and guide table on articulator movements.

infraocclusion: *n* malocclusion in which the occluding surfaces of teeth are below the normal plane of occlusion.

initial occlusal contact: the first or initial contact of opposing teeth.

interocclusal distance: the distance between the occluding surfaces of the maxillary and mandibular teeth when the mandible is in a specified position.

labioversion: *n* labial position of a tooth beyond normal arch form.

leaf gauge: a set of blades or leaves of increasing thickness used to measure the distance between two points or to provide metered separation.

local etiologic factors: the environmental influences that may be implicated in the causation, modification, and/or perpetuation of a disease entity.

low lip line: *1:* the lowest position of the inferior border of the upper lip when it is at rest. *2:* the lowest position of the superior border of the lower lip during smiling or voluntary retraction.

mandibular hinge position: *obs* the position of the mandible in relation to the maxilla at which opening and closing movements can be made on the hinge axis (GPT-4).

mandibular trismus: reduced mobility of the mandible resulting from tonic contracture of the masticatory muscles.

masticatory force: the force applied by the muscles of mastication during chewing.

muscle spasm: a sudden involuntary contraction of a muscle or group of muscles attended by pain and interference with function. It differs from muscle splinting in that the contraction is sustained even when the muscle is at rest and the pain/dysfunction is present with passive and active movements of the affected part—also called *myospasm.*

muscle splinting: *(slang)* involuntary contraction (rigidity) of muscles occurring as a means of avoiding the pain caused by movement of the part (resistance to passive stretch). The involved muscle(s) relaxes at rest.

musculoskeletal pain: deep, somatic pain that originates in skeletal muscles, facial sheaths, and tendons (myogenous pain); bone and periosteum (osseous pain); joint, joint capsules, and ligaments (arthralgic pain); and in soft connective tissues.

myofascial trigger point: a hyperirritable spot, usually within a skeletal muscle or in the muscle fascia, that is painful on compression and can give rise to characteristic referred pain, tenderness (secondary hyperalgesia), and autonomic phenomena.

NMR: acronym for Nuclear Magnetic Resonance; a radiologic procedure that provides images in any plane without radiation or any biologic after-effect by picking up signals from resonating hydrogen nuclei.

nonworking side interference: undesirable contacts of the opposing occlusal surfaces on the nonworking side.

occlude: *vb* **occluded; occluding:** *vt* (1597) *1:* to bring together; to shut. *2:* to bring or close the mandibular teeth into contact with the maxillary teeth.

occlusal force: the result of muscular force applied on opposing teeth; the force created by the dynamic action of the muscles during the physiologic act of mastication; the result of muscular activity applied to opposing teeth.

overhang: *n* (1864) excess restorative material projecting beyond a cavity or preparation margin.

palpate: *vt* **palpated; palpating:** (1849) to examine by touch.

panoramic radiograph: a radiograph produced by a panoramic machine—also called *orthopantograph.*

percussion: *n* (1544) *1:* the act of striking a part with sharp blows to help diagnose the condition of the underlying parts by means of the sound obtained. *2:* in dentistry, striking a part with short, sharp blows as a diagnostic aid in evaluation of a tooth or dental implant by the sound obtained.

periapical: *adj* relating to tissues surrounding the apex of a tooth, including the alveolar bone and periodontal ligament.

periradicular: *adj* around or surrounding a tooth root.

PFM: acronym for Porcelain Fused to Metal.

physical elasticity of muscle: *obs* the physical quality of being elastic; (i.e., yielding to active or passive physical stretch) (GPT-4).

preoperative records: *obs* any record(s) made for the purpose of study or treatment planning (GPT-4).

pretreatment records: any records made for the purpose of diagnosis, recording of the patient history, or treatment planning before therapy.

prosthetic restoration: *obs* an artificial replacement for an absent part of the human body (GPT-4).

pulpitis: *n* inflammation of the dental pulp.

radiograph: *n* (1880) an image produced on any sensitive surface by means of electromagnetic radiation other than light; an x-ray photograph.

radiolucent: permitting the passage of radiant energy with relatively little attenuation by absorption.

radiopaque: (1917) a structure that strongly inhibits the passage of radiant energy

range of motion: the range, measured in degrees of a circle, through which a joint can be extended or flexed. The range of the opening, lateral, and protrusive excursions of the temporomandibular joint.

reciprocal click: a pair of clicks emanating from the temporomandibular joint, one of which occurs during opening movements and the other during closing movements.

1 record: *vb* (14c) *1:* to register data relating to specific conditions that exist currently or previously *2:* to register permanently by mechanical means (i.e., jaw relationships)

2 record: *n* (14c) *1:* an official document. *2:* a body of known or recorded facts about someone or something.

reduced interarch distance: an occluding vertical dimension that results in an excessive interocclusal distance when the mandible is in rest position and in a reduced interridge distance when the teeth are in contact—also called *overclosure.*

retruded contact position: that guided occlusal relationship occurring at the most retruded position of the condyles in the joint cavities. A position that may be more retruded than the centric relation position.

reverse articulation: an occlusal relationship in which the mandibular teeth are located facial to the opposing maxillary teeth; the maxillary buccal cusps are positioned in the central fossae of the mandibular teeth.

root fracture: a microscopic or macroscopic cleavage of the root in any direction.

tinnitus: *n* (1843) a noise in the ears, often described as ringing or roaring.

tomograph: *n* a radiograph produced from a machine that has the source of radiation moving in one direction and the film moving in the opposite direction.

tomography: *n* a general term for a technique that provides a distinct image of any selected plane through the body, while the images of structures that lie above and below that plane are blurred. The term *body-section radiography* has been applied to the procedure, although the several methods to accomplish it have been given distinguishing names.

torus: *n; pl* **tori:** (1563) a smooth, rounded anatomical protuberance.

trigger point: a focus of hyperirritability in tissue, which, when palpated, is locally tender and leads to heterotopic pain.

unstrained jaw relation: *obs* *1:* the relation of the mandible to the skull when a state of balanced tonus exists among all the muscles involved *2:* any jaw relation that is attained without undue or unnatural force and that causes no undue distortion of the tissues of the temporomandibular joints (GPT-4).

xerostomia: *n* dryness of the mouth from lack of normal secretions.

REFERENCES

1. Bouquot JE, Seime RJ: Bulimia nervosa: dental perspectives, *Pract Periodont Aesthet Dent* 9:655, 1997.

2. Milosevic A: Eating disorders and the dentist, *Br Dent J* 186:109, 1999.

3. Cope MR: Metoclopramide-induced masticatory muscle spasm, *Br Dent J* 154:335, 1983.

4. Pajukoski H et al: Salivary flow and composition in elderly patients referred to an acute care geriatric ward, *Oral Surg* 84:265, 1997.

5. Hunter KD, Wilson WS: The effects of antidepressant drugs on salivary flow and content of sodium and potassium ions in human parotid saliva, *Arch Oral Biol* 40:983, 1995.

6. American Dental Association: Infection control recommendations for the dental office and laboratory, *J Am Dent Assoc* (Suppl) 1, 1992.

7. Epstein O et al: *Clinical examination*, ed 2, St Louis, 1997, Mosby.

8. Little JW et al: *Dental management of the medically compromised patient*, ed 5, St Louis, 1997, Mosby.

9. Solberg WK: Occlusion-related pathosis and its clinical evaluation. In Clark JW, editor: *Clinical dentistry*, vol 2, ch 35, Hagerstown, Md, 1976, Harper & Row.

10. Pullinger AG et al: Differences between sexes in maximum jaw opening when corrected to body size, *J Oral Rehabil* 14:291, 1987.

11. Krogh-Poulsen WG, Olsson A: Occlusal disharmonies and dysfunction of the stomatognathic system, *Dent Clin North Am* 10:627, 1966.

12. Moskowitz ME, Nayyar A: Determinants of dental esthetics: a rational for smile analysis and treatment, *Compend Contin Educ Dent* 16:1164, 1995.

13. Crispin BJ, Watson JF: Margin placement of esthetic veneer crowns. I. Anterior tooth visibility, *J Prosthet Dent* 45:278, 1981.

14. Lombardi RE: The principles of visual perception and their clinical application to denture esthetics, *J Prosthet Dent* 29:358, 1973.

15. Matthews TG: The anatomy of a smile, *J Prosthet Dent* 39:128, 1978.

16. The American Academy of Periodontology: Epidemiology of periodontal diseases, *J Periodontol* 67:935, 1996.

17. The American Academy of Periodontology: Guidelines for periodontal therapy, *J Periodontol* 69:405, 1998.

18. Carranza FA Jr, Newman MG: *Clinical periodontology*, ed 8, Philadelphia, 1996, WB Saunders.

19. Goodson JM: Selection of suitable indicators of periodontitis. In Bader JD, editor: *Risk assessment in dentistry*, Chapel Hill, N.C., 1989, University of North Carolina Dental Ecology.

20. The American Academy of Periodontology: *Parameters of care*, Chicago, 1998, The American Academy of Periodontology.

21. Van Sickels JE et al: Transcranial radiographs in the evaluation of craniomandibular (TMJ) disorders, *J Prosthet Dent* 49:244, 1983.

22. Blaschke DD et al: Arthrography of the temporomandibular joint: review of current status, *J Am Dent Assoc* 100:388, 1980.

23. Fava C, Preti G: Lateral transcranial radiography of temporomandibular joints. II. Image formation studied with computerized tomography, *J Prosthet Dent* 59:218, 1988.

24. Laurell KA et al: Magnetic resonance imaging of the temporomandibular joint. I. Literature review, *J Prosthet Dent* 58:83, 1987.

25. Laurell KA et al: Magnetic resonance imaging of the temporomandibular joint. II. Comparison with laminographic, autopsy, and histologic findings, *J Prosthet Dent* 58:211, 1987.

26. Laurell KA et al: Magnetic resonance imaging of the temporomandibular joint. III. Use of a cephalostat for clinical imaging, *J Prosthet Dent* 58:355, 1987.

27. Kapa SF et al: Assessing condylar changes with digital subtraction radiography, *Oral Surg* 75:247, 1993.

CHAPTER TWO

DIAGNOSTIC CASTS AND RELATED PROCEDURES

KEY TERMS

anterior guide table
arbitrary facebow
arcon
articulator
articulator controls
centric relation (CR)
centric relation record
diagnostic impressions

diagnostic waxing
hinge axis
irreversible hydrocolloid
kinematic facebow
nonarcon
pantograph
programming device
third reference point

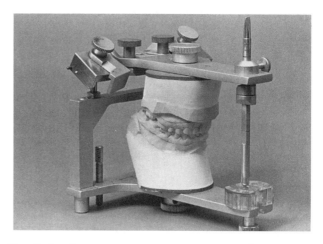

Fig. 2-1. Diagnostic casts mounted on a Whip Mix articulator.

Accurate diagnostic casts (Fig. 2-1) transferred to a semiadjustable **articulator** are essential in planning fixed prosthodontic treatment. This permits static and dynamic relationships of the teeth to be examined without interference from protective neuromuscular reflexes, and unencumbered views from all directions reveal aspects of the occlusion not always easily detectable intraorally (e.g., the relationship of the lingual cusps in the occluded position). If the maxillary cast has been transferred with a facebow, a **centric relation (CR)** interocclusal record has been used for articulation of the mandibular cast, and the condylar elements have been appropriately set (such as with protrusive and/or excursive interocclusal records), reproducing the patient's movements with reasonable accuracy is possible. If the casts have been articulated in CR, assessing both the CR and the MI position is possible, because any slide can then be reproduced. Other critical information not immediately apparent during the clinical examination includes the occlusocervical dimension of edentulous spaces. On an articulator, these are readily assessed in the occluded position and throughout the entire range of mandibular movement. Relative alignment and angulation of proposed abutment teeth are easier to evaluate on casts than intraorally, as are many other subtle changes in individual tooth position. Articulated diagnostic casts permit a detailed analysis of the occlusal plane and the occlusion, and diagnostic procedures can be performed for a better diagnosis and treatment plan; tooth

preparations can be "rehearsed" on the casts, and **diagnostic waxing** procedures allow evaluation of the eventual outcome of proposed treatment.

IMPRESSION MAKING FOR DIAGNOSTIC CASTS

Accurate impressions of both dental arches are required. Flaws in the impressions will result in inaccuracies in the casts that easily compound. For instance, a small void in the impression caused by trapping an air bubble on one of the occlusal surfaces will result in a nodule on the occlusal table. If it is not recognized and carefully removed, it will lead to an inaccurate articulator mounting, and the diagnostic data will be incorrect.

As long as the impression extends several millimeters beyond the cervical line of the teeth, the borders of **diagnostic impressions** are usually not of great concern for fixed prosthodontic purposes, unless a removable prosthesis also is to be fabricated. Properly manipulated irreversible hydrocolloid (alginate) is sufficiently accurate and offers adequate surface detail for planning purposes. However, the material does not reproduce sufficient surface detail for suitable working casts and dies on which actual fixed prostheses are fabricated (see Chapter 17).

IRREVERSIBLE HYDROCOLLOID

The **irreversible hydrocolloids,** or alginates, are essentially sodium or potassium salts of alginic acid and are therefore water soluble. They react chemically with calcium sulfate to produce insoluble calcium alginate. These materials contain other ingredients, chiefly diatomaceous earth (for strength and body), trisodium phosphate (Na_3PO_4), and similar compounds to control the setting rate as they react preferentially with calcium sulfate. When this reaction is complete and the retarder is consumed, gel formation begins. The clinician can control the reaction rate by varying the temperature of the mixing water. Because set irreversible hydrocolloid is largely water, it will readily absorb (by imbibition) as well as give off (by syneresis) liquid to the atmosphere, causing distortion of the impression. Alginate impressions must therefore be poured immediately.

DIAGNOSTIC IMPRESSION TECHNIQUE

Armamentarium

- Impression trays
- Modeling compound
- Mixing bowl
- Mixing spatula
- Gauze squares
- Irreversible hydrocolloid
- ADA Type IV or V stone
- Vacuum mixer
- Humidor
- Disinfectant

Tray Selection

All impression materials require retention in the impression tray. This can be provided for irreversible hydrocolloid by using an adhesive or by making perforations or undercuts around the rim of the tray. All types of trays are capable of producing impressions with clinically acceptable accuracy.[1] For irreversible hydrocolloids, the largest tray that will fit comfortably in the patient's mouth should be selected. A greater bulk of material will produce a more accurate impression (i.e., a bulky impression has a more favorable surface area/volume ratio and is less susceptible to water loss or gain and therefore unwanted dimensional change). In contrast, elastomeric impression materials work well with a relatively tightly fitting custom impression tray in which a relatively uniform thin layer of material is used. This produces the most accurate impression (see Chapter 14).

Distortion of irreversible hydrocolloid can occur if any part of the impression is unsupported by the tray or if there is movement of the tray during setting. For these reasons, the tray may need to be extended and its perimeter modified with modeling compound (Fig. 2-2).

Impression Making

For optimum results the teeth should be cleaned and the mouth thoroughly rinsed. Some drying is necessary, but excessively dried tooth surfaces will cause the irreversible hydrocolloid impression material to adhere. The material is mixed to a homogeneous consistency, loaded into the tray, and its surface smoothed with a moistened, gloved finger.[2] Concurrently, a small amount of material is wiped into the crevices of the occlusal surfaces (Fig. 2-3, *A, B*) before the tray is seated (Fig. 2-3, *C*). Also, a small amount can be applied by wiping it into the mucobuccal fold. As the tray is inserted into the patient's mouth and seated, the patient is reminded to relax the cheek muscles. If a patient continues to stretch wide open while the tray is being fully seated, impression material is often squeezed out of the mucobuccal fold or from underneath the upper lip.

A loss of tackiness of the material (gelation) implies initial set. The tray should be removed quickly 2 to 3 minutes after gelation. Teasing or wiggling the set impression from the mouth causes excessive distortion due to viscous flow. Also, certain irreversible hydrocolloid materials distort if held in the mouth more than 2 or 3 minutes after gelation.[3] Following removal, the impression should be rinsed and disinfected, dried slightly with a gentle air stream, and poured immediately. For disinfection, spraying with

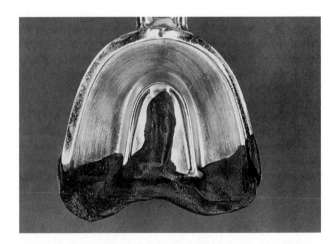

Fig. 2-2. Stock impression trays can be readily modified with modeling compound to provide better support for the alginate. Typically the posterior border needs extension. If the patient has a high palate, the alginate should be supported here too, although it should not block out the retentive area of the tray.

a suitable glutaraldehyde and placement in a self-sealing plastic bag for approximately 10 minutes is recommended, after which it can be poured. Alternatively, the impression can be immersed in iodophor or glutaraldehyde disinfectant. The disinfection protocol is an essential precaution for preventing cross-infection and protecting laboratory personnel (see Chapter 14). It should be noted that irreversible hydrocolloid impressions carry significantly higher numbers of bacteria than elastomeric materials.[4] There is no significant loss of accuracy or surface detail due to the disinfection procedure.[5,6] To ensure accuracy, pouring should be completed within 15 minutes of the time the impression is removed from the mouth. Keeping an impression in a moist towel is no substitute for pouring within the specified time. Trimming off gross excess impression material before setting the tray down on the bench top is helpful. A vacuum-mixed ADA Type IV or Type V stone is recommended. The choice of the brand of stone is important because of the harmful surface interactions between specific irreversible hydrocolloid materials and gypsum products.[7]

After mixing, a small amount of stone is added in one location (e.g., the posterior aspect of one of the molars). Adding small amounts consistently in the same location will minimize bubble formation (see the section on pouring stone dies in Chapter 17). If air is trapped, bubbles can be eliminated by poking at them with a small instrument (e.g., a periodontal probe or a wax spatula). While setting, the poured impressions must be stored tray side down, not inverted. Inverting freshly poured impressions results in a cast with a rough and grainy surface.[8] Stone is added to create a sufficient base that provides adequate retention for mounting on the articulator. To achieve maximum strength and surface detail, the poured impression should be covered with wet paper and stored in a humidor for 1 hour. This minimizes distortion of the irreversible hydrocolloid during the setting period. The setting gypsum cast should *never* be immersed in water. If this is done, setting expansion of plaster, stone, or die stone will double or even triple through the phenomenon of hygroscopic expansion (see Chapter 22). For best results, the cast should be separated 1 hour after pouring.

Evaluation

Although it is apparently a simple procedure, diagnostic cast fabrication is often mishandled. Seemingly minor inaccuracies can lead to serious diagnostic errors. Questionable impressions and casts should be discarded and the process repeated (Fig. 2-4). Voids in the impression create nodules on the poured cast. These can prevent proper articulation and effectively render useless a subsequent occlusal analysis or other diagnostic procedure.

Articulator Selection

Handheld casts can provide information concerning alignment of the individual arches but do not permit analysis of functional relationships. For an analysis, the diagnostic casts need to be attached to an articulator, a mechanical device that simulates mandibular movement. Articulators can simulate the movement of the condyles in their corresponding fossae. They are classified according to how closely

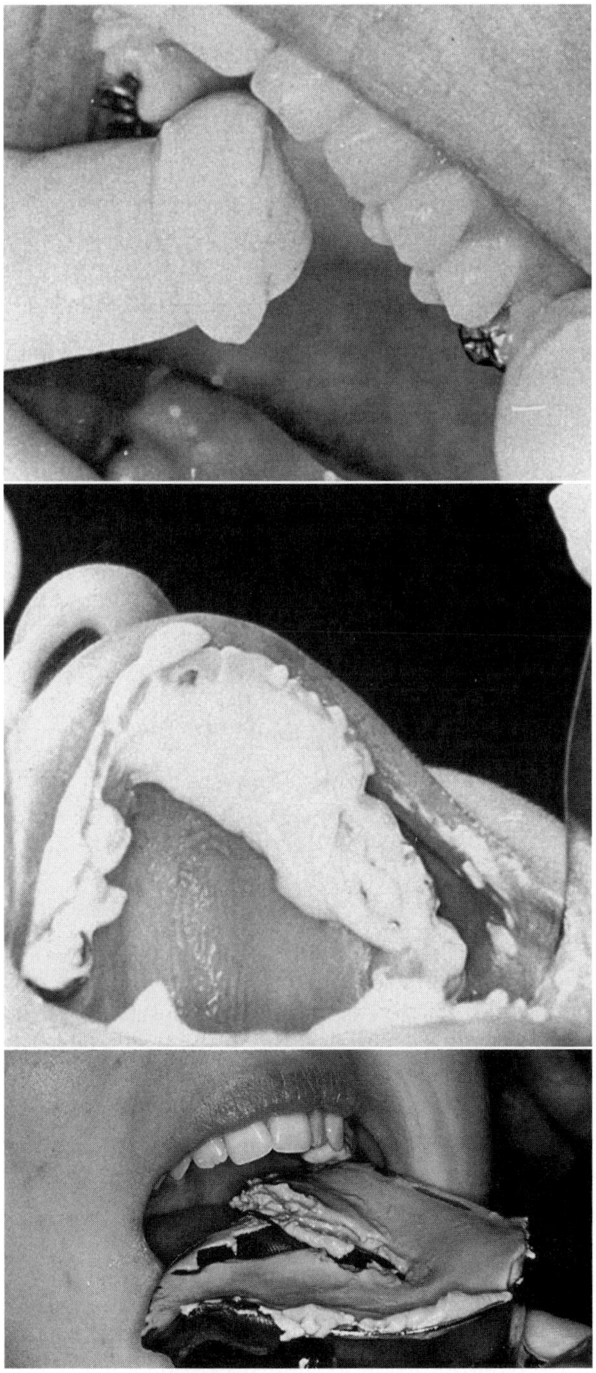

Fig. 2-3. **A** to **C,** Making an alginate impression for diagnostic casts.

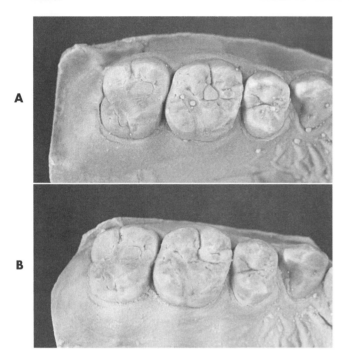

Fig. 2-4. Diagnostic casts must be accurate if they are to articulate properly. **A,** Occlusal nodules may make proper occlusal analysis impossible. **B,** Proper technique will ensure a satisfactory cast.

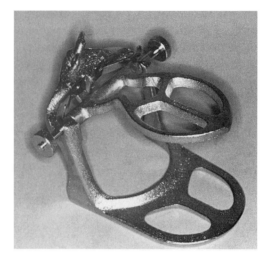

Fig. 2-5. A small nonadjustable articulator.

they can reproduce mandibular border movements. Because the movements are governed by the bones and ligaments of the TMJs, they are relatively constant and reproducible. Most articulators use mechanically adjustable posterior controls to simulate these movements, although some use plastic premilled or customized fossa analogs. If an articulator closely reproduces the actual border movements of a given patient, this will significantly reduce chair time because the dental laboratory can then design the prosthesis to be in functional harmony with the patient's movements. In addition, less time will be needed for adjustments at delivery.

On some instruments, the upper and lower members are permanently attached to each other, while on others they can be readily separated. The latter group may have a latch or clamplike feature that locks the two components together in the hinge position. Instrument selection depends on the type and complexity of treatment needs, the demands for procedural accuracy, and general expediency. For instance, when waxing a fixed partial denture, it is advantageous to be able to separate the instrument into two more easily handled parts. Use of the proper instrument for a given procedure can translate into significant time-saving during subsequent stages of treatment.

SMALL NONADJUSTABLE ARTICULATORS

Many cast restorations are made on small nonadjustable articulators (Fig. 2-5). Their use often leads to restorations with occlusal discrepancies, because these instruments do not have the capacity to reproduce the full range of mandibular movement. Some discrepancies can be corrected intraorally, but this is often time consuming and frustrating, leading to increased inaccuracy. If discrepancies are left uncorrected, occlusal interferences and associated neuromuscular disorders may result.

Of practical significance are differences between the hinge closure of a small articulator and that of the patient. The distance between the hinge and the tooth to be restored is significantly less on most nonadjustable articulators than in the patient. This can lead to restorations with premature tooth contacts because cusp position is affected. This type of arcing motion on the nonadjustable articulator results in steeper travel than occurs clinically, resulting in premature contacts subsequently on fabricated restorations between the distal mandibular inclines and the mesial maxillary inclines of posterior teeth (Fig. 2-6).

Depending on the specific design of the articulator, ridge and groove direction may be affected in accordance with the same principle. This is important to note, because resulting prematurities are likely on the nonworking side (see Chapters 1 and 4).

SEMIADJUSTABLE ARTICULATORS

For most routine fixed prostheses, the use of a semiadjustable articulator (Fig. 2-7) is a practical approach to providing the necessary diagnostic information while minimizing the need for clinical adjustment during treatment. Semiadjustable instruments do not require an inordinate amount of time or expertise. They are about the same size as the anatomic structures they represent. Therefore, the articulated casts can be positioned with sufficient accuracy so that arcing errors will be minimal and usually of minimal clinical significance (i.e.,

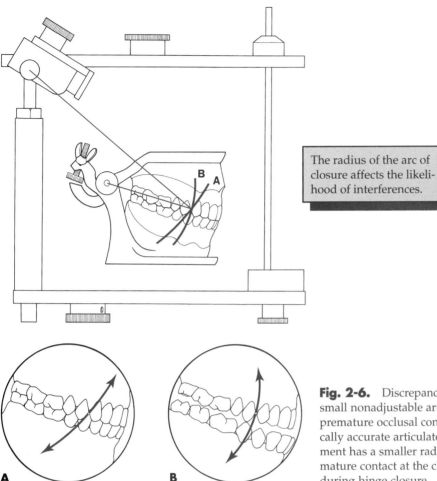

The radius of the arc of closure affects the likelihood of interferences.

Fig. 2-6. Discrepancies in the path of closure when using a small nonadjustable articulator can lead to restorations with premature occlusal contacts. **A,** Path of closure of an anatomically accurate articulator. **B,** The small nonadjustable instrument has a smaller radius closure path, which results in premature contact at the clinical try-in between the premolars during hinge closure.

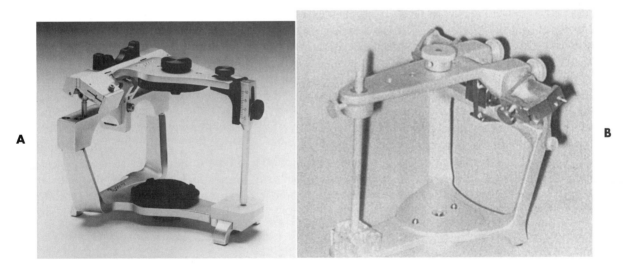

Fig. 2-7. Semiadjustable arcon articulators. **A,** The Denar Mark II. **B,** The Whip Mix model 2240. (*A Courtesy Denar Corporation.*)

minimal time should be required for chairside adjustments of fabricated prostheses).

There are two basic designs of the semiadjustable articulator: the **arcon** (for **ar**ticulator and **con**dyle) (Fig. 2-8, *A, C*) and the **nonarcon** (Fig. 2-8, *B, D*). Nonarcon instruments gained considerable popular-

ity in complete denture prosthodontics because the upper and lower members are rigidly attached, permitting easier control when positioning artificial teeth. As a consequence of their design, however, certain inaccuracies occur in cast restorations, which led to the development of the arcon-type instrument.

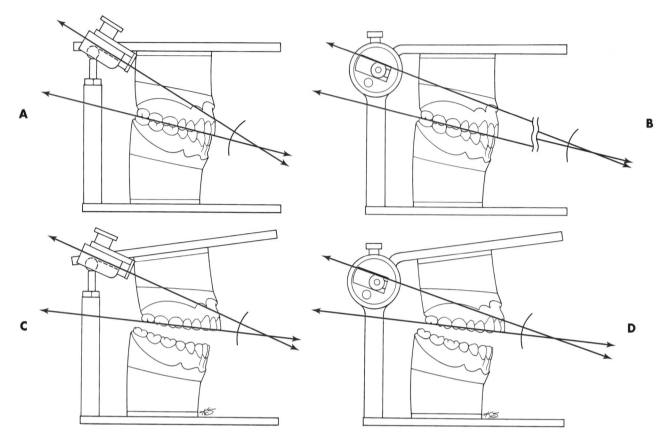

Fig. 2-8. **A** and **C** show an arcon; **B** and **D** show a nonarcon articulator. An advantage of the arcon design is that the condylar inclination of the mechanical fossae is at a fixed angle to the maxillary occlusal plane. With the nonarcon design, the angle changes as the articulator is opened, which can lead to errors when a protrusive record is being used to program the articulator.
(Redrawn from Shillingburg HT et al: Fundamentals of fixed prosthodontics, *ed 2, Chicago, 1981, Quintessence Publishing.)*

In an arcon articulator, the condylar spheres are attached to the lower component of the articulator, and the mechanical fossae are attached to the upper member of the instrument. Thus, the arcon articulator is anatomically "correct," which makes understanding of mandibular movements easier, as opposed to the nonarcon articulator (whose movements are confusingly "backward"). The angulation of the mechanical fossae of an arcon instrument is fixed relative to the occlusal plane of the maxillary cast; in the nonarcon design, it is fixed relative to the occlusal plane of the mandibular cast.

Most semiadjustable articulators permit adjustments to the condylar inclination and progressive and/or immediate side shift. Some have straight condylar inclined paths, although more recent instruments have curved condylar housings, which are more anatomically correct.

The mechanical fossae on semiadjustable articulators can be adjusted to mimic the movements of the patient through the use of interocclusal records. These consist of several thicknesses of wax or another suitable material in which the patient has closed. Because these records can be several millimeters thick, an error is introduced when setting nonarcon articulators with protrusive wax records, because its condylar path is not fixed relative to the maxillary occlusal plane. As the protrusive record used to adjust the instrument is removed from the nonarcon articulator, the maxillary occlusal plane and the condylar inclination become more parallel to each other, leading to reduced cuspal heights in subsequently fabricated prostheses (see Table 4-3).

FULLY ADJUSTABLE ARTICULATORS

A fully (or highly) adjustable articulator (Fig. 2-9) has a wide range of positions and can be set to follow a patient's border movements. The accuracy of reproduction of movement depends on the care and skill of the operator, the errors inherent in the articulator and recording device, and any malalignments due to slight flexing of the mandible and the nonrigid nature of the TMJs.

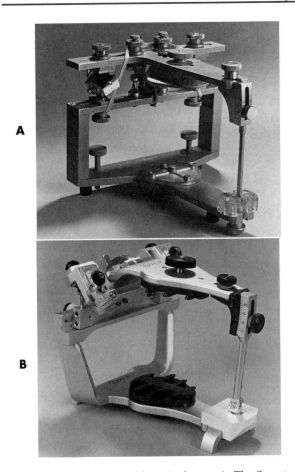

Fig. 2-9. Fully adjustable articulators. **A,** The Stuart. **B,** The Denar D5A.

Rather than relying on wax records to adjust the instrument, special pantographic tracings are used to record the patient's border movements in a series of tracings. The armamentarium used to generate these tracings is then transferred to the articulator, and the instrument is adjusted so the articulator replicates the tracings, essentially reproducing the border movements of the patient. The ability of fully adjustable instruments to track irregular pathways of movement throughout entire trajectories permits the fabrication of complex prostheses, requiring minimal adjustment at the try-in and delivery appointment.

Fully adjustable articulators are not often required in general practice. Using and adjusting them can be time consuming and requires a high level of skill and understanding from the dentist and the technician. Once this skill has been acquired, however, the detailed information they convey can save considerable chairside time. They can be very useful as treatment complexity increases (e.g., when all four posterior quadrants are to be restored simultaneously or when it is necessary to restore an entire dentition, especially in the presence of atypical mandibular movement).

FACEBOWS

TRANSVERSE HORIZONTAL AXIS

The mandibular hinging movement around the transverse horizontal axis is repeatable. That makes this imaginary "**hinge axis**" around which the mandible may rotate in the sagittal plane of considerable importance when fabricating fixed prostheses. Facebows are used to record the anteroposterior and mediolateral spatial position of the maxillary occlusal surfaces relative to this transverse opening and closing axis of the patient's mandible. The facebow is then attached to the articulator to transfer the recorded relationship of the maxilla by ensuring that the corresponding cast is attached in the correct position relative to the hinge axis of the instrument. After the maxillary cast has been attached to the articulator with mounting stone or plaster, the mandibular cast is subsequently related to the maxillary cast through the use of an interocclusal record. If the patient's casts are accurately transferred to an instrument, considerable time is saved in the fabrication and delivery of high-quality prostheses.

Most facebows are rigid, caliper-like devices that permit some adjustments. Two types of facebows are recognized: arbitrary and kinematic. **Arbitrary facebows** are less accurate than the kinematic type, but they suffice for most routine dental procedures. **Kinematic facebows** are indicated when it is critical to precisely reproduce the exact opening and closing movement of the patient on the articulator. For instance, when a decision to alter the vertical dimension of occlusion is to be made in the dental laboratory during the fabrication of fixed prostheses, the use of a kinematic facebow transfer in conjunction with an accurate CR interocclusal record is indicated.

KINEMATIC HINGE AXIS FACEBOW

Hinge Axis Recording. The hinge axis of the mandible can be determined to within 1 mm by observing the movement of kinematic facebow styli positioned immediately lateral to the TMJ close to the skin. A clutch (Fig. 2-10, *A*), which is essentially a segmented impression traylike device, is attached onto the mandibular teeth with a suitable rigid material such as impression plaster. The kinematic facebow consists of three components: a transverse component and two adjustable side arms. The transverse rod is attached to the portion of the clutch that protrudes from the patient's mouth. The side arms are then attached to the transverse member and adjusted so that the styli are as close to the joint area as possible. The mandible is then manipulated to produce a terminal hinge movement, and the stylus locations are adjusted with thumbscrews (superiorly and inferiorly, anteriorly and posteriorly) until they make a purely rotational

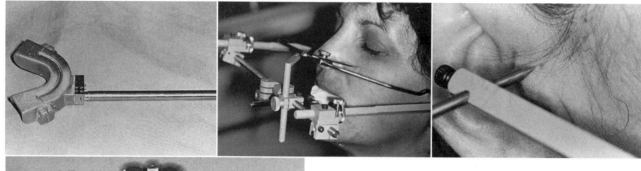

Fig. 2-10. Kinematic hinge axis facebow. **A,** Mandibular clutch. The clutch separates for removal into two components by loosening the screws on left and right sides. **B,** Transferring the position of the mandibular hinge axis. **C,** Pointers aligned with the previously marked hinge axis location. **D,** Kinematic facebow aligned on the articulator.

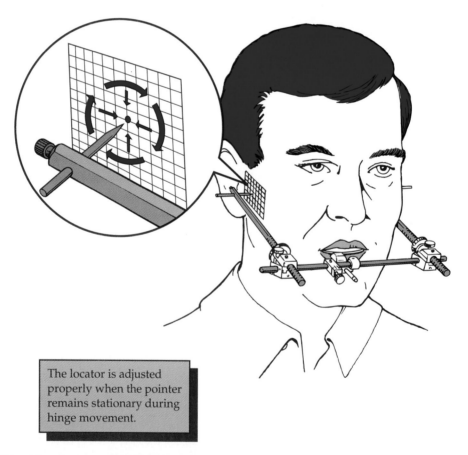

The locator is adjusted properly when the pointer remains stationary during hinge movement.

Fig 2-11. Hinge axis recording: Left and right styli are attached via a facebow to a clutch affixed to the mandibular teeth. When the mandible makes a strictly rotational movement, the stylus will remain stationary if aligned with the actual axis of rotation. If the stylus is positioned forward or backward, above or below the actual axis, it will travel one of the arcs indicated by the arrows when the mandible makes a rotational movement. Thus, the arc indicates in what direction an adjustment should be made to the stylus position.

movement (Fig. 2-11). Because the entire assembly is rigidly attached to the mandible, a strictly rotational movement signifies that stylus position coincides with the hinge axis. When this purely rotational movement is verified, the position of the hinge axis is marked with a dot on the patient's skin, or it may be permanently tattooed if future use is anticipated or required.

Kinematic Facebow Transfer. An impression of the maxillary cusp tips is obtained in a suitable recording medium on a facebow fork. The facebow is attached to the protruding arm of the fork. The side arms are adjusted until the styli are aligned with the hinge axis marks on the patient's skin. The patient must be in the same position that was used when the axis was marked to prevent skin movement from introducing any inaccuracy. A pointer device is usually attached to the bow and adjusted to a repeatable reference point selected by the clinician. The reference point is used later for reproducibility. The kinematic facebow recording is then transferred to the articulator, and the maxillary cast is attached.

The kinematic facebow technique is time consuming, so it is generally limited to extensive prosthodontics, particularly when a change in the vertical dimension of occlusion is to be made. A less precisely derived transfer would then lead to unacceptable errors and a compromised result.

ARBITRARY HINGE AXIS FACEBOW

Arbitrary hinge axis facebows (Fig. 2-12) approximate the horizontal transverse axis and rely on anatomic average values. Manufacturers design these facebows so the relationship to the true axis falls within an acceptable degree of error. Typically, an easily identifiable landmark such as the external acoustic meatus is used to stabilize the bow, which is aligned with earpieces similar to those on a stethoscope. Such facebows can be used single-handedly because they are self-centering and do not require complicated assembly. They give a sufficiently accurate relationship for most diagnostic and restorative procedures. However, regardless of which arbitrary position is chosen, a minimum error of 5 mm from the axis can be expected.[9] When coupled with the use of a thick interocclusal record made at an increased vertical dimension, this factor can lead to considerable inaccuracy.

Anterior Reference Point (Fig. 2-13). The use of an anterior reference point enables the clinician to duplicate the recorded position on the articulator at future appointments. This saves time, because previously recorded articulator settings can be used again. An anterior reference point, such as the inner canthus of the eye or a freckle or mole on the skin, is selected. After this has been marked, it is used, along with the two points of the hinge axis, to define the position of the maxillary cast in space. This has the following advantages:

- After the posterior controls have been adjusted initially, subsequent casts can be mounted on the articulator without repeating the facebow determinations and having to reset the posterior **articulator controls.**
- Because the maxillary arch is properly positioned relative to the axis, average values for posterior articulator controls can be used without having to readjust the instrument on the basis of eccentric records.
- When the articulator has been adjusted, the resulting numerical values for the settings can be compared with known average values to provide information about the patient's individual variations and the likelihood of encountering difficulties during restorative procedures.

Facebow Transfer
Armamentarium
- Arbitrary-type hinge axis facebow
- Modeling compound
- Cotton rolls

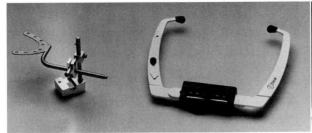
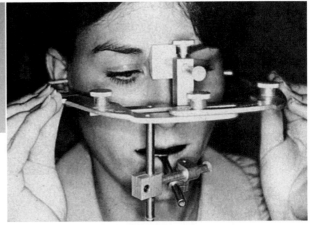

Fig. 2-12. **A,** The Denar Slidematic and, **B,** Whip Mix Quick Mount arbitrary hinge axis facebows. Note the nasion relator as the **third reference point.** *(A Courtesy Denar Corporation.)*

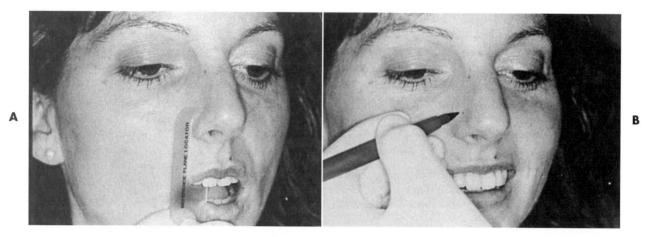

Fig. 2-13. A, B, The Denar Slidematic facebow uses a mark 43 mm superior to the incisal edge of the maxillary central incisor as an anterior reference point. Other systems use the infraorbital foramen or nasion. The mark serves as a reference to average anatomic values. It also allows subsequent casts to be mounted without a repeat recording.

Step-by-step Procedure

1. Add modeling compound to the facebow fork (Fig. 2-14, *A*).
2. Temper in water and seat the fork, making indentations of the maxillary cusp tips. The facebow fork is positioned in the patient's mouth, and an impression is made of the maxillary cusp tips. The impression must be deep enough to permit accurate repositioning of the maxillary cast after the facebow fork has been removed from the mouth. Only the cusp tips should be recorded. It is not necessary to get an impression of every cusp, or even an entire cusp—just one that is sufficient to position the diagnostic cast accurately. If the impression is too deep, accurate repositioning of the cast can become problematic because the diagnostic casts are not absolutely accurate reproductions of the teeth. In general, the tips are reproduced more accurately than the fossae.
3. Remove the fork from the mouth. Chill and reseat the fork, and check that no distortion has occurred (Fig. 2-14, *B*). The inclusion of details of pits and fissures in the recording medium will lead to inaccuracies when trying to seat the stone cast. Trim the recording medium as necessary before reseating. After reseating, check for stability.
4. Have the patient stabilize the facebow fork by biting on cotton rolls. As an alternative, wax can be added to the mandibular incisor region of the fork. The mandibular anterior teeth will stabilize the fork as they engage the wax.

5. Slide the universal joint onto the fork and position the caliper to align with the anterior reference mark (Fig. 2-14, *C*).
6. Tighten the screws securely in the correct sequence (Fig. 2-14, *D*).
7. If the articulator has an adjustable intercondylar width, record this measurement (Fig. 2-14, *E*). Remove the facebow from the mouth.

The technique is slightly different with other arbitrary facebows (Fig. 2-14, *F to K*).

Centric Relation Record. A **centric relation record** (Fig. 2-15) provides the orientation of mandibular to maxillary teeth in CR in the terminal hinge position, where opening and closing are purely rotational movements. *Centric relation* is defined as the maxillomandibular relationship in which the condyles articulate with the thinnest avascular portion of their respective disks with the condyle-disk complex in the anterior-superior position against the articular eminences. This position is independent of tooth contact.

Maximum intercuspation may or may not occur coincident with the centric relation position. The centric relation record is transferred to the maxillary cast on the articulator and is used to relate the mandibular cast to the maxillary cast. Once the mandibular cast is attached to the articulator with mounting stone, the record is removed. The casts will then occlude in precisely the CR position as long as the maxillary cast is correctly related to the hinge axis with a facebow (see Fig. 2-14). When the articulator controls are set properly, using appropriate excursive records, translated mandibular

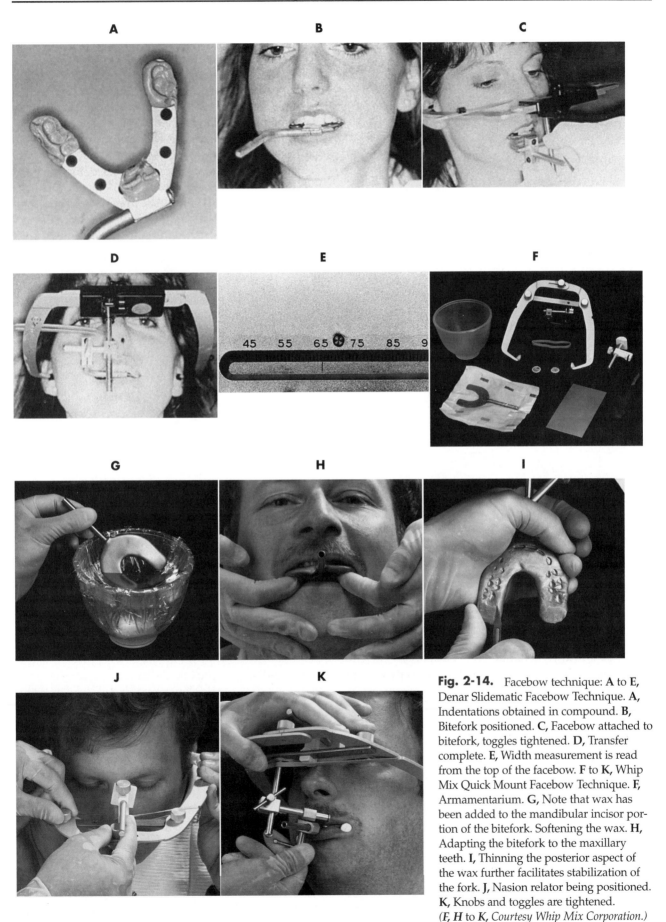

Fig. 2-14. Facebow technique: **A** to **E,** Denar Slidematic Facebow Technique. **A,** Indentations obtained in compound. **B,** Bitefork positioned. **C,** Facebow attached to bitefork, toggles tightened. **D,** Transfer complete. **E,** Width measurement is read from the top of the facebow. **F** to **K,** Whip Mix Quick Mount Facebow Technique. **F,** Armamentarium. **G,** Note that wax has been added to the mandibular incisor portion of the bitefork. Softening the wax. **H,** Adapting the bitefork to the maxillary teeth. **I,** Thinning the posterior aspect of the wax further facilitates stabilization of the fork. **J,** Nasion relator being positioned. **K,** Knobs and toggles are tightened. (*F, H* to *K, Courtesy Whip Mix Corporation.*)

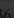

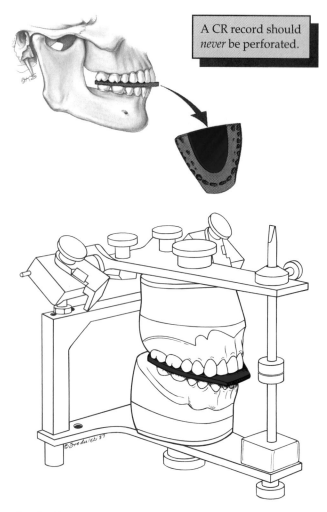

A CR record should *never* be perforated.

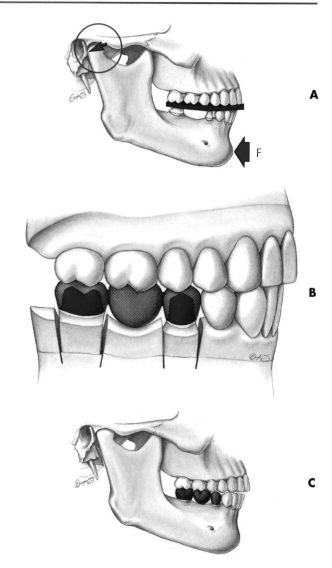

A

F

B

C

Fig. 2-15. A CR record transfers the tooth relationships at CR from the patient to the articulator.

Fig. 2-16. Incorrect CR recording. **A,** If the mandible is forced backward *(F)*, the condyles will not be in their most superior position but will be moved backward and downward *(arrow)*. **B,** Any restorations made on casts related with this CR record will be in supraclusion when tried in the mouth. **C,** Note the relationship of the anterior teeth.

positions can be reproduced from CR. A CR/MI slide will be readily reproducible on casts that have been articulated in CR. Thus, premature tooth contacts (deflective contacts) can be observed, and it can be determined whether an occlusal correction is necessary or appropriate before fixed prosthodontic treatment. Casts articulated in the maximum intercuspation (MI) position do not permit the evaluation of CR and retruded contact relationships. Therefore, the articulation of diagnostic casts in CR is of greater diagnostic value.

When using a kinematic facebow, in theory, the thickness of a terminal hinge record is unimportant; a thicker record merely increases the amount of rotation. When using an arbitrary facebow, any arcing movement will result in some degree of inaccuracy. Both techniques are subject to small errors, which can be minimized by keeping the record thin.[10,11] However, it is essential that the teeth not perforate the record. Any tooth contact during record fabrication can cause mandibular translation due to neuromuscular protective reflexes governed

by mechanoreceptors in the periodontium, rendering the resulting articulation useless.

Jaw Manipulation. Accurately mounted casts depend on precise manipulation of the patient's mandible by the dentist. The condyles should remain in the same place throughout the opening-closing arc. Trying to force the mandible backward will lead to downward translation of the condyles, and restorations made to such a mandibular position will be in supraclusion at the try-in stage (Fig. 2-16).

The load-bearing surfaces of the condylar processes, which face anteriorly, should be manipulated into apposition with the mandibular fossae of the temporal bones, with the disk properly interposed. The ease with which this can be accomplished depends on the degree of the patient's neuromuscular relaxation

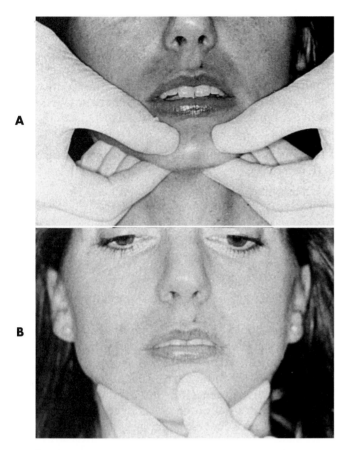

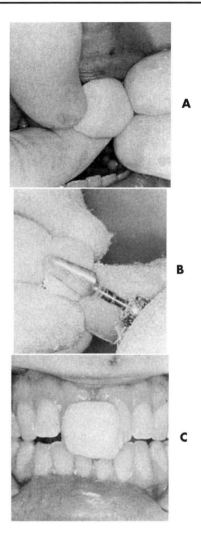

Fig. 2-17. Manipulating a patient's mandible into centric relation. Note the position of the examiner's thumbs and fingers on the mandibular border. The bimanual (**A**) and the single-handed technique (**B**).

and on sound technique. The latter, in turn, depends on the patient permitting the dentist to control the mandible. Attempts to force or shake the mandible will lead to a protective muscle response by the patient.

The bimanual manipulation technique described by Dawson[12] is recommended as a reproducible technique[13] that can be reliably learned.[14] In this technique, the dental chair is reclined and the patient's head is cradled by the examiner. With both thumbs on the chin and the fingers resting firmly on the inferior border of the mandible (Fig. 2-17, *A*), the examiner exerts gentle downward pressure on the thumbs and upward pressure on the fingers, manipulating the condyle-disk assemblies into their fully seated positions in the mandibular fossae. Next, the mandible is carefully hinged along the arc of terminal hinge closure. *Note*: It is more difficult to ensure that the condyles will be properly located when the single-handed approach (Fig 2-17, *B*) is used with the fingers exerting upward pressure, although this technique does allow the other hand to hold the record.

Anterior Programming Device (Fig. 2-18). In some patients in whom CR does not coincide with IP,

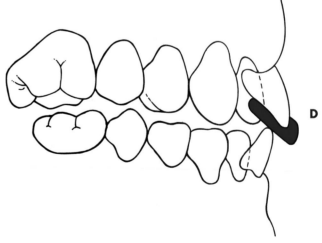

Fig. 2-18. An anterior programming device is used to facilitate centric relation recording. **A,** Autopolymerizing resin is adapted to the maxillary central incisors. The patient is guided into closure and stopped when the posterior teeth are about 1 mm apart. The indentations are used as a guide during trimming of the device (**B**). The completed device (**C**) should allow the patient to make smooth lateral and protrusive movements. An inclined contact area must be avoided, because it will tend to retrude the mandible excessively. **D,** Cross section through device.

protective reflexes may be encountered. Because of well-established protective reflexes that are reinforced every time the teeth come together, such patients will not allow their mandible to be manipulated and hinged easily. If tooth contact can be prevented, they will "forget" these reflexes, and manipulation becomes easier. The teeth can be kept apart with cotton rolls, a plastic leaf gauge, or a small anterior **programming device** made of autopolymerizing acrylic resin (also known as a *Lucia jig*).[15]

If the mandible cannot be manipulated satisfactorily after an anterior programming device has been in place for 30 minutes, marked neuromuscular dysfunction is likely. Normally this is relieved by providing an occlusal device (whose fabrication and adjustment are described in Chapter 4).

Centric Relation Recording Technique. Different techniques can be used to make a CR record. The choice of recording medium is to some degree a function of the casts to be articulated. For instance, very accurate casts made from elastomeric impression materials can be articulated with a high-accuracy interocclusal record material such as polyvinyl siloxane. On the other hand, less accurate diagnostic casts poured from irreversible hydrocolloid are better articulated using a more "forgiving" material such as interocclusal wax, provided that the record is properly reinforced. Most studies have shown considerable variability among various registration materials and techniques,[16] so particular care is needed with this procedure.

Reinforced Aluwax Record. The reinforced Aluwax record is a "forgiving" method for recording the CR position. It is a reliable technique, originally described by Wirth[17] and Wirth and Aplin,[18] and has provided consistent results.[19,20]

Armamentarium (Fig. 2-19, *A*)
- Heat-retaining wax sheet (i.e., Aluwax)*
- Soft metal sheet (Ash's metal)*
- Sticky wax
- Scissors
- Ice water

Step-by-step Procedure
1. Soften half a sheet of occlusal wax in warm water and adapt it to the maxillary cusp tips. Allow the patient to close lightly and make cuspal indentations of the mandibular teeth (Fig. 2-19, *B*). These indentations form no part of the record, but they thin the wax slightly and indi-

cate the approximate positions of the mandibular teeth for later reference.
2. Add baseplate wax to the mandibular anterior region of the record and seal along the periphery (Fig. 2-19, *C, D*).
3. Readapt the record to the maxillary teeth, resoftening if necessary. Guide the patient into centric closure, making shallow indentations in the baseplate wax. Verify that no posterior tooth contact occurs. If it does, add an additional layer of baseplate wax (Fig. 2-19, *E, F*).
4. Remove the record carefully and verify that no distortion has occurred. Then chill it thoroughly in ice water.
5. Reseat the record on the maxillary teeth and evaluate it for stability. If the maxillary cast is available, evaluate the fit on this as well.
6. Add heat-retaining wax in the mandibular incisor region only (Fig. 2-19, *G*) and manipulate the mandible as previously described. Having the patient in a supine position for this manipulation allows better control.
7. Make indentations of the mandibular incisor tips in the wax, repeating several times to ensure reproducibility. Remove the wax record and rechill it in ice water until the anterior indentations are hard (Fig. 2-19, *H, I*).
8. Add a small amount of heat-retaining wax in the mandibular posterior region and reseat the record (Fig. 2-19, *J, K*). Then guide the mandibular teeth into the anterior indentations and have the patient close lightly. The baseplate wax will prevent excessive closure. Excessive force may distort the record or flex the mandible.[21] The elevator muscles of the mandible will ensure that the most superior position of the condylar processes is recorded.
9. Remove the record and chill it (Fig. 2-19, *L*). If there is difficulty in obtaining an undistorted record, the palatal area can be reinforced with the soft metal sheet (Fig. 2-19, *D*). Be sure that it is kept away from the indentations. Also remember that when new wax is added, the record should be dried; otherwise, the wax will not adhere and may become detached.

The advantage of this sequential technique is that the CR position is reproduced multiple times as the record is generated. The heat-retaining Aluwax is soft and distorts easily. Therefore, if the patient is not guided into exactly the same position, this problem will become readily apparent. Once the completed record has been obtained with adequate but fairly shallow indentations for all cusps, the same arcing motion has been reproduced four times, confirming that the CR position has been accurately captured.

*See Appendix A.

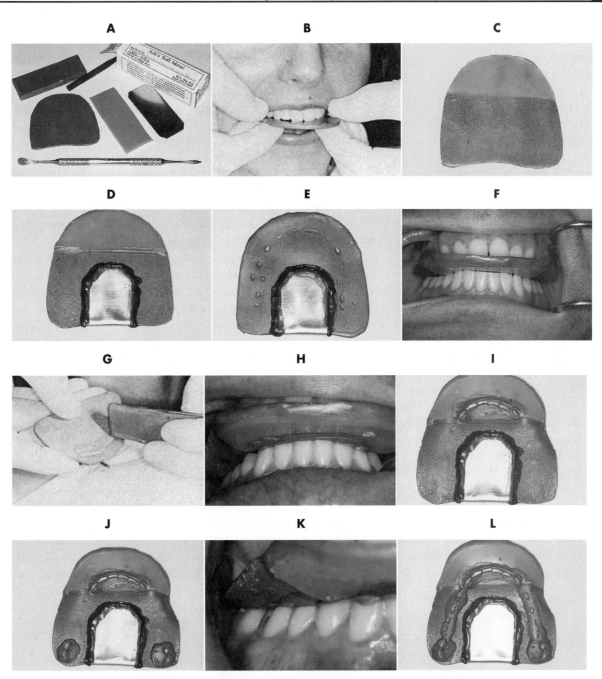

Fig. 2-19. CR recording technique. The reproducibility of the CR position is verified because CR has to be reproduced several times while the record is made. **A,** Armamentarium. **B,** A sheet of soft Aluwax is adapted to the maxillary arch. **C,** A piece of hard pink wax is added to the lower anterior portion of the wafer. **D,** Some Ash's Metal #7 is folded around the posterior border and luted to the wafer with sticky wax to increase rigidity. **E,** Note that the maxillary indentations capture only the cusp tips. **F,** The reinforced sheet is repositioned and the mandible is guided into CR until the pink wax provides a stop for vertical closure. **G,** Some Aluwax is added to the lower incisor indentations. **H,** The record is repositioned and the CR closure repeated. **I,** The incisor indentations are reproduced in the Aluwax. **J,** After additional wax is added to the area of the first molars, hinge closure is repeated. The molar indentations are clearly visible. The incisor indentations should have been reproduced. Any "double" indentation indicates inaccuracy. **K,** The CR closure is repeated one more time after additional Aluwax is added to the premolar regions. **L,** The completed CR record.
(Courtesy Dr. J. N. Nelson.)

Anterior Programming Device with Elastomeric or ZOE Record

Armamentarium

- Self-curing resin
- Petroleum jelly
- Elastomeric material
- Syringe
- Scalpel blade

Step-by-step Procedure

1. Fabricate an anterior programming device from self-curing resin. The resin should be mixed to the consistency of putty and, after lubrication of the central incisors with petroleum jelly, adapted to the teeth. The lingual aspect of the anterior programming device should follow the lingual contours of the teeth. After trimming, it should result in separation of the posterior teeth (see Fig. 2-18, *D*). When the patient closes on the anterior programming device, no translation should occur.

2. Verify that no posterior contact remains and that the only occlusal contact is on the anterior programming device. The device should be stable and remain in position. If necessary, some petroleum jelly can be applied to its internal surface.

3. Rehearse the closing of the mandible with the patient until a reproducible CR position is obtained.

4. Verify that the syringe tip is large enough to permit free flow of the elastomeric material. Enlarge the opening of the syringe tip if necessary by trimming it with a scalpel blade.

5. Dispense and mix the elastomeric material according to the manufacturer's instructions (Fig. 2-20, *A*). (The Automix materials are convenient.)

6. Blow the occlusal surfaces of the teeth dry, and syringe the material onto the occlusal of the mandibular arch (Fig. 2-20, *B*).

7. Guide the patient's mandible into hinge movement until the mandible comes to rest on the anterior programming device. Maintain this position until the material has set (Fig. 2-20, *C*).

8. Remove the record from the mouth and trim with the scalpel blade following the buccal cusps (Fig. 2-20, *D*).

9. Verify that the mandibular and maxillary casts seat fully in the record.

As an alternative to the use of elastomeric material, a gauze mesh with zinc oxide-eugenol occlusal registration paste can be used (Fig. 2-21). The step-by-step procedure follows the one described for the elastomeric technique. However, rather than syringing the material onto the mandibular arch, the practitioner should coat the interocclusal cloth forms outside the mouth and interpose them, after which the patient can be guided into CR. Care must be taken, however, to position the frame that holds the cloth form so it does not interfere with the closure movement.

Other alternatives include using impression plaster or autopolymerizing resin as the recording medium. In all these techniques, accuracy depends on complete seating of the casts into the recording medium. Seating is often prevented by better detail reproduction in the record than in the casts, especially around the fossa.

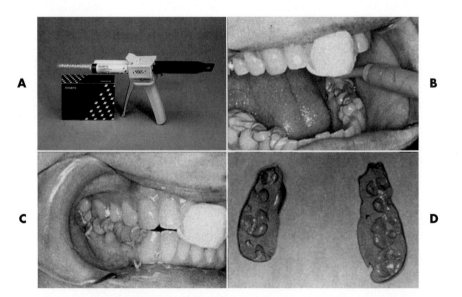

Fig. 2-20.   **A,** Elastomeric material for CR recording. **B,** Mandibular quadrants coated. **C,** The patient remains occluded until the material has set. **D,** The completed record must be evaluated after trimming. (**A** *Courtesy Sullivan-Schein Dental.*)

This additional detail needs to be carefully trimmed until the cast is completely seated in the record.

Recording Jaw Relationships in Partially Edentulous Dentitions (Fig. 2-22). When there are insufficient teeth to provide bilateral stability, obtaining a CR record as described may not be possible. As a result, acrylic resin record bases must be fabricated. To avoid errors caused by soft tissue displacement, which prevents accurate transfer of rigid materials from one set of casts to another, these bases should be made on the casts that are to be articulated. If breakage of the casts is a concern, it may be advisable to make record bases on an accurate duplicate cast made with reversible agar hydrocolloid impression material in a flask designed for that purpose.

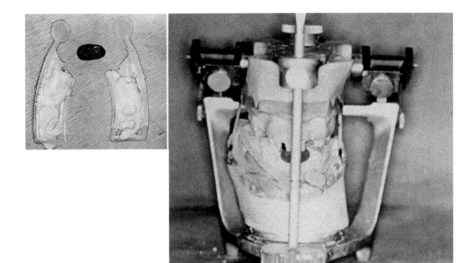

Fig. 2-21. Gauze mesh cloth forms with plastic holders, and ZOE paste can be used instead of elastomeric paste.

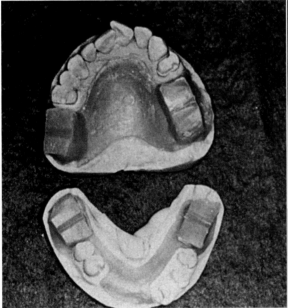

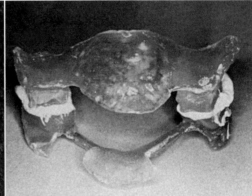

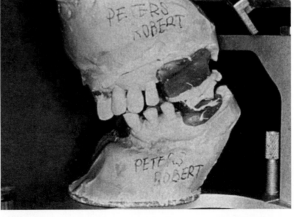

Fig. 2-22. Acrylic resin record base for mounting a partially edentulous cast.

Articulating the Diagnostic Casts

Maxillary Cast (Fig. 2-23). The maxillary cast is seated in the indentations on the facebow fork after the facebow is attached to the articulator. Wedges or specially designed braces can be used to support the weight of the cast and to prevent the fork from flexing or moving. After it has been scored and wetted, the cast is attached to the mounting ring of the articulator with a low-expansion, fast-setting mounting stone or plaster.

Mandibular Cast (Fig. 2-24). To relate the mandibular cast properly to the maxillary cast, the incisal guide pin should be lowered sufficiently to compensate for the thickness of the centric relation record. The articulator is inverted, and the record is seated on the maxillary cast. The mandibular cast is then carefully seated in the record, and each cast is checked for stability. The maxillary and mandibular casts can be luted together with metal rods, or pieces of wooden tongue blade, and sticky wax. The mandibular member of the articulator is closed into mounting stone; the condylar balls should be fully seated in the corresponding fossae. If the articulator has a centric latch, this step is simplified. Otherwise, the articulator should be held until the stone has reached its initial set. No attempt should be made to smooth the stone until it has fully set.

Evaluation (Fig. 2-25)

Accuracy is critical in both centric relation and the intercuspal position. Before the articulator controls are adjusted, the accuracy of CR must be confirmed by comparing the tooth contacts on the casts with those in the mouth. During the clinical examination, the position of tooth contacts in CR can be marked with thin articulating film. Normally, the markings will be on the mesial inclines of maxillary cusps and the distal inclines of mandibular cusps. Their exact location can be transferred by having the patient close through thin occlusal indicator wax. The articulated casts are closed and the retruded tooth contacts marked with articulating film. When the indicator wax is transferred to the casts, the perforations should correspond exactly to these marks.

For additional verification, the intercuspal position of the articulated casts should be examined. Maximum intercuspation is usually a translated mandibular position that may not be reproducible with absolute accuracy on a semiadjustable articulator. However, any substantive discrepancy invariably indicates an incorrect mounting. If further confirmation of mounting accuracy is required (as may be the case when working casts are being articulated), additional CR records can be made and compared with a split cast mounting system or a measuring device such as the Denar Vericheck (Fig. 2-26).

Posterior Articulator Controls

The advantages and disadvantages of the different articulators are summarized in Table 2-1. The more sophisticated (fully adjustable) articulators have a large range of adjustments that can be programmed to follow the condylar paths precisely. Their posterior controls are designed to permit simulation of movement of the condylar processes, duplicating protrusive and lateral tooth contacts. The semiadjustable instruments can be adjusted to a lesser extent. Their posterior controls are designed to replicate the most clinically significant features of mandibular movement (e.g., condylar inclination and mandibular side shift). These instruments can be programmed from eccentric interocclusal records or a simplified pantograph. An alternative technique is to use average values for the control settings. It is important to note that no method used to program an articulator to reproduce eccentric jaw movements is without error.[22]

Arbitrary Values. Based on clinical investigations, certain generally applicable average anatomic values have evolved for condylar inclination, immediate and progressive sideshift. These values have been described relative to the Frankfort horizontal plane and the midsagittal plane. For instance, an average value of 1.0 mm has been reported[23] for immediate sideshift.

When arbitrary values are used to adjust posterior articulator controls, the actual instrument settings will vary from one manufacturer to another. However, depending on the degree of adjustability of the articulator, using arbitrary values is not necessarily less accurate than alternative techniques (e.g., eccentric interocclusal records to program a semiadjustable articulator, particularly when the instrument can execute only a straight protrusive path).

Eccentric Interocclusal Recordings. Eccentric interocclusal records (check-bites) have been recommended[24] for setting the posterior controls of a semiadjustable articulator. These consist of wax or another recording material interposed between the maxillary and mandibular arches; they record the position of the condyles in eccentric mandibular positions. Static positional records are made in translated jaw positions: a protrusive record and two lateral records. The protrusive record can be used to adjust both condylar inclinations on the articulator, and the lateral records are used to adjust the side shift on semiadjustable articulators.

An articulator set by an eccentric record is accurate in only two positions: at CR and at the position recorded by the record (Fig. 2-27). This occurs because the path taken between these may differ significantly on the articulator from what is actually performed by the mandible. A semiadjustable instrument may have a protrusive and a sideshift

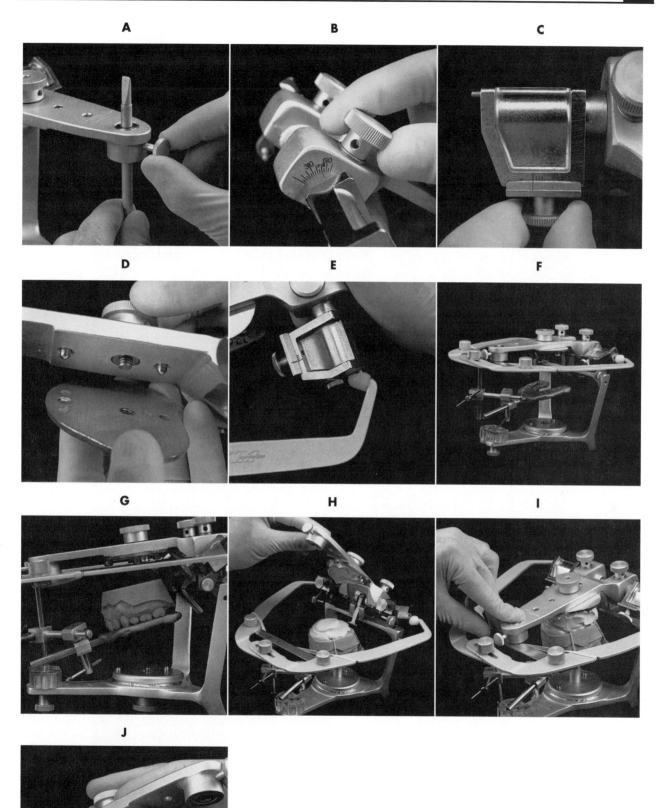

Fig. 2-23. Mounting the maxillary cast on a Whip Mix articulator. **A,** Remove the incisal pin. **B,** Adjust the condylar inclination to the facebow setting. **C,** Set the sideshift to zero. **D,** Attach a mounting plate. **E,** Attach the facebow earpieces to the condylar elements. **F,** Facebow attached to the articulator. **G,** Position the scored maxillary cast on the bitefork and prewet the cast. **H,** Mounting stone is applied to the cast and the mounting plate. **I,** Close the upper member of the articulator until it contacts the cross bar of the facebow. **J,** Add additional stone as needed. *(Courtesy Whip Mix Corporation.)*

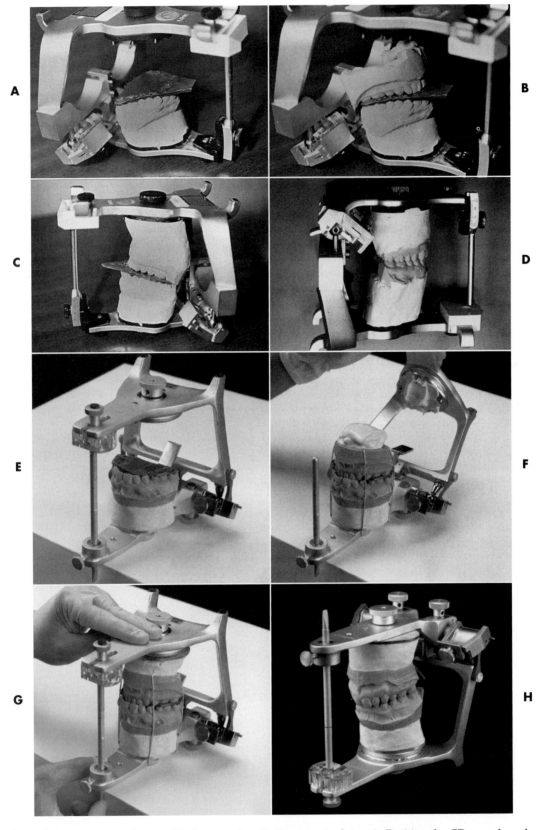

Fig. 2-24. Mounting the mandibular cast. **A** to **D**, Denar articulator. **A**, Position the CR record on the inverted maxillary cast. **B**, Adjust the incisal guide pin and orient the mandibular cast in the record. **C**, Attach the cast with mounting stone. **D**, When the pin is raised, the casts will contact in CR closure. **E** to **H**: Whip Mix articulator. **E**, Position the CR record. **F**, The incisal guidepin is adjusted, the cast is stabilized, and plaster is applied to the prewetted cast and the mandibular mounting plate. **G**, Close the articulator. **H**, Completed mounting.
(E to H Courtesy Whip Mix Corporation.)

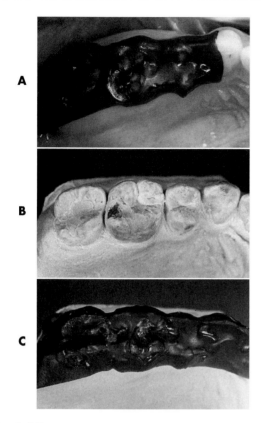

Fig. 2-25.   Verifying mounting accuracy. **A,** Occlusal indicator wax is adapted to the maxillary teeth, and the patient is guided into CR closure. **B,** The cast contacts are marked with thin articulating film. **C,** If the mounting is accurate, the markings will correspond to perforations in the wax.

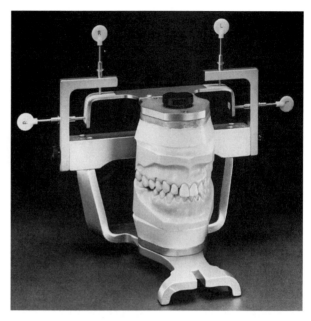

Fig. 2-26.   The Denar Vericheck. The casts are positioned in the same relationship as on the articulator, but the condylar elements are replaced by four styli. Each marks graph paper attached to the maxillary half of the articulator. Successive CR records can be compared by examining these marks.
(Courtesy Denar Corporation.)

Articulator Selection for Fixed Prosthodontics							TABLE 2-1
Fully Adjustable	Semiadjustable		Nonadjustable			Unmounted Casts	
	Arcon	Nonarcon	Large	Small		Arch	Quadrant
Denar D5-A	Denar Mark II	Hanau 96H20					
Stuart	Whip Mix	Dentatus					
TMJ	Hanau 183-2						
More ←——————————— Diagnostic information provided ←——————————— Less							
More ←——————————— Occlusal information conveyed to laboratory ←——————————— Less							
More ←——————————— Time and skill needed at initial appointment ←——————————— Less							
Less ——————————→ Chair time needed before cementation ——————————→ More							
Multiple opposing restorations	Diagnostic assessment and treatment of most patients requiring fixed prosthodontics		Larger articulators for single restorations; some adjustment necessary			Only when occlusal influence minimal	
No anterior guidance							
Extensive occlusal pathology			Small hinge articulator only when occlusal influence minimal				

Modified slightly from Rosenstiel SF: In Rayne J, editor: *General dental treatment,* London, 1983, Kluwer Publishing.

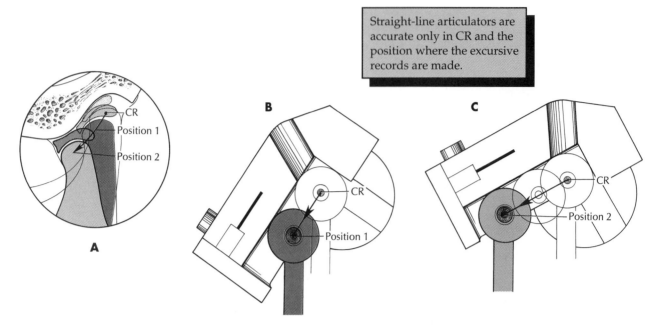

Straight-line articulators are accurate only in CR and the position where the excursive records are made.

Fig. 2-27. **A,** The typical condylar path is curved, with its steepest inclination near CR. If a semiadjustable articulator with a straight condylar path is programmed from an eccentric record, very different values will be obtained (depending on where the record is made) from what is actually performed by the mandible. **B,** Record made at Position 1. **C,** Record made at Position 2.

path that are straight lines, whereas the true paths will invariably be curved. In an attempt to minimize errors, many contemporary semiadjustable articulators come with curved fossae.

Armamentarium
- Interocclusal wax record material

Step-by-step Technique
1. Practice the three excursive positions with the patient until they can be reproduced. The patient can be guided into an anterior end-to-end position and left and right lateral positions where the canines are end-to-end when viewed from the front. We have found guiding the patient helpful in obtaining the records easily, although unguided records have been equally accurate.[25]
2. Adapt a wax record to the maxillary arch (Fig. 2-28, *A*) and guide the patient into a protrusive position. Have the patient close to form indentations in the recording medium (Fig. 2-28, *B*). Verify that the midline remains properly aligned and that when viewed from the side, the maxillary and mandibular incisors are end to end.

3. For the lateral records, add additional wax to one posterior quadrant of a wax record to compensate for the additional space on the patient's nonworking side.
4. Adapt this to the patient's maxillary arch and guide the patient's mandible into an excursive position, again verifying that the canines are end to end (Fig. 2-28, *C, D*).
5. Repeat this step for the other lateral excursion.
6. Mark each record to facilitate its identification when using it to adjust the posterior articulator controls (Fig. 2-28, *E*).

Simplified Pantographs (Fig. 2-29). A simplified **pantograph** measures only certain components of mandibular movement thought to be of greatest clinical significance, usually the condylar inclinations and mandibular sideshift. This device can be quickly assembled. Numerical values are measured directly from the recording and are used to set a semiadjustable articulator to provide useful diagnostic information.

Simplified pantographs may reveal an excessively shallow condylar inclination or an exaggerated mandibular sideshift. If either of these conditions are identified, restoration of the posterior teeth is likely to be complex, and the use of a fully adjustable articulator is recommended. Some manu-

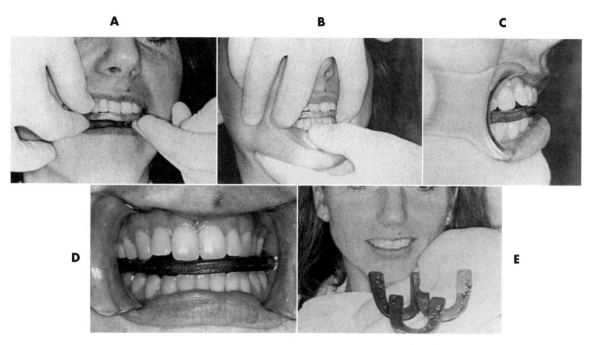

Fig. 2-28. Eccentric interocclusal records. **A,** Adaptation of wax to the maxillary arch. **B,** Protrusive record. **C** and **D,** The patient is guided into left and right lateral excursive movements. Records are made in the left and right canine edge-to-edge positions. **E,** The completed records.

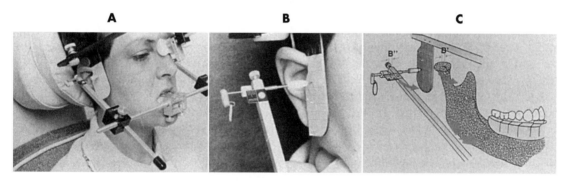

Fig. 2-29. **A,** The Panadent Axi-Path Recorder. **B,** An axis stylus traces the condylar-path and measures the amount of Bennett movement while the patient is guided into an eccentric border movement **(C).** *(A to C courtesy Panadent Corporation.)*

facturers offer inserts of standard "fossae" of varying configuration, whose selection depends on the measurements obtained with a simplified pantograph (Fig. 2-30).

Pantographic Recordings (Fig. 2-31). Fully adjustable articulators are usually programmed on the basis of a pantographic recording. Jaw movements are registered by directional tracings on recording plates. The plates are rigidly attached to one jaw, and the recording styli are attached to the other. A total of six plates are needed to achieve a precise movement record of the mandible. Left and right lateral border and protrusive tracings are made on each plate. The pantograph is then attached to the articulator, and

the controls are adjusted and modified until the instrument can faithfully reproduce the movements of the styli on the tracings (Fig. 2-32). A simpler, though less accurate, procedure is to measure the tracings directly and adjust the condylar controls without transferring the recordings.

Electronic Pantograph (Fig. 2-33). The Axiograph* is an electronic pantograph designed to record and measure functional and border movements. It consists of upper and lower bows that record and measure mandibular movements.

---

*Great Lakes Orthodontics: Tonawanda, N.Y.

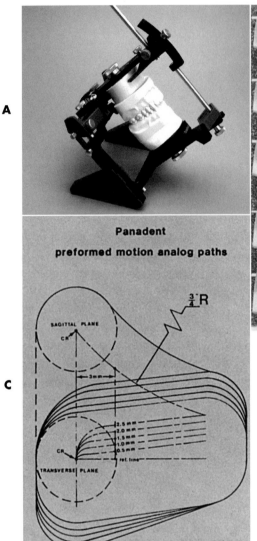

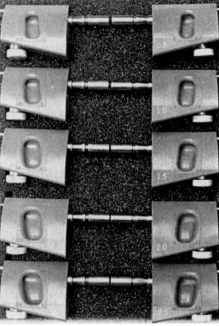

Panadent

preformed motion analog paths

Fig. 2-30. **A,** The Panadent PCH Articulator with support Legs. **B,** Fossa blocks (motion analogs) with different amounts of Bennett movement are selected from the simplified recorder or lateral check bites. The blocks are rotated to the correct condylar inclination. **C,** Schematic showing the sagittal and transverse planes of the available motion analogs blocks.
(A to C courtesy Panadent Corporation.)

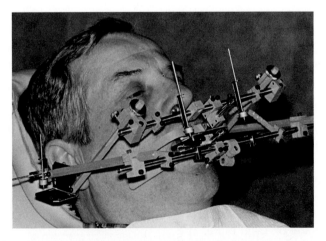

Fig. 2-31. Pantographic recording with the Stuart instrument.
(Courtesy Drs. R. Giering and J. Petrie.)

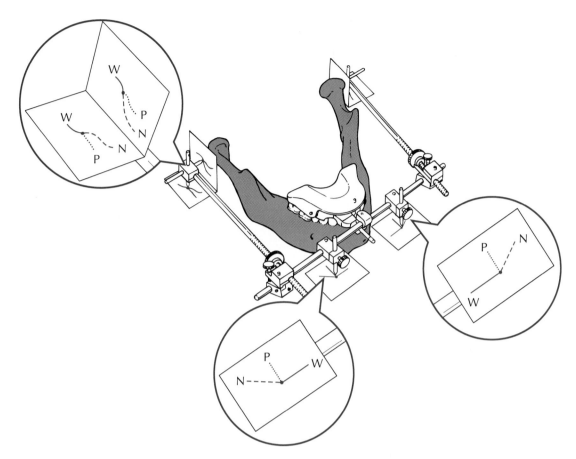

Fig. 2-32. Pantographic tracings represent information that could only be obtained with an infinite number of excursive records: This simplified schematic shows the relative orientation of six recording plates (attached to the maxillary bow, omitted for clarity) to the scribing styli, attached to the mandibular bow. *W*, Working movement; *N*, nonworking or balancing movement; *P*, protrusive movement. The CR position is represented by the intersection of the paths marked by the dot.

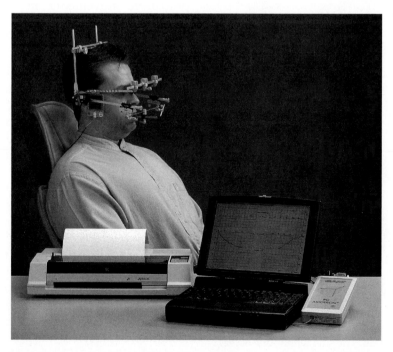

Fig. 2-33. Electronic jaw recording system. The Axiotron is an electronic recording system that attaches to the Axiograph pantograph.
(Courtesy Great Lakes Orthodontics.)

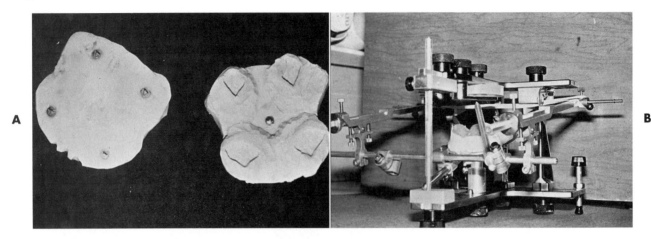

Fig. 2-34. A, B, The TMJ articulator is programmed from three-dimensional acrylic resin recordings. *(Courtesy Dr. A. Peregrina.)*

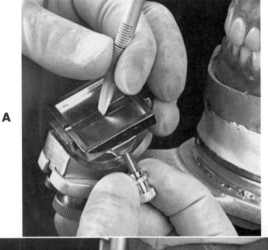

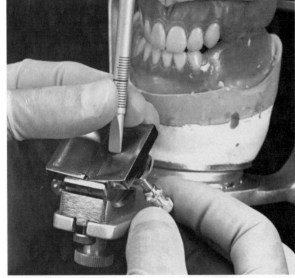

Fig. 2-35. Mechanical anterior guide table. **A,** The protrusive path has been adjusted. The side screw adjusts the lateral flange. **B,** Lateral flange adjusted to the right working movement.

Stereograms (Fig. 2-34). Another approach to reproducing posterior condylar controls is to cut or mold a three-dimensional recording of the jaw movements. This "stereogram" is then used to form custom-shaped fossae for the condylar heads.

Anterior Guidance

Border movements of the mandible are governed by tooth contacts and by the shape of the left and right temporomandibular joints. In patients with normal jaw relationships, the vertical and horizontal overlap of anterior teeth and the lingual concavities of the maxillary incisors are highly significant during protrusive movements. In lateral excursions, the tooth contacts normally existing between the canines are usually dominant, although the posterior teeth may also be involved (see Chapter 4). Restorative procedures that change the shape of the anterior teeth can have a profound effect on excursive tooth contacts. For this reason, when preparation of anterior teeth is contemplated, the exact nature of the anterior contacts should be transferred to the articulator, where it can be studied and stored before these teeth are prepared.

Mechanical Anterior Guidance Table (Fig. 2-35). Most articulator manufacturers supply a mechanical anterior guidance (incisal guidance) table. Such tables can be pivoted anteriorly and posteriorly to simulate protrusive guidance, and they have lateral wings that can be adjusted to approximate lateral guidance. However, the sensitivity of these adjustments is insufficient for successfully transferring the existing lingual contours of natural teeth to newly fabricated restorations. Therefore, the principal use for these mechanical tables is in the fabrication of complete dentures and occlusal devices (see Chapter 4).

Custom Acrylic Anterior Guidance Table. This simple device is used for accurately transferring to an articulator the contacts of anterior teeth when determining their influence on border movements of the mandible. Acrylic resin is used to record and preserve this information, even after the natural lingual contours of the teeth have been altered during preparation for complete coverage restorations. The technique is similar to that for stereographic recording used in setting the posterior controls of some articulators.

Custom Guide Table Fabrication

Armamentarium (Fig. 2-36, *A*)
- Plastic incisal table
- Tray and fossa acrylic resin
- Petrolatum

Step-by-step Procedure
1. After raising and lubricating the pin, moisten the plastic incisal table with acrylic resin monomer to ensure a good bond (Fig. 2-36, *B* to *D*).
2. Mix a small quantity of resin and mold it to the table (Fig. 2-36, *E, F*).
3. Raise the incisal pin about 2 mm from the table, cover its tip with petrolatum, and close it into the soft resin (Fig. 2-36, *G*).
4. Manipulate the articulator in hinge, lateral, and protrusive movements while the resin is in the doughy stage of polymerization (Fig. 2-36, *H* to *J*). As the pin moves through these excursions, its tip will push into and mold the doughy acrylic resin lying in its path, ultimately creating an accurate and rigid three-dimensional record of the mandibular movements and their lateral and protrusive limits through the functional range (Fig. 2-36, *K*).
5. Continue these closures until the resin is no longer plastic, being careful not to abrade or damage the casts during the process. A thin film of plastic foil placed between the casts will help minimize abrasion without significantly affecting the accuracy of the guide table.

Evaluation

When the custom anterior guidance table has been completed, the incisal pin should contact the table in all excursive movements. This can be checked with thin Mylar strips (shim stock). If contact is deficient, a small mix of new resin is added and the process repeated. If too much resin has been used, the table may interfere with the hinge opening-closing arc of the articulator (Fig. 2-37). Excess can be easily trimmed away.

Diagnostic Cast Modification

One advantage of having accurately articulated diagnostic casts is that proposed treatment procedures can be rehearsed on the stone cast before making any irreversible changes in the patient's mouth. These diagnostic procedures are essential when attempting to solve complicated problems. Even the most experienced clinician may have difficulty deciding between different treatment plans. Even in apparently simple situations, time that the practitioner spends rehearsing diagnostic procedures on the casts is usually well rewarded.

Diagnostic cast modifications include the following:

1. Changing the arch relationship preparatory to orthognathic procedures when surgical correction of skeletal jaw discrepancy is to be performed
2. Changing the tooth position before orthodontic procedures (Fig. 2-38)
3. Modifying the occlusal scheme before attempting any selective occlusal adjustment
4. Trial tooth preparation and waxing (Fig. 2-39) before fixed restorative procedures. (This is one of the most useful diagnostic techniques for patients seeking fixed prosthodontics. It enables the practitioner to rehearse a proposed restorative plan and to test it on a stone cast, providing considerable information in advance of the actual treatment and helping to explain the intended procedure to the patient.)

On many occasions it will be necessary to combine two or more of these options. In fact, most treatment planning decisions (e.g., preparation design, choice of abutment teeth, selection of an optimum path of withdrawal of a fixed partial denture, or deciding to treat a patient with an FPD or an RPD) can be simplified by adhering to these diagnostic techniques.

SUMMARY

Diagnostic casts provide valuable preliminary information and a comprehensive overview of the patient's needs often not apparent during the clinical examination. They are obtained from accurate irreversible hydrocolloid impressions and should be transferred to a semiadjustable articulator using a facebow transfer and interocclusal record. For most routine fixed prosthodontic diagnostic purposes, the use of an arbitrary hinge axis facebow is sufficient. If special concerns apply, such as a change in vertical dimension, a kinematic facebow transfer is needed. Two types of articulators are recognized: arcon and nonarcon. For highly complex treatment

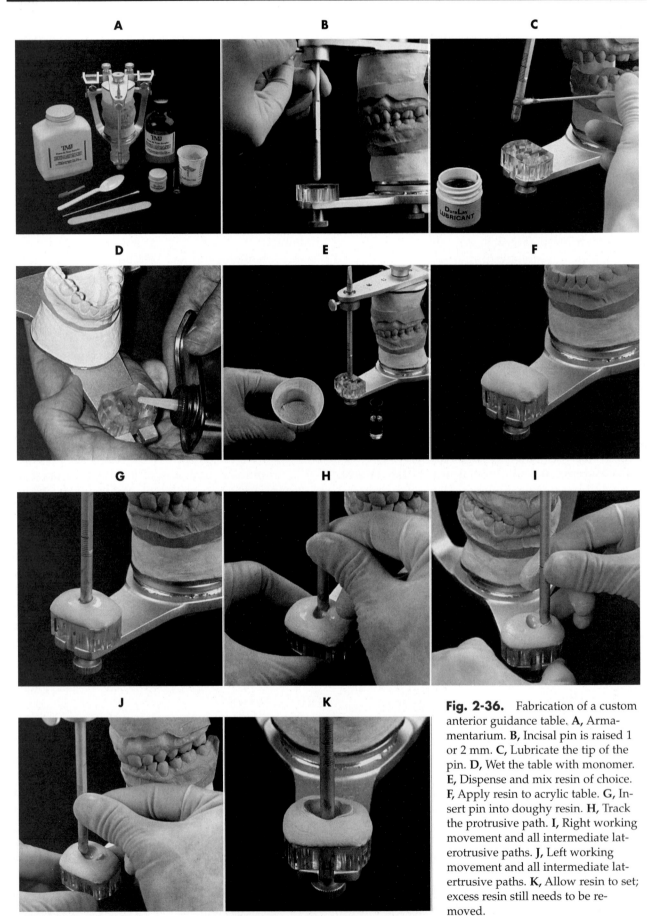

Fig. 2-36. Fabrication of a custom anterior guidance table. **A,** Armamentarium. **B,** Incisal pin is raised 1 or 2 mm. **C,** Lubricate the tip of the pin. **D,** Wet the table with monomer. **E,** Dispense and mix resin of choice. **F,** Apply resin to acrylic table. **G,** Insert pin into doughy resin. **H,** Track the protrusive path. **I,** Right working movement and all intermediate laterotrusive paths. **J,** Left working movement and all intermediate latertrusive paths. **K,** Allow resin to set; excess resin still needs to be removed.
(Courtesy Whip Mix Corporation.)

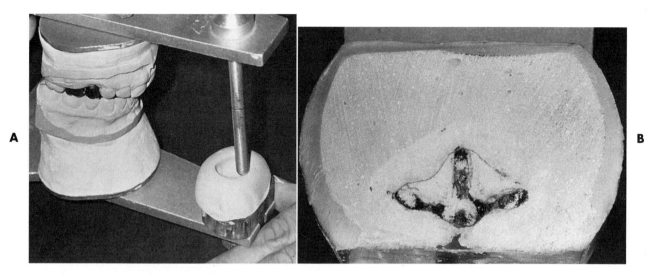

Fig. 2-37. **A,** A custom anterior guidance table made with excess resin. This must be trimmed if it interferes with the path of closure of the incisal pin. **B,** The completed table with excess resin ground away. Note the lateral and protrusive paths.

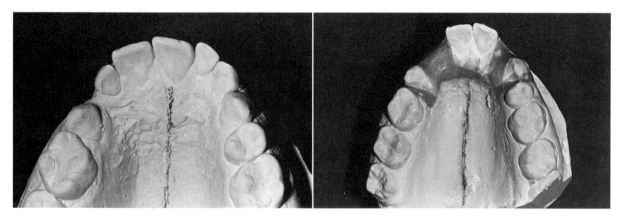

Fig. 2-38. Diagnostic cast modifications in advance of orthodontic treatment.

needs, a fully adjustable articulator may be indicated. Such articulators are adjusted by using a pantographic tracing.

Diagnostic casts should be articulated in centric relation to enable observation of deflective tooth contact and to assess any slide that may be present from CR to IP. *Centric relation* is defined as the maxillomandibular relationship in which the condyles articulate with the thinnest avascular portion of their respective disks with the complex in the anterior-superior position against the shapes of the articular eminences. This position is independent of tooth contact. It is recorded with a suitable medium interposed between the maxillary and mandibular teeth and by guiding the patient into the CR position. This can be accomplished through bimanual manipulation. If many teeth are absent, record bases

with wax rims may need to be fabricated to obtain a centric relation record.

If a patient's mandible is difficult to manipulate into a reproducible hinge movement, a deprogramming device is helpful. These can be used to help minimize "muscle memory," resulting in easier replication of the rotational hinge movement of the mandible.

Posterior articulator controls can be adjusted on the basis of arbitrary values based on anatomic averages, by means of eccentric records, simplified pantographs, pantographs, or stereographs.

Anterior guidance can be approximated on articulators with a mechanical guide table. As an alternative, a custom acrylic guide table can be generated from the diagnostic casts. The latter is useful when anterior teeth are to be restored.

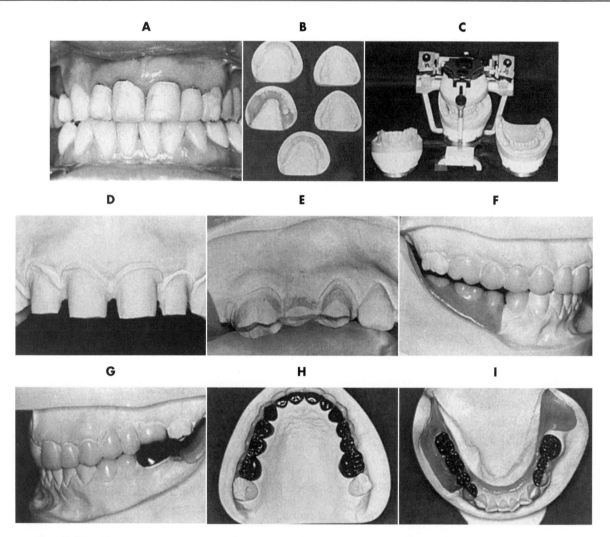

Fig. 2-39. Diagnostic waxing procedure. Diagnostic tooth preparation and waxing help simplify complex prosthodontic treatment planning for predictable results. **A,** Before treatment. The patient needs extensive fixed and removable treatment. **B** and **C,** Cross-mounted diagnostic casts. A record base is used to articulate the partially edentulous mandibular cast. **D** and **E,** Diagnostic tooth preparations determine the correct reduction for esthetics and function. **F** to **I,** Diagnostic waxing, done in conjunction with diagnostic denture tooth arrangement.
(Courtesy Dr. J. Bailey.)

Study Questions

1. Discuss the uses and limitations of irreversible hydrocolloid and include an overview of its material properties.
2. Why are diagnostic casts articulated in centric relation? Why aren't they articulated in the intercuspal position?
3. List five items that are easier to determine on diagnostic casts rather than intraorally.
4. What is accomplished with a facebow transfer? How do arbitrary facebows differ from kinematic facebows? When would one be selected over the other?
5. Describe the differences between arcon and nonarcon articulators. When would use of a simple hinge instrument be acceptable and when would it be contraindicated? Why?
6. What is the role of excursive records in adjusting the articulator?
7. What does a simplified pantograph record? What does a pantograph record? When would either be indicated?
8. For what purpose is a custom acrylic guide table fabricated, and when is its use necessary?
9. Give two examples when a diagnostic waxing procedure is indicated.

Diagnostic procedures such as diagnostic waxing, tooth preparation, and diagnostic cast modification can greatly enhance diagnosis and treatment planning.

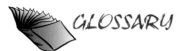

GLOSSARY

adjustable anterior guidance: an anterior guide on an articulator whose surface may be altered to provide desired guidance of the articulator's movement mechanism: the guide may be programmed (calibrated) to accept eccentric interocclusal records.

agar: *n* (1889) a complex sulfated polymer of galactose units, extracted from *Gelidium cartilagineum, Gracilaria confervoides*, and related red algae. It is a mucilaginous substance that melts at approximately 100°C and solidifies into a gel at approximately 40°C. It is not digested by most bacteria and is used as a gel in dental impression materials and solid culture media for microorganisms.

anterior guidance: *1:* the influence of the contacting surfaces of anterior teeth on tooth-limiting mandibular movements. *2:* the influence of the contacting surfaces of the guide pin and anterior guide table on articular movements. *3:* the fabrication of a relationship of the anterior teeth preventing posterior tooth contact in all eccentric mandibular movements.

anterior guide pin: that component of an articulator, generally a rigid rod attached to one member, contacting the anterior guide table on the opposing member. It is used to maintain the established vertical separation. The anterior guide pin and table, together with the condylar elements, direct the movements of the articulator's separate members.

anterior guide table: that component of an articulator on which the anterior guide pin rests to maintain the occlusal vertical dimension and influence articulator movements. The guide table influences the degree of separation of the casts in all relationships.

anterior programming device: an individually fabricated anterior guide table that allows mandibular motion without the influence of tooth contacts and facilitates the recording of maxillomandibular relationships; also used for deprogramming.

anterior reference point: any point located on the midface that, together with two posterior reference points, establishes a reference plane.

arbitrary face-bow: a device used to arbitrarily relate the maxillary cast to the condylar elements of an articulator. The position of the transverse horizontal axis is estimated on the face before using this device.

arcon: *n* a contraction of the words *articulator* and *condyle*, used to describe an articulator containing the condylar path elements within its upper member and the condylar elements within the lower member.

arcon articulator: an articulator that applies the arcon design. This instrument maintains anatomic guidelines by the use of condylar analogs in the mandibular element and fossae assemblies within the maxillary element.

arrow point tracer: *1:* a mechanical device used to trace a pattern of mandibular movement in a selected plane—usually parallel to the occlusal plane. *2:* a mechanical device with a marking point attached to one jaw and a graph plate or tracing plane attached to the other jaw. It is used to record the direction and range of movements of the mandible.

articulator: *n* a mechanical instrument that represents the temporomandibular joints and jaws, to which maxillary and mandibular casts may be attached to simulate some or all mandibular movements—usage: articulators are divisible into four classes. Class I articulator: a simple holding instrument capable of accepting a single static registration. Vertical motion is possible. Class II articulator: an instrument that permits horizontal as well as vertical motion but does not orient the motion to the temporomandibular joints. Class III articulator: an instrument that simulates condylar pathways by using averages or mechanical equivalents for all or part of the motion. These instruments allow orientation of the casts relative to the joints and may be arcon or nonarcon instruments. Class IV articulator: an instrument that will accept three-dimensional dynamic registrations. These instruments allow orientation of the casts to the temporomandibular joints and replication of all mandibular movements.

average axis face-bow: a face-bow that relates the maxillary teeth to the average location of the transverse horizontal axis.

average value articulator: an articulator that is fabricated to permit motion based on mean mandibular movements—also called Class III articulator.

centric relation: *1:* The maxillomandibular relationship in which the condyles articulate with the thinnest avascular portion of their respective disks with the complex in the anterior-superior position against the shapes of the articular eminences. This position is independent of tooth contact. This position is clinically discernible when the mandible is directed superior and anteriorly. It is restricted to a purely rotational movement about the transverse horizontal axis (GPT 5) *2:* The most retruded physiologic relation of the mandible to the maxillae to and from which the individual can make lateral movements. It is a condition that can exist at various degrees of jaw separation. It occurs around the terminal hinge axis (GPT-3) *3:* The most retruded relation of the mandible to the maxillae when the condyles are in the most posterior unstrained position in the glenoid fossae from which lateral movement can be made, at any given degree of jaw separation (GPT-1) *4:* The most posterior relation of the lower to the upper jaw from which lateral movements can be made at a given vertical dimension (Boucher) *5:* A maxilla to mandible relationship in which the condyles and disks are thought to be in the midmost uppermost position. The position has been difficult to define anatomically but is determined clinically by assessing when the jaw can hinge on a fixed terminal axis (up to 25 mm). It is a clinically determined relationship of the mandible to the maxilla when the condyle disk assemblies are positioned in their most superior position in the mandibular fossa and against the distal slope of the articular eminence (Ash) *6:* The relation of the mandible to the maxillae when the condyles are in the uppermost and rearmost position in the glenoid fossae. This position may not be able to be recorded in the presence of dysfunction of the masticatory system *7:* A clinically determined position of the mandible placing both condyles into their anterior uppermost position. This can be determined in patients without pain or derangement in the TMJ (Ramsfjord) Boucher CO. Occlusion in prosthodontics. J Prosthet Dent 1953; 3:633-56. Ash MM. Personal communication, July 1993. Lang BR, Kelsey CC. International prosthodontic workshop on complete denture occlusion. Ann Arbor: The University of Michigan School of Dentistry; 1973. Ramsfjord SP. Personal communication, July 1993.

centric relation record: a registration of the relationship of the maxilla to the mandible when the mandible is in centric relation. The registration may be obtained either intraorally or extraorally.

condylar hinge position: *obs* the position of the condyles of the mandible in the glenoid fossae at which hinge axis movement is possible (GPT-4).

deprogrammer: *n* various types of devices or materials used to alter the proprioceptive mechanism during mandibular closure.

diagnostic cast: a life-size reproduction of a part or parts of the oral cavity and/or facial structures for the purpose of study and treatment planning.

face-bow: a caliper-like instrument used to record the spatial relationship of the maxillary arch to some anatomic reference point or points, which then transfers this relationship to an articulator; it orients the dental cast in the same relationship to the opening axis of the articulator. Customarily, the anatomic references are the mandibular condyle's transverse horizontal axis and one other selected anterior point; also called *hingebow.*

face-bow fork: that component of the face-bow used to attach the occlusion rim to the face-bow.

face-bow record: the registration obtained by means of a face-bow.

Frankfort horizontal plane: *1:* eponym for a plane established by the lowest point in the margin of the right or left bony orbit and the highest point in the margin of the right or left bony auditory meatus. *2:* a horizontal plane represented in profile by a line between the lowest point on the margin of the orbit to the highest point on the margin of the auditory meatus; adopted at the 13th General Congress of German Anthropologists (the Frankfurt Agreement) at Frankfurt am Main, 1882, and finally by the International Agreement for the Unification of Craniometric and Cephalometric Measurements in Monaco in 1906; also called auriculo-orbital plane, eye-ear plane, Frankfurt horizontal (FH), Frankfurt horizontal line.

fully adjustable articulator: an articulator that allows replication of three-dimensional movement of recorded mandibular motion—also called Class IV articulator.

fully adjustable gnathologic articulator: an articulator that allows replication of three dimensional movement plus timing of recorded mandibular motion—also called Class IV articulator.

horizontal plane of reference: a horizontal plane established on the face of the patient by one anterior reference point and two posterior reference points from which measurements of the posterior anatomic determinants of occlusion and mandibular motion are made.

hydrocolloid: *n* (1916) a colloid system in which water is the dispersion medium; those materials described as colloid sols with water that are used in dentistry as elastic impression materials.

incisal guidance: *1:* the influence of the contacting surfaces of the mandibular and maxillary anterior teeth on mandibular movements *2:* the influence of the contacting surfaces of the guide pin and guide table on articulator movements.

interocclusal record: a registration of the positional relationship of the opposing teeth or arches; a record of the positional relationship of the teeth or jaws to each other.

irreversible hydrocolloid: a hydrocolloid consisting of a sol of alginic acid having a physical state that is changed by an irreversible chemical reaction forming insoluble calcium alginate—called also alginate, dental alginate.

kinematic face-bow: a face-bow with adjustable caliper ends used to locate the transverse horizontal axis of the mandible.

lateral interocclusal record: a registration of the positional relationship of opposing teeth or arches made in either a right or left lateral position of the mandible.

leaf gauge: a set of blades or leaves of increasing thickness used to measure the distance between two points or to provide metered separation.

Lucia jig: [Victor O. Lucia, U.S. prosthodontist]: eponym—see anterior programming device (Lucia

VO. *Treatment of the edentulous patient.* Chicago: Quintessence, 1986.)

maxillomandibular relationship record: a registration of any positional relationship of the mandible relative to the maxillae. These records may be made at any vertical, horizontal, or lateral orientation.

mounting: *v* the laboratory procedure of attaching a cast to an articulator or cast relator.

mounting plate: removable metal or resin devices that attach to the superior and inferior members of an articulator, which are used to attach casts to the articulator.

nonadjustable articulator: an articulator that does not allow adjustment to replicate mandibular movements.

occlude: *b* occluded; occluding: *vt* (1597) **1:** to bring together; to shut **2:** to bring or close the mandibular teeth into contact with the maxillary teeth.

occluding centric relation record: *obs* a registration of centric relation made at the established occlusal vertical dimension (GPT-4).

occlusal device: any removable artificial occlusal surface used for diagnosis or therapy affecting the relationship of the mandible to the maxillae. It may be used for occlusal stabilization, for treatment of temporomandibular disorders, or to prevent wear of the dentition.

pantograph: *n* (1723) **1:** an instrument used for copying a planar figure to any desired scale. **2:** in dentistry, an instrument used to graphically record paths of mandibular movements and to provide information for the programming instead of adjustment of an articulator.

pantographic tracing: a graphic record of mandibular movement in three planes as registered by the stylii on the recording tables of a pantograph; tracings of mandibular movement recorded on plates in the horizontal and sagittal planes.

preliminary cast: a cast formed from a preliminary impression for use in diagnosis or the fabrication of an impression tray.

preliminary impression: a negative likeness made for the purpose of diagnosis, treatment planning, or the fabrication of a tray.

preoperative wax-up: a dental diagnostic procedure in which planned restorations are developed in wax on a diagnostic cast to determine optimal clinical and laboratory procedures necessary to achieve the desired esthetics and function—also called *diagnostic wax-up, preoperative waxing.*

protrusive interocclusal record: a registration of the mandible in relation to the maxillae when both condyles are advanced in the temporal fossa.

reciprocal click: a pair of clicks emanating from the temporomandibular joint, one of which occurs during opening movements and the other during closing movements.

1 record: *vb* (14c) **1:** to register data relating to specific conditions that exist currently or previously. **2:** to register permanently by mechanical means (i.e., jaw relationships).

2 record: *n* (14c) **1:** an official document **2:** a body of known or recorded facts about someone or something.

record base: an interim denture base used to support the record rim material for recording maxillomandibular records.

semiadjustable articulator: an articulator that allows adjustment to replicate average mandibular movements—also called *Class III articulator.*

stereographic record: an intra- or extraoral recording of mandibular movement. Viewed in three planes in which the registrations are obtained by engraving, milling, or burnishing the recording medium by means of studs, rotary instruments, styli, teeth, or abrasive rims.

REFERENCES

1. Mendez AJ: The influence of impression trays on the accuracy of stone casts poured from irreversible hydrocolloid impressions, *J Prosthet Dent* 54:383, 1985.

2. Lim PF et al: Adaptation of finger-smoothed irreversible hydrocolloid to impression surfaces, *Int J Prosthodont* 8:117, 1995.

3. Khaknegar B, Ettinger RL: Removal time: a factor in the accuracy of irreversible hydrocolloid impressions, *J Oral Rehabil* 4:369, 1977.

4. al-Omari WM et al: A microbiological investigation following the disinfection of alginate and addition cured silicone rubber impression materials, *Eur J Prosthodont Restor Dent* 6:97, 1998.

5. Matyas J et al: Effects of disinfectants on dimensional accuracy of impression materials, *J Prosthet Dent* 64:25, 1990.

6. Johnson GH et al: Dimensional stability and detail reproduction of irreversible hydrocolloid and elastomeric impressions disinfected by immersion, *J Prosthet Dent* 79:446, 1998.

7. Reisbick MH et al: Irreversible hydrocolloid and gypsum interactions, *Int J Prosthodont* 10:7, 1997.

8. Young JM: Surface characteristics of dental stone: impression orientation, *J Prosthet Dent* 33:336, 1975.

9. Palik JF et al: Accuracy of an earpiece face-bow, *J Prosthet Dent* 53:800, 1985.

10. Piehslinger E et al: Computer simulation of occlusal discrepancies resulting from different mounting techniques, *J Prosthet Dent* 74:279, 1995.

11. Adrien P, Schouver J: Methods for minimizing the errors in mandibular model mounting on an articulator, *J Oral Rehabil* 24:929, 1997.

12. Dawson PE: Temporomandibular joint pain-dysfunction problems can be solved, *J Prosthet Dent* 29:100, 1973.

13. Tarantola GJ et al: The reproducibility of centric relation: a clinical approach, *J Am Dent Assoc* 9:1245, 1997.

14. McKee JR: Comparing condylar position repeatability for standardized versus nonstandardized methods of achieving centric relation, *J Prosthet Dent* 77:280, 1997.

15. Lucia VO: A technique for recording centric relation, *J Prosthet Dent* 14:492, 1964.

16. Gross M et al: The effect of three different recording materials on the reproducibility of condylar guidance registrations in three semi-adjustable articulators, *J Oral Rehabil* 25:204, 1998.

17. Wirth CG: Interocclusal centric relation records for articulator mounted casts, *Dent Clin North Am* 15:627, 1971.

18. Wirth CG, Aplin AW: An improved interocclusal record of centric relation, *J Prosthet Dent* 25:279, 1971.

19. Lundeen HC: Centric relation records: the effect of muscle action, *J Prosthet Dent* 31:244, 1974.

20. Kepron D: Variations in condylar position relative to central mandibular recordings. In Lefkowitz W, editor: *Proceedings of the Second International Prosthodontic Congress*, St Louis, 1979, Mosby, p 210.

21. Teo CS, Wise MD: Comparison of retruded axis articular mountings with and without applied muscular force, *J Oral Rehabil* 8:363, 1981.

22. Tamaki K et al: Reproduction of excursive tooth contact in an articulator with computerized axiography data, *J Prosthet Dent* 78:373, 1997.

23. Lundeen HC, Wirth CG: Condylar movement patterns engraved in plastic blocks, *J Prosthet Dent* 30:866, 1973.

24. Bell LJ, Matich JA: A study of the acceptability of lateral records by the Whip-Mix articulator, *J Prosthet Dent* 38:22, 1977.

25. Celar AG et al: Guided versus unguided mandibular movement for duplicating intraoral eccentric tooth contacts in the articulator, *J Prosthet Dent* 81:14, 1999.

TREATMENT PLANNING

KEY TERMS

abutment
Ante's law
cantilever
complete dentures
crown
fixed partial denture (FPD)
nonrigid connectors

removable partial denture
  (RPD)
residual ridge
span length
supraclusion
treatment sequence

Treatment planning consists of formulating a logical sequence of treatment designed to restore the patient's dentition to good health, with optimal function and appearance. The plan should be presented in written form and should be discussed in detail with the patient. Good communication with the patient is essential when formulating the plan. Most dental disorders can be corrected with several different procedures; the patient's preferences are paramount in establishing a suitable treatment plan. An appropriate plan informs the patient about the present conditions, the extent of dental treatment proposed, the time and cost of treatment, and the level of home care and professional follow-up needed for success. In addition, before any irreversible procedures are undertaken, the patient should understand that some details may need to be altered during the course of treatment.

This chapter outlines the decisions that will be necessary when planning treatment for fixed prosthodontics. Foremost among these is the identification of patients' needs and their preferences, which must be correlated with the range of treatments available. For long-term success, when a **fixed partial denture (FPD)** is being considered, the **abutment** teeth must be carefully assessed. Finally, the treatment plan must be properly sequenced as part of an ongoing program of comprehensive dental care.

■ IDENTIFICATION OF PATIENT NEEDS

Successful treatment planning is based on proper identification of the patient's needs. If an attempt is made to have the patient conform to the "ideal"

treatment plan rather than have the treatment plan conform to the patient's needs, success is unlikely. Frequently, several treatment plans are presented and discussed, each with advantages and disadvantages. Indeed, failing to explain and present alternatives may be legally negligent.

Treatment is required to accomplish one or more of the following objectives: correcting an existing disease, preventing future disease, restoring function, and improving appearance.

CORRECTION OF EXISTING DISEASE

Existing disease will be revealed during the clinical examination. The disease process can usually be arrested by identification and reduction of the initiating factors, identification and improvement of the resistive factors, or both (Fig. 3-1). For example, oral hygiene instruction will reduce the amount of residual plaque, an initiating factor, and thus will reduce the likelihood of further dental caries. It will also improve gingival health, and the resulting healthy tissue will be more resistant to disease. Additional fluoride intake (e.g., mouth rinses) is also recommended in a patient with a caries problem. Restorative care will replace damaged or missing tooth structure, but additional treatment is essential for controlling the disease that caused the damage.

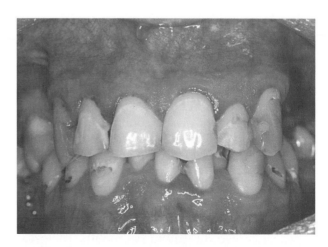

Fig. 3-1. Poor plaque control with dental caries.

PREVENTION OF FUTURE DISEASE

The likelihood of future disease can be predicted by evaluating the patient's disease experience and by knowing the prevalence of the disease in the general population. Treatment should be proposed if future disease seems likely in the absence of such intervention.

RESTORATION OF FUNCTION

Although objective measurement may be difficult, the level of function is assessed during the examination. Treatment may be proposed to correct impaired function (e.g., mastication or speech).

IMPROVEMENT OF APPEARANCE

Patients often seek dental treatment because they are dissatisfied with their appearance. However, it is difficult to objectively assess dental esthetics. The dentist should develop expertise in this area and should be prepared to appraise the appearance of the patient's dentition and listen carefully to the patient's views. If the appearance is far outside socially accepted values, the feasibility of corrective procedures should be brought to the patient's attention. Long-term dental health should not be compromised by unwise attempts to improve appearance. Patients should always be made aware of the possible adverse consequences of treatment.

AVAILABLE MATERIALS AND TECHNIQUES

All existing restorative materials and techniques have limitations and cannot exactly match the properties of natural tooth structure. Before the clinician selects the appropriate procedure, he or she should understand these limitations. This will help prevent an experimental approach to treatment.

PLASTIC MATERIALS

Plastic materials (e.g., silver amalgam or composite resin) are the most commonly used dental restoratives. They allow simple and conservative restoration of damaged teeth. However, their mechanical properties are inferior to cast metal or metal-ceramic restorations. Their continued service depends on the strength and integrity of the remaining tooth structure. When the remaining tooth substance needs reinforcement, a cast metal restoration should be fabricated, usually with amalgam as the foundation or core (see Chapter 6).

Large amalgam restorations (Fig. 3-2, *A*) are shaped or carved directly in the mouth. The great degree of difficulty associated with this direct approach often results in defective contours and poor

occlusion. The indirect procedure, used in making cast metal **crowns** (Fig. 3-2, *B*), facilitates the fabrication of more accurately shaped restorations.

CAST METAL

Cast metal crowns are fabricated outside the mouth and are cemented with a luting agent. To minimize exposure of the luting agent to oral fluids, a long-lasting restoration must have good marginal adaptation. The highly refined techniques for overcoming the problem of marginal fit also permit the manufacture of cast metal crowns with precisely shaped axial and occlusal surfaces. This ensures continued periodontal health and good occlusal function. The internal dimensions of a casting must seat without binding against the walls while remaining stable and not becoming displaced during function. Preparation design for cast metal restorations is critical and is discussed in detail in Chapter 7.

Intracoronal Restorations (Fig. 3-3).   An intracoronal cast metal restoration or inlay relies on the strength of the remaining tooth structure for support and retention, just as a plastic restoration does. However, greater tooth bulk is needed to resist any wedging effect on the preparation walls. Therefore, this restoration is contraindicated in a significantly weakened tooth. When fabricated correctly, it is extremely durable because of the strength and corro-

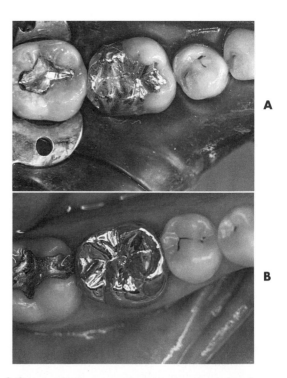

Fig. 3-2.   **A,** The large amalgam restoration is hard to condense and contour accurately. **B,** The complete cast crown is stronger and can be shaped by an indirect procedure in the dental laboratory.

sion resistance of the gold casting alloy; in a tooth with a minimal proximal carious lesion, however, it usually requires greater removal of tooth structure than an amalgam preparation. Inlays do not have sufficient resistance or retention to be used as abutment retainers for fixed partial dentures.

Extracoronal Restorations (Fig. 3-4). An extracoronal cast metal restoration or crown encircles all or part of the remaining tooth structure. As such, it can strengthen and protect a tooth weakened by caries or trauma. To provide the necessary bulk of material for strength, considerably more tooth structure must be removed than for an intracoronal

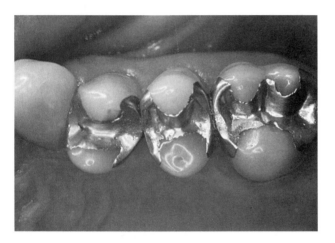

Fig. 3-3. The MOD inlay is generally contraindicated because there is the risk of tooth fracture. However, it can be a very long-lasting restoration. These, placed in 1948, are still satisfactory after 52 years.

restoration. The margins of an extracoronal restoration often must be near the free gingiva, which can make maintenance of tissue health difficult. Tooth preparation for an extracoronal restoration may be combined with intracoronal features (e.g., grooves and pinholes) to gain resistance and retention.

METAL-CERAMIC

Metal-ceramic restorations (Fig. 3-5) consist of a tooth-colored layer of porcelain bonded to a cast metal substructure. They are used when a complete crown is needed to restore appearance as well as function. Sufficient reduction of tooth structure is necessary to provide space for the bulk of porcelain needed for a natural appearance. Thus the preparation design for a metal-ceramic crown is among the least conservative, although tooth structure can be conserved if only the most visible part of the restoration is veneered.

The labial margins of a metal-ceramic restoration are often discernible and may detract from its appearance. They can be hidden by subgingival placement, although they then have the potential for increasing gingival inflammation; this should be avoided when possible.[1] Appearance can be improved by omitting the metal shoulder and making the labial margin in porcelain. As discussed in Chapter 24, this is a more demanding laboratory procedure.

RESIN-VENEERED

Resin-veneered restorations were popular before the metal-ceramic technique was fully developed,

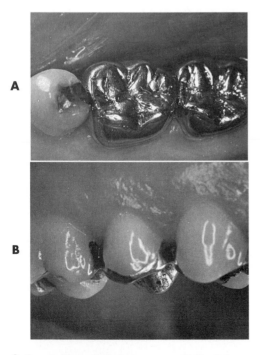

Fig. 3-4. **A,** Complete cast crowns. **B,** Partial veneer crown on a second premolar.

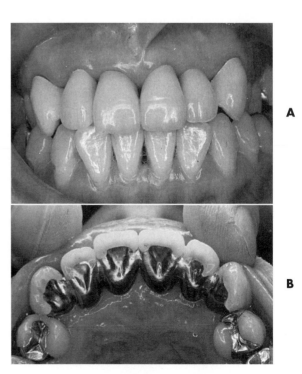

Fig. 3-5. **A, B,** Metal-ceramic restorations.

but problems with wear and discoloration of the polymethyl methacrylate veneer (Fig. 3-6) limited their use to long-term provisional restorations. Current resin-veneer techniques[2] incorporate bis-GMA–based materials (bisphenol-A glycidyl dimethacrylates), which have better physical properties than the earlier acrylic resins, and adhesive techniques to improve the bond to the supporting metal.[3,4]

FIBER-REINFORCED RESIN

Advances in composite resin technology, especially the introduction of glass and polyethylene fibers,[5-7] have prompted the use of indirect composite resin restorations for inlays, crowns, and FPDs. Excellent marginal adaptation and esthetic results are achievable (Fig 3-7), but because these are newer technologies, little is known about their longer-term performance (see Chapter 27).

COMPLETE CERAMIC

Crowns, inlays, and laminate veneers made entirely of dental porcelain can be the most esthetically pleasing of all fixed restorations (Fig. 3-8). Drawbacks include a comparative lack of strength and the difficulties associated with achieving an acceptable marginal fit. The current focus in improving strength lies with either veneering a high-strength alumina, zirconia, or spinel core[8,9] with a more translucent porcelain or using a leucite-reinforced translucent material[10-12] (see Chapter 25). Complete ceramic restorations are fabricated by an indirect technique and generally retained with composite resin. Acid etching is used to provide retention "keys."

FIXED PARTIAL DENTURES

An FPD (Fig. 3-9) is often indicated where one or more teeth require removal or are missing. Such teeth are replaced by pontics that are designed to fulfill the functional and often the esthetic requirements of the missing teeth (see Chapter 19). Pontics are connected to retainers, which are the restorations on prepared abutment teeth.

All the components of an FPD are fabricated and assembled in the laboratory before cementation in the mouth. This requires precise alignment of tooth preparations. Because unseating forces on individual retainers can be considerable, highly retentive restorations are essential. The predictable long-term success of an FPD is ensured by controlling the magnitude and direction of forces and by making sure the patient practices appropriate oral hygiene measures.

IMPLANT-SUPPORTED PROSTHESES

Single or multiple missing teeth can be replaced with an implant-supported prosthesis (Fig. 3-10). For the successful "osseointegrated" technique, the bone is atraumatically drilled to receive precisely fitting titanium cylinders.[13] These are left in place without loading for some months until they are invested with bone. Only then are function and esthetics restored with a prosthesis (see Chapter 13).

REMOVABLE PARTIAL DENTURES

A **removable partial denture (RPD)** (Fig. 3-11) is designed to replace missing teeth and their supporting structures. Forces applied to a well-designed prosthesis are distributed to the remaining teeth and the residual alveolar ridges. These forces are most accurately controlled if the abutment teeth are provided with fixed cast restorations that have carefully contoured guide planes and rest seats (see Chapter 20).

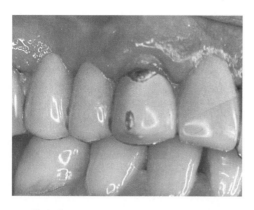

Fig. 3-6. Worn acrylic resin veneer.

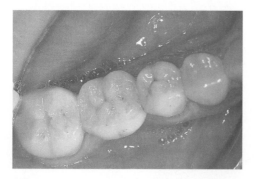

Fig. 3-7. Fiber-reinforced fixed partial denture.

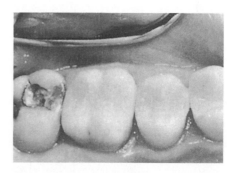

Fig. 3-8. Complete ceramic restoration.

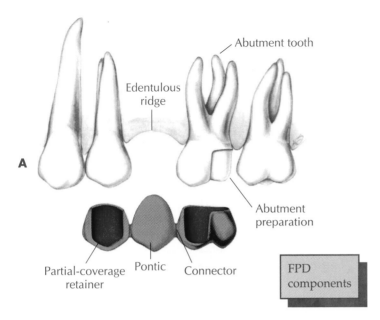

Abutment tooth

Edentulous ridge

Abutment preparation

Partial-coverage retainer

Pontic

Connector

FPD components

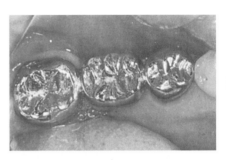

B

Fig. 3-9. **A,** A three-unit FPD showing the main components. **B,** The pontic rigidly attached to crowns on the abutment teeth. The connectors should occupy the normal interproximal contact area and be large enough for strength but not so large as to impede plaque control.

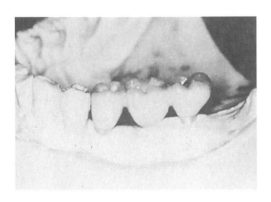

Fig. 3-10. Three-unit FPD supported by two dental implants.

Reciprocal arm

Minor connector

Retentive arm

Retentive arm

Denture base

Occlusal rest

Occlusal rest

Reciprocal arm

Major connector

Fig. 3-11. The component parts of an RPD.

RPDs must be sturdy to withstand stresses generated during insertion, function, and removal.

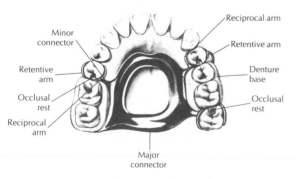

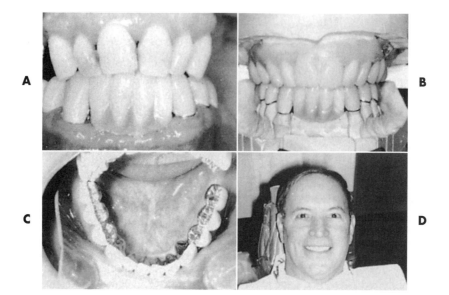

Fig. 3-12.   Special planning is required when a combination of a complete maxillary denture is planned opposing a fixed mandibular prosthesis. In general, a trial maxillary denture is indicated so the fixed prosthesis can be fabricated to a well-aligned occlusal plane. **A,** Preoperative appearance. **B,** Trial denture articulated with diagnostic waxing. **C** and **D,** Completed restoration. *(Courtesy Dr. K.A. Laurell.)*

COMPLETE DENTURES

Some of the difficulties encountered with **complete dentures** relate to the lack of denture stability and a gradual loss of supporting bone. Stability is enhanced if the denture has a carefully designed occlusion. Problems with stability can be especially severe when the mandibular incisors are the only teeth retained, with ensuing damage to the opposing premaxilla,[14] although any treatment plan that involves a complete denture opposing fixed restorations requires careful planning of the occlusion (Fig. 3-12). For selected patients, providing an overdenture that rests on endodontically treated roots may help preserve the **residual ridge** and enhance the stability of the complete denture.[15]

◼ TREATMENT OF TOOTH LOSS

A treatment plan involving fixed prosthodontics will generally include the replacement of missing teeth. Most teeth are lost as a result of dental caries or periodontal disease. More rarely they may be congenitally absent or lost as a result of trauma or neoplastic disease.

DECISION TO REMOVE A TOOTH

The decision to remove a tooth is part of the treatment-planning process and is made after assessing the advantages and disadvantages associated with retention of the tooth. Sometimes it is possible to retain a tooth with an apparently hopeless prognosis by us-

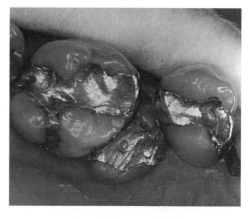

Fig. 3-13.   Poor treatment planning. The displaced premolar should never have been restored under these circumstances. *(Courtesy Dr. P.B. Robinson.)*

ing highly specialized and complex techniques. At other times, removing the tooth will be the treatment of choice. A decision about replacing a missing tooth is best made at the time its removal is recommended, rather than months or years after the fact (Fig. 3-13).

CONSEQUENCES OF REMOVAL WITHOUT REPLACEMENT

The stability of an individual tooth depends on a balance of the forces exerted on that tooth by the adjacent and opposing teeth and supporting tissues and by the soft tissues of the cheeks, lips, and tongue. When a single tooth is not replaced, this balance is upset (Fig. 3-14). The consequences may be **supra-**

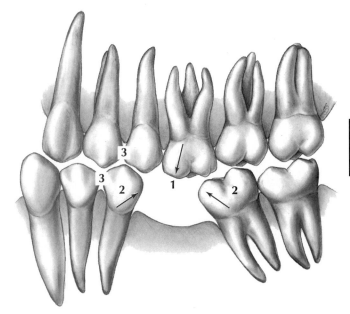

Over time, loss of arch integrity will result in tooth movement.

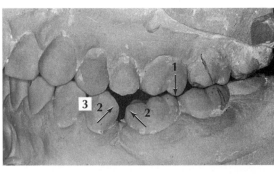

Fig. 3-14. Loss of a mandibular first molar not replaced with an FPD. The typical consequences are supraclusion of opposing teeth *(1)*, tilting of adjacent teeth *(2)*, and loss of proximal contacts *(3)*. *(Redrawn from Rosenstiel SF: In Rayne J, editor: General dental treatment, London, 1983, Kluwer Publishing.)*

clusion of the opposing tooth or teeth, tilting of the adjacent teeth, and loss of proximal contact (with resulting disturbances in the health of the supporting structures and the occlusion). Although simple replacement of the missing tooth at this late stage may prevent further disruption, it may be insufficient to return the dentition to full health. Extended treatment plans, including orthodontic repositioning and additional cast restorations (to correct the disturbed occlusal plane), may be needed to compensate for the lack of treatment at the time of tooth removal.

◼ SELECTION OF ABUTMENT TEETH

Whenever possible, FPDs should be designed as simply as possible, with a single well-anchored retainer fixed rigidly at each end of the pontic. The use of multiple splinted abutment teeth, **nonrigid connectors**, or intermediate abutments makes the procedure much more difficult, and often the result compromises the long-term prognosis (Fig. 3-15).

REPLACEMENT OF A SINGLE MISSING TOOTH

Unless bone support has been weakened by advanced periodontal disease, a single missing tooth

can almost always be replaced by a three-unit FPD having one mesial and one distal abutment tooth. An exception is when the FPD is replacing a maxillary or mandibular canine. Under these circumstances, the small anterior abutment tooth needs to be splinted to the central incisor to prevent lateral drift of the FPD.

Cantilever Fixed Partial Dentures. FPDs in which only one side of the pontic is attached to a retainer are referred to as *cantilevered*. An example would be a lateral incisor pontic attached only to an extracoronal metal-ceramic retainer on a canine. Their use remains popular because some of the difficulties encountered in making a three-unit FPD are lessened. Also, many clinicians are reluctant to prepare an intact central incisor, preferring instead to use a **cantilever.**

However, the long-term prognosis of the single-abutment cantilever is poor.[16] Forces are best tolerated by the periodontal supporting structures when directed in the long axes of the teeth.[17] This is the case when a simple three-unit FPD is used. A cantilever will induce lateral forces on the supporting tissues, which may be harmful and lead to tipping,

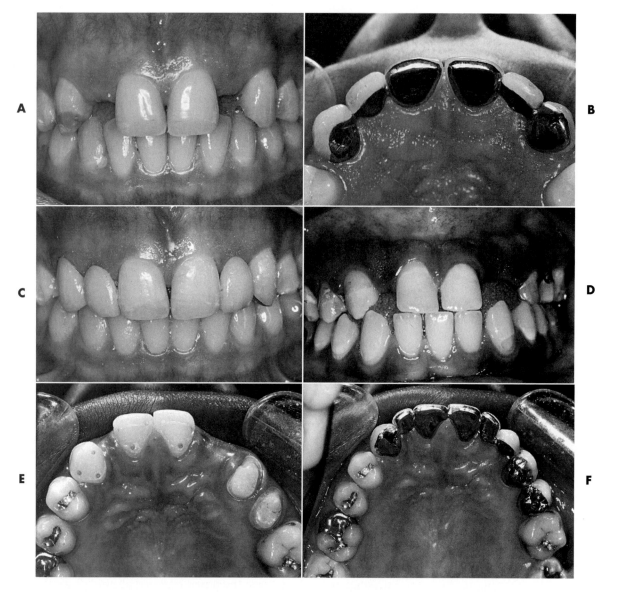

Fig. 3-15. **A** to **C,** Congenitally missing lateral incisors replaced with two simple three-unit FPDs. **D** to **F,** This patient had a missing canine as well as two congenitally missing laterals. Here, there is a much greater restorative challenge than in **A,** requiring an eight-unit prosthesis.

rotation, or drifting of the abutment (Fig. 3-16). Laboratory analysis[18,19] has confirmed the potential harmful nature of such fixed partial dentures. However, clinical experience with resin-retained FPDs has suggested that cantilever designs may be preferred, especially since readhesion after failure is greatly facilitated and often leads to predictable long-term success[20] (see Chapter 26).

When multiple missing teeth are replaced, cantilever FPDs have considerable application (see p. 70). The harmful tipping forces are resisted by multiple abutment teeth, and movement of the abutments is unlikely. Cantilevers are also successfully used with implant-supported prostheses (see Chapter 13).

Assessment of Abutment Teeth. Considerable time and expense are spared, and loss of a patient's

confidence can be avoided, by thoroughly investigating each abutment tooth before proceeding with tooth preparation. Radiographs are made, and pulpal health is assessed by evaluating the response to thermal and electrical stimulation. Existing restorations, cavity liners, and residual caries are removed[21] (preferably under a rubber dam), and a careful check is made for possible pulpal exposure. Teeth in which pulpal health is doubtful should be endodontically treated before the initiation of fixed prosthodontics. Although a direct pulp cap may be an acceptable risk for a simple amalgam or composite resin, conventional endodontic treatment is normally preferred for cast restorations, especially where the later need for endodontic treatment would jeopardize the overall success of treatment.

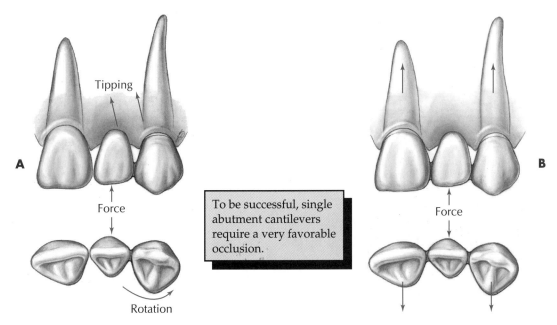

> To be successful, single abutment cantilevers require a very favorable occlusion.

Fig. 3-16. **A,** Forces applied to a cantilever FPD are resisted on only one side, leading to imbalance. Vertical forces can cause tipping, and horizontal forces, rotation, of abutment teeth. **B,** By including both adjacent teeth in the prosthesis, it is possible to resist forces much better since the teeth have to be moved bodily rather than merely rotated or tipped.
(Redrawn from Rosenstiel SF: In Rayne J, editor: General dental treatment, *London, 1983, Kluwer Publishing.)*

Endodontically Treated Abutments. If a tooth is properly treated endodontically, it can serve well as an abutment with a post and core foundation for retention and strength (see Chapter 12). Failures occur, however, particularly on teeth with short roots or little remaining coronal tooth structure. Care is needed to obtain maximum retention for the post and core. Sometimes it is better to recommend removal of a badly damaged tooth rather than to attempt endodontic treatment.

Unrestored Abutments. An unrestored, caries-free tooth is an ideal abutment. It can be prepared conservatively for a strong retentive restoration with optimum esthetics (Fig. 3-17). The margin of the retainer can be placed without modifications to accommodate existing restorations or caries. In an adult patient, an unrestored tooth can be safely prepared without jeopardizing the pulp as long as the design and technique of tooth preparation are wisely chosen. Certain patients are reluctant to have a perfectly sound tooth cut down to provide anchorage for a fixed partial denture. In these cases, the overall dental health of the patient should be emphasized rather than looking at each tooth individually.

Mesially Tilted Second Molar. Loss of a permanent mandibular first molar to caries early in life is still relatively common (Fig. 3-18). If the space is ignored, the second molar will tilt mesially, espe-

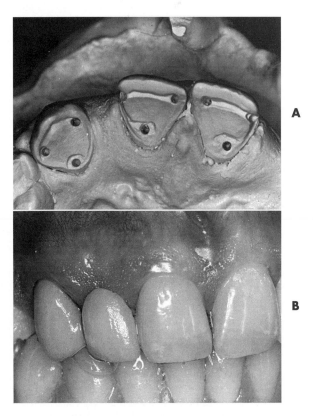

Fig. 3-17. **A,** Unrestored abutment teeth can be prepared for conservative retainers. **B,** An esthetic FPD replacing a maxillary incisor.

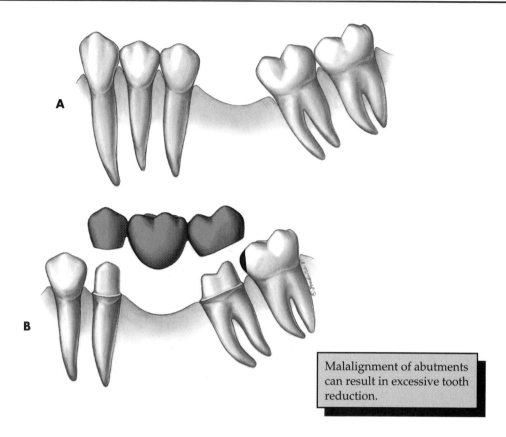

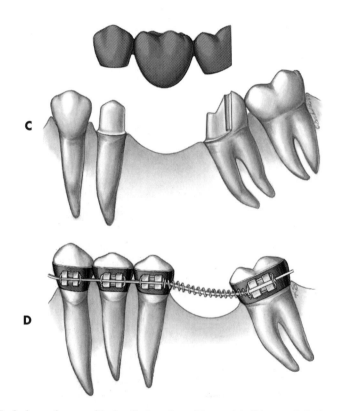

Malalignment of abutments can result in excessive tooth reduction.

Fig. 3-18.   **A,** Early loss of a mandibular first molar with mesial tilting and drifting of the second and third molars. **B,** A conventional three-unit FPD will fail because its seating is prevented by the third molar. **C,** A modified preparation design can be used on the distal abutment. **D,** A better treatment plan would be to remove the third molar and upright the second molar orthodontically before fabricating an FPD. *(Redrawn from Rosenstiel SF: In Rayne J, editor:* General dental treatment, *London, 1983, Kluwer Publishing.)*

cially with eruption of the third molar. It then becomes difficult or impossible to make a satisfactory fixed partial denture, because the positional relationship no longer allows for parallel paths of insertion without interference from the adjacent teeth. In such circumstances, an FPD is sometimes made with modified preparation designs or with a nonrigid connector, or a straightforward solution[22] may be considered: uprighting the tilted abutment orthodontically with a simple fixed appliance. However, the problem can be avoided altogether if a space-maintainer appliance (Fig. 3-19) is fabricated when the first molar is removed. This device may be as simple as a square section of orthodontic wire bent to follow the edentulous ridge and anchored with small restorations in adjacent teeth.

REPLACEMENT OF SEVERAL MISSING TEETH

Fixed prosthodontics becomes more difficult when several teeth must be replaced. Problems will be encountered when restoring a single long, uninterrupted edentulous area or multiple edentulous areas with intermediate abutment teeth (Fig. 3-20), especially when anterior and posterior teeth are to be replaced with a single fixed prosthesis. Underestimation of the problems involved in extensive prosthodontics can lead to failure. One key to ensuring a successful result is to plan the prostheses by waxing the intended restorations on articulated diagnostic casts. This is essential for complex fixed prosthodontic treatments, particularly where an irregular occlusal plane is to be corrected, the vertical dimension of occlusion is to be altered, an implant-supported prosthesis is recommended, or a combination of fixed and removable prostheses are to be used. The precise end point of such complicated treatments can be far from evident, even to an experienced prosthodontist (see Fig. 2-39).

Overloading of Abutment Teeth. The ability of the abutment teeth to accept applied forces without drifting or becoming mobile must be estimated and has a direct influence on the prosthodontic treatment plan. These forces can be particularly severe during parafunctional grinding and clenching (see Chapter 4), and the need to eliminate them becomes obvious during the restoration of such a damaged dentition. Although it may be hoped that a well-reconstructed occlusion will reduce the duration and strength of any parafunctional activity, there is little scientific evidence to support this. It is unwise to initiate treatment on the assumption that new restorations will reduce parafunctional activity, unless this has been demonstrated with treatment appliances over a significant period.[23]

Direction of Forces. Whereas the magnitude of any applied force is difficult to regulate, a well-fabricated fixed partial denture can distribute these forces in the most favorable way, directing them in the long axis of the abutment teeth. Potentially damaging lateral forces can be confined to the anterior teeth, where they are reduced by the longer lever arm (see Chapter 4).

Root Surface Area. The root surface area of potential abutment teeth must be assessed when planning treatment for fixed prosthodontics. Ante[24] suggested in 1926 that it was unwise to provide a fixed partial denture when the root surface area of the abutment was less than the root surface area of the teeth being replaced; this has been adopted and reinforced by other authors[25-27] as **Ante's law.** Average values for the root surface area of permanent teeth are given in Table 3-1.[28] As an example of Ante's law, consider the patient who has lost a first molar and second premolar (Fig. 3-21). In this situation, a four-unit FPD is an acceptable risk, as long as there has not been bone loss from periodontal disease, because the second molar and first premolar abutments have root surface areas approximately equal to those of the missing teeth. If the first molar and both premolars are missing, however, an FPD is not considered a good risk because the missing teeth have a greater total root surface area than the potential abutments.

Nyman and Ericsson,[29] however, cast doubt on the validity of Ante's law by demonstrating that teeth with considerably reduced bone support can be successfully used as fixed partial denture abutments. The majority of the treatments presented by

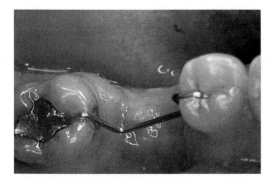

Fig. 3-19. Square section orthodontic wire can be used as a simple stabilizing appliance to prevent drifting of abutment teeth after exodontia. The wire is retained by placing small restorations. As an alternative, orthodontic bands can be used as the retainer. NOTE: These simple stabilizers do not prevent supraeruption of opposing teeth; in areas where this is anticipated, a provisional FPD is needed.

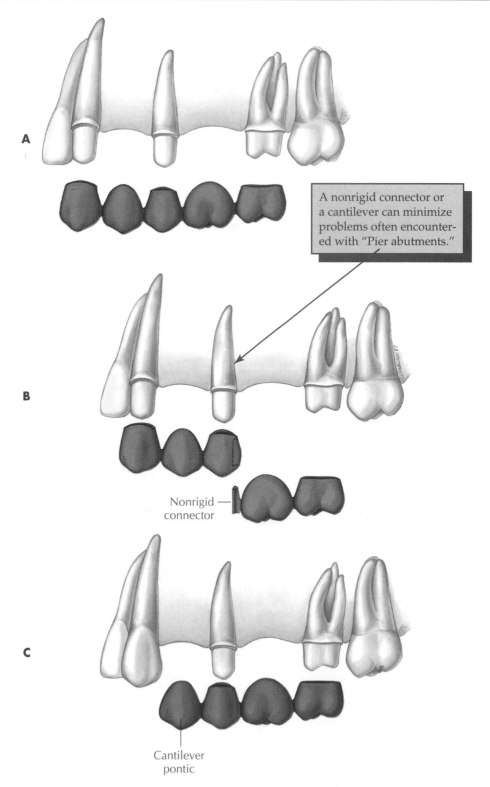

A nonrigid connector or a cantilever can minimize problems often encountered with "Pier abutments."

Nonrigid connector

Cantilever pontic

Fig. 3-20.   **A,** A five-unit FPD replacing the maxillary first molar and first premolar. The middle abutment can act as a fulcrum during function, with possible unseating of one of the other abutments. To be successful, this type of FPD needs extremely retentive retainers. **B,** An alternative approach is a nonrigid dovetail connector between the molar pontic and the second premolar. **C,** Where periodontal support is adequate, a much simpler approach would be to cantilever the first premolar pontic.
(Redrawn from Rosenstiel SF: In Rayne J, editor: General dental treatment, *London, 1983, Kluwer Publishing.)*

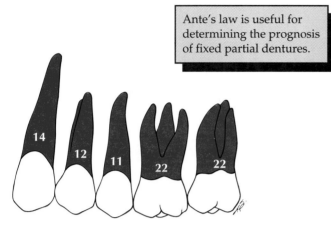

Ante's law is useful for determining the prognosis of fixed partial dentures.

Fig. 3-21. To assess the support of a fixed partial denture, Ante's law has been invoked. It proposes a relationship between the root surface areas of the missing teeth and those of the potential abutment teeth. (The numbers represent root surface area percentages.) If the first molar (22) and second premolar (11) are missing, the abutments for a four-unit FPD will have slightly greater total root surface area (34%) than the teeth being replaced. Then, in the absence of other detrimental factors, an FPD's prognosis will be favorable. However, if the first premolar (12) is also missing, the loss of potential abutment root surface area will comprise 45%, whereas the remaining abutments have only 36%, which is much less favorable.

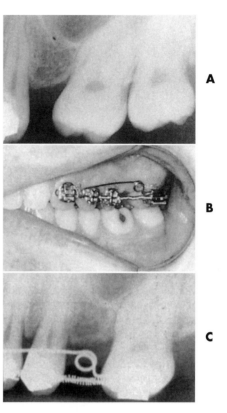

Fig. 3-22. **A,** A misaligned abutment tooth may be difficult or impossible to prepare for an FPD abutment and provides poor support. **B** and **C,** Where possible, this should be corrected with orthodontic treatment before restoration. *(Courtesy Dr. G. Gruendeman.)*

Root Surface Area (mm²) of Abutment		TABLE 3-1
		Percentage Root Surface Area in Quadrant
MAXILLARY		
Central	204	10
Lateral	179	9
Canine	273	14
First premolar	234	12
Second premolar	220	11
First molar	433	22
Second molar	431	22
MANDIBULAR		
Central	154	8
Lateral	168	9
Canine	268	15
First premolar	180	10
Second premolar	207	11
First molar	431	24
Second molar	426	23

Data from Jepsen A: *Acta Odontol Scand* 21:35, 1963.

these authors had an abutment root surface area less than half that of the replaced teeth, and there was no loss of attachment after 8 to 11 years. They attributed this success to meticulous root planing during the active phase of treatment, proper plaque control during the observed period, and the oc-

clusal design of the prostheses. Others have confirmed that abutment teeth with limited periodontal bone can successfully support fixed prostheses.[30,31]

Root Shape and Angulation. When tooth support is borderline, the shape of the roots and their angulation should be considered. A molar with divergent roots will provide better support than a molar with conical roots and little or no interradicular bone. A single-rooted tooth with an elliptic cross-section will offer better support than a tooth with similar root surface area but a circular cross-section. Similarly, a well-aligned tooth will provide better support than a tilted one. Alignment can be improved with orthodontic uprighting (Fig. 3-22).

Periodontal Disease. After horizontal bone loss from periodontal disease, the PDL-supported root surface area can be dramatically reduced.[32] Because of the conical shape of most roots (Fig. 3-23), when one third of the root length has been exposed, half the supporting area is lost. In addition, the forces applied to the supporting bone are magnified because of the greater leverage associated with the lengthened clinical crown. Thus potential abutment

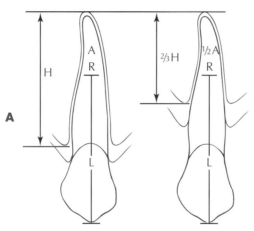

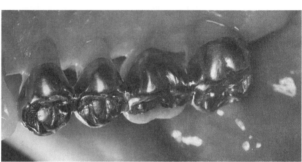

Horizontal bone loss can be deceptive. A little can result in a considerable loss of bone support because of root morphology.

Fig. 3-23. **A,** Because of the conical shape of most roots, the actual area of support *(A)* diminishes more than might be expected from the height of the bone *(H)*. In addition, the center of rotation *(R)* moves apically and the lever arm *(L)* increases, magnifying the forces on the supportive structure. **B,** A fixed partial denture replacing a maxillary first molar. The first premolar is an abutment providing additional stabilization for this FPD on abutment teeth with compromised bone support. *(A redrawn from Rosenstiel SF: In Rayne J, editor:* General dental treatment, *London, 1983, Kluwer Publishing.)*

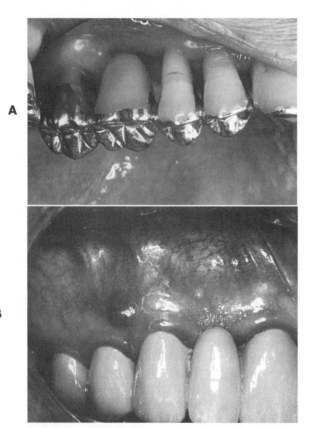

Fig. 3-24. **A,** Supragingival margins and large gingival embrasures facilitate plaque control in a periodontally compromised patient. **B,** Poor prosthetic contours and margins have contributed to this failure.

teeth need very careful assessment where significant bone loss has occurred.

In general, successful fixed prostheses can be fabricated on teeth with severely reduced periodontal support, provided the periodontal tissues have been returned to excellent health, and long-term maintenance has been ensured[33,34] (Fig. 3-24). When extensive reconstruction is attempted without complete control over the health of the periodontal tissues, the results can be disastrous.

Healthy periodontal tissues are a prerequisite for all fixed restorations. If the abutment teeth have normal bone support, an occasional lapse in plaque removal by the patient is unlikely to affect the long-term prognosis. However, when teeth with severe bone loss resulting from periodontal disease are used as abutments, there is very little tolerance. It then becomes imperative that excellent plaque-removal technique be implemented and maintained at all times.

Span Length. Excessive flexing under occlusal loads may cause failure of a long-span fixed partial denture (Fig. 3-25). It can lead to fracture of a porcelain veneer, breakage of a connector, loosening of a retainer, or an unfavorable soft tissue response and thus render a prosthesis useless. All FPDs flex slightly when subjected to a load—the longer the span, the greater the flexing. The relationship be-

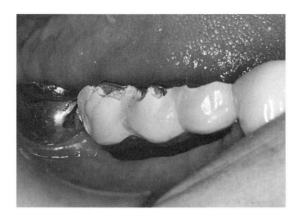

Fig. 3-25. Failure of a long-span fixed partial denture.

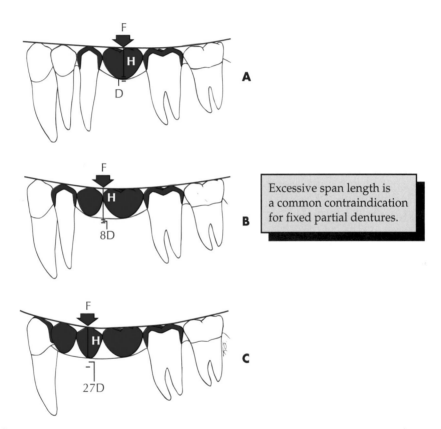

Excessive span length is a common contraindication for fixed partial dentures.

Fig. 3-26. The deflection of a fixed partial denture is proportional to the cube of the length of its span. **A,** A single pontic will deflect a small amount *(D)* when subjected to a certain force *(F)*. **B,** Two pontics will deflect 2^3 times as much *(8 D)* to the same force. **C,** Three pontics will deflect 3^3 times as much *(27 D)*.

tween deflection and length of span is not simply linear but varies with the cube of the length of the span. Thus, other factors being equal, if a span of a single pontic is deflected a certain amount, a span of two similar pontics will move 8 times as much, and three will move 27 times as much[35] (Fig. 3-26).

Replacing three posterior teeth with an FPD rarely has a favorable prognosis, especially in the mandibular arch. Under such circumstances it is usually better to recommend an implant-supported prosthesis or a removable partial denture.

When a long-span FPD is fabricated, pontics and connectors should be made as bulky as possible to ensure optimum rigidity without jeopardizing gingival health. In addition, the prosthesis should be made of a material that has high strength and rigidity (see Chapter 16).

Replacing Multiple Anterior Teeth. Special considerations in this situation include problems with appearance and the need to resist laterally directed tipping forces.

The four mandibular incisors can usually be replaced by a simple fixed partial denture with retainers on each canine. It is not usually necessary to include the first premolars. If a lone incisor remains, it should be removed because its retention will unnecessarily complicate the design and fabrication of the FPD and can jeopardize the long-term result. Mandibular incisors, because of their small size, generally make poor abutment teeth. It is particularly important not to have overcontoured restorations on these teeth because plaque control will be nearly impossible. Thus the clinician may have to make a choice between (1) compromised esthetics from too thin a ceramic veneer and (2) pulpal exposure during tooth preparation. A third alternative would be selective tooth removal.

The loss of several maxillary incisors presents a much greater problem in terms of restoring appearance and providing support. Because of the curvature of the arch, forces directed against a maxillary incisor pontic will tend to tip the abutment teeth. Unlike the mandibular incisors, the maxillary incisors are not positioned in a straight line (particularly in patients with narrow or pointed dental arches). Tipping forces must be resisted by means of two abutment teeth at each end of a long span anterior FPD. Thus, when replacing the four maxillary incisors, the clinician should generally use the canines and first premolars as abutment teeth.[36]

There may be considerable difficulty in achieving a good appearance when several maxillary incisors are being replaced with a fixed partial denture. Obtaining the best tooth contours and position for appearance and phonetics can be a challenge. A good attempt can be made with the diagnostic waxing procedure, evaluating any esthetic problems. As treatment progresses, a provisional restoration is provided (see Chapter 15). This may be used to test appearance and phonetics. It may also be readily shaped and modified to suit the patient, and the final restoration can be made as a copy of it, thereby avoiding any embarrassing misunderstandings when the finished fixed prosthesis is delivered.

If anterior bone loss has been severe, as can happen when teeth are lost due to trauma or periodontal disease, there may be a ridge defect (Fig. 3-27). In these patients, a removable partial denture should be considered, especially when the person has a high smile line, since a fixed partial denture generally replaces only the missing tooth structure, not the supporting tissues. Again, a provisional restoration may help the patient determine the most appropriate treatment. A surgical ridge augmentation procedure[37] may also be an option, although the results can be unpredictable.

INDICATIONS FOR REMOVABLE PARTIAL DENTURES

Whenever possible, edentulous spaces should be restored with fixed rather than removable partial den-

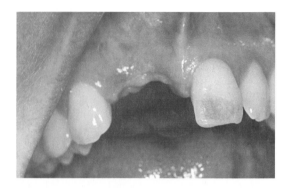

Fig. 3-27. This patient lost two incisors in an accident. Considerable alveolar bone has also been lost. An aesthetic fixed prosthesis would be very difficult or impossible to fabricate without surgical ridge augmentation. *(Courtesy Dr. N. Archambo.)*

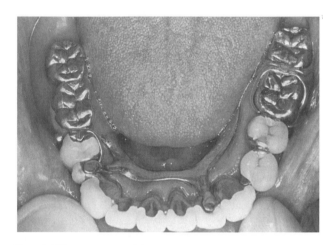

Fig. 3-28. A removable partial denture replacing the mandibular right first and second molars.

tures. A well-fabricated FPD will provide better health and better function than an RPD and is preferred by most patients. Under the following circumstances, however, a removable partial denture is indicated:

1. Where vertical support from the edentulous ridge is needed; for example, in the absence of a distal abutment tooth (Fig. 3-28)
2. Where resistance to lateral movement is needed from contralateral teeth and soft tissues; for example, to ensure stability with a long edentulous space
3. When there is considerable bone loss in the visible anterior region and an FPD would have an unacceptable appearance (Fig. 3-29)

Multiple edentulous spaces often are best restored with a combination of fixed and removable partial dentures (Fig. 3-30).

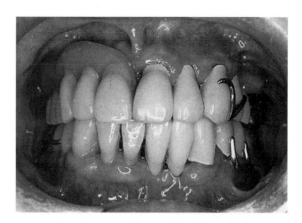

Fig. 3-29. Where there has been considerable bone loss, an RPD has a more natural appearance than an FPD.

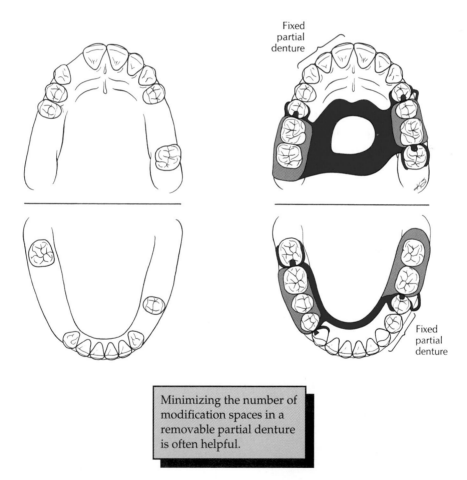

Fixed
partial
denture

Fixed
partial
denture

Minimizing the number of
modification spaces in a
removable partial denture
is often helpful.

Fig. 3-30. Treatment planning for multiple edentulous spaces. A combination of fixed and removable prostheses may provide the best replacement when several teeth are missing. In the maxillary arch, the missing lateral has been restored with a simple three-unit FPD, which is more easily cleaned than an RPD. In the mandibular arch, the single remaining premolar is splinted to the canine with a three-unit FPD. An RPD that fits around a lone-standing premolar usually does not have a good prognosis.
(Redrawn from Rosenstiel SF: In Rayne J, editor: General dental treatment, *London, 1983, Kluwer Publishing.)*

SEQUENCE OF TREATMENT

When patient needs have been identified and the appropriate corrective measures have been determined, a logical sequence of steps must be decided on—including the treatment of symptoms, stabilization of deteriorating conditions, definitive therapy, and a program of follow-up care. The importance of proper sequencing is stressed, since mistakes can lead to compromised effort or unnecessary and expensive remakes.

TREATMENT OF SYMPTOMS

The relief of discomfort accompanying an acute condition is a priority item in planning treatment (Fig. 3-31). Discomfort can be due to one or more of the following: a fractured tooth or teeth, acute pulpitis, acute exacerbation of a chronic pulpitis, dental abscess, an acute pericoronitis or gingivitis, and myofascial pain dysfunction.

The clinician needs only sufficient diagnostic information to ascertain the nature of a particular condition and to form a diagnosis; treatment is instituted without delay. A full examination is neither desirable nor generally possible until the symptoms of the acute condition have been addressed.

Urgent Treatment of Nonacute Problems. Fortunately, most potential candidates for fixed prosthodontics do not seek treatment for acute conditions; however, they may have a specific problem that should receive immediate attention, such as a lost anterior crown, a cracked or broken porcelain veneer, or a fractured removable prosthesis (Fig. 3-32).

STABILIZATION OF DETERIORATING CONDITIONS

The second phase of treatment involves stabilizing conditions such as dental caries or periodontal disease by removing the etiologic factors, increasing the patient's resistance, or doing both.

Dental Caries. Treatment of carious lesions is approached in a conventional manner, and the teeth are restored with properly contoured plastic materials. These may serve as a foundation for fixed castings during a subsequent phase of treatment (see Chapter 6). However, cast restorations are best avoided in a patient with active caries because the results of such extensive treatment would be jeopardized by recurrence of the disease. This can be prevented by a combination of dietary advice, oral hygiene measures, and fluoride treatment.

Periodontal Disease. Chronic periodontitis with continuing irreversible bone loss should be treated as early as possible by effective daily plaque control. The proper removal of plaque is possible only if the teeth are smooth and their contours allow unimpeded access to the gingival sulci. Therefore, the following are essential (Fig. 3-33):

* Replacement of defective restorations
* Removal of carious lesions
* Recontouring of overcontoured crowns (especially near furcation areas)
* Proper oral hygiene instruction adequately implemented at home

DEFINITIVE THERAPY

When the stabilization phase has been completed, successful elective long-term treatment aimed at promoting dental health, restoring function, and improving appearance can begin. On occasion, this will take considerable time. Several therapeutic proposals may be applicable to a single patient and may range in complexity from minimum restorative treatment with regular maintenance to full mouth prosthodontic reconstruction preceded by orthognathic surgery and orthodontic treatment. The advantages and disadvantages of each should be thoroughly explained to the patient, with diagnostic casts and waxings used as guides. When a definitive plan is established, it should attempt to minimize the possibility of having to repeat earlier treatment if problems later occur. Usually oral surgical procedures are scheduled first, followed by periodontics,

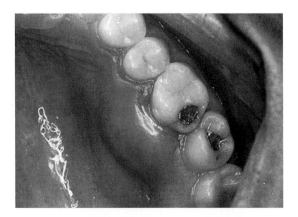

Fig. 3-31. Swelling from an acute periapical abscess. (*Courtesy Dr. P.B. Robinson.*)

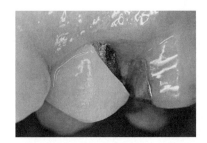

Fig. 3-32. For both appearance and comfort, fractured porcelain often necessitates urgent treatment.

endodontics, orthodontics, fixed prosthodontics, and finally, removable prosthodontics.

Oral Surgery. The treatment plan should allow time for healing and ridge remodeling. Therefore, teeth with a hopeless prognosis, unerupted teeth, and residual roots and root tips should be removed early. All preprosthetic surgical procedures (e.g., ridge contouring) should be undertaken during the early phase of treatment.

Periodontics. Most periodontal procedures should (or will) have been accomplished as part of the stabilization phase of treatment. Any surgery, pocket elimination, mucogingival procedure, guided tissue regeneration, or root resection is performed at this time (see Chapter 5).

Endodontics. Some endodontic treatment may have been accomplished as part of the relief of discomfort and stabilization of conditions. Elective endodontics may be needed to provide adequate space for a cast restoration or to provide retention for a badly damaged or worn tooth.

If a tooth with doubtful pulpal health is to be used as an abutment for an FPD, it should be endodontically treated prophylactically, despite the consideration that periodic recall may be more appropriate treatment if a single restoration is planned.

Orthodontics. Minor orthodontic tooth movement is a common adjunct to fixed prosthodontics. A tooth can be uprighted, rotated, moved laterally, intruded, or extruded to improve its relationship before fixed prosthodontic treatment. Orthodontics should always be considered when a treatment plan is being proposed, especially if tooth loss has been neglected and drifting has occurred.

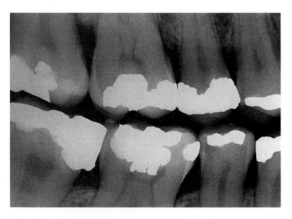

Fig. 3-33. Overhangs and defective restorations impede proper plaque control and should be corrected as part of the stabilization process.

Fixed Prosthodontics. Fixed prosthodontic treatment is initiated only after the preceding modalities have been completed. This will permit modification of the original plan if unforeseen difficulties surface during treatment. For example, a tooth scheduled for endodontic treatment might prove to be untreatable, requiring considerable modification of the restorative treatment plan.

Occlusal Adjustment. Occlusal adjustments are often necessary before the initiation of fixed prosthodontics. Where extensive fixed prosthodontics is to be provided, an accurate and well-tolerated occlusal relationship may be obtainable only if a discrepancy between intercuspal position and centric relation is eliminated first (see Chapter 4). When less extensive treatment is planned, it may be acceptable to conform the fixed prosthesis to the existing occlusion, provided the patient is functioning satisfactorily. However, any supraeruption or drifting should be corrected rather than be allowed to compromise the patient's occlusal scheme.

Anterior Restorations. If both anterior and posterior teeth are to be restored, the anterior teeth are usually done first because they influence the border movements of the mandible and thus the shape of the occlusal surfaces of the posterior teeth (see Chapter 4). If the posterior teeth were restored first, a subsequent change in the lingual contour of the anterior teeth could require considerable adjustment of the posterior restorations.

Posterior Restorations. Restoring opposing posterior segments at the same time is often advantageous. This permits the development of an efficient occlusal scheme through the application of an additive wax technique (see Chapter 18). One side of the mouth should be completed before the other side is treated; restoring all four posterior segments at the same time might lead to considerably more complications for the patient and dentist, including fracture or breaking of provisional restorations, discomfort with bilateral local anesthesia, and difficulties in confirming the accuracy of jaw relationship recordings.

Complex Prosthodontics. Carefully planned treatment sequencing is particularly important when complex prosthodontic treatments involving alteration of the vertical dimension or a combination of fixed and removable prostheses are required. One recommended approach is illustrated in Figure 3-34. Two sets of diagnostic casts are accurately mounted so they can be precisely interchanged on the articulator. One set is prepared and waxed to the intended end point of treatment, with denture teeth

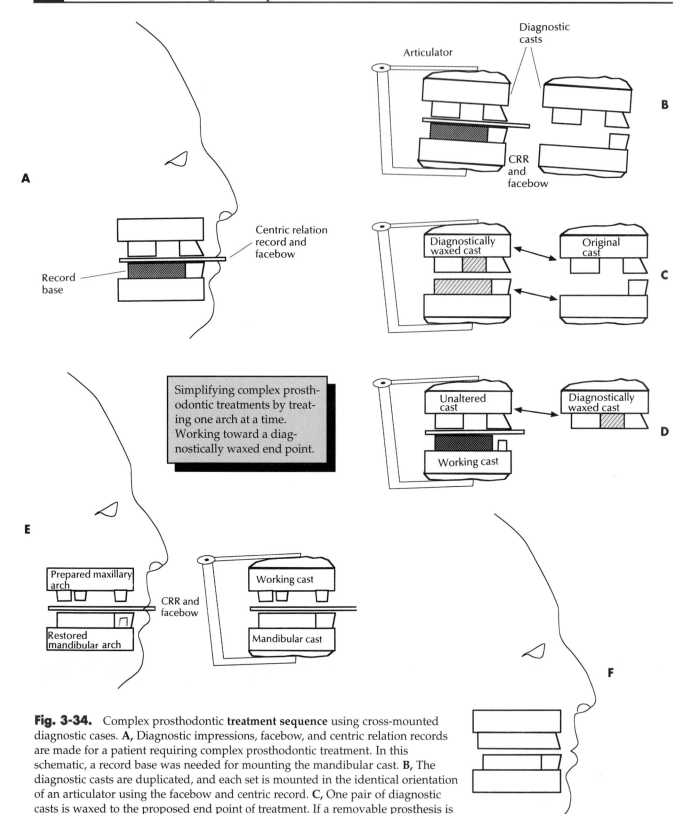

Fig. 3-34. Complex prosthodontic **treatment sequence** using cross-mounted diagnostic cases. **A,** Diagnostic impressions, facebow, and centric relation records are made for a patient requiring complex prosthodontic treatment. In this schematic, a record base was needed for mounting the mandibular cast. **B,** The diagnostic casts are duplicated, and each set is mounted in the identical orientation of an articulator using the facebow and centric record. **C,** One pair of diagnostic casts is waxed to the proposed end point of treatment. If a removable prosthesis is planned, denture teeth are set for this step. The other pair of casts is left unaltered. **D,** One arch is treated at a time. For this patient, the mandibular arch has been prepared for crowns. The working cast is mounted on the articulator with a centric record made against the (unaltered) maxillary teeth. This record is used to mount the working cast against the (unaltered) maxillary cast. Then the maxillary cast is removed and replaced with the cross-mounted diagnostically waxed cast. The mandibular restorations are fabricated against this cast to ensure an optimal occlusal plane. **E,** Once the mandibular arch has been restored, the maxillary teeth are prepared and mounted against a cast of the newly restored mandibular arch. **F,** The completed restoration conforms to the diagnostic waxing.

inserted where removable prostheses are to be used. The waxing is carefully evaluated on the articulator in relation to occlusion and appearance. When anterior teeth are to be replaced, they can be assessed for appearance and phonetics directly in the mouth if they are mounted on a removable record base. Definitive tooth preparation starts in one arch only, preserving the occlusal surfaces of the opposing arch to act as an essential reference for mounting the working cast. The definitive restorations are waxed against the diagnostically waxed cast, establishing optimal occlusion. When one arch has been completed, the opposing cast can be restored, achieving the predicted result.

FOLLOW-UP

A specific program of follow-up care and regular recall is an essential part of the treatment plan. The aim is to monitor dental health, identify the signs of disease early, and initiate prompt corrective measures as necessary (see Chapter 32). Restorations do not last forever, are subject to wear, and may need replacement. Adequate follow-up will help maintain long-term health.

SUMMARY

The basis of logical treatment planning consists of identifying the patient's needs, eliciting his or her expectations and wishes, and comparing these with the available corrective materials and techniques. It also involves evaluating whether a technique has a good prognosis. Then a rational sequence of treatment may be initiated for symptomatic relief, stabilization, definitive therapy, and follow-up care. The extent of treatment is modified throughout and is dictated by the patient's attitude and by the objectives for that patient.

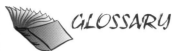

GLOSSARY

abfraction: *n* (1991) the pathologic loss of hard tooth substance caused by biomechanical loading forces. Such loss is thought to be due to flexure and ultimate fatigue of enamel and/or dentin at some location distant from the actual point of loading.

abutment: *n* (1634) *1:* that part of a structure that directly receives thrust or pressure; an anchorage. *2:* a tooth, a portion of a tooth, or that portion of a dental implant that supports and/or retains a prosthesis.

Ante's Law: [Irvin H. Ante, Toronto, Ontario Canada, dentist]: an eponym in fixed partial prosthodontics for the observation that the combined pericemental area of all abutment teeth supporting a fixed partial denture should be equal to or greater in pericemental area than the tooth or teeth to be replaced; as formulated for removable partial prosthodontics, the combined pericemental area of the abutment teeth plus the mucosa area of the denture base should be equal to or greater than the pericemental area of the missing teeth (From Ante IH: The fundamental principles, design, and construction of crown and bridge prosthesis, *Dent Item Int* 50:215-232, 1928.)

artificial crown: a metal, plastic, or ceramic restoration that covers three or more axial surfaces and the occlusal surface or incisal edge of a tooth.

buccolingual relationship: any position of reference relative to the tongue and cheeks.

cantilever: *n* (1667) a projecting beam or member supported on one end.

Study Questions

1. Discuss 12 considerations that affect the design of a fixed partial denture and their general impact on FPD design.
2. Discuss at least four different indications for a removable partial denture as opposed to a fixed partial denture.
3. When would a nonrigid connector be indicated in a fixed partial denture? When would it be contraindicated?
4. If a patient has a multitude of needs involving all clinical disciplines, in what typical sequence would treatment be conducted? Why? How are the various stages of occlusal therapy sequenced? Why?
5. Contrast the replacement of all the maxillary incisors by an FPD with the replacement of all the mandibular incisors by an FPD. How would you treat each situation?
6. Which occlusal forces are of least concern? Why? Which forces/loading should be avoided? Why?
7. How do span length and FPD design influence flexure? When is rigidity essential? Why?
8. List the steps in treating a patient with extensive restorative needs using the cross-mounted cast method of treating complex prosthodontic patients. Explain briefly the importance of treatment sequence.

cantilever fixed partial denture: a fixed partial denture in which the pontic is cantilevered, (i.e., retained and supported only on one end by one or more abutments).

clinical crown: the portion of a tooth that extends from the occlusal table or incisal edge to the free gingival margin.

complete crown: a restoration that covers all the coronal tooth surfaces (mesial, distal, facial, lingual, and occlusal).

complete denture: a removable dental prosthesis that replaces the entire dentition and associated structures of the maxillae or mandible.

connector: *n* in fixed prosthodontics, the portion of a fixed partial denture that unites the retainer(s) and pontics.

1 crown: *n* (12c) *1:* the highest part, as the topmost part of the skull, head or tooth; the summit; that portion of a tooth occlusal to the dentinoenamel junction or an artificial substitute for this. *2:* an artificial replacement that restores missing tooth structure by surrounding part or all of the remaining structure with a material such as cast metal, porcelain, or a combination of materials such as metal and porcelain.

2 crown: *vt* (12c) to place on the head, as to place a crown on a tooth, dental implant, or tooth substitute—usage: implies fabrication of a restoration for a tooth on a natural tooth or dental implant.

crown fracture: micro- or macroscopic cleavage in the coronal portion of a tooth.

crown-root ratio: the physical relationship between the portion of the tooth within alveolar bone compared with the portion not within the alveolar bone, as determined by radiograph.

demineralization: *n* (ca. 1903) *1:* loss of minerals (as salts of calcium) from the body. *2:* in dentistry, decalcification.

extracoronal retainer: that part of a fixed partial denture uniting the abutment to the other elements of a fixed partial denture that surrounds all or part of the prepared crown.

fixed partial denture: a partial denture that is luted or otherwise securely retained to natural teeth, tooth roots, and/or dental implant abutments that furnish the primary support for the prosthesis—usage: with respect to a fixed partial denture retained on dental implants, adjectives may be used to describe the means of attachment, such as *screw retained f.p.d., cement retained f.p.d*—also called *fixed prosthesis.*

fixed partial denture retainer: the part of a fixed partial denture that unites the abutment(s) to the remainder of the restoration.

frenulum: *n pl -la* (1706) a connecting fold of membrane serving to support or retain a part.

high lip line: the greatest height to which the inferior border of the upper lip is capable of being raised by muscle function.

horizontal overlap: the projection of teeth beyond their antagonists in the horizontal plane.

hydroxyapatite ceramic: a composition of calcium and phosphate in physiologic ratios to provide a dense, nonresorbable, and biocompatible ceramic used for dental implants and residual ridge augmentation.

immediate denture: a complete denture or removable partial denture fabricated for placement immediately following the removal of natural teeth.

incisal guidance: *1:* the influence of the contacting surfaces of the mandibular and maxillary anterior teeth on mandibular movements. *2:* the influence of the contacting surfaces of the guide pin and guide table on articulator movements.

indirect retainer: the component of a removable partial denture that assists the direct retainer(s) in preventing displacement of the distal extension denture base by functioning through lever action on the opposite side of the fulcrum line when the denture base moves away from the tissues in pure rotation around the fulcrum line.

indirect retention: the effect achieved by one or more indirect retainers of a removable partial denture that reduces the tendency for a denture base to move in an occlusal direction or rotate about the fulcrum line.

intermediate abutment: a natural tooth located between terminal abutments that supports a fixed or removable prosthesis.

interim denture: see *interim prosthesis.*

interim prosthesis: a fixed or removable prosthesis, designed to enhance esthetics, stabilization, and/or function for a limited period of time, after which it is to be replaced by a definitive prosthesis. Often such prostheses are used to assist in determination of the therapeutic effectiveness of a specific treatment plan or the form and function of the planned definitive prosthesis—*synonym: provisional prosthesis, provisional restoration.*

interproximal contact: the area of a tooth that is in close association, connection, or touch with an adjacent tooth in the same arch.

keyway: *n* an interlock using a matrix and patrix between the units of a fixed partial denture. It may serve two functions: *1)* to hold the pontic in the proper relationship to the edentulous ridge and the opposing teeth during occlusal adjustment on the working cast (during application of any veneering material) and *2)* to reinforce the connector after soldering.

low lip line: *1:* the lowest position of the inferior border of the upper lip when it is at rest. *2:* the lowest position of the superior border of the lower lip during smiling or voluntary retraction.

masticatory force: the force applied by the muscles of mastication during chewing.

mesial drift: movement of teeth toward the midline.

nonrigid connector: any connector that permits limited movement between otherwise independent members of a fixed partial denture.

occlusal analysis: an examination of the occlusion in which the interocclusal relations of mounted casts are evaluated.

occlusal device: any removable artificial occlusal surface used for diagnosis or therapy affecting the relationship of the mandible to the maxillae. It may be used for occlusal stabilization, for treatment of temporomandibular disorders, or to prevent wear of the dentition.

occlusal equilibration: the modification of the occlusal form of the teeth with the intent of equalizing occlusal stress, producing simultaneous occlusal contacts, or harmonizing cuspal relations.

occlusal stability: the equalization of contacts that prevents tooth movement after closure.

patrix: *n pl* **patrices:** *1:* a pattern or die used in type founding to form a matrix. *2:* the extension of a dental attachment system that fits into the matrix.

PFM: acronym for *porcelain fused to metal.*

plunger cusp: a cusp that tends to force food interproximally.

residual bone: that component of maxillary or mandibular bone, once used to support the roots of the teeth, that remain after the teeth are lost.

residual ridge: the portion of the residual bone and its soft tissue covering that remains after the removal of teeth.

span length: the length of a beam between two supports.

splinting: *v 1:* in dentistry, the joining of two or more teeth into a rigid unit by means of fixed or removable restorations or devices. *2:* in physiology, prolonged muscle spasms that inhibit or prevent movement.

stress breaker: see *stress director.*

stress director: a device or system that relieves specific dental structures of part or all of the occlusal forces and redirects those forces to other bearing structures or regions.

supraeruption: *n* movement of a tooth or teeth above the normal occlusal plane.

supraocclusion: *n* malocclusion in which the occluding surfaces of teeth extend beyond the normal occlusal plane—also called *overeruption.*

sympathetic nervous system: the part of the autonomic nervous system that responds to dangerous or threatening situations by preparing a person physiologically for "fight or flight."

tooth supported: a term used to describe a prosthesis or part of a prosthesis that depends entirely on natural teeth for support.

transitional prosthesis: see *interim prosthesis.*

up-right *adj* the movement of a tooth into an erect or normal position.

working articulation the occlusal contacts of teeth on the side toward which the mandible is moved.

REFERENCES

1. Palomo F, Peden J: Periodontal considerations of restorative procedures, *J Prosthet Dent* 36:387, 1976.
2. Jones RM et al: A comparison of the physical properties of four prosthetic veneering materials, *J Prosthet Dent* 61:38, 1989.
3. Vojvodic D et al: The bond strength of polymers and metal surfaces using the 'silicoater' technique, *J Oral Rehabil* 22:493, 1995.
4. Rothfuss LG et al: Resin to metal bond strengths using two commercial systems, *J Prosthet Dent* 79:270, 1998.
5. Karmaker AC et al: Continuous fiber reinforced composite materials as alternatives for metal alloys used for dental appliances, *J Biomater Appl* 11:318, 1997.
6. Rosenthal L et al: A new system for posterior restorations: a combination of ceramic optimized polymer and fiber-reinforced composite, *Pract Periodont Aesthet Dent* 9(suppl 5):6, 1997.
7. Zanghellini G: Fiber-reinforced framework and Ceromer restorations: a technical review, *Signature* 4(1):1, 1997.
8. Claus H: Vita In-Ceram, a new procedure for preparation of oxide-ceramic crown and bridge framework, *Quintessenz Zahntech* 16:35, 1990.
9. Magne P, Belser U: Esthetic improvements and in vitro testing of In-Ceram Alumina and Spinell ceramic, *Int J Prosthodont* 10:459, 1997.
10. Denry IL: Recent advances in ceramics for dentistry, *Crit Rev Oral Biol Med* 7:134, 1996.
11. Sorensen JA et al: IPS Empress crown system: three-year clinical trial results, *J Calif Dent Assoc* 26:130, 1998.
12. Denry IL et al: Effect of cubic leucite stabilization on the flexural strength of feldspathic dental porcelain, *J Dent Res* 75:1928, 1996.
13. Adell R et al: A 15-year study of osseointegrated implants in the treatment of the edentulous jaw, *Int J Oral Surg* 10:387, 1981.
14. Saunders TR et al: The maxillary complete denture opposing the mandibular bilateral distal-extension partial denture: treatment considerations, *J Prosthet Dent* 41:124, 1979.
15. Brewer AA, Morrow RM: *Overdentures,* ed 2, St Louis, 1980, Mosby.
16. Cheung GS et al: A clinical evaluation of conventional bridgework, *J Oral Rehabil* 17:131, 1990.
17. Glickman I et al: Photoelastic analysis of internal stresses in the periodontium created by occlusal forces, *J Periodontol* 41:30, 1970.
18. Wright KWJ, Yettram AL: Reactive force distributions for teeth when loaded singly and when

used as fixed partial denture abutments, *J Prosthet Dent* 42:411, 1979.

19. Yang HS et al: Stress analysis of a cantilevered fixed partial denture with normal and reduced bone support, *J Prosthet Dent* 76:424, 1996.

20. Briggs P et al: The single unit, single retainer, cantilever resin-bonded bridge, *Br Dent J* 181:373, 1996.

21. Christensen GJ: When to use fillers, build-ups or posts and cores, *J Am Dent Assoc* 127:1397, 1996.

22. Miller TE: Orthodontic therapy for the restorative patient. I. The biomechanic aspects, *J Prosthet Dent* 61:268, 1989.

23. Holmgren K et al: The effects of an occlusal splint on the electromyographic activities of the temporal and masseter muscles during maximal clenching in patients with a habit of nocturnal bruxism and signs and symptoms of craniomandibular disorders, *J Oral Rehabil* 17:447, 1990.

24. Ante IH: The fundamental principles of abutments, *Mich State Dent Soc Bull* 8:14, July 1926.

25. Dykema RW et al: *Johnston's modern practice in fixed prosthodontics*, ed 4, Philadelphia, 1986, WB Saunders, p 4.

26. Tylman SD, Malone WFP: *Tylman's theory and practice of fixed prosthodontics*, ed 7, St Louis, 1978, Mosby, p 15.

27. Shillingburg HT et al: *Fundamentals of fixed prosthodontics*, ed 2, Chicago, 1981, Quintessence Publishing, p 20.

28. Jepsen A: Root surface measurement and a method for x-ray determination of root surface area, *Acta Odontol Scand* 21:35, 1963.

29. Nyman S, Ericsson I: The capacity of reduced periodontal tissues to support fixed bridgework, *J Clin Periodontol* 9:409, 1982.

30. Freilich MA et al: Fixed partial dentures supported by periodontally compromised teeth, *J Prosthet Dent* 65:607, 1991.

31. Decock V et al: 18-year longitudinal study of cantilevered fixed restorations, *Inter J Prosthodont* 9:331, 1996.

32. Penny RE, Kraal JH: Crown-to-root ratio: its significance in restorative dentistry, *J Prosthet Dent* 42:34, 1979.

33. Nyman S et al: The role of occlusion for the stability of fixed bridges in patients with reduced periodontal tissue support, *J Clin Periodontol* 2:53, 1975.

34. Laurell L et al: Long-term prognosis of extensive polyunit cantilevered fixed partial dentures, *J Prosthet Dent* 66:545, 1991.

35. Smyd ES: Dental engineering, *J Dent Res* 27:649, 1948.

36. Dykema RW: Fixed partial prosthodontics, *J Tenn Dent Assoc* 42:309, 1962.

37. Olin PS et al: Improved pontic/tissue relationships using porous coralline hydroxyapatite block, *J Prosthet Dent* 66:234, 1991.

PRINCIPLES OF OCCLUSION

KEY TERMS

anterior guidance	interference
articular disk	malocclusion
attrition	mandibular movement
Bennett movement	mandibular sideshift
border movement	mutual protection
bruxism	nonworking side
capsule	occlusal device
clenching	parafunction
determinants of occlusion	pathogenic occlusion
disocclusion	Posselt
eccentric	speaking space
excursion	temporomandibular joint
group function	terminal hinge axis
guidance	translation
horizontal overlap	vertical overlap
intercondylar distance	working side

Most restorative procedures affect the shape of the occlusal surfaces. Proper dental care ensures that functional contact relationships are restored in harmony with both dynamic and static conditions. Maxillary and mandibular teeth should contact to allow optimum function, minimal trauma to the supporting structures, and an even load distribution throughout the dentition. Positional stability of the teeth is critical if arch integrity and proper function are to be maintained over time.

As an aid to the diagnosis of occlusal dysfunction, it is helpful to evaluate the condition of specific anatomic features and functional aspects of a patient's occlusion with reference to a concept of "optimum" or "ideal" occlusion. Deviation from this concept can then be measured objectively and may prove to be a useful guide during treatment planning and active treatment phases.

Over time, many concepts of "ideal" occlusion have been proposed. In the literature, the concept of what is "ideal," "acceptable," and "harmful" continues to evolve.

This chapter reviews the anatomic structures important to the study of occlusion and includes a discussion of **mandibular movement.** The concepts of ideal versus pathologic occlusion are introduced, as is the history of occlusal theory. The chapter concludes with guidelines for the initial phase of occlusal treatment.

◼ ANATOMY

TEMPOROMANDIBULAR JOINTS

The major components of the **temporomandibular joints** are the cranial base, the mandible, and the muscles of mastication with their innervation and vascular supply. Each joint can be described as ginglymoarthrodial, meaning that it is capable of both a hinging and a gliding articulation. An **articular disk** separates the mandibular fossa and articular tubercle of the temporal bone from the condylar process of the mandible.

The articulating surfaces of the condylar processes and fossae are covered with avascular fibrous tissue (in contrast to most other joints, which have hyaline cartilage). The articular disk consists of dense connective tissue; it also is avascular and devoid of nerves in the area where articulation normally occurs. Posteriorly it is attached to loose vascularized connective tissue, the retrodiscal pad or bilaminar zone*, which connects to the posterior wall of the articular **capsule** surrounding the joint (Fig. 4-1). Medially and laterally the disk is attached firmly to the poles of the condylar process. Anteriorly it fuses with the capsule and with the superior lateral pterygoid muscle. Superior and inferior to the articular disk are two spaces, the superior and inferior synovial cavities. These are bordered peripherally by the capsule and the synovial membranes and are filled with synovial fluid. Because of its firm attachment to the poles of each condylar process, the disk follows condylar movement during both hinging and translation, which is made possible by the loose attachment of the posterior connective tissues.

---

*Called *bilaminar* because it consists of two layers: an elastic superior layer and a collagenous inelastic inferior layer.

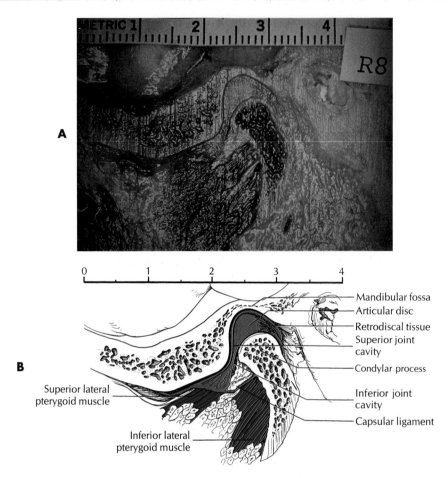

Fig. 4-1. Temporomandibular joint (lateral section). The mandible is open.
(A courtesy Dr. K.A. Laurell.)

Mandibular Ligaments

TABLE **4-1**

	Origin	Insertion	Function
Temporomandibular			
Superficial	Outer surface of articular eminence	Posterior aspect of neck of condylar process	Limits mandibular rotation on opening
Medial	Crest of articular eminence	Lateral aspect of neck of condylar process	Limits posterior movement
Sphenomandibular	Spine of sphenoid	Inferior to lingula	Accessory to temporomandibular articulation; influence on mandibular movement disputed
Stylomandibular	Styloid process	Mandibular angle and fascia of medial pterygoid muscle	Limits extreme protrusion of the mandible; influence on mandibular movement disputed

LIGAMENTS

The body of the mandible is attached to the base of the skull by muscles and also by three paired ligaments (Table 4-1): the temporomandibular (also called the lateral), the sphenomandibular, and the stylomandibular. Ligaments cannot be stretched significantly, so they limit the movement of joints. The temporomandibular ligaments limit the amount of rotation of the mandible and protect the structures of the joint, limiting **border movements**.[1] The spheno-mandibular and stylomandibular ligaments (Fig. 4-2) limit separation between the condylar process and the disk; the stylomandibular ligaments also limit protrusive movement of the mandible.

MUSCULATURE

Several muscles are responsible for mandibular movements. These can be grouped into the muscles of mastication and the suprahyoid muscles (Fig. 4-3). The former include the temporal, the masseter,

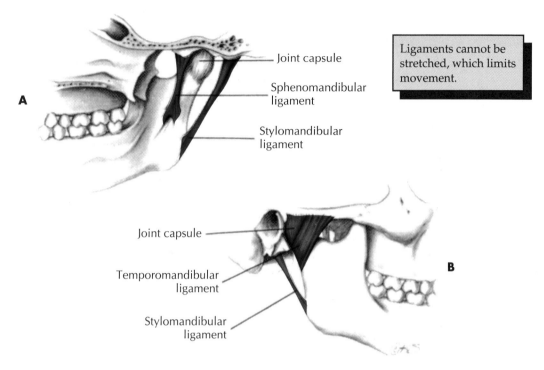

A

Joint capsule

Sphenomandibular ligament

Stylomandibular ligament

Ligaments cannot be stretched, which limits movement.

Joint capsule

Temporomandibular ligament

Stylomandibular ligament

B

Fig. 4-2. Ligaments of the temporomandibular joint. **A,** Mesial view. **B,** Lateral view.

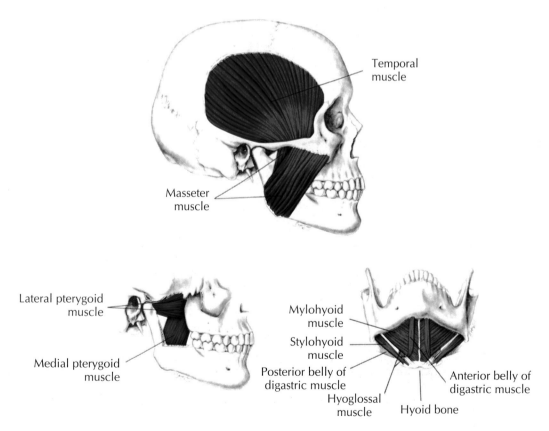

Temporal muscle

Masseter muscle

Lateral pterygoid muscle

Medial pterygoid muscle

Mylohyoid muscle

Stylohyoid muscle

Posterior belly of digastric muscle

Hyoglossal muscle

Anterior belly of digastric muscle

Hyoid bone

Fig. 4-3. The muscles of mastication and the suprahyoids.

and the medial and lateral pterygoids; the latter are the geniohyoid, the mylohyoid, and the digastrics. Their respective origins, insertions, and innervation and vascular supply are summarized in Table 4-2.

Muscular Function. The functions of the mandibular muscles are well-coordinated, complex events.

The three paired muscles of mastication provide elevation and lateral movement of the mandible.

Muscles of Mastication

TABLE **4-2**

	Origin	Insertion	Innervation	Vascular Supply	Function
Temporal	Lateral surface of skull	Coronoid process and anterior border of ramus	Temporal nerve (branch of mandibular)	Middle and deep temporal arteries (branches of superficial temporal and maxillary)	Elevates and retracts jaw, assists in rotation, active in clenching
Masseter	Zygomatic arch	Angle of mandible	Masseteric nerve (division of trigeminal)	Masseteric artery (branch of maxillary)	Elevates and protracts jaw, assists in lateral movement, active in clenching
Medial pterygoid	Pterygoid fossa and medial surface of lateral pterygoid plate	Medial surface of angle of mandible	Medial pterygoid nerve (division of trigeminal)	Branch of maxillary artery	Elevates jaw, causes lateral movement and protrusion
Superior lateral pterygoid	Infratemporal surface of greater wing of sphenoid	Articular capsule and disc, neck of condyle	Branch of masseteric or buccal nerve	Branch of maxillary artery	Positions disc in closing
Inferior lateral pterygoid	Lateral surface of lateral pterygoid plate	Neck of condyle	Branch of masseteric or buccal nerve	Branch of maxillary artery	Protrudes and depresses jaw, causes lateral movement
Mylohyoid	Inner surface of mandible	Hyoid and mylohyoid raphe	Branches of mylohyoid nerve (division of trigeminal)	Submental artery	Elevates and stabilizes hyoid
Geniohyoid	Genial tubercle	Hyoid	First cervical via hypoglossal nerve	Branch of lingual artery	Elevates and draws hyoid forward
Anterior belly of digastric	Tendon linked to hyoid by fascia	Digastric fossa (lower border of mandible)	Branch of mylohyoid nerve (division of trigeminal)	Branch of facial artery	Elevates hyoid, depresses jaw

These are the temporals, the masseters, and the medial pterygoids. The lateral pterygoid muscles, each with two bellies (which some suggest should be considered as two separate muscles), function horizontally during opening and closing; the inferior belly (or inferior lateral pterygoid) is active during protrusion, depression, and lateral movement; the superior belly (or superior lateral pterygoid) is active during closure. The last is thought to assist in maintaining the integrity of the condyle-disk assembly by pulling the condylar process firmly against the disk, because the superior belly has been shown to attach to the disk and the neck of the condyle.

The muscles of the suprahyoid group have a dual function. They can elevate the hyoid bone or depress the mandible. The movement that results when they contract depends on the state of contraction of the other muscles of the neck and jaw region. When the muscles of mastication are in a state of contraction, the suprahyoids will elevate the hyoid bone. However, if the infrahyoid muscles (which anchor the hyoid bone to the sternum and clavicle) are contracted, the suprahyoids will depress and retract the mandible. The geniohyoid and mylohyoid initiate the opening movements, and the anterior belly of the digastric completes mandibular depression. Although the stylohyoid muscle (which also belongs to the suprahyoid group) may contribute indirectly to mandibular movement through fixation of the hyoid bone, it does not play a significant role in mandibular movement.

DENTITION

The relative positions of the maxillary and mandibular teeth influence mandibular movement. Many "ideal" occlusions have been described.[2] In most of these, the maxillary and mandibular teeth contact simultaneously when the condylar processes are fully seated in the mandibular fossae and the teeth

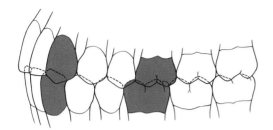

Fig. 4-4. The Angle Class I occlusal relationship.

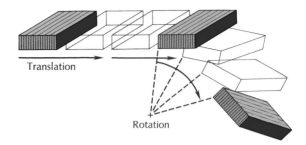

Fig. 4-5. Three-dimensional movement of a body can be defined by a combination of translation (all points within the body having identical movement) and rotation (all points turning around an axis).

do not interfere with harmonious movement of the mandible during function. In the fully bilateral seated position of the condyle-disk assemblies, the maxillary and mandibular teeth ideally exhibit maximum intercuspation. This means that the maxillary lingual and mandibular buccal cusps of the posterior teeth are in evenly distributed and stable contact with the opposing occlusal fossae. These centric cusps can then act as stops for vertical closure without excessively loading any one tooth.

If the mesiobuccal cusp of the maxillary first molar is aligned with the buccal groove of the mandibular first molar, an Angle Class I orthodontic relationship (Fig. 4-4) exists; this is considered normal (see glossary). In such a relationship, the anterior teeth overlap both horizontally and vertically. Orthodontic textbooks[3] have traditionally described an arbitrary 2 mm for horizontal and vertical overlap as being ideal. For most patients, however, greater vertical overlap of the anterior teeth is desirable to prevent undesirable posterior tooth contact as a result of flexing of the mandible during mastication. Empirically, dentitions with greater vertical overlap of the anterior teeth appear to have a better long-term prognosis in comparison to dentitions with minimal vertical overlap.

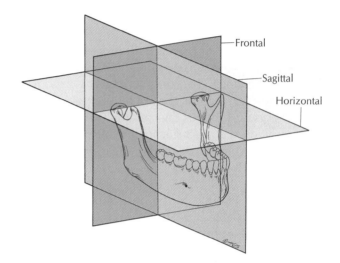

Fig. 4-6. Reference planes.

CENTRIC RELATION

Centric relation is considered the optimal mandibular position in which the bilateral condyle-disk assemblies are fully seated in their corresponding glenoid fossae, with the condyles positioned along the anterior slope of the articular eminence. Centric relation is considered a reliable and reproducible reference position. If the intercuspal position coincides with the centric relation position, restorative treatment is often straightforward. When the intercuspal position does not coincide with centric relation, it is necessary to determine whether corrective occlusal therapy is needed before restorative treatment.

MANDIBULAR MOVEMENT

As for any other movement in space, complex three-dimensional mandibular movement can be broken down into two basic components: translation, when all points within a body have identical motion, and rotation, when the body is turning about an axis (Fig. 4-5). Every possible three-dimensional movement can be described in terms of these two components. In addition, it is easier to understand mandibular movement when the components are described as projections in three perpendicular planes: sagittal, horizontal, and frontal (Fig. 4-6).

REFERENCE PLANES

Sagittal Plane (Fig. 4-7). In the sagittal plane, the mandible is capable of a purely rotational movement as well as translation. Rotation occurs around the **terminal hinge axis,** an imaginary horizontal line through the rotational centers of the left and right condylar processes. The rotational movement is limited to about 12 mm of incisor separation before the temporomandibular ligaments and

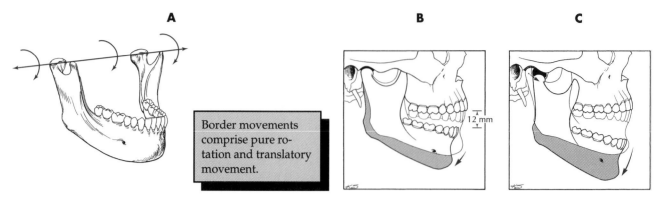

A   **B**   **C**

Border movements comprise pure rotation and translatory movement.

12 mm

Fig. 4-7. **A,** Rotation of the mandible in a sagittal plane can be made around the terminal hinge axis. **B,** After about 12 mm of incisal opening, the mandible is forced to translate. **C,** Maximum opening; the condyles have translated forward.

structures anterior to the mastoid process force the mandible to translate. The initial rotation or hinging motion is between the condyle and the articular disk. During translation, the lateral pterygoid muscle contracts and moves the condyle-disk assembly forward along the posterior incline of the tubercle. Condylar movement is similar during protrusive mandibular movement.

Horizontal Plane. In the horizontal plane, the mandible is capable of rotation around several vertical axes. For example, lateral movement consists of rotation around an axis situated in the working (laterotrusive) condylar process (Fig. 4-8) with relatively little concurrent translation. A slight lateral translation—known as **Bennett movement,**[4] **mandibular sideshift,** or *laterotrusion* (Fig. 4-9)—is frequently present. This may be slightly forward or slightly backward (lateroprotrusion or lateroretrusion). The orbiting (nonworking) condyle travels forward and medially as limited by the medial aspect of the mandibular fossa and the temporomandibular ligament. Finally, the mandible can make a straight protrusive movement (Fig. 4-10).

Frontal Plane. When observing a lateral movement in the frontal plane, the mediotrusive (or nonworking) condyle moves down and medially while the laterotrusive (or working) condyle rotates around the sagittal axis perpendicular to this plane (Fig. 4-11). Again, as determined by the anatomy of the medial wall of the mandibular fossa on the mediotrusive side, transtrusion may be observed: as determined by the anatomy of the mandibular fossa on the laterotrusive side, this may be lateral and upward or lateral and downward (laterosurtrusion and laterodetrusion). A straight protrusive movement observed in the frontal plane, with both condylar processes moving downward as they

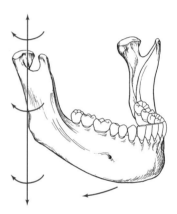

Fig. 4-8. Rotation in the horizontal plane occurs during lateral movement of the mandible. (The vertical axis is situated in the condylar process.) Normally there is relatively little translation (sideshift).

slide along the tubercular eminences, is shown in Figure 4-12.

BORDER MOVEMENTS

Mandibular movements are limited by the temporomandibular joints and ligaments, the neuromuscular system, and the teeth. Posselt[5] was the first to describe the extremes of mandibular movement, which he called *border movements* (Fig. 4-13). His classic work is well worth reviewing as one attempts to understand how the determinants control the extent to which movement can occur.

Posselt used a three-dimensional representation of the extreme movements the mandible is capable of (Fig. 4-13, *B*). All possible mandibular movements occur within its boundaries. At the top of both illustrations, a horizontal tracing represents the protrusive movement of the incisal edge of the mandibular incisors.

Starting at the intercuspal positions in the protrusive pathway, the lower incisors are initially guided

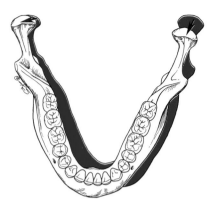

Fig. 4-9. Right lateral mandibular movement in the horizontal plane.

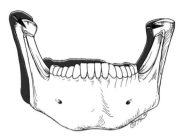

Fig. 4-11. Lateral movement in the frontal plane.

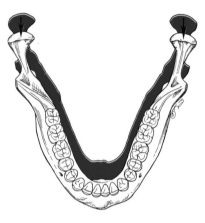

Fig. 4-10. Protrusive mandibular movement in the horizontal plane.

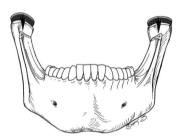

Fig. 4-12. Protrusive movement in the frontal plane.

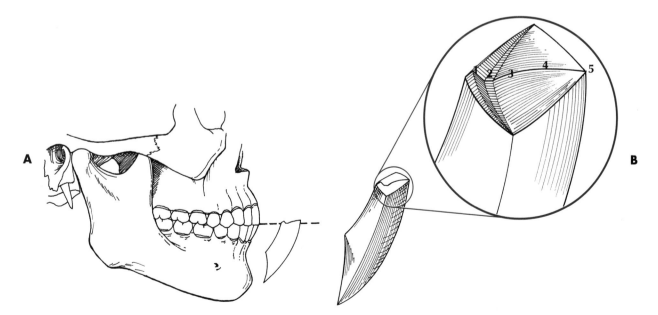

Fig. 4-13. **A,** Mandibular border movement in the sagittal plane. **B,** Posselt's three-dimensional representation of the total envelope of mandibular movement. *1,* Mandibular incisors track along the lingual concavity of the maxillary anterior teeth. *2,* Edge-to-edge position. *3,* Incisors move superiorly until posterior tooth contact recurs. *4,* Protrusive path. *5,* Most protrusive mandibular position.

Impact of Selected Variables on Occlusal Form of Restorations   TABLE 4-3

POSTERIOR DETERMINANTS	VARIATION	IMPACT ON RESTORATION
Inclination of articular eminence	Steeper	Posterior cusps *may* be taller
	Flatter	Posterior cusps *must* be shorter
Medial wall of glenoid fossa	Allows more lateral translation	Posterior cusps *must* be shorter
	Allows minimal lateral translation	Posterior cusps *may* be taller
Intercondylar distance	Greater	Smaller angle between laterotrusive and mediotrusive movement
	Lesser	Increased angle between laterotrusive and mediotrusive movement
ANTERIOR DETERMINANTS		
Horizontal overlap of anterior teeth	Increased	Posterior cusps *must* be shorter
	Reduced	Posterior cusps *may* be taller
Vertical overlap of anterior teeth	Increased	Posterior cusps *may* be taller
	Reduced	Posterior cusps *must* be shorter
OTHER		
Occlusal plane	More parallel to condylar guidance	Posterior cusps *must* be shorter
	Less parallel to condylar guidance	Posterior cusps *may* be longer
Curve of Spee	More convex (shorter radius)	The most posterior cusps *must* be shorter
	Less convex (larger radius)	The most posterior cusps *may* be longer

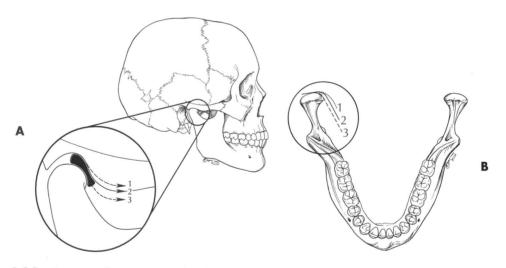

Fig. 4-14. Posterior **determinants of occlusion. A,** Angle of the articular eminence (condylar guidance angle). *1,* Flat; *2,* average; *3,* steep. **B,** Anatomy of the medial walls of the mandibular fossae. *1,* Greater than average; *2,* average; *3,* minimal sideshift.

by the lingual concavity of the maxillary anterior teeth. This leads to gradual loss of posterior tooth contact as the incisors reach the edge-to-edge position. This is represented in Posselt's diagram by the initial downward slope. As the mandible moves farther protrusively, the incisors slide over a horizontal trajectory representing the edge-to-edge position (the flat portion in the diagram), after which the lower incisors move upward until new posterior tooth contact occurs. Further protrusive movement of the mandible typically takes place without significant tooth contact.

The border farthest to the right of **Posselt's** solid (see Fig. 4-13, *B*) represents the most protruded opening and closing stroke. The maximal open position of the mandible is represented by the lowest point in the diagram. The left border of the diagram represents the most retruded closing stroke. This movement occurs in two phases: The lower portion consists of a combined rotation and translation, until the condylar processes return to the fossae. The second portion of the most retruded closing stroke is represented by the top portion of the border that is farthest to the left in Posselt's diagram. It is strictly rotational.

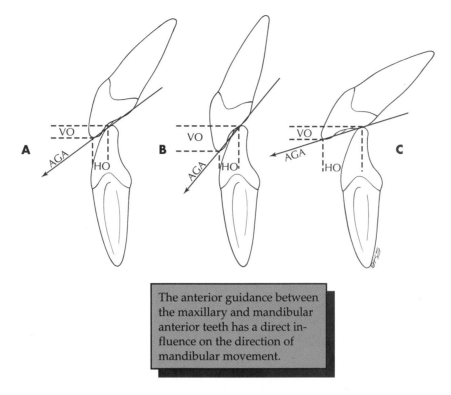

The anterior guidance between the maxillary and mandibular anterior teeth has a direct influence on the direction of mandibular movement.

Fig. 4-15. Anterior determinants of occlusion. Different incisor relationships with differing horizontal and vertical overlaps (*HO* and *VO*) produce different anterior guidance angles (*AGA*). **A,** Class I. **B,** Class II, Division 2 (increased VO; steep AGA). **C,** Class II, Division 1 (increased HO; flat AGA).

Posterior and Anterior Determinants (Table 4-3). The characteristics of mandibular movement are established posteriorly by the morphology of the temporomandibular joints and anteriorly by the relationship of the anterior teeth.

The *posterior determinants* (Fig. 4-14)—shape of the articular eminences, anatomy of the medial walls of the mandibular fossae, configuration of the mandibular condylar processes—cannot be controlled, nor is it possible to influence the neuromuscular responses of the patient, unless it is done by indirect means (e.g., through changes in the configuration of the contacting teeth or by the provision of an occlusal appliance). If a patient has steeply sloped eminences, there will be a large downward component of condylar movement during lateral and protrusive **excursions.** Similarly, the anatomy of the medial wall of each fossa normally will allow the condyle to move slightly medially as it travels forward (mandibular sideshift, or transtrusion). The sideshift will become greater as the extent of medial movement increases. However, the anatomy of the joint dictates the actual path and timing of condylar movement. Movement of the laterotrusive or working condylar process is influenced predominantly by the anatomy of the lateral wall of the mandibular fossa. The amount of the sideshift is, of course, a function of the mediotrusive or nonworking

condyle; on the **working side**, however, it is the anatomy of the lateral aspect of the fossa that guides the working condyle straight out or upward and downward. The amount of sideshift does not appear to increase as the result of a loss of occlusion.[6]

The *anterior determinants* (Fig. 4-15) are the vertical and **horizontal overlaps** and the maxillary lingual concavities of the anterior teeth. These can be altered by restorative and orthodontic treatment. A greater vertical overlap causes the direction of mandibular opening to be more vertical during the early phase of protrusive movement and creates a more vertical pathway at the end of the chewing stroke. Increased horizontal overlap allows a more horizontal jaw movement.

Although the posterior and anterior determinants combine to affect mandibular movement, no correlation has been established[7]; that is, patients with steep **anterior guidance** angles do not necessarily have a steep posterior disclusion, and vice versa.

FUNCTIONAL MOVEMENTS

Most functional movement of the mandible (as occurs during mastication and speech) takes place inside the physiologic limits established by the teeth, the temporomandibular joints, and the muscles and ligaments of mastication; therefore, these movements are rarely coincident with border movements.

Chewing. When incising food, adults open their mouth a comfortable distance and move the mandible forward until they incise, with the anterior teeth meeting approximately edge to edge. The food bolus is then transported to the center of the mouth as the mandible returns to its starting position, with the incisal edges of the mandibular anterior teeth tracking along the lingual concavities of the maxillary anterior teeth (Fig. 4-16). The mouth then opens slightly, the tongue pushes the food onto the occlusal table, and after moving sideways, the mandible closes into the food until the guiding teeth (typically the canines) contact.[8] The cycle is completed as the mandible returns to its starting position.[9] This pattern repeats itself until the food bolus has been reduced to particles that are small enough to be swallowed, at which point the process can start over. The direction of the mandibular path of closure is influenced by the inclination of the occlusal plane with the teeth apart and by the occlusal guidance as the jaw approaches intercuspal position.[10]

The chewing pattern observed in children differs from that found in adults. Until about age 10, children begin the chewing stroke with a lateral movement. After the age of 10, they start to chew increasingly like adults, with a more vertical stroke[11] (Fig. 4-17). Stimuli from the pressoreceptors play an important role in the development of functional chewing cycles.[12]

Mastication is a learned process. At birth no occlusal plane exists, and only after the first teeth have erupted far enough to contact each other is a message sent from the receptors to the cerebral cortex, which controls the stimuli to the masticatory musculature. Stimuli from the tongue and cheeks, and perhaps from the musculature itself and from the periodontium, may influence this feedback pattern.

Speaking. The teeth, tongue, lips, floor of the mouth, and soft palate form the resonance chamber that affects pronunciation. During speech, the teeth are generally not in contact, although the anterior teeth may come very close together during "C," "CH," "S," and "Z" sounds, forming the "**speaking space.**"[13] When pronouncing the fricative "F," the inner vermilion border of the lower lip traps air against the incisal edges of the maxillary incisors. Phonetics is a useful diagnostic guide for correcting vertical dimension and tooth position during fixed and removable prosthodontic treatment.[14-17]

PARAFUNCTIONAL MOVEMENTS

Parafunctional movements of the mandible may be described as sustained activities that occur beyond the normal functions of mastication, swallowing, and speech. There are many forms of parafunctional activities, including **bruxism**, **clenching**, nail biting, and pencil chewing, among others. Typically, **parafunction** is manifested by long periods of increased muscle contraction and hyperactivity. Concurrently, excessive occlusal pressure and prolonged tooth contact occur, which is inconsistent with the normal chewing cycle. Over a protracted period this can result in excessive wear, widening of the periodontal ligament (PDL), and mobility, migration, or fracture of the teeth. Muscle dysfunction such as myospasms,

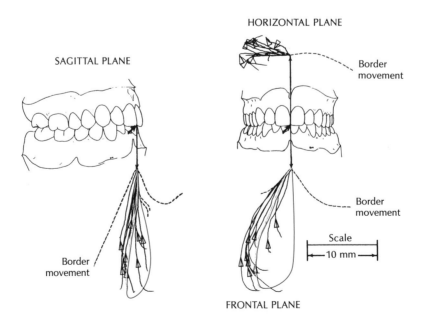

Fig. 4-16. Comparison of border and chewing movements for soft food at the central incisor. Sagittal, frontal, and horizontal views in an orthographic projection.
(*From Gibbs CH et al: J Prosthet Dent 46:308, 1981.*)

myositis, myalgia, and referred pain (headaches) from trigger point tenderness may also occur. The degree of symptoms varies considerably among individuals. The two most common forms of parafunctional activities are bruxism and clenching. Increased radiographic bone density is often seen in patients with a history of sustained parafunctional activity.

Bruxism. Sustained grinding, rubbing together, or gnashing of the teeth with greater-than-normal chewing force is known as *bruxism* (Fig. 4-18). This activity may be diurnal, nocturnal, or both. Although bruxism is initiated on a subconscious level, nocturnal bruxism is potentially more harmful because the patient is not aware of it while sleeping. Therefore, it can be difficult to detect, but it should be suspected in any patient exhibiting abnormal tooth wear or pain. The prevalence of bruxism is about 10% and is less common with age.[18] The etiology of bruxism is often unclear. Some theories relate bruxism to **malocclusion,** neuromuscular disturbances, responses to emotional distress, or a combination of these factors.[19] A study on cohort twins has demonstrated substantial genetic effects,[20] the condition has been related to sleep disturbance,[21] and the symptoms of bruxism are three times more common in smokers.[22] Altered mastication has been observed in subjects who brux[23,24] and may be due to an attempt to avoid premature occlusal contacts (occlusal interferences). There may also be a neuromuscular attempt to "rub out" an interfering cusp. The fulcrum effect of rubbing on posterior interferences will create a protrusive or laterotrusive movement that can cause overloading of the anterior teeth, with resultant excessive anterior wear. It is common for wear on anterior teeth to progress from initial faceting on the canines to the central and lateral incisors. Once vertical overlap diminishes as the result of wear, posterior wear facets are commonly observed. However, the chewing patterns of normal subjects can be quite varied, and the relationship, if any, between altered mastication and occlusal dysfunction is not clear.[25]

The causes of bruxism are difficult to determine. One theory[26] states that bruxism is performed on a subconscious reflex-controlled level and is related to emotional responses and occlusal interferences. In certain malocclusions, the neuromuscular system exerts fine control during chewing to avoid particular occlusal interferences. As the degree of muscle activity necessary to avoid the interferences becomes greater, an increase in muscle tone may

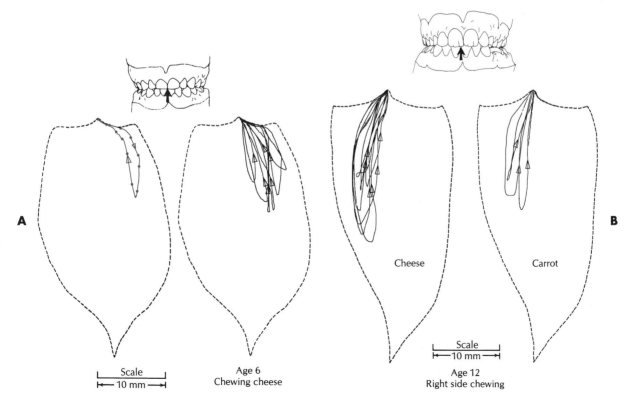

Fig. 4-17. Frontal views of chewing on the left side. The dashed lines are border movements. **A,** Chewing in a young person, characterized by a wide lateral movement on opening and decreased lateral movement on closing. **B,** In an older child, the chewing pattern resembles that of an adult. *(From Wickwire NA et al: Angle Orthod 51:48, 1981.)*

result, with subsequent pain in the hyperactive musculature, which in turn can lead to restricted movement. The relationship, if any, between bruxism and temporomandibular disorders is still unclear.[27]

Patients who brux can exert considerable forces on their teeth, and much of this may have a lateral component. Posterior teeth do not tolerate lateral forces as well as vertical forces in their long axes. Buccolingual forces, in particular, appear to cause rapid widening of the periodontal ligament space and increased mobility.

Clenching. *Clenching* is defined as forceful clamping together of the jaws in a static relationship. The pressure thus created can be maintained over a considerable time with short periods of re-laxation in between. The etiology can be associated with stress, anger, physical exertion, or intense concentration on a given task, rather than an occlusal disorder. As opposed to bruxism, clenching does not necessarily result in damage to the teeth because the concentration of pressure is directed more or less through the long axes of the posterior teeth without the involvement of detrimental lateral forces. Abfractions—cervical defects at the CEJ—may result from sustained clenching.[28,29] Also, the increased load may result in damage to the periodontium, temporomandibular joints, and muscles of mastication. Typically, the elevators will become overdeveloped. A progression of muscle splinting, myospasm, and myositis may occur, causing the patient to seek treatment. As with bruxism, clenching can be difficult to diagnose and difficult if not impossible for the patient to voluntarily control.

HISTORY OF OCCLUSAL STUDIES

Historically, the study of occlusion has undergone an evolution of concepts. These can be broadly categorized as bilaterally balanced,[30] unilaterally balanced, and mutually protected. Current emphasis in teaching fixed prosthodontics and restorative dentistry has been on the concept of **mutual protection** (Fig. 4-19). However, since restorative treatment requirements vary, the clinician should understand possible combinations of occlusal schemes and their advantages, disadvantages, and indications.

In most patients, maximum tooth contact occurs anterior to the centric relation position of the mandible. Often, this maximum intercuspation position anterior to centric relation is referred to as *centric occlusion*, although the term is also used to refer to occlusal contact in centric relation. To avoid con-

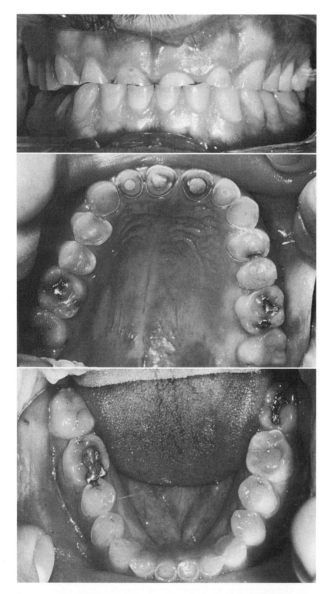

Fig. 4-18. Extensive abrasion (tooth wear) resulting from parafunctional grinding in a 23-year-old patient.

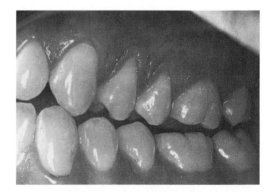

Fig. 4-19. Canine-guided or mutually protected occlusion. During lateral excursions, there are no contacts on the mediotrusive (nonworking) side; all contacts are between the laterotrusive (working side) canines.

fusion, *maximum intercuspation (MI)* and *centric relation (CR)* are the terms used in this text.

BILATERALLY BALANCED ARTICULATION

Early work in removable prosthodontics centered around the concept of a bilaterally balanced articulation. This requires having a maximum number of teeth in contact in maximum intercuspation and all excursive positions. In complete denture fabrication, this tooth arrangement helps maintain denture stability because the nonworking contact prevents the denture from being dislodged. However, as the principles of bilateral balance were applied to the natural dentition and in fixed prosthodontics, it proved to be extremely difficult to accomplish, even with great attention to detail and sophisticated articulators. In addition, high rates of failure resulted. An increased rate of occlusal wear, increased or accelerated periodontal breakdown, and neuromuscular disturbances were commonly observed. The last were often relieved when posterior contacts on the mediotrusive side were eliminated in an attempt to eliminate unfavorable loading. Thus the concept of a unilaterally balanced occlusion **(group function)** evolved[31] (Fig. 4-20).

UNILATERALLY BALANCED ARTICULATION (GROUP FUNCTION)

In a unilaterally balanced articulation, excursive contact occurs between all opposing posterior teeth on the laterotrusive (working) side only. On the mediotrusive (nonworking) side, no contact occurs until the mandible has reached centric relation. Thus, in this occlusal arrangement the load is distributed among the periodontal support of all posterior teeth on the working side. This can be advantageous if, for instance, the periodontal support of

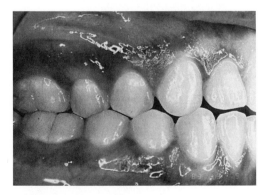

Fig. 4-20. Group function or unilaterally balanced occlusion. During lateral excursions, there are no contacts between teeth on the mediotrusive (nonworking) side, but even excursive contacts occur on the laterotrusive (working) side.

the canine is compromised. While on the working side, occlusal load is distributed during excursive movement, and the posterior teeth on the **nonworking side** do not contact. In the protrusive movement, no posterior tooth contact occurs.

Long Centric. As the concept of unilateral balance evolved, it was suggested that allowing some freedom of movement in an anteroposterior direction is advantageous. This concept is known as *long centric.* Schuyler[32] was one of the first to advocate such an occlusal arrangement. He thought that it was important for the posterior teeth to be in harmonious gliding contact when the mandible translates from centric relation forward to make anterior tooth contact. Others[33] have advocated long centric because centric relation only rarely coincides with the maximum intercuspation position in healthy natural dentitions. However, its length is arbitrary. At given vertical dimensions, long centric ranges from 0.5 to 1.5 mm in length have been advocated. This theory presupposes that the condyles can translate horizontally in the fossae over a commensurate trajectory before beginning to move downward. It also necessitates a greater horizontal space between the maxillary and mandibular anterior teeth (deeper lingual concavity), allowing horizontal movement before posterior **disocclusion.**

MUTUALLY PROTECTED OCCLUSION

During the early 1960s, an occlusal scheme called *mutually protected occlusion* was advocated by Stuart and Stallard,[34] based on earlier work by D'Amico.[35] In this arrangement, centric relation coincides with the maximum intercuspation position. The six anterior maxillary teeth, together with the six anterior mandibular teeth, guide excursive movements of the mandible, and no posterior occlusal contacts occur during any lateral or protrusive excursions.

The relationship of the anterior teeth, or anterior guidance, is critical to the success of this occlusal scheme. In a mutually protected occlusion, the posterior teeth come into contact only at the very end of each chewing stroke, minimizing horizontal loading on the teeth. Concurrently, the posterior teeth act as stops for vertical closure when the mandible returns to its maximum intercuspation position. Posterior cusps should be sharp and should pass each other closely without contacting to maximize occlusal function. Investigations of the neuromuscular physiology of the masticatory apparatus indicate advantages associated with a mutually protected occlusal scheme.[8] However, in studies involving unrestored dentitions, relatively few occlusions can be classified as mutually protected.[36]

Optimum Occlusion

In an ideal occlusal arrangement, the load exerted on the dentition should be distributed optimally. Occlusal contact has been shown[37] to influence muscle activity during mastication. Any restorative procedures that adversely affect occlusal stability may affect the timing and intensity of elevator muscle activity. Horizontal forces on any teeth should be avoided or at least minimized, and loading should be predominantly parallel to the long axes of the teeth. This is facilitated when the tips of the centric cusps are located centrally over the roots and when loading of the teeth occurs in the fossae of the occlusal surfaces rather than on the marginal ridges. Horizontal forces are also minimized if posterior tooth contact during excursive movements is avoided. Nevertheless, to enhance masticatory efficiency, the cusps of the posterior teeth should have adequate height.

The chewing and grinding action of the teeth is enhanced if opposing cusps on the laterotrusive side interdigitate at the end of the chewing stroke. The mutually protected occlusal scheme probably meets this criterion better than the other occlusal arrangements. The features of a mutually protected occlusion are as follows[38]:

1. Uniform contact of all teeth around the arch when the mandibular condylar processes are in their most superior position
2. Stable posterior tooth contacts with vertically directed resultant forces
3. Centric relation coincident with maximum intercuspation (intercuspal position) (CR = MI)
4. No contact of posterior teeth in lateral or protrusive movements
5. Anterior tooth contacts harmonizing with functional jaw movements

In achieving these criteria, it is assumed that (1) a full complement of teeth exists, (2) the supporting tissues are healthy, (3) there is no cross bite, and (4) the occlusion is Angle Class I.

Rationale. At first glance it might seem illogical to load the single-rooted anterior teeth as opposed to the multirooted posterior teeth during chewing. However, the canines and incisors have a distinct mechanical advantage over the posterior teeth[39]: the effectiveness of the force exerted by the muscles of mastication is notably less when the loading contact occurs farther anteriorly.

The mandible is a lever of the class III type (Fig. 4-21), which is the least efficient of lever systems. An example of another class III lever would be a fishing pole. The longer the pole, the more effort it takes to pull a fish out of the water. The same holds true for the muscles of mastication and the teeth: the farther anteriorly initial tooth-to-tooth contact occurs (i.e., the longer the lever arm), the less effective will be the forces exerted by the musculature and the smaller the load to which the teeth are subjected. The canine—with its long root, significant amount of periodontal surface area, and strategic position in

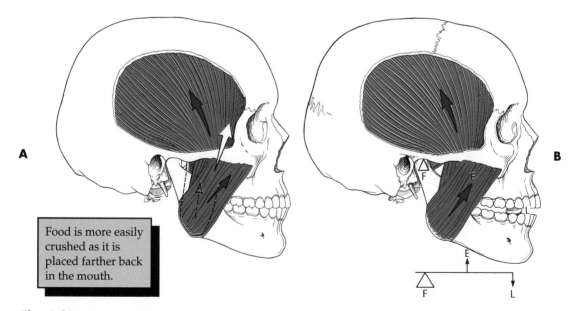

Food is more easily crushed as it is placed farther back in the mouth.

Fig. 4-21. Lever system of the mandible. **A,** The elevator muscles of the mandible insert anterior to the TMJs and posterior to the teeth, forming a class III lever system. **B,** The fulcrum *(F)* is the TMJ, the force or effort *(E)* is applied by the muscles of mastication, and the resistance or load *(L)* is food placed between the teeth. The load will diminish as the lever arm increases. Therefore less load is placed on the anterior than on the posterior teeth.

the dental arch—is well adapted to guiding excursive movements. This function is governed by pressoreceptors in the periodontal ligament, receptors that are very sensitive to mechanical stimulation.[40]

The elimination of posterior contacts during excursions reduces the amount of lateral force to which posterior teeth are subjected. Therefore, molars and premolars in group function are subjected to greater horizontal and potentially more pathologic force than the same teeth in a mutually protected occlusion.

PATIENT ADAPTABILITY

There are significant differences in the adaptive response of patients to occlusal abnormalities. Some individuals are unable to tolerate seemingly trivial occlusal deficiencies, whereas others are able to sustain distinct malocclusions without obvious symptoms. Most patients seem able to adapt to small occlusal deficiencies without exhibiting acute symptoms.

LOWERED THRESHOLD
Patients with a low pain threshold generally do not present much difficulty in diagnosis. They readily identify every pain. A lowered threshold, however, is not to be confused with hypochondria; it is merely an indication of poor adaptability to occlusal discrepancies. NOTE: The tolerance or adaptability of an individual patient will likely vary—it will be lower at times of emotional stress and general malaise, when clinical symptoms such as severe headaches, muscle spasm, and pain may surface.

RAISED THRESHOLD
Individuals who have adapted to existing malocclusions may report being quite comfortable with their dentition, although considerable symptoms are evident. Even in the absence of pain, however, occlusal treatment may be advised to prevent or minimize wear on the teeth and damage to the musculature or temporomandibular joints.

PATHOGENIC OCCLUSION

A **pathogenic occlusion** is defined as an occlusal relationship capable of producing pathologic changes in the stomatognathic system. In such occlusions sufficient disharmony exists between the teeth and the TMJs to result in symptoms that require intervention.

SIGNS AND SYMPTOMS
There are many indications that a pathogenic occlusion may be present. Diagnosis is often complicated because patients almost always have a combination of symptoms. Although it is often not possible to prove a direct correlation between specific symptoms and malocclusion, the following symptoms can help confirm this diagnosis.

Teeth. The teeth may exhibit hypermobility, open contacts, or abnormal wear. Hypermobility of an individual tooth or opposing pair of teeth is often an indication of excessive occlusal force. This may be due to premature contact in centric relation or during excursive movements. Such contacts frequently can be detected by placing the tip of the index finger on the crown portion of the mobile tooth and asking the patient to repeatedly tap the teeth together. Small amounts of movement (fremitus) that otherwise might not be readily seen often can be felt this way.

Open proximal contacts may be the result of tooth migration because of an unstable occlusion and should prompt further investigation (Fig. 4-22). Diagnostic casts made during previous treatment will help assess any changes in the stability of the occlusion. Abnormal tooth wear, cusp fracture, or chipping of incisal edges may be signs of parafunctional activity.[41,42] However, extensive tooth destruction is often due to a combination of acid erosion and **attrition**[43-45] In these cases, the acid may be from the diet (e.g., excessive citrus fruit consumption) or endogenous (due to regurgitation or frequent vomiting).

Periodontium. There is no convincing evidence that chronic periodontal disease is caused directly by occlusal overload. However, a widened periodontal ligament space (detected radiographically) may indicate premature occlusal contact and is often associated with tooth mobility (Fig. 4-23). Similarly, isolated or circumferential periodontal defects are often associated with occlusal trauma. In patients with advanced periodontal disease who

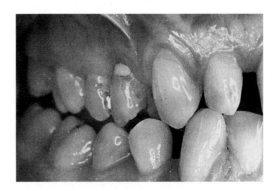

Fig. 4-22. Unstable occlusion. Removal of a tooth without replacement has led to tilting and drifting.

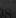

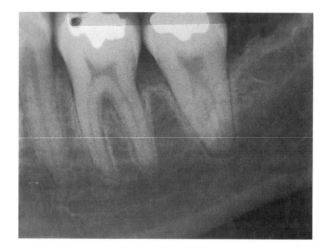

Fig. 4-23. Widened periodontal ligament space and increased mobility of mandibular molars. Occlusal premature contacts were noted in lateral and protrusive movements.

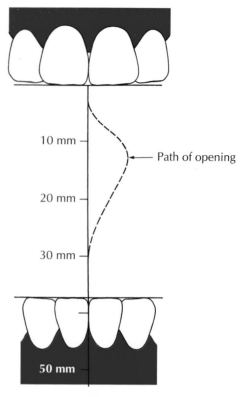

Fig. 4-24. Midline deviation during opening and closing movements can be indicative of asymmetric muscle activity or joint derangement. Here, during opening, less than optimal translation occurs on the patient's left side.

have extensive bone loss, rapid tooth migration may occur with even minor occlusal discrepancies. Tooth movement may make it difficult for these patients to institute proper oral hygiene measures, and the result may be a recurrence of periodontal disease. Precise adjustment of the occlusion is probably more critical in patients with a compromised crown/root ratio than in those with better periodontal support (see Chapter 32).

Musculature. Acute or chronic muscular pain on palpation can indicate habits associated with tension such as bruxing or clenching. Chronic muscle fatigue can lead to muscle spasm and pain. In one study,[46] subjects were instructed to grind their teeth for approximately 30 minutes. They experienced muscle pain that typically peaked 2 hours after parafunctioning and lasted as long as 7 days. Asymmetric muscle activity can be diagnosed by observing a patient's opening and closing movements in the frontal plane. A deviation of a few millimeters is quite common, but anything beyond this calls for further examination (Fig. 4-24) and may be a sign of dysfunction.[47] Restricted opening, or trismus, may be due to the fact that the mandibular elevator muscles are not relaxing.

Temporomandibular Joints. Pain, clicking, or popping in the TMJs can indicate TM disorders. Clicking and popping may be present without the patient's awareness. A stethoscope is a useful diagnostic aid; a recent study found joint sounds are generally reliable indicators of temporomandibular disorders.[48] The patient may complain of TMJ pain that is actually of muscular origin and is referred to the joints.

Clicking may also be associated with internal derangements of the joint. A patient with unilateral clicking when opening and closing (reciprocal click) in conjunction with a midline deviation may have a displaced disk. The midline deviation will typically occur toward the side of the affected joint because the displaced disk can prevent (or slow down) the normal anterior translatory movement of the condyle.

Myofascial Pain Dysfunction. The myofascial pain dysfunction (MPD) syndrome presents as diffuse unilateral pain in the preauricular area, with muscle tenderness, clicking, or popping noises in the contralateral TMJ and limitation of jaw function. Often the muscles, and not the TMJ, are the primary site, but over time the functional problem may lead to organic changes in the joint. Three major theories relative to the cause of MPD are recognized: The psychophysiologic theory[49] states that MPD results from bruxing and clenching, with chronic muscle fatigue leading to muscle spasm and altered mandibular movement. Tooth movement may follow, and the malocclusion becomes apparent when spasm is relieved. According to this theory, treatment should focus on emotional rather than physical therapy.

The muscle theory[50] states that continuous muscle hyperactivity is responsible for MPD, with pain referred to the TMJ and other areas of the head and neck region.

The mechanical displacement theory[51] states that malocclusion of the teeth displaces the condyles, and the feedback from the dentition is altered, which results in muscle spasm.

Correct diagnosis and management is often complicated by the concurrent presence of multiple etiologies. Patients with MPD may require multidisciplinary treatment involving occlusal therapy, medications, biofeedback, and physical therapy. Extensive fixed prosthodontic treatment should be postponed until the patient's condition(s) have been stabilized at acceptable levels.

OCCLUSAL TREATMENT

When a patient exhibits signs and symptoms that appear correlated to occlusal interferences (see also p. 157), occlusal treatment should be considered.[52] Such treatment can include tooth movement through orthodontics, elimination of deflective occlusal contacts through selective reshaping of the occlusal surfaces of teeth, or the restoration and replacement of missing teeth resulting in more favorable distribution of occlusal force.

The objectives of occlusal treatment are as follows:

1. To direct the occlusal forces along the long axes of the teeth
2. To attain simultaneous contact of all teeth in centric relation
3. To eliminate any occlusal contact on inclined planes to enhance the positional stability of the teeth
4. To have centric relation coincide with the maximum intercuspation position
5. To arrive at the occlusal scheme selected for the patient (e.g., unilateral balanced versus mutually protected)

In the short term, these objectives can be accomplished with a removable **occlusal device** (Fig. 4-25) fabricated from clear acrylic resin that overlays the occlusal surfaces of one arch. On a more permanent basis, this can be accomplished through selective occlusal reshaping, tooth movement, the placement of restorations, or a combination of these. Definitive occlusal treatment involves accurate manipulation of the mandible, particularly in centric relation. Because the patient may resist such manipulation as a result of protective muscular reflexes, some type of deprogramming device may be needed (e.g., an occlusal device).

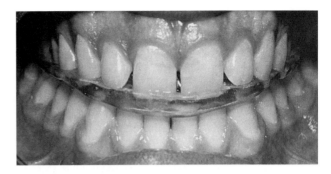

Fig. 4-25. Occlusal device. *(Courtesy Dr. W.V. Campagni.)*

OCCLUSAL DEVICE THERAPY

Occlusal devices (sometimes referred to as *occlusal splints, occlusal appliances,* or *orthotics*) are extensively used in the management of TM disorders and bruxism.[53] In controlled clinical trials, they have effectively controlled myofascial pain (i.e., the patient's perceived positive changes as a result of the device therapy). However, no clear hypothesis about the mechanism of action has been proved, and none of the various hypotheses (repositioning of condyle and/or the articular disk, reduction in masticatory muscle activity, modification of "harmful" oral behavior, and changes in the patient's occlusion) has been consistently supported by scientific studies.[54] Occlusal devices are particularly helpful in determining whether a proposed change in a patient's occlusal scheme will be tolerated. The proposed scheme is created in an acrylic resin overlay, which allows testing of the scheme through reversible means, although at a slightly increased vertical dimension. If a patient responds favorably to an occlusal device, the response to restorative treatment should be positive as well. Thus, occlusal device therapy can serve as an important diagnostic procedure before initiation of fixed prosthodontic treatment. The device can be made for either maxillary or mandibular teeth. Some clinicians express a preference for one or the other and cite advantages; however, both maxillary and mandibular devices have proved satisfactory.

FABRICATION OF DEVICE

There are several satisfactory methods for making an occlusal device.[44] One made from heat-polymerized acrylic resin will have the advantage of durability, but autopolymerizing resin used alone or in conjunction with a vacuum-formed matrix can serve equally well. Box 4-1 compares the indirect and direct techniques.

Direct Procedure Using a Vacuum-Formed Matrix

1. Adapt a sheet of clear thermoplastic resin to a diagnostic cast using a vacuum-forming machine. Hard resin (1 mm thick) is suitable. Be sure that excessive undercuts have been blocked out. Trim the excess resin so all facial soft tissues are exposed. On the facial surfaces of the teeth, the device must be kept well clear of the gingival margins (Fig. 4-26, A). On the lingual surface of maxillary devices, the matrix should cover the anterior third of the hard palate for rigidity.

2. Try in the matrix for fit and stability. Add a small amount of autopolymerizing acrylic resin in the incisal region. Guide the mandible into CR using the bimanual manipulation technique (see Chapter 2). Hinge the mandible to make shallow indentations in the resin (Fig. 4-26, B).

3. Add more resin to the incisor and canine regions and guide the patient to retrusive, protrusive, and lateral closures in the soft resin. Allow the resin to polymerize. NOTE: The resin should be allowed to polymerize on the cast or with the appliance in place in the mouth. Otherwise, the heat generated by polymerization may distort the thermoplastic matrix.

4. With the help of marking ribbon, adjust the resin to give smooth, even contacts during protrusive and lateral excursions as well as a definite occlusal stop for each incisor in centric relation (Fig. 4-26, C). Confine protrusive contacts to the incisors and lateral contacts to the laterotrusive canines (Fig. 4-26, D). All posterior contacts should be relieved at this stage.

5. Have the patient wear the device for a few minutes in the office. Repeated protrusive and lateral movements will overcome most problems in jaw manipulation. Occasionally it will be necessary for the patient to wear the device overnight before the acquired protective muscle patterns are overcome. NOTE: In such cases, if posterior tooth eruption is to be avoided, the patient must be seen again within 24 to 48 hours.

6. Add autopolymerizing acrylic resin to the posterior region of the device and guide the patient into centric relation. Hold CR until the acrylic resin has polymerized.

7. Remove the device and examine the impressions of the opposing arch in the resin (Fig. 4-26, E). Polymerization can be accelerated by placing the device on the cast in warm water in a pressure pot (Fig. 4-26, F).

8. Place pencil marks in the depressions formed by the opposing centric cusps. If a cusp registration is missing, new resin can be added and the device reseated.

9. Remove excess resin with a bur or wheel to leave only the pencil marks (Fig. 4-26, G). All other contacts must be eliminated if posterior disclusion is to be achieved.

10. Check the device in the mouth for CR contacts, marking them with a ribbon. Relieve heavy contacts by continued adjustment until each centric cusp has an even mark.

11. Identify protrusive and lateral excursions using different-colored tape. Adjust excursive contacts as necessary, being careful not to remove the centric cusp stops.

12. Smooth and polish the device, again being careful not to alter the functional surfaces (Fig. 4-26, H).

13. After a period of satisfactory use, the device can be duplicated in heat-polymerized resin using a standard denture reline technique.

Indirect Procedure Using Autopolymerizing Acrylic Resin

Accurately mounted diagnostic casts are essential for this procedure. A relatively small mounting er-

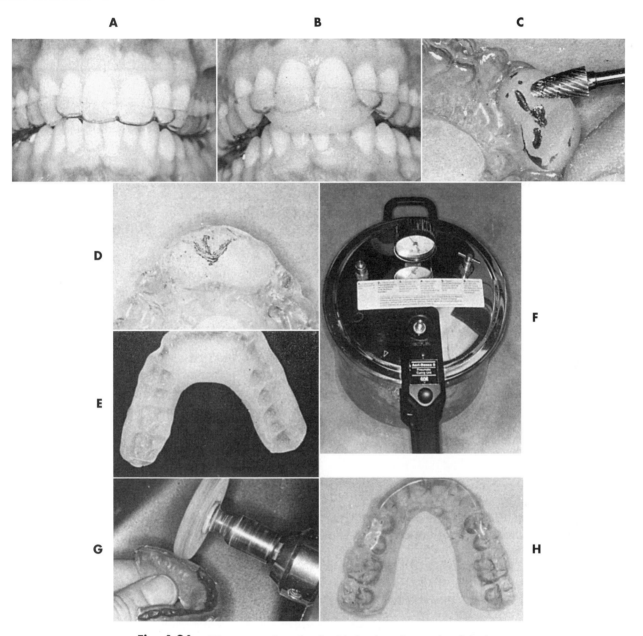

Fig. 4-26. Direct procedure for the fabrication of an occlusal device.

ror can lead to considerable loss of time at try-in. Particular attention must be given to occlusal defects or interfering soft tissue projections on the casts, which could cause errors during mounting.

1. Be sure that the device is made at the same vertical dimension of occlusion as the CR record. This will reduce mounting errors derived from using an arbitrary facebow.
2. Fit the articulator with a mechanical incisal guidance table initially set flat.
3. Lower the incisal guide pin until there is approximately 1 mm of clearance between the posterior teeth (Fig. 4-27, *A*). This should be the same vertical dimension of occlusion as the one at which the CR record was made.

4. Depending on the type of articulator used, it may be necessary to reposition the incisal guide table after step 3.
5. Check the clearance between opposing casts during protrusive movement of the articulator. Where this is less than 1 mm, increase it by tilting the incisal guidance table.
6. Raise the platform wings of the incisal guidance table so there is at least 1 mm of clearance in all lateral excursions (Fig. 4-27, *B*). It may be necessary to raise the incisal pin occasionally to ensure adequate clearance.
7. Mark the height of contour of each tooth on the cast and block out undercuts with wax (Fig. 4-27, *C*).

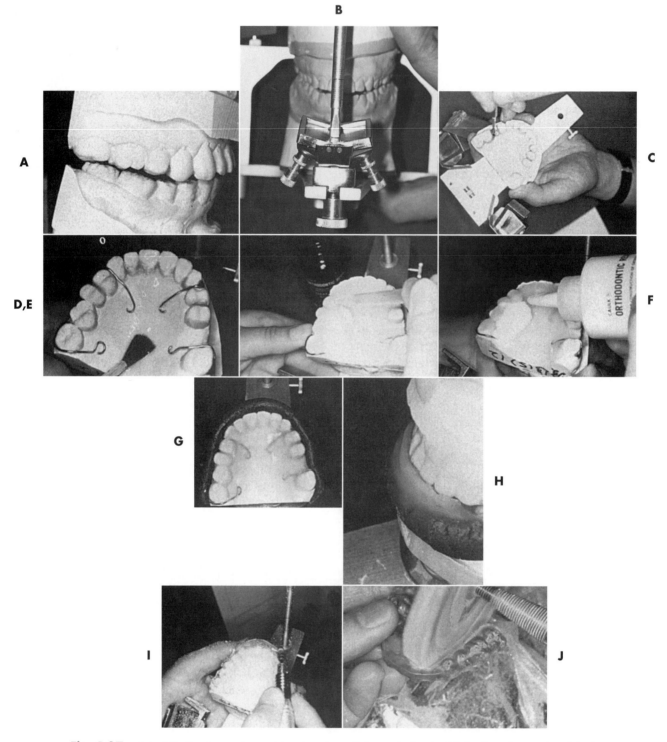

Fig. 4-27. A to J, Indirect procedure with autopolymerizing resin for the fabrication of an occlusal device.

8. Form wire clasps to engage facial under-cuts and seal the cast with a separating medium (e.g., Al-Cote) and allow it to dry (Fig. 4-27, *D*). The opposing cast can be soaked in water to prevent the acrylic resin from sticking to it.

9. Fabricate the device with autopolymerizing clear acrylic resin (Fig. 4-27, *E*) applied by alternating liquid and powder (Fig. 4-27, *F*). To avoid porosities, the resin should always be kept wet with monomer and added in small increments (Fig. 4-27, *G*).

10. While the resin is still soft, close the articulator (Fig. 4-27, *H*). Add resin where necessary until a slight depression is formed by each centric cusp.

11. Again, while the resin is still soft, close the articulator into protrusive and lateral excursions. Add or remove resin until it is in constant contact with the anterior teeth when the incisal guide pin contacts the incisal guidance table. This adjustment need only be approximate because the working time of the acrylic resin is limited and the occlusal contacts will be refined after the resin has polymerized.

12. Place the device and cast in warm water in a pressure vessel to polymerize. When this is complete, flush wax from the cast with boiling water.

13. Refine the occlusion on the articulator (Fig. 4-27, *I*).
    a. There should be even contact for each centric cusp in centric relation.
    b. A stop should exist for each anterior tooth in CR.
    c. Protrusive contact on the incisors should be smooth and even.
    d. There should also be smooth and even lateral contact on the laterotrusive (working-side) canines.

14. Remove the device from the cast and smooth and polish it, taking care not to alter the functional surfaces (Fig. 4-27, *J*).

15. At try-in, check for fit and stability. Also check the occlusal contacts and adjust as necessary, using different-colored marking ribbon for centric and **eccentric** contacts.

Indirect Procedure Using Heat-polymerized Acrylic Resin

A more durable device can be made with heat-polymerized acrylic resin. The desired occlusal surface is shaped in wax on articulated diagnostic casts, or the direct device made with a vacuum-formed matrix can be used as a pattern. This is flasked and processed in a manner similar to that for a complete denture. Because of processing errors, it is important to remount the cast and make necessary adjustments before finishing and polishing are completed.

1. Articulate the casts in CR. Allow for a remount procedure by notching the base of the cast on which the device will be processed.
2. Create the desired configuration of the device in wax, obtaining centric stops and anterior guidance. Use the mechanical anterior guidance table as for an autopolymerizing resin device.
3. Separate the cast from its mounting and flask as for conventional processing of complete dentures.

4. Process in clear, heat-cured resin.
5. Rearticulate and adjust the occlusion.
6. Remove the stone cast with a shell blaster. Polish the external surfaces on a lathe with pumice and an appropriate polishing compound.
7. Store in 100% humidity.

Attention to Detail

Regardless of the device chosen, success depends very much on meticulous attention to detail during the fabrication. When making a direct device, use a well-adapted and stable vacuum-formed base and follow the procedure exactly. For example, be sure that the anterior guidance is properly established and that the patient's jaw can be easily manipulated before adding resin to the posterior region. When the indirect procedure is used, be sure that the casts articulate to an accurate CR record made at the correct vertical dimension of occlusion. Inaccurate mounting is probably the most common cause for frustration and results in excessive adjustments at delivery.

FOLLOW-UP

After delivery to the patient, the occlusion must be verified and corrected as necessary. The patient is instructed to wear the device 24 hours a day, removing it only for oral hygiene, and to return at regular weekly and biweekly intervals (or sooner if a problem is anticipated) for modification. A reduction in discomfort suggests that definitive occlusal adjustment (see Chapter 5) or restorative dentistry, or both, will likely be successful. If device therapy fails to relieve the discomfort, further evaluation and diagnosis of the etiology and parameters of the chief complaint should be pursued.

SUMMARY

Mandibular movement depends on certain anatomic limitations. The extremes, called *border movements*, are subject to restriction by the temporomandibular joints and ligaments and the teeth. Speech and mastication are examples of *functional movements*. Bruxism and clenching are examples of *parafunctional movements*. These accomplish no purposeful objective and are potentially harmful.

A balanced occlusion provides complete denture patients with stability, because there is even contact between all the teeth in each excursion. This is potentially destructive in dentate patients and is not indicated for fixed prosthodontic treatment. In a unilaterally balanced occlusion (group function), eccentric occlusal contact occurs only between posterior teeth on the laterotrusive (working) side. This may be indicated when it is important to distribute the occlusal load over multiple teeth. The mutually protected occlusion offers the most desirable distribution of occlusal load. Centric relation coincides with the maximum intercuspation position, and the relationship of the maxillary and mandibular anterior teeth (the anterior guidance) is instrumental to its success.

In the presence of pathology that is potentially related to malocclusion, occlusal therapy may be indicated. Occlusal devices can serve as useful diagnostic and therapeutic adjuncts to treatment. For such patients, occlusal therapy should be initiated and completed before any substantial restorative care is undertaken.

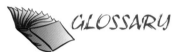

GLOSSARY

Angle's classification of occlusion: [Edward Harley Angle, American orthodontist, 1855-1930]: eponym for a classification system of occlusion based on the interdigitation of the first molar teeth originally described by Angle as four major groups depending on the anteroposterior jaw relationship. Class IV is no longer used. Class I (normal occlusion or neutrocclusion): the dental relationship in which there is normal anteroposterior relationship of the jaws, as indicated by correct interdigitation of maxillary and mandibular molars, but with crowding and rotation of teeth elsewhere, i.e., a dental dysplasia or arch length deficiency. Class II (distocclusion): the dental relationship in which the mandibular dental

arch is posterior to the maxillary dental arch in one or both lateral segments; the mandibular first molar is distal to the maxillary first molar. Further subdivided into two divisions. Division 1: bilateral distal retrusion with a narrow maxillary arch and protruding maxillary incisors. Subdivisions include right or left (unilaterally distal with other characteristics being the same). Division 2: bilateral distal with a normal or square-shaped maxillary arch, retruded maxillary central incisors, labially malposed maxillary lateral incisors, and an excessive vertical overlap. Subdivisions include right or left (unilaterally distal with other characteristics the same). Class III (mesiocclusion): the dental relationship in which the mandibular arch is anterior to the maxillary arch in one or both lateral segments; the mandibular first molar is mesial to the maxillary first molar. The mandibular incisors are usually in anterior cross-bite. Subdivisions include right or left (unilaterally mesial with other characteristics the same). Class IV: the dental relationship in which the occlusal relations of the dental arches present the peculiar condition of being in distal occlusion in one lateral half and in mesial occlusion in the other (no longer used). (Angle EH. Classification of malocclusion. Dental Cosmos 1899; 41:248-64, 350-7.)

anterior open occlusal relationship: the lack of anterior tooth contact in any occluding position of the posterior teeth

arc of closure: the circular or elliptic arc created by closure of the mandible, most often viewed in the mid-sagittal plane, using a reference point on the mandible (frequently either mandibular central incisors' mesial incisal edge).

Study Questions

1. Discuss the various functions of the mandibular ligaments and relate them to their respective origins and insertions.
2. Discuss the various functions of the mandibular muscles and relate them to their respective origins and insertions.
3. What are border movements? Draw and label Posselt's solid.
4. What are the determinants of occlusion and what do they determine?
5. Give examples of pathologic occlusion and list five categories with multiple associated symptoms for each category.
6. Describe a mutually protected occlusal scheme, its advantages, and indications. When is a mutually protected occlusion undesirable? Why?
7. Discuss typical mandibular movement during normal function and during parafunction. What is the influence of age on chewing patterns?
8. What is the difference between a bilateral balanced occlusion, a unilateral balanced occlusion, and mutual protection?
9. What are the purposes of an occlusal device? Describe a scenario justifying its use, and explain how the device should be designed. Explain your rationale for this design.

arthrodial joint: a joint that allows gliding motion of the surfaces.

attrition: *(n) (14c)* **1:** the act of wearing or grinding down by friction **2:** the normal mechanical wear resulting from mastication, limited to contacting surfaces of the teeth

balanced articulation: the bilateral, simultaneous, anterior, and posterior occlusal contact of teeth in centric and eccentric positions.

Bennett angle: *obs:* the angle formed between the sagittal plane and the average path of the advancing condyle as viewed in the horizontal plane during lateral mandibular movements (GPT-4).

border movement: mandibular movement at the limits dictated by anatomic structures, as viewed in a given plane.

bruxism: *(n) (ca. 1940)* **1:** the parafunctional grinding of teeth **2:** an oral habit consisting of involuntary rhythmic or spasmodic nonfunctional gnashing, grinding, or clenching of teeth, in other than chewing movements of the mandible, which may lead to occlusal trauma—called also tooth grinding, occlusal neurosis.

canine protected articulation: a form of mutually protected articulation in which the vertical and horizontal overlap of the canine teeth disengage the posterior teeth in the excursive movements of the mandible.

capsular ligament: within the temporomandibular joint, a ligament that scparately encapsulates the superior and inferior synovial cavities of the temporomandibular articulation.

capsule: *(n) (1693):* a fibrous sac or ligament that encloses a joint and limits its motion. It is lined with synovial membrane.

clenching: *(vt) (13c):* the pressing and clamping of the jaws and teeth together, frequently associated with acute nervous tension or physical effort.

determinants of mandibular movement: those anatomic structures that dictate or limit the movements of the mandible. The anterior determinant of mandibular movement is the dental articulation. The posterior determinants of mandibular movement are the temporomandibular articulations and their associated structures.

disk: *n (1664):* with respect to the temporomandibular joint, the avascular interarticular tissue (spelled also disc).

elevator muscle: one of the muscles that, on contracting, elevates or closes the mandible.

envelope of motion: the three-dimensional space circumscribed by mandibular border movements within which all unstrained mandibular movement occurs.

frontal plane: any plane parallel with the long axis of the body and at right angles to the median plane, thus dividing the body into front and back parts. So called because this plane roughly parallels the frontal suture of the skull.

group function: multiple contact relations between the maxillary and mandibular teeth in lateral movements on the working side whereby simultaneous contact of several teeth act as a group to distribute occlusal forces.

horizontal overlap: the projection of teeth beyond their antagonists in the horizontal plane

incisal guidance: **1:** the influence of the contacting surfaces of the mandibular and maxillary anterior teeth on mandibular movements **2:** the influence of the contacting surfaces of the guide pin and guide table on articulator movements.

intercondylar distance: the distance between the rotational centers of two condyles or their analogues.

laterotrusion: *(n):* condylar movement on the working side in the horizontal plane. This term may be used in combination with terms describing condylarmovement in other planes, for example, laterodetrusion, lateroprotrusion, lateroretrusion, and laterosurtrusion.

malocclusion: *(n) (1888)* **1:** any deviation from a physiologically acceptable contact of opposing dentitions **2:** any deviation from a normal occlusion.

mandibular hinge position: *(obs):* the position of the mandible in relation to the maxilla at which opening and closing movements can be made on the hinge axis (GPT-4).

mandibular translation: the translatory (medio-lateral) movement of the mandible when viewed in the frontal plane. While this has not been demonstrated to occur as an immediate sideward movement when viewed in the frontal plane, it could theoretically occur in an essentially pure translatory form in the early part of the motion or in combination with rotation in the latter part of the motion or both.

masticatory cycle: a three dimensional representation of mandibular movement produced during the chewing of food.

mutually protected articulation: an occlusal scheme in which the posterior teeth prevent excessive contact of the anterior teeth in maximum intercuspation, and the anterior teeth disengage the posterior teeth in all mandibular excursive movements.

occlusal balance: a condition in which there are simultaneous contacts of opposing teeth or tooth analogues (i.e., occlusion rims) on both sides of the opposing dental arches during eccentric movements within the functional range

occlusal contact: **1:** the touching of opposing teeth on elevation of the mandible **2:** any contact relation of opposing teeth.

open occlusal relationship: the lack of tooth contact in an occluding position.

opening movement: *(obs)* movement of the mandible executed during jaw separation (GPT-1).

parafunction: *(adj):* disordered or perverted function.

pathogenic occlusion: an occlusal relationship capable of producing pathologic changes in the stomatognathic system.

posterior border movement: movements of the mandible along the posterior limit of the envelope of motion.

protrusion: *(n)* (1646): a position of the mandible anterior to centric relation.

retrodiscal tissue: a mass of loose connective tissue attached to the posterior edge of the articular disk and extending to and filling the loose folds of the posterior capsule of the temporomandibular joint-called also bilaminar zone.

retruded contact position: that guided occlusal relationship occurring at the most retruded position of the condyles in the joint cavities. A position that may be more retruded than the centric relation position.

rotation: *(n)* (1555) *1:* the action or process of rotating on or as if on an axis or center *2:* the movement of a rigid body in which the parts move in circular paths with their centers on a fixed line called the axis of rotation. The plane of the circle in which the body moves is perpendicular to the axis of rotation.

sagittal plane: any vertical plane or section parallel to the median plane of the body that divides a body into right and left portions.

synovial fluid: a viscid fluid contained in joint cavities and secreted by the synovial membrane

temporomandibular joint: *1:* the articulation between the temporal bone and the mandible. It is a diarthrodial, bilateral ginglymus arthrodial joint *2:* the articulation of the condylar process of the mandible and the interarticular disk with the mandibular fossa of the squamous portion of the temporal bone; a diarthrodial, sliding hinge (ginglymus) joint. Movement in the upper joint compartment is mostly translational, whereas that in the lower joint compartment is mostly rotational. The joint connects the mandibular condyle to the articular fossa of the temporal bone with the temporomandibular disk interposed.

translation: *(n)* (14c): that motion of a rigid body in which a straight line palling through any two points always remains parallel to its initial position. The motion may be described as a sliding or gliding motion.

transverse horizontal axis: an imaginary line around which the mandible may rotate within the sagittal plane.

vertical overlap: *1:* the distance teeth lap over their antagonists as measured vertically; especially the distance the maxillary incisal edges extend below those of the mandibular teeth. It may also be used to describe the vertical relations of opposing cusps *2:* the vertical relationship of the incisal edges of the maxillary incisors to the mandibular incisors when the teeth are in maximum intercuspation.

working side the side toward which the mandible moves in a lateral excursion.

REFERENCES

1. Okeson JP: *Management of temporomandibular disorders and occlusion*, ed 4, St Louis, 1998, Mosby, p 13.
2. Schweitzer JM: Concepts of occlusion: a discussion, *Dent Clin North Am* 7:649, 1963.
3. Proffit WR, Fields HW Jr: *Contemporary orthodontics*, ed 3, St Louis, 1999, Mosby.
4. Bennett NG: A contribution to the study of the movements of the mandible, *Odontol Sec R Soc Med Trans* 1:79, 1908. (Reprinted in *J Prosthet Dent* 8:41, 1958.)
5. Posselt U: Movement areas of the mandible, *J Prosthet Dent* 7:375, 1957.
6. Goldenberg BS et al: The loss of occlusion and its effect on mandibular immediate side shift, *J Prosthet Dent* 63:163, 1990.
7. Pelletier LB, Campbell SD: Evaluation of the relationship between anterior and posterior functionally disclusive angles. II. Study of a population, *J Prosthet Dent* 63:536, 1990.
8. Hayasaki H et al: A calculation method for the range of occluding phase at the lower incisal point during chewing movements using the curved mesh diagram of mandibular excursion (CMDME), *J Oral Rehabil* 26:236, 1999.
9. Lundeen HC, Gibbs CH: *Advances in occlusion*, Boston, 1982, John Wright PSG.
10. Ogawa T et al: Inclination of the occlusal plane and occlusal guidance as contributing factors in mastication, *J Dent* 26:641, 1998.
11. Wickwire NA et al: Chewing patterns in normal children, *Angle Orthod* 51:48, 1981.
12. Lavigne G et al: Evidence that periodontal pressoreceptors provide positive feedback to jaw closing muscles during mastication, *J Neurophysiol* 58:342, 1987.
13. Burnett CA, Clifford TJ: Closest speaking space during the production of sibilant sounds and its value in establishing the vertical dimension of occlusion, *J Dent Res* 72:964, 1993.
14. Pound E: The mandibular movements of speech and their seven related values, *J Prosthet Dent* 16:835, 1966.
15. Pound E: Let /S/ be your guide, *J Prosthet Dent* 38: 482, 1977.
16. Howell PG: Incisal relationships during speech, *J Prosthet Dent* 56:93, 1986.
17. Rivera-Morales WC, Mohl ND: Variability of closest speaking space compared with interocclusal distance in dentulous subjects, *J Prosthet Dent* 65:228, 1991.
18. Duckro PN et al: Prevalence of temporomandibular symptoms in a large United States metropolitan, *Cranio* 8:131, 1990.
19. Hathaway KM: Bruxism. Definition, measurement, and treatment. In Fricton JR, Dubner RB,

editors: *Orofacial pain and temporomandibular disorders,* New York, 1995, Raven Press.

20. Hublin C et al: Sleep bruxism based on self-report in a nationwide twin cohort, *J Sleep Res* 7: 61, 1998.

21. Macaluso GM et al: Sleep bruxism is a disorder related to periodic arousals during sleep, *J Dent Res* 77:565, 1998.

22. Madrid G et al: Cigarette smoking and bruxism, *Percept Mot Skills* 87:898 1998.

23. Mongini F, Tempia-Valenta G: A graphic and statistical analysis of the chewing movements in function and dysfunction, *J Craniomandib Pract* 2:125, 1984.

24. Faulkner KD: Preliminary studies of some masticatory characteristics of bruxism, *J Oral Rehabil* 16:221, 1989.

25. Mohl ND et al: Devices for the diagnosis and treatment of temporomandibular disorders. I. Introduction, scientific evidence, and jaw tracking, *J Prosthet Dent* 63:198, 1990.

26. Rugh JD, Solberg WK: Electromyographic studies of bruxist behavior before and during treatment, *J Calif Dent Assoc* 3(9):56, 1975.

27. Lobbezoo F, Lavigne GJ: Do bruxism and temporomandibular disorders have a cause-and-effect relationship? *J Orofac Pain* 11:15, 1997.

28. Grippo JO: Abfractions: a new classification of hard tissue lesions of teeth, *J Esthet Dent* 3:14, 1991.

29. Owens BM, Gallien GS: Noncarious dental "abfraction" lesions in an aging population, *Compend Contin Educ Dent* 16:552, 1995.

30. Sears VH: Balanced occlusions, *J Am Dent Assoc* 12:1448, 1925.

31. Schuyler CH: Considerations of occlusion in fixed partial dentures, *Dent Clin North Am* 3:175, 1959.

32. Schuyler CH: An evaluation of incisal guidance and its influence in restorative dentistry, *J Prosthet Dent* 9:374, 1959.

33. Mann AW, Pankey LD: Concepts of occlusion: the P.M. philosophy of occlusal rehabilitation, *Dent Clin North Am* 7:621, 1963.

34. Stuart C, Stallard H: Concepts of occlusion, *Dent Clin North Am* 7:591, 1963.

35. D'Amico A: Functional occlusion of the natural teeth of man, *J Prosthet Dent* 11:899, 1961.

36. Ogawa T et al: Pattern of occlusal contacts in lateral positions: canine protection and group function validity in classifying guidance patterns, *J Prosthet Dent* 80:67, 1998.

37. Bakke M et al: Occlusal control of mandibular elevator muscles, *Scand J Dent Res* 100:284, 1992.

38. Dawson PE: *Evaluation, diagnosis, and treatment of occlusal problems,* ed 2, St Louis, 1989, Mosby.

39. Stuart CE, Stallard H: Diagnosis and treatment of occlusal relations of the teeth, *Texas Dent J* 75:430, 1957.

40. Ramfjord S, Ash MM: *Occlusion,* ed 4, Philadelphia, 1994, WB Saunders.

41. Ekfeldt A: Incisal and occlusal tooth wear and wear of some prosthodontic materials: an epidemiological and clinical study, *Swed Dent J* (suppl) 65:1, 1989.

42. Imfeld T: Dental erosion. Definition, classification and links, *Eur J Oral Sci* 104:151, 1996.

43. Lewis KJ, Smith BGN: The relationship of erosion and attrition in extensive tooth loss. Case reports, *Br Dent J* 135:400, 1973.

44. Rytomaa I et al: Bulimia and tooth erosion, *Acta Odontol Scand* 56:36, 1998.

45. Simmons JJ, Hirsh M: Role of chemical erosion in generalized attrition, *Quintessence Int* 29:793, 1998.

46. Christensen LV: Facial pain and internal pressure of masseter muscle in experimental bruxism in man, *Arch Oral Biol* 16:1021, 1971.

47. Ishigaki S et al: Clinical classification of maximal opening and closing movements, *Int J Prosthod* 2:148, 1989.

48. Leader JK et al: The influence of mandibular movements on joint sounds in patients with temporomandibular disorders, *J Prosthet Dent* 81:186, 1999.

49. Mikami DB: A review of psychogenic aspects and treatment of bruxism, *J Prosthet Dent* 37:411, 1977.

50. Schwartz LL: A temporomandibular joint pain-dysfunction syndrome, *J Chron Dis* 3:284, 1956.

51. Gelb H: An orthopedic approach to occlusal imbalance and temporomandibular dysfunction, *Dent Clin North Am* 23:181, 1979.

52. Dawson PE: Position paper regarding diagnosis, management, and treatment of temporomandibular disorders, *J Prosthet Dent* 81: 174, 1999.

53. Okeson JP: *Management of temporomandibular disorders and occlusion,* ed 4, St Louis, 1998, Mosby, ch 15.

54. Dao TT, Lavigne GJ: Oral splints: the crutches for temporomandibular disorders and bruxism? *Crit Rev Oral Biol Med* 9:345, 1998.

CHAPTER FIVE

PERIODONTAL CONSIDERATIONS

Robert F. Baima

KEY TERMS

attached gingiva	interdental papillae
bifurcation	marginal gingiva
debridement	mucogingival junction (MGJ)
gingiva	occlusal trauma
guided tissue regeneration	reflection
hemisection	Sharpey's fibers

In the fabrication of any fixed prosthesis, the practitioner must determine the periodontal status of the involved abutment teeth. This allows a reliable and accurate prognosis for the restoration. Because periodontal disease is a major cause of tooth loss in adults, the practitioner must be aware of the basic concepts and clinical modes of therapy available in periodontics to be able to develop an appropriate diagnosis and treatment plan.

This chapter reviews these concepts and treatment modalities and gives the practitioner a better understanding of periodontics and how it relates to restorative dentistry.

◼ ANATOMY

The lining of the oral cavity consists of three types of mucosa, each with a different function[1]:

1. Masticatory (keratinized) mucosa—covering the **gingiva** and hard palate
2. Lining or reflecting mucosa—covering the lips, cheeks, vestibule, alveoli, floor of the mouth, and soft palate
3. Specialized (sensory) mucosa—covering the dorsum of the tongue and taste buds

GINGIVA

Normal gingiva (Fig. 5-1)—exhibiting no fluid exudate or inflammation due to bacterial plaque—is pink and stippled. It varies in width from 1 to 9 mm and extends from the free margin of the gingiva to the alveolar mucosa. The gingivae and alveolar mucosa are separated by a demarcation called the **mucogingival junction (MGJ)**, which marks the differentiation between stippled keratinized tissue and smooth, shiny mucosa; the latter contains more elastic fibers in its connective tissue. Apical to the MGJ, the alveolar mucosa then forms the vestibule and attaches to the muscles and fascia of the lips and cheeks.

The gingiva (Fig. 5-2) consists of three parts:

1. Free **(marginal) gingiva**—extending from the most coronal aspect of the gingiva to the epithelial attachment with the tooth

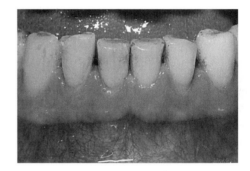

Fig. 5-1. Normal gingiva.

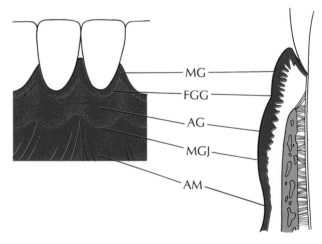

Fig. 5-2. Normal gingival structure and anatomic landmarks. *MG,* Marginal gingiva; *FGG,* free gingival groove; *AG,* attached gingiva; *MGJ,* mucogingival junction; AM, alveolar mucosa. *(Redrawn from Schluger S et al: Periodontal disease, ed 2, Philadelphia, 1990, Lea & Febiger.)*

2. **Attached gingiva**—extending from the level of the epithelial attachment to the junction between the gingiva and the alveolar mucosa (the MGJ)

3. **Interdental papillae**—triangular projections of gingivae filling the area between adjacent teeth and consisting of a buccal and a lingual component separated by a central concavity (the col)

A V-shaped depression on the labial or buccal surface of the gingiva at or somewhat apical to the level of the epithelial attachment to the tooth is called the *free gingival groove*. It is not always readily apparent clinically but can be seen histologically and may serve as a reference point for dividing the free gingiva from the labial or buccal-attached gingiva.[2,3]

The gingiva consists of dense collagen fibers, sometimes referred to as the *gingivodental ligament*, which can be divided into alveologingival, dentogingival, circular, dentoperiosteal, and transseptal groups. These fibers firmly bind the gingiva to the teeth and are continuous with the underlying alveolar periosteum. A more detailed description can be found in standard periodontal texts.[4-8]

PERIODONTIUM

The periodontium is a connective tissue structure attached to the periosteum of both the mandible and the maxillae that anchors the teeth in the mandibular and maxillary alveolar processes. It provides attachment and support, nutrition, synthesis and resorption, and mechanoreception. The main element of the periodontium is the periodontal ligament (PDL), which consists of collagenous fibers embedded in bone and cementum, giving support to the tooth in function (Fig. 5-3). These fibers, also known as **Sharpey's fibers,** follow a wavy course and terminate in either cementum or bone. There are five principal fiber groups in the PDL that traverse the space between the tooth root and alveolar bone, providing attachment and support.[4]

1. Transseptal fibers—extending interproximally between adjacent teeth (Their ends are embedded in cementum.)

2. Alveolar crest fibers—beginning just apical to the epithelial attachment and extending from cementum to the alveolar crest

3. Horizontal fibers—coursing at right angles from cementum to the alveolar bone

4. Oblique fibers—extending in an oblique direction apically, attaching cementum to the alveolar bone (They are the most numerous fibers.)

5. Apical fibers—radiating from cementum into the alveolar bone at the apex of the root

There are also smaller, irregularly arranged collagen fibers interspersed between the principal fiber groups. In addition, the PDL contains elastic fibers[9] as well as oxytalan fibers.[10]

Cellular elements found in the PDL include fibroblasts (the main synthetic cell, producing collagen and other proteoglycans), cementoblasts and cementoclasts, osteoblasts and osteoclasts (maintaining the viability of their respective tissues), and mast cells and epithelial rests (playing a role in pathologic conditions of the periodontium).[1]

DENTOGINGIVAL JUNCTION

At the base of the gingival sulcus (crevice) is the epithelium-tooth interface, also known as the *dentogingival junction (DGJ)*. This structural relationship between hard and soft tissues is unique in the body. At the ultrastructural level, it is made up of hemidesmosomes and a basal lamina, which anchor the epithelial cells to the enamel and cemental surfaces.[4,11]

The depth of the sulcus varies in healthy individuals, averaging 1.8 mm.[12] In general, the shallower it is, the more likely the gingiva will be in a state of health. Sulcular depths up to 3 mm are considered maintainable. The continued maintenance of the gingiva in a state of health depends on tight, shallow sulci, which in turn depend on optimal plaque control, and will ensure the success of periodontal therapy as well as affording a good prognosis for subsequent restorative treatment.

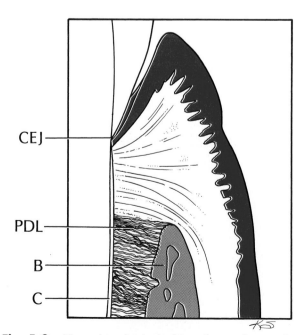

Fig. 5-3. Normal tooth-gingival interface and coronal periodontium. *CEJ,* Cementoenamel junction; *PDL,* periodontal ligament; *B,* bone; *C,* cementum.

▍DISEASES OF THE PERIODONTIUM

The general term *periodontal disease* is used to describe any condition of the periodontium other than normal. It covers such pathologic states as gingival hyperplasia, juvenile periodontitis (also known as *periodontosis*), and acute necrotizing ulcerative gingivitis—all distinct clinical entities that warrant specific treatment. For information concerning these disease states, refer to any of the standard periodontal texts.[4-8] Periodontal disease must be recognized and treated before fixed prosthodontics so that the gingival tissue levels can be determined to proper margin placement, esthetics, and gingival displacement (with an $AlCl_3$-impregnated or plain cord, see Chapter 14). Only when the gingiva and periodontium are in an optimal state of health can these determinations be made with ease or predictability.

This discussion is limited to the etiology and progression of the inflammatory gingivitis-periodontitis lesion, which affects the majority of adults[13] and constitutes the bulk of pathologic disorders needing treatment before restorative dentistry.

ETIOLOGY

Most gingival and periodontal diseases result from microbial plaque, which causes inflammation and its subsequent pathologic processes. Other contributors to inflammation include calculus, acquired pellicle, materia alba, and food debris.[5, 14]

Terminology

Microbial Plaque.   Microbial plaque (Fig. 5-4) is a sticky substance composed of bacteria and their by-products in an extracellular matrix; it also contains substances from the saliva, diet, and serum. It is basically a product of the growth of bacterial colonies and is the initiating factor in gingival and periodontal disease. If left undisturbed, it will grad-

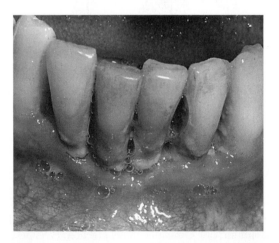

Fig. 5-4.   Gross plaque and calculus accumulation on the mandibular anterior teeth.

ually cover an entire tooth surface and can be removed only by mechanical means.

Calculus.   Dental calculus is a chalky or dark deposit attached to the tooth structure. It is essentially microbial plaque that has undergone mineralization over time. Calculus can be found on tooth structure in a supragingival and/or a subgingival location.

Acquired Pellicle.   Pellicle is a thin, brown or gray film of salivary proteins that develops on teeth after they have been cleaned. It frequently forms the interface between the tooth surface and dental deposits.

Materia alba.   Materia alba is a white coating composed of microorganisms, dead epithelial cells, and leukocytes that adheres loosely to the tooth. It can be removed from the tooth surface by water spray or by rinsing.

Structure of the Dental Plaque.   Dental plaque consists mainly of microorganisms, scattered leukocytes, enzymes, food debris, epithelial cells, and macrophages in an intracellular matrix. Bacteria make up 70% of the solid portion of the mass. The remainder is an intracellular matrix consisting of carbohydrates, proteins, and calcium and phosphate ions.[15-17]

As the plaque mass increases and matures, the flora progresses apically from a supragingival position, facilitated by the presence of gingival crevicular fluid. The flora also changes from a predominantly gram-positive, aerobic, and facultatively anaerobic population of coccoid morphology to a mix relatively high in gram-negative, anaerobic, and rodlike or filamentous organisms, along with increasing numbers of spirochetes.[18,19] Evidence[5] indicates that an increase in gram-negative organisms leads to an increase in disease activity within the periodontium and causes both direct and indirect tissue damage.

As the plaque colony matures and increases its mineral content, calculus forms within the plaque mass. Although gingival inflammation is often most severe in areas where calculus is present, the calculus itself is not the most significant source of inflammation; rather, it provides a nidus for plaque accumulation and retains the plaque in proximity to the gingiva. Dental plaque is the etiologic agent of the inflammation.[20]

PATHOGENESIS

The pathogenesis or sequence of events in the development of a gingivitis-periodontitis lesion is very complex. It involves not only local phenomena in the gingiva, PDL, tooth surface, and alveolar bone but also a number of complex host response mechanisms modified by the bacterial infection and behavioral factors.[21] Implicated in the pathogenic mechanism are phagocytic cells, the lymphoid system, antibodies and immune complexes, complement and clotting cascades, immune reactions, and the microcirculation. Detailed descriptions of host response in the gingivitis-periodontitis lesion can be obtained by referring to standard periodontal texts.[5-7]

The chronic plaque-induced lesion has been investigated[5, 22] in great detail clinically, histopathologically, and ultrastructurally, and the model of disease activity has remained consistent over time. From these analyses, an indistinct division into initial, early, established, and advanced stages has been put forth. The salient features and approximate time frame for each stage are presented here.

Initial Lesion.   The initial lesion (Fig. 5-5) is localized in the region of the gingival sulcus and is evident after approximately 2 to 4 days of undisturbed plaque accumulation from a baseline of gingival health. The vessels of the gingiva become enlarged, and vasculitis occurs, allowing a fluid exudate of polymorphonuclear leukocytes to form in the sulcus. Collagen is lost perivascularly, and the resultant space is filled with proteins and inflammatory cells. The most coronal portion of the junctional epithelium becomes altered.

Early Lesion.   Although there is no distinct division between the stages of lesion formation, the early lesion (Fig. 5-6) generally appears within 4 to 7 days of plaque accumulation. This stage of devel-

opment exhibits further loss of collagen from the marginal gingiva. In addition, an increase in gingival sulcular fluid flow occurs with increased inflammatory cells and the accumulation of lymphoid cells subjacent to the junctional epithelium. The basal cells of the junctional epithelium begin to proliferate, and significant alterations are seen in the connective tissue fibroblasts.

Established Lesion.   Within 7 to 21 days the lesion enters the established stage (Fig. 5-7). It is still

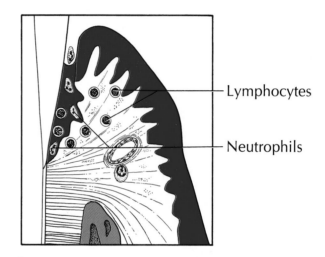

Fig. 5-6. Early lesion of gingivitis-periodontitis. The predominant inflammatory cells are lymphocytes subjacent to the junctional epithelium. The epithelium is beginning to proliferate into rete ridges.
(Redrawn from Schluger S et al: Periodontal disease, *ed 2, Philadelphia, 1990, Lea & Febiger.)*

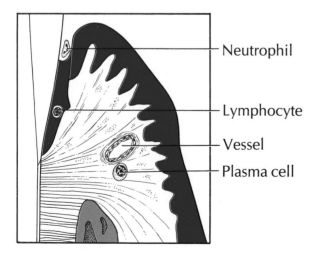

Fig. 5-5. Initial lesion of gingivitis-periodontitis. There is a predominance of polymorphonuclear leukocytes in the beginning stages of inflammation.
(Redrawn from Schluger S et al: Periodontal disease, *ed 2, Philadelphia, 1990, Lea & Febiger.)*

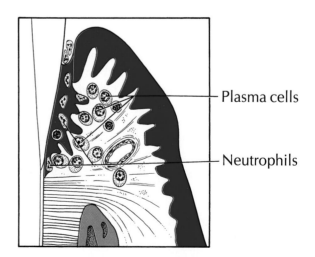

Fig. 5-7. Established lesion of gingivitis-periodontitis. The junctional epithelium is converted into pocket epithelium. Pocket formation may begin. The predominant inflammatory cells are plasma cells.
(Redrawn from Schluger S et al: Periodontal disease, *ed 2, Philadelphia, 1990, Lea & Febiger.)*

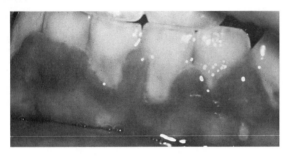

Fig. 5-8. Gingivitis.   The interproximal gingiva is bulbous and inflamed. Note the erythematous and edematous tissue extending onto the labial portions of the lateral incisors.

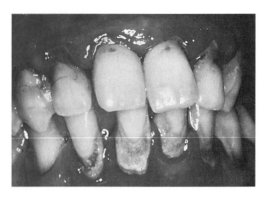

Fig. 5-10.   Periodontitis. Plaque and calculus accumulation has resulted in a loss of connective tissue attachment apical to the CEJ.

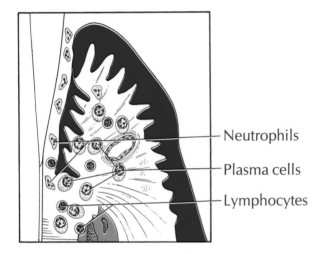

Neutrophils

Plasma cells

Lymphocytes

Fig. 5-9.   Advanced lesion of gingivitis-periodontitis. Pocket formation has begun, with a loss of connective tissue attachment apical to the CEJ. Bone is converted into fibrous connective tissue and is subsequently lost. The predominant inflammatory cells are plasma cells, and there are scattered lymphocytes present.
(Redrawn from Schluger S et al: Periodontal disease, ed 2, Philadelphia, 1990, Lea & Febiger.)

located at the apical portion of the gingival sulcus, and the inflammation is centered in a relatively small area. There is continuing loss of connective tissue, with persistence of the features of the early lesion. This stage exhibits a predominance of plasma cells, the presence of immunoglobulins in the connective tissue, and a proliferation of the junctional epithelium (Fig. 5-8). Pocket formation, however, does not necessarily occur.

Advanced Lesion.   It is difficult to pinpoint the time at which the established lesion of gingivitis results in a loss of connective tissue attachment to the tooth structure and becomes an advanced lesion or overt periodontitis (Fig. 5-9). Upon conversion to the advanced stage, the features of an established lesion persist. The connective tissue continues to

lose collagen content, and fibroblasts are further altered. Periodontal pockets are formed, with increased probing depths, and the lesion extends into alveolar bone. The bone marrow converts to fibrous connective tissue, with a significant loss of connective tissue attachment to the root of the tooth. This is accompanied by the manifestations of immunopathologic tissue reactions and inflammatory responses in the gingiva.

Periodontitis.   When a loss of connective tissue attachment occurs, the lesion transforms from gingivitis into periodontitis (Fig. 5-10), a disease that may be characterized by alternating periods of quiescence and exacerbation. The extent to which the lesion progresses before it is treated will determine the amount of bone and connective tissue attachment loss that occurs. It will subsequently affect the prognosis of the tooth with regard to restorative demands.

EXAMINATION, DIAGNOSIS, AND TREATMENT PLANNING

Before treatment is rendered, all facts and findings related to the patient's disease state should be recorded.[23,24] These data can then be used to formulate a precise working blueprint for the proposed treatment. The diagnosis and treatment-planning stages should be completed before therapy is initiated. In general practice, the data collection, diagnosis, and treatment-planning for a patient's restorative needs are accomplished at approximately the same time.

The treatment plan should be concise, logical, and rational—a realistic approach to therapy. It should not be a rigid or inflexible sequence of events, because often it will need to be amended as new information or changing circumstances dictate. The timing and sequencing of treatment are important to correcting the patient's dental problems as efficiently as possible.

The following is a viable working model for periodontal treatment:

INITIAL THERAPY
   Control of microbial plaque
     Toothbrushing
     Flossing
     Other aids
   Scaling and polishing
   Correction of defective and/or overhanging restorations
   Root planing
   Strategic tooth removal
   Stabilization of mobile teeth
   Minor tooth movement
EVALUATION OF INITIAL THERAPY
SURGICAL THERAPY
   Soft tissue procedures
     Gingivectomy
     Open debridement
     Mucosal repair (see Chapter 6)
   Hard tissue procedures
     Bone induction
     Osseous resection
   Treatment of furcation involvements
     Odontoplasty-osteoplasty
     Root amputation
     Hemisection
     Provisionalization
     Restoration
EVALUATION OF SURGICAL THERAPY
GUIDED TISSUE REGENERATION
(HARD AND SOFT TISSUE PROCEDURES)
   Technique
   Restoration
MAINTENANCE
PROGNOSIS

INITIAL THERAPY

Initial therapy consists of all treatment carried out in advance of evaluation for the surgical phases of periodontal therapy. A number of procedures in each patient's treatment regimen may be accomplished before more definitive or invasive approaches are undertaken.

Control of Microbial Plaque. The most critical aspect of periodontal therapy is the control of microbial flora in the sulcular area. If the patient does not maintain excellent oral hygiene and thereby the optimum condition of soft and hard tissues, subse-

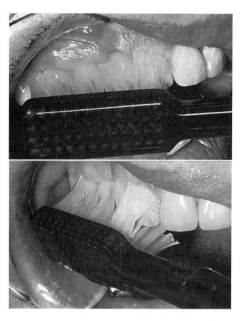

Fig. 5-11. Bass sulcular method of toothbrushing.

quent periodontal and restorative treatments will be jeopardized.

Bacterial plaque occurs on all surfaces of the teeth but is especially prevalent on the gingival third.[25] It is strongly adherent to the tooth structure, which means that it is not removed by the chewing of fibrous foods.[26] The prevention of plaque accumulation, by either mechanical or chemical means, is critical to the prevention of hard and soft tissue pathosis. Although there are chemical means for removing plaque accumulation, only mechanical methods will be considered in this text. For excellent reviews of the subject of chemical plaque removal, refer to standard periodontal texts.[5,7]

Toothbrushing. Plaque removal is accomplished with a toothbrush and other orophysiotherapy aids. Many types of toothbrushes can be used and are classified according to their size, shape, length, bristle arrangement, and whether they are manually or electrically powered. Reviews of the many types of brushes and alternate techniques can be reviewed in standard periodontal textbooks.[4-7] The soft-bristle brush is particularly effective for cleaning in the gingival sulci and at buccal and lingual surfaces of interproximal areas[27,28] without causing gingival damage and tooth abrasion that can result from a hard-bristle brush.[29]

Technique. In toothbrushing, effective placement of the bristles is more important than the amount of energy expended. The Bass sulcular method of brushing (Fig. 5-11) is preferred for most fixed prosthodontics patients because it cleans the sulci, where the margins of restorations are often placed.

The bristles are placed in the sulci at an angle of approximately 45 degrees to the tooth surface, directed gingivally, and moved back and forth with short scrubbing motions under light pressure. The brush is applied in a similar manner throughout the mouth on all buccal and lingual or palatal surfaces of the teeth. In the anterior area, where interproximal spaces are small and where it may seem impossible to place the brush horizontally against the gingiva, the brush can be turned vertically for better access. After the sulcular areas have been cleansed, the occlusal surfaces are brushed, as is the dorsal surface of the tongue. For excellent descriptions and illustrations of toothbrush placement, refer to standard periodontal texts.[5-7]

Flossing. Interproximal plaque can be controlled with dental floss.[30,31] Both waxed and unwaxed types will clean proximal surfaces, but the unwaxed floss has several advantages[32]:

1. It is smaller in diameter and thus more easily passed through interproximal contact areas.

2. It flattens out under tension, and thus each separate thread effectively covers a larger surface area.

3. It makes a squeaking noise when applied to a clean tooth surface, which can be used as a guide to effective performance.

Technique. A generous length of floss is cut and wrapped around the middle fingers of each hand. The forefingers and thumbs are used for placement (Fig. 5-12). The floss is slipped past the contact area to the base of the sulcus and is moved up and down on each proximal tooth surface until both surfaces are free of plaque. The floss is then removed and inserted in the next proximal area, systematically progressing until all the proximal surfaces have been cleaned.

Other Aids. Plaque may also be controlled effectively by orophysiotherapy aids such as dental tape, yarn, rubber and wooden tips, toothpicks, interdental stimulators, interproximal brushes, and electric toothbrushes.

When plaque is removed around a fixed partial denture or a restoration involving splinted teeth, a floss threader may be needed. Alternatively, special

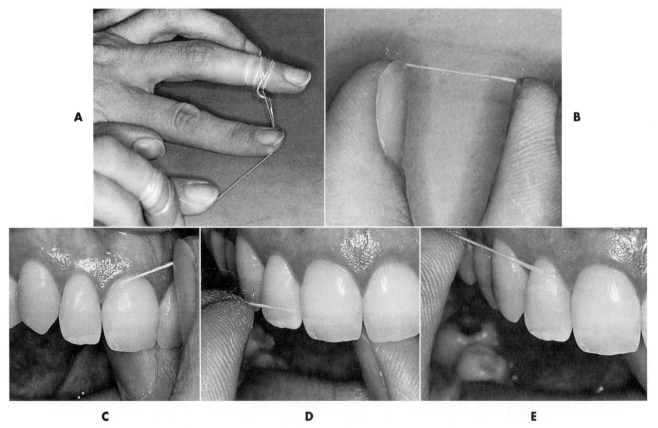

Fig. 5-12.   Proper use of dental floss. **A,** Forefinger grip for positioning. **B,** Thumb grip for positioning. **C,** The floss is placed apical to the contact area and is gently worked to the base of the sulcus. **D,** After cleaning the mesial portion of the proximal sulcus, the floss is moved coronally and placed at the distal portion of the sulcus. **E,** Cleaning the distal portion of the proximal sulcus (i.e., mesial of the adjacent tooth).

lengths of floss with stiffened ends are available and have been shown to be quite effective.

Disclosing agents may be used to provide better visualization of areas where plaque control is difficult or deficient. Erythrosin dye in tablet or liquid form stains plaque and is readily observable. Ultraviolet light has been used in combination with fluorescein dye to reveal plaque deposits, bypassing the undesirable red stain that remains after erythrosin use.

All the previously mentioned items are useful in removing and controlling inflammation-inducing microbial plaque. However, the most important aspect of plaque control is *patient motivation.* Without motivation, all orophysiotherapy aids and the knowledge to apply them are useless.

Scaling and Polishing.   Removal of supragingival calculus (scaling) and polishing of the coronal portion of the tooth are the first definitive steps in debridement of the teeth. Scaling consists of the removal of deposits and accretions from the crowns of teeth and from tooth surfaces slightly subgingival. This is accomplished with the use of sharp scalers or curettes. The gingiva responds to this removal of supragingival and slightly subgingival calculus with a decrease in inflammation and bleeding. Thus the patient is able to observe the first signs of therapeutic gain, especially when part or half of the mouth is instrumented at one appointment, and the remainder is done after a short amount of time has elapsed.

Correction of Defective and/or Overhanging Restorations.   Overhanging restorations, open interproximal contacts, and areas of food impaction contribute to local irritation of the gingiva and (of greater importance) impede proper plaque control. These deficiencies (Fig. 5-13) should be corrected

during the initial therapy phase of treatment by either replacement or reshaping and/or removal of the overhang (Fig. 5-14). Close cooperation and communication between the periodontist and the restorative dentist are essential during this treatment phase.

Root Planing.   Root planing (Fig. 5-15) is the process of debriding the root surface with a curette. It is a more deliberate and more delicately executed procedure than scaling and requires the administration of a local anesthetic in most instances. At

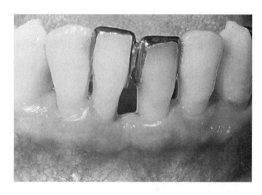

Fig. 5-14.   Recontouring of the interproximal space of the castings seen in Fig. 5-13 allows the patient to clean the area. Note the excellent gingival health between the central incisors as a result of good oral hygiene techniques.

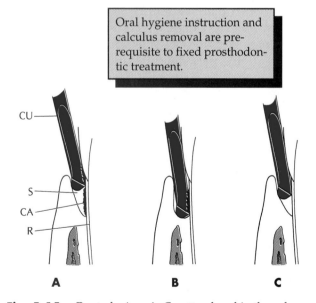

Oral hygiene instruction and calculus removal are prerequisite to fixed prosthodontic treatment.

Fig. 5-15.   Root planing. **A,** Curette placed in the sulcus to address calculus. **B,** The curette, initially placed apical to the calculus, moves coronally to dislodge the calculus. **C,** Accretions removed and the root planed to a smooth finish. *CU,* Curette; *CA,* calculus; *S,* sulcus; *R,* root surface. *(Redrawn from Carranza FA Jr: Glickman's clinical periodontology, ed 7, Philadelphia, 1990, WB Saunders.)*

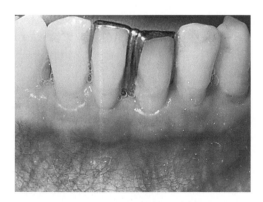

Fig. 5-13.   Overhanging splinted restoration connecting the mandibular right and left central incisors, with obliteration of the interproximal space by the castings. The patient's inability to clean this area properly has resulted in iatrogenic loss of attachment.

present it constitutes the primary mode of initial therapy in periodontics, and evidence suggests that disease progression will continue without root planing, even with effective oral hygiene.[33]

The curette is a spoon-shaped instrument well suited to cleaning and smoothing root surfaces. It is applied apically on the root with respect to the accretion and is moved coronally to lift deposits off the root surface and to plane it to a glasslike smoothness. As the patient's plaque-control techniques improve, the changes observed when root planing is completed may necessitate changing or modifying the treatment plan, and further therapy may not be indicated.

Root planing and the incidental curettage of soft tissue that accompanies it may be an end point of active periodontal therapy. In many cases the combination of root planing and improved oral hygiene on the part of the patient leads to manageable probing depths, and no further treatment is necessary. For this reason the initial therapy requires careful evaluation.

Strategic Tooth Removal.   An important part of treatment sequencing is the elimination of teeth that are hopelessly involved periodontally or are nonrestorable. Although no hard-and-fast rules exist regarding the timing of such extractions, removing teeth early in therapy is often more advantageous, when the patient has recently been informed of the prognosis and is prepared for treatment.

Extractions can be accomplished during initial therapy when the quadrant being instrumented is anesthetized. The operator can make an excellent determination of questionable teeth at this time by "sounding" the periodontium and can inform the patient of the verdict immediately. The patient is thus prepared psychologically (and also pharmacologically) for the removal. Teeth can also be removed during periodontal surgery, when the same conditions exist.

Early extraction of teeth and/or roots will allow the socket areas to heal and can provide better access for plaque control of adjacent tooth surfaces. A transitional or provisional RPD or FPD can also be fabricated and will stabilize the arch and potentially maintain or improve occlusion, function, and esthetics.[5, 7]

Stabilization of Mobile Teeth.   Tooth mobility occurs when a tooth is subjected to excessive forces, especially when bony support is lacking. It is not necessarily a sign of disease, because it may be a normal response to abnormal forces, and it does not always need corrective treatment. However, it is sometimes a source of discomfort to the patient, and

in these cases it should be treated by reduction of the abnormal forces after occlusal evaluation. Depending on the patient's need, the teeth may also be treated by splinting with provisional restorations (see Chapter 15) or an acid-etch resin technique (see Chapter 26) in conjunction with occlusal adjustment (see Chapter 6). Such restorations should be carefully designed so they do not impede plaque control or future periodontal treatment. Close communication between the periodontist and the restorative dentist is critical in this phase of treatment.

Minor Tooth Movement.   Orthodontics can be of major benefit to periodontal therapy. Malposed teeth may be realigned to make them more receptive to periodontal treatment and to improve the efficacy of plaque-control measures. As seen in Chapter 6, restorative procedures can also be aided by minor tooth movement. Thus, for the best treatment of a patient with complex dental problems, good communication among consulting dentists is essential.

EVALUATION OF INITIAL THERAPY

The periodontium recovering from active disease should be regularly reexamined and reevaluated to determine the efficacy of treatment. Soft tissue responses to the initial therapy are observed along with the patient's motivation and ability to maintain a relatively inflammation-free state. Probing depths should be recorded again, and the location of the mucogingival junction noted in relation to the teeth. Changes must be assessed in regard to the necessity of further periodontal treatment.

Reevaluation gives the practitioner a firmer grasp on the progress of treatment, and if necessary, it allows revision of the initial treatment plan. At this time, the gingiva is healthier, probing depths may have decreased because of better plaque control and root planing, and an improved working knowledge of the patient's abilities and desires should exist. The combination of these factors facilitates decisions regarding further treatment of the periodontium and allows a more informed prognosis.

SURGICAL THERAPY

There are a number of surgical procedures for the improvement of plaque removal aimed primarily at reducing or eliminating probing depths. Accurately diagnosing and choosing the most appropriate surgical regimen is crucial for maximum results.

Soft Tissue Procedures
Gingivectomy.   Gingivectomy is the removal of diseased or hypertrophied gingiva. Introduced by G.V. Black,[34, 35] it was the first periodontal surgical

approach to gain widespread acceptance. Gingivectomy is essentially the resection of keratinized gingiva only, and it may be applied to the treatment of suprabony pockets[36] and to fibrous or enlarged gingiva, particularly when they result from diphenylhydantoin (Dilantin) therapy[37] (see Fig 1-4). However, it is unsuitable for the treatment of infrabony defects.

Technique. The surgical technique consists of establishing bleeding points (Fig. 5-16) at the base of the gingival sulcus with a pocket marker or periodontal probe to serve as a guide for the gingival excision. The initial incision (Fig. 5-17) is made to these points in a beveled fashion with firm, continuous strokes from the gingivectomy knife. The interproximal tissue is freed by sharp excision and is removed from the site. The resulting ledge of tissue at the buccal and lingual or palatal terminations of the incision (Fig. 5-18) is then smoothed with the knife or a rotary instrument to a margin continuous with the remaining tissue.

After vigorous debridement of the newly accessible tooth surfaces, a surgical dressing is applied for protection and hemostasis; it remains in place for 7 to 10 days. When it is removed, oral hygiene procedures are immediately resumed (Fig. 5-19).

Contraindications. The major contraindication to gingivectomy-gingivoplasty is the absence of attached keratinized tissue. The procedure should be confined to areas of keratinized tissue to prevent leaving gingival margins that consist of alveolar mucosa (which is ill-suited to resisting the trauma of restorative procedures and mastication).

Open Debridement (Modified Widman Procedure). Open debridement or curettage is a surgical procedure designed to gain better access to root surfaces for complete debridement and root planing. The modified Widman approach[38] has been advocated in recent years, because it allows good soft tissue flap control, minimum surgical trauma, and good postoperative integrity without excessive loss of osseous tissue or connective tissue attachment.

Technique. A sulcular or minimal internal bevel incision (Fig. 5-20) is made on the buccal or the lingual surfaces of the mandibular teeth. Next, a scalloped internal bevel incision is made on the palatal surfaces of maxillary teeth. The palatal flap is then thinned and the underlying connective tissue removed. The resulting flaps are reflected minimally yet sufficiently to allow access for complete debridement of the root surfaces and degranulation of any osseous lesions in the field. No osseous resection is accomplished, except where necessary for proper flap placement. The flaps are then carefully coapted and sutured to promote healing by primary intention (Fig. 5-21).

Mucosal Repair. Mucosal reparative surgery is used to increase the width of the band of keratinized gingiva. It is particularly useful where

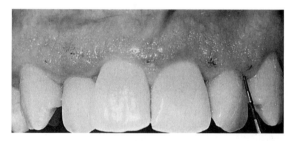

Fig. 5-16. Demarcation of pocket depth before the initial incision of a gingivectomy.

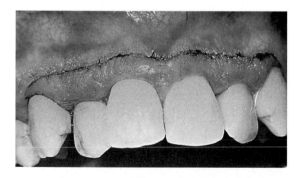

Fig. 5-17. Initial incision for the gingivectomy.

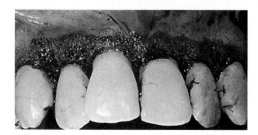

Fig. 5-18. Final gingival contours after removal of the coronal tissue and beveling of the incised area.

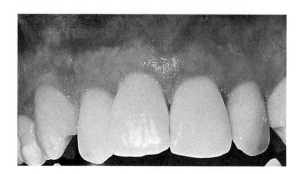

Fig. 5-19. Result of the gingivectomy, 6 months after surgery. Note the excellent gingival health and contours.

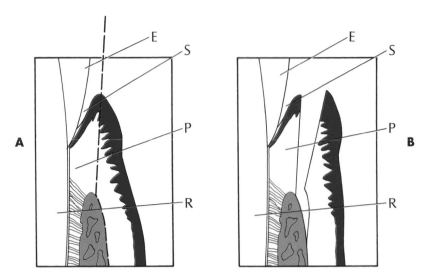

Fig. 5-20.   Internal bevel incision. **A,** Ending on the bone, to allow reflection of the flap. **B,** Flap reflected. The supracrestal connective tissue and epithelium are to be removed. *E,* Enamel; *S,* sulcus; *P,* supracrestal periodontium; *R,* root.
(Redrawn from Carranza FA Jr: Glickman's clinical periodontology, ed 7, Philadelphia, 1990, WB Saunders.)

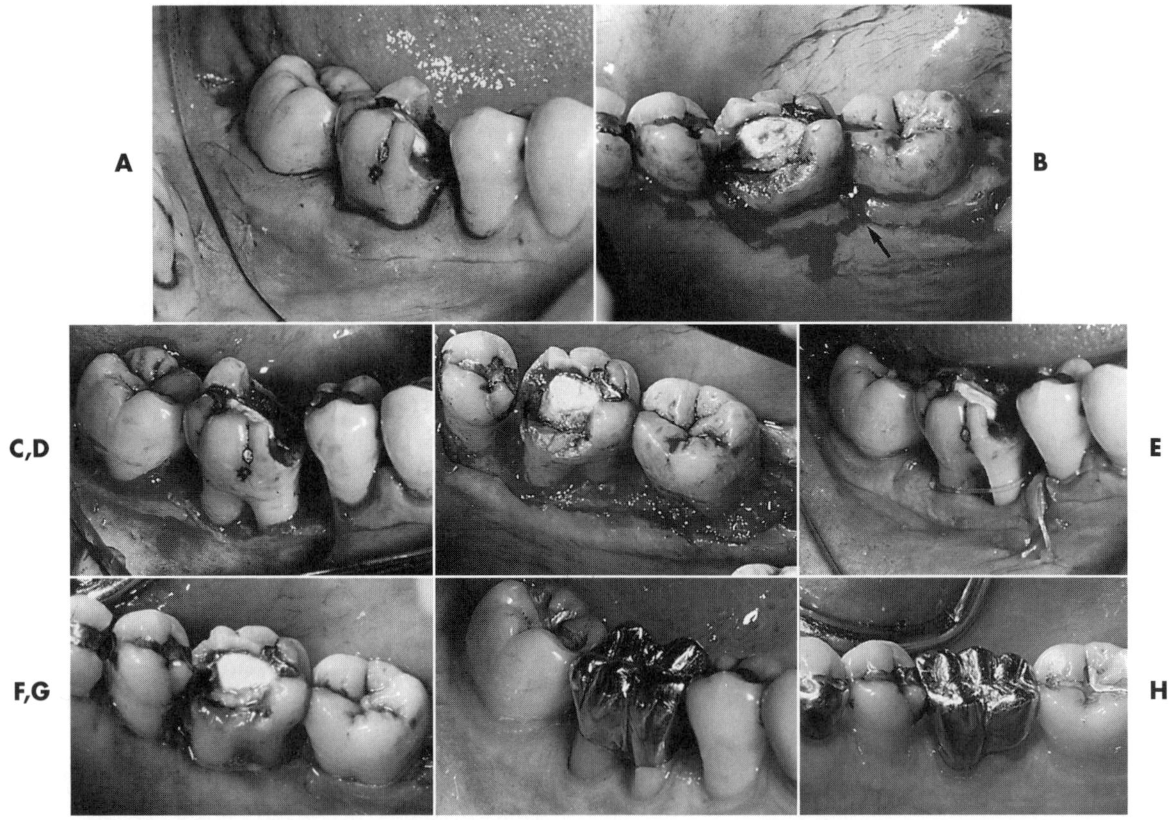

Fig. 5-21.   **A,** Initial thinning incision on the buccal for open debridement. **B,** Lingual flap thinned. **C,** Roots planed to remove subgingival accretions. **D,** Roots debrided and planed. **E and F,** Flaps coapted and sutured. **G and H,** The completed restoration, with a healthy periodontium.

complete-coverage restorations are planned (see Chapter 6 for a more detailed discussion).

Hard Tissue Procedures

Hard tissue therapy is aimed at modifying the topography of areas where plaque control is difficult or impossible. Two examples are obvious:

1. In areas where an irregular pattern of bone loss has led to intrabony pockets.
2. Around root furcations (hard tissue procedures may include techniques for the induction of new bone formation, for the judicious removal of bone by surgery, and for tooth modification or root resection.)

Bone Induction. Intrabony lesions (Fig. 5-22) are categorized as one-walled, two-walled, or three-walled, depending on the remaining osseous topography. The three-walled defect responds best to inductive or degranulation procedures, with resulting new attachment and resolution of all or part of the lesion. The one-walled and two-walled (crater) defects respond better to pocket elimination procedures.[39]

Many materials have been used to fill osseous defects: ceramic,[40] sclera,[41] cartilage,[42] bone chips,[43] cementum and dentin,[44] osseous coagulum,[45] freeze-dried bone,[46] iliac crest marrow,[47,48] hydroxylapatite,[49] tricalcium phosphate,[50] and bioactive glass materials.[51,52] Results have been mixed, and no currently available alloplastic grafting material is clearly superior to any other in the regeneration of periodontal defects.

Technique. After the flaps have been reflected and the lesion thoroughly degranulated, the grafting material is packed firmly into the lesion until it is slightly overfilled. The flaps are then coapted, and interrupted sutures are placed (Fig. 5-23). A surgical dressing is applied and removed after 7 to 10 days.

Osseous Resection with Apically Positioned Flaps. Chronic inflammatory periodontitis results in the loss of osseous tissue, destruction of osseous architecture, and creation of an intrabony lesion. The osseous tissue has no predictable or simple pattern of loss; the resorption may take the form of craters, hemiseptal defects, or well-like (troughlike) shapes. Craters in the interproximal areas (Fig. 5-24) are the most common type of lesion.[4]

The objective of osseous resection is to shape the bone to form even contours. This is accomplished by leveling interproximal lesions, reducing osseous recontour lesions that are too wide and/or shallow for predictable repair or bony fill, thinning bony ledges, and eliminating or ramping crater defects. The result is intended to be a sound osseous base for gingival attachment and the elimination of pockets and excessive sulcular depth. Long-term studies[53-55] have shown that although osseous resection surgery results in attachment loss and gingival recession, it is the most effective therapy for decreasing pocket depth, which can subsequently be maintained by the patient.

Technique. Before **reflection** of the flaps, the osseous topography of the lesion is assessed. After the area to be treated has been anesthetized, a periodontal probe is inserted into the pocket and forced through the epithelial attachment and connective tissue to the osseous crest. Multiple probings are made and the surface morphology is observed. This "sounding" of the bone provides a reasonable representation of the width and depth of the lesion and is helpful in designing the incision.

Inverse bevel incisions are made on the buccal and lingual or palatal surfaces, and full-thickness mucoperiosteal flaps are reflected to expose the osseous tissue. After the flaps are thinned and the lesions are thoroughly degranulated, the roots of the teeth are planed vigorously. Osseous resection is then accomplished by the combination of rotary instrumentation with carbide and/or diamond burs, chisels, and bone files. When osteoplasty of the interproximal sluiceways, furcation areas, and buccal and lingual bone is completed, the flaps are positioned at the crest of the bone in an apical position on the tooth. Surgical dressings are applied, and in 7 to 10 days, the patient is seen again for suture removal and dressing removal or change.

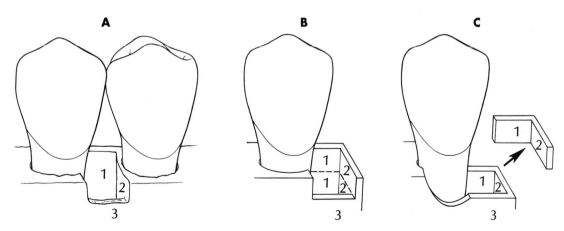

Fig. 5-22. Osseous defects. **A,** Three walls of bone present: at the lingual *(1)*, distal *(2)*, and buccal *(3)*. **B,** Two walls of bone *(1* and *2)* in the coronal portion of the defect and three walls *(1, 2,* and *3)* in the apical portion. **C,** The two coronal walls have been removed and the buccal surface of the bone recontoured, leaving the apical three-walled defect to fill with bone after degranulation.
(Redrawn from Carranza FA Jr: Glickman's clinical periodontology, ed 7, Philadelphia, 1990, WB Saunders.)

A   B   C

D   E   F

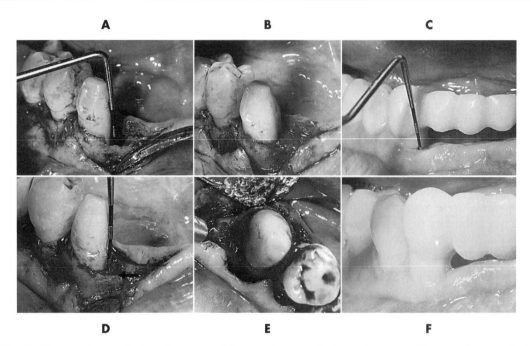

Fig. 5-23. **A,** Degranulation of a mesial defect on the mandibular right canine. This is a three-walled defect, with approximately 9 mm of intrabony lysis. **B,** The defect has been filled (slightly overfilled) with autogenous iliac crest marrow coagulum. **C,** Sulcular depth of approximately 3 mm 4 months after surgery. **D,** Osseous fill at reentry 1 year after surgery. Note the rim of bone at the margin of a previously existing defect *(arrow).* **E,** 1 year after surgery there is a near-total fill of the defect. The rim of bone demarcates the margin of the previous intrabony lesion. **F,** Result of osseous grafting at the mesial of the canine 15 months after surgery. The gingival health and contours are excellent. Note the acrylic resin provisional restoration in place before the final restoration.

A   B   C

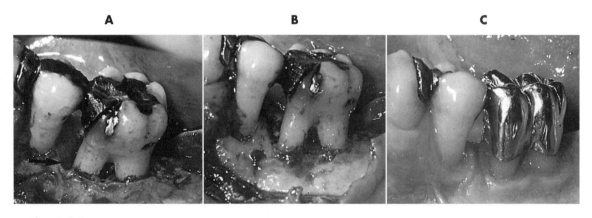

Fig. 5-24. **A,** Osseous ledge and a crater defect. **B,** Osseous recontouring. **C,** Final restoration 3 months after apical positioning of the flap.

Postsurgical Healing. Postsurgically, the healing of the periodontium must be considered before any restorative procedures are performed. Initial connective tissue and epithelial healing is complete at 4 to 6 weeks. Final tissue maturation and sulcus reformation, however, may not be complete until 6 months to 1 year after surgery.

If the margins of the restorations are to be placed intrasulcularly (subgingivally) or at the gingival crest or if gingival displacement procedures are to be used in making the impression, waiting as long as possible postsurgically before attempting these procedures is recommended. If the restorative margins are to be placed at a suprasulcular (supragingival) position (which may not necessitate the use of a gingival displacement cord), these restorations may be started when the gingiva exhibits initial reepithelialization and a return to clinical health (approximately 4 to 6 weeks).

Treatment of Furcation Involvement
Diagnosis and treatment of furcation involvement of multirooted teeth is one of the more difficult

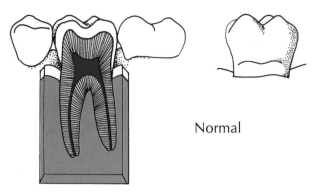

Fig. 5-25. Normal relationship of the CEJ and the osseous crest.
(From Baima RF: J Prosthet Dent 56:138, 1986.)

problems encountered in the periodontal-restorative dentistry continuum. Familiarity with the furcation's anatomic and morphologic variations is essential when formulating a treatment plan and prognosis for multirooted teeth.

Classification of Involvements. Furcation involvements can be classified as Class (or Grade) I, II, III, and IV. Because these classifications are arbitrary, however, the reader should refer to periodontal textbooks and other readings[5-7, 56] for further detail and clarification.

The normal position of the osseous crest (Fig. 5-25) is approximately 1.5 mm apical to the cementoenamel junction (CEJ) in a young, healthy adult. If vertical loss of periodontal support is less than 3 mm apical to the CEJ, this is considered to be Class I involvement (Fig. 5-26, *A*). There is no gross or radiographic evidence of bone loss. Clinically the furca can be probed up to 1 mm horizontally. If vertical loss is greater than 3 mm but the total horizontal width of the furcation is not involved, Class II involvement (Fig. 5-26, *B*) exists. A portion of the bone and periodontium remains intact, but osseous loss is evident on radiographs. The furca is penetrable more than 1 mm horizontally but does not extend through-and-through.

A horizontal through-and-through lesion that is occluded by gingiva but allows passage of an instrument from the buccal, lingual, or palatal surface is defined as a Class III involvement (Fig. 5-26, *C*). The degree of osseous loss is grossly evident on radiographs. A horizontal through-and-through lesion that is not occluded by gingiva is defined as a Class IV involvement (Fig. 5-26, *D*).

Review of Root Anatomy. The discussion of root anatomy is logically divided into maxillary and mandibular teeth.

Most maxillary molars have three roots—mesiobuccal, distobuccal, and palatal—although

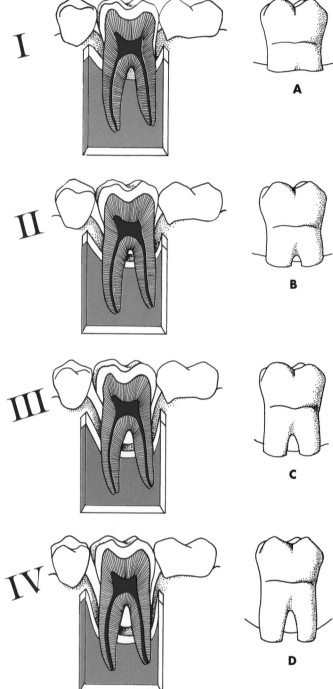

Fig. 5-26. Furcation involvements. **A,** Class I. **B,** Class II. **C,** Class III. **D,** Class IV.
(From Baima RF: J Prosthet Dent 56:138, 1986.)

there may be variations, such as fused roots or fewer roots, particularly with second and third molars. The mesiobuccal root of most maxillary molars, especially the first molar, is usually biconcave and curves to the distal. The distobuccal root also is biconcave and somewhat less curved. The palatal root is wide buccolingually and mesiodistally and palatally diverges from the crown of the tooth. This configuration is unique to human dentition and may pose special problems when preparing, restoring, and designing restorations. The distobuccal and palatal roots tend to be in the same plane distally, and the distal furcation is more apical on the tooth than the mesial furcation. In spite of this anatomy, the distal furca is more often involved in periodontal lesions than the mesial furca. From the apical perspective, a groove tends to unite the buccal and mesiopalatal openings of the trifurcation and can be probed when there is furca involvement.

Most mandibular molars have two roots—mesial and distal—although, as with maxillary molars, there may be variations. The mesial root is flattened buccolingually, with concave surfaces on each proximal side. It curves distally, especially in first molars. The distal root is wider buccolingually than the mesial root and is concave on its mesial side. Its apex is often curved distally with a flat or convex distal aspect. Both root surfaces of mandibular molars facing the furca are concave, resulting in an osseous chamber that is wider mesiodistally than either the buccal or the lingual furcation opening. The roof of the furcation is difficult to maintain because of mesiodistal **bifurcation** ridges.

NOTE: Maxillary and mandibular second and third molars often have more apically placed furcas than first molars and often exhibit fused roots with little or no furcation.[57-59]

Maxillary premolars, particularly first premolars and (at times) mandibular premolars, also have furcations. However, because they are rarely amenable to treatment by odontoplasty-osteoplasty or root amputation procedures,[5] they will not be discussed here. Students should refer to oral anatomy and morphology textbooks[60, 61] for further clarification and study of molar root anatomy.

Odontoplasty-osteoplasty. Lesser degrees of furcation involvement can often be controlled by root planing and scaling, adequate oral hygiene, and/or gingivectomy-gingivoplasty. However, when the involvement is more extensive, recontouring of the tooth or bone may be necessary.

Class I and incipient Class II lesions (Fig. 5-27) can be treated by reflecting the soft tissue in the fur-

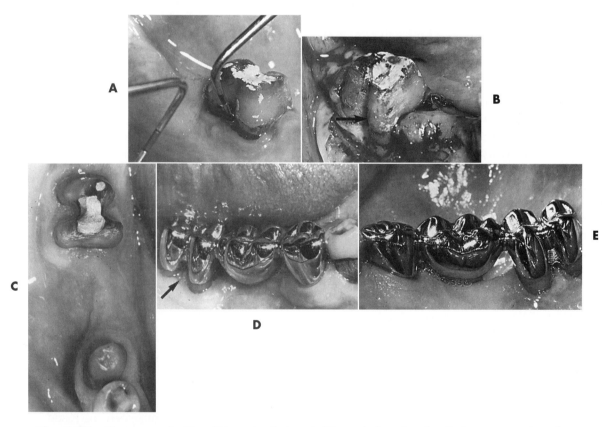

Fig. 5-27. Treatment of a Class II furcation lesion. **A,** The periodontal probe discloses approximately 3 mm of horizontal involvement. **B,** The lesion reduced to Class I by odontoplasty-osteoplasty. Note the contours of the tooth at the coronal portion of the buccal furcation *(arrow).* **C,** Preparations for a fixed partial denture to be placed in the right mandibular quadrant. Note the figure-8 shape of the molar preparation. **D,** Final restoration of the molar. There is excellent gingival health in the furcation area *(arrow).* **E,** Restoration of the quadrant. Note the slight contact of pontic on ridge and the open embrasures for access by oral hygiene instruments.
(Courtesy Dr. H.J. Gulbransen.)

cation area and recontouring both the tooth structure and the supporting bone to improve access for cleaning.[4,57] Pocket elimination in this manner provides the best results and the fairest prognosis. A minimal amount of tooth structure and bone is lost, and the patient can easily maintain it.

Class II and Class III involvements can be treated by a procedure known as *tunneling*.[6,7] The osseous structure is completely removed in the furcation, converting the lesion to a through-and-through defect. Teeth suitable for tunneling must have long, divergent roots, which will facilitate penetration by an oral hygiene aid (e.g., a proximal brush or a pipe cleaner). Patient selection is particularly important, because oral hygiene and patient motivation are critical. Failure to maintain the furcation in a relatively plaque-free state may lead to caries, which are often impossible to correct. The common location of accessory canals in the roof of the furca can also be a problem. Because of irreversible pulp damage, endodontic treatment may be needed at a later date.[57, 58, 62-64]

Root Amputation. In many patients, Class II and Class III furcation lesions are most effectively treated by root amputation (Fig. 5-28), which eliminates the furcation completely. The indications are as follows[5, 7, 63, 65-67]:

1. Severe vertical bone loss involving one root of a mandibular molar or one or two roots of a maxillary molar
2. Furcation involvement that is not treatable by odontoplasty-osteoplasty
3. Vertically or horizontally fractured roots or teeth from trauma or endodontic procedures
4. Unfavorable root proximity precluding treatment by conservative measures
5. Severe caries
6. Internal or external resorption
7. Inability to treat one root canal successfully
8. Severe dehiscence and sensitivity of a root that precludes grafting procedures
9. Failure of an abutment in a long-span splint or FPD

10. Strategic removal of a root to improve the prognosis of an adjacent tooth

Certain roots will not be suitable for amputation. Individual considerations include the extent of furcation involvement, the anatomy and topography of the supporting bone, the anatomy of the root canal, and the periapical health of the tooth. The major contraindications to root resection are teeth exhibiting any of the following[5, 63, 67]:

1. Closely approximated or fused roots
2. Significantly decreased general osseous support or an increased crown/root ratio
3. Remaining structure that will not provide adequate resistance against the forces of mastication
4. Excessive loss of supporting root structure
5. Inability to be treated endodontically
6. Remaining structure that cannot be restored

Before the gingiva is reflected, the furca is probed with a curved furcation instrument so that the precise location of the bur cut can be determined (Fig. 5-29). The cut is then made over the center of the furca but slightly toward the root to be removed. This will protect the residual root and/or tooth body. Whenever possible, the cut should be made before reflecting the flap so the field will be cleaner when the osseous tissue is exposed. When the cut is made into the root to be removed, the operator is able to inspect the residual root and remaining furcation area. A lip is often created in the furcation area, however (Fig. 5-30), and after the root to be extracted has been delivered, the furcation lip is removed and the tooth is finally contoured and finished. Removing the lip from the root of the furca is crucial to the treatment's success. If this is not done, the osseous tissue will not be recontoured properly (Figs. 5-31 and 5-32), plaque control will be impaired, and, in effect, the furca will still be present.[4, 67, 68]

There are few surgical problems with root resection. The ones most frequently encountered are fracture of the root[69] and loss of a root tip in the

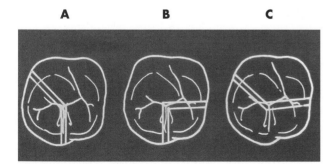

Fig. 5-28. Types of root amputation. **A,** Mesiobuccal. **B,** Distobuccal. **C,** Palatal or mesiobuccal and distobuccal.

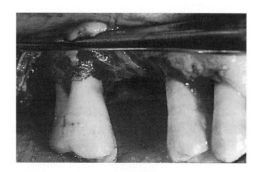

Fig. 5-29. Mesiobuccal root amputation. A full-thickness flap has been reflected to reveal Class I buccal furcation involvement and a Class II lesion in the mesiopalatal furca.

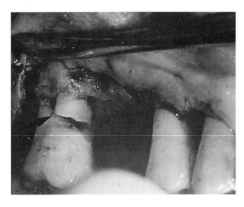

Fig. 5-30. The mesiobuccal root is sectioned at approximately 45 degrees to the tooth trunk. The section has been made into the root that is to be removed, and the result is a lip at the buccal furca.

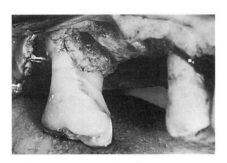

Fig. 5-31. Final osseous contours after removal of the mesiobuccal root and osteoplasty-ostectomy. The furcation lip has also been removed.

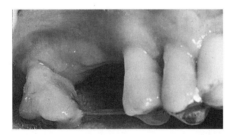

Fig. 5-32. Mesiobuccal root amputation, 2 months after surgery. The remaining tooth structure is stabilized with a wire-and-acrylic resin provisional splint.

maxillary sinus.[70, 71] Osseous anatomic features like a flat mandibular shelf and a flat palatal area can make access to the surgical site difficult and may complicate flap placement. Root proximity may complicate flap placement. Root proximity can pose a problem for separation and removal of the sectioned fragment from the surgical site. Mucogingival anatomy must be considered, because any flap procedure is contraindicated if there is a lack of keratinized attached gingiva.

Hemisection.[4,65-68] *Hemisection* means cutting a tooth in half. In the case of mandibular molars, hemisection is followed by removal and subsequent

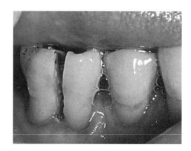

Fig. 5-33. Initial bur cut for hemisection and removal of the mesial root of a mandibular right first molar. The cut was made before reflection of the flap.

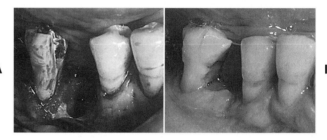

Fig. 5-34. **A,** Removal of the mesial root of a mandibular right first molar and final osseous contouring. **B,** Hemisection and removal of the mesial root, 2 months after surgery. The remaining tooth structure has been stabilized with a wire-and-acrylic resin provisional restoration.

restoration of one root or restoration of each half of the tooth. The latter procedure is sometimes called *premolarization* or *bicuspidization*.[68]

The technical procedures of hemisection and root amputation are similar (Fig. 5-33). If one hemisected root is to be extracted, osteoplasty-osteoectomy and removal of the furcation lip are performed as previously described (Fig. 5-34). If the roots are to be maintained and restored separately, the furca requires special attention for removal of furcation lips from each root. The individual roots may then be separated orthodontically, if necessary, to gain new interseptal osseous area.[62, 72]

Provisionalization. Provisional stabilization is indicated in many cases of root resection to allow proper healing of the surgical site before definitive restorations are placed and to stabilize the remaining tooth structure against masticatory forces[57, 73] (Fig. 5-35).

Normally, an acrylic resin provisional restoration (Fig. 5-35, *A*) is provided (as described in Chapter 15), although on occasion an existing restoration can be successfully modified as a provisional (Fig. 5-35, *D*). Acid-etch retained composite resin or amalgam with orthodontic wire (Fig. 5-35, *B, C*) can also be used on an interim basis to maintain space and stabilize remaining tooth structure.

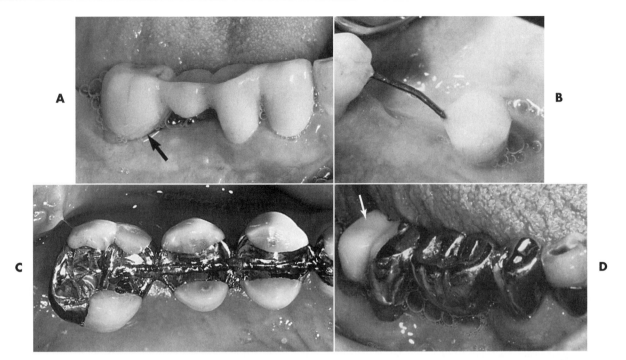

Fig. 5-35. Provisional restorations. **A,** Acrylic resin with an overcontoured area corresponding to the mesial root of the mandibular right second molar. Ideal contouring of such a provisional would remove excess resin where the root had been amputated *(arrow).* **B,** Wire-and-acrylic resin splint stabilizing the mandibular right quadrant. **C,** Wire-and-amalgam splint. **D,** Existing restoration lined with acrylic resin *(arrow).* This can serve adequately as a provisional restoration.
(**A** *courtesy Dr. S.B. Ross;* **C** *courtesy Dr. K.G. Palcanis;* **D** *courtesy Dr. H.J. Gulbransen.)*

Restoration. Teeth with a resected root or roots may be restored in a variety of ways.[57, 66, 73-75] They may be involved in a treatment plan as single units, as fixed or removable partial denture abutments, or as vertical stops for an overdenture.

The most common types of restorations for teeth with resected roots involve:

1. The remaining root restored as an individual tooth (Fig. 5-36)
2. The tooth used as an abutment for a fixed or removable partial denture[74, 76] (Fig. 5-37)
3. Premolarization—individual roots of a molar restored with premolar morphology[66] (Fig. 5-38)
4. Minimum treatment—amalgam placed in the root(s) and the occlusion adjusted[77]

EVALUATION OF SURGICAL THERAPY

The prognosis for a tooth whose root(s) have been resected and/or amputated depends on many factors. The manner in which the tooth is to be used in the restorative plan—as an abutment for a partial denture or as a single crown—has a bearing on prognosis.[7, 65] The amount of residual osseous structure to support the remaining tooth also influences the outlook. Most important, however, are the moti-

vation and oral hygiene of the patient. Long-term studies considering all of these factors have reported results ranging from 4% to 38% loss of residual roots with up to 53 years of postsurgical service.[62, 78, 79] With careful diagnosis, treatment planning, and good surgical technique, the tooth with resected roots may have a favorable prognosis. Plaque control is critical. For this reason, the patient has the final word about whether the tooth will ultimately be lost or remain as a healthy functioning unit in the dentition.

GUIDED TISSUE REGENERATION (HARD AND SOFT TISSUE PROCEDURES)

It has long been a goal of periodontal therapists to replace lost connective tissue attachment and bone. As previously described, many materials have been used in the quest for reattachment to diseased root surfaces. In the recent past, regaining lost attachment with cells from the host has been successful. Through the use of physical barriers that prevent cells from the gingival connective tissue and apically migrating oral epithelium from contacting the root surface, space is created over the root surface, which allows selective repopulation of this space by cells from the residual periodontal ligament. These

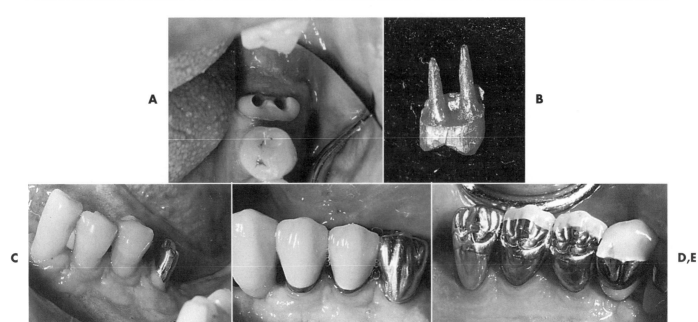

Fig. 5-36. Mesial root of a mandibular left first molar prepared for a single crown restoration. **A,** Canals have been made parallel for a dowel and core. **B,** Casting with parallel dowels. **C,** Dowel and core restoration cemented and the root prepared for a single crown. **D** and **E,** Single nonsplinted restoration of the mesial root of a mandibular left first molar.

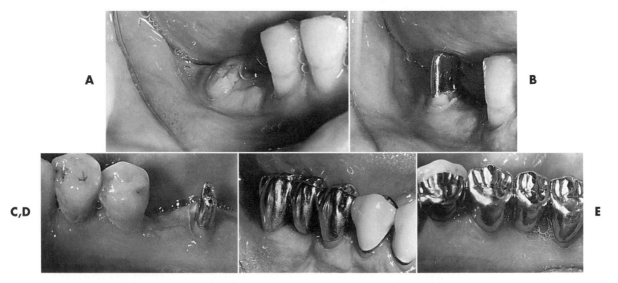

Fig. 5-37. Distal root of a mandibular right first molar prepared for a dowel and core restoration. **A,** The root will be used as an abutment for a fixed partial denture. **B** and **C,** Dowel and core restoration of the root. **D,** Final restoration, with the root used as the distal abutment for a fixed partial denture. Note the excellent gingival health and contours. **E,** Final restoration of the mandibular right quadrant, lingual view. The point contact of the totally convex pontic and the wide embrasure spaces allow optimum oral hygiene and excellent gingival health.

cells become the regenerated periodontal ligament.[80, 81]

Several types of barriers,[82-85] both resorbable and nonresorbable, as well as native periosteum,[86] have been used to regenerate the periodontium about root surfaces,[87] in furcations,[88-91] and with dental implants.[92-94] The most significant evidence has been attained by the use of a nonresorbable, polytetrafluoroethylene (PTFE) barrier (Gore-Tex Periodontal Material). Although long-term, follow-up results are not conclusive, coronal movement of the connective tissue attachment has been impressive in

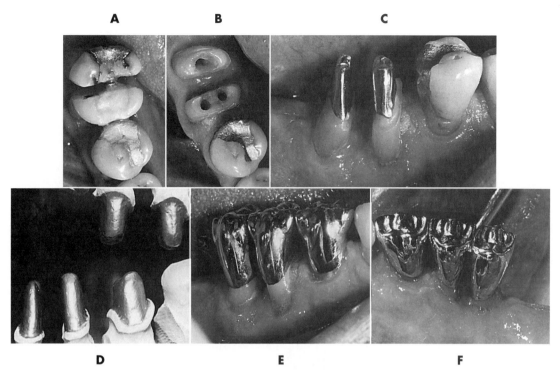

Fig. 5-38. Premolarization. Mesial and distal roots of a mandibular right first molar after hemisection. **A,** A wire-and-acrylic resin provisional is in place. **B,** The mesial and distal roots have been prepared for a dowel and core. Each will be restored as an individual premolar. Note that the distal root has been moved (orthodontically) 4 mm to the distal before the restoration was fabricated to provide room in the newly created interproximal area for the dowel and core and crown restorations. **C,** The dowel and cores in place. Note the space between the roots created by the orthodontic movement. **D,** Dies with die relief placed and mounted on a suitable articulator for fabrication of the final restoration. **E** and **F,** Final result. The open interproximal areas and flat emergence profiles from the gingival area will permit optimum oral hygiene and assist in the preservation of gingival health.

many clinical and laboratory investigations. Although **guided tissue regeneration** is a technique-sensitive mode of therapy and has yet to be viewed as widely successful, it may prove to be the most promising approach to regeneration.

Technique (Fig. 5-39 and 5-40). Following diagnosis of the lesion and any initial therapy deemed appropriate, full-thickness flaps are reflected in an attempt to maintain the maximum amount of tissue for coverage of the barrier. The lesion is completely debrided of granulation tissue, and the roots are planed thoroughly.

The barrier is placed at the CEJ and secured with sutures placed in a suspensory (sling)-type fashion, maintaining a position covering the entire root surface. The full-thickness flap is mobilized to cover the entire surface of the barrier in an apicocoronal as well as a mesiodistal direction. Antibiotic coverage and an antibacterial mouthrinse may be prescribed for the postoperative interval. Weekly monitoring for possible infection is recommended.

After a healing period of 4 to 6 weeks, a full-thickness flap is again reflected and is teased away from the external portion of the barrier. The barrier is then carefully removed to reveal a glossy and very vascular surface of new connective tissue. After the internal surface of the flap is stripped of epithelium by either sharp or rotary excision, the flap is placed to cover the entire surface of the new connective tissue. A periodontal dressing and systemic antibiotics or antibacterial mouthrinse may be used at the operator's discretion.

Recent studies[95-97] have favorably demonstrated the use of calcium sulfate (plaster of paris) as a resorbable barrier. In addition to a significantly reduced cost versus a PTFE barrier, the main advantage of this type of barrier is that the desired guided tissue regeneration may be accomplished without the need for a second surgical procedure. The technique of flap reflection, degranulation of the defect(s), and wound closure are similar to those used in other barriers (Fig. 5-41), with primary wound closure over the barrier being the surgery's main objective.

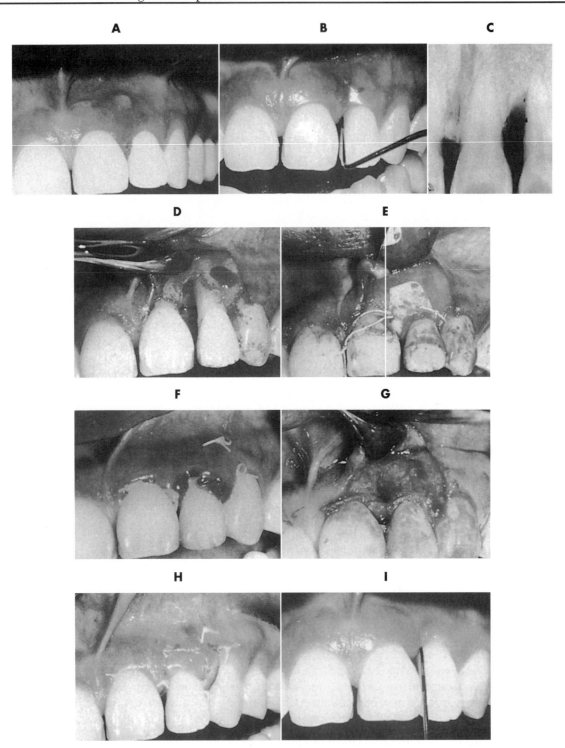

Fig. 5-39. Guided tissue regeneration about an anterior tooth. **A,** Abscess at the mesial of the left lateral incisor. **B,** After initial debridement and 3 days of antibiotic therapy. Probing depth is 8 mm. **C,** Radiograph taken at the time of barrier placement. **D,** The mesial surface after degranulation. Note the degree of bone loss. **E,** The PTFE barrier placed at the CEJ completely covers the defect. **F,** Healing at 5 weeks. Note the new connective tissue coronal to the barrier and the CEJ. **G,** When the barrier is removed, the new connective tissue can be seen at the mesial and buccal surfaces. **H,** Healing 10 days after barrier removal. **I,** Healing at 9 months. Note the minimal sulcular depth with excellent tissue health. There is slight recession of the CEJ.

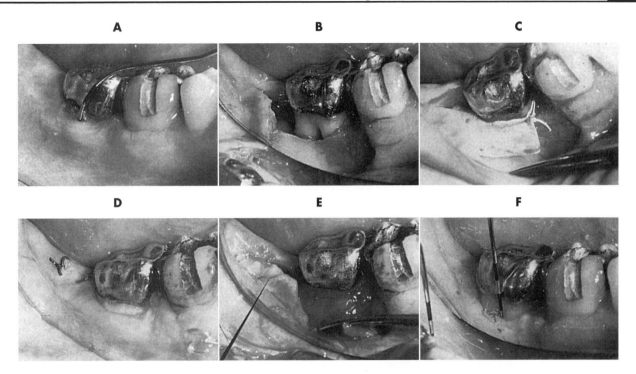

Fig. 5-40. Guided tissue regeneration in a furcation defect. **A,** Buccal aspect of a mandibular second molar showing the defect. A curved furcation probe reveals 6 mm of vertical bone loss and 3 mm of horizontal loss. **B,** With reflection of the flap, the Class II defect can be seen. **C,** PTFE barrier in place at the CEJ. **D,** Healing at 6 weeks. Note the recession of the flap at the coronal surface of the barrier. **E,** After barrier removal. Note the new connective tissue apical to the margin of the gold crown. **F,** Healing at 10 weeks. Despite minimum pocket depth, some loss of connective tissue is apparent.

Restoration. Following the completion of guided tissue regeneration procedures, a period of healing is necessary that depends on the restorative needs of the patient. As a general guideline, 6 to 8 weeks should be allowed before using displacement cord in the sulcus; this will allow tissue maturation. The subsequent restorative procedures are accomplished as described earlier.

MAINTENANCE

Continued reexamination and evaluation of periodontal status are necessary to verify the treatment's success. Of particular importance is the identification of areas where oral hygiene measures are partially effective or ineffective. The patient and the dentist must work together to preserve the health of the soft and hard tissues and prevent further periodontal breakdown or the recurrence of active disease.

There is no standard maintenance schedule for patients requiring periodontal therapy. Some should be recalled only at 5- to 6-month intervals; others should be seen by the dentist (or periodontist) *and* the hygienist every 2 or 3 months. The maintenance regimen varies greatly among individuals and requires close coordination between the patient and the involved professionals.

PROGNOSIS

The progress, course, and outcome of gingival and periodontal disease are critically dependent on the patient. *Without the ability and desire of the patient to maintain his or her teeth and periodontium, any treatment will ultimately fail.* Determining a prognosis for the teeth and periodontium debilitated from moderate disease is therefore quite difficult. Unfortunately, failure is often the best teacher.

There are many factors involved when one attempts to arrive at a prognosis for a tooth or an arch. With optimal intentions and the best technique, a favorable result can be expected (even in the absence of good host resistance). Without them, treatment is doomed to ultimate failure. The age of the patient may help in predicting the success or failure of the treatment. Generally speaking, the prognosis is better for an older patient with a given amount of lost bone or tissue attachment than for a younger one. The older individual will often be more resistant to disease, and the disease will have less effect. The amount of residual alveolar bone, the number of remaining teeth and their overall condition, any tooth mobility, and the patient's general occlusion and systemic integrity all can influence the outcome of therapy.

Also important to the long-term stability and function of the dentition are the condition of the

A   **B**   **C**

D   **E**

F   **G**

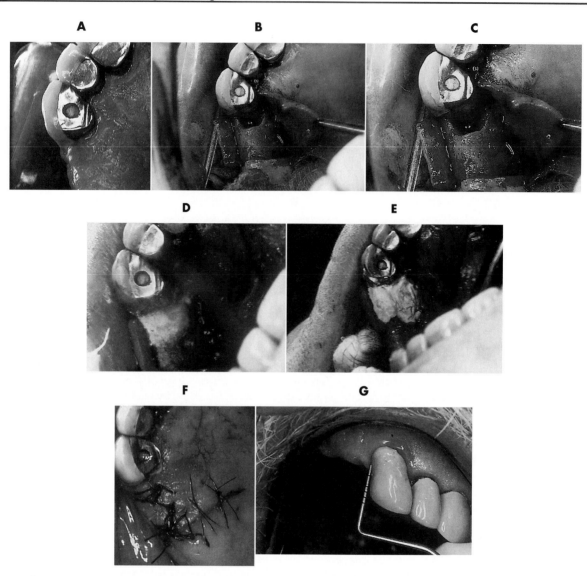

Fig. 5-41.   Guided tissue regeneration with a resorbable calcium sulfate barrier. **A,** Preoperative view of the maxillary right canine to be restored with a new crown. **B,** Flaps reflected and granulomatous tissue removed from the defect at the distal surface. **C,** Three-walled intrabony defect prepared for barrier placement. **D,** Defect is filled with dense calcium sulfate graft. **E,** Calcium sulfate slurry placed to act as a barrier and facilitate guided tissue regeneration. **F,** Minimal probing depths before final restoration. **G,** Favorable tissue contours after the elimination of the intrabony defect. *(Courtesy Dr. V. Ng.)*

arches to be restored and the ability of the restorative dentist to execute complex treatment plans without iatrogenically disturbing the gingiva and periodontium. This is a delicate undertaking and will adversely affect a periodontally unstable arch if not skillfully performed.

◼SUMMARY

The periodontium is the most important anatomic structure of the oral cavity in fixed prosthodontics. Its main component, the periodontal ligament, anchors the teeth in the alveolar processes and provides attachment, nutrition, tissue synthesis and resorption, and mechanoreception. The practitioner embarking on a restorative program must therefore first make an accurate periodontal diagnosis and then institute effective treatment of any periodontal disease—whose main etiologic factor is neglected accumulations of plaque. Allowing the proper time for healing after periodontal surgery is also very important. The healing time required depends on the design of the restoration and is critical to the correct placement of restorations near the free gingival margin.

Study Questions

1. Discuss the different types of fibers that make up the periodontal ligament.
2. Describe and discuss the processes and sequence in the development of an advanced lesion of gingivitis-periodontitis. What specifically occurs at the cellular level?
3. What are the classifications for furcation involvement?
4. List at least eight indications for root amputation. Describe the contraindications for root resection.
5. List soft tissue surgical procedures that are primarily aimed at reducing probing depths.
6. What is the typical sequence for periodontal therapy?

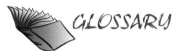

GLOSSARY

bifurcation: *(n)* (1615) *1:* division into two branches *2:* the site where a dingle structure divides into two parts, as in two roots of a tooth.

crevicular epithelium: the nonkeratinized epithelium of the gingival crevice.

crown-root ratio: the physical relationship between the portion of the tooth within alveolar bone compared with the portion not within the alveolar bone, as determined radiographically.

debridement: *(n)* (ca. 1842): the removal of inflamed, devitalized, contaminated tissue or foreign material from or adjacent to a lesion.

etiologic factors: the elements or influences that can be assigned as the cause or reason for a disease or lesion.

free gingiva: the part of the gingiva that surrounds the tooth and is not directly attached to the tooth surface.

free gingival margin: the unattached gingiva surrounding the teeth in a collar-like fashion and demarcated from the attached gingiva by a shallow linear depression, termed the *free gingival groove.*

fremitus: *(n)* (1879): a vibration perceptible on palpation; in dentistry, a vibration palpable when the teeth come into contact.

gingiva: *(n, pl)* -e: the fibrous investing tissue, covered by epithelium, which immediately surrounds a tooth and is contiguous with its periodontal membrane and with the mucosal tissues of the mouth.

hemisection: *(n):* the surgical separation of a multi-rooted tooth, especially a mandibular molar, through the furcation in such a way that a root and the associated portion of the corn may be removed.

lengthening of the clinical crown: a surgical procedure designed to increase the extent of supragingival tooth structure for restorative or esthetic purposes by apically positioning the gingival margin, removing supporting bone, or both.

marginal gingiva: the most coronal portion of the gingiva; often used to refer to the free gingiva that forms the wall of the gingival crevice in health.

mucogingival junction: the junction of gingiva and alveolar mucosa.

primary occlusal trauma: the effects induced by abnormal or excessive occlusal forces acting on teeth with normal periodontal support.

reattachment: *n:* in periodontics, the reunion of epithelial and connective tissues with root surfaces and bone such as occurs after incision or injury.

secondary occlusal trauma: the effects induced by occlusal forces (normal or abnormal) acting on teeth with decreased periodontal support.

REFERENCES

1. Bhaskar SN: *Orban's oral histology and embryology,* ed 11, St Louis, 1991, Mosby.
2. Bowers GM: A study of the width of the attached gingiva, *J Periodontol* 34:210, 1963.
3. Ainamo J, Loe H: Anatomic characteristics of gingiva: a clinical and microscopic study of the free and attached gingiva, *J Periodontol* 37:5, 1966.
4. Carranza FA Jr, Newman MG: *Clinical periodontology,* ed 8, Philadelphia, 1996, WB Saunders.
5. Schluger S et al: *Periodontal disease: basic phenomena, clinical management, and occlusal and restorative interrelationships,* ed 2, Philadelphia, 1990, Lea & Febiger.
6. Lindhe J: *Textbook of clinical periodontology,* Copenhagen, 1989, Munksgaard.
7. Genco RJ et al: *Contemporary periodontics,* St Louis, 1990, Mosby.
8. Shafer WG et al: *A textbook of oral pathology,* ed 4, Philadelphia, 1983, WB Saunders.
9. Thomas NG: Elastic fibers in periodontal membrane and pulp, *J Dent Res* 7:325, 1965.
10. Fullmer HM: A critique of normal connective tissues of the periodontium and some alterations with periodontal disease, *J Dent Res* 41(suppl 1):223, 1962.
11. Schroeder HE, Listgarten MA: Fine structure of the developing epithelial attachment of human teeth, *Monogr Dev Biol* 2:1, 1971.

12. Orban B, Kohler J: The physiologic gingival sulcus, *Z Stomatol* 22:353, 1924.

13. U.S. Public Health Service, National Institute of Dental Research, *Oral Health of United States Adults; National Findings,* NIH Publ No 87-2868 Bethesda; NIDR, 1987.

14. Schwartz RS, Massler M: Tooth accumulated materials: a review and classification, *J Periodontol* 40:407, 1969.

15. Mandel ID: Dental plaque: nature, formation, and effects, *J Periodontol* 37:357, 1966.

16. Loe HE et al: Experimental gingivitis in man, *J Periodontol* 36:177, 1965.

17. Newman HN: Calcium, matrix polymers, and plaque formation, *J Periodontol* 53:101, 1982.

18. Ritz HL: Microbial population shifts in developing human dental plaque, *Arch Oral Biol* 12:1561, 1967.

19. Slots J et al: Microbiota of gingivitis in man, *Scand J Dent Res* 86:174, 1978.

20. Allen D, Kerr D: Tissue response in the guinea pig to sterile and non-sterile calculus, *J Periodontol* 36:121, 1965.

21. Wolff L, Dahlen G, Aeppli D: Bacteria as risk markers for periodontitis, *J Periodontol* 65:498, 1994.

22. Page RC, Schroeder HE: Pathogenesis of inflammatory periodontal disease: a summary of current work, *Lab Invest* 34:235, 1976.

23. The American Academy of Periodontology: *Parameters of care. Ad Hod Committee on Parameters of Care,* Chicago, 1996, The American Academy of Periodontology.

24. The American Academy of Periodontology: Guidelines for periodontal therapy, *J Periodontol* 69:405, 1998.

25. Turesky S et al: Histologic and histochemical observations regarding early calculus formation in children and adults, *J Periodontol* 32:7, 1961.

26. Fine DH, Baumhammers A: Effect of water pressure irrigation on stainable material on the teeth, *J Periodontol* 41:468, 1970.

27. Bass CC: The optimum characteristics of tooth brushes for personal oral hygiene, *Dent Items Interest* 70:696, 1948.

28. Bass CC: The necessary personal oral hygiene for prevention of caries and periodontoclasia, *J Louisiana Med Soc* 101:52, 1948.

29. O'Leary TJ et al: *The incidence of recession in young males: relationship to gingival and plaque scores,* SAM-TR-67-97:1, July, 1967, USAF School of Aerospace Medicine.

30. Gjermo P, Flotra L: The plaque removing effect of dental floss and toothpicks: a group comparison study, *J Periodont Res* 4:170, 1969.

31. Graves R, Disney J, Stamm J: Comparative effectiveness of flossing and brushing in reducing interproximal bleeding, *J Periodontol* 60:243, 1989.

32. Arnim SS: The use of disclosing agents for measuring tooth cleanliness, *J Periodontol* 34:277, 1963.

33. Westfelt E et al: The effect of supragingival plaque control on the progression of advanced periodontal disease, *J Clin Periodontol* 25:536, 1998.

34. Black GV: *A work on special dental pathology devoted to the diseases and treatment of the investing tissues of the teeth and dental pulp,* Chicago, 1915, Medico-Dental Publishing.

35. Black AD: Treatment of chronic suppurative pericementitis, *Natl Dent Assoc J* 7:134, 1920.

36. Benjamin EM: The quantitative comparison of subgingival curettage and gingivectomy in the treatment of periodontitis simplex, *J Periodontol* 27:144, 1956.

37. Hassell TM: Epilepsy and the oral manifestations of phenytoin therapy, *Monogr Oral Sci* 9:1, 1981.

38. Ramfjord SP, Nissle RR: The modified Widman flap, *J Periodontol* 45:601, 1974.

39. Prichard J: Gingivoplasty, gingivectomy, and osseous surgery, *J Periodontol* 32:275, 1961.

40. Levin MP et al: Healing of periodontal defects with ceramic implants, *J Clin Periodontol* 1:197, 1974.

41. Klingsberg J: Periodontal scleral grafts and combined grafts of sclera and bone: two year appraisal, *J Periodontol* 45:262, 1974.

42. Boyne PJ, Cooksey DE: Use of cartilage and bone implants in the restoration of edentulous ridges, *J Am Dent Assoc* 71:1426, 1965.

43. Forsberg H: Transplantation of os purum and bone chips in the surgical treatment of periodontal disease, *Acta Odontol Scand* 13:235, 1956.

44. Schaffer EM: Cementum and dentine implants in a dog and a rhesus monkey, *J Periodontol* 28:125, 1957.

45. Robinson RE: The osseous coagulum for bone induction technique: a review, *J Calif Dent Assoc* 46:18, 1970.

46. Mellonig JT et al: Clinical evaluation of freeze-dried bone allografts in periodontal osseous defects, *J Periodontol* 47:125, 1976.

47. Dragoo MK, Sullivan HC: A clinical and histological evaluation of autogenous iliac bone grafts in humans. I. Wound healing 2 to 8 months, *J Periodontol* 44:599, 1973.

48. Schallhorn RG: Present status of osseous grafting procedures, *J Periodontol* 48:570, 1977.

49. Kenney EB et al: Bone formation within porous hydroxylapatite implants in human periodontal defects, *J Periodontol* 57:76, 1986.

50. Stahl SS, Froum S: Histological evaluation of human intraosseous healing responses to the placement of tricalcium phosphate ceramic implants, *J Periodontol* 57:211, 1986.

51. Schepers EJG, Ducheyne P: The application of bioactive glass particle of narrow size range as a filler material for bone lesions, *Bioceramics* 6:401, 1993.

52. Ong MMA et al: Evaluation of a bioactive glass alloplast in treating periodontal intrabony defects, *J Periodontol* 69:1346, 1998.

53. Olsen C, Ammons W, van Belle G: A longitudinal study comparing apically positioned flaps, with and without osseous surgery, *Int J Periodont Rest Dent* 5:11, 1985.

54. Becker W et al: A longitudinal study comparing scaling, osseous surgery and modified Widman procedures: results after one year, *J Periodontol* 59:351, 1988.

55. Kaldahl W et al: Evaluation of four modalities of periodontal therapy. Mean probing depth, probing attachment level and recession changes, *J Periodontol* 59:783, 1988.

56. Baima RF: Considerations for furcation treatment. I. Diagnosis and treatment planning, *J Prosthet Dent* 56:138, 1986.

57. Abrams L, Trachtenberg DI: Hemisection—technique and restoration, *Dent Clin North Am* 18:415, 1974.

58. Highfield JE: Periodontal treatment of multirooted teeth, *Aust Dent J* 23:91, 1978.

59. Gher ME, Vernino AR: Root anatomy: a local factor in inflammatory periodontal disease, *Int J Periodont Rest Dent* 1(5):52, 1981.

60. Cohen S, Burns RC: *Pathways of the pulp,* ed 5, St Louis, 1991, Mosby.

61. Ash MM: *Wheeler's dental anatomy, physiology, and occlusion,* ed 8, Philadelphia, 1993, WB Saunders.

62. Hamp SE et al: Periodontal treatment of multirooted teeth. Results after 5 years, *J Clin Periodontol* 2:126, 1975.

63. Ross IF, Thompson RH: A long-term study of root retention in the treatment of maxillary molars with furcation involvement, *J Periodontol* 49:238, 1978.

64. Hellden LB et al: The prognosis of tunnel preparations in treatment of class III furcations, *J Periodontol* 60:182, 1989.

65. Amen CR: Hemisection and root amputations, *Periodontics* 4:197, 1966.

66. Newell DH, Morgano SM, Baima RF: Fixed prosthodontics with periodontally compromised dentitions. In Malone WF, Koth DL, editors: *Tylman's theory and practice of fixed prosthodontics,* ed 8, Tokyo, 1989, Ishiyaku-EuroAmerica.

67. Baima RF: Considerations for furcation treatment. II. Periodontal therapy, *J Prosthet Dent* 57:400, 1987.

68. Bergenholtz A: Radiectomy of multirooted teeth, *J Am Dent Assoc* 85:870, 1972.

69. Haskell EW, Stanley HR: A review of vital root resection, *Int J Periodont Rest Dent* 2(6):28, 1982.

70. Lee FMS: The displaced root in the maxillary sinus, *Oral Surg* 29:491, 1970.

71. Waldrep AC Jr: Management of fractured root fragments, *Dent Clin North Am* 17:549, 1973.

72. Langer B et al: An evaluation of root resections: a ten year study, *J Periodontol* 52:719, 1981.

73. Basaraba N: Root amputation and tooth hemisection, *Dent Clin North Am* 13:121, 1969.

74. Polson AM: Periodontal considerations for functional utilization of a retained root after furcation management, *J Clin Periodontol* 4:223, 1977.

75. Baima RF: Considerations for furcation treatment. III. Restorative therapy, *J Prosthet Dent* 58:145, 1987.

76. Caplan CM: Fixed bridge placement following endodontic therapy and root hemisection, *Dent Surv* 54(6):28, 1978.

77. Haskell EW, Stanley HR: Resection of two vital roots, *J Endodont* 1:36, 1975.

78. Carnevale G, Pontoriero R, Hurzeler M: Management of furcation involvement, *Periodontol 2000* 9:69, 1995.

79. Carnevale G, Ponrotiero R, di Febo G: Long-term effects of root-resective therapy in furcation-involved molars: a 10-year longitudinal study, *J Clin Periodontol* 25:209, 1998.

80. Melcher AH: On the repair potential of periodontal tissues, *J Periodont Res* 47:256, 1976.

81. Aukhil I et al: Periodontal wound healing in the absence of periodontal ligament cells, *J Periodontol* 58:71, 1987.

82. Nyman S et al: The regenerative potential of the periodontal ligament: an experimental study in the monkey, *J Clin Periodontol* 9:257, 1982.

83. Magnusson I et al: New attachment formation following controlled tissue regeneration using biodegradable membranes, *J Periodontol* 59:1, 1988.

84. Pitaru S et al: Collagen membranes prevent the apical migration of epithelium during periodontal wound healing, *J Periodont Res* 22:331, 1988.

85. Cortellini P et al: Guided tissue regeneration with different materials, *Int J Peridont Rest Dent* 10:136, 1990.

86. Kwan SK et al: The use of autogenous periosteal grafts as barriers for the treatment of intrabony defects in humans, *J Periodont* 69:1203, 1998.

87. Tonetti MS et al: Generalizability of the added benefits of guided tissue regeneration in the treatment of deep intrabony defects: evaluation in a multi-center randomized controlled clinical trial, *J Periodontol* 69:1184, 1998.

88. Pontoriero R et al: Guided tissue regeneration in the treatment of furcation defects in man, *J Clin Periodont* 14:618, 1987.

89. Caffesse RG et al: Class II furcations treated by guided tissue regeneration in humans: case reports, *J Periodontol* 61:510, 1990.

90. Vernino AR et al: Use of biodegradable polylactic acid barrier materials in the treatment of grade II periodontal furcation defects in humans. I. A multicenter investigative clinical study, *Int J Periodont Rest Dent* 18:573, 1998.

91. De Deonardis D et al: Clinical evaluation of the treatment of class II furcation involvements with bioabsorbable barriers alone or associated with demineralized freeze-dried bone allografts, *J Periodontol* 70:8, 1999.

92. Becker W et al: Bone formation at dehisced dental implant sites treated with implant augmentation material: a pilot study in dogs, *Int J Periodont Rest Dent* 10:92, 1990.

93. Dahlin C et al: Membrane-induced bone augmentation at titanium implants: a report on ten fixtures followed from 1 to 3 years after loading, *Int J Periodont Rest Dent* 11:273, 1991.

94. Becker W, Becker BE: Guided tissue regeneration for implants placed into extraction sockets and for implant dehiscences: surgical techniques and case reports, *Int J Periodont Rest Dent* 10:376, 1990.

95. Sottosanti J: Calcium sulfate: a biodegradable and biocompatible barrier for guided tissue regeneration, *Compend Contin Educ Dent* 13:226, 1992.

96. Payne JM et al: Migration of human gingival fibroblasts over guided tissue regeneration barrier materials, *J Periodontol* 67:236, 1996.

97. Kim C-K et al: Periodontal repair with intrabony defects treated with a calcium sulfate implant and calcium sulfate barrier, *J Periodontol* 69:1317, 1998.

MOUTH PREPARATION

KEY TERMS

definitive periodontal
   treatment
foundation restorations
minor tooth movement

multidisciplinary
   considerations
occlusal adjustment
treatment sequence

As the scope of fixed prosthodontics has expanded, it has become increasingly clear that failures are often attributable to inadequate mouth preparation. In this case, mouth preparation refers to the dental procedures that need to be accomplished before fixed prosthodontics can be properly undertaken. Rarely are crowns or fixed partial dentures provided without initial therapy of a multidisciplinary and often extensive nature, because the etiologic factors that lead to the need for fixed prosthodontics also promote other pathologic conditions (caries and periodontal disease are the most common). These must be corrected as an early phase of treatment. Fixed prosthodontics will be successful only if restorations are placed on well-restored teeth in a healthy environment, a fact that can become obscured in the misguided attempt to try to help a patient by accelerating treatment; unfortunately, such action often leads to unforgivable failure.

This chapter reviews the ways in which treatment by the different dental disciplines relates to fixed prosthodontics. Obviously, detailed descriptions of the particular procedures are beyond the scope of this text.

Comprehensive treatment planning will ensure that mouth preparation is undertaken in a logical and efficient sequence aimed at bringing the teeth and their supporting structures to optimum health. Equally important is the need to educate and motivate the patient to maintain long-term dental health through meticulous oral hygiene practices. As a general plan, the following sequence of treatment procedures in advance of fixed prosthodontics should be adhered to:

1. Relief of symptoms (chief complaint)
2. Removal of etiologic factors (e.g., excavation of caries, removal of deposits)
3. Repair of damage
4. Maintenance of dental health

The following list describes a typical sequence in the treatment of a patient with extensive dental disease—including missing teeth, retained roots, caries, and defective restorations:

Preliminary assessment (Fig. 6-1, *A*)

Emergency treatment of presenting symptoms (Fig. 6-1, *B*)

Oral surgery (Fig. 6-1, *C*)

Caries control and replacement of existing restorations (Fig. 6-1, *D*)

Endodontic treatment (Fig. 6-1, *E*)

Definitive periodontal treatment, possibly in conjunction with preliminary occlusal therapy (Fig. 6-1, *F*)

Orthodontic treatment

Definitive occlusal treatment

Fixed prosthodontics (Fig. 6-1, *G, H*)

Removable prosthodontics (Fig. 6-1, *I*)

Follow-up care

However, the sequence of preparatory treatment should be flexible. Two or more of these phases are often performed concurrently. Carious lesions or defective restorations will often prevent proper oral hygiene measures, and their elimination or correction must be a part of preparatory treatment. If caries control results in a pulpal exposure or exacerbates an existing chronic pulpitis, endodontic treatment may be needed earlier than anticipated. When the primary symptoms have been eliminated, the occlusal needs of the patient are carefully evaluated through clinical examination and the study of articulated diagnostic casts. Extensive treatment of both arches simultaneously may be beyond the scope of the nonspecialist, and the use of cross-mounted diagnostically mounted casts should be considered (see p. 75). This enables treatment of each arch to be accomplished predictably and independently. Only when preparatory occlusal treatment is completed will the patient be ready for definitive restorative care.

A   B   C

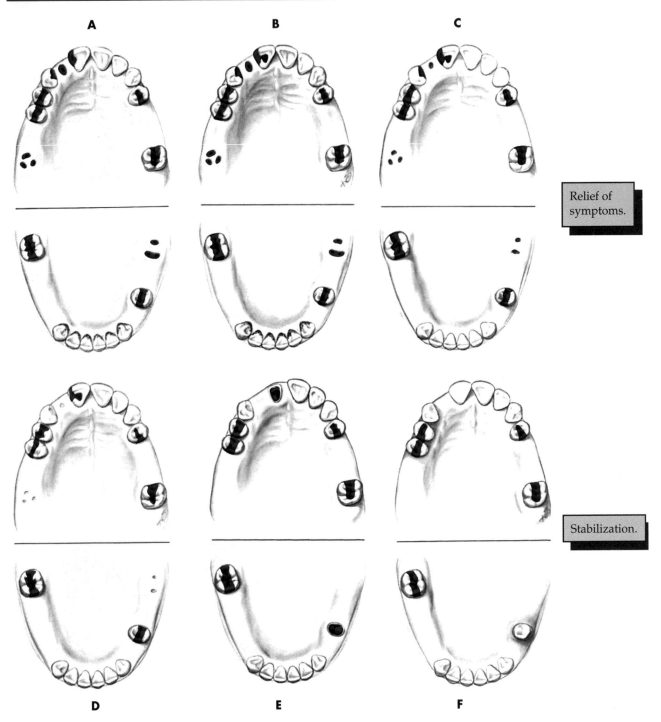

Relief of symptoms.

Stabilization.

D   E   F

Fig. 6-1. Sequence of treatment. **A,** The patient has pain that seems to originate from the maxillary right central incisor. In addition, there are several missing teeth, retained roots, caries, calculus, and defective restorations. **B,** Relief of the acute problem by endodontic treatment of the incisor. **C,** Removal of deposits and unrestorable teeth. **D,** Caries are controlled, and defective restorations are replaced. The progress of ongoing disease has been halted. **E,** Endodontic treatment is undertaken, and post-and-cores and a provisional restoration are placed. **F,** Definitive periodontal treatment is performed.

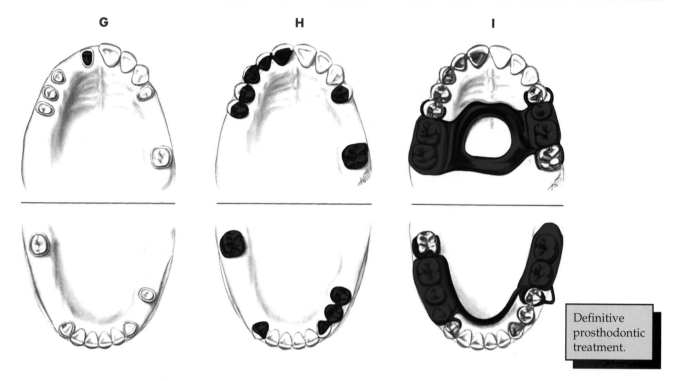

G   H   I

Definitive prosthodontic treatment.

Fig. 6-1, cont'd.   G, Teeth are prepared for the final restoration. **H,** The fixed restorations are completed. **I,** Active phase of the treatment has been accomplished. NOTE: predictable management of complex prosthodontics involving fixed and removable prostheses can be facilitated by adopting the technique described on p. 78.

ORAL SURGERY

SOFT TISSUE PROCEDURES

Any soft tissue abnormalities that may require surgical intervention should be recognized during the initial or radiographic examination. If necessary, the patient can be referred to an oral surgeon for further consultation and/or treatment. Diagnosis of pathologic conditions can be difficult, and the general practitioner should make the appropriate referral to a specialist when there is doubt.

Elective soft tissue surgery may include alteration of muscle attachments, removal of a wedge of soft tissue distal to the molars, increase of the vestibular depth, or modification of edentulous ridges to accommodate fixed or removable partial prostheses (Fig. 6-2).

HARD TISSUE PROCEDURES

Simple tooth removal is the most common surgical procedure involving hard tissue. It should be performed as early during treatment as possible for maximum healing time and osseous recontouring.

Tuberosity reduction (Fig. 6-3) is also common, especially when there is inadequate space to accommodate a prosthesis. Although maxillary or mandibular tori (Fig. 6-4) seldom interfere with the fabrication of a fixed partial denture, their excision may make it easier to design a removable partial denture and occasionally will improve access for oral hygiene measures.

Impacted or unerupted supernumerary teeth should be removed if damage to adjacent structures can be avoided.

ORTHOGNATHIC SURGERY

Candidates for orthognathic surgery require careful restorative evaluation and attention before treatment. Otherwise, an expected improvement in the facial skeleton may be accompanied by unexpected occlusal dysfunction. After surgery, the connection between plaque control, caries prevention, and periodontal health should be stressed to the patient.

IMPLANT-SUPPORTED FIXED PROSTHESES

Successful implant dentistry requires meticulous selection of the patient and skillful execution of the chosen technique. A team approach to treatment is strongly recommended with close cooperation between the specialties (see Chapter 13).

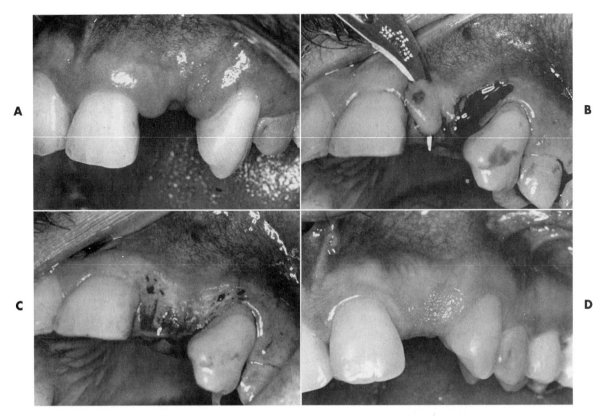

Fig. 6-2.   **A** to **D,** Soft tissue surgery to correct an unfavorable edentulous ridge before FPD fabrication.

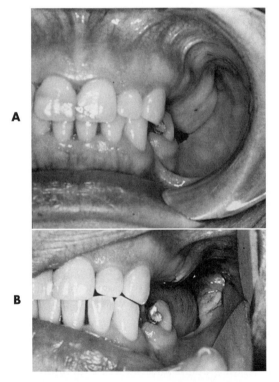

Fig. 6-3.   Tuberosity reduction was indicated for this patient to accommodate a mandibular removable partial denture. **A,** Preoperative and, **B,** postoperative appearances. *(Courtesy Dr. J. Bergamini.)*

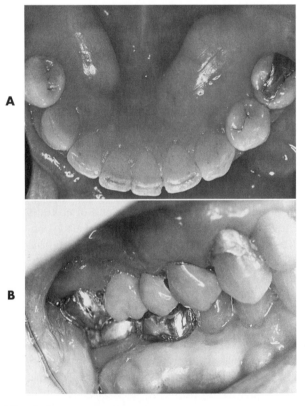

Fig. 6-4.   **A,** Mandibular torus requiring surgical reduction before the fabrication of an RPD. **B,** Buccal torus that was interfering with oral hygiene.

CARIES AND EXISTING RESTORATIONS

Crowns and fixed partial dentures are definitive restorations. They are time-consuming and expensive treatment options and should not be recommended unless an extended lifetime of the restoration is anticipated. Often, teeth requiring crowns are severely damaged or have large existing restorations. Any restoration on such teeth must be carefully examined and a determination made regarding its serviceability. If doubt exists, the restoration should be replaced. Time spent replacing an existing restoration that in retrospect might have been serviceable is a modest price to pay for the assurance that the foundation will be caries free and well restored. Studies have shown that accurately detecting caries beneath a restoration without its complete removal can be very difficult.[1-3] Even on caries-free teeth, an existing restoration may not be a suitable foundation. Preparation design is different for a foundation than for a conventional restoration, particularly regarding the placement of retention. Generally, when a crown is needed, the dentist should plan to replace any existing restorations. Although most teeth will require **foundation restorations,** small defects resulting from less extensive lesions can often be incorporated in the design of a cast restoration or can be blocked out with cement (Fig. 6-5). The latter is recommended on axial walls where an undercut would otherwise result. If a small defect is present on the occlusal surface, however, it may be better to incorporate it into the final restoration than to block it out. The difficulty, of course, is anticipating this during the preparatory phase of treatment. Assessment is more difficult when an existing crown or FPD is being replaced. Then the extent of damage can be seen only after the defective restoration has been removed.

FOUNDATION RESTORATIONS

A foundation restoration, or core, is used to build a damaged tooth to ideal anatomic form before it is prepared for a crown. With extensive treatment plans, the foundation may have to serve for an extended time. It should provide the patient with adequate function and should be contoured and finished to facilitate oral hygiene. Subsequent tooth preparation is greatly simplified if the tooth is built up to ideal contour. Then it can be prepared essentially as if it were intact. Guide grooves can be used to facilitate accurate occlusal and axial reduction (see Chapter 8), and the preparation design will be consistent from tooth to tooth. The skills learned

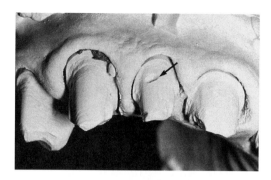

Fig. 6-5. Small defects *(arrow)* that would create undercuts are best blocked out intraorally with cement or resin.

preparing preclinical manikins with "ideal" teeth can be readily transferred to clinical practice.

SELECTION CRITERIA

Selection of the foundation material depends on the extent of tooth destruction, the overall treatment plan, and operator preference (Fig. 6-6). The effect of subsequent tooth preparation for the cast restoration on the retention and resistance of the foundation should be considered. Retention features such as grooves or pinholes should be placed sufficiently pulpal to allow adequate room for the definitive restoration. Adhesive retention may be helpful in preventing loss of the foundation during tooth preparation.

Dental Amalgam. Despite its limitations, amalgam is still the material of choice for most foundation restorations on posterior teeth. It has good resistance to microleakage and is therefore recommended when the crown preparation will not extend more than 1 mm beyond the foundation-tooth junction.[4] It can be shaped to ideal restoration form and serves well as an interim. It has better strength than the glass ionomers, and retention can be provided by undercuts, pins, or slots. Adhesive bonding systems such as those based on 4-META* are also available,[5-8] and may reduce leakage of the restoration.[9,10] Additional retention may be provided with the use of polymeric beads supplied with the Amalgambond system.[11] Amalgam requires an absolutely rigid matrix for proper condensation. Otherwise the foundation will break. Matrix placement can be demanding when restoring a tooth with little remaining coronal tissue. This is discussed in the step-by-step procedure on p. 140. Amalgam has a longer setting time than the other

---

*4-Methacryloxyethyl trimellitate anhydride.

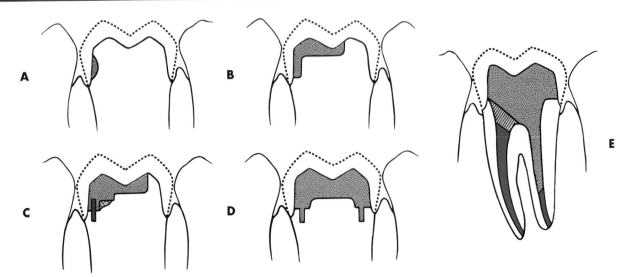

Fig. 6-6. The placement of a foundation restoration depends on the extent of damage to the tooth and should always be designed with the definitive restoration in mind. **A,** Cement. This is suitable when damage is minimal. **B,** Amalgam. **C,** Pin-retained amalgam. **D,** Cast gold. **E,** Post-and-core. (See Chapter 12.)

foundation materials. This normally delays crown preparation to a subsequent patient visit. When this presents a problem, a rapid-setting, high-copper, spherical alloy should be chosen. These can be prepared for a crown about 30 minutes after placement. Spherical amalgams are advantageous for foundation restorations because they have greater early strength than admixed materials, which makes fracture soon after placement less of a problem.[12]

Glass Ionomer Cement. This is a suitable choice for a small lesion. The material sets rapidly, enabling crown preparation to be performed with limited delay. When placed correctly, it exhibits adhesion to dentin, although conventional undercut retention is needed to supplement this. Glass ionomers designed for use as a core or **base** are radiopaque; restoration formulations are more radiolucent than dentin and should not be used as a core, because their radiographic appearance may suggest recurrent caries.[13] The presence of fluoride in glass ionomers may help prevent recurrent caries. The chief disadvantage of glass ionomers is their comparatively low strength, although newer formulations have improved properties. At this time, glass ionomers are inferior to amalgam or composite resin for the restoration of extensive lesions.[14,15]

Composite Resin. Composite resin exhibits many of the advantages of glass ionomers. It does not require condensation and sets rapidly. Formulations are available that release fluoride, which may provide an anticariogenic benefit.[16] Bonding is achieved with a dentinal bonding agent or by etching a glass ionomer liner. Neither method develops the bond strengths needed to withstand high masticatory forces, and conventional undercut retention is also needed. There are concerns about continued polymerization of the resin and its high thermal expansion coefficient, which may lead to microleakage of the crown.[17] Also of concern is the moisture sorption properties of composite resin that causes delayed expansion and may lead to axial binding of crowns made on composite resin cores.[18,19] Delayed expansion is not a problem with traditional glass ionomer,[20] but it is a problem with the resin-ionomer hybrids and the compomer materials.[19] Conventional tooth-colored composite resin is not recommended as a foundation material, because it is difficult to discern the composite-tooth junction. Special colored core materials should be used.

Pin-retained Cast Metal Core. A cast metal core should be considered for an extensively damaged tooth. The cemented foundation is retained by tapered pins. The preparation requires careful location and placement of the pinholes but otherwise is straightforward. The foundation is fabricated in the laboratory as an indirect procedure. This increases the complexity and expense of treatment but facilitates obtaining good preparation form.

Advantages and disadvantages of the available materials are summarized in Table 6-1.

Step-by-step Procedures
Amalgam Core (Fig. 6-7)
1. Isolate the tooth. Rubber dam isolation is strongly recommended for moisture control,

Foundation Restoration Materials

TABLE 6-1

	Advantages	Disadvantages	Recommended Use	Precautions
Amalgam	Good strength Intermediate restoration	Preparation delay Condensation Corrosion No bonding*	Most foundations	Well-supported matrix
Glass ionomer	Rapid setting Adhesion Fluoride	Low strength Moisture sensitive†	Smaller lesions	Moisture control
Composite resin	Rapid setting Ease of use Bonding	Thermal expansion Setting contraction Delayed expansion	Smaller lesions Anterior teeth	Moisture control
Cast gold	Highest strength Indirect procedure	Two-visit procedure Provisional needed	Extensive lesions	Alignment of pinholes

*Bonding can be achieved with 4-META products.
†Resin-modified formulations are less sensitive.

infection control, and optimum visibility. Placement follows techniques developed for conventional amalgam restorations, although with extensively damaged teeth, placing the dam can be a problem. Sometimes cotton roll isolation must suffice.

2. Design the tooth preparation with the intended cast restoration in mind. Be sure that the cast restoration does not eliminate retention of the foundation. The preparation will differ somewhat from a conventional amalgam restoration. The ensuing discussion highlights these differences.[21]

3. Limit the extent of the outline form. In contrast to conventional amalgam preparations, which are extended to include unsupported enamel and the deep occlusal fissures, a less extensive outline is recommended for foundation restorations, because the fissures and contacts are removed during crown preparation. Although minimizing foundation outline can help conserve supporting tooth structure, the foundation should be adequate for the detection of any carious lesions (Fig. 6-7, A).

4. Retain unsupported enamel if convenient. For a conventional amalgam tooth preparation, unsupported enamel must always be removed; otherwise, the enamel may fracture during function and leave a deficient margin. However, for a foundation restoration, the unsupported enamel may be preserved most effectively if it is substantial enough to withstand condensation forces and if it can be determined whether the enamel-dentin junc-

tion is caries free. Preserving unsupported enamel may facilitate matrix placement and improve amalgam condensation (Fig. 6-7, B).

5. Finish the cavosurface margins. For conventional amalgam restorations, cavosurface margins of 90 degrees are needed to minimize the potential for fracturing the enamel and amalgam during function. However, for foundation restorations, the amalgam-tooth interface will not be subjected to high stresses (they are protected by the crown), and marginal fracture is not likely to be a problem. Therefore, a 46- to 136-degree margin is acceptable. Furthermore, such a margin will conserve useful tooth substance and improve condensation (Fig. 6-7, C).

6. Remove any carious dentin carefully and thoroughly with a hand excavator or large round bur in a low-speed handpiece. Discolored but hard dentin can be left on the pulpal wall, but caries-affected areas at the enamel-dentin junction should be removed completely. If a pulp exposure occurs during the preparation, whether carious or mechanical, endodontics or tooth removal will be necessary. A direct pulp cap is not a good choice for a tooth requiring an FPD; however, if endodontics is elected and the pulp cannot be extirpated immediately, a suitable sedative dressing should be placed.

7. Create optimum resistance form. Good resistance to masticatory forces is as critical for a foundation as for a conventional restoration. Whenever possible, the tooth preparation should be perpendicular to the occlusal

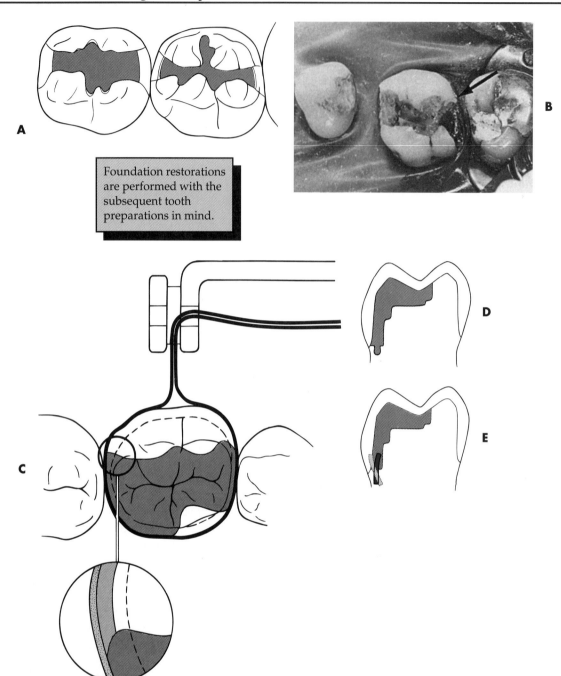

Foundation restorations are performed with the subsequent tooth preparations in mind.

Fig. 6-7. The principles of preparation design for an amalgam foundation restoration differ slightly from those for a conventional extensive amalgam restoration. **A,** The outline form of a foundation need not include fissures or proximal or occlusal contacts, provided complete caries removal can be accomplished. **B,** Unsupported enamel *(arrow)* can sometimes be left when preparing a foundation restoration. It may facilitate matrix placement and is removed when the crown is prepared. **C,** Acute cavosurface margins are acceptable for a foundation restoration but not for a definitive amalgam. **D,** Resistance form is improved by preparing the tooth in a series of steps perpendicular to the direction of occlusal force. **E,** When pin retention is used, pinholes should be drilled slightly pulpal and at an angle to the root surface *(solid line)* as compared to the way they are placed for a conventional extensive amalgam restoration *(dashed line)*. This will ensure retention for the foundation remains after crown preparation.

forces. If a sloping axial wall exists, it should be modified into a series of steps to enhance resistance form.

8. Be sure that the foundation restoration has adequate retention (augmented if necessary by pins, slots, or wells). Proper placement of retention features is essential to the preparation of a successful foundation. The features must be incorporated into the design so they are not eliminated during preparation of the crown (Fig. 6-7, *D, E*).

This can be a particular problem with the extensive reduction necessary for a metal-ceramic restoration. Pin placement is dictated by root furcations and the size of the pulp chamber. Generally, pins should be placed further pulpally than when conventional extensive pin amalgams are being provided; to prevent pulp perforation, they should be positioned at a slight angle to the long axis of the tooth. If a pin is slightly exposed during crown preparation, this may not be a problem—in contrast to the conventional pin-amalgam restoration. With a foundation restoration, the pin-amalgam interface receives little stress during function.

Retention can also be provided by slots or wells. These will create less residual stress in the dentin and will thus reduce the risk of pulp exposure or damage.[22-26] They should be placed pulpal to the intended crown margin, at a depth of about 1 mm, with a small carbide bur. Careful condensation of amalgam into the slots will ensure good restoration retention.

Bonding agents can assist amalgam retention, but adhesion is not adequate to resist occlusal loading. Currently retention is best provided by conventional means. An example of the use of bonding agents appears in Figure 6-8. If bonding agents are used, the clinician should follow the manufacturer's directions about storage and manipulation.

Bases and Varnishes. A base is necessary to prevent thermal irritation if the preparation extends close to the pulp. A material with good physical properties, such as glass ionomer or zinc phosphate, should be chosen, because weaker materials are likely to fracture during amalgam condensation. Excessively thick bases should be avoided if they would leave inadequate thickness of amalgam foundation after tooth preparation. Postoperative sensitivity can be prevented with two or more coats of cavity varnish or a dentin bonding agent. The coats should be placed after any pinholes are drilled but before the pins are placed to avoid material at the pin-amalgam interface.

Calcium hydroxide liners should be reserved for use in deep cavities when a microscopic pulp exposure is suspected. They generally have low strength and do not resist condensation forces well. Macroscopic exposures should receive endodontic treatment or, if direct pulp-capping is the only option, a conventional pin-amalgam should be placed as the definitive restoration, at least until the success of the pulp-capping can be guaranteed.

Matrix Placement. A rigid, well-contoured matrix allows the amalgam to be properly condensed and facilitates carving. However, it can present a problem when much tooth structure is missing. Conventional matrix retainers, such as the Tofflemire, are unstable if both the lingual and the buccal walls are missing. A circumferential matrix (e.g., the Automatrix*) is useful for extensive restorations. Alternatives include copper bands or orthodontic bands. These are removed by cutting with a bur after the amalgam has set. Stability of the matrix is improved by proximal wedging, by crimping to shape, and by using modeling plastic or autopolymerizing acrylic resin for external stabilization[27,28] (Fig. 6-9).

Condensation. Condensation follows conventional practice, with particular attention paid to condensing into wells and around pins. If the foundation is prepared during the same visit, a high-copper spherical alloy is chosen. A mechanical condenser is useful for large amalgam restorations.

Contouring and Finishing. Care is needed to prevent amalgam fracture during matrix removal. After allowing time for setting, the dentist trims the amalgam away from the occlusal edge of the matrix and removes the wedges and matrix retainer. At this stage it is helpful to cut the buccal ends of the matrix band with scissors close to the tooth. Then the band can be pulled through the proximal contacts toward the lingual. Pulling the band occlusally is more likely to fracture the freshly placed amalgam.

Contouring follows conventional practice if the foundation is to serve for a significant period. Such a foundation should also be finished to facilitate plaque control. If the foundation is to be prepared shortly after placement, a more rudimentary occlusal contour is acceptable. However, the occlusal contour should be adequate to provide proper tooth stability. Moreover, all margins should be carved properly, because flash will lead to plaque retention and will make crown margin placement difficult.

---

*Caulk, Dentsply.

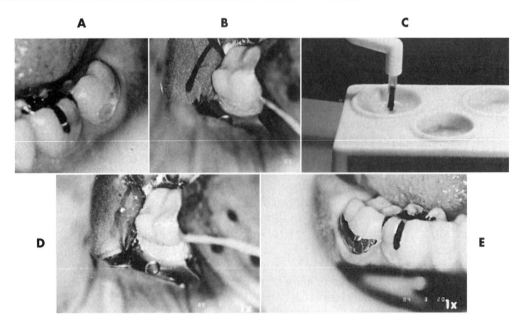

Fig. 6-8.   Adhesives such as AmalgamBond, a 4-META product, may be helpful in retaining shallow amalgams. **A,** Class V caries in a mandibular second molar. **B,** Shallow Class V cavity is prepared and dentin conditioned. Good isolation is essential when using adhesives. **C,** After rinsing and drying, the adhesive agent is brushed into the prepared cavity. This is followed by the mixed adhesive liner. **D,** The amalgam is condensed while the liner is still wet. **E,** The finished restoration. *(Courtesy Parkell Products, Inc.)*

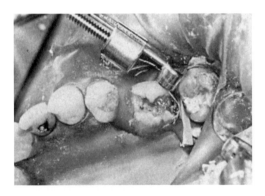

Fig. 6-9.   Autopolymerizing resin can help stabilize the matrix for an amalgam foundation restoration.

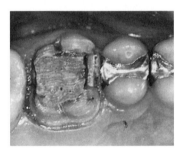

Fig. 6-10.   The foundation restoration for this crown was a silver-containing glass ionomer.

Glass Ionomer Core (Fig. 6-10)
1. Isolate the tooth. As with amalgam preparations, moisture control is critical with glass ionomer preparations. The setting material is very sensitive to moisture. When it is set, it must not be allowed to dry out or it will deteriorate rapidly. The light-cured, resin-modified glass-ionomers are less sensitive to early moisture.[29]
2. Prepare the tooth for a casting; then remove any existing restorations and bases, excavate caries, and create the undercut retention. Glass ionomer is best for small foundations on teeth with at least two axial walls of sound dentin remaining. Presently available glass

ionomers are not strong enough to be used for large pin-retained foundations. (Often they are chosen when the foundation and crown preparation are completed during one visit.) After tooth preparation and the creation of undercuts, glass ionomer is used to build the tooth up to ideal preparation form, provided any defects are relatively small. Adhesion to dentin can be enhanced by removing some of the smear layer with a chemical agent. However, excessive removal of the smear layer is not recommended, because it could lead to pulp irritation. A 20-second application with a dentin-conditioning agent that contains 10% polyacrylic acid should be sufficient. Dry the tooth with a cotton pledget before placing the ionomer; do not use an air syringe.

3. Syringe the glass ionomer onto the tooth, being careful not to create voids at the cement-tooth interface. Remember: With the conventional self-hardening formulations, adhesion of glass ionomer to tooth structure occurs only if the cement is placed rapidly after mixing; 10 seconds should be allowed for loading the syringe and 10 seconds for placement and manipulation. Some manufacturers provide an encapsulated delivery system that helps place the cement rapidly. A matrix is not normally needed for a small cavity, since the core materials do not slump. After injection, the cement can be rapidly manipulated to shape. However, manipulation beyond 3 or 4 seconds will disturb the developing bond and should be avoided. It is better to overfill slightly and reprepare the tooth after it has set (under 5 minutes for the metal-containing cements). If a resin-modified glass-ionomer is used, this is light-cured according to the manufacturer's recommendations.

4. Finish the preparation as for other types of cores. Conventional glass ionomers are extremely sensitive to drying, even when they are set, a fact that should be kept in mind when fabricating the crown preparation, making the provisional, or making the impression. Resin-modified formulations are less moisture sensitive. Vital teeth are also sensitive to desiccation, so this consideration should not modify normal practice.

Composite Resin

Composite resin foundations are much stronger than glass ionomer foundations, a difference that correlates with the higher diametral tensile strength of the composite.[30] They are strong enough for larger pin-retained cores. However, the current materials have disadvantages, particularly their absorption of moisture and high thermal expansion, which has led many dentists to avoid composite resin foundations entirely.

Moisture Control. Composite resins are sensitive to moisture contamination, and rubber dam isolation is strongly recommended.

Preparation. Because the material sets rapidly (about 5 minutes), composite resin is generally chosen if the dentist wishes to place the foundation and prepare the tooth during the same visit. The crown is prepared to approximate shape first, and then ex-

isting restorations and caries are removed. A glass ionomer is an appropriate choice of liner, with additional retention being provided by pins. For convenient access, the pinholes can be prepared and the liner placed before the pins are seated.

Placement. Both light-cured and chemically cured core composites are available. Light-cures have the convenience of extended working time, but there is concern about the adequacy of polymerization, especially around the pins.[31] The autopolymerizing materials need to be mixed and placed quickly, preferably with the aid of a composite syringe.* A Mylar matrix is used to confine them and provide good adaptation.

Finishing. Composite resin core materials are easily prepared with conventional tooth preparation diamonds.

Pin-retained Cast Core (Fig. 6-11)

As with glass ionomer and composite resin cores, cast cores are used to build a tooth to ideal preparation form without the need for matrix placement or condensation. However, they require the additional steps of an indirect procedure.

1. Prepare the tooth to approximate shape for a crown, removing any existing restorations and caries. Remove or block out all undercuts, and evacuate any weakly supported dentin.

2. Make pinholes using the small-diameter twist drill that comes with self-threading pins. The locations for these pins will be similar to those of self-threading pins, but all restorations using cast pins must have a common path of withdrawal. Prepare a flat area around each pin location with a large tapered carbide, and make the starting point for the pinhole with a small round bur. Pilot holes 2 mm deep are made for each pin, with the small-diameter twist drill carefully oriented in the planned path of withdrawal. Using a mouth mirror to observe the angulation of the drills helps ensure correct alignment. Plastic patterns are available for both tapered and parallel-sided cast pins. We prefer the tapered pins because they allow some leeway in paralleling the holes, and their tapered shape provides strength where needed. However, the parallel design is more retentive. The plastic patterns are manufactured to match specific bur sizes, which are used to

---

*Centrix Inc., Milford, Conn.

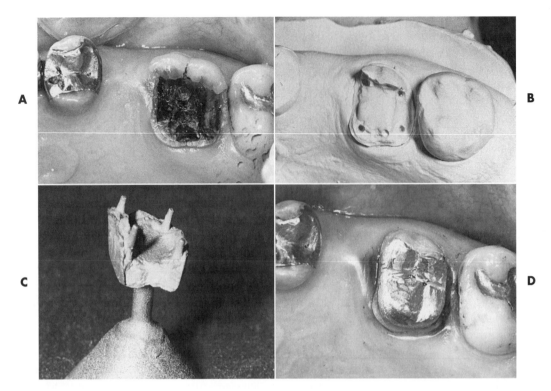

Fig. 6-11. Pin-retained cast core. **A,** Badly damaged maxillary molar. The pulp is healthy. **B,** Caries excavated and the tooth prepared for a pin-retained cast core. **C,** Four tapered pins provide retention. **D,** The completed foundation.

enlarge the pilot holes. To avoid overheating, always use low rotational speeds when drilling pinholes. Finally, a small countersink is created where the pinhole meets the gingival floor; this will facilitate forming a die that is free of defects and will help prevent pin fracture.

3. Make the impression with an elastomeric material, using a lentulo to fill the pinholes. Place a small quantity of mold-release substance (e.g., die lubricant) into each pinhole with a paper point to prevent tearing of the impression. As an alternative, use the plastic pattern for the impression.

4. Fabricate a provisional restoration. This procedure is described in Chapter 15. Place loose-fitting pins in the pinholes to provide retention. If retention is not a problem, avoid introducing luting agent into the pinholes when cementing the provisional.

5, 6, and **7.** Dies, waxing, and casting. These steps present no special problems. Plastic patterns are used to form the pins. If a tapered pin fits loosely, it can be shortened with a scalpel until it fits properly. Retention of pins in the wax pattern is accomplished by flattening the heads of the pins with a heated instrument. The foundation should be waxed as exactly as possible to final preparation form, with particular attention paid to the occlusal reduction. If

it is properly performed, a cast core should require minimum finishing in the mouth. If necessary, the die can be sectioned, trimmed, and mounted to facilitate this. The pattern is then invested and cast with the same regimen as for inlay castings (which generally require slightly less expansion than crowns). Factors that affect casting expansion are described in Chapter 22.

8. For try-in and cementation, do all grinding or adjustment of the casting before the cementation. The newly set cement may be damaged by vibration. To be acceptable, the fit of the cast foundation should be good, with complete seating and no discernible rock. A small marginal defect can be tolerated, provided it is not indicative of incomplete seating, because the margins will be completely covered by the definitive restoration. During cementation, completely fill the pinholes with cement; this can be done with a lentulo.

ENDODONTICS

ASSESSMENT

During the initial data collection, attention must be directed toward potential endodontic needs of the patient. The clinical examination should include vitality testing of all teeth in the dental arch. This may be done with an electric pulp tester, an "ice pencil" (conveniently made by filling an anesthetic needle cap with water and freezing), an aerosol cryogen spray, or heated gutta-percha. Tenderness to percussion should also be noted. Any abnormal sensitivity, soft tissue swellings, fistulous tracts, or discolored teeth will prompt a suspicion of pulpal involvement.

Patients who have definite symptoms seldom present problems in diagnosis, because pain is generally their chief complaint. When there is doubt concerning pulpal health, however, patients should be examined radiographically during the mouth preparation phase, and the films should be carefully inspected for signs of periapical disease (a radiolucency or widening of the PDL space). When there is doubt regarding the endodontic prognosis of a tooth, radiographic findings (Fig. 6-12) should always be evaluated in reference to the results of percussion and vitality tests.

TREATMENT

As a general rule, conventional (or orthograde) rather than surgical (or retrograde) endodontics should be performed if possible—not only because additional trauma results from the surgical approach but also because apicoectomy adversely affects the crown/root ratio and thus the support of the planned prosthesis. If an existing post prevents access to a recurrent periapical lesion, the post can usually be removed. (A Masserann kit has shown some success with this—see Chapter 12.) When a post-and-core restoration is needed in an endodon-

tically treated tooth, 3 to 5 mm of apical seal should be retained (see Chapter 12).

Performing elective endodontics may be desirable in the following situations: when there are problems in obtaining a compatible line of draw between multiple abutments, when it is impossible to gain adequate retention in a badly worn or damaged tooth, and when the endodontic prognosis of an abutment tooth is compromised and additional preparation is likely to further jeopardize its longevity.

DEFINITIVE PERIODONTAL TREATMENT

Robert F. Baima

Unless a patient's existing periodontal disease has been properly diagnosed and treated, fixed prosthodontics is doomed to failure. The treatment modalities presented in Chapter 5 form the basis for an effective approach to chronic periodontal disease. In addition, certain specific periodontal procedures may be indicated to improve the prognosis of a restoration. They are presented in the ensuing paragraphs.

MUCOSAL REPARATIVE THERAPY

The width of the band of attached keratinized gingiva may be increased by surgical grafting as part of mouth preparation before restorative treatment. Although the amount of gingiva necessary for long-term periodontal health is open to debate and definite conclusions are difficult to draw, comprehensive evaluation of the amount of attached keratinized tissue is always advised.[32,33] It is recommended[34,35] that a tooth to be treated with a restoration extending into the gingival sulcus should have approximately 5 mm of keratinized gingiva, at least 3 mm of which is attached gingiva. Where less keratinized gingiva is present, or in areas of localized gingival recession, a grafting or other gingival augmentation procedure should be considered.

FREE AUTOGENOUS GINGIVAL GRAFT (FIG. 6-13)

A free (detached) autogenous gingival graft is used to increase the width of attached gingiva in areas where it is deemed inadequate. The donor site most commonly used is the hard palate, although any area of keratinized tissues, such as an edentulous ridge or the retromolar pad, may be suitable.

The recipient bed site is prepared by making a horizontal split-thickness incision just coronal to the mucogingival junction. As the incision passes apical to the junction, it may become either split thickness

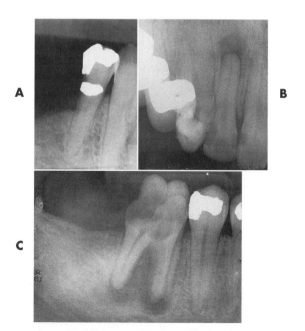

Fig. 6-12.   Commonly seen periapical lesions. **A,** Widened periodontal ligament space. **B** and **C,** Large radiolucencies (established granulomas or cysts). *(Courtesy Dr. G. Taylor.)*

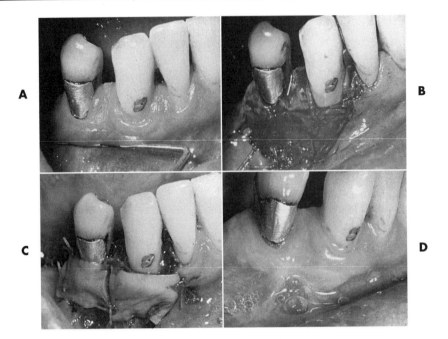

Fig. 6-13.   Free autogenous gingival graft. **A,** The location of the mucogingival junction is determined by moving the edge of a probe coronally. **B,** The recipient site is prepared. **C,** The graft is sutured to place. Some apical adjustment will be needed around the premolar before application of the surgical dressing. **D,** The healed graft. (Compare the width of attached keratinized gingiva here with that in **A.**) The defective restoration can be treated at this stage.

or full thickness.[36,37] The recipient bed is trimmed of tissue tags and thinned. (A template of tinfoil may be used as a guide for the correct size and shape of the graft.) The graft is then carefully removed from the donor site, and any fat or glandular tissue is excised, leaving a maximum thickness of 1 mm. Sterile saline is used to keep the graft moist until it is placed on the recipient bed for a check of size and shape, and it is then further shaped if necessary. When the proper dimensions have been attained, the graft is sutured into place. Finally, the graft site and the donor site may be covered with a surgical dressing. Complete healing requires approximately 6 weeks,[38,39] at which time the donor site and the grafted site should appear normal.

LATERALLY POSITIONED PEDICLE GRAFT (FIG. 6-14)

The laterally positioned pedicle graft[40,41] is used for an area of recession or lack of attached gingiva on a single tooth when there are adequate amounts of keratinized gingiva in adjacent teeth or edentulous spaces. Although several studies have proposed techniques that use free (detached) autogenous gingival grafts for root coverage,[42-44] the pedicle graft can be a more predictable treatment due to maintenance of the blood supply to the pedicle.

The recipient site is prepared by excising 1 to 3 mm of split-thickness marginal gingiva bordering the recession area. At the donor site, oblique vertical

incisions are placed in the mucosa as far apically as possible to ensure adequate blood supply for the graft. The apical area of the donor tissue is made wider than the coronal area. The flap is mobilized and placed on the recipient site and sutured into place. A free gingival graft may be needed to cover the donor site. A surgical dressing is placed over the site.

There are certain limitations of laterally positioned pedicle grafts:

1. Some recession always occurs at the donor site (an average of about 1 mm) when the free margin of the gingiva is involved.[45]
2. Severe recession is possible if the donor site uncovers any bony fenestration or dehiscence. However, because the graft retains its vascularity, it may be used to cover areas of recession rather than just to increase the band of attached keratinized gingiva. Success in covering areas of previously denuded root surface may be limited, depending on the amount and morphology of the recession,[46,47] and the attachment between graft and root will often be epithelial rather than connective tissue.

CORONALLY POSITIONED PEDICLE GRAFT (FIG. 6-15)

A coronally positioned pedicle graft[48,49] is used when a single tooth exhibits gingival recession and

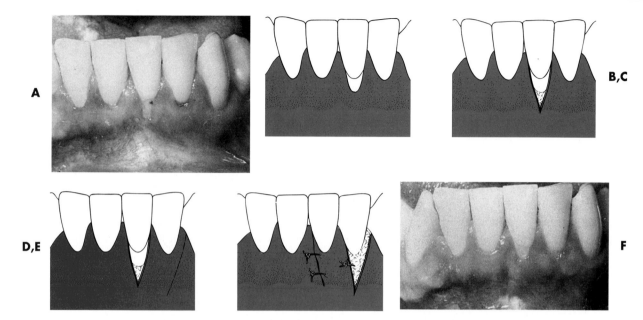

Fig. 6-14. Laterally positioned pedicle graft. **A** and **B** show localized recession around a mandibular incisor. The lateral incisor has an adequate band (width) of keratinized tissue, so it is suitable as a donor site. **C,** Bed preparation of the recipient site. An incision is made obliquely toward the site. **D,** Releasing incision at the distal of the donor site. The graft is rotated into position over the recipient site. **E,** Flap sutured in position. A free autogenous gingival graft may be used to cover the donor site. **F,** The healed graft. There will almost always be some loss of attachment at the donor site (average 1 mm).

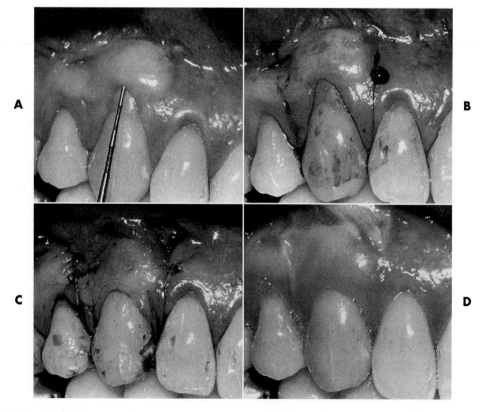

Fig. 6-15. Coronally positioned pedicle graft. **A,** The position of the free gingival margin after autogenous graft placement. There is approximately 4 mm of recession. **B,** Incisions for the pedicle. Divergence of the incisions will ensure an adequate blood supply because the base of the flap is broad. **C,** The pedicle is coronally positioned and sutured snugly to place at the CEJ with horizontal and suspension sutures. **D,** The healed graft.
(Courtesy Dr. S.B. Ross.)

sensitivity. If the width of the attached keratinized gingiva is inadequate, a free autogenous gingival graft may be placed to increase it before the coronal positioning.

Although there are various techniques,[50, 51] divergent vertical incisions are most commonly placed as far apically as possible into the mucosa. This results in a broader apical than coronal portion of the flap and ensures that the flap will have an adequate blood supply. The root surface is planed to a glasslike finish, and the graft is sutured in a coronal position to obtain maximum root coverage. Recent studies have used an alternative guided tissue regeneration technique to promote reattachment before suturing the graft.[52,53] After the graft has been held in position with pressure to decrease hemorrhage and to obtain proper placement, it is covered with a surgical dressing.

SUBEPITHELIAL CONNECTIVE TISSUE GRAFT

Connective tissue that does not carry epithelium has also been used for gingival grafting purposes. This technique involves the use of subepithelial connective tissue harvested from the palate in a split-thickness fashion, which allows the wound to be closed after removal of the graft. This approach minimizes patient discomfort at the donor site.

The graft is placed at the recipient site between a minimally reflected split-thickness flap and the periosteum, covering the root. This "sandwich" placement of the connective tissue supplies the graft with blood from two different sources.[43,54] A "tunnel" placement may be used as an alternative technique,[55] and up to 100% coverage of root recession has been reported.

CROWN-LENGTHENING PROCEDURES (FIG. 6-16)

Surgical crown lengthening or extension may be indicated to improve the appearance of an anterior tooth or when the clinical crown is too short to provide adequate retention without the restoration's impinging on the normal soft tissue attachment[56] or biologic width.* This attachment averages approximately 2 mm in width, and any restoration that impinges on it may cause bone loss because of the effort of the host to maintain the 2 mm distance. If impingement occurs in an interproximal area, it can lead to problems with plaque control and possible osseous resorption.[57-59] Therefore, from the stand-

---

*The term *biologic width* refers to the combined connective tissue–epithelial attachment from the crest of the alveolar bone to the base of the gingival sulcus.[34]

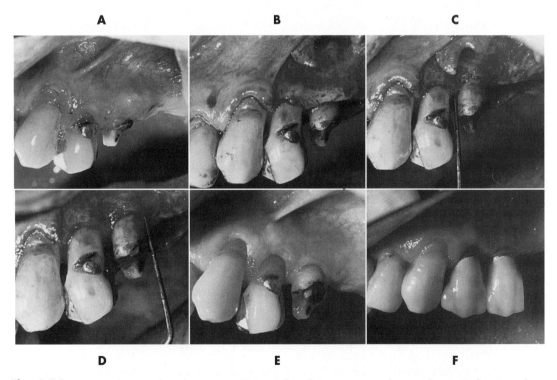

Fig. 6-16. Surgical crown lengthening. **A,** Fractured and carious second premolar. **B,** Reflection of a flap and removal of granulation tissue. **C,** Bone removed on the mesial to increase the distance to the fracture site to 3.5 mm. **D,** Distally the bone is removed so there will be 3.5 mm from the caries to the alveolar crest. **E,** Healing after the surgical crown lengthening. **F,** Final crown restoration after cementation, before restoration of the sextant with a removable partial denture.

point of prognosis, the biologic width should never be compromised.

In some patients, an apparently hopeless tooth with extensive subgingival caries, a subgingival fracture, or root perforation resulting from endodontics can be successfully restored after crown lengthening. Crown lengthening increases the crown/root ratio, however, and a pretreatment decision must be made about whether the tooth should be removed or restored.

Crown lengthening may be accomplished either surgically or with combined orthodontic-periodontic[60-64] techniques, depending on the patient and the dental situation.

Surgical Crown Lengthening (see Fig. 6-16)
It is sometimes possible to achieve an effective increase in crown length by gingivectomy or removal of gingiva by electrosurgery alone, although most often osseous recontouring is needed to prevent encroachment of the prosthesis on the biologic width. For these procedures, a full thickness mucoperiosteal flap is reflected, and the osseous resection creates 3.5 to 4.0 mm of space between the gingival crest and the margin of the existing restoration or carious lesion.[56, 65] In these instances, however, the following factors should be considered:

1. *Esthetics.* When surgical crown lengthening (Fig. 6-17) is indicated, it may be difficult to achieve a harmonious transition from the tissue around the lengthened tooth to that around adjacent teeth. Alternatives include orthodontic extrusion or removal and replacement with a prosthesis. If surgery is undertaken, most of the osseous reduction should be on the lingual or palatal side, where there is usually no esthetic problem, with blending on the labial or buccal side only as necessary.

2. *Root length within bone.* If there is limited osseous support, it may be better to remove the tooth and replace it with a prosthesis than to have the patient undergo surgery on a tooth with a doubtful prognosis.

3. *Effect on adjacent teeth.* Often a fracture or defect will be of such depth that it cannot be eliminated without severely endangering the adjacent teeth. In these instances removal or orthodontic extrusion may be preferable.

4. *Root furcation exposure in a posterior tooth.* If this situation cannot be remedied by osteoplasty and/or odontoplasty, the tooth may require removal.

5. *Mobility.* Postsurgical mobility of a tooth with small or conical roots is a valid concern. If such a tooth cannot support itself or cannot be supported by the adjacent teeth, then removal may be necessary.

6. *Extent of the defect.* The severity and complications of any fracture, root caries, or cervical wear must be carefully evaluated during the treatment planning phase.

7. *Root perforation.* This is uncommon, but if it occurs during endodontic therapy, its location will determine whether to remove, orthodontically extrude, or lengthen the tooth surgically.[66]

Although surgical crown lengthening may not be a panacea for fractured, perforated, or badly decayed teeth, it can help solve difficult and/or complex restorative problems when used with proper clinical judgment.

MAINTENANCE AND RECONSTRUCTION OF THE INTERDENTAL PAPILLA (FIGS. 6-18 TO 6-20)
The presence or absence of the interproximal papilla, especially in the maxillary anterior area, is a concern to the restorative dentist, the periodontist, and the patient. Multiple techniques have been

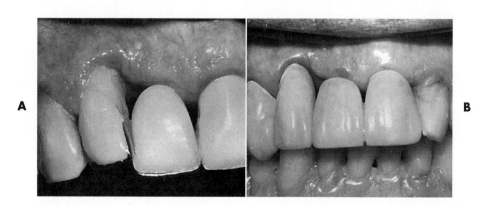

Fig. 6-17. Esthetic problems can occur after surgical crown lengthening of an anterior tooth. **A,** Lateral incisor is lengthened to include a mesial periodontal defect. **B,** Esthetics would have been better if the distal had been included and the gingival contour gradually sloped.

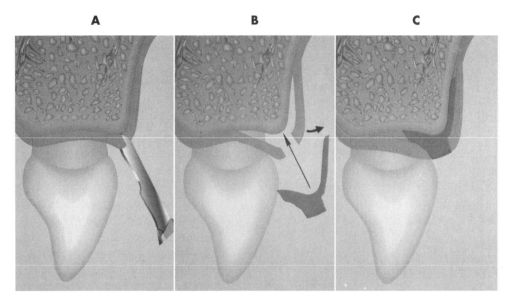

Fig. 6-18. Technique for surgical reproduction of the interdental papilla. **A,** Intrasulcular incision and buccal incision placed in the interdental papilla, leaving the existing papilla attached to the palatal flap. **B,** Split-thickness flap is elevated buccally and palatally. Connective tissue graft is prepared for placement under the buccal and palatal flaps. **C,** Buccal and palatal flaps are sutured after connective tissue from the retromolar area is placed under the flap.
(From Azzi R, Etienne D, Carranza F: Int J Periodontol Rest Dent 18:467, 1998.)

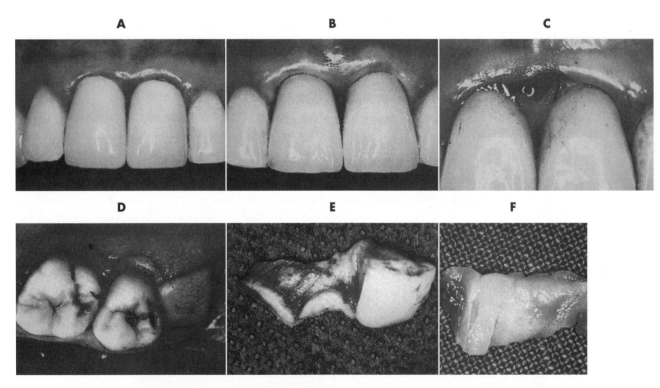

Fig. 6-19. Reconstruction of the interdental papilla. **A,** Poorly contoured and bulky crowns on maxillary central incisors with loss of interdental papilla. **B,** Replaced crowns 1 year after cementation with improved tissue contours. However, interdental papilla remains in an apical position. **C,** Papillary incisions. **D,** Incisions to harvest retromolar connective tissue combined with incisions to the thin palatal flap. **E,** Connective tissue harvested in bulk. **F,** Connective tissue graft trimmed for placement into the papillary area.
(From Azzi R, Etienne D, Carranza F: Int J Periodontol Rest Dent 18:467, 1998.)

G   **H**   **I**

J

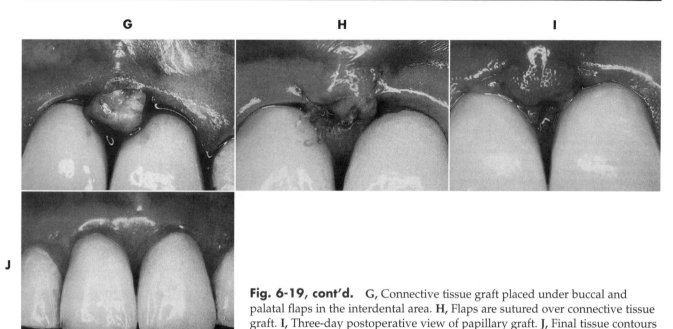

Fig. 6-19, cont'd. **G,** Connective tissue graft placed under buccal and palatal flaps in the interdental area. **H,** Flaps are sutured over connective tissue graft. **I,** Three-day postoperative view of papillary graft. **J,** Final tissue contours around replacement crowns.

A   **B**

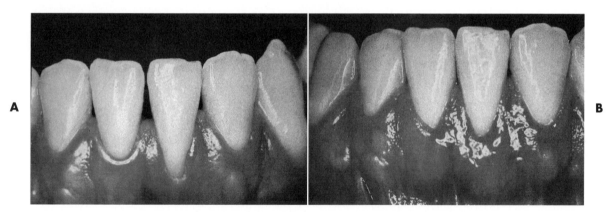

Fig. 6-20. Reconstruction of the interdental papilla. **A,** Preoperative view of papillary deficiency in the interproximal area of teeth #24 and #25. **B,** Results of papillary graft and final tissue contour. *(From Azzi R, Etienne D, Carranza F: Int J Periodontol Rest Dent 18:467, 1998.)*

used, with and without the use of guided tissue or bone regeneration, to maintain and reconstruct the interdental papilla.[67-72] The results of these procedures have not been predictable or reproducible. The reconstruction or preservation of the papilla is dependent on multiple factors such as the amount of attachment lost in the area, the blood supply available for the newly created papilla,[68] and the distance from the contact area to the crest of the interproximal bone.[73] The majority of the techniques used for restoration or reconstruction of the interdental papilla are surgical in nature and therefore involve coordination and co-therapy with surgical or periodontal colleagues. Consultation with the appropriate surgeon before planning the final restoration of the area is crucial.

ORTHODONTIC-PERIODONTIC EXTRUSION (FIG. 6-21)

Orthodontic extrusion[60,61,74] may be considered whenever a fracture or carious lesion extends apical to the free margin of the gingiva. However, it is especially important where esthetics is a prime concern. The margin of the fracture or lesion is moved away from the alveolar crest orthodontically (with brackets, wires, and/or elastic bands), and the gingiva often requires surgical repositioning when orthodontic therapy is completed.

• • •

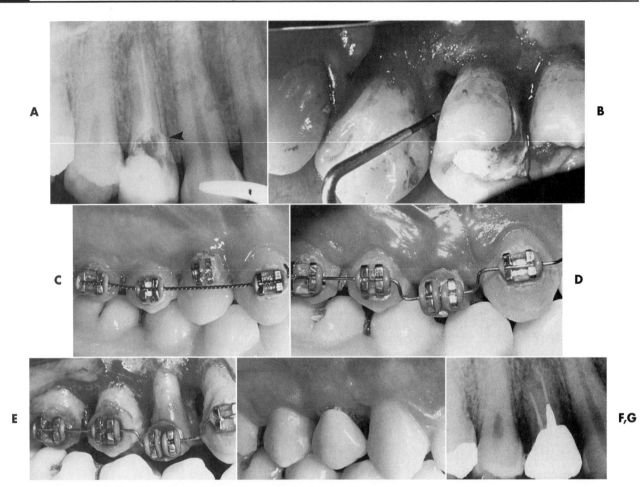

Fig. 6-21. Orthodontic extrusion before restoring a badly damaged tooth. **A,** This maxillary first premolar has been perforated mesially *(arrow).* A surgical crown lengthening was contraindicated because of the level of the perforation apical to the osseous crest. **B,** A flap was reflected to debride the perforation and associated lesion. **C,** Orthodontic brackets cemented with rebounding wire initially. When the wire is placed in the premolar bracket, it will impart an occlusally directed force. (The occlusion must be relieved periodically as the tooth moves.) **D,** Completion of the extrusion. **E,** Osseous recontouring at this stage ensures a harmonious bony and gingival contour. **F** and **G,** Coronal tooth structure restored with a metal-ceramic crown. *(Courtesy Dr. S.B. Ross.)*

ORTHODONTIC TREATMENT

Minor orthodontic tooth movement[75-78] can significantly enhance the prognosis of subsequent restorative treatment. Uprighting malpositioned abutment teeth can improve axial alignment, create more favorable pontic spaces, and improve embrasure form in the fixed prosthesis. It can also direct occlusal forces along the long axes of the teeth and often leads to a substantial conservation of tooth structure (see Fig. 7-11, *B, C*).

ASSESSMENT

The clinical examination should focus on tooth malpositioning both buccolingually and mesiodistally. Abnormal tooth relationships such as anterior or posterior cross bites should alert the dentist to the possible need for orthodontic treatment. In particular, attempts to correct abnormal tooth relationships

with fixed prosthodontics alone are rarely successful; orthodontic preparation is normally preferred.

The need for orthodontic treatment is determined through a careful analysis of articulated diagnostic casts, whose usefulness can be enhanced with a dental surveyor (Fig. 6-22). One helpful procedure[79] is to section a duplicate cast (Fig. 6-23) and reassemble it according to the proposed orthodontic modifications. This facilitates assessing the validity of any **minor tooth movement** (e.g., closing diastemas, uprighting molars, aligning tilted teeth) and is especially valuable when explaining the treatment proposal to the patient. Diagnostic preparations and waxing procedures made on these altered casts often clearly illustrate the benefits of minor tooth movement. Many dentists are now using computer imaging technology to optimize esthetic treatment planning and improve patient communication[80-83] (Fig. 6-24).

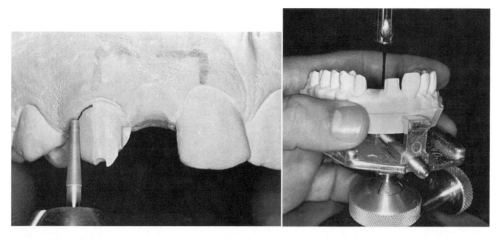

Fig. 6-22. Use of diagnostic preparations and a dental surveyor in assessing the need for orthodontic treatment before fixed prosthodontics.

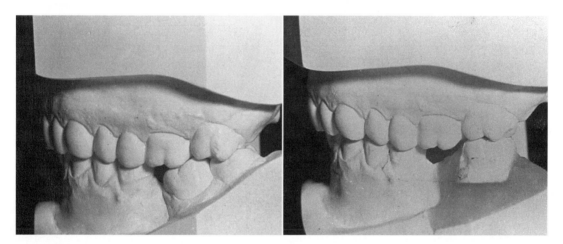

Fig. 6-23. Diagnostic cast sectioning for determination of desired orthodontic tooth movement. *(Courtesy Dr. P. Ngan.)*

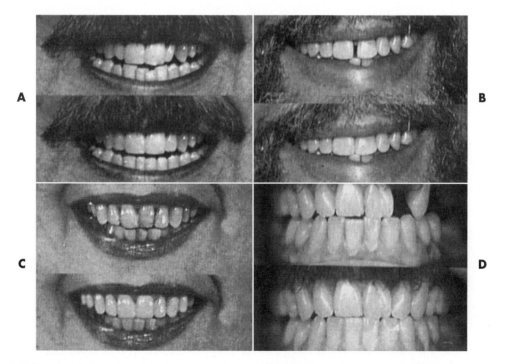

Fig. 6-24. Computer imaging technology can assist in treatment planning and communicating to the patient the esthetic changes that are envisioned. The equipment consists of a video camera, a monitor, and a computer. The software allows the video image to be manipulated to ascertain the post-treatment appearance.

(Courtesy Envision International, Inc.)

TREATMENT

In general practice it is often possible to perform minor tooth movement before fixed prosthodontic treatment without referral to an orthodontist. However, a specialist should be consulted if treatment is more complex than the straightforward tipping, uprighting, or extruding of an abutment tooth.

For tipping or extruding a single anterior tooth, acid-etch brackets can be used with a multistrand elastic wire ligated in place to attain the desired po-

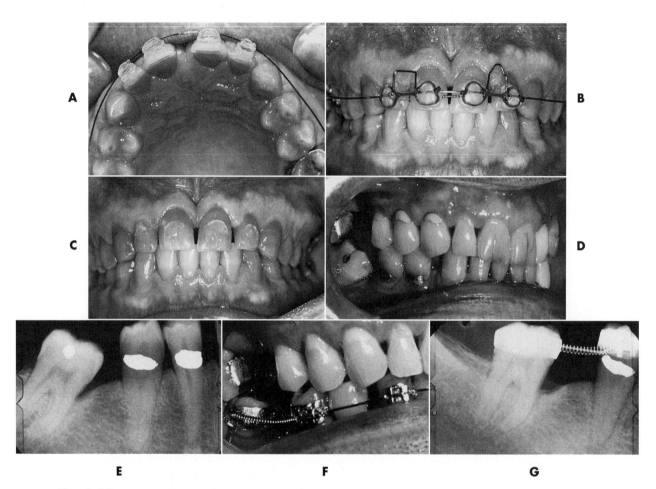

Fig. 6-25. Orthodontic tooth movement as an adjunct to fixed prosthodontics. **A** to **C,** Minor tooth movement before correction of a diastema. **D** to **G,** A mesially tilted molar uprighted with a coil spring before the provision of a fixed partial denture. (**D** to **G** courtesy Dr. P. Ngan.)

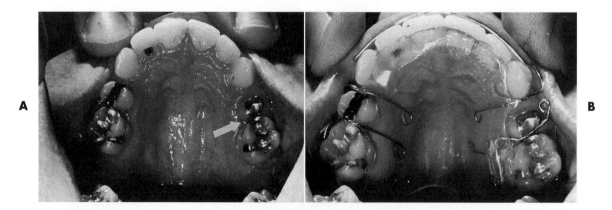

Fig. 6-26. **A,** The maxillary premolar (*arrow*) was prepared for a metal-ceramic crown but was inadequately provisionalized. Unfortunately, the patient failed to return when the provisional became dislodged. The tooth had moved distally and was in contact with the first molar, making crown placement impossible. **B,** A removable appliance was used to reposition the tooth before impression making. (*Courtesy Dr. P. Ngan.*)

sition. When moving any anterior tooth, however, the amount of labial bone should be carefully evaluated and found to be adequate. Orthodontic treatment should also be considered when restorations are being used to correct a diastema. Often esthetics can be dramatically improved by distributing the space of a midline diastema around all the anterior teeth (Fig. 6-25, *A* to *C*). A diagnostic waxing procedure will help determine the optimum tooth position. Uprighting a mesially tilted molar can be accomplished with a coil spring (Fig. 6-25, *D* to *G*), but the tooth should first be adjusted out of occlusion. A neglected crown preparation can be salvaged with a simple orthodontic appliance (Fig. 6-26). All orthodontic movement requires adequate anchorage so that inadvertent movement of other teeth will be avoided.

DEFINITIVE OCCLUSAL TREATMENT

Mouth preparation often involves reorganization of the patient's occlusion, typically to make intercuspal position coincident with centric relation and remove eccentric interferences (see Chapter 4). This may be done therapeutically, principally to relieve symptoms of occlusal dysfunction, or as a prerequisite to extensive restorative treatment. The coincidence of CR and MI greatly facilitates accurately transferring the patient's casts to an articulator. **Occlusal adjustment** as a therapeutic modality is fraught with controversy. The current balance of research places a low priority on the influence of occlusion in disorders of the temporomandibular joints and associated musculature.[84] Also, there is clinical evidence to the contrary.[85-87] However, these disorders should be diagnosed and alleviated before definitive fixed prosthodontics is undertaken. This can generally be achieved by noninvasive, reversible means.[88] The role of occlusal forces in the progress of periodontal disease is also controversial. The balance of current research indicates that occlusal forces do not initiate periodontitis but may modify attachment loss caused by plaque-induced inflammatory periodontal disease.[89]

When selective reshaping of the natural dentition is being considered, it is important to remember that this is a purely subtractive procedure (tissue is removed), and it is limited by the thickness of the enamel. Obviously, before any irreversible changes are made in the dentition, a careful diagnosis must establish whether restorations will be needed.

DIAGNOSTIC ADJUSTMENT

Two sets of articulated diagnostic casts (Fig. 6-27) are required for diagnostic occlusal adjustment. One set will serve as a reference; the other will be used to

evaluate how much tooth structure has been removed and how much more must be removed to meet the objectives of the procedure. This will reveal the efficacy of the treatment plan before anything is done clinically.

The occlusal surfaces of each cast are painted with poster paint (which will not soak into the stone) to demonstrate the extent of any planned corrective reshaping. The pin setting on the articulator is recorded before adjustment so the operator can judge the amount of enamel that must be removed. Each step of the adjustment is recorded sequentially on a reshaping list. When completed, the procedure is reviewed carefully. Areas where enamel is likely to be penetrated are identified so that the patient can be advised of the likely need for additional restrictions on these teeth.

The primary objectives of selective occlusal reshaping are as follows:

- To redistribute forces parallel to the long axes of the teeth by eliminating contacts on inclined planes and creating cusp-fossa occlusion
- To eliminate deflective occlusal contacts: centric relation coincides with the intercuspal position
- To improve worn occlusal anatomy, enhance cuspal shape, narrow occlusal tables, and reemphasize proper developmental and supplemental grooves in otherwise flat surfaces
- To correct marginal ridge discrepancies and extrusions so oral hygiene will be easier
- To correct tooth malalignment through selective reshaping

It will not always be possible to achieve every one of these goals. If a choice must be made, corrective therapy should not be at the expense of functional surfaces and should not destroy any functional contact.

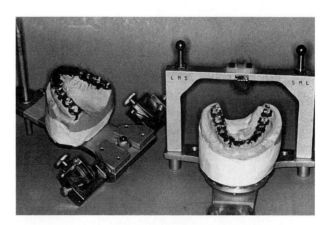

Fig. 6-27. Diagnostic occlusal adjustment on articulated casts.

CLINICAL OCCLUSAL ADJUSTMENT

Patient Selection. Careful analysis of the diagnostic occlusal adjustment is necessary to determine whether the patient is a good candidate for such irreversible subtractive treatment. Precise reduction and close attention to the sequence are essential. A written record of each reduction is also recommended. If too much is ground off a tooth, it cannot be put back on. The following should be considered as contraindications to definitive occlusal adjustment:

1. A bruxer whose habit cannot be controlled
2. A diagnostic correction that indicates that too much tooth structure will be removed
3. A complex spatial relationship (e.g., an Angle Class II and a skeletal Class III)
4. Maxillary lingual cusps contacting mandibular buccal cusps
5. An open anterior occlusal relationship
6. Excessive wear
7. Before orthodontic or orthognathic treatment
8. Before physical or occlusal appliance therapy
9. A patient with temporomandibular pain
10. A patient whose jaw movements cannot be manipulated easily

Occlusal adjustment needs to be undertaken in a logical sequence to avoid repetition and improve the efficacy of treatment. Although different sequences have been proposed, we find the one described next to be successful.

Elimination of Centric Relation Interferences. As the mandible rotates around the terminal hinge axis, each mandibular tooth follows its own arc of closure. If the intercuspal and CR positions do not coincide, premature contacts will be unavoidable.

Step-by-Step Procedure

1. Manipulate the mandible and mark the teeth so both the initial contact in centric relation and the extent and direction of jaw movement to intercuspation are seen. This movement, or slide, can be in either an anterior or a lateral direction.
2. Find any interferences that cause the condylar processes to be displaced anteriorly (protrusive interferences). These will usually be between the mesial inclines of maxillary teeth and the distal inclines of mandibular teeth (Fig. 6-28).
3. Continue the adjustment until all teeth contact evenly (except possibly the incisors). If excursive movements are guided adequately by the canines, it may be better to stop when bilateral canine-to-canine contact has been reestablished.
4. When dealing with a laterally displacing prematurity, adjust the buccal-facing inclines of the maxillary and the lingual-facing inclines of the mandibular teeth. The premature contact will usually be on either the laterotrusive or the mediotrusive side of the mandible (lateral slide or medial slide).
5. When dealing with a lateral slide, adjust the buccal inclines of the maxillary lingual cusps and the lingual inclines of the mandibular buccal cusps until there is contact on the cusp tips (Fig. 6-29).
6. When dealing with a medial slide, adjust the buccal inclines of the mandibular buccal cusps or the lingual inclines of the maxillary lingual cusps until there is contact on the cusp tips. At this time, any further adjustments can be made through widening of the opposing central grooves by reduction of the internal inclines of

This prematurity will result in the mandible sliding forward as the teeth come together in maximum intercuspation (MI).

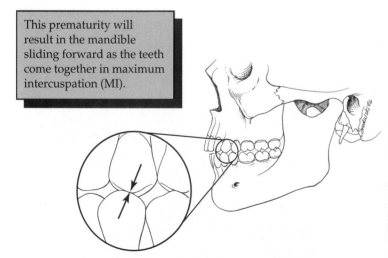

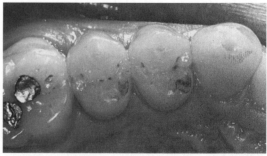

Fig. 6-28. Interferences that deflect the mandible anteriorly (protrusive interferences) are found between the mesial inclines of maxillary teeth and the distal inclines of mandibular teeth.

the maxillary buccal and mandibular lingual cusps (Fig. 6-30).

Evaluation. The foregoing rules for occlusal adjustment should be followed as closely as possible while maintaining the normal anatomic form of the tooth. When the discrepancy between CR and MI has been corrected, there will be uniform contact between all posterior teeth. This can be verified with thin Mylar shim stock held in forceps (Fig. 6-31).

Elimination of Lateral and Protrusive Interferences. The second phase of occlusal adjustment concentrates on laterotrusive, mediotrusive, and protrusive interferences. Use red and blue marking ribbons to distinguish between centric and eccentric contacts.

The goals of this second phase of adjustment are to eliminate contact between all posterior teeth during protrusive movements and to eliminate any interferences on the nonworking (mediotrusive) as well as the working (laterotrusive) side. In certain patients, group function of the working side contacts should be considered rather than the more

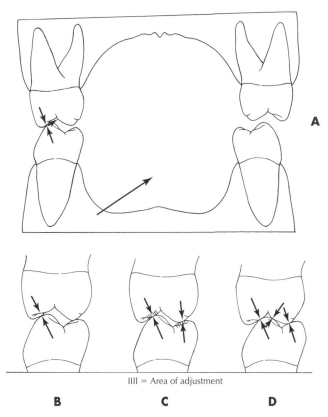

IIII = Area of adjustment

B   **C**   **D**

Fig. 6-30. Correcting a medial slide by selective grinding. **A,** The contacting inclines are adjusted until the cusp tips are in contact (**B**). The opposing central grooves are then widened (**C** and **D**).

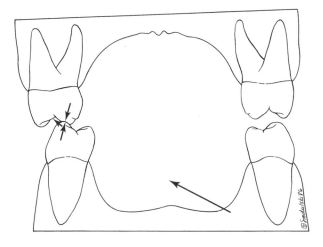

> The premature contact occurs on opposing cuspal inclines and will cause the mandible to shift in the direction of the arrow as the teeth slide into their MI position.

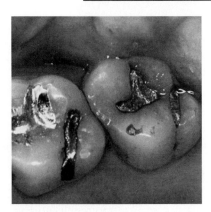

Fig. 6-29. Laterally displacing contact between the buccal incline of a maxillary lingual cusp and the lingual incline of a mandibular buccal cusp.

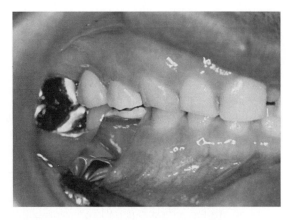

Fig. 6-31. Verifying occlusal contacts with thin Mylar shim stock.

ideal mutually protected occlusion (e.g., when there is mobility or poor bone support of the canines). In other patients, group function may be retained because of wear or malpositioning of the canines.

During this phase of adjustment, it is essential that no centric contacts be removed. In general, lateral and protrusive interferences are eliminated by creating a groove that permits escape of the centric cusp during eccentric movement (Fig. 6-32).

◼SUMMARY

A logical **treatment sequence** should be planned before beginning any fixed prosthodontic intervention. Such planning will normally be multidisciplinary—it will incorporate oral surgery; operative dentistry; and endodontic, periodontic, orthodontic, and/or occlusal therapies. Mouth preparation is particularly important to fixed prosthodontics, which, like all dental disciplines, is facilitated and enhanced by meticulous preparatory treatment.

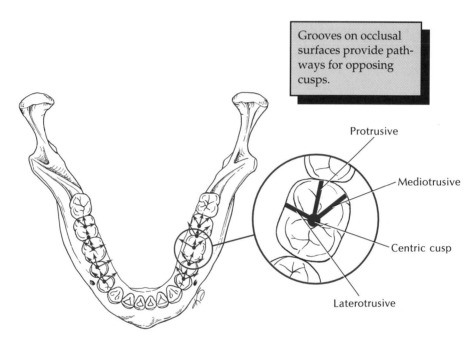

Grooves on occlusal surfaces provide pathways for opposing cusps.

Protrusive

Mediotrusive

Centric cusp

Laterotrusive

Fig. 6-32.   Detection of eccentric interferences is facilitated by understanding where they normally occur. The arrows represent the paths of opposing centric cusps during each excursion (mediotrusive, protrusive, and laterotrusive). Look, for example, to find a mediotrusive interference distobuccal to a centric contact. In the maxillary arch, the pattern is reversed.

Study Questions

1. Discuss in detail the recommended sequence of preparatory treatment procedures before initiation of definitive fixed prosthodontic treatment.
2. Discuss the advantages, disadvantages, indications, and any applicable precautions for the various foundation restoration materials.
3. How does the tooth preparation for an extensive amalgam foundation restoration differ from a conventional extensive amalgam restoration? Why?
4. Discuss three types of periodontal grafting procedures, their indications, and their limitations.
5. What are the indications for minor tooth movement before initiating fixed prosthodontic treatment?
6. What are the indications and contraindications for comprehensive occlusal reshaping? If indicated, what is the recommended procedure and sequence of events?

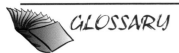
GLOSSARY

1 base: *vt* (1587): the act of placing a lining material under a dental restoration.

2 base: *n* (14c): any substance placed under a restoration that blocks out undercuts in the preparation, acts as a thermal or chemical barrier to the pulp, and/or controls the thickness of the overlying restoration—called also base material—usage: adjectives such as insulating b., therapeutic b may also be used.

creep: *n* (1818): the slow change in dimensions of an object due to prolonged exposure to high temperature or stress.

debridement: *n* (ca. 1842): the removal of inflamed, devitalized, contaminated tissue or foreign material from or adjacent to a lesion.

deflective occlusal contact: a contact that displaces a tooth, diverts the mandible from its intended movement, or displaces a removable denture from its basal seat.

exposure: *n* (1606) *1:* the act of laying open, as a surgical or dental exposure *2:* in radiology, a measure of the roentgen rays or gamma radiation at a certain place based on its ability to cause ionization. The unit of exposure is the roentgen, called also exposure dose.

extrusion: *n* (1540): the movement of teeth beyond the natural occlusal plane that may be accompanied by a similar movement of their supporting tissues.

graft: *n* (14c): a tissue or material used to repair a defect or deficiency.

maximal intercuspal position: the complete intercuspation of the opposing teeth independent of condylar position, sometimes referred to as the best fit of the teeth regardless of the condylar position—called also maximal intercuspation.

mouth guard: a resilient intraoral device useful in reducing mouth injuries and protecting the teeth and surrounding structures from injury.

protrusive deflection: a continuing eccentric displacement of the midline incisal path on protrusion, symptomatic of a restriction of movement.

pulp capping: application of a material to protect the pulp from external influences and promote healing, done either directly or indirectly.

REFERENCES

1. DeSchepper EJ et al: Clinical predictability of caries beneath restorations, *Oper Dent* 11:136, 1986.

2. Kidd EM: Caries diagnosis within restored teeth, *Oper Dent* 14:149, 1989.

3. Nair MK et al: The effects of restorative material and location on the detection of simulated recurrent caries: a comparison of dental film, direct digital radiography and tuned aperture computed tomography, *Dentomaxillofac Radiol* 27:80, 1998.

4. Tjan AHL, Chiu J: Microleakage of core materials for complete cast gold crowns, *J Prosthet Dent* 61:659, 1989.

5. Fischer GM et al: Amalgam retention using pins, boxes, and Amalgambond, *Am J Dent* 6:173, 1993.

6. Ramos JC, Perdigao J: Bond strengths and SEM morphology of dentin-amalgam adhesives, *Am J Dent* 10:152, 1997.

7. Diefenderfer KE, Reinhardt JW: Shear bond strengths of 10 adhesive resin/amalgam combinations, *Oper Dent* 22:50, 1997.

8. 4-Methacryloxyethyl trimellitate anhydride.

9. Tarim B et al: Marginal integrity of bonded amalgam restorations, *Am J Dent* 9:72, 1996.

10. Korale ME, Meiers JC: Microleakage of dentin bonding systems used with spherical and admixed amalgams, *Am J Dent* 9:249, 1996.

11. Ratananakin T et al: Effect of condensation techniques on amalgam bond strengths to dentin, *Oper Dent* 21:191, 1996.

12. Schulte GA et al: Early fracture resistance of amalgapin-retained complex amalgam restorations, *Oper Dent* 23:108, 1998.

13. Prevost AP et al: Radiopacity of glass ionomer dental materials, *Oral Surg* 70:231, 1990.

14. DeWald JP et al: Evaluation of glass-cermet cores under cast crowns, *Dent Mater* 6:129, 1990.

15. Lloyd CH, Butchart DG: Retention of core composites, glass ionomers, and cermets by a self-threading dentin pin: the influence of fracture toughness upon failure, *Dent Mater* 6:185, 1990.

16. Cohen BI et al: A five year study: fluoride release of four reinforced composite resins, *Oral Health* 88:81, 1998.

17. Hormati AA, Denehy GE: Microleakage of pin-retained amalgam and composite resin bases, *J Prosthet Dent* 44:526, 1980.

18. Oliva RA, Lowe JA: Dimensional stability of composite used as a core material, *J Prosthet Dent* 56:554, 1986.

19. Martin N, Jedynakiewicz N: Measurement of water sorption in dental composites, *Biomaterials* 19:77, 1998.

20. Cooley RL et al: Dimensional stability of glass ionomer used as a core material, *J Prosthet Dent* 64:651, 1990.

21. Lambert RL, Goldfogel MH: Pin amalgam restoration and pin amalgam foundation, *J Prosthet Dent* 54:10, 1985.

22. Outhwaite WC et al: Pin versus slot retention in extensive amalgam restorations, *J Prosthet Dent* 41:396, 1979.

23. Shavell HM: The amalgapin technique for complex amalgam restorations, *J Calif Dent Assoc* 8:48, 1980.

24. Bailey JH: Retention design for amalgam restorations: pins versus slots, *J Prosthet Dent* 65:71, 1991.

25. Irvin AW et al: Photoelastic analysis of stress induced from insertion of self-threading retentive pins, *J Prosthet Dent* 53:311, 1985.

26. Felton DA et al: Pulpal response to threaded pin and retentive slot techniques: a pilot investigation, *J Prosthet Dent* 66:597, 1991.

27. Bonilla ED et al: A customized acrylic resin shell for fabricating an amalgam core on the coronally debilitated, endodontically treated posterior tooth, *Quintessence* 26:317, 1995.

28. Livaditis GJ: Crown foundations with a custom matrix, composites, and reverse carving, *J Prosthet Dent* 77:540, 1997.

29. Nicholson JW, Croll TP: Glass-ionomer cements in restorative dentistry, *Quintessence* 28:705, 1997.

30. Kerby RE, Knobloch L: Strength characteristics of conventional and silver-reinforced glass-ionomer cements, *Oper Dent* 17:170, 1992.

31. Butchart DGM, Lloyd CH: The retention of self-threading pins embedded in visible light-cured composites, *J Dent* 15:253, 1987.

32. American Academy of Periodontology: Guidelines for periodontal therapy, *J Periodontol* 69:405, 1998.

33. American Academy of Periodontology: *Parameters of care*, 1996, The American Academy of Periodontology Scientific and Educational Affairs Department.

34. Maynard JG, Wilson RDK:Physiologic dimensions of the periodontium significant to the restorative dentist, *J Periodontol* 50:170, 1979.

35. Wilson RDK, Maynard JG: Intracrevicular restorative dentistry, *Int J Periodont Rest Dent* 1:34, 1981.

36. Sullivan HC, Atkins JH: Free autogenous gingival grafts. I. Principles of successful grafting, *Periodontics* 6:121, 1968.

37. Dordick B et al: Clinical evaluation of free autogenous gingival grafts placed on alveolar bone. I. Clinical predictability, *J Periodontol* 47:559, 1976.

38. Oliver RC et al: Microscopic evaluation of the healing and revascularization of free gingival grafts, *J Periodontol Res* 3:84, 1968.

39. Staffileno H Jr, Levy S: Histological and clinical study of mucosal (gingival) transplants in dogs, *J Periodontol* 40:311, 1969.

40. Grupe HE, Warren RF: Repair of gingival defects by a sliding flap operation, *J Periodontol* 29:92, 1956.

41. Bjorn H: Coverage of denuded root surfaces with a lateral sliding flap: use of free gingival grafts, *Odontol Rev* 22:37, 1971.

42. Holbrook T, Ochsenbien C: Complete coverage of the denuded root surface with a one-stage gingival graft, *Int J Periodont Rest Dent* 3:9, 1983.

43. Miller PD Jr: Root coverage using the free soft tissue autograft following citric acid application. III. A successful and predictable procedure in areas of deep wide recession, *Int J Periodont Rest Dent* 5:15, 1985.

44. Raetzke PB: Covering localized areas of root exposure employing the "envelope" technique, *J Periodontol* 56:397, 1985.

45. Caffesse RG, Guinard EA: Treatment of localized gingival recessions. IV. Results after three years, *J Periodontol* 51:167, 1980.

46. Sullivan HC, Atkins JH: Free autogenous gingival grafts. III. Utilization of grafts in the treatment of gingival recession, *Periodontics* 6:152, 1968.

47. Miller PD Jr: A classification of marginal tissue recession, *Int J Periodont Rest Dent* 5:9, 1985.

48. Bernimoulin JP et al: Coronally repositioned periodontal flap: clinical evaluation after one year, *J Clin Periodontol* 2:1, 1975.

49. Maynard JG: Coronal positioning of a previously placed autogenous gingival graft, *J Periodontol* 48:151, 1977.

50. Tarnow DP: Semilunar coronally repositioned flap, *J Clin Periodontol* 13:182, 1986.

51. Allen EP, Miller PD Jr: Coronal positioning of existing gingiva: short-term results in the treatment of shallow marginal tissue recession, *J Periodontol* 60:316, 1989.

52. Pini Prato GP et al: Guided tissue regeneration versus mucogingival surgery in the treatment of human buccal recessions, *J Periodontol* 67:1216, 1996.

53. Matarasso MD et al: Guided tissue regeneration versus coronally repositioned flap in the treatment of recession with double papillae, *Int J Periodontol Rest Dent* 18:445, 1998.

54. Langer B, Langer L: Subepithelial connective tissue graft technique for root coverage, *J Periodontol* 56:715, 1985.

55. Zabalegui I et al : Treatment of multiple gingival recessions with the tunnel subepithelial connective tissue graft: a clinical report, *Int J Periodontol Rest Dent* 19:199, 1999.

56. Davarpanah M et al: Restorative and periodontal considerations of short clinical crowns, *Int J Periodontol Rest Dent* 18:5, 1998.

57. Palomo F, Kopczyk RA: Rationale and methods for crown lengthening, *J Am Dent Assoc* 96:257, 1978.

58. Ochsenbien C, Ross SE: A reevaluation of osseous surgery, *Dent Clin North Am* 13:87, 1969.

59. Maynard JG: Personal communication, 1993.

60. Ross SB et al: Orthodontic extrusion: a multidisciplinary treatment approach, *J Am Dent Assoc* 102:189, 1981.

61. Brown IS: The effect of orthodontic therapy on certain types of periodontal defects: clinical findings, *J Periodontol* 44:742, 1973.

62. Ingber JS: Forced eruption. I. A method of treating isolated one and two wall infrabony osseous defects: rationale and case report, *J Periodontol* 45:199, 1974.

63. Delivanis P et al: Endodontic-orthodontic management of fractured anterior teeth, *J Am Dent Assoc* 97:483, 1978.

64. Potashnik SR, Rosenberg ES: Forced eruption: principles in periodontics and restorative dentistry, *J Prosthet Dent* 48:141, 1982.

65. Baima RF: Extension of clinical crown length, *J Prosthet Dent* 55:547, 1986.

66. Rosenberg ES et al: Tooth lengthening procedures, *Compend Contin Educ Dent* 1:11, 1980.

67. Shapiro A: Regeneration of interdental papilla using periodic curettage, *Int J Periodont Rest Dent* 5:27, 1985.

68. Evian C, Corn H, Rosenberg E: Retained interdental procedure for maintaining anterior esthetics, *Comp Contin Educ Dent* 6:5, 1985.

69. Han TJ, Takei HH: Progress in gingival papilla reconstruction, *Periodontol 2000* 11:65, 1996.

70. Cortellini P, Pini Prato G, Tonetti MS: The modified papilla preservation technique with bioresorbable barrier membranes in the treatment of intrabony defects. *Case reports, Int J Periodont Rest Dent* 16:547, 1996.

71. Beagle JR: Surgical reconstruction of the interdental papilla: case report, *Int J Periodontol Rest Dent* 12:145, 1992.

72. Azzi R, Etienne D, Carranza F: Surgical reconstruction of the interdental papilla, *Int J Periodontol Rest Dent*, 18:467, 1998.

73. Tarnow DP, Magner AW, Fletcher P: The effect of the distance from the contact point to the crest of bone on the presence or absence of the interproximal papilla, *J Periodontol* 63:995, 1992.

74. Johnson GK, Sivers JE: Forced eruption in crown-lengthening procedures, *J Prosthet Dent* 56:424, 1986.

75. Tuncay OC: Orthodontic tooth movement as an adjunct to prosthetic therapy, *J Prosthet Dent* 46:41, 1981.

76. Miller TE: Orthodontic therapy for the restorative patient. I. The biomechanic aspects, *J Prosthet Dent* 61:268, 1989.

77. Celenza F, Mantzikos TG: Periodontal and restorative considerations of molar uprighting, *Compendium* 17:294, 1996.

78. Shaughnessy TG: Implementing adjunctive orthodontic treatment, *J Am Dent Assoc* 126:679, 1995.

79. Proffit WR: *Contemporary orthodontics,* ed 2, St Louis, 1993, Mosby.

80. Ackerman JL, Proffit WR: Communication in orthodontic treatment planning: bioethical and informed consent issues, *Angle Orthod* 65:253, 1995.

81. Grubb JE et al: Clinical and scientific applications/advances in video imaging, *Angle Orthod* 66:407, 1996.

82. Levine JB: Esthetic diagnosis, *Curr Opin Cosmet Dent* 9, 1995.

83. Goldstein RE, Miller MC: The role of high technology in maintaining esthetic restorations, *J Esthet Dent* 8:39, 1996.

84. Clark GT et al: The validity and utility of disease detection methods and of occlusal therapy for temporomandibular disorders, *Oral Surg* 83:101, 1997.

85. Kirveskari P: The role of occlusal adjustment in the management of temporomandibular disorders, *Oral Surg* 83:87, 1997.

86. Kirveskari P et al: Occlusal adjustment and the incidence of demand for temporomandibular disorder treatment, *J Prosthet Dent* 79:433, 1998.

87. Kerstein RB et al: A comparison of ICAGD (immediate complete anterior guidance development) to mock ICAGD for symptom reductions in chronic myofascial pain dysfunction patients, *Cranio* 15:21, 1997.

88. McNeill C: Craniomandibular disorders: guidelines for evaluation, diagnosis, and management. In American Academy of Craniomandibular Disorders: *Oral and facial pain,* Chicago, 1990, Quintessence Publishing.

89. Gher ME: Changing concepts. The effects of occlusion on periodontitis, *Dent Clin North Am* 42:285, 1998.

CLINICAL PROCEDURES PART I

PRINCIPLES OF TOOTH PREPARATION

KEY TERMS

causes of injury	path of insertion
conservation of tooth structure	resistance
diagnostic preparations	retention
margin designs	taper
margin placement	undercut

Teeth do not possess the regenerative ability found in most other tissues. Therefore, once enamel or dentin is lost as a result of caries, trauma, or wear, restorative materials must be used to reestablish form and function. Teeth require preparation to receive restorations, and these preparations must be based on fundamental principles from which basic criteria can be developed to help predict the success of prosthodontic treatment. Careful attention to every detail is imperative during tooth preparation. A good preparation will ensure that subsequent techniques (e.g., provisionalization, impression making, pouring of dies and casts, waxing) can be accomplished.

The principles of tooth preparation may be divided into three broad categories:

1. Biologic considerations, which affect the health of the oral tissues
2. Mechanical considerations, which affect the integrity and durability of the restoration
3. Esthetic considerations, which affect the appearance of the patient

Successful tooth preparation and subsequent restoration depend on simultaneous consideration of all these factors. Often improvement in one area will adversely affect another, and striving for perfection in one may lead to failure in another. For example, in the fabrication of a metal-ceramic crown (see Chapter 24), sufficient thickness of porcelain is necessary for a lifelike appearance. However, if too much tooth structure is removed to accommodate a greater thickness of porcelain for esthetic reasons, the pulpal tissue may be damaged (biologic consideration) and the tooth unduly weakened (mechanical consideration). An in-depth knowledge and understanding of the various criteria are prerequisites to the development of satisfactory tooth preparation skills. Predictable accomplishment of optimum tooth preparation (Fig. 7-1) often entails finding the best

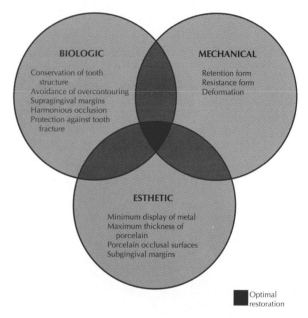

Fig. 7-1. The optimum restoration should satisfy biologic, mechanical, and esthetic requirements.

combination of compromises among the prevalent biologic, mechanical, and esthetic considerations.

■ BIOLOGIC CONSIDERATIONS

Surgical procedures involving living tissues must be carefully executed to avoid unnecessary damage. The adjacent teeth, soft tissues, and the pulp of the tooth being prepared are easily damaged in tooth preparation. If poor preparation leads to inadequate marginal fit or deficient crown contour, plaque control around fixed restorations will become more difficult. This will impede the long-term maintenance of dental health.

PREVENTION OF DAMAGE DURING TOOTH PREPARATION

Adjacent Teeth. Iatrogenic damage to an adjacent tooth is a common error in dentistry. Even if a damaged proximal contact area is carefully reshaped and polished, it will be more susceptible to dental caries than the original undamaged tooth surface. This is presumably because the original surface enamel contains higher fluoride concentrations and the interrupted layer is more prone to plaque **retention**. The technique of tooth preparation must avoid and prevent damage to the adjacent tooth surfaces.

A metal matrix band around the adjacent tooth for protection may be helpful; however, the thin band can still be perforated and the underlying enamel damaged. The preferred method is to use the proximal enamel of the tooth being prepared for protection of the adjacent structures. Teeth are 1.5 to 2 mm wider at the contact area than at the cementoenamel junction (CEJ), and a thin, tapered diamond can be passed through the interproximal contact area (Fig. 7-2) to leave a slight lip or fin of enamel without causing excessive tooth reduction or undesirable angulation of the rotary instrument.

Soft Tissues. Damage to the soft tissues of the tongue and cheeks can be prevented by careful retraction with an aspirator tip, mouth mirror (Fig. 7-3), or flanged saliva ejector. Great care is needed to protect the tongue when the lingual surfaces of mandibular molars are being prepared.

Pulp. Great care also is needed to prevent pulpal injuries during fixed prosthodontic procedures, especially complete crown preparation. Pulpal degeneration that occurs many years after tooth preparation has been documented.[1] Extreme temperatures, chemical irritation, or microorganisms can cause an irreversible pulpitis,[2] particularly when they occur on freshly sectioned dentinal tubules. Prevention of pulpal damage necessitates selection of techniques and materials that will reduce the risk of damage while preparing tooth structure.[3]

Tooth preparations must take into consideration the morphology of the dental pulp chamber. Pulp size, which can be evaluated on a radiograph, decreases with age. Average pulp dimensions have been related to coronal contour[4] and are presented in Table 7-1 and Figure 7-4.

Causes of Injury

Temperature. Considerable heat is generated by friction between a rotary instrument and the surface being prepared (Fig. 7-5). Excessive pressure, higher rotational speeds, and the type, shape, and condition of the cutting instrument (Fig. 7-6) may all increase generated heat.[5] With a high-speed handpiece, a feather-light touch allows efficient removal of tooth material with minimal heat generation. Nevertheless, even with the lightest touch, the tooth will be overheated unless a water spray is used. This must be accurately directed at the area of contact between tooth and bur. It will also remove debris (important because clogging reduces cutting efficiency) and prevent desiccation of the dentin (a cause of severe pulpal irritation[1,6]). If the spray prevents adequate visibility, as may be the case when finishing a lingual margin, a slow-speed handpiece or hand instrumentation should be used. Relying on air cooling with a high-speed handpiece is hazardous, because it can easily overheat a tooth and damage the pulp.[7]

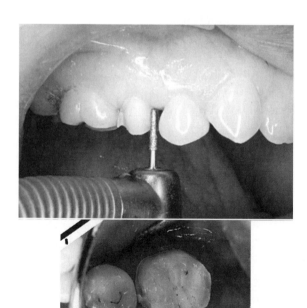

Fig. 7-2. Damage to adjacent teeth is prevented by making a thin "lip" of enamel as the bur passes through a proximal contact.

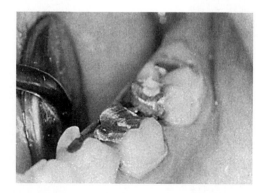

Fig. 7-3. Mouth mirror protecting the soft tissues during tooth preparation.

TABLE 7-1 Dimensions of Pulp and the Coronal Contour

Maxillary Central Incisor

Age Range (yr)	Coronal Length (mm)	Incisal to MPH (mm)	Incisal to DPH (mm)	Mesial Surface to MPH (mm)	Distal Surface to DPH (mm)	Labial Surface to MPH (mm)	Labial Surface to DPH (mm)	Palatal Surface to MPH (mm)	Palatal Surface to DPH (mm)
10-19	12.1	4.7	4.8	1.7	2.1	1.8	1.8	1.4	1.3
20-29	11.5	4.8	5.1	2.2	2.3	1.9	1.9	1.4	1.2
30-39	11.2	5.3	5.5	2.1	2.5	2.3	2.4	2.1	2.0
40-49	10.8	6.3	6.2	2.5	2.9	2.0	2.1	2.0	1.8
50-59	12.3	6.3	6.2	2.6	2.6	2.8	2.3	2.2	2.1
Mean ± SD	11.58 ± 0.34	5.5 ± 0.25	5.6 ± 0.28	2.2 ± 0.16	2.5 ± 0.14	2.2 ± 0.12	2.1 ± 0.12	1.8 ± 0.16	1.7 ± 0.19
Range	9.70-14.00	4.0-6.2	4.0-6.2	1.2-3.3	1.4-3.5	1.5-2.9	1.5-2.9	1.0-2.9	1.1-2.9

Maxillary Lateral Incisor

Age Range (yr)	Coronal Length (mm)	Incisal to MPH (mm)	Incisal to DPH (mm)	Mesial Surface to MPH (mm)	Distal Surface to DPH (mm)	Labial Surface to MPH (mm)	Labial Surface to DPH (mm)	Palatal Surface to MPH (mm)	Palatal Surface to DPH (mm)
10-19	10.1	3.9	4.3	2.4	2.6	2.0	2.1	1.3	1.3
20-29	10.2	4.8	5.2	2.5	3.2	2.4	2.4	1.9	1.9
30-39	10.0	4.8	—	2.4	3.2	2.1	2.3	2.0	1.7
40-49	9.0	4.8	5.2	1.9	2.2	2.1	2.1	1.7	1.5
50-59	9.7	6.0	—	2.2	2.3	2.3	2.3	2.6	2.5
Mean ± SD	8.84 ± 0.23	4.9 ± 0.40	4.9 ± 0.32	2.3 ± 0.20	2.7 ± 0.19	2.2 ± 0.04	2.2 ± 0.15	1.9 ± 0.11	1.8 ± 0.17
Range	7.90-11.91	3.6-6.2	3.6-6.4	1.2-3.2	1.8-3.6	1.7-2.7	1.8-2.7	1.2-3.2	1.1-2.9

Maxillary Canine

Age Range (yr)	Coronal Length (mm)	Incisal to PH (mm)	Mesial Surface to PH (mm)	Distal Surface to PH (mm)	Labial Surface to PH (mm)	Palatal Surface to PH (mm)
10-19	10.7	4.4	3.4	4.0	2.7	2.3
20-29	10.6	4.6	3.3	3.7	3.1	2.6
30-39	10.5	4.8	3.0	4.0	2.9	2.5
40-49	9.5	4.8	3.0	3.6	2.8	2.8
50-59	9.9	5.4	2.8	3.4	2.9	3.0
Mean ± SD	10.23 ± 0.26	4.8 ± 0.20	3.1 ± 0.13	3.7 ± 0.12	2.9 ± 0.11	2.6 ± 0.15
Range	8.29-12.20	3.8-1.2	2.3-3.6	2.9-4.8	2.5-3.5	1.9-3.7

From Ohashi Y: *Shikagakuho* 68:726, 1968.
MPH, Mesial pulp horn; *DPH,* distal pulp horn; *PH,* pulp horn.

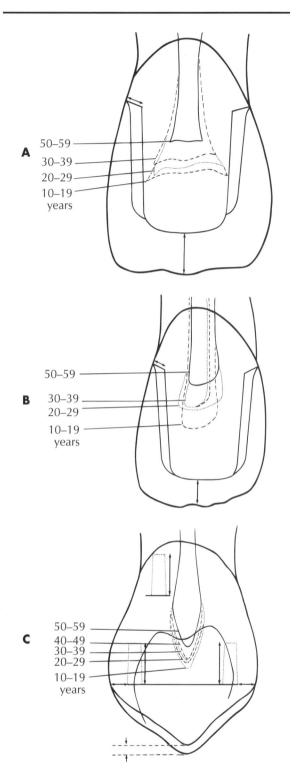

Fig. 7-4. Relationship between tooth preparation and pulp chamber size. The dotted lines represent pulp chamber morphology at various ages. **A,** Maxillary central incisor with a metal-ceramic crown preparation. **B,** Maxillary lateral incisor with a metal-ceramic crown preparation. **C,** Maxillary canine with a pinledge preparation.
(From Ohashi Y: Shikagakuho 68:726, 1968.)

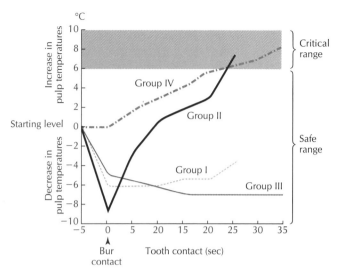

Fig. 7-5. Pulpal temperature rise during tooth preparation. Group I, air turbine, water cooled. Group II, air turbine, dry. Group III, low speed, water cooled. Group IV, low speed, dry.
(From Zach L, Cohen G: Oral Surg 19:515, 1965.)

Particular care is needed when preparing grooves or pinholes, because coolant cannot reach the cutting edge of the bur. To prevent heat buildup, these retention features should always be prepared at low rotational speed.

Chemical Action. The chemical action of certain dental materials (bases, restorative resins, solvents, and luting agents) can cause pulpal damage,[8] particularly when they are applied to freshly cut dentin. Cavity varnish or dentin bonding agents will form an effective barrier in most instances, but their effect on the retention of a cemented restoration is controversial.[9-11]

Chemical agents are sometimes used for cleaning and degreasing tooth preparations. However, they have been shown[12] to be pulpal irritants. Thus their use is generally contraindicated, particularly because they do not improve the retention of cemented restorations.[13]

Bacterial Action. Pulpal damage under restorations has been attributed[14,15] to bacteria that either were left behind or gained access to the dentin because of microleakage. However, many dental materials, including zinc phosphate cement, have an antibacterial effect[16]; because vital dentin seems to resist infection,[17] the routine use of antimicrobials may not be advantageous. Many dentists now use an antimicrobial agent, such as Consepsis,* after tooth

---

*Ultradent Products, Inc.

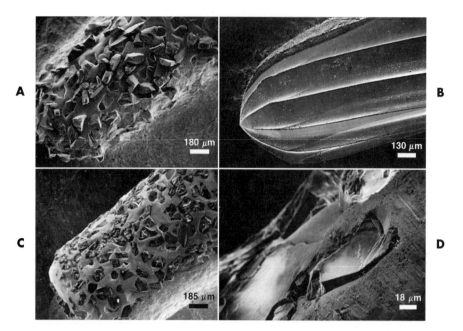

Fig. 7-6. Scanning electron micrographs of a rotary instrument. **A,** Unused diamond. **B,** Unused carbide. **C,** Worn diamond. **D,** Diamond particles have fractured at the level of the binder. *(Courtesy Dr. J.L. Sandrik.)*

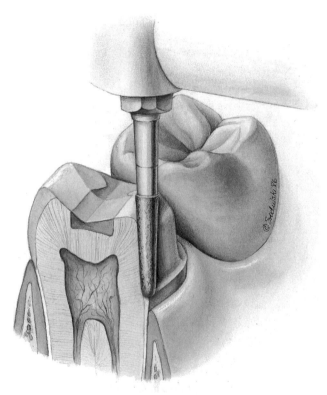

Fig. 7-7. A considerable amount of care is needed when preparing a tooth for a complete crown because of the extensive nature of the reduction, with many dentinal tubules sectioned. Each tubule communicates directly with the dental pulp.

preparation and before cementation, although the benefit has not been documented in clinical trials.[18]

NOTE: All carious dentin should be removed before placing a restoration that will serve as a foundation for a fixed prosthesis. An indirect pulp cap is not recommended, because its later failure is likely to jeopardize extensive prosthodontic treatment.

CONSERVATION OF TOOTH STRUCTURE

One of the basic tenets of restorative dentistry is to conserve as much tooth structure as possible consistent with the mechanical and esthetic principles of tooth preparation. This will reduce the harmful pulpal effects of the various procedures and materials used. The thickness of remaining dentin has been shown[19] to be inversely proportional to the pulpal response, and tooth preparations extending deeply toward the pulp should be avoided. Dowden[20] has argued that any damage to the odontoblastic processes will adversely affect the cell nucleus at the dentin-pulp interface, no matter how far from the nucleus it occurs. For this reason, when assessing likely adverse pulpal response, the amount of dentin removed is important; particular care must be exercised when preparing vital teeth for complete-coverage restorations (Fig. 7-7).

Tooth structure is conserved by using the following guidelines:

1.   Use of partial-coverage rather than complete-coverage restorations (Fig. 7-8)

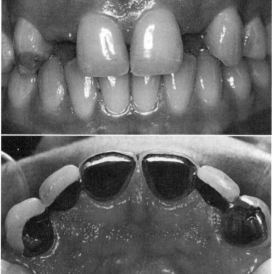

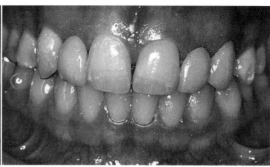

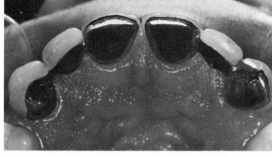

Fig. 7-8. Conservation of tooth structure by using partial-coverage restorations. In this case, they are used as FPD abutments to replace congenitally missing lateral incisors.

2. Preparation of teeth with the minimum practical convergence angle **(taper)** between axial walls (Fig. 7-9)
3. Preparation of the occlusal surface so reduction follows the anatomic planes to give uniform thickness in the restoration (Fig. 7-10)
4. Preparation of the axial surfaces so tooth structure is removed evenly; if necessary, teeth should be orthodontically repositioned (Fig. 7-11)
5. Selection of a conservative margin compatible with the other principles of tooth preparation (Fig. 7-12)
6. Avoidance of unnecessary apical extension of the preparation (Fig. 7-13)

CONSIDERATIONS AFFECTING FUTURE DENTAL HEALTH

An improperly prepared tooth may have an adverse effect on long-term dental health. For example, insufficient axial reduction inevitably results in an overcontoured restoration that hampers plaque control. This may cause periodontal disease[21] or dental caries. Alternatively, inadequate occlusal reduction may result in occlusal dysfunction, and poor margin placement may lead to chipped enamel or cusp fracture.

Axial Reduction. Gingival inflammation is commonly associated with crowns and FPD abutments having excessive axial contours, probably because it is more difficult for the patient to maintain plaque control around the gingival margin.[22] A tooth preparation must provide sufficient space for

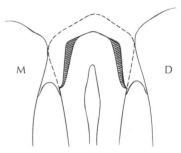

Fig. 7-9. Excessive taper results in considerable loss of tooth structure *(shaded area).*

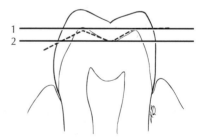

Minimally required clearances:
Buccal cusp—1.5 mm
Lingual cusp—1.0 mm
Marginal ridges and fossae—1.0 mm

Fig. 7-10. An anatomically prepared occlusal surface results in adequate clearance without excessive tooth reduction. A flat occlusal preparation will result in either *(1)* insufficient clearance or *(2)* an excessive amount of reduction.

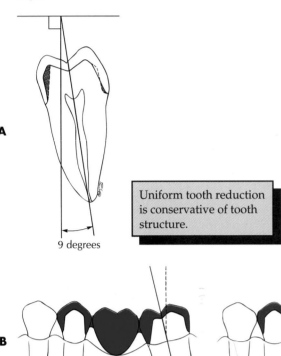

A

9 degrees

Fig. 7-11. To conserve tooth structure, the preparation of axial surfaces should be as uniform as possible. **A,** The path of withdrawal should coincide with the long axis of the tooth, which for a mandibular premolar is typically inclined 9 degrees lingually. Preparing the tooth perpendicular to the occlusal plane is a commonly seen error and results in additional tooth reduction *(shaded area)*. **B** and **C,** Tooth structure is conserved by uprighting a tilted FPD abutment.

Uniform tooth reduction is conservative of tooth structure.

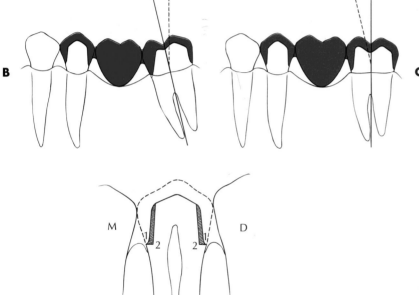

B

C

M   D

Fig. 7-12. A shoulder margin *(2)* is less conservative than a chamfer *(1)*.

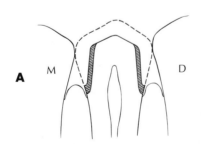

A   M   D

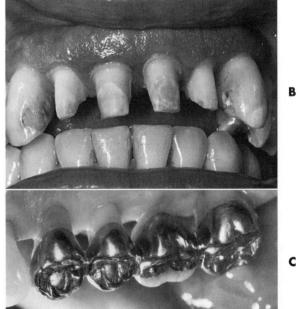

B

C

Fig. 7-13. **A,** Apical extension of the preparation can necessitate additional tooth reduction. **B,** Preparations for periodontally involved teeth may necessitate considerable reduction if the margins are to be placed subgingivally for esthetic reasons. **C,** Supragingival margins are preferred where applicable.

the development of good axial contours. This will enable the junction between the restoration and the tooth to be smooth and free of any ledges or abrupt changes in direction.

Under most circumstances a crown should duplicate the contours and profile of the original tooth (unless the restoration is needed to correct a malformed or malpositioned tooth). If an error is made, a slightly undercontoured flat restoration is better because it is easier to keep free of plaque; however, increasing proximal contour on anterior crowns to maintain the interproximal papilla[23] (see Chapter 5) may be beneficial. Sufficient tooth structure must be removed to allow the development of correctly formed axial contours (Fig. 7-14), particularly in the interproximal and furcation areas of posterior teeth, where periodontal disease often begins.

Margin Placement. Whenever possible, the margin of the preparation should be **supragingival**. Subgingival margins of cemented restorations have been identified[24-29] as a major factor in periodontal disease, particularly where they encroach on the ep-

ithelial attachment (see Chapter 5). Supragingival margins are easier to prepare accurately without trauma to the soft tissues. They can usually also be situated on hard enamel, whereas subgingival margins are often on dentin or cementum.

Other advantages of supragingival margins include the following:

1. They can be easily finished.
2. They are more easily kept clean.
3. Impressions are more easily made, with less potential for soft tissue damage.
4. Restorations can be easily evaluated at recall appointments.

However, a subgingival margin (Fig. 7-15) is justified if any of the following pertain:

1. Dental caries, cervical erosion, or restorations extend subgingivally, and a crown-lengthening procedure (see Chapter 6) is not indicated.
2. The proximal contact area extends to the gingival crest.
3. Additional retention is needed.
4. The margin of a metal-ceramic crown is to be hidden behind the labiogingival crest.

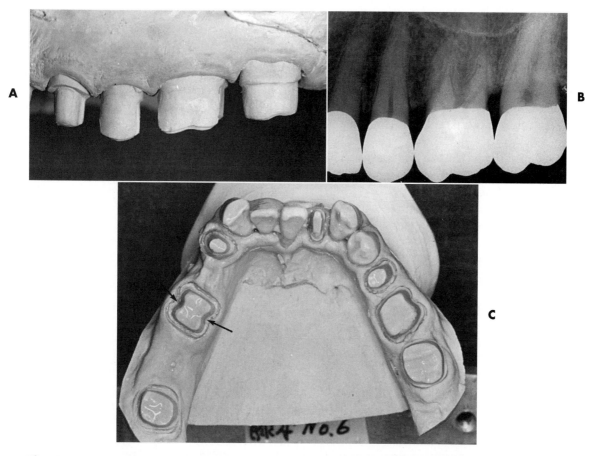

Fig. 7-14. A and B, Tooth preparations with adequate axial reduction allow the development of properly contoured embrasures. Tissue is conserved by using partial coverage and supragingival margins where possible. C, Preparing furcation areas adequately is important; otherwise, the restoration will be excessively contoured, making plaque control difficult.

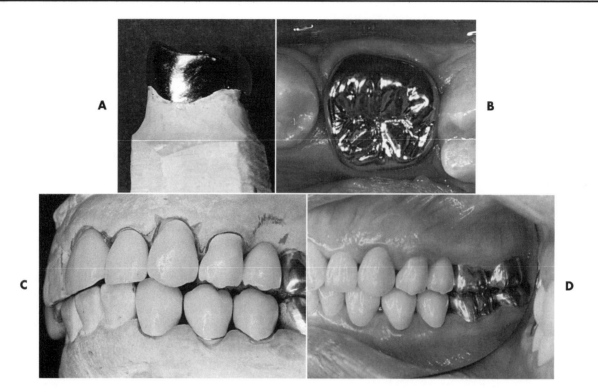

Fig. 7-15. Examples where subgingival margins are indicated. **A,** To include an existing restoration. **B,** To extend apical to the proximal contact (adequate proximal clearance). **C** and **D,** To hide the metal collar of metal-ceramic crowns.

5. Root sensitivity cannot be controlled by more conservative procedures, such as the application of dentin bonding agents.
6. Modification of the axial contour is indicated.

Margin Adaptation. The junction between a cemented restoration and the tooth is always a potential site for recurrent caries because of dissolution of the luting agent and inherent roughness. The more accurately the restoration is adapted to the tooth, the lesser the chance of recurrent caries or periodontal disease.[30] Although a precise figure for acceptable margin adaptation is not available, a skilled technician can make a casting that fits to within 10 μm[31] and a porcelain margin that fits to within 50 μm,[32] provided the tooth is properly prepared. A well-designed preparation has a smooth and even margin. Rough, irregular, or "stepped" junctions greatly increase the length of the margin and substantially reduce the adaptation of the restoration (Fig. 7-16). The importance of preparing smooth margins cannot be overemphasized. Time spent obtaining a smooth margin will make the subsequent steps of tissue displacement, impression making, die formation, waxing, and finishing much easier and will ultimately provide the patient with a longer-lasting restoration.

Margin Geometry. The cross-sectional configuration of the margin has been the subject of much analysis and debate.[33-40] Different shapes have been described and advocated.[41,42] For evaluation, the following guidelines for margin design should be considered:
1. Ease of preparation without overextension or unsupported enamel
2. Ease of identification in the impression and on the die
3. A distinct boundary to which the wax pattern can be finished
4. Sufficient bulk of material (to enable the wax pattern to be handled without distortion and to give the restoration strength and, when porcelain is used, esthetics)
5. Conservation of tooth structure (provided the other criteria are met)

Proposed **margin designs** are presented in Table 7-2.

Although they are conservative of tooth structure, featheredge or shoulderless crown preparations (Fig. 7-17, *A*) should be avoided because they fail to provide adequate bulk at the margins. Overcontoured restorations often result from featheredge margins because the technician can handle the wax pattern without distortion only by increas-

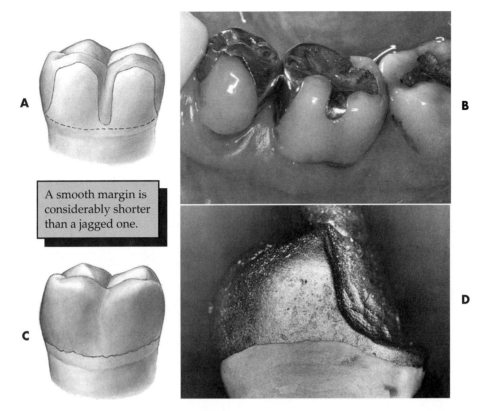

A smooth margin is considerably shorter than a jagged one.

Fig. 7-16. **A** and **B,** Poor preparation design, leading to increased margin length. **C,** A rough, irregular margin will make the fabrication of an accurately fitted restoration almost impossible. **D,** An accurately fitting margin is possible only if it is prepared smoothly.

Advantages and Disadvantages of Different Margin Designs   TABLE 7-2

	Advantages	Disadvantages	Indications
Featheredge	Conservative of tooth structure	Does not provide sufficient bulk	Not recommended
Chisel edge	Conservative of tooth structure	Location of margin difficult to control	Occasionally on tilted teeth
Bevel	Removes unsupported enamel, allows finishing of metal	Extends preparation into sulcus if used on apical margin	Facial margin of maxillary partial-coverage restorations and inlay/onlay margins
Chamfer	Distinct margin, adequate bulk, easier to control	Care needed to avoid unsupported lip of enamel	Cast metal restorations, lingual margin of metal-ceramic crowns
Shoulder	Bulk of restorative material	Less conservative of tooth structure	Facial margin of metal-ceramic crowns, complete ceramic crowns
Sloped shoulder	Bulk of material, advantages of bevel	Less conservative of tooth structure	Facial margins of metal-ceramic crowns
Shoulder with bevel	Bulk of material, advantages of bevel	Less conservative, extends preparation apically	Facial margin of posterior metal-ceramic crowns with supragingival margins

ing its bulk beyond the original contours. A variation of the featheredge, the chisel edge margin (Fig. 7-17, *B*), is formed when there is a larger angle between the axial surfaces and the unprepared tooth structure. Unfortunately, this margin is frequently associated with an excessively tapered preparation or one in which the axial reduction is not correctly aligned with the long axis of the tooth.

Under most circumstances, featheredges and chisel edges are unacceptable. Historically their main advantage was that they facilitated the making of impressions with rigid modeling compound in copper bands (a technique rarely used today), because there was no ledge on which a band could catch. A chamfer margin (Fig. 7-17, *C*) is particularly suitable for cast metal crowns and the

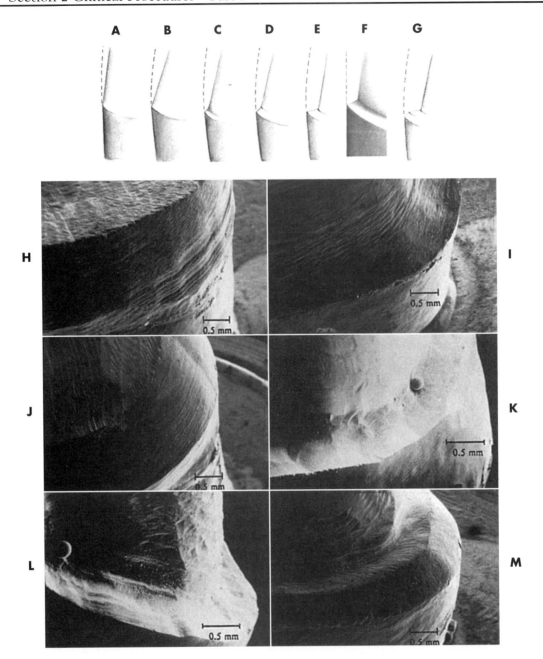

Fig. 7-17. Margin designs: **A,** Featheredge. **B,** Chisel. **C,** Chamfer. **D,** Bevel. **E,** Shoulder. **F,** Sloped shoulder. **G,** Beveled shoulder. Scanning electron micrographs. **H,** Feather-chisel edge. **I,** Chamfer. **J,** Bevel. **K,** Shoulder. **L,** Sloped shoulder. **M,** Beveled shoulder. *(Courtesy Dr. H. Lin.)*

metal-only portion of metal-ceramic crowns (Fig. 7-18). It is distinct and easily identified, provides room for adequate bulk of material, and can be placed with precision, although care is needed to avoid leaving a ledge of unsupported enamel.

Probably the most suitable instrument for making a chamfer margin is the tapered diamond with a rounded tip; the margin formed is the exact image of the instrument (Fig. 7-19). Marginal accuracy depends on having a high-quality diamond and a true-running handpiece. The gingival margin is prepared with the diamond held precisely in the in-tended path of withdrawal of the restoration (Fig. 7-20). Tilting it away from the tooth will create an **undercut,** whereas angling it toward the tooth will lead to overreduction and loss of retention. The chamfer should never be prepared wider than half the tip of the diamond; otherwise, an unsupported lip of enamel could result (Fig. 7-21). Some authorities have recommended the use of a diamond with a noncutting guide tip to aid accurate chamfer placement.[43] However, the guide has been shown to damage tooth structure beyond the intended preparation margin.[44]

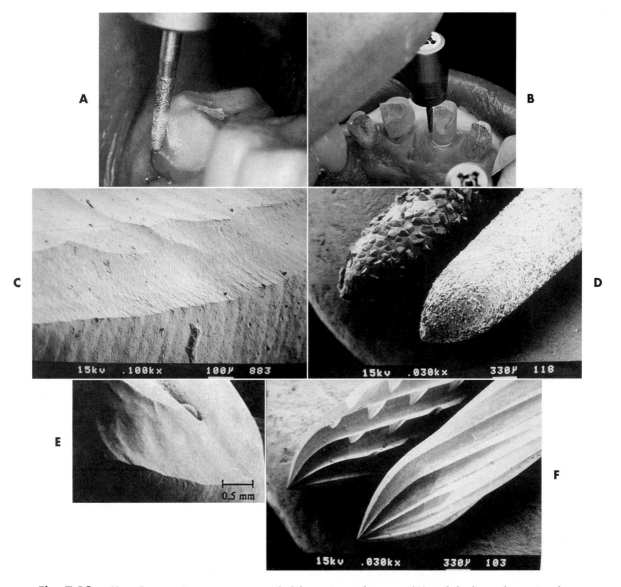

Fig. 7-18. Chamfer margins are recommended for cast metal crowns **(A)** and the lingual margin of a metal-ceramic crown **(B)**. Compare the scanning electron micrographs of a chamfer **(C)** achieved with a fine-grit diamond after initial preparation with a coarser instrument **(D)** and a chamfer achieved with finishing carbides **(E and F)**.
(C to F courtesy Dr. H. Lin.)

Under some circumstances a beveled margin (Fig. 7-17, *D*) is more suitable for cast restorations, particularly if a ledge or shoulder already exists, possibly from dental caries, cervical erosion, or a previous restoration. The objective in beveling is threefold: (1) to allow the cast metal margin to be bent or burnished against the prepared tooth structure; (2) to minimize the marginal discrepancy[33] caused by a complete crown that fails to seat completely (however, Pascoe[38] has shown that when an oversized crown is considered, the discrepancy is increased rather than decreased [Fig. 7-22]); and (3) to protect the unprepared tooth structure from chipping (e.g., by removing unsupported enamel). NOTE: When access for burnishing is limited, there is little advantage in beveling. This applies particularly to a

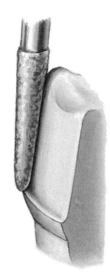

Fig. 7-19. A chamfer margin is formed as the negative image of a round-ended tapered diamond.

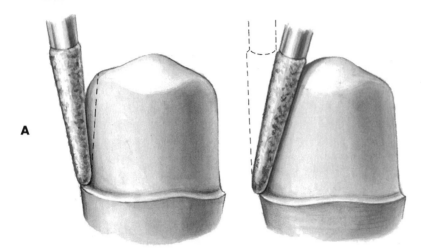

A

B

At left, the diamond is tipped away from the path of placement, resulting in an undercut; at right, the diamond is tipped into the tooth too far, leading to an excessively tapered preparation.

Fig. 7-20.   Precise control of the orientation of the diamond is very important. **A,** Tilting away from the tooth creates an undercut. **B,** Tilting toward the tooth results in excessive convergence.

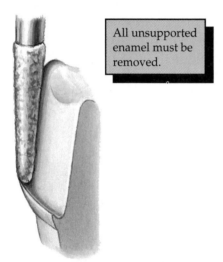

All unsupported enamel must be removed.

Fig. 7-21.   A chamfer should not be wider than half the bur used to form it. Otherwise, a lip of unsupported enamel will be left.

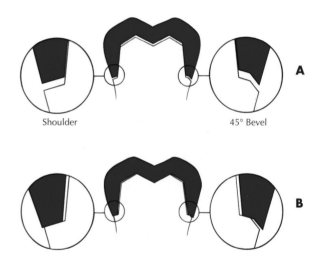

Shoulder   45° Bevel

A

B

Properly seated castings should have minimal marginal gap widths.

Fig. 7-22.   Effect on marginal fit of beveling the gingival margin. **A,** If the internal cross section of a crown is the same as or less than that of the prepared tooth, a 45-degree bevel will decrease the marginal discrepancy by 70%. **B,** If the internal diameter is slightly larger than the prepared tooth, beveling will increase the marginal discrepancy. In practice, crowns are made slightly larger than the prepared tooth to allow for the luting agent.

gingival margin, where beveling would lead to subgingival extension of the preparation or placement of the margin on dentin rather than on enamel. Facial margins of maxillary partial-coverage restorations should be beveled to protect the remaining tooth structure and to allow for burnishing.

Because a shoulder margin (Fig. 7-17, *E*) allows room for porcelain, it is recommended for the facial part of metal-ceramic crowns, especially when the porcelain margin technique is used. It should form a 90-degree angle with the unprepared tooth surface. An acute angle is likely to chip (Fig. 7-23, *A*). In practice, dentists tend to underprepare the facial shoulder,[45] leading to restorations with inferior esthetics or poor axial contour.

Some authorities[46] have recommended a heavy chamfer rather than a shoulder margin, and some find a chamfer easier to prepare with precision. Earlier work[36,37] found less distortion of the metal framework during porcelain application, although with modern alloys, this doesn't appear to be a problem (see Chapter 19).

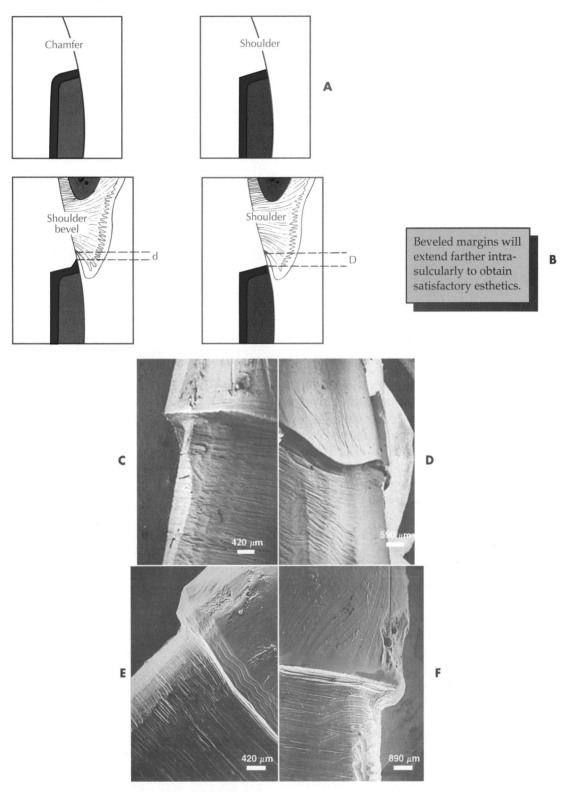

Fig. 7-23. **A,** A shoulder provides more bulk of metal than a heavy chamfer, which may facilitate the laboratory steps. **B,** A disadvantage of the shoulder bevel is that its margin must be placed deeper in the gingival sulcus so that the wider band of metal will be hidden (compare *d* with *D*). **C,** Scanning electron micrograph of a shoulder margin prepared with a high-speed diamond. **D,** This margin has been refined with a sharp chisel. **E,** This has been beveled with a tungsten carbide bur. **F,** This bevel was placed with a sharp hand instrument.

(Microscopy by Dr. J. Sandrik; teeth prepared by Dr. G. Byrne.)

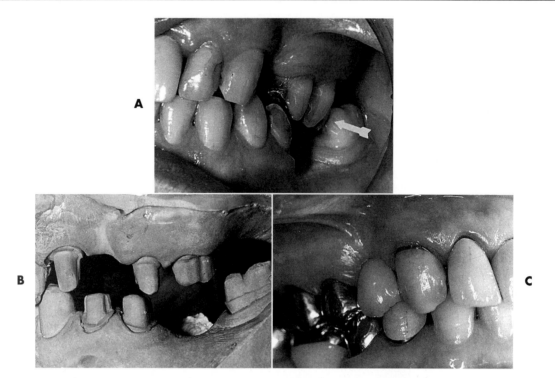

Fig. 7-24. **A,** Nonreplacement of missing teeth has led to supraocclusion and a protrusive interference (*arrow*). **B,** Teeth reduced with the help of trial tooth preparations and diagnostic waxing. **C,** Restorations with anterior guidance.

A 120-degree sloped shoulder margin (Fig. 7-17, *F*) is used as an alternative to the 90-degree shoulder for the facial margin of a metal-ceramic crown. The sloped shoulder reduces the possibility of leaving unsupported enamel and yet leaves sufficient bulk to allow thinning of the metal framework to a knife-edge for acceptable esthetics.

A beveled shoulder margin (Fig. 7-17, *G*) is often recommended for the facial surface of a metal-ceramic restoration where a metal collar (as opposed to a porcelain labial margin) is used. The beveling removes unsupported enamel and may allow some finishing of the metal. However, a shoulder or sloped shoulder is preferred for biologic and esthetic reasons. This allows improved esthetics because the metal margin can be thinned to a knife edge and hidden in the sulcus without the need for positioning the margin closer to the epithelial attachment (Fig. 7-23, *B*).

Occlusal Considerations. A satisfactory tooth preparation should allow sufficient space for developing a functional occlusal scheme in the finished restoration. Sometimes a patient's occlusion is disrupted by supraerupted or tilted teeth (Fig. 7-24). When these teeth are prepared for restoration, the

eventual occlusal plane must be carefully analyzed and the teeth reduced accordingly. Often considerable reduction is needed to compensate for the supraeruption of abutment teeth.

Sometimes even endodontic treatment is necessary to make enough room. However, under these circumstances, violating the principle of conservation of tooth structure is preferable to the potential harm from a traumatic occlusal scheme. Obviously, careful judgment is needed, and diagnostic tooth preparations and waxing procedures are essential to determining the exact amount of reduction required to develop an optimum occlusion.

Preventing Tooth Fracture. No tooth is unbreakable. If teeth are smashed together (as in an automobile accident, sport injury, or biting on a hard object unexpectedly), a cusp may break. Cuspal fracture also can occur from parafunctional habits such as bruxism.

The likelihood that a restored tooth will fracture can be lessened if the tooth preparation is designed to minimize potentially destructive stresses (Fig. 7-25). For example, an intracoronal cast restoration (inlay) has a greater potential for fracture because when occlusal forces are applied to the restoration,

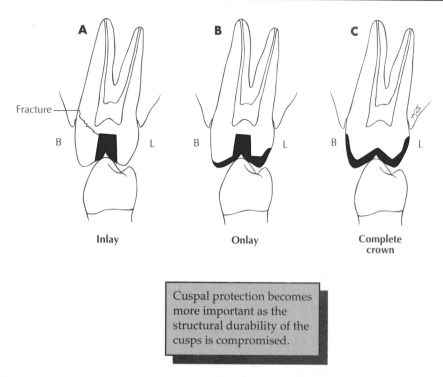

Fig. 7-25. **A,** An intracoronal cast restoration (inlay) can act as a wedge during cementation or function. If the cusps are weakened, fracture will occur. **B,** A cuspal-coverage onlay provides better protection but often lacks retention. **C,** A complete crown provides the best protection against fracture. It also has the best retention, but it can be associated with periodontal disease and poor esthetics. *(Redrawn from Rosenstiel SF: In Rayne J, editor:* General dental treatment, *London, 1983, Kluwer Publishing.)*

it tends to wedge opposing walls of the tooth apart. This wedging must be resisted by the remaining tooth structure; if the structure is thin (as with a wide preparation isthmus), the tooth may fracture during function. Providing a cuspal coverage restoration (onlay) rather than an inlay lessens the chance of such fracture.[47] However, although not conservative of tooth structure, a complete crown is often a better solution, because it offers the greatest protection against tooth fracture, tending to "hold" the cusps of the tooth together.

MECHANICAL CONSIDERATIONS

The design of tooth preparations for fixed prosthodontics must adhere to certain mechanical principles; otherwise, the restoration may become dislodged or may distort or fracture during service. These principles have evolved from theoretical and clinical observations and are supported by experimental studies.

Mechanical considerations can be divided into three categories:
1. Providing retention form
2. Providing **resistance** form
3. Preventing deformation of the restoration

RETENTION FORM

Certain forces (e.g., when the jaws are moved apart after biting on very sticky food) act on a cemented restoration in the same direction as the path of withdrawal. The quality of a preparation that prevents the restoration from becoming dislodged by such forces parallel to the path of withdrawal is known as *retention.* Only dental caries and porcelain failure outrank lack of retention as a cause of failure of crowns and fixed partial dentures.[48,49]

The following factors must be considered when deciding whether retention is adequate for a given fixed restoration:
1. Magnitude of the dislodging forces
2. Geometry of the tooth preparation
3. Roughness of the fitting surface of the restoration
4. Materials being cemented
5. Film thickness of the luting agent

Magnitude of the Dislodging Forces. Forces that tend to remove a cemented restoration along its path of withdrawal are small compared to those that tend to seat or tilt it. A fixed partial denture or splint can be subjected to such forces by pulling with floss under the connectors; however, the greatest removal forces generally arise when exceptionally sticky food (e.g., caramel) is eaten. The magnitude of the dislodging forces depends on the stickiness of the food and the surface area and texture of the restoration being pulled.

Geometry of the Tooth Preparation. Most fixed prostheses depend on the geometric form of the preparation rather than on adhesion for retention because most of the traditional cements (e.g., zinc phosphate) are nonadhesive (i.e., they act by increasing the frictional resistance between tooth and restoration). The grains of cement prevent two surfaces from sliding, although they do not prevent one surface from being lifted from another. This is analogous to the effect of particles of sand or dust within machinery. They do not have a specific adhesion to metal, but they increase the friction between sliding metal parts. If sand or dust gets into an old-fashioned, mechanical camera or watch, the increase in friction can effectively jam the mechanism.

Cement is effective only if the restoration has a single path of withdrawal (i.e., the tooth is shaped to restrain the free movement of the restoration). The relationship between a nut and a bolt is an example of restrained movement (Fig. 7-26). The nut is not free to move in any direction but can move only along the precisely determined helical path of the threads on the bolt.

The relationship between two bodies, one (in this case a tooth preparation) restraining movement of

> Minimizing taper effectively limits the number of directions in which a cast crown can be dislodged.

the other (a cemented restoration), has been studied mathematically and is known in analytical mechanics as a *closed lower pair of kinematic elements.*[50] In fixed prosthodontics, a *sliding pair* is the only pair that has relevance. It is formed by two cylindrical* surfaces constrained to slide along one another. The elements are constrained if the curve that defines the cylinder is closed or shaped to prevent movement at right angles to the axis of the cylinder (Fig. 7-27).

A tooth preparation will be cylindrical if the axial surfaces are prepared by a cylindrical bur held at a constant angle. The gingival margin of the preparation becomes the fixed curve of the mathematical definition, and the occlusoaxial line angle of the tooth preparation should be a replica of the gingival margin geometry. The curve of a complete crown preparation is closed, whereas the grooves of a partial crown preparation prevent movement at right angles to the long axis of the cylinder. However, if one wall of the complete crown preparation is over-

---

Cylinder is defined in its mathematical sense as the solid generated by a straight line parallel to another straight line and moving so that its ends describe a fixed curve.

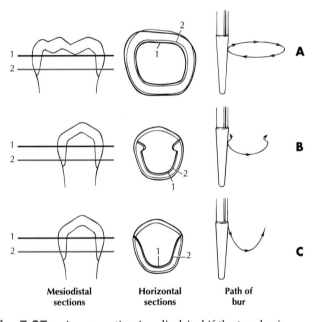

Fig. 7-27. A preparation is cylindrical if the two horizontal cross sections of the prepared axial tooth surface (1 and 2) are coincident. **A,** This complete crown is cylindrical and therefore retentive. **B,** A partial crown will be retentive if its sections are coincident and perpendicular movement is prevented by grooves. **C,** This preparation is cylindrical (1 and 2 coincide) but not retentive, because it can move perpendicularly to the axis of the cylinder. *(Redrawn from Rosenstiel E: Br Dent J 103:388, 1957.)*

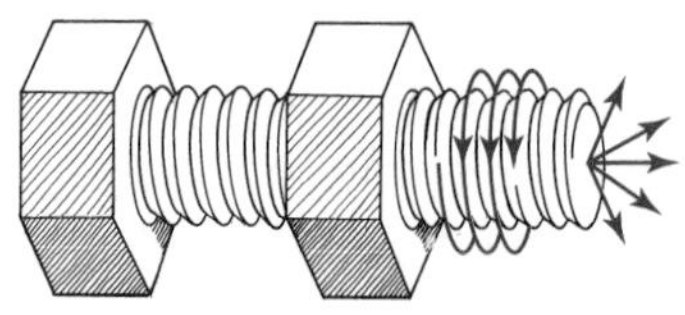

Mesiodistal sections   Horizontal sections   Path of bur

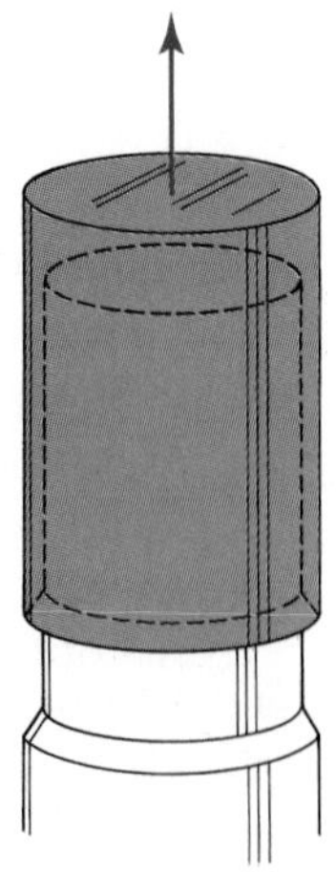

Fig. 7-26. A, The relationship of a nut and a bolt is an example of restrained movement; the nut must move along a precisely defined helical path *(arrows).* **B,** For effective retention, a tooth preparation must constrain the movement of a restoration. For this to occur, it must be cylindrical. (See Figure 7-27.)

tapered, it will no longer be cylindrical, and the cemented restoration will not be constrained by the preparation because the restoration then has multiple paths of withdrawal. Under these circumstances, the cement particles will tend to lift away from rather than slide along the preparation, and the only retention will be a result of the cement's limited adhesion (Fig. 7-28).

Taper. Theoretically, maximum retention is obtained if a tooth preparation has parallel walls. However, it is impossible to prepare a tooth this way using current techniques and instrumentation; slight undercuts are created that prevent the restoration from seating.

An undercut is defined as a divergence between opposing axial walls, or wall segments, in a cervical-occlusal direction (Fig. 7-29, *A*). For instance, if the cervical diameter of a tooth preparation at the margin is narrower than at the occlusoaxial junction (reverse taper), it will be impossible to seat a complete cast crown of similar geometry (Fig. 7-29, *B*). Undercuts can be present whenever two axial walls face in opposite directions (Fig. 7-29, *C*). Thus the mesial wall of a complete cast crown preparation can be undercut relative to the distal wall; in addi-

tion, the buccal wall can be undercut relative to the lingual wall; finally, in a partial veneer preparation, the lingual wall of a proximal groove can be undercut relative to the lingual wall of the preparation.

A slight convergence, or taper, is necessary in the completed preparation. As long as this taper is small, the movement of the cemented restoration will be effectively restrained by the preparation and will have what is known as a *limited path of withdrawal*. As the taper increases, however, so does the free movement of the restoration, and retention will be reduced.

The relationship between the degree of axial wall taper and the magnitude of retention was first demonstrated experimentally by Jørgensen[51] in 1955. He cemented brass caps on Galalith cones of different tapers and measured retention with a tensile-testing machine. The relationship was found to be hyperbolic, with retention rapidly becoming less as taper increased (Fig. 7-30), although the relation-

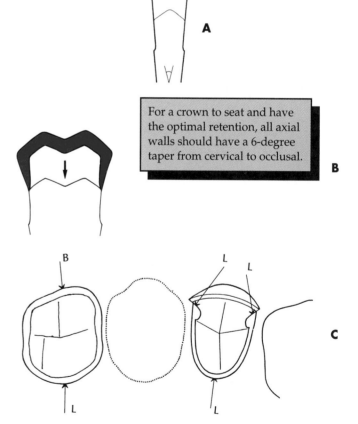

For a crown to seat and have the optimal retention, all axial walls should have a 6-degree taper from cervical to occlusal.

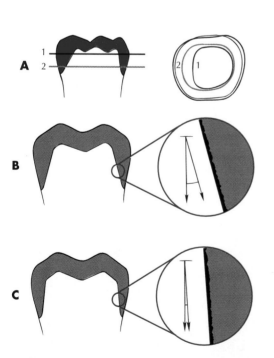

Fig. 7-28. **A,** Cross sections *1* and *2* do not coincide, and the preparation thus has little retention. **B,** Under these circumstances, very little friction develops between the cement and the axial walls, and the cement is subjected to tensile stress. **C,** A retentive near-parallel preparation with frictional resistance. The cement is placed under shear stress.
(**A** *redrawn from Rosenstiel E:* Br Dent J 103:388, 1957.)

Fig. 7-29. **A,** An undercut is formed if opposing walls diverge. **B,** A crown is prepared, because an undercut preparation cannot "seat," since it cannot pass over the divergent walls. **C,** Undercuts are possible in other locations when fixed partial dentures or restorations with preparation features such as grooves or boxes are prepared. Here one buccal facing wall *(B)* can be undercut relative to (four) lingual facing walls *(L)*.

ship was no longer hyperbolic when the internal surfaces of the caps were roughened. The retention of a cap with 10 degrees of taper* was approximately half that of a cap with 5 degrees. Similar results have been reported by other workers.[52-54]

Selection of the appropriate degree of taper for tooth preparation involves compromise. Too small a taper may lead to unwanted undercuts; too large will no longer be retentive. The recommended convergence between opposing walls is 6 degrees, which has been shown to optimize retention for zinc phosphate cement.[55] Recognizing this angle is important (Fig. 7-31), although there is no need to deliberately tilt a rotary cutting instrument to create a taper, since this will invariably lead to overpreparation. Rather, teeth are readily prepared with a rotary instrument of the desired taper held at a constant angulation. The rotary instrument should be moved through a cylindrical path as the tooth is prepared, and the taper of the instrument should produce the desired axial wall taper on the completed preparation. In practice, many dentists experience difficulty consistently avoiding excessively tapered preparations, particularly when preparing posterior teeth with limited access.[56] Some authorities recommend the routine use of grooves to reduce the incidence of restoration displacement. It is unclear, however, whether accurate groove alignment is more easily achieved than axial wall convergence, and skillfully prepared axial walls at a minimal convergence are very conservative of tooth structure.

Surface Area. Provided the restoration has a limited path of withdrawal, its retention depends on the length of this path or, more precisely, on the surface area in sliding contact. Therefore, crowns with long axial walls are more retentive than those with short axial walls,[57] and molar crowns are more retentive than premolar crowns of similar taper. Surfaces where the crown is essentially being pulled away from rather than sliding along the tooth, such as the occlusal surface, do not add much to total retention.

Stress Concentration. When a retentive failure occurs, cement often adheres to both the tooth preparation and the fitting surface of the restoration. In these cases, cohesive failure occurs through the cement layer because the strength of the cement is less than the induced stresses. A computerized analysis of these stresses[58] reveals that they are not uniform throughout the cement but are concentrated around the junction of the axial and occlusal surfaces. Changes in the geometry of the preparation (e.g., rounding the internal line angles) may reduce stress concentrations and thus increase the retention of the restoration.

Type of Preparation. Different types of preparation have different retentive values that correspond fairly closely to the surface area of the axial

---

*In this discussion, as is generally the case in the dental literature, *taper* and *convergence* are used interchangeably and refer to the angle between diametrically opposed axial walls.

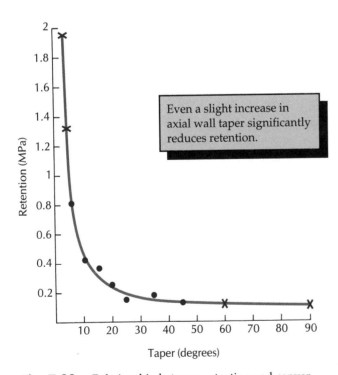

Fig. 7-30. Relationship between retention and convergence angle. •, Experimental values; x, calculated values outside the experimental range.
(*Redrawn from Jorgensen KD:* Acta Odontol Scand *13:35, 1955.*)

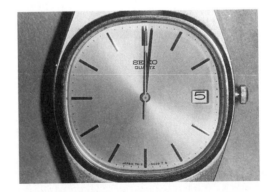

Fig. 7-31. The recommended convergence angle is 6 degrees. This is a very slight taper. (The angle between the hands of a clock showing 12:01 is 5½ degrees.)

walls, as long as other factors (e.g., taper) are kept constant. Thus the retention of a complete crown is about double that of partial-coverage restorations[59] (Fig. 7-32).

Adding grooves or boxes (Fig. 7-33) to a preparation with a limited path of withdrawal does not markedly affect its retention because the surface area is not increased significantly. However, where the addition of a groove limits the paths of withdrawal, retention is increased.[60,61]

Roughness of the Surfaces Being Cemented. When the internal surface of a restoration is very smooth, retentive failure occurs not through the cement but at the cement-restoration interface. Under these circumstances, retention will be increased if the

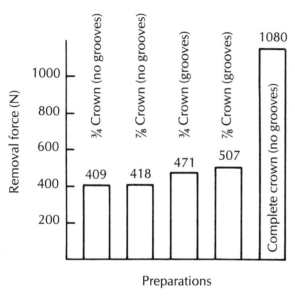

Fig. 7-32. Retention of different preparation designs. *(From Potts RG et al: J Prosthet Dent 43:303, 1980.)*

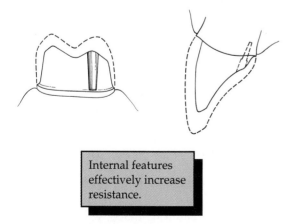

Internal features effectively increase resistance.

Fig. 7-33. Retention form of an excessively tapered preparation can be increased by adding grooves or pinholes, because these will limit the paths of withdrawal.

restoration is roughened or grooved.[62-64] The casting is most effectively prepared by air-abrading the fitting surface with 50 μm of alumina. This should be done carefully to avoid abrading the polished surfaces or margins. Airborne particle abrasion has been shown[65] to increase in vitro retention by 64%.

Failure rarely occurs at the cement-tooth interface. Therefore, deliberately roughening the tooth preparation hardly influences retention and is not recommended, because roughness adds to the difficulty of impression making and waxing.

Materials Being Cemented. Retention is affected by both the casting alloy and the core or buildup material. Laboratory testing results have yet to be confirmed by longer-term clinical studies, but it appears that the more reactive the alloy is, the more adhesion there will be with certain luting agents. Therefore, base metal alloys are better retained than less reactive high-gold content metals.[66] The effect of adhesion to different core materials also has been tested, with conflicting results. One laboratory study[67] examining adhesion between cements and core materials found that the cement adhered better to amalgam than to composite resin or cast gold. However, when crowns were tested for retention, higher values were found with the composite resin than with amalgam cores.[68] The differences may have been due to dimensional changes of the core materials, although the clinical implications of this finding are not clear.

Type of Luting Agent. The type of luting agent chosen affects the retention of a cemented restoration.[69-71] However, the decision regarding which agent to use is also based on other factors. In general, the data suggest that adhesive resin cements are the most retentive[72,73] (Fig 7-34), although long-term clinical evidence about the durability of the bond is not available.

Film Thickness of the Luting Agent. There is conflicting evidence[74-77] about the effect of increased thickness of the cement film on retention of a restoration. This may be important if a slightly oversized casting is made (as when the die-spacer technique is used).

The factors that influence the retention of a cemented restoration are summarized in Table 7-3.

RESISTANCE FORM

Certain features must be present in the preparation to prevent dislodgment of a cemented restoration. Mastication and parafunctional activity may subject a prosthesis to substantial horizontal or oblique

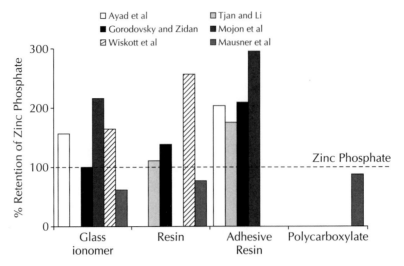

Fig. 7-34. Crown retention studies. Effect of luting agent. These six in vitro studies evaluated the effect of luting agent on crown retention.[11,71,73,90-92] The data were normalized as a percentage of the retention value with zinc phosphate cement. Adhesive resins had consistently greater retention than zinc phosphate. Conventional resins and glass ionomers yielded less consistent results.
(From Rosenstiel SF et al: J Prosthet Dent 80:280, 1998.)

forces. These forces are normally much greater than the ones overcome by retention, especially if the restoration is loaded during eccentric contact between posterior teeth. Lateral forces tend to displace the restoration by causing rotation around the gingival margin. Rotation is prevented by any areas of the tooth preparation that are placed in compression, called *resistance areas* (Fig. 7-35). Multiple resistance areas cumulatively make up the resistance form of a tooth preparation.

Adequate resistance depends on the following:
1. Magnitude and direction of the dislodging forces
2. Geometry of the tooth preparation
3. Physical properties of the luting agent

Magnitude and Direction of the Dislodging Forces. Some patients can develop enormous biting forces. Gibbs et al[78] discovered one individual (Fig. 7-36) who had a biting force of 4340 N (443 kg).* Although this is considered extraordinary, restorations should nevertheless be designed to withstand forces approaching such magnitude. In one laboratory study,[58] a complete crown cemented on a nickel-chromium test die was found to be capable of withstanding over 13,500 N (1400 kg)—a far greater force than would occur in the mouth—before becoming displaced (Fig. 7-37).

When quantifying resistance, ask yourself the following question: How much tooth structure needs to break, or how much does the crown have to deform in order to dislodge this restoration?

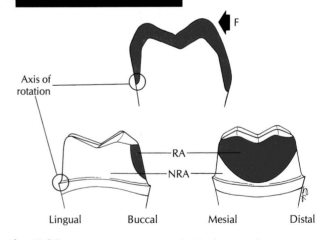

Fig. 7-35. The resistance area *(RA)* of a complete crown is placed under compression when a lateral force *(F)* is applied. *NRA,* Nonresisting area.
(Redrawn from Hegdahl T, Silness J: J Oral Rehabil 4:201, 1977.)

In a normal occlusion, biting force is distributed over all the teeth; most of it is axially directed. If a fixed prosthesis is carefully made with a properly designed occlusion, the load should be well distributed and favorably directed (see Chapter 4). However, if a patient has a biting habit such as pipe smoking or

---

*This compares with the world record super heavyweight (105+ kg) snatch of 205.5 kg.

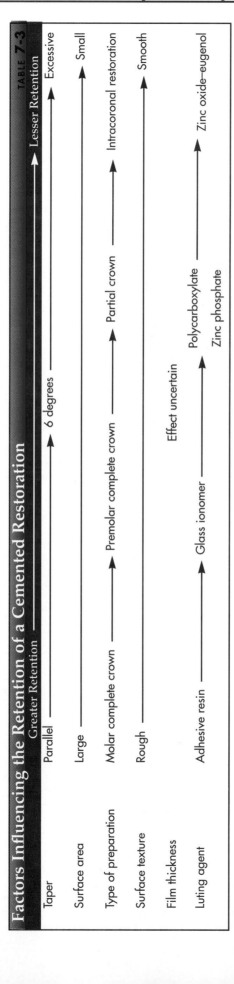

TABLE 7-3 Factors Influencing the Retention of a Cemented Restoration

	Greater Retention ←	→ Lesser Retention
Taper	Parallel ←——— 6 degrees	———→ Excessive
Surface area	Large ←———	———→ Small
Type of preparation	Molar complete crown ←——— Premolar complete crown ←———	Partial crown ———→ Intracoronal restoration
Surface texture	Rough ←———	———→ Smooth
Film thickness	Effect uncertain	
Luting agent	Adhesive resin ←——— Glass ionomer ←———	Polycarboxylate ———→ Zinc oxide–eugenol
		Zinc phosphate

bruxing, it may be difficult to prevent fairly large oblique forces from being applied to a restoration. Consequently the completed tooth preparation and restoration must be able to withstand considerable oblique forces as well as the normal axial ones.

Geometry of the Tooth Preparation.   As with retention, preparation geometry plays a key role in attaining desirable resistance form. The tooth preparation must be shaped so that particular areas of the axial wall will prevent rotation of the crown.

Hegdahl and Silness[79] analyzed how these resisting areas alter as changes are made in the geometry of the tooth preparation. They demonstrated that increased preparation taper and rounding of axial angles tend to reduce resistance. Short tooth preparations with large diameters were found to have very little resistance form. In general, molar teeth require more parallel preparation than premolar or anterior teeth to achieve adequate resistance form.[80] The relationship between preparation height, or diameter, and resistance to displacement is approximately linear.[81]

A partial-coverage restoration may have less resistance (Fig. 7-38) than a complete crown because it

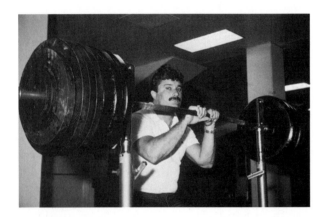

Fig. 7-36. Mr. H. sitting beside 443 kg of gymnasium weights to illustrate the magnitude of his biting strength. *(Reproduced from Gibbs CH et al: J Prosthet Dent 56:226, 1986.)*

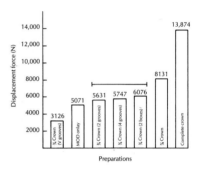

Fig. 7-37. Resistance of different preparation designs. The line connects preparations with statistically similar displacement forces ($p > 0.05$). *(Modified from Kishimoto M et al: J Prosthet Dent 49:188, 1983.)*

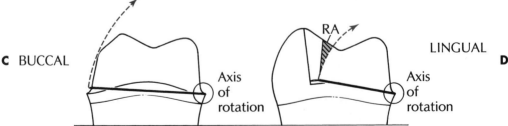

Fig. 7-38. Resistance form of partial and complete crowns. **A,** The buccoaxial wall *(RA)* of a complete crown should provide good resistance to rotation around a lingual axis. **B,** In a partial crown, resistance must be furnished by mesial and distal grooves. **C,** In a short or excessively tapered complete crown, resistance form is minimal because most of the buccal wall is missing. A mesiodistal groove should be placed to increase resistance form. **D,** Poor resistance form is less a problem in a short partial crown, provided the grooves have sufficient definition. However, lack of retention form may indicate the need for complete coverage.

has no buccal resistance areas. Resistance must be provided by boxes or grooves (Fig. 7-39) and will be greatest if they have walls that are perpendicular to the direction of the applied force. Thus U-shaped grooves or flared boxes provide more resistance than V-shaped ones.[59] The resistance form of an excessively tapered preparation can be improved by adding grooves or pinholes, because these interfere with rotational movement and in so doing subject additional areas of the luting agent to compression.

Physical Properties of the Luting Agent. Resistance to deformation is affected by physical properties of the luting agent, such as compressive strength and modulus of elasticity. To satisfy ADA/ANSI specification no. 96 (ISO 9917), the compressive strength of zinc phosphate cement must exceed 70 MPa* at 24 hours (Fig. 7-40). Glass

---

*One megapascal (MPa) equals 1 million newtons per square meter.

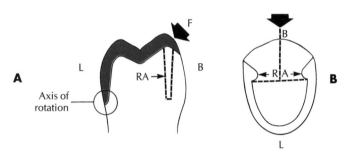

Fig. 7-39. **A,** The grooves of a partial crown should provide the maximum resistance to rotation around an axis situated at the linguogingival margin. **B,** The lingual walls of the groove—the resistance areas *(RA)*—should be prepared perpendicular to the direction of force *(F).*

ionomer cements and most resins have higher compressive strength, whereas polycarboxylates have similar values.[82]

Increasing temperature has a dramatic effect on the compressive strength of luting agents, particularly weakening reinforced zinc oxide–eugenol cement (Fig. 7-41). An increase from room temperature (23° C) to body temperature (37° C) halves the compressive strength of reinforced zinc oxide–eugenol cements, and a rise in temperature to 50° C (equivalent to hot food) reduces the compressive strength by over 80%.[83] Equivalent testing of more modern cements has not been reported.

Zinc phosphate cements have a higher modulus of elasticity than do polycarboxylate cements, which exhibit relatively large plastic deformation.[84] This may account for the observation that the retentive ability of polycarboxylate cement is more dependent on the taper of the preparation than is the retention with zinc phosphate cement.[85]

The factors that affect the resistance to displacement of a cemented restoration are summarized in Table 7-4.

DEFORMATION

A restoration must have sufficient strength to prevent permanent deformation during function (Fig. 7-42). Otherwise, it will fail (typically at the restoration-cement, or the metal-porcelain, interface). This may be a result of inappropriate alloy selection, inadequate tooth preparation, or poor metal-ceramic framework design.

Alloy Selection. Although Type I and Type II gold alloys (see Chapter 22) are satisfactory for intracoronal cast restorations, they are too soft for

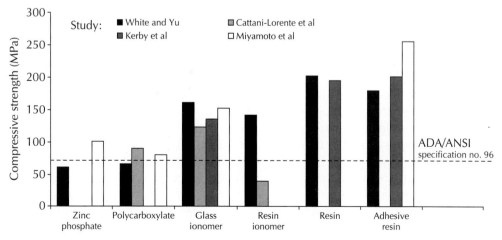

Fig. 7-40. Compressive strength of luting agents. Higher-strength values were reported in these studies[94-97] with the resin cements and glass ionomers than with zinc phosphate or polycarboxylate. Resin-modified glass ionomer exhibited greater variation than other cements.
(From Rosenstiel SF et al: J Prosthet Dent 80:280, 1998)

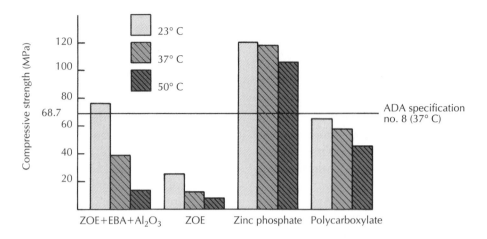

Fig. 7-41. Compressive strength of luting agents at different temperatures. *(Redrawn from Mesu FP: J Prosthet Dent 49:59, 1983.)*

Factors Influencing the Resistance of Cemented Restorations			TABLE 7-4
	Higher Resistance ━━━━━━━━━━━━━━━━━━━━━━━━━━━━━▶ Lower Resistance		
Dislodging forces	Habits ━━━━━━━━▶ Eccentric interferences ━━━━━━━━▶		Anterior guidance
Taper	Minimum ━━━━━━▶ 6 degrees ━━━━━━━━━━━━━━━━━▶		Excessive
Diameter	Small (premolar) ━━━━━━━━━━━━━━━━━━━━━━━━▶		Large (molar)
Height	Long ━━━━━━━━━▶ Average ━━━━━━━━━━━━━━━▶		Short
Type of preparation	Complete coverage ━━━━━━━▶ Partial coverage ━━━━▶		Onlay
Luting agent	Adhesive resin ➤ Glass ionomer ➤ Zinc phosphate ➤ Polycarboxylate ➤ Zinc oxide–eugenol		

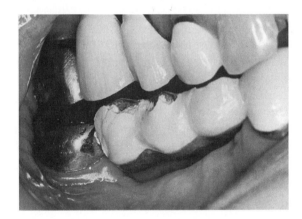

Fig. 7-42. Ceramic failure resulting from deformation of the metal substructure.

crowns and fixed partial dentures, for which Type III or Type IV gold alloys (or an appropriate low-gold alternative) are chosen. These are harder, and their strength and hardness can be increased by heat treatment.

High-noble metal content metal-ceramic alloys have a hardness equivalent to that of Type IV golds, whereas nickel-chromium alloys are considerably harder. These may be indicated when large forces are anticipated, such as with a long-span FPD, although their use presents certain problems (see Chapter 16).

Adequate Tooth Reduction. Even the stronger alloys need sufficient bulk if they are to withstand occlusal forces. Largely based on empirical data, there should be a minimum alloy thickness of about 1.5 mm over centric cusps (buccal in the mandible, lingual in the maxillae). The less stressed noncentric cusps can be protected with less metal (1 mm is adequate in most circumstances) for a strong and long-lasting restoration. Occlusal reduction should be as uniform as possible, following the cuspal planes of the teeth; this will ensure that sufficient occlusal **clearance** is combined with preservation of as much tooth structure as possible. In addition, an anatomically prepared occlusal surface (Fig. 7-43) will give rigidity to the crown because of the "corrugated effect"[86] of the planes.

When teeth are malaligned or overerupted, the occlusal surface needs to be prepared with the eventual restoration in mind. For example, a supraerupted tooth may need considerably more than 1.5 mm of reduction to result in adequate clearance to reestablish an ideal occlusal plane (Fig. 7-44). Diagnostic tooth preparation and waxing are helpful in determining the correct tooth reduction.

Margin Design. Distortion of the restoration margin is prevented by designing the preparation

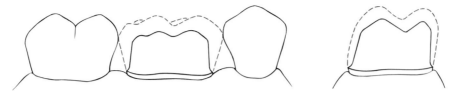

Fig. 7-43. Anatomic occlusal reduction is conservative of tooth structure and gives rigidity to the restoration.

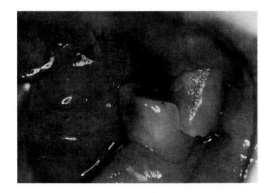

Fig. 7-44. This molar relationship is a result of extreme occlusal wear. When designing a tooth preparation, consideration of the eventual occlusal plane is essential. This is done with the aid of a diagnostic waxing procedure.

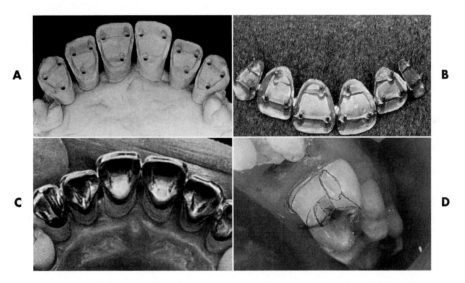

Fig. 7-45. Grooves and ledges provide rigidity in pinledges (**A** to **C**) and partial-coverage restorations (**D**).

outline to avoid occlusal contact in this area. Also, tooth reduction should provide sufficient room for bulk of metal at the margin to prevent distortion. As discussed earlier, one disadvantage of the feather-edge preparation is that the resulting thin layer of gold is not as strong as the comparatively thicker restoration of a chamfer preparation.

The grooves and ledges incorporated in a partial-coverage restoration provide essential strengthening for the casting, particularly an anterior pinledge retainer (Fig. 7-45).

ESTHETIC CONSIDERATIONS

The restorative dentist should develop skill in determining the esthetic expectations of the patient. Patients prefer their dental restorations to look as natural as possible. However, care must be taken that esthetic considerations are not pursued at the expense of a patient's long-term oral health or functional efficiency.

At the initial examination it is important to make a full assessment of the appearance of each patient, noting which areas of which teeth show during smiling, talking, and laughing. The patient's esthetic requirements must be discussed and related to oral hygiene needs and the potential for disease. The final decision regarding an appropriate restoration can then be made with the full cooperation and informed consent of the patient.

METAL-CERAMIC RESTORATIONS

The poor appearance of some metal-ceramic restorations is often due to insufficient porcelain thickness. On the other hand, adequate porcelain thickness is sometimes obtained at the expense of proper axial contour (such overcontoured restorations almost invariably lead to periodontal disease). In addition, the labial margin of a metal-ceramic crown is not always accurately placed. To correct all these deficiencies, certain principles are recommended during tooth preparation that will ensure sufficient room for porcelain and accurate placement of the margins. Otherwise, good appearance would be achievable only at the expense of periodontal health.

Facial Tooth Reduction. If there is to be sufficient bulk of porcelain for appearance and metal for strength, adequate reduction of the facial surface is essential. The exact amount of reduction will depend to some extent on the physical properties of the alloy used for the substructure as well as on the manufacturer and the shade of the porcelain. A minimum reduction of 1.5 mm typically is required for optimal appearance. Adequate thickness of porcelain (Fig. 7-46) is needed to create a sense of color depth and translucency. Shade problems are frequently encountered in maxillary incisor crowns at the incisal and cervical thirds of the restoration,

where direct light reflection from the opaque layer can make the restoration appear very noticeable. Because opaque porcelains generally have a different shade from body porcelains, they often need to be modified with special stains in these areas.[87]

With very thin teeth (e.g., mandibular incisors) it may be impossible to achieve adequate tooth reduction without exposing the pulp or leaving a severely weakened tooth preparation. Under these circumstances a less than ideal appearance may have to be accepted.

The labial surfaces of anterior teeth should be prepared for metal-ceramic restorations in two distinct planes (Fig. 7-47). If they are prepared in a single plane, insufficient reduction in either the cervical or the incisal area of the preparation will result.

Incisal Reduction. The incisal edge of a metal-ceramic restoration has no metal backing and can be made with a translucency similar to that of natural tooth structure. An incisal reduction of 2 mm is recommended for good esthetics. Excessive incisal reduction must be avoided because it reduces the resistance and retention form of the preparation.

Proximal Reduction. The extent of proximal reduction is contingent on exact predetermination of the location of the metal-ceramic junction in the completed restoration. The proximal surfaces of anterior teeth will look most natural if they are restored as the incisal edges, without metal backing. This will allow some light to pass through the restoration in a manner similar to what occurs on a natural tooth (Fig. 7-48). Obviously, if the restoration is part of a fixed partial denture, the need for connectors will make this impossible.

Labial Margin Placement. Supragingival margin placement has many biologic advantages. The restorations are easier to prepare properly and eas-

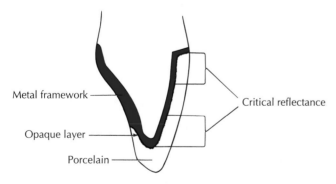

Fig. 7-46. Adequate porcelain thickness is essential for preventing direct light reflection from the highly pigmented opaque porcelain. The most critical areas are the gingival and incisal thirds; in practice, opaque modifying stains are often used in these areas.
(*Redrawn from McLean JW: The science and art of dental ceramics, vol 1, Chicago, 1979, Quintessence Publishing.*)

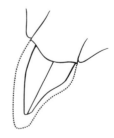

Fig. 7-47. Recommended tooth preparation for a metal-ceramic restoration. The facial reduction has two distinct planes.

ier to keep clean. Nevertheless, subgingival margins may be indicated for esthetic reasons, particularly when the patient has a high lip line and the use of a metal collar labial margin is contemplated.

The patient's smile is observed as part of the initial examination (see Chapter 1). It is important to record which teeth and which parts of each tooth are exposed. Patients with a high lip line, which exposes considerable gingival tissue, present the greatest problem if complete crowns are needed. Where the root surface is not discolored, appearance can be restored with a metal-ceramic restoration having a supragingival porcelain labial margin—sometimes called a "collarless" design (see Chapter 24). If the patient has a low lip line, a metal supragingival collar may be placed because the metal is not seen during normal function. Metal margins generally have a more accurate fit than porcelain margins.

However, it cannot be assumed that the patient will be happy with a supragingival metal collar just because the metal is not visible during normal function. Some patients have reservations about exposed metal, and the advantages of such supragingival margins must be carefully explained before treatment.

Metal collars can be hidden below the gingival crest, although there will be some discoloration if the gingival tissue is thin. Successful margin placement within the gingival sulcus requires care to ensure that inflammation and/or recession, with resulting metal exposure, are avoided or minimized. The periodontium must be healthy before the tooth is prepared. If periodontal surgery is needed, the sulcular space should not be eliminated completely; rather, a postsurgical depth of about 2 mm should be the objective. Sufficient time should be allowed after surgery for the periodontal tissues to stabilize. Wise[88] found that the gingival crest does not stabilize until 20 weeks after surgery.

Margins should not be placed so far apically that they encroach on the attachment; extension to within 1.5 mm of the alveolar crest will lead to bone resorption.[89] The margin should follow the contour of the free gingiva, being further apical in the middle of the tooth and further incisal interproximally. A common error (Fig. 7-49) is to prepare the tooth so the margin lies almost in one plane, with exposure of the collar labially and irreversible loss of bone and papilla proximally.

PARTIAL-COVERAGE RESTORATIONS

Whenever possible, accomplishment of an esthetically acceptable result without the use of metal-ceramic crowns is preferred, not only because tooth structure is conserved but also because no restorative material can approach the appearance of intact tooth enamel. Esthetic partial-coverage restorations depend on accurate placement of the potentially visible facial and proximal margins. Understandably, many patients will not readily accept a visible display of metal. If a partial-coverage restoration is poorly prepared, the patient may demand that it be replaced by a metal-ceramic crown, and the result will be unnecessary loss of tooth structure and a greater potential for tissue damage.

Proximal Margin. Placement of the proximal margins (particularly the mesial, generally more visible, margin) is critical to the esthetic result of a partial-coverage restoration. The rule here is to

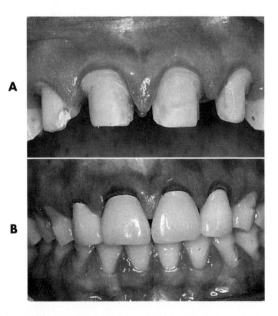

Fig. 7-49. A, Poor preparation design. The apical margin of the preparation does not follow the free gingival contours. B, The restoration displays a metal collar labially, and the deep proximal margins have led to periodontal disease.

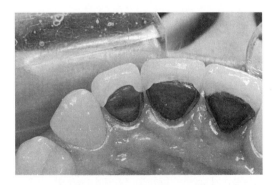

Fig. 7-48. The proximal surfaces of these anterior metal-ceramic crowns are restored in porcelain, which allows light to be transmitted for maximum esthetics.

place the margin just buccal to the proximal contact area, where metal will be hidden by the distal line angle of the neighboring tooth. Tooth preparation angulation is critical and should normally follow the long axes of posterior teeth and the incisal two thirds of the facial surface of anteriors. If a buccal or lingual tilt is given to the tooth preparation, metal may be visible (Fig. 7-50).

The distal margin of posterior partial-coverage restorations is less visible than the mesial margin. Often in this area it is advantageous to extend the preparation farther beyond the contact point for easier preparation and finishing of the restoration and better access for oral hygiene.

Facial Margin.   The facial margin of a maxillary partial-coverage restoration should be extended just

beyond the occlusofacial line angle. A short **bevel** is needed to prevent enamel chipping. A chamfer can be placed where appearance is less important (e.g., on molars) because this will provide greater bulk of metal for strength.

If the buccal margin of metal is correctly shaped (Fig. 7-51), it will not reflect light to an observer. As a result, the tooth will appear to be merely a little shorter than normal and not as though its buccal cusp is outlined in metal. If the buccal margin is skillfully placed following the original cuspal contour, the final restoration will have an acceptable appearance.

When mandibular partial cast crowns are made, metal display is unavoidable because the occlusal surface of mandibular teeth can be seen during speech. A chamfer, rather than a bevel, is recom-

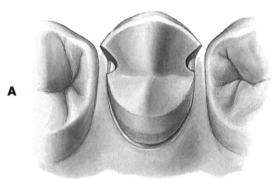

A

Clearance must be sufficient to permit fabrication of a die system but should minimize the display of metal.

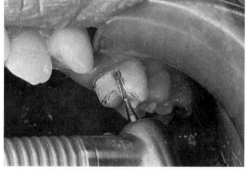

B

Fig. 7-50.   **A,** Correct placement of the mesial margin of a partial-coverage restoration is essential to good esthetics. To allow proper access for finishing, the restoration must extend just beyond the contact area, but the metal must remain hidden from the casual observer. **B,** The tooth should be prepared in its long axis; otherwise, metal will be displayed.

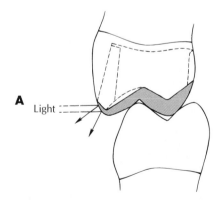

A

Light

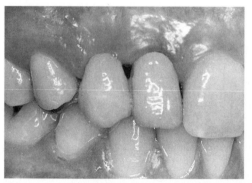

B

Fig. 7-51.   **A,** The facial margin of a partial crown should be shaped so that light is not reflected directly to the observer. **B,** A three-unit FPD. The mesial abutment is canine shaped to look like a lateral incisor. The distal abutment is a partial crown, which proved to be esthetically acceptable because the facial surface had been correctly contoured.

mended for the buccal margin because it provides a greater bulk of metal around the highly stressed centric cusp (Fig. 7-52). If the appearance of metal is unacceptable to the patient, a metal-ceramic restoration with porcelain coverage on the occlusal surface can be made.

Anterior partial-coverage restorations can be fabricated to show no metal (Fig. 7-53), but their preparation requires considerable care. The facial margin is extended just beyond the highest contour of the incisal edge but not quite to the incisolabial line angle. Here the metal will protect the tooth from chipping but will not be visible.

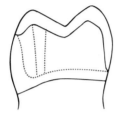

Fig. 7-52. A substantial chamfer is recommended for the centric buccal cusp of a mandibular partial cast crown. It will provide greater bulk of metal in a stressed area.

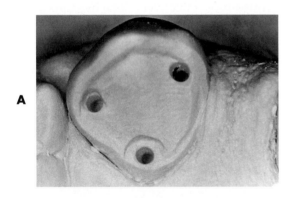
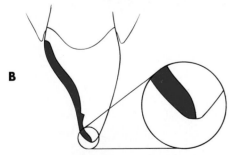

Fig. 7-53. **A,** Teeth can be prepared for partial-coverage restorations that do not show any metal. Success depends on very careful margin placement. **B,** The incisal edge is not completely covered. The restoration margin is located between the highest point of the incisal contour and the incisofacial angle.

PLANNING AND EVALUATING TOOTH PREPARATIONS

Tooth preparation is a technically complicated and irreversible procedure. Thus it is the practitioner's responsibility to carry it out properly every time. Mistakes are often difficult, if not impossible, to correct.

DIAGNOSTIC TOOTH PREPARATIONS

Diagnostic tooth preparations are performed on articulated casts before the actual clinical preparation. They yield information with regard to the following:
- Selecting the appropriate path of withdrawal for a fixed partial denture, particularly when the abutment teeth are tilted or have an atypical coronal contour (Fig. 7-54)
- Determining the best location for the facial and proximal margins of a partial-coverage restoration so the metal will not be visible (Fig. 7-55)
- Deciding on the amount of tooth reduction necessary to accomplish a planned change in the occlusion

Another advantage of diagnostic tooth preparations is that the operator can practice each step of the intended restoration. Mistakes are not permanently destructive. Additionally, **diagnostic preparations** can be used in the prefabrication of provisional restorations, significantly reducing the appointment time at tooth preparation (the indirect/direct technique is described in Chapter 15).

Diagnostic Waxing Procedures (Fig. 7-56). For all but the most straightforward prosthodontic treatment plans, a diagnostic waxing procedure should be performed. This is done on diagnostic tooth preparations and establishes the optimum contour and occlusion of the eventual prosthesis. The procedure is of particular benefit if the patient's occlusal scheme or anterior (incisal) guidance requires alteration.

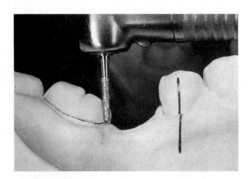

Fig. 7-54. Selecting the best path of withdrawal for a fixed partial denture with the aid of diagnostic tooth preparations.

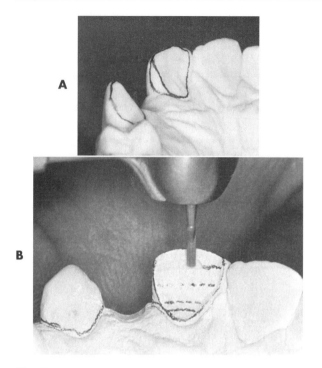

Fig. 7-55. Diagnostic tooth preparations are extremely helpful in determining the ideal reduction for esthetic partial-coverage restorations.

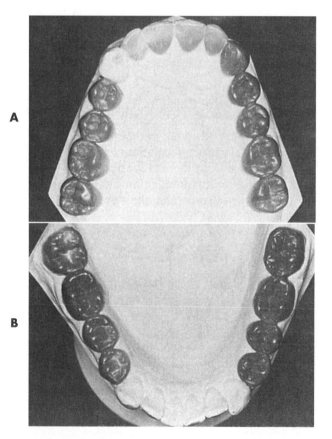

Fig. 7-56. A, B, Diagnostic waxing procedure. *(Courtesy Dr. M. Padilla.)*

Evaluative Procedures during Tooth Preparation. Each step of a tooth preparation should be carefully evaluated with direct vision or indirectly with a dental mirror. Alignment of multiple abutment teeth can be a special problem, and using the mirror helps to superimpose the image of adjacent abutment teeth. Complex preparations should be evaluated by making an alginate impression and pouring it in fast-setting stone. A dental surveyor (Fig. 7-57) can then be used to precisely measure the **axial inclinations** of the tooth preparation. The less experienced dentist may hesitate to make such an impression for fear of losing time. However, the information obtained often saves time in subsequent procedures by identifying problems that can then be addressed immediately. During tooth preparation, it is useful to learn to use the contraangle handpiece as both a measuring and a cutting instrument. This is done by concentrating on the top surface of the turbine head, which is perpendicular to the shank of the bur. If the top surface is kept parallel to the occlusal surface of the tooth being prepared, the bur will automatically be in the correct orientation (Fig. 7-58). To prevent undercuts or excessive convergence during axial reduction, the handpiece must be maintained at the same angulation. The correct taper is imparted by the diamond instrument. Keeping the turbine head at its correct angulation initially is often most effectively done by supporting it with a finger of the opposite hand.

PATIENT AND OPERATOR POSITIONING

Learning the proper patient and operator positions is as beneficial as learning the proper preparation

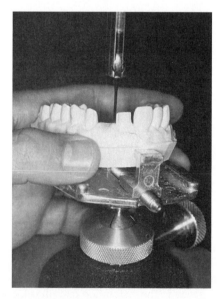

Fig. 7-57. A dental surveyor can be used to evaluate the axial alignments of a tooth preparation.

steps. Of particular importance are the advantages of obtaining a direct view of the preparation, which is always preferred to an indirect or mirror view. However, certain areas (e.g., the distal surfaces of maxillary molars) cannot be seen directly.

Inexperience, coupled with a hesitation to move the patient's head into a more favorable position, can unnecessarily complicate tooth preparation. For instance, having the patient rotate the head to the left or right side can considerably improve the visibility of molar teeth that are being prepared. In most instances a direct view can be obtained by subtly changing the operator's or the patient's position. Having the patient open maximally does not necessarily provide the best view. If the jaw is partially open, the cheek may be retracted more easily (Fig. 7-59), and if the patient is encouraged to make a lateral excursion, the distobuccal line angle, together with the buccal third of the distal wall, may be seen

directly. In practice, the mirror is essential only to visualizing a small portion of the distal surface. When preparing a complete crown, the parts of the tooth most easily seen should be prepared first, leaving the other areas for preparation with the help of the mirror as a final stage.

◼ SUMMARY

The principles of tooth preparation can be categorized into biologic, mechanical, and esthetic considerations. Often these principles conflict, and the practitioner must decide how the restoration should be designed. One area may be given too much emphasis, and the long-term success of the procedure may be limited by a lack of consideration of other factors.

Experience will help in determining whether preparations are "complete." Each tooth preparation must be measured by clearly defined criteria, which can be used to identify and correct problems. Diagnostic tooth preparations and evaluative impressions are often very helpful. The types of preparation described in the following chapters are explained in a step-by-step format. Understanding the pertinent theories underlying each step is crucial. Successful preparation can be obtained most easily by systematically following the steps. It is critical to refrain from "jumping ahead" before the previous step has been evaluated and, if necessary, corrected. If the clinician proceeds too rapidly, precious chair time will be lost, and the quality of the preparation will probably suffer.

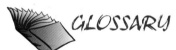

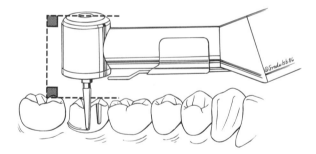

> The correct taper is established by moving the tapered diamond parallel to itself around the tooth.

Fig. 7-58. Top surface of the handpiece held parallel to the occlusal surface. The bur is in correct axial alignment.

GLOSSARY

axial inclination: *1:* the relationship of the long axis of a body to a designated plane *2:* in dentistry, the alignment of the long axis of a tooth to a horizontal plane.

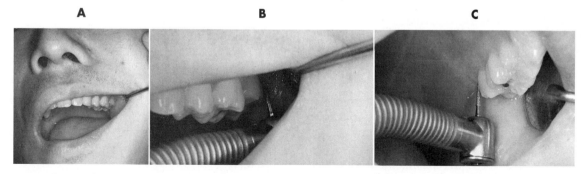

A   **B**   **C**

Fig. 7-59. Careful patient positioning can help obtain a direct view during tooth preparation. **A,** Often access is better if the mouth is not open maximally, because partial opening allows the cheek to be more easily retracted. **B,** Access to the buccal surface. **C,** Access to the lingual surface. A direct view is obtained by tilting the patient's head.

Study Questions

1. Discuss how the manipulation and condition of the armamentarium being used can contribute to injury.
2. Discuss optimal occlusocervical margin placement. What are some reasons for deviating from the ideal? Why?
3. Discuss the difference between retention and resistance. What can be done to enhance retention, and what can be done to improve the resistance form of a tooth preparation?
4. Discuss six different finish line configurations. Discuss their advantages, disadvantages, indications, and contraindication as applicable.
5. What is an undercut? How is an undercut eliminated? Can a buccal and lingual wall be undercut relative to each other? Why or why not?
6. What are the differences in retention and resistance form between a partial veneer crown preparation and complete cast crown preparation on the same tooth? How does clinical crown length and tooth size influence either? Why?
7. List six different means of conserving tooth structure during tooth preparation design and explain why they result in the objective.
8. What is the purpose of diagnostic waxing? Give four indications for a diagnostic waxing procedure.

axis of preparation: the planned line or path of placement and removal for a dental restoration.

1 bevel: *n* (1611): a slanting edge.

2 bevel: *vt:* the process of slanting or sloping the finish lines and curves of a tooth preparation.

chamfer: *n 1:* a finish line design for tooth preparation in which the gingival aspect meets the external axial surface at an obtuse angle *2:* a small groove or furrow *3:* the surface found by cutting away the angle of intersection of two faces of a piece of material (i.e., stone, metal, wood): a beveled edge.

clearance: *n obs:* a condition in which bodies may pass each other without hindrance. Also, the distance between bodies (GPT-4).

clinical crown: the portion of a tooth that extends from the occlusal table or incisal edge to the free gingival margin.

divergence: *n* (1656) *1:* a drawing apart as a surface extends away from a common point *2:* the reverse taper of walls of a preparation for a restoration—divergency n, pl -cies (1709).

draw: *vt:* the taper or convergence of walls of a preparation for a restoration; slang—DRAFT, DRAUGHT.

finish line: *n* (1899) *1:* a line of demarcation *2:* the peripheral extension of a tooth preparation *3:* the planned junction of different materials *4:* the terminal portion of the prepared tooth.

groove: *n:* a long narrow channel or depression, such as the indentation between tooth cusps or the retentive features placed on tooth surfaces to augment the retentive characteristics of crown preparations.

interocclusal clearance: *1:* the arrangement in which the opposing occlusal surfaces may pass one another without any contact *2:* the amount of reduction achieved during tooth preparation to provide for an adequate thickness of restorative material.

margin: *n (14c):* the outer edge of a crown, inlay, onlay, or other restoration. The boundary surface of a tooth preparation and/or restoration is termed the finish line or finish curve.

path of placement: the specific direction in which a prosthesis is placed on the abutment teeth.

resistance form: the features of a tooth preparation that enhance the stability of a restoration and resist dislodgment along an axis other than the path of placement.

retention form: the feature of a tooth preparation that resists dislodgment of a crown in a vertical direction or along the path of placement.

REFERENCES

1. Zoellner A et al: Histobacteriology and pulp reactions to long-term dental restorations, *J Marmara Univ Dent Fac* 2:483, 1996.
2. Langeland K, Langeland LK: Pulp reactions to crown preparation, impression, temporary crown fixation, and permanent cementation, *J Prosthet Dent* 15:129, 1965.
3. Baldissara P et al: Clinical and histological evaluation of thermal injury thresholds in human teeth: a preliminary study, *J Oral Rehabil* 24:791, 1997.
4. Ohashi Y: Research related to anterior abutment teeth of fixed partial denture, *Shikagakuho* 68:726, 1968.
5. Morrant GA: Dental instrumentation and pulpal injury. II. Clinical considerations, *J Br Endod Soc* 10:55, 1977.
6. Brännström M: Dentinal and pulpal response. II. Application of an air stream to exposed dentine, short observation period: an experimental study, *Acta Odontol Scand* 18:17, 1960.

7. Laforgia PD et al: Temperature change in the pulp chamber during complete crown preparation, *J Prosthet Dent* 65:56, 1991.

8. Hume WR, Massey WL: Keeping the pulp alive: the pharmacology and toxicology of agents applied to dentine, *Aust Dent J* 35:32, 1990.

9. Johnson GH et al: Crown retention with use of a 5% glutaraldehyde sealer on prepared dentin, *J Prosthet Dent* 79:671, 1998.

10. Felton DA et al: Effect of cavity varnish on retention of cemented cast crowns, *J Prosthet Dent* 57:411, 1987.

11. Mausner IK et al: Effect of two dentinal desensitizing agents on retention of complete cast coping using four cements, *J Prosthet Dent* 75:129, 1996.

12. Going RE: Status report on cement bases, cavity liners, varnishes, primers and cleansers, *J Am Dent Assoc* 85:654, 1972.

13. Dahl BL: Effect of cleansing procedures on the retentive ability of two luting cements to ground dentin in vitro, *Acta Odontol Scand* 36:137, 1978.

14. Brännström M, Nyborg H: Cavity treatment with a microbicidal fluoride solution: growth of bacteria and effect on the pulp, *J Prosthet Dent* 30:303, 1973.

15. Watts A: Bacterial contamination and the toxicity of silicate and zinc phosphate cements, *Br Dent J* 146:7, 1979.

16. Dahl BL: Antibacterial effect of two luting cements on prepared dentin in vitro and in vivo, *Acta Odontol Scand* 36:363, 1978.

17. Mjör IA: Bacteria in experimentally infected cavity preparations, *Scand J Dent Res* 85:599, 1977.

18. Quarnstrom F et al: A randomized clinical trial of agents to reduce sensitivity after crown cementation, *Gen Dent* 46(1):68, 1998.

19. Seltzer S, Bender IB: The dental pulp: biologic considerations in dental procedures, ed 2, Philadelphia, 1975, JB Lippincott, p 180.

20. Dowden WE: Discussion of methods and criteria in evaluation of dentin and pulpal responses, *Int Dent J* 20:531, 1970.

21. Sorensen JA: A rationale for comparison of plaque-retaining properties of crown systems, *J Prosthet Dent* 62:264, 1989.

22. Perel ML: Axial crown contours, *J Prosthet Dent* 25:642, 1971.

23. Han TJ, Takei HH: Progress in gingival papilla reconstruction, *Periodontology 2000* 1165, 1996.

24. Silness J: Periodontal conditions in patients treated with dental bridges. III. The relationship between the location of the crown margin and the periodontal condition, *J Periodont Res* 5:225, 1970.

25. Karlsen K: Gingival reactions to dental restorations, *Acta Odontol Scand* 28:895, 1970.

26. Newcomb GM: The relationship between the location of subgingival crown margins and gingival inflammation, *J Periodontol* 45:151, 1974.

27. Bader JD et al: Effect of crown margins on periodontal conditions in regularly attending patients, *J Prosthet Dent* 65:75, 1991.

28. Block PL: Restorative margins and periodontal health: a new look at an old perspective, *J Prosthet Dent* 57:683, 1987.

29. Ackerman MB: The full coverage restoration in relation to the gingival sulcus, *Compendium* 18:1131, 1997.

30. Felton DA et al: Effect of in vivo crown margin discrepancies on periodontal health, *J Prosthet Dent* 65:357, 1991.

31. Byrne G et al: Casting accuracy of high-palladium alloys, *J Prosthet Dent* 55:297, 1986.

32. Belser UC et al: Fit of three porcelain-fused-to-metal marginal designs in vivo: a scanning electron microscope study, *J Prosthet Dent* 53:24, 1985.

33. Rosner D: Function, placement, and reproduction of bevels for gold castings, *J Prosthet Dent* 13:1160, 1963.

34. Rosenstiel E: The marginal fit of inlays and crowns, *Br Dent J* 117:432, 1964.

35. Hoard RJ, Watson J: The relationship of bevels to the adaptation of intracoronal inlays, *J Prosthet Dent* 35:538, 1976.

36. Shillingburg HT et al: Preparation design and margin distortion in porcelain-fused-to-metal restorations, *J Prosthet Dent* 29:276, 1973.

37. Faucher RR, Nicholls JI: Distortion related to margin design in porcelain-fused-to-metal restorations, *J Prosthet Dent* 43:149, 1980.

38. Pascoe DF: Analysis of the geometry of finishing lines for full crown restorations, *J Prosthet Dent* 40:157, 1978.

39. Gavelis JR et al: The effect of various finish line preparations on the marginal seal and occlusal seat of full crown preparations, *J Prosthet Dent* 45:138, 1981.

40. Hunter AJ, Hunter AR: Gingival crown margin configurations: a review and discussion. I. Terminology and widths, *J Prosthet Dent* 64:548, 1990.

41. Dykema RW et al: *Johnston's modern practice in crown and bridge prosthodontics*, ed 4, Philadelphia, 1986, WB Saunders, p 27.

42. Shillingburg HT et al: *Fundamentals of fixed prosthodontics*, ed 3, Chicago, 1997, Quintessence Publishing, p 128.

43. Dimashkieh MR: Modified rotary design instruments for controlled finish line crown preparation, *J Prosthet Dent* 69:120, 1993.

44. Ramp MH et al: Tooth structure loss apical to preparations for fixed partial dentures when

using self-limiting burs, *J Prosthet Dent* 79:491, 1998.

45. Seymour K at al: Assessment of shoulder dimensions and angles of porcelain bonded to metal crown preparations, *J Prosthet Dent* 75:406, 1996.

46. Hoffman EJ: How to utilize porcelain fused to gold as a crown and bridge material, *Dent Clin North Am* 9:57, 1965.

47. Farah JW et al: Effects of design on stress distribution of intracoronal gold restorations, *J Am Dent Assoc* 94:1151, 1977.

48. Walton JN et al: A survey of crown and fixed partial denture failures: length of service and reasons for replacement, *J Prosthet Dent* 56:416, 1986.

49. Lindquist E, Karlsson S: Success rate and failures for fixed partial dentures after 20 years of service. I. *Int J Prosthod* 11:133, 1998.

50. Rosenstiel E: The retention of inlays and crowns as a function of geometrical form, *Br Dent J* 103:388, 1957.

51. Jørgensen KD: The relationship between retention and convergence angle in cemented veneer crowns, *Acta Odontol Scand* 13:35, 1955.

52. Kaufman EG et al: Factors influencing the retention of cemented gold castings, *J Prosthet Dent* 11:487, 1961.

53. Dodge WW et al: The correlation of resistance and retention to convergence angle, *J Dent Res* 62:267, 1983 (abstract no. 880).

54. Hovijitra S et al: The relationship between retention and convergence of full crowns when used as fixed partial denture retainers, *J Indiana Dent Assoc* 58(4):21, 1979.

55. Wilson AH, Chan DC: The relationship between preparation convergence and retention of extracoronal retainers, *J Prosthod* 3:74, 1994.

56. Nordlander J et al: The taper of clinical preparations for fixed prosthodontics, *J Prosthet Dent* 60:148, 1988.

57. Reisbick MH, Shillingburg HT: Effect of preparation geometry on retention and resistance of cast gold restorations, *Calif Dent Assoc J* 3:51, 1975.

58. Nicholls JI: Crown retention. I. Stress analysis of symmetric restorations, *J Prosthet Dent* 31:179, 1974.

59. Potts RG et al: Retention and resistance of preparations for cast restorations, *J Prosthet Dent* 43:303, 1980.

60. Kishimoto M et al: Influence of preparation features on retention and resistance. II. Three-quarter crowns, *J Prosthet Dent* 49:188, 1983.

61. Galun EA et al: The contribution of a pinhole to the retention and resistance form of veneer crowns, *J Prosthet Dent* 56:292, 1986.

62. Worley JL et al: Effects of cement on crown retention, *J Prosthet Dent* 48:289, 1982.

63. Smith BGN: The effect of the surface roughness of prepared dentin on the retention of castings, *J Prosthet Dent* 23:187, 1970.

64. Arcoria CJ et al: Effect of undercut placement on crown retention after thermocycling, *J Oral Rehabil* 17:395, 1990.

65. O'Connor RP et al: Effect of internal microblasting on retention of cemented cast crowns, *J Prosthet Dent* 64:557, 1990.

66. Saito C et al: Adhesion of polycarboxylate cements to dental casting alloys, *J Prosthet Dent* 35:543, 1976.

67. Chan KC et al: Bond strength of cements to crown bases, *J Prosthet Dent* 46:297, 1981.

68. DeWald JP et al: Crown retention: a comparative study of core type and luting agent, *Dent Mater* 3:71, 1987.

69. McComb D: Retention of castings with glass ionomer cement, *J Prosthet Dent* 48:285, 1982.

70. Arfaei AH, Asgar K: Bond strength of three cements determined by centrifugal testing, *J Prosthet Dent* 40:294, 1978.

71. Tjan AHL, Li T: Seating and retention of complete crowns with a new adhesive resin cement, *J Prosthet Dent* 67:478, 1992.

72. el-Mowafy OM et al: Retention of metal ceramic crowns cemented with resin cements: effects of preparation taper and height, *J Prosthet Dent* 76:524, 1996.

73. Ayad MF et al: Influence of tooth surface roughness and type of cement on retention of complete cast crowns, *J Prosthet Dent* 77:116, 1997.

74. Jørgensen KD, Esbensen AL: The relationship between the film thickness of zinc phosphate cement and the retention of veneer crowns, *Acta Odontol Scand* 26:169, 1968.

75. Hembree JH, Cooper EW: Effect of die relief on retention of cast crowns and inlays, *Oper Dent* 4:104, 1979.

76. Gegauff AG, Rosenstiel SF: Reassessment of die-spacer with dynamic loading during cementation, *J Prosthet Dent* 61:655, 1989.

77. Carter SM, Wilson PR: The effect of die-spacing on crown retention, *Int J Prosthod* 9:21, 1996.

78. Gibbs CH et al: Limits of human bite strength, *J Prosthet Dent* 56:226, 1986.

79. Hegdahl T, Silness J: Preparation areas resisting displacement of artificial crowns, *J Oral Rehabil* 4:201, 1977.

80. Parker MH et al: New guidelines for preparation taper, *J Prosthod* 2:61, 1993.

81. Wiskott HW et al: The effect of tooth preparation height and diameter on the resistance of complete crowns to fatigue loading, *Int J Prosthodont* 10:207, 1997.

82. Rosenstiel SF et al:Dental luting agents: a review of the current literature, *J Prosthet Dent* 80:280, 1998.

83. Mesu FP: The effect of temperature on compressive and tensile strengths of cements, *J Prosthet Dent* 49:59, 1983.

84. Branco R, Hegdahl T: Physical properties of some zinc phosphate and polycarboxylate cements, *Acta Odontol Scand* 41:349, 1983.

85. McLean JW: Polycarboxylate cements: five years' experience in general practice, *Br Dent J* 132:9, 1972.

86. Guyer SE: Multiple preparations for fixed prosthodontics, *J Prosthet Dent* 23:529, 1970.

87. McLean JW: *The science and art of dental ceramics,* vol 1, Chicago, 1979, Quintessence Publishing, p 136.

88. Wise MD: Stability of gingival crest after surgery and before anterior crown placement, *J Prosthet Dent* 53:20, 1985.

89. Palomo F, Kopczyk RA: Rationale and methods for crown lengthening, *J Am Dent Assoc* 96:257, 1978.

90. Gorodovsky S, Zidan O: Retentive strength, disintegration, and marginal quality of luting cements, *J Prosthet Dent* 68:269, 1992.

91. Wiskott HW et al: The relationship between abutment taper and resistance of cemented crowns to dynamic loading, *Int J Prosthod* 9:117, 1996.

92. Mojon P et al: Maximum bond strength of dental luting cement to amalgam alloy, *J Dent Res* 68:1545, 1989.

93. White SN, Yu Z: Compressive and diametral tensile strengths of current adhesive luting agents, *J Prosthet Dent* 69:568, 1993.

94. Kerby RE et al: Some physical properties of implant abutment luting cements, *Int J Prosthodont* 5:321, 1992.

95. Cattani-Lorente M-A et al: Early strength of glass ionomer cements, *Dent Mater* 9:57, 1993.

96. Miyamoto S et al: Study on fatigue toughness of dental materials. I. Compressive strength on various luting cements and composite resin cores, *Nippon Hotetsu Shika Gakkai Zasshi* 33:966, 1989.

CHAPTER EIGHT

THE COMPLETE CAST CROWN PREPARATION

Although esthetic factors may limit its application, the all-metal complete cast crown should always be offered to patients requiring restoration for badly damaged posterior teeth. The complete cast crown has the best longevity of all fixed restorations. It can be used to rebuild a single tooth or as a retainer for a fixed partial denture (FPD). It involves all axial walls as well as the occlusal surface of the tooth being restored (Fig. 8-1).

Preparation for a complete cast crown requires that adequate tooth structure be removed to allow restoration of the tooth to its original contours. Tooth structure should be preserved when possible, but reduction should produce a crown of acceptable strength.

ADVANTAGES

Because all axial surfaces of the tooth are included in the preparation, the complete cast crown has greater retention than a more conservative restoration on the same tooth (e.g., a seven-eighths or three-quarter crown [see Fig. 7-32]).

Normally a complete cast crown preparation also has greater resistance form than a partial-coverage restoration on the same tooth. For a partial veneer crown to rotate off the tooth, only the tooth structure immediately lingual to the occlusal portion of the proximal groove or box need fail. However, if the axial walls of a complete cast crown have been prepared with the proper degree of taper or convergence, a significant amount of tooth structure must fail before the crown can be torqued off.

The strength of a complete cast crown is superior to that of other restorations. Its cylinder-like configuration encircles the tooth and is reinforced by a corrugated occlusal surface. Just as an O-shaped link in a chain resists deformation better than a C-shaped link, this restoration is less easily deformed than its counterparts, which are more conservative of tooth structure.

A complete cast crown allows the operator to modify axial tooth contour. This can be of special

significance when dealing with malaligned teeth, although the extent of possible recontouring is limited by periodontal considerations. Similarly, it is possible to allow better access to furcations for improved patient oral hygiene through recontouring of buccal and lingual walls (Fig. 8-2). When special requirements exist for axial contours, such as where retainers are needed for removable partial dentures, a complete crown is often the only restoration that will allow the necessary modifications for the creation of properly shaped survey lines, guide planes, and occlusal rests (Fig. 8-3). (See Chapter 21.)

The restoration permits easy modification of the occlusion, which is often difficult to accomplish if a more conservative restoration is made. This is

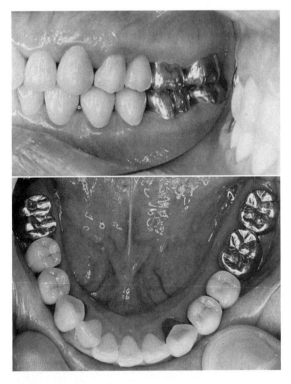

Fig. 8-1. Complete cast crowns used to restore the molar teeth. The canines and premolars, which are more visible because of their more anterior arch position, have been restored with metal-ceramic crowns.

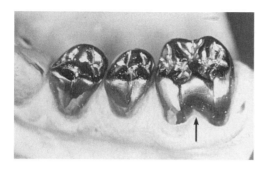

Fig. 8-2. Fluting of the axial walls of a molar complete cast crown *(arrow)* will allow better access to the furcation area for oral hygiene and will improve the long-term prognosis of the restoration.

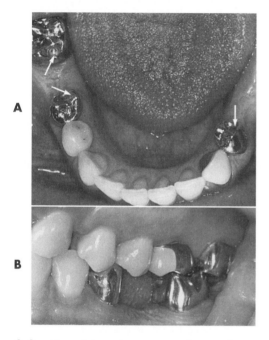

Fig. 8-3. Complete cast crowns used as retainers to accommodate a mandibular removable partial denture. Metal-ceramic crowns have been placed on the mandibular left canine **(A)** and the maxillary first molar **(B).** Note the occlusal rests **(A,** *arrows)* and the survey contours **(B),** which extend to form reciprocating guide planes. (See Chapter 21.)

especially important when supraerupted teeth are present or when the occlusal plane needs to be reestablished.

DISADVANTAGES

Because all coronal surfaces are involved in the preparation for a complete cast crown, removal of tooth structure is extensive and can have adverse effects on the pulp and periodontium. Because of the proximity of the margin to the gingiva, it is not uncommon to see inflammation of gingival tissues (al-

though a properly fitting complete cast crown with good axial contour should minimize this).

After cementation, it is no longer feasible to perform electric vitality testing of an abutment tooth. The conductivity of the metal interferes with the test. This can be a disadvantage if future complications occur, although thermal tests occasionally will yield the necessary information.

Patients may object to the display of metal associated with complete cast crowns, and in those with a normal smile line, the restoration may be restricted to maxillary molars and mandibular molars and premolars.

INDICATIONS

The complete cast crown is indicated on teeth that exhibit extensive coronal destruction by caries or trauma. It is the restoration of choice whenever maximum retention and resistance are needed. On short clinical crowns or when high displacement forces are anticipated, such as for the retainer of a long-span FPD, grooves should be included as additional retentive features.

This restoration is fabricated when correction of axial contours is not feasible with a more conservative technique. The restoration also may be used to support a removable partial denture, because obtaining the necessary contours with a partial-coverage restoration is more difficult. Although proximal guide planes can sometimes be prepared through simple enamel modification, arriving at properly inclined reciprocal guide planes and survey contours is often impractical. The minimum dimensions required for occlusal rests of an RPD framework necessitate removing significant amounts of enamel and, if the dentin is exposed, restoring the tooth with a cast crown.*

The complete cast crown is indicated on endodontically treated teeth. Its superior strength compensates for the loss of tooth structure that results from previous restorations, carious lesions, and endodontic access.

CONTRAINDICATIONS

The complete cast crown is contraindicated if treatment objectives can be met with a more conservative restoration. Wherever an intact buccal or lingual wall exists, use of a partial-coverage restoration

---

*On mandibular premolars, a rest can sometimes be placed on top of the modified occlusal surface without interfering with the occlusion or articulation.

should be considered. In particular, if less than maximum retention and resistance are needed (e.g., on a short-span fixed partial denture), a preparation more conservative of tooth structure is called for. Similarly, if an adequate buccal contour exists or can be obtained through enamel modification (enameloplasty), a complete crown is not indicated. If a high esthetic need exists (e.g., anterior teeth), a complete cast crown is also contraindicated.

CRITERIA

The occlusal reduction must allow adequate room for the restorative material from which the cast crown is to be fabricated: Type III or IV gold casting alloy or their low-gold content equivalent. Minimum recommended clearance is 1 mm on noncentric cusps and 1.5 mm on centric cusps. The occlusal reduction should follow normal anatomic contours to remain as conservative of tooth structure as possible. Axial reduction should parallel the long axis of the tooth while allowing for the recommended 6-degree taper or convergence between opposing axial surfaces.

The margin should have a chamfer configuration and should ideally be located supragingivally. Sometimes crown lengthening is indicated to obtain a supragingival margin, rather than risk future periodontal disease (see Chapter 6). The chamfer should be smooth and distinct and allow for approximately 0.5 mm of metal thickness at the margin. Typically it will be an exact replica of half the rotary instrument that was used to prepare it. (The recommended dimensions for reduction are shown in Figure 8-4.)

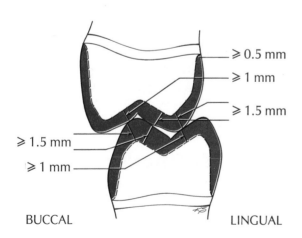

Fig. 8-4. Recommended dimensions for a complete cast crown. On functional cusps (buccal mandibular and lingual maxillary) the occlusal clearance should be equal to or greater than 1.5 mm. On nonfunctional cusps, a clearance of at least 1 mm is needed. The chamfer should allow for approximately 0.5 mm of metal thickness at the margin.

SPECIAL CONSIDERATIONS

Functional (Centric) Cusp Bevel. Proper tooth preparation for a complete cast crown will result in the reduction being directly beneath the cusps of the crown (see Fig. 7-43). This is important for ensuring optimum restoration contour with maximum durability and conservation of tooth structure. Proper placement of the functional cusp bevel will achieve it. Because additional reduction is needed for the functional cusps (to give 1.5 mm of occlusal clearance), the bevel must be angled flatter than the external surface (Fig. 8-5). On most teeth the functional cusp bevel will be placed at about 45 degrees to the long axis.

Nonfunctional (Noncentric) Cusp Bevel. All complete crown preparations should be assessed for adequate reduction at the occlusoaxial line angles of the nonfunctional cusps. A minimum of 0.6 mm of clearance is needed here for adequate strength. Maxillary molars in particular often require an additional reduction bevel in this area (Fig. 8-6). Without it, an overcontoured restoration that does not follow normal configuration may result. Such additional reduction is often unnecessary for mandibular molars, however, because they are lingually inclined and their profile is relatively straight.

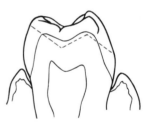

Fig. 8-5. The functional cusp bevel is prepared by slanting the bur at a flatter angle than the cuspal angulation. This will ensure additional reduction for the functional cusp.

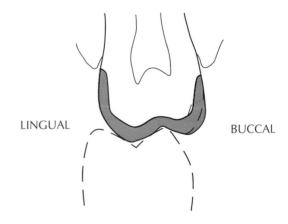

Fig. 8-6. The configuration of the facial wall of the maxillary molars may require slight additional reduction in the occlusal third to prevent an overcontoured restoration.

Chamfer Width. Increasing the faciolingual width of a complete crown is a common fault in practice and is a leading cause of periodontal disease associated with restorations. Adequate chamfer width (minimum 0.5 mm) is important for developing optimum axial contour. However, on small premolars it may be advantageous to prepare a slightly narrower chamfer to conserve tooth structure and retention form. This requires increasingly careful manipulation of the wax pattern during fabrication of the restoration and careful assessment to ensure that the crown is not excessively contoured.

PREPARATION

The clinical procedure to prepare a tooth for a complete cast crown consists of the following steps:
- Occlusal guiding grooves
- Occlusal reduction
- Axial alignment grooves
- Axial reduction
- Finishing and evaluation
- Armamentarium (Fig. 8-7 and Table 8-1)

STEP-BY-STEP PROCEDURE

The tooth preparation steps have been illustrated for a mandibular second molar. Depending on the tooth to be prepared (e.g., a premolar versus a molar) the exact number of guiding grooves may vary. The recommended sequence remains identical, however.

Guiding Grooves for Occlusal Reduction. A tapered carbide or a narrow, tapered diamond is recommended to place the guiding grooves for occlusal reduction.*
1. Place depth holes approximately 1 mm deep in the central, mesial, and distal fossae and connect them so that a channel runs the length of the central groove and extends into the mesial and distal marginal ridge.
2. Place guiding grooves in the buccal and lingual developmental grooves and in each tri-

---

*The use of guiding grooves for occlusal reduction is helpful only if the tooth is in good occlusal relationship before preparation. On most teeth this can be achieved with a foundation restoration and is done as part of the mouth preparation phase of treatment. Where this is not practical (e.g., when correcting occlusal discrepancies or replacing existing crowns), a matrix is made from the diagnostic waxing procedure, and this is used to assess optimal reduction (see Fig. 15-14, A).

angular ridge extending from the cusp tip to the center of its base (Figs. 8-8 and 8-9).
3. Because the centric or functional cusp is to be protected by an adequate thickness of metal,

Armamentarium	TABLE 8-1
Instrument	Use
Tapered carbide bur or diamond	Occlusal guiding grooves Additional retentive features
Narrow, round-tipped, tapered diamond (regular grit) (0.8 mm)	Occlusal reduction Axial alignment grooves Axial reduction Chamfer preparation
Wide, round-tipped, tapered diamond (fine grit) (1.2 mm)	Finishing
Utility wax and wax caliper Occlusal reduction gauge High- and low-speed friction grip contra-angles	Verification of occlusal clearance

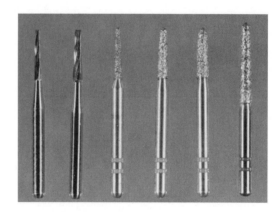

Fig. 8-7. Armamentarium for the complete cast crown preparation.

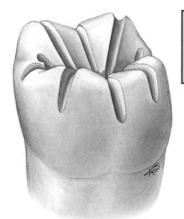

Note that the grooves are deeper for the functional cusp.

Fig. 8-8. Guiding grooves are placed on the occlusal surface. They are deeper on the functional cusp, and for the functional cusp bevel they diminish in depth from the cusp tip to the cervical margin.

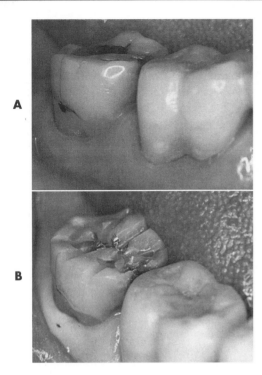

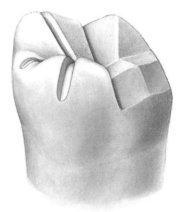

Half of the occlusal reduction is performed; the other half is maintained for reference purposes.

Fig. 8-10. After the guiding grooves are placed, the occlusal reduction is performed. Either the mesial or the distal half is maintained initially as a reference.

Fig. 8-9. **A,** A complete cast crown is indicated on this mandibular second molar with occlusal, proximal, and cervical lesions as well as a buccal longitudinal fracture. **B,** Initial depth grooves placed for occlusal reduction. Note that they have not yet been extended onto the buccal surface, where the functional cusp bevel will be placed.

place a functional cusp bevel to ensure this in the area of contact with the opposing tooth. The depth of this guiding groove should be slightly less than 1.5 mm (to allow for smoothing) in the area of the centric stop, and it should gradually diminish in a cervical direction.

4. Use the guiding grooves to ensure that occlusal reduction follows anatomic configuration and thus minimizes the loss of tooth structure while ensuring adequate reduction, as dictated by the mechanical properties of the alloy from which the restoration is to be fabricated. The guiding grooves must be placed with accuracy; the practitioner should concentrate on the position, depth, and angulation of each groove. A groove should be placed in the low point and high point of each cusp. The low points are the central and developmental grooves; the high points are the cusp tips and triangular ridges. Correct depth (0.8 mm* for the central groove and nonfunctional cusps, 1.3 mm* for the functional cusps) is achieved by knowledge of the

instruments being used. The practitioner should memorize the diameters of the rotary instruments; this will facilitate assessing the adequacy of the reduction in progress. If necessary, a periodontal probe can be used to measure the extent of reduction. Correct angulation of the grooves is needed to ensure that the occlusal reduction is correctly situated beneath the occlusal surface of the restoration. On the nonfunctional cusp, the groove should parallel the intended cuspal inclination; on the functional cusp, it should be angled slightly flatter to ensure the additional reduction of the functional cusp.

Occlusal Reduction. Once the guiding grooves have been deemed satisfactory, the tooth structure that remains between the grooves is removed with the carbide or the narrow, round-end, tapered diamond. Proper placement of the grooves automatically results in adequate occlusal clearance.

5. Complete the occlusal reduction in two steps (Fig. 8-10). Half the occlusal surface is reduced first so that the other half can be maintained as a reference. When the necessary reduction of the first half has been accomplished, reduction of the remaining half can be completed (Fig. 8-11).

6. On completion, check that a minimum clearance of 1.5 mm has been established on functional cusps and at least 1.0 mm on nonfunctional cusps. This clearance must be verified

---

*Allowing 0.2 mm for smoothing the preparation.

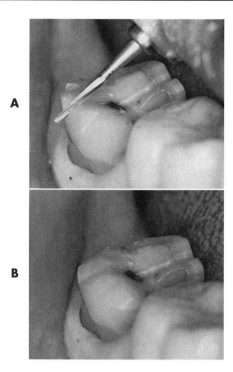

Fig. 8-11. **A,** Note the angulation of the bur as the functional cusp bevel is placed. **B,** Completed occlusal reduction. Note that it follows normal occlusal form. Three distinct planes can be seen buccolingually.

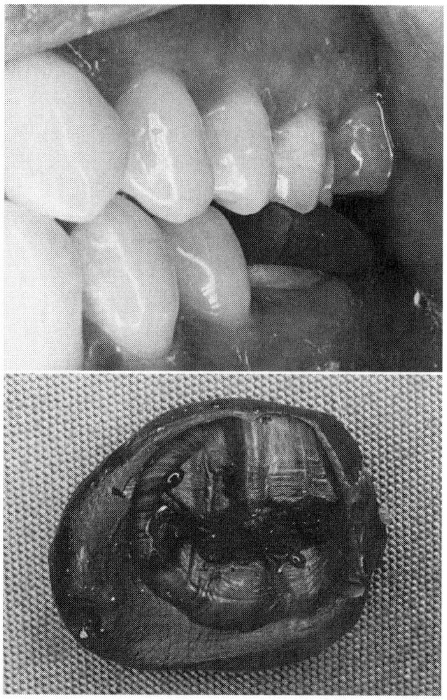

Fig. 8-12. Evaluation of the adequacy of occlusal clearance. **A,** The patient closes into softened wax. **B,** The thickness of the wax is assessed visually and measured with a wax caliper after it has been removed from the mouth.

in all excursive movements that the patient can make. The patient should close into several layers of dark-colored utility wax in maximum intercuspation (Fig. 8-12).

7. Remove the wax from the mouth and evaluate it for thin spots, which can be measured with a wax caliper.

8. Place the wax back in the patient's mouth and have the patient move the mandible into protrusive and excursive positions. On removal, the thickness of the utility wax is again measured, this time to verify that adequate clearance exists in the dynamic range as well as the intercuspal position. A convenient alternative is to use an occlusal reduction gauge* (Fig 8-13).

Alignment Grooves for Axial Reduction. After the occlusal reduction is completed, three alignment grooves are placed in each buccal and lingual wall with a narrow, round-end, tapered diamond. One is placed in the center of the wall, and one in each mesial and distal transitional line angle (Fig. 8-14).

1. When these guiding grooves are placed, be sure that the shank of the diamond is parallel

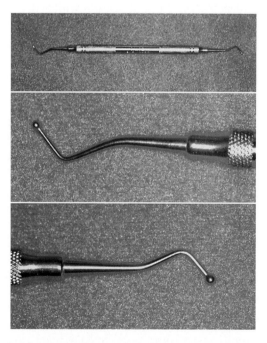

Fig. 8-13. Occlusal clearance can be judged intraorally with a reduction gauge. This instrument has 1-mm- and 1.5-mm-diameter spherical tips.

*Thompson Dental Mfg. Co., Inc: Missoula, Montana.

to the proposed path of withdrawal of the restoration. This automatically produces a convergence between the axial walls of the alignment grooves that is identical to the

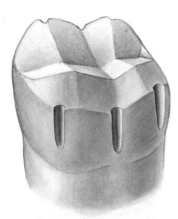

When placing these grooves, keep reduction to a minimum at the tip of the diamond.

Fig. 8-14.   Alignment grooves for axial reduction are placed in the buccal and lingual surfaces parallel to the long axis of the tooth buccolingually and mesiodistally.

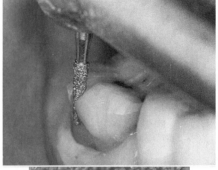

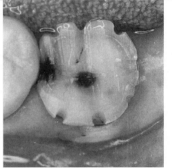

Fig. 8-15.   **A,** The diamond is aligned parallel to the long axis of the tooth as the buccal guiding grooves for axial alignment are placed. **B,** After all six grooves have been placed. Note that they are deep occlusally but shallower toward the cervical margin.

taper of the diamond. If a diamond with a 6-degree taper is used, an identical axial convergence on the preparation wall will result.

2. Do not let the diamond cut into the tooth beyond the point where its tip is buried in tooth structure up to the midpoint; otherwise, a lip of unsupported tooth enamel will be created (see Fig. 7-21). Gingivally the resulting depth of the alignment grooves therefore should be no more than one half the width of the tip of the diamond. Occlusocervically, the placement of the tip of the instrument will determine the location of the margin (Fig. 8-15).

3. Note that the alignment grooves determine the path of withdrawal of the restoration. They should be placed parallel to the proposed path of withdrawal, typically the long axis of the tooth.

4. Use a periodontal probe to assess the relative parallelism of the alignment grooves with one another or with the proposed path of withdrawal of a secondary retainer if the prepared tooth is to serve as a fixed partial denture abutment. When uncertainty exists regarding the correct placement of alignment grooves (as is likely on long-span fixed partial denture abutments), making an impression with irreversible hydrocolloid (alginate) is especially helpful. This can be poured in rapid-setting stone, and the resulting cast can be analyzed

with a dental surveyor.* At this time, corrections may still be easily made before unnecessary tooth reduction has occurred.

Axial Reduction.   The technique for axial reduction is similar to that for occlusal reduction. The remaining islands of tooth structure between the alignment grooves are removed while the chamfer margin is being placed, and the same narrow, round-tipped diamond is used for the procedure (Figs. 8-16 and 8-17).

5. As with the occlusal reduction, perform the axial reduction for half the tooth at a time, maintaining the other half as a reference for assessing adequacy of the preparation.

6. Pay special attention to the interproximal areas to prevent unintentional damage to the adjacent teeth. This often results if the practitioner is impatient and attempts to force the diamond into the area. Sufficient time must be allowed for the cutting instrument to create its own space (Fig. 8-18). Typically, if the

---

*The same cast can be used to fabricate the provisional restoration (see Chapter 15).

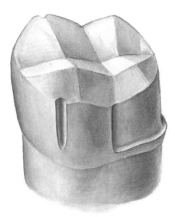

Fig. 8-16. If axial reduction is completed first on either the distal or the mesial half of the tooth, evaluation is simplified because the remaining intact tooth can serve as a reference.

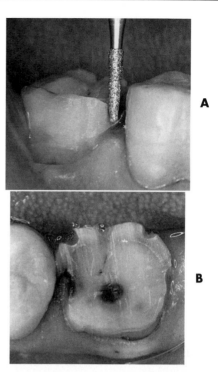

Fig. 8-18. **A,** As the mesiobuccal axial reduction is performed, a cervical chamfer is placed. **B,** Make the chamfer of relatively even width and maintain the somewhat angular preparation outline form to maximize resistance form.

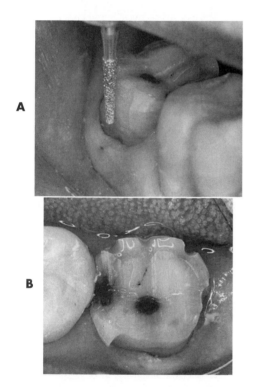

Fig. 8-17. **A,** Note the alignment of the diamond as tooth structure between the alignment grooves is removed. **B,** Axial reduction. The distobuccal axial reduction has been completed.

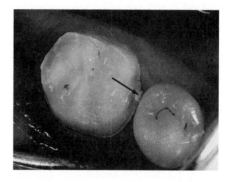

Fig. 8-19. A lip of enamel *(arrow)* protects the adjacent tooth from iatrogenic damage as the axial reduction is completed.

proper cervical placement of the margin has been selected with proper axial alignment of the instrument, a lip of tooth enamel will be maintained between the diamond and the adjacent tooth that protects it from any damage (Fig. 8-19).

7. If desired, protect the adjacent teeth by placing a metal matrix band. The most difficult interproximal areas to reduce are those with significant buccolingual dimension and those with root proximity. Typically, however, the critical area will be only a few millimeters in length.

8. Cut into the proximal area from both sides until only a few millimeters of interproximal island remain (Fig. 8-20). This area can then be removed and contact broken by using thinner, tapered diamonds. If the adjacent proximal surface is damaged, it must be

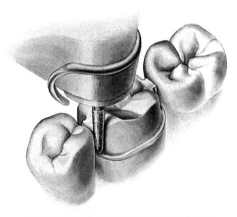

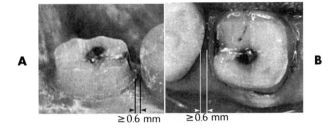

Fig. 8-21. **A,** Note that adequate clearance (≥ 0.6 mm) exists between the external surface of the proximal chamfer and the adjacent tooth. **B,** Occlusal view of the preparation.

> As the axial reduction is performed, eventually a small island of tooth structure will remain in the interproximal area. When removing this, maintain a narrow "lip" of tooth structure between the diamond and the adjacent tooth to protect the latter from damage.

Fig. 8-20. Preparation of the proximal contact area.

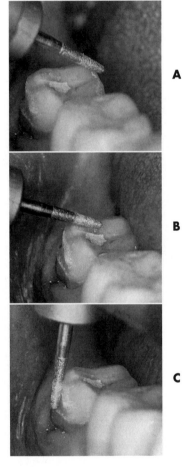

Fig. 8-22. **A,** The transition from lingual to occlusal is rounded with a fine-grit diamond. **B,** All sharp line angles between occlusal reduction and functional cusp bevel are similarly rounded. **C,** The margin is refined, and any minor irregularities are removed.

polished with white stones, silicone points, and prophylaxis paste before impression making. Ideally a fluoride application should be given for improved resistance and to prevent demineralization of the surface enamel.

9. Place the cervical chamfer concurrently with axial reduction. Its width should be approximately 0.5 mm, which will allow adequate bulk of metal at the margin. This chamfer must be smooth and continuous mesiodistally, and a distinct resistance against vertical displacement should be detected when probed with the tip of an explorer (Fig. 8-21). Unsupported enamel cannot be tolerated because it is likely to fracture when the restoration is tried in or cemented, which will result in an open margin and early failure of the restoration.

Finishing. A smooth surface finish and continuity of all prepared surfaces will aid most phases of fabrication of the restoration. Smooth transitions from occlusal to axial surfaces facilitate impression making, waxing, investing, and casting because bubble formation is reduced (Fig. 8-22).

1. Use a fine-grit diamond or carbide bur of slightly greater diameter for finishing the chamfer margin. This should be done as

smoothly as possible, with the handpiece operating at reduced speed. NOTE: Some practitioners favor using a low-speed contraangle for the finishing. A properly finished margin should be glassy smooth when touched by the tine of an explorer.

2. Finish all prepared surfaces and slightly round all line angles. If necessary, place a

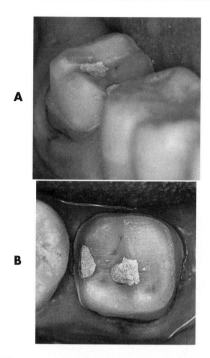

Fig. 8-23. Completed preparation. The carious lesions have been excavated and the resulting irregularities blocked out with amalgam. **A,** Buccal appearance. **B,** Occlusal appearance.

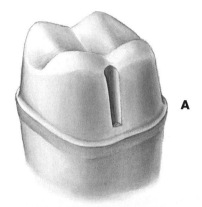

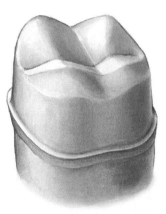

Fig. 8-24. **A,** When opposing axial walls are excessively tapered, internal features such as this buccal groove can be used to improve retention and resistance form. **B,** Mesially tipped molars and short premolars often benefit from grooves and/or boxes incorporated in the preparation design.

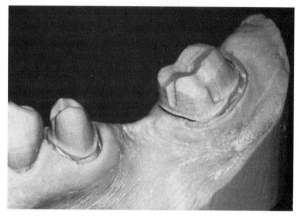

Fig. 8-25. The completed preparation is characterized by a smooth, even chamfer; a 6-degree taper; and gradual transitions between all prepared surfaces.

nonfunctional cusp bevel at this time (Fig. 8-23). During finishing of the chamfer, the use of air cooling alone is recommended to improve visibility. However, when only air cooling is used, a water spray should be applied from time to time to prevent the tooth from dehydrating, and the possible development of pulpal damage, as well as to wash away debris. The wider diamond is recommended because it will smooth out any unwanted ripples that may have been created during axial reduction and will eliminate any unsupported enamel at the margin.

3. Place additional retentive features as needed (e.g., grooves or boxes) with the tapered carbide bur (Fig. 8-24).

The criteria used to determine the need for such features to enhance retention and resistance are described in Chapter 7.

Evaluation. Upon completion, the preparation is evaluated to assess whether all the criteria have been fulfilled (Fig. 8-25).

One of the more common errors in complete cast crown preparations is overtapering of the opposing axial walls. This significantly reduces the retention of the completed restoration. If a tooth preparation has been inadvertently overreduced through exces-

sive tapering of axial walls, it should be carefully evaluated to determine how it can be corrected. If a band of several millimeters of tooth structure can be prepared circumferentially with a restricted taper of approximately 6 degrees, it is probably unnecessary to modify the preparation further to compensate for areas of excessive reduction in the occlusal third. If this is not the case, an approach slightly less conservative of tooth structure may be warranted: (1) uprighting overtapered axial walls to obtain the mechanical advantage of increased retention or (2) using grooves, boxes, or pinholes as needed.

No undercuts between any opposing axial walls can be accepted. When the diamond is placed against the axial surface of the prepared tooth, parallel to the path of withdrawal, it should be possible to move the instrument around the tooth so the entire height of the preparation is touching the diamond at all times. The tip of the diamond should rest on the chamfer throughout this movement, and no light should be visible between the instrument and the axial surface.

Finally, occlusal and proximal clearances are assessed. They should be adjusted if inadequate provision has been made for the restorative material. Any problems must be corrected before provisionalization (Fig. 8-26) and impression making.

SUMMARY

The complete cast crown, an all-metal restoration often used on single posterior teeth as a retainer for a fixed partial denture, provides greater retention and resistance than any other type of restoration. It is not indicated for every restorative circumstance, however. It is unnecessary if the buccal and/or lingual walls of a tooth are intact or if less than maximum retention is needed. The rather extensive removal of tooth structure required in its preparation can have adverse pulpal and periodontal effects. Its high strength makes it especially suitable for restoring an endodontically treated tooth, although in patients who find visible metal a significant drawback, the metal-ceramic or a more conservative partial-coverage restoration may be preferred.

A well-organized approach to preparation for a complete cast crown should be based on the selective use of guiding grooves of predetermined depth correlated with specific properties of the restorative material. Adequate occlusal reduction is necessary,

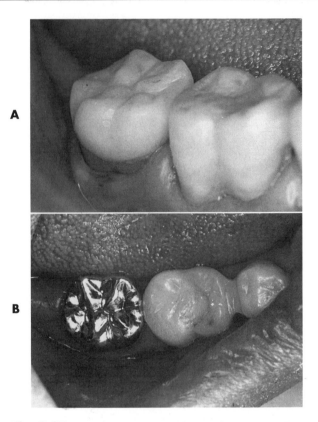

Fig. 8-26.   **A,** Acrylic resin provisional restoration is cemented. **B,** Complete cast crown is cemented.

following the normal anatomic tooth contours, and the axial reduction should also conform to the normal configuration of the tooth, with minimum taper (6 degrees). Under no circumstances should undercuts remain in the proximal walls. These must be removed by additional tooth preparation or blocked out with a suitable base material. The chamfer is the margin of choice for a complete cast crown. It should be distinct and of adequate width. No unsupported enamel can be permitted. Occlusocervically, the margin should be supragingival, and it should be smooth and continuous mesiodistally. When assessing the adequacy of the chamfer, one should be able to feel distinct resistance against vertical displacement by an explorer or periodontal probe.

Study Questions

1. What are the indications and contraindications for complete cast crowns?
2. What are the advantages and disadvantages of complete cast crowns?
3. What is the recommended armamentarium, and in what sequence should a mandibular molar be prepared, for a complete cast crown?
4. What are the minimum criteria for each step described in question 3?

SUMMARY CHART

Indications	Contraindications	Advantages	Disadvantages
Extensive destruction from caries or trauma	Less than maximum retention necessary	Strong	Removal of large amount of tooth structure
Endodontically treated teeth	Esthetics	High retentive qualities	Adverse effects on tissue
Existing restoration		Usually easy to obtain adequate resistance form	Vitality testing not readily feasible
Necessity for maximum retention and strength		Option to modify form and occlusion	Display of metal
To provide contours to receive a removable appliance			
Other recontouring of axial surfaces (minor corrections of malinclinations)			
Correction of occlusal plane			

COMPLETE CAST CROWN

Preparation Steps	Recommended Armamentarium	Criteria
Depth grooves for occlusal reduction	Tapered carbide or diamond	Minimum clearance on noncentric cusps: 1 mm Minimum clearance on centric cusps: 1.5 mm
Functional cusp bevel	Same	Flatter than cuspal plane, to allow additional reduction at functional cusp
Occlusal reduction (half at a time)	Regular-grit, round-tipped, tapered diamond	Should follow normal anatomic configuration of occlusal surface
Alignment grooves for axial reduction	Same	Chamfer allows 0.5 mm of thickness of wax at margins
Axial reduction (half at a time)	Same	Reduction performed parallel to long axis
Finishing of chamfer	Wide, round-tipped diamond or carbide	Smooth mesiodistally and buccolingually; resistance to vertical displacement by tip of explorer or periodontal probe
Additional retentive features if needed	Tapered carbide	Grooves, boxes, pinholes as described for partial-coverage restorations
Finishing	Fine-grit diamond or carbide	Rounding of all sharp line angles to facilitate impression making, die pouring, waxing, and casting

THE METAL-CERAMIC CROWN PREPARATION

In many dental practices the metal-ceramic crown is one of the most widely used fixed restorations. This has resulted in part from technologic improvements in the fabrication of restoration by dental laboratories and in part from the growing amount of cosmetic demands that challenge dentists today.

The restoration consists of a complete-coverage cast metal crown (or substructure) that is veneered with a layer of fused porcelain to mimic the appearance of a natural tooth. The extent of the veneer can vary.

To be successful, a metal-ceramic crown preparation requires considerable tooth reduction wherever the metal substructure is to be veneered with dental porcelain. Only with sufficient thickness can the darker color of the metal substructure be masked and the veneer duplicate the appearance of a natural tooth. The porcelain veneer must have a certain minimum thickness for esthetics. Consequently, much tooth reduction is necessary, and the metal-ceramic preparation is one of the least conservative of tooth structures (Fig. 9-1).

Historically, attempts to veneer metal restorations with porcelain had several problems. A major challenge was the development of an alloy and a ceramic material with compatible physical properties that would provide adequate bond strength. In addition, it was initially difficult to obtain a natural appearance.

The technical aspects of the fabrication of this restoration are discussed more in Chapter 24. For now, only a brief description is provided. The metal substructure is waxed and then cast in a special metal-ceramic alloy having a higher fusing range and a lower thermal expansion than conventional gold alloys. After preparatory finishing procedures, this substructure, or framework, is veneered with dental porcelain. The porcelain is fused onto the framework in much the same manner as household articles are enameled. Modern dental porcelains fuse at a temperature of about 960° C (1760° F). Because conventional gold alloys would melt at this temperature, the special alloys are necessary.

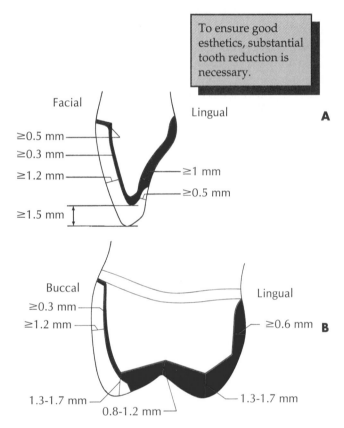

To ensure good esthetics, substantial tooth reduction is necessary.

Fig. 9-1. Recommended minimum dimensions for a metal-ceramic restoration on an anterior tooth **(A)** and a posterior tooth **(B).** Note the significant reduction needed compared to that for a complete cast or partial veneer crown.

INDICATIONS

The metal-ceramic crown is indicated on teeth that require complete coverage, where significant esthetic demands are placed on the dentist (e.g., the anterior teeth). It should be recognized, however, that, if esthetic considerations are paramount, an all-ceramic crown (see Chapters 11 and 25) has distinct cosmetic advantages over the metal-ceramic restoration; nevertheless, the metal-ceramic crown is more durable than the all-ceramic crown and generally has superior marginal fit. Furthermore, it can serve as a retainer for a fixed partial denture because its metal substructure can accommodate cast or soldered connectors. Whereas the all-ceramic restoration cannot accommodate a rest for a removable prosthesis, the metal-ceramic crown may be successfully modified to incorporate occlusal and cingulum rests as well as milled proximal and reciprocal guide planes in its metal substructure (see Chapter 21).

Typical indications are similar to those for all-metal complete crowns: extensive tooth destruction as a result of caries, trauma, or existing previous restorations that precludes the use of a more conservative restoration; the need for superior retention and strength; an endodontically treated tooth in conjunction with a suitable supporting structure (a post-and-core); and the need to recontour axial surfaces or correct minor malinclinations. Within certain limits this restoration can also be used to correct the occlusal plane.

CONTRAINDICATIONS

Contraindications for the metal-ceramic crown, as for all fixed restorations, include patients with active caries or untreated periodontal disease. In young patients with large pulp chambers, the metal-ceramic crown is also contraindicated because of the high risk of pulp exposure (see Fig. 7-4). If at all possible, a more conservative restorative option such as a composite resin or porcelain laminate veneer (see Chapter 25) is preferred.

A metal-ceramic restoration should not be considered whenever a more conservative retainer is feasible, unless maximum retention is needed—as for a long-span FPD. If the facial wall is intact, the practitioner should decide whether it is truly necessary to involve all axial surfaces of the tooth in the proposed restoration. Although perhaps technically more demanding and time consuming, a more conservative solution usually can be found to satisfy the patient's needs that may provide superior long-term service.

ADVANTAGES

The metal-ceramic restoration combines, to a large degree, the strength of cast metal with the esthetics of an all-ceramic crown. The underlying principle is to reinforce a brittle, more cosmetically pleasing material through support derived from the stronger metal substructure. Natural appearance can be closely matched by good technique and if desired through characterization of the restoration with internally or externally applied stains. Retentive qualities are excellent because all axial walls are included in the preparation, and it is usually quite easy to ensure adequate resistance form during tooth preparation. The complete-coverage aspect of the restoration permits easy correction of axial form. In addition, the required preparation often is much less demanding than for partial-coverage retainers. Generally, the degree of difficulty of a metal-ceramic preparation is comparable to that of preparing a posterior tooth for a complete cast crown.

DISADVANTAGES

The preparation for a metal-ceramic crown requires significant tooth reduction to provide sufficient space for the restorative materials. To achieve better esthetics, the facial margin of an anterior restoration is often placed subgingivally, which increases the potential for periodontal disease. However, a supragingival margin can be used if significant cosmetic concerns do not prohibit it or if the restoration incorporates a porcelain labial margin (see Chapter 24).

Compared to an all-ceramic restoration, the metal-ceramic crown may have slightly inferior esthetics, but it can be used in higher-stress situations or on teeth that would not provide adequate support for an all-ceramic restoration.

Because of the glasslike nature of the veneering material, a metal-ceramic crown is subject to brittle fracture (although such failure can usually be attributed to poor design or fabrication of the restoration). A frequent problem is the difficulty of accurate shade selection and of communicating it to the dental ceramist. This is often underestimated by the novice. Since many procedural steps are required for both metal casting and porcelain application, laboratory costs generally place the metal-ceramic restoration among the more expensive of dental procedures.

PREPARATION

The recommended sequence of preparation is illustrated for a maxillary right central incisor (Fig. 9-2); however, the same step-by-step approach can be applied to other teeth (Fig. 9-3). As with all tooth preparations, a systematic and organized approach to tooth reduction will save time.

Armamentarium (Fig. 9-4). The instruments needed to prepare teeth for a metal-ceramic crown include:
- Round-tipped rotary diamonds (regular grit for bulk reduction, fine grit for finishing) or carbides

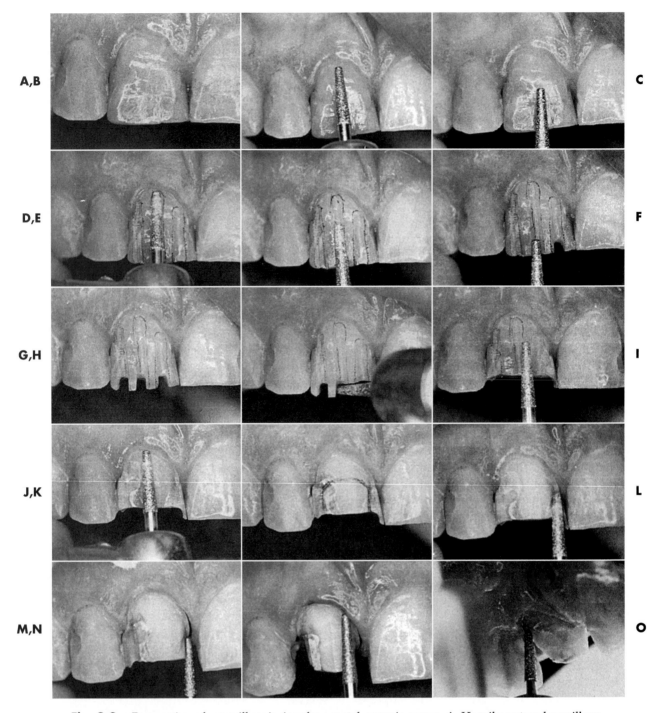

Fig. 9-2.   Preparation of a maxillary incisor for a metal-ceramic crown. **A,** Heavily restored maxillary central incisor. **B** and **C,** Rotary instrument aligned with the cervical one third and incisal two thirds to gauge correct planes of reduction. **D** and **E,** Guiding grooves placed in the two planes. The cervical groove is made parallel to the path of withdrawal, which usually coincides with the long axis of the tooth. The incisal depth groove is prepared parallel to the facial contour of the tooth. **F** and **G,** Incisal guiding grooves are placed. **H,** Incisal edge reduction. **I** to **K,** Facial reduction accomplished in two planes. **L,** Breaking proximal contact, maintaining a lip of enamel to protect the adjacent tooth from inadvertent damage. **M** and **N,** Proximal reduction. **O,** Placing a 0.5-mm lingual chamfer.

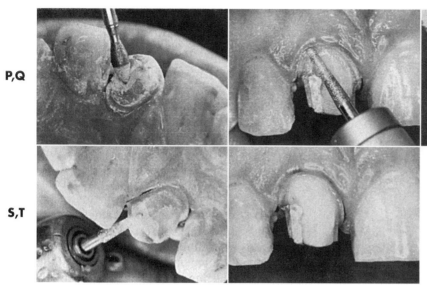

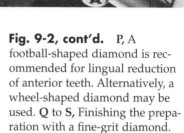

P,Q

S,T

R

Fig. 9-2, cont'd. P, A football-shaped diamond is recommended for lingual reduction of anterior teeth. Alternatively, a wheel-shaped diamond may be used. **Q** to **S**, Finishing the preparation with a fine-grit diamond. **T**, The completed preparation.

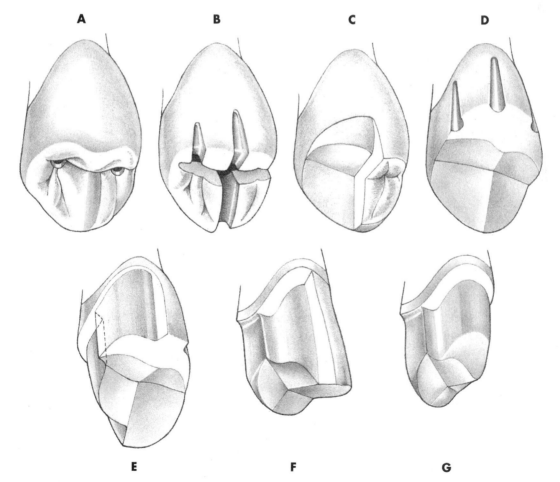

Fig. 9-3. Preparation of a maxillary premolar for a metal-ceramic crown. **A**, Depth holes. **B**, Occlusal depth cuts. **C**, Half of the occlusal reduction is completed. **D**, Occlusal reduction is complete. Guiding grooves are placed for axial reduction. **E** and **F**, Lingual chamfer and facial shoulder are prepared on half the tooth. **G**, Completed preparation.
(A to E, Lingual view; F and G, buccal view.)

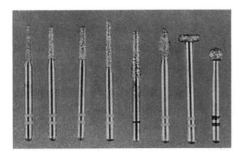

Fig. 9-4. Armamentarium for the metal-ceramic crown preparation.

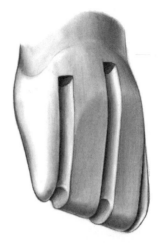

Fig. 9-5. Depth grooves in the facial wall are placed in two directions: incisally, parallel to the tooth contour; cervically, parallel to the path of withdrawal. The grooves should be 1.3 mm deep.

- Football- or wheel-shaped diamond (for lingual reduction of anterior teeth)
- Flat-ended, tapered diamond (for shoulder preparation)
- Finishing stones
- Explorer and periodontal probe
- Hatchet and chisel

The actual sequence of steps can be varied slightly depending on operator preference.

Step-By-Step Procedure. The preparation is divided into five major steps: guiding grooves, incisal or occlusal reduction, labial or buccal reduction in the area to be veneered with porcelain, axial reduction of the proximal and lingual surfaces, and final finishing of all prepared surfaces.

Guiding Grooves

1. Place three depth grooves (Fig. 9-5), one in the center of the facial surface and one each in the approximate locations of the mesiofacial and distofacial line angles (see Fig. 9-2, *A* to *E*). These will be in two planes: the cervical portion to parallel the long axis of the tooth, the incisal (occlusal) portion to follow the normal facial contour (see Fig. 9-2, *D* and *E*).
2. Perform the facial reduction in the cervical and incisal planes. The cervical plane will determine the path of withdrawal of the completed restoration. The incisal or occlusal plane will provide the space needed for the porcelain veneer; it should be approximately 1.3 mm deep to allow for additional reduction during finishing. The incisal grooves usually extend halfway down the facial surface, although (depending on the shape of the tooth) they may extend to include the incisal two thirds. Cervical grooves are generally made parallel to the long axis of the tooth. However, they can be adjusted slightly to create a more desirable path of withdrawal; in particular, some labial inclination will im-

prove retention on a tooth with little cingulum height. On small teeth it may be advisable to keep the cervical grooves somewhat shallower near the margin.

3. Place three depth grooves (about 1.8 mm deep) in the incisal edge of an anterior tooth. This will provide the needed reduction of 2 mm and allow finishing (see Fig. 9-2, *F* and *G*). Verify the depth of these grooves can be verified with a periodontal probe. On posterior teeth where the occlusion is to be established in porcelain, 2 mm of clearance must exist. If the occlusion is to be established in metal, the same minimum clearances are needed as for a complete cast crown. Posterior occlusal reduction incorporates a functional cusp bevel on the lingual cusp, similar to that for a complete cast crown. When initially positioning the diamond for anterior teeth, it may be helpful to observe the long axis of the opposing tooth in the intercuspal position and to orient the instrument perpendicular to that (Fig. 9-6). The grooves must not be too deep; otherwise, an overreduced and undulating surface will result.

Incisal (Occlusal) Reduction. The completed reduction of the incisal edge on an anterior tooth should allow 2 mm for adequate material thickness to permit translucency in the completed restoration. Posterior teeth generally require less (1.5 mm) because esthetics is not as critical. Caution must be used, however, because excessive occlusal reduction shortens the axial walls and thus is a common cause of inadequate retention and resistance form in

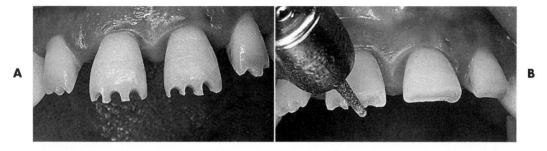

Fig. 9-6. **A,** Depth grooves 1.8 mm deep placed in the incisal edges to ensure adequate and even reduction. **B,** Incisal reduction completed on the left central and lateral incisors. Note the angulation of the diamond, perpendicular to the direction of loading by the mandibular anterior teeth.

the completed preparation. This can be particularly problematic on anterior teeth (where as a consequence of tooth form, most of the retention is derived from the proximal walls).

4. Remove the islands of remaining tooth structure. On anterior teeth, access is usually unrestricted, and the thickest portion of the cutting instrument can be used to maximize cutting efficiency (see Fig. 9-2, *H*). On posterior teeth, the same pattern is followed as in preparing depth grooves for a complete cast crown (see Chapter 8). This will include the use of a centric cusp bevel, although additional occlusal reduction will be needed where the porcelain is to be applied (see Fig. 9-3, *A* to *C*).

Labial (Buccal) Reduction. When completed, the reduction of the facial surface should have produced sufficient space to accommodate the metal substructure and porcelain veneer. A minimum of 1.2 mm is necessary to permit the ceramist to produce a restoration with satisfactory appearance (1.5 mm is preferable). This requires significant tooth reduction. For comparison, the cervical diameter of a maxillary central incisor averages between 6 and 7 mm.

In the cervical area of small teeth, obtaining optimal reduction is not always feasible (see Fig. 7-4.) Often a compromise is made with lesser reduction in the area where the cervical shoulder margin is prepared.

5. Remove the remaining tooth structure between depth grooves (see Fig. 9-2, *I* to *L*), creating a shoulder at the cervical margin (Fig. 9-7). If a restoration with a narrow subgingival metal collar is to be fabricated and sufficient sulcular depth is present, place the shoulder approximately 0.5 mm apical to the crest of the free gingiva at this time. Additional finishing will then result in a margin that is 0.75 to 1 mm subgingival. Use adequate water spray during the entire phase of

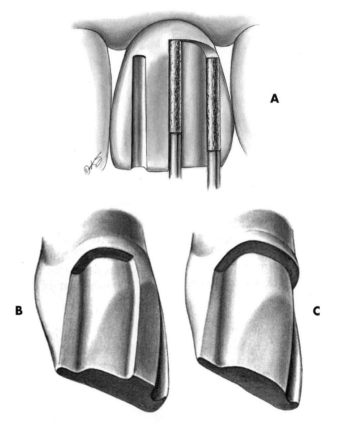

Fig. 9-7. **A,** The cervical shoulder is established as the tooth structure between the depth grooves is removed. The rotary instrument is moved parallel to the intended path of withdrawal during this procedure. **B,** The facial reduction should be completed in two phases, initially maintaining one half intact for assessment of the adequacy of reduction. Note the two distinct planes of reduction on the facial. The proximal aspect parallels the cervical reduction on the facial wall. **C,** Facial reduction completed. A 6-degree taper has been established between the proximal walls.

preparation, because a significant amount of tooth structure is being removed and copious irrigation (along with intermittent strokes) will expedite the preparation process. Such a cautious approach will prevent unnecessary trauma to the pulp. The resulting shoulder should be approximately 1 mm wide and should extend well into the proximal embrasures when viewed from the incisal (occlusal) side (Fig. 9-8). Where access permits, establishing this shoulder from the proximal gingival crest toward the middle of the facial wall is preferred. This will minimize placement of the initial shoulder preparation too close to the epithelial attachment. If the margin is established from facial to proximal, a tendency exists to "bury" the instrument and encroach on the epithelial attachment. A conscious effort to maintain proper margin position relative to the crest of the free gingiva is critical (see Fig. 7-49). The location and specific configuration of the facial margin depend on several factors: the type of metal-ceramic restoration selected, the cosmetic expectations of the patient, and operator preference.

From a periodontal point of view, a supragingival margin is always preferred. Its application is restricted, however, because patients often object to a visible metal collar or discolored root surface. Such objections are common, even when the gingival margin is not visible during normal function, as in patients with a low lip line. This generally limits the use of supragingival margins to posterior teeth (Fig. 9-9) and to un-discolored anterior teeth (in which case a porcelain labial margin is preferred; see Chapter 24). The optimum location of the margin should be carefully determined with the full cooperation of the patient. Where a subgingival margin is to be placed, careful tissue manipulation is essential; otherwise, there will be damage that leads to permanent gingival recession and subsequent exposure of the metal collar. This is most effectively avoided through meticulous gingival displacement with a cord before finishing (Fig. 9-10). The configuration of the margin is also finalized at this time (Fig. 9-11).

Axial Reduction of the Proximal and Lingual Surfaces. (see Fig. 9-2, *M* to *P*). Sufficient tooth structure must be removed to provide a distinct, smooth chamfer of about 0.5 mm width.

6. Reduce the proximoaxial and linguoaxial surfaces with the diamond held parallel to the intended path of withdrawal of the restoration. These walls should converge slightly from cervical to incisal or occlusal. A taper of approximately 6 degrees is recommended. On anterior teeth, a lingual concavity is prepared for adequate clearance for the restorative material(s). Typically, 1 mm is required if the centric contacts in the completed restoration are to be located on metal. When contact is on porcelain, additional reduction will be necessary. For anterior teeth, usually only one groove is placed, in the center of the lingual surface. For molars, three grooves can be placed in a manner similar to that described for the all-metal complete cast crown.

> To ensure esthetics, the shoulder margin must extend into the interproximal area.

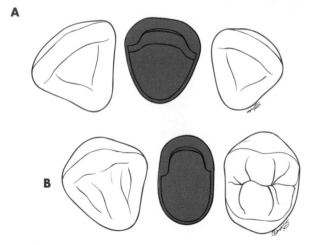

Fig. 9-8. **A,** The facial shoulder preparation should wrap around into the interproximal embrasure and extend at least 1 mm lingual to the proximal contact. **B,** The shoulder preparation extends adequately to the lingual side of the proximal contact. Note that on the mesial (visible) side, the preparation extends slightly farther than on the distal (cosmetically less critical) side.

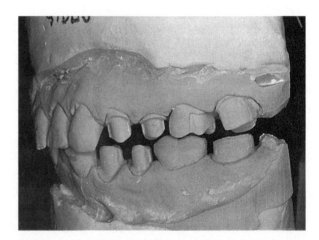

Fig. 9-9. Supragingival margins on the maxillary premolars. They were possible because of a favorable lip line hiding the cervical aspect of these posterior teeth. The subgingival margins on the mandibular premolars were prepared only because of previously existing restorations.

7. Make a lingual alignment groove by positioning the diamond parallel to the cervical plane of the facial reduction. When the round-tipped diamond of appropriate size and shape is aligned properly, it will be almost halfway submerged into tooth structure. Verify the alignment of the groove, and carry the axial reduction from the groove along the lingual surface into the proximal; maintain the originally selected alignment of the diamond at all times.

8. As the lingual chamfer is developed, extend it buccally into the proximal to blend with the interproximal shoulder placed earlier (Fig. 9-12). Alternatively, a facial approach may be used. Although this is slightly more difficult initially, after some practice it should be easy to eliminate the lingual guiding groove and to perform the proximal and lingual axial reduction in one step; however, this requires that the diamond be held freehand parallel to the path of withdrawal. The proximal flange

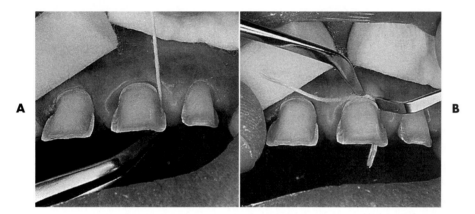

Fig. 9-10. **A,** A gingival displacement cord (under tension) is placed in the interproximal sulcus. **B,** A second instrument can be used to prevent it from rebounding from the sulcus after it has been packed.

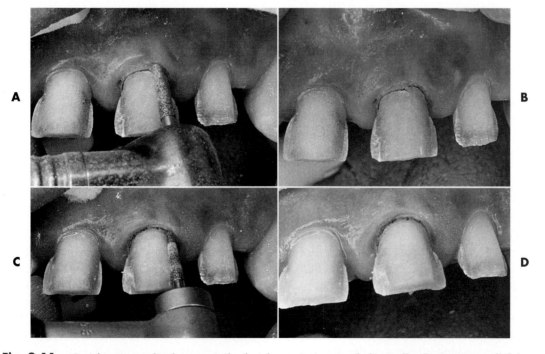

Fig. 9-11. **A,** After tissue displacement, the facial margin is extended apically. Caution is needed, because if the diamond inadvertently grabs the cord, it may be ripped out of the sulcus and traumatize the epithelial attachment. **B,** Note the additional apical extension of the shoulder on the distal aspect. **C,** The entire facial shoulder is placed at a level that will be subgingival after the tissue rebounds. **D,** The facial margin has been prepared to the level of the previously placed cord.

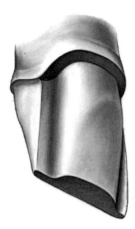

Fig. 9-12. A lingual chamfer is prepared to allow adequate space for metal. A smooth transition from interproximal shoulder to chamfer is essential.

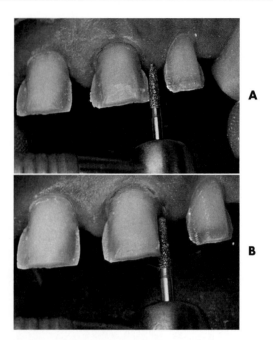

Fig. 9-13. **A,** Proximal reduction of the flange with a facial approach. **B,** Once sufficient tooth structure has been removed, the cervical chamfer is prepared simultaneously with the lingual axial surface. After the distolingual preparation has been completed, the mesial chamfer is blended into a smooth transition with the shoulder.

that resulted from the shoulder preparation can be used as a reference for judging alignment of the rotary instrument (Fig. 9-13). The interproximal margin should not be inadvertently placed too far gingivally and thereby infringe on the attachment apparatus. It must follow the soft tissue contour (see p. 150). On posterior teeth, the lingual wall reduction blends into the functional cusp bevel placed during the occlusal reduction. Anterior teeth require an additional step: After preparation of the cingulum wall, one or more depth grooves are placed in the lingual surface. These are approximately 1 mm deep.

9. Use a football-shaped diamond to reduce the lingual surface of anterior teeth (see Fig. 9-2, *P*). It is helpful to stop when half this reduction has been completed to evaluate clearance in the intercuspal position and all excursions. The remaining intact tooth structure can serve as a reference.

Finishing. The margin must provide distinct resistance to vertical displacement of an explorer tip, and it must be smooth and continuous circumferentially. (A properly finished margin should feel like smooth glass slab.) All other line angles should be rounded, and the completed preparation should have a satin finish free from obvious diamond scratch marks. Tissue displacement is particularly helpful when finishing subgingival margins (Fig. 9-14). Sometimes this step is postponed until just before impression making after tissue displacement.

10. Finish the margins with diamonds, hand instruments, or carbides (see Fig. 9-2, *Q* and *R*). All internal line angles should be radiused to facilitate the impression-making and die-pouring steps (see Fig. 9-2, *S*). The

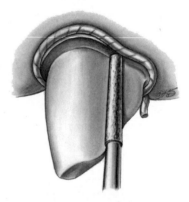

Fig. 9-14. Controlled tissue displacement can be helpful when finishing the margin with a fine-grit diamond or another rotary instrument.

finishing steps for the facial margin depend on the design of margin chosen (see Table 7-2 and Fig. 9-15). A porcelain labial margin requires proper support for the porcelain. A shoulder with a 90-degree cavosurface angle is recommended. This type of shoulder can also be used for a crown with a conventional metal collar and offers the advantage of allowing the collar to be kept narrow. However, there is then the risk of leaving unsupported enamel. For this reason, the margin is often beveled or sloped to create a more obtuse cavosurface angle (Fig. 9-16). A

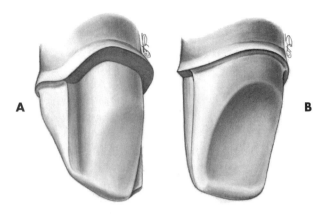

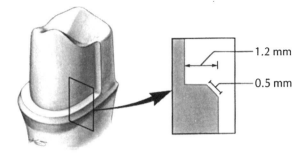

Fig. 9-17. The shoulder bevel.

Fig. 9-15. **A,** Completed preparation. Note that the transition from incisal to axial walls is rounded, and a distinct 90-degree or slightly sloping shoulder has been established. **B,** Even chamfer width and a smooth transition between lingual and axial surfaces. The chamfer is distinct and blends smoothly into the facial shoulder.

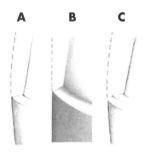

Fig. 9-16. **A,** 90-degree shoulder. **B,** 120-degree shoulder. **C,** Shoulder bevel.

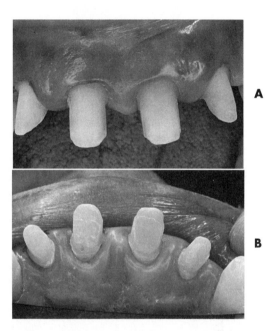

Fig. 9-18. **A,** Facial and **B,** lingual views of metal-ceramic preparations.

flat-ended diamond in a low-speed handpiece creates the 90-degree shoulder. Any unsupported enamel must be removed subsequently by careful planing with a sharp chisel. Care must also be taken to orient the rotary instrument as it moves around the tooth if inadvertent undercuts are to be avoided. When a metal-collar design of ceramic restoration is planned, the need for a 90-degree shoulder is less critical. A sloping shoulder has been advocated to ensure the elimination of unsupported enamel and to minimize marginal gap width (see Chapter 7). Such a shoulder (cavosurface angle of about 120 degrees) can be accomplished with a flat-ended diamond by changing its alignment, paying particular attention to the configuration of the tooth structure cervical to the margin. Alternatively, a hatchet can be used to plane the margin to the correct angulation. Again, be careful to avoid undercutting the axial wall of the preparation where it meets the shoulder during finishing. A shoulder-bevel margin is most effectively achieved with a flame-shaped carbide

bur or hand instrument, depending on the length of bevel required (Fig. 9-17). Generally a short bevel with a cavosurface angle of 135 degrees is advocated, although longer bevels have been recommended for improved marginal fit. Special care must be exerted where the bevel meets the interproximal chamfer. The chamfer and bevel should be continuous with each other. Care must be taken not to damage the epithelial attachment during beveling; tissue displacement before preparation of subgingival bevels is recommended.

11. After a satisfactory facial margin has been obtained, round all sharp line angles within the preparation (see Fig. 9-2, S). This will facilitate surface wetting and expedite subsequent procedures (impression making, pouring of casts, waxing, and investing). A fine-grit diamond operating at low speed is

particularly useful. However, where access allows, a slightly larger tapered diamond may be preferred because the greater diameter of its tip prevents "ditching" of the chamfer. Blend all surfaces together, and re-

move any sharp transitions (see Figs. 9-2, *T*; 9-18; and 9-19).

Evaluation. Areas often missed during finishing are the incisal edges of anterior preparations and the transition from occlusal to axial wall of posterior preparations. The completed chamfer should provide 0.5 mm of space for the restoration at the margin. The chamfer must be smooth and continuous, and when evaluated, a distinct resistance to vertical displacement of the tip of an explorer or periodontal probe should be felt. The chamfer should be continuous with the interproximal shoulder or beveled shoulder. The cavosurface angle of the chamfer should be slightly obtuse or 90 degrees. Under no circumstances should any unsupported tooth structure remain, especially at the facial margin. Care is also needed to avoid creating an undercut between the facial and lingual walls. This aspect of the preparation should be thoroughly evaluated. Excessive convergence should also be avoided, because this may lead to pulpal exposure. All residual debris is removed with thorough irrigation. (Various examples of metal-ceramic preparations are shown in Figs. 9-20 and 9-21.)

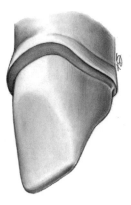

Fig. 9-19. The "wingless" variation does not exhibit the defined transition from chamfer to shoulder seen in Fig. 9-15. Rather, the shoulder gradually narrows toward the lingual side. Interproximally, the same criteria for minimum extension of the shoulder apply as for the wing-type or flange preparation.

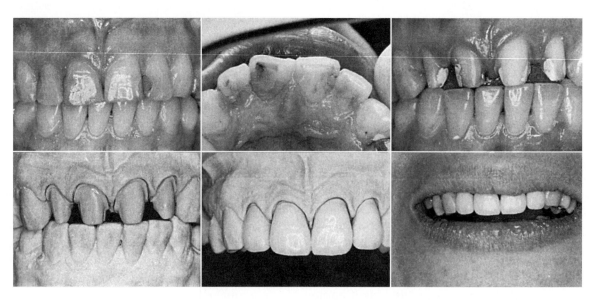

Fig. 9-20. Metal-ceramic crowns used to restore maxillary incisor teeth.

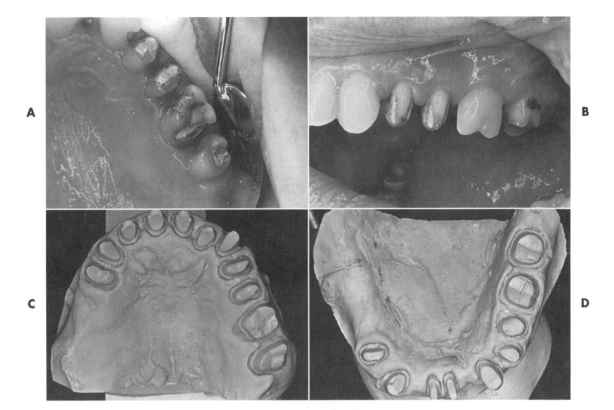

Fig. 9-21. **A,** Metal-ceramic preparations on the maxillary premolars in conjunction with more conservative preparations on the molars. **B,** Buccal view of the preparations. Note that, by comparison, considerable tooth reduction was needed on the premolars to accommodate metal-ceramic restorations. **C,** Except for the molars, all remaining teeth in this patient have been prepared for metal-ceramic restorations. Note the subtle variations and modifications of the same underlying theme: wing-type preparations on the anterior teeth, wingless on the premolars. **D,** Mandibular arch of the same patient. Many of the smaller mandibular teeth were prepared with wingless restorations. Because of previously existing restorations, excessively heavy shoulderlike chamfers resulted on some of the posterior teeth.

Study Questions

1. What are the indications and contraindications for metal-ceramic crowns?
2. What are the advantages and disadvantages of metal-ceramic crowns?
3. What is the recommended armamentarium, and in what sequence should a maxillary central incisor be prepared, for a metal-ceramic crown?
4. What are the minimal criteria for each step described above. Why?
5. What are the differences between wing-type and wingless preparations? When would one be used over the other? Why?
6. Discuss how to determine the buccolingual position of a proximal groove to precisely obtain the desired position of the facial finish line.

SUMMARY CHART

Indications	Contraindications	Advantages	Disadvantages
Esthetics	Large pulp chamber	Superior esthetics as compared to complete cast crown	Removal of substantial tooth structure
If all-ceramic crown is contraindicated	Intact buccal wall		Subject to fracture because porcelain is brittle
Gingival involvement	When more conservative retainer is technically feasible		Difficult to obtain accurate occlusion in glazed porcelain
			Shade selection can be difficult
			Inferior esthetics compared to all-ceramic crown
			Expensive

METAL-CERAMIC CROWN

Preparation Steps	Recommended Armamentarium	Criteria
Incisal (occlusal) reduction guide grooves	Tapered, round-tipped diamond	1.5 to 2 mm of clearance in intercuspal positions and all excursions
Incisal (occlusal) reduction	Tapered, round-tipped diamond	
Labial reduction guide grooves (two plane)	Tapered, round-tipped diamond	1.2 to 1.5 mm of reduction for metal and porcelain (see Fig. 9-1)
Labial reduction (two plane)	Tapered, flat-tipped diamond	
Axial reduction	Tapered, round-tipped diamond	6 degrees of convergence
Lingual reduction	Football-shaped diamond	Should provide 1 mm of clearance in all excursions and IP ($\geq$1.5 mm if occlusal is porcelain)
Finishing of shoulder (or beveled shoulder)	Tapered, flat-tipped diamond Hand instrument	Shoulder must extend at least 1 mm lingual to proximal contact area; bevel, if selected, should be as far incisal as possible relative to epithelial attachment
Finishing	Tapered, round-tipped diamond or carbide	All line angles rounded and preparation surfaces smooth

CHAPTER TEN

THE PARTIAL VENEER CROWN, INLAY, AND ONLAY PREPARATIONS

An extracoronal metal restoration that covers only part of the clinical crown is considered to be a partial veneer crown. It can also be referred to as a *partial-coverage restoration.* An intracoronal cast metal restoration is called an *inlay* or an *onlay* if one or more cusps are restored. Examples of these restorations are presented in Figure 10-1. Partial veneer crowns generally include all tooth surfaces except the buccal or labial wall in the preparation. Whenever feasible, a partial-coverage restoration should be selected rather than a complete veneer because it preserves more of the tooth's coronal surface. However, the preparation is more demanding and is not routinely provided by practitioners. Buccolingual displacement of the restoration is prevented by internal features (e.g., proximal boxes and grooves). The partial veneer can be used as a single-tooth restoration, or it may serve as a retainer for a fixed partial

denture (FPD). It can be used on both anterior and posterior teeth. Because it does not cover the entire coronal surface, it tends to be less retentive than a complete crown and is less resistant to displacement. Unless the partial veneer is very carefully prepared, the reduced retention may contraindicate its use. Inlays and onlays are even less retentive than partial veneer crowns and are not recommended for FPD abutment retainers. However, they provide the advantages of a casting, with less enamel removal than a crown. When carefully performed, they can produce an exceptionally long-lasting restoration.

◼ PARTIAL VENEER CROWNS

Several types of partial veneers exist: for posterior teeth—three-quarter, modified three-quarter, and seven-eighths crowns; for anterior teeth—three-quarter crowns and pinledges.

The indications, contraindications, advantages, and disadvantages of partial veneer crowns will be considered first, and any specific deviations that pertain to a given preparation will be identified as that type is discussed.

INDICATIONS

Partial veneer crowns often can be used to restore posterior teeth that have lost moderate amounts of tooth structure, provided the buccal wall is intact and well supported by sound tooth structure. They are also commonly used as retainers for a fixed partial denture or where restoration or alteration of the occlusal surface is needed. Anterior partial veneers are rarely suitable for restoring damaged teeth, but they can be used as retainers, to reestablish anterior guidance, and to splint teeth. They are particularly suitable for teeth with sufficient bulk because they can accommodate the necessary retentive features.

CONTRAINDICATIONS

Partial veneer restorations are contraindicated on teeth that have a short clinical crown because

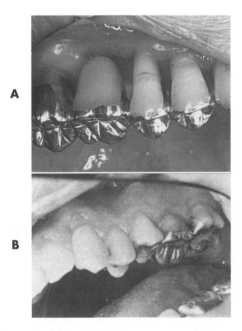

Fig. 10-1 **A,** Partial veneer crowns serving as retainers on the premolars for a four-unit FPD replacing the maxillary first molar. **B,** Maxillary premolars restored with gold inlays, molar restored with gold onlay. These restorations have served for about 30 years.

retention may not be adequate. They are also contraindicated as retainers for long-span FPDs. They are rarely suitable for endodontically treated teeth, especially anteriors, because insufficient supporting tooth structure remains for the retentive features. Likewise, they should not be used on endodontically treated posterior teeth if the buccal cusps are weakened by the access cavity or on teeth with an extensively damaged crown. As is true of all cast restorations, partial veneers are contraindicated in dentitions with active caries or periodontal disease.

The shape and alignment of teeth are important determinants of the feasibility of partial veneer crowns. The alignment of axial surfaces should be evaluated, and partial veneers should not be placed on teeth that are proximally bulbous. Making the necessary proximal grooves on these teeth is likely to leave unsupported enamel. Similarly it may be impossible to prepare adequate grooves on thin teeth of restricted faciolingual dimension.

Partial veneers are usually prepared parallel to the long axis of the tooth, and poorly aligned abutment teeth may not be suitable. When poorly aligned teeth are being prepared for a partial-coverage restoration, problems with unsupported enamel often result.

ADVANTAGES

The primary advantage associated with partial veneer crowns is conservation of tooth structure. Another advantage is reduced pulpal and periodontal insult during tooth preparation. Access to supragingival margins is rather easy and allows the operator to perform selected finishing procedures that are more difficult or impossible with complete-coverage restorations. Access is also better for oral hygiene. Because less of the margin approximates the soft tissues subgingivally, there is less gingival involvement than with complete coverage.

During cementation of a partial veneer, the luting agent can escape more easily, which produces relatively good seating of the restoration. Because of direct visibility, verification of seating and cement removal are simple. After cementation, the remaining intact facial or buccal tooth structure permits electric vitality testing.

DISADVANTAGES

Partial veneer restorations have less retention and resistance than complete cast crowns. Preparing the tooth for this type of coverage is difficult, primarily because only limited adjustments can be made in the path of withdrawal. The placement of grooves, boxes, and pinholes requires dexterity from the operator. Some metal is displayed in the completed

restoration, which may be unacceptable to patients with high cosmetic expectations.

PREPARATION

The following discussions will cover the teeth most commonly prepared for partial veneer restorations. It should be noted that the use of partial veneers on anterior teeth has declined because of the difficulty in achieving an esthetic result. The technique illustrated may be suitable for posterior teeth and, with minimal variation, for other teeth. On both posterior and anterior teeth, meticulous care and precision are required if partial veneers are to be a successful (conservative) alternative to complete-coverage restorations.

Armamentarium (Fig. 10-2). The necessary instruments for a partial veneer crown preparation include the following:

- Narrow (approximately 0.8 mm), round-tipped, tapered diamond (regular or coarse grit)
- Regular-size, (approximately 1.2 mm), round-tipped, tapered diamond (fine grit) or carbide
- Football-shaped or wheel-shaped diamond (regular grit)
- Tapered and straight carbide fissure burs
- Small, round carbide bur
- Small-diameter twist drill
- Inverted-cone carbide bur
- Finishing stones
- Mirror
- Explorer and periodontal probe
- Chisels

This is the typical armamentarium for a partial veneer crown preparation. Depending on operator preference, additional instruments can be used. The regular- or coarse-grit diamonds are used for bulk reduction, and the fine-grit diamonds or carbides are used for finishing. Pinholes are prepared with the twist drill and finalized with a tapered carbide. The fissure burs are recommended for preparing

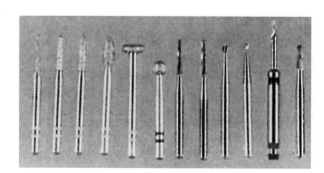

Fig. 10-2. Armamentarium for a partial veneer crown preparation.

boxes and ledges, and the inverted-cone carbide is recommended for preparing incisal offsets. Hand instruments can be used to finish proximal flares and bevels. A periodontal probe is invaluable when assessing the direction and dimension of the various steps.

POSTERIOR PARTIAL VENEER CROWN PREPARATIONS

Maxillary Premolar Three-quarter Crown (Fig. 10-3). The three-quarter crown preparation derives its name from the number of axial walls involved.

Except for a slight bevel or chamfer placed along the buccocclusal line angle, the buccal tooth surface remains intact. The other surfaces (including the occlusal surface) are prepared to accommodate a casting in the same manner as a complete crown preparation (see Chapter 8), differing only in the need for axial retention grooves.

Occlusal Reduction. Upon the completion of occlusal reduction, a clearance of at least 1.5 mm should exist on the centric cusp and at least 1.0 mm

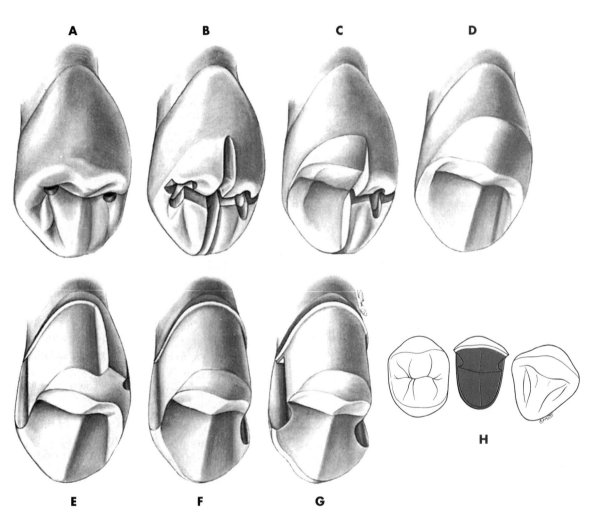

Fig. 10-3.   The maxillary premolar three-quarter crown. **A,** Initial depth holes are placed in the mesial and distal fossae approximately 0.8 mm deep. **B,** They are connected by a guiding groove that extends through the central groove. Additional guiding grooves are placed on the lingual cusp similar to those for a complete cast crown (see Fig. 8-8). The depth cut placed on the triangular ridge of the buccal cusp becomes shallower as it approaches the cusp tip. **C,** Half the occlusal reduction is completed. Note the centric cusp bevel. The occlusocervical height of the buccal surface is not reduced at this stage. **D,** Occlusal reduction completed. **E,** After guiding grooves are placed in the lingual surface of the tooth parallel to the proposed path of withdrawal, the proximoaxial and linguoaxial reductions are initiated. Simultaneously a smooth and even-width cervical chamfer is created. **F,** When the axial reduction of the first half is considered acceptable, the other half can begin. **G,** Proximal grooves are placed perpendicular to the prepared surface, and the buccal wall of each groove is flared to leave no unsupported enamel. The proximal flares are connected with a narrow contrabevel. After rounding of the line angles, the preparation is complete. **H,** The interproximal clearance relative to adjacent teeth extends cervically as well as near the occlusal aspect of the buccal flares of the proximal grooves.

on the noncentric cusp and in the central groove. Simultaneously, the tooth should be prepared so that the restoration displays a minimum of metal, with preservation of the buccal wall outline.

1. Before any partial veneer crown preparation, mark the proposed location of the margin of the completed preparation on the tooth with a pencil (Fig. 10-4).

2. Place depth grooves for the occlusal reduction. These should be made with a tapered carbide or narrow diamond in the developmental grooves of the mesial and distal fossae and on the crest of the triangular ridge. In the central groove they should be slightly less (about 0.2 mm) than 1 mm deep to allow for finishing; on the centric (lingual) cusp they should be slightly less than 1.5 mm deep in the location of the occlusal contacts.

3. Place three depth grooves on the lingual incline of the buccal cusp. Initially, these should be kept somewhat shallow as they approach the buccal cusp ridge (Fig. 10-3, *B*). In the area of occlusal contact, the groove should be about 0.8 mm deep so that there will be at least 1 mm of clearance after finishing.

4. Verify groove depth with a periodontal probe. When this is found to be acceptable, remove the islands of tooth structure remaining between the grooves (Fig. 10-3, *C* and *D*).

5. Assess the amount of occlusal clearance in the intercuspal position and in all excursive movements of the mandible (Fig. 10-5). Grinding a small concavity on the incline of the buccal cusp may help obtain sufficient clearance while maintaining the original occlusocervical dimension of the buccal tooth surface (Fig. 10-6).

Axial Reduction

6. Place grooves for axial alignment in the center of the lingual surface and in the mesiolingual and distolingual transitional line angles. These should be parallel to the long axis of the tooth and should not exceed half the width of the tip of the diamond used to place them.

7. Because the path of withdrawal of a partial veneer is critical, assess these grooves carefully when correction is still possible. A common error is to incline the path of withdrawal toward the buccal. This either reduces retention or leads to an excessive display of metal. A periodontal probe placed in each groove should be carefully viewed in both planes (mesiodistal and buccolingual). It often helps to pour an irreversible hydrocolloid (alginate) impression in fast-setting plaster and to evaluate the cast with a dental surveyor, particularly if multiple partial veneers are being used as retainers for an FPD.

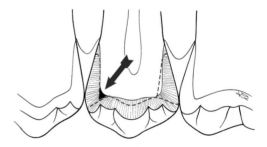

Fig. 10-5. A common error is insufficient reduction of tooth structure in the marginal ridge area (*arrow*).

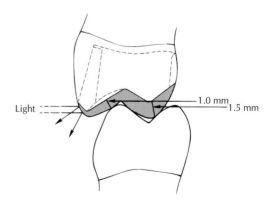

Fig. 10-6. Recommended minimum clearances for reduction of a partial veneer crown preparation. Slight hollow grinding of the lingual incline of the buccal cusp results in an acceptable clearance with the least display of metal. Also, the final restoration retains the normal contours of the cuspal ridge, so incident light is not reflected, and the restoration is less evident.

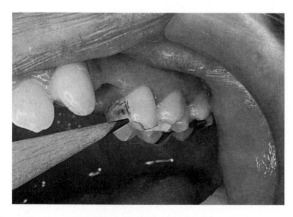

Fig. 10-4. The anticipated location of the completed preparation is marked with a pencil.

8. After verifying the alignment, remove tooth structure between the guide grooves (with a smooth continuous motion) and place a cervical chamfer (Fig. 10-7).

9. Carry the diamond into the proximal embrasure and reduce the proximal wall (Fig. 10-3, *E* and *F*). For proper reduction of the axial tooth surface, it is important to understand the factors that determine correct positioning of the proximal groove. A proximal groove is placed parallel to the path of withdrawal. Normally, unsupported tooth structure will remain on the buccal side of the groove, and this side is flared to remove it. Figure 10-8 illustrates the relationship among the initial axial reduction, groove placement, and location of the cavosurface angle where the flare meets the intact buccal wall. The cavosurface angle is especially significant when preparing a tooth for a partial veneer that should display a minimum of metal; the further to the buccal the margin is, the more gold will be visible. A subtle but extremely important variable that determines the final location of the cavosurface angle is the apical extension of the preparation. As the cervical chamfer extends closer to the cementoenamel junction, more axial tooth structure is removed. Consequently, the deepest portion of the groove (its pulpal wall) will be located slightly closer to the center of the tooth. This results in a flare that can extend farther onto the facial or buccal surface than desirable. Marking the location of the intended facial flare on the tooth with a pencil before initiating the proximoaxial reduction is helpful. The intersection of this mark with the reduced occlusal surface is a convenient reference point.

10. Stop the proximal reduction well short of the pencil mark and usually slightly short of breaking the proximal contact (Fig. 10-9). The resulting flange should be parallel to the linguoaxial preparation, with the chamfer placed sufficiently cervical to provide at least 0.6 mm of clearance with the adjacent tooth and the axial wall allowing for a proximal groove of at least 4 mm of length occlusocervically (see Fig. 10-3, *F*).

Groove Placement. Preparation of the proximal grooves is best done with a tapered carbide bur.

11. Position the bur against the interproximal flange parallel to the path of withdrawal and make a groove perpendicular to the axial surface. The groove need not be deeper than 1 mm at its cervical end but may be deeper near its occlusal end (Fig. 10-10). During this stage, the bur must be held precisely parallel to the selected path of withdrawal. Allowing it to tip axially will result in excessive taper between opposing proximal grooves, which is a common error. The

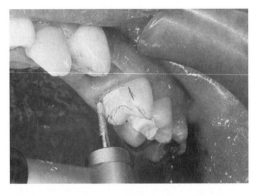

Fig. 10-7. Proximal and lingual axial reduction is performed with a round-tipped diamond. The proximal reduction is stopped short of the proposed location of the buccal margin.

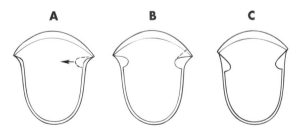

Fig. 10-8. **A,** Upon completion of the proximal axial reduction, a groove is placed perpendicular to the prepared surface. **B,** Note that some unsupported tooth structure remains at the cavosurface angle. **C,** After the buccal wall of the proximal groove is flared, no unsupported tooth structure remains. NOTE: It is important to anticipate in advance the influence of the buccal extent of the proximoaxial reduction (**A**) on the ultimate location of the margin.

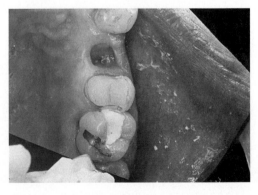

Fig. 10-9. The distal proximal reduction is stopped before breaking proximal contact. After groove placement and subsequent flaring, interproximal clearance will result.

criteria that need to be met consist of the following (see Figs. 10-9 and 10-11):

The grooves should resist lingual displacement of a periodontal probe or explorer.

The walls of the grooves should not be undercut relative to the selected path of withdrawal.

The walls should be flared toward the intact buccal surface of the tooth (see Fig. 10-3, *G* and *H*).

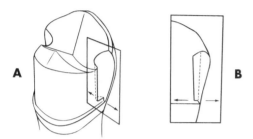

Fig. 10-10. Because of the rotary instrument's taper **(A)**, the proximal groove is deeper near the occlusal table. The floor of the groove should be flat and smooth. Often the proximal chamfer will extend slightly cervically to the floor of the groove. If only minimal difference exists, as in **B**, the cervical margin adjacent to the groove can be beveled. The recommended occlusocervical height for a proximal groove is 4 mm.

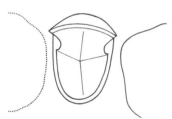

Fig. 10-11. The 90-degree angle between the lingual walls of the proximal grooves will resist lingual displacement. Because the buccal aspect of the grooves has been adequately flared, no unsupported tooth structure remains.

Depending on available access, it may be feasible to complete the flaring with the same rotary instrument that was used to place the groove (Fig. 10-12). However, removing the last lip of unsupported tooth structure with a chisel is often a better option, because this minimizes the risk of damage to the adjacent tooth.

Buccocclusal Contrabevel

12.   Connect the mesial and distal flares with a narrow contrabevel that follows the buccal cusp ridges. This can be placed with a diamond, a carbide, or even a hand instrument. Its primary purpose is to remove any unsupported enamel and thereby protect the buccal cusp tip from chipping during function. If group function is planned (as opposed to a mutually protected occlusion), a heavier bevel, chamfer, or occlusal offset will be needed, because tooth contact occurs in this area during excursive movement. The bevel should remain within the curvature of the cusp tip rather than extend onto the buccal wall (Fig. 10-13). This will result in a convex shape of the restoration, and light will be prevented from reflecting back to a casual observer (see Fig. 10-6). Thus the restoration will be less obvious, and the outline form of remaining buccal enamel will be perceived as the shape of the tooth.

Occlusal Offset. If additional bulk is needed to ensure rigidity of the restoration, it can be provided with an occlusal offset. This V-shaped groove extends from the proximal grooves along the buccal cusp. It is not usually necessary for posterior partial veneer crowns but is essential for the structural durability of anterior partial veneer crowns. This is described in detail on p. 243.

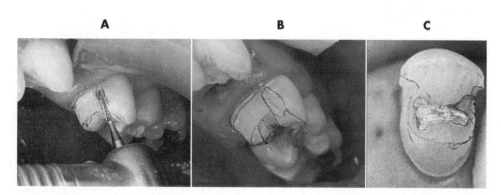

Fig. 10-12. **A,** Initial preparation of the mesial proximal groove. Note that the carbide is oriented parallel to the path of withdrawal as dictated by the lingual surface of the tooth. **B,** Initial flaring has resulted in elimination of most unsupported tooth structure. **C,** Hand or rotary instruments will be used to refine these proximal flares and remove all unsupported enamel.

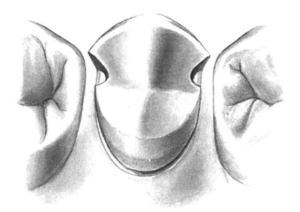

Fig. 10-13. The buccocclusal contrabevel remains within the curvature of the cusp tip rather than extending onto the buccal surface.

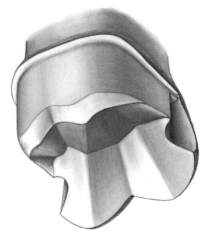

Fig. 10-15. Three-quarter crown preparation on a maxillary molar. Note that the occlusal reduction follows normal anatomic form.

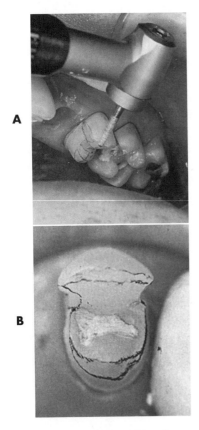

Fig. 10-14. A fine-grit diamond in a low-speed contraangle is used to place the buccocclusal contrabevel connecting the mesioproximal and distoproximal flares.

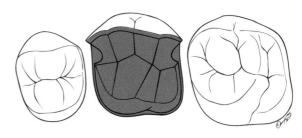

Fig. 10-16. The three-quarter crown preparation on a maxillary first molar.

Finishing

13. Round all sharp internal line angles to facilitate subsequent procedures. A fine-grit diamond or carbide can be used to blend the surfaces (Fig. 10-14).

14. Reevaluate the flares, paying particular attention to any remaining undercuts, which must be removed. The flares should be straight and smooth, with sufficient clear-

ance between them and the adjacent tooth. A minimum clearance of 0.6 mm is recommended. The mesial flare cannot extend beyond the transitional line angle. However, because the distal margin is less visible, it may extend slightly farther to the buccal, allowing better access for oral hygiene.

Maxillary Molar Three-quarter Crown (Fig. 10-15 and Fig. 10-16). The principles used in a premolar preparation also apply for a maxillary molar. However, some additional leeway may exist for groove placement because more tooth structure is present on molars than on premolars. Also, because of their less prominent position in the dental arch, molars are less visible. As a result, the mesioproximal flare can sometimes be extended onto the buccal surface without incurring esthetic liability.

Maxillary Molar Seven-eighths Crown (Fig. 10-17). The seven-eighths crown preparation includes, in addition to the surfaces covered by the three-quarter crown, the distal half of the buccal surface. Therefore the mesial aspect of this preparation resembles that for a three-quarter crown; the

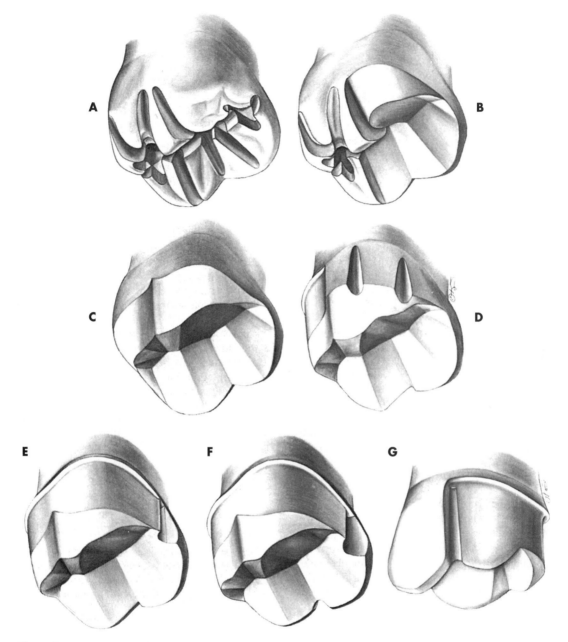

Fig. 10-17. The maxillary molar seven-eighths crown preparation. **A,** Occlusal depth grooves. On the lingual of the mesiobuccal cusp, they are identical to grooves for any centric cusp. On the buccal, note their difference from grooves placed on the triangular ridges. The mesial groove becomes shallower as it approaches the cuspal ridge; the distal extends through the cuspal ridge. **B,** Mesial half of the occlusal reduction is completed. Normal occlusal form can be recognized in the reduced area. **C,** Occlusal reduction completed. **D,** Distal half of the axial reduction completed. This is comparable to the preparation for a complete cast crown. The rotary instrument is moved parallel to the guiding grooves placed in the lingual tooth surface. **E,** Mesial half of the axial reduction completed and a proximal groove placed. **F,** The buccal groove, with flaring of the mesial groove. Note the monoplane of the flare, extending from the deepest portion of the groove to the cavosurface angle. **G,** A contrabevel connects the mesial flare with the buccal groove. The mesial wall of the buccal groove is smooth and has a 90-degree cavosurface angle, leaving no unsupported enamel.

distal aspect resembles that for a complete crown. The mesial half of the buccal tooth surface remains intact and is protected by a narrow contrabevel or chamfer similar to the one used in the three-quarter crown preparation. A distal groove may be placed, although generally this is not necessary. A groove in the middle of the buccal surface is placed parallel to the path of withdrawal. Distal to this groove the buccal surface is reduced in two planes, cervical and occlusal, with the cervical paralleling the path of withdrawal and the occlusal following the normal anatomic contour. The lingual surface of the tooth also is reduced in two planes, and centric cusp bevels are incorporated.

Occlusal Reduction. Upon completion of the occlusal reduction, adequate clearance should exist in all excursive movements of the mandible. Minimum measurements are the same as for the three-quarter crown preparation.

1. Place depth grooves in the central and developmental grooves as well as on the crests of the triangular ridges. To delineate the extent of the lingual centric cusp bevel, they should extend onto the lingual surface of the tooth. On the lingual incline of the mesiobuccal cusp they will resemble depth cuts for the three-quarter crown preparation. On the distobuccal cusp they should be approximately 0.8 mm deep to provide sufficient occlusal clearance for this noncentric cusp (see Fig. 10-17, *A*).

2. Remove the tooth structure between the depth grooves. Concave shaping of the resulting mesiobuccal incline may again prove useful because it will permit the occlusocervical height of the cusp to be maintained. When completed, this bevel should provide 1.5 mm of clearance in the intercuspal position as well as throughout all excursive movements of the mandible (see Fig. 10-17, *B* and *C*).

Axial Reduction. In principle, the steps for axial reduction follow those for occlusal reduction.

3. Place three alignment grooves in the lingual wall and transfer the selected path of withdrawal to the distobuccal transitional line angle area, where a fourth alignment groove can be placed.

4. Start the reduction in the middle of the lingual surface. The mesial half is prepared like a three-quarter crown and the distal half like a complete crown (see Fig. 10-17, *D*).

5. Carry the facial reduction sufficiently mesial to include the buccal groove. Although the occlusal half of the buccal surface of maxillary molars is rather flat, some additional reduction may be necessary in the occlusal third. This follows the normal anatomic configuration of the tooth and often resembles a small version of the centric cusp bevel. If correctly performed, the reduction will allow for contouring of the restoration so that when viewed from the mesial, the distal half of the restoration is hidden behind the mesiobuccal cusp. A frequent error is to overtaper the

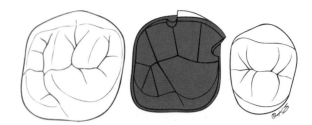

Fig. 10-18. The seven-eighths crown preparation. Note that adequate clearance has been established. From this perspective it is evident why little or no flaring is necessary for the buccal groove as opposed to the considerable flaring needed for the mesial groove.

buccal wall segment, with resulting loss of retention.

Groove Placement, Flaring, and Contrabevel

6. Prepare the mesial groove like the three-quarter crown (see Fig. 10-17, *E* and *F*).

7. Place the buccal groove parallel to the mesial groove and perpendicular to the buccoaxial wall. Often it is not necessary to flare the buccal groove because the flat configuration of this area of the tooth precludes any unsupported enamel after the groove is placed. The buccal groove should resist mesiodistal displacement of a probe.

8. Connect the two grooves with a smooth contrabevel that follows the ridge of the mesiobuccal cusp (see Fig. 10-17, *G*). This bevel should meet the same criteria as described in the three-quarter crown preparation. Adequate clearance must be established interproximally upon completion (Fig. 10-18). All surfaces are finished to the same specifications as the preceding preparations (Fig. 10-19).

Mandibular Premolar Modified Three-quarter Crown (Fig. 10-20). Mandibular partial veneer preparations are made more often on premolars than on molars. They differ from maxillary molar three-quarter crown preparations in two respects:

Additional retention is required because of the shorter crown lengths of mandibular teeth. This can be obtained by extending the preparation buccally, although because of their rather prominent position in the dental arch, these teeth should be modified only distal to their height of contour (Fig. 10-21).

The axial surface that is not prepared (the buccal) includes the functional cusp. This means that additional tooth structure must be removed to provide sufficient bulk of metal for strength.

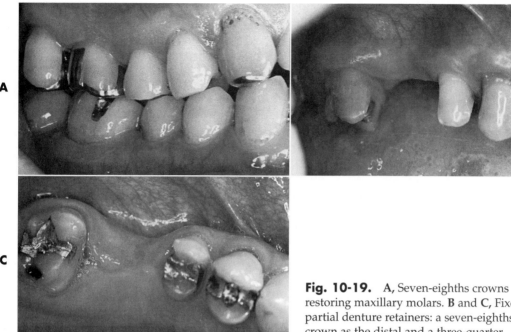

Fig. 10-19. **A,** Seven-eighths crowns restoring maxillary molars. **B** and **C,** Fixed partial denture retainers: a seven-eighths crown as the distal and a three-quarter crown as the mesial.

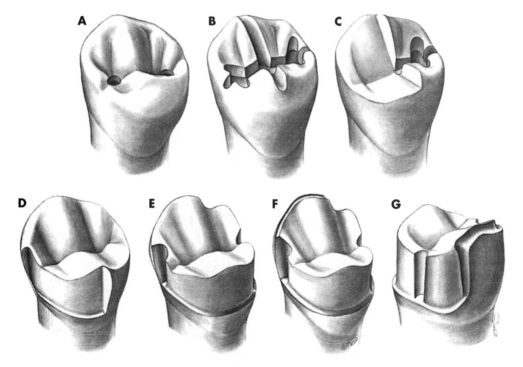

Fig. 10-20. The mandibular premolar modified three-quarter crown preparation. **A,** Depth holes placed in the mesial and distal fossae approximately 0.8 mm deep. **B,** The holes are connected by a guiding groove that extends through the central groove and the mesial and distal marginal ridges. Guiding grooves are also placed in the buccal and lingual triangular ridges, extending through the cuspal ridges on both sides. **C,** Half the occlusal reduction is completed. **D,** Occlusal reduction and mesial half of the axial reduction are completed. **E,** Axial reduction is completed. The proximal grooves have been placed. Note that the distal groove is located close to the buccolingual center of the tooth. This permits retention of considerable tooth structure in the area of the distobuccal line angle, enhancing the resistance form of the preparation. **F,** The mesial groove has been flared and the centric cusp chamfer placed. **G,** Facial view. There is considerable width of the chamfer on the centric cusp. Note that the distobuccal cervical margin angles occlusally as it progresses mesially. This permits a more conservative tooth preparation in the area of the distobuccal modification that is placed to improve resistance form.

A   **B**   **C**

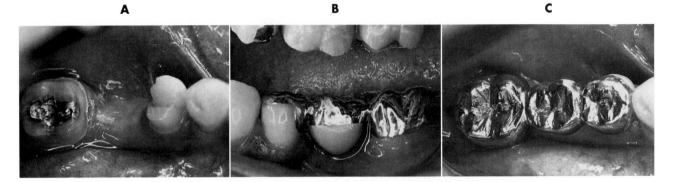

Fig. 10-21. Modified three-quarter crown restoring a mandibular second premolar. It is serving as the anterior retainer for a three-unit FPD. Because the distobuccal modification remains in the distal fourth of the buccal preparation, it is hidden behind the normal height of contour of the buccal tooth surface. Note the considerable thickness of gold that protects the buccal cusp.

Occlusal Reduction

1. Place 0.8-mm depth grooves on the buccal inclines of the lingual cusp and 1.3-mm grooves on the lingual inclines of the buccal cusp (see Fig. 10-20, *A* and *B*). These guiding grooves are once again placed to follow the basic groove and fissure pattern of the occlusal surface. Only one depth cut needs to be placed to accommodate the functional cusp bevel on the distal aspect of the distal ridge.

2. Reduce the occlusal surface by removing the tooth structure between the grooves (see Fig. 10-20, *C*).

Axial Reduction

3. Place guiding grooves on the lingual surface to parallel the proposed path of withdrawal and the long axis of the tooth.

4. Prepare the mesial as already described for the three-quarter and seven-eighths crown (see Fig. 10-20, *D*).

5. Reduce the distal surface as for a complete crown, extending the preparation to the transitional line angle and onto the buccal surface. However, it should not extend mesially beyond the middle of the distal half of the buccal surface, and the chamfer should not extend too far cervically; otherwise, the distobuccal line angle will be unnecessarily reduced, which would decrease the resistance form (see Fig. 10-20, *E*).

Finishing. The modified three-quarter crown preparation can include two or three grooves.

6. Place the mesial and buccal grooves as described for the seven-eighths crown (see Fig. 10-20, *F*). Another distal groove may be placed. In general, to gain as much length as

possible, the grooves of the three-quarter crown should be slightly buccal. Care must be taken so that the distal groove is slightly closer to the center of the distal wall (so the distobuccal line angle will not be undermined).

7. Connect the mesial and buccal grooves with a centric cusp chamfer after the grooves and mesial flare have been placed and evaluated. The chamfer must be heavy enough to allow 1.5 mm of clearance in the area of occlusal contact (see Fig. 10-20, *G*). A regular or thick diamond is used to place the chamfer, which should connect the grooves and provide a protective "staple" linkage of alloy in the completed restoration. Insufficient tooth reduction where this chamfer meets the mesial flare is a common error. Finally, all prepared surfaces are smoothed and the internal line angles rounded.

ANTERIOR PARTIAL VENEER CROWN PREPARATIONS

As stated, with the advent of metal-ceramic restorations, the use of partial veneers on anterior teeth has become rare. Nevertheless, two anterior partial veneer crown preparations are worthy of consideration (Figs. 10-22 and 10-23).

Maxillary Canine Three-quarter Crown (Figs. 10-24 and 10-25). The three-quarter crown on a maxillary canine is probably one of the most demanding of all tooth preparations. As with such preparations on other teeth, on a maxillary canine it involves the proximal and lingual surfaces and leaves the facial surface intact. However, the greater degree of difficulty stems from the different shape of the canine tooth. Unless the placement of grooves is determined very precisely in advance, there will be

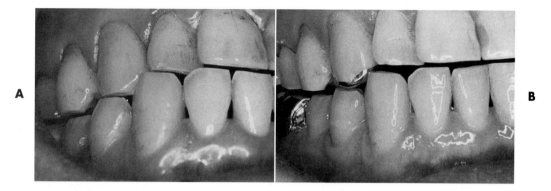

Fig. 10-22. **A,** Deficient anterior guidance resulting from years of parafunctional activity. **B,** An anterior partial veneer crown has reestablished it, allowing the intact sound labial tooth structure to be retained as a conservative alternative to a metal-ceramic restoration.

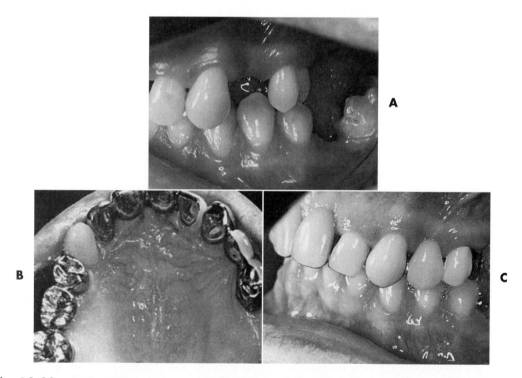

Fig. 10-23. **A,** Caries-free canine and lateral incisor of adequate bulk—excellent candidates for anterior partial veneer crowns. **B,** The canine restored with a three-quarter crown, serving as the anterior retainer for a three-unit FPD to replace the first premolar. The lateral incisor has been restored with a modified pinledge that serves as a retainer for an anterior four-unit FPD. Satisfactory esthetics **(C)** with minimal display of metal are apparent.

an undesirable display of metal in the interproximal embrasures (see Fig. 10-25, *A* and *B*). The relatively short proximal walls do not allow much correction after initial groove placement. Similarly, the greater degree of curvature in each proximal wall immediately adjacent to the contact area significantly influences the location of the preparation's facial margin.

Incisal and Lingual Reduction

1. Remove enough enamel to allow 1 mm of metal thickness. The design of the incisal bevel should prevent contact between opposing teeth and the incisal margin. However, the original configuration of the facial surface should be preserved without significant

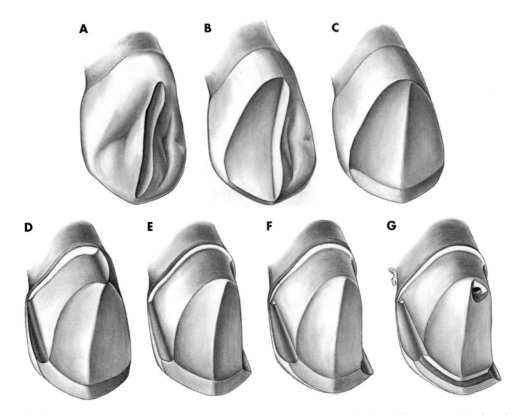

Fig. 10-24. The maxillary canine three-quarter crown preparation. **A,** A guiding groove is placed on the lingual surface. **B,** Half the lingual surface is reduced. Clearance is verified before reduction of the other half. **C,** Lingual reduction is completed, with an incisal bevel placed. No significant change has occurred in the incisocervical height. **D,** After an alignment groove is placed in the center of the cingulum wall, half the axial reduction is complete. Note that the path of withdrawal parallels the incisal or middle third of the labial surface. As a result, the lingual chamfer is quite wide, perhaps even resembling a shoulder. This permits paralleling of the cingulum wall, with the proximal grooves and pinhole providing additional retention. **E,** Axial reduction is completed. Any final modification of the path of withdrawal is done at this time before groove placement. **F,** Proximal grooves. The visible mesial groove has been flared, but unsupported enamel remains on both grooves where they meet the incisal bevel. **G,** Completed preparation. The lingual pinhole is surrounded by adequate dentin. Note the horizontal ledge prepared before pinhole placement.

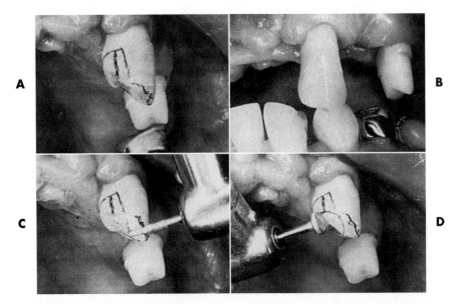

Fig. 10-25. **A,** Proposed margin location outlined on the tooth with a pencil. **B,** Careful assessment of the anticipated outline from as many directions as possible is valuable at this time. **C,** Preparing the incisal bevel. Typically a lingually tilted bevel is prepared at a 45-degree angle to the long axis of the tooth. **D,** The lingual surface is reduced with a wheel- or football-shaped diamond.

incisal reduction of the tooth. Outlining the anticipated location of the margin with a pencil can be helpful.

2. Place depth grooves for both the incisal bevel and the lingual reduction (see Fig. 10-24, *A*). The direction of the bevel may vary somewhat depending on the configuration of the tooth. Generally it will make an angle of approximately 45 degrees with the long axis of the tooth.

3. After the depth has been verified, perform the reduction. A football- or wheel-shaped diamond is used to reduce the concave lingual wall (see Figs. 10-24, *B*, and 10-25, *D*). The lingual reduction should not extend onto the cingulum itself, which will be prepared as part of the axial reduction. (The completed reduction is shown in Fig. 10-24, *C*.)

Axial Reduction and Groove Placement. The path of withdrawal of the restoration must be accurately determined before axial reduction. Mesiodistally it should parallel the long axis of the tooth; buccolingually it should parallel the middle third or incisal two thirds of the facial surface. This will permit the preparation of proximal grooves of optimum length in an area of the tooth where sufficient bulk is present.

4. To enhance the retention and resistance form of the preparation, place a slightly exaggerated chamfer on the lingual aspect of the tooth (see Fig. 10-24, *D*) and a guiding groove in the

middle of the lingual wall. When alignment has been verified, the axial reduction can be performed in the same manner as the other preparations (Fig. 10-26). It is important to understand the difference between this phase of the preparation on a canine, with little bulk of lingual tooth structure as opposed to a premolar or molar. After completion, a proximal flange should result that will guide the rotary instrument during groove placement (see Figs. 10-24, *E*, and 10-26, *B*). The technical aspects of the preparation of proximal grooves are like those described for the other partial veneer preparations (Figs. 10-27 and 10-28). The primary difference is the direction in which the groove is prepared. Because the groove is placed perpendicular to the proximal wall, its deepest portion will be slightly labial to the proximal flange that results when proximoaxial reduction is completed. As a result, the proximal flares will extend slightly farther onto the facial surface. This is even more accentuated by the curvature of the proximal wall (Fig. 10-29). Meticulous assessment of the needed extent of the initial axial reduction is a prerequisite for successful preparation (see Fig. 10-24, *F*, and 10-30). (The required interproximal clearance is illustrated in Fig. 10-31.)

Incisal Offset and Lingual Pinhole. Anterior partial veneer crowns require a means of reinforcement for preserving the casting's integrity. Posterior three-quarter crowns usually do not need as much additional reinforcement because the solid "corrugated" occlusal surface provides rigidity. For an anterior tooth, an incisal offset or groove is needed to create a band of thicker metal to provide a "staple"

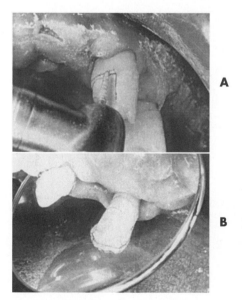

Fig. 10-26. **A,** A regular-grit diamond is used to complete the axial reduction. Mesiodistally the diamond is oriented parallel to the long axis of the tooth. **B,** When completed, a mesial and distal flange results that will serve as a guide during preparation of the proximal groove.

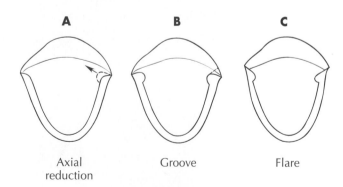

Axial reduction   Groove   Flare

Fig. 10-27. **A,** Because the groove is prepared perpendicular to the proximal surface of the tooth, its deepest portion will be slightly buccal to where axial reduction was halted. **B,** The dotted line indicates the proposed flare. Note that the curvature of the tooth causes the final margin to be located a considerable distance buccal to where the initial axial reduction stopped. **C,** Completed flares.

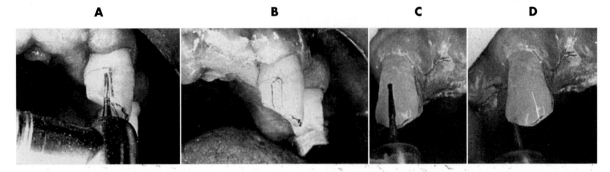

Fig. 10-28. **A,** A tapered carbide is used to place the proximal groove. **B,** Initial groove preparation is completed. **C,** The carbide is moved parallel to itself. **D,** Mesial and distal grooves must be prepared in strict alignment.

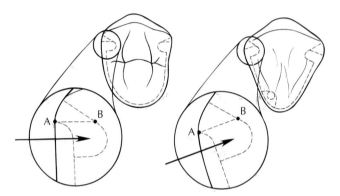

Fig. 10-29. Differences between the proximal flares on premolars and canines. **A** designates where the initial proximal reduction is halted. Because a facial component is present in the direction of groove placement on the canine, as opposed to the premolar, the starting point **(B)** for the flare is located farther to the facial. In conjunction with the greater degree of proximal curvature of canines, it is critical that the initial axial reduction not be carried too far facially; otherwise, the final margin will extend too far onto the labial surface of the tooth and result in excessive display of metal.

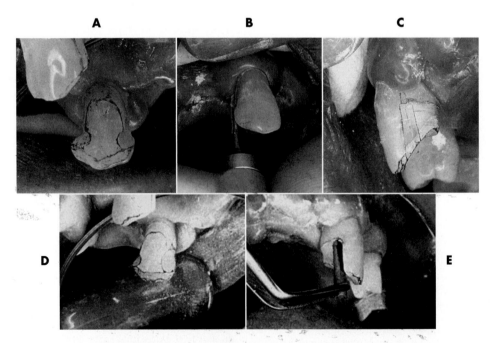

Fig. 10-30. **A,** Unsupported enamel remaining after initial groove placement. **B,** A carbide bur can be used to flare the grooves. **C,** The flared groove. Note the irregularity of the margin near the cervical aspect of the groove. **D,** After the flaring. Note that a mesial box, rather than a groove, has been prepared. This restoration is designed to contain an intracoronal removable partial denture rest; hence, the box. Nevertheless, there is adequate resistance to lingual displacement. **E,** A special mandrel is placed in the box to ensure that it fits within its confines. It is identical in size to the male attachment of the RPD.

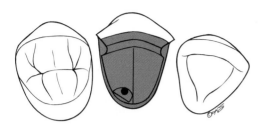

Fig. 10-31. Completed three-quarter crown preparation. Note the location of the facial margin relative to the adjacent teeth. Sufficient interproximal clearance has been established, but unnecessary display of metal is avoided.

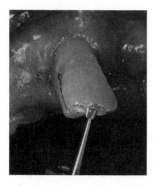

Fig. 10-32. An inverted-cone diamond or carbide can be used to prepare the incisal offset. Note the faciolingual inclination of the rotary instruments.

configuration. This provides additional rigidity and resistance against bending of the casting.

5. Connect the mesial and distal grooves with an incisal offset. It should improve the general resistance form of the preparation against lingual displacement and should have a V configuration. Sufficient dentin must be preserved facially to the offset to prevent the metal from being visible through the translucent tooth enamel. This is most effectively accomplished with an offset that is slightly narrower labiolingually than incisocervically. The offset should follow the normal configuration of the incisal edge, and its transition into the proximal flares should be smooth and continuous. An inverted-cone diamond or carbide (Fig. 10-32) can be used to prepare the offset.

6. Place a pinhole in the cingulum area slightly off center to improve the retention and resistance form of this preparation. The pinhole is prepared in five stages: first, a small horizontal ledge is made with a large, tapered carbide bur; second, a slight "dimple" is created with a round bur at the intended pinhole location; third, a pilot hole is prepared with a small-di-

ameter twist drill* (it must be parallel to the precise path of withdrawal of the restoration); fourth, the preparation is completed with a tapered carbide bur to a pinhole depth of approximately 2 mm; finally, a larger, round bur is used to countersink or bevel the junction between pinhole and ledge.

The technical aspects of pinhole preparation are described in the ensuing paragraphs. The completed preparation (Fig. 10-33) is carefully assessed for any remaining undercuts. The flares are a common area for undercuts, and all surfaces should be smoothed as previously described.

PINLEDGE PREPARATIONS

A pinledge (Fig. 10-34) is occasionally used as a single restoration, generally to reestablish anterior guidance, in which case only the lingual surface is prepared. More commonly, however, it is used as a retainer for a fixed partial denture (Fig. 10-35) or to splint periodontally compromised teeth (Fig. 10-36). In these cases, one or more of the proximal surfaces are included in the preparation design to accommodate the required connector(s). Retention and resistance are provided primarily by pins that extend to a depth of 2 mm into dentin. Compared to other retainers, the pinledge preparation is very conservative of tooth structure.

The preparation steps themselves are not difficult, but advance planning and a thorough understanding of the various steps are prerequisites to success. Diagnostic preparation on an accurate cast is particularly useful during the planning phase. Preparation of a number of parallel pinholes with a common path of withdrawal can be intimidating. With some practice, however, this can be accomplished freehand by most operators, especially when a tapered bur is used. Paralleling devices are available for practitioners who do not feel comfortable preparing multiple pinholes. Generally, pinledges are highly esthetic restorations. Plaque control after treatment is easier because of short margin length and largely supragingival margin location.

Indications. The pinledge is indicated for undamaged anterior teeth in dentitions with a low caries experience. The presence of a small proximal carious lesion, however, does not preclude its use. If a high esthetic requirement exists, the advantage of this restoration is that the labial tooth surface

---

*The twist drills supplied with threaded pin kits for amalgam retention are suitable.

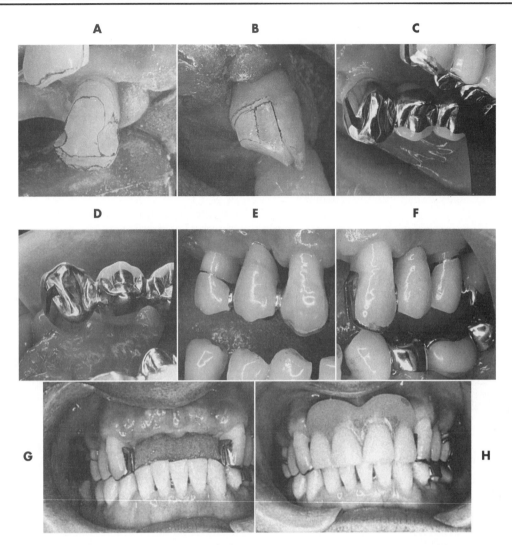

Fig. 10-33. **A,** Completed three-quarter crown preparation on a maxillary canine. **B,** The contralateral canine. **C,** A three-quarter crown serves as the anterior retainer for a three-unit FPD; its female intracoronal RPD rest is incorporated in the mesial box. **D,** Note the connector and the open embrasures on the contralateral side. **E** to **G,** Labial views of the cemented FPDs. **H,** The definitive RPD.

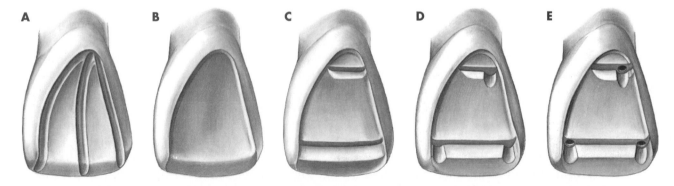

Fig. 10-34.   The pinledge preparation on a maxillary central incisor. **A,** Guiding grooves placed for lingual reduction. **B,** The lingual reduction completed and an incisal bevel placed. **C,** Incisal and cervical ledges prepared. **D,** Indentations have been made. Note the spacing of the ledges relative to each other and to the pulp. All pinholes will be in sound dentin. **E,** Pinholes prepared to a depth of 2 mm. The junction between the ledge and the pinholes has been countersunk.

A   **B**   **C**

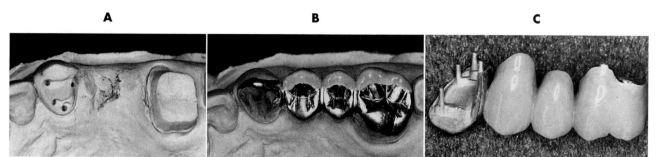

Fig. 10-35. **A,** Modified pinledge serving as a retainer for a four-unit FPD. An additional pinhole was placed in the cingulum and in the cervical aspect of the proximal groove; in the latter instance, this was done because insufficient tooth structure remained to provide resistance against lingual displacement. **B,** The FPD on the master cast. **C,** A four-unit FPD consisting of a modified pinledge, two metal-ceramic pontics, and a metal-ceramic crown.

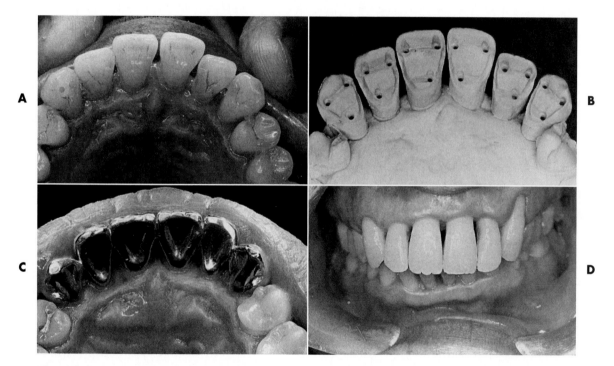

Fig. 10-36. **A,** Periodontally compromised but caries-free teeth of adequate buccolingual width are excellent candidates for a pinledge retained fixed splint. **B,** The master cast. **C,** Pinledge splint consisting of six separate castings that were soldered together and seated. **D,** A minimum display of metal results. The pinledge preparations permit retention of the intact labial enamel of all six anterior teeth.

remains intact, although this is sometimes offset by the display of a slight amount of metal along the incisal edge. Pinledges can be prepared on bulbous teeth that are unsuitable for three-quarter crowns, which would result in a significant amount of unsupported enamel interproximally. The lingual concavity of a maxillary anterior tooth can be modified successfully with a pinledge restoration (see Fig. 10-22) to establish the desired anterior guidance.

Contraindications. Patients with poor oral hygiene or a high caries rate are not good candidates for this type of restoration. Young patients with large pulps generally are better served by a resin-retained FPD (see Chapter 26). Often it is not possible to place pinholes of adequate size and length in teeth that are thin labiolingually (Fig. 10-37). Pinledges are contraindicated on nonvital teeth and when the alignment of the abutment will conflict with the proposed path of withdrawal of the fixed partial denture. Because less surface area is involved in the preparation, pinledges are not as retentive as their less conservative counterparts. Therefore they should not be used when optimum retention is needed.

Maxillary Central Incisor Pinledge. Three designs of pinledge preparations are discussed here: the conventional pinledge (see Fig. 10-34), involving only the lingual surface of the tooth; the pinledge

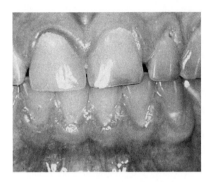

Fig. 10-37. Where incisors are thin labiolingually and insufficient dentin remains facial to the casting, appearance is compromised by a pinledge restoration.

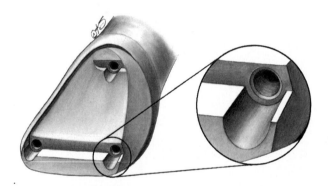

Fig. 10-38. Pinledge preparation with a proximal slice. The slice provides room for an FPD connector. Sufficient tooth structure should remain between the slice and the pinhole adjacent to it. Note that the junction between pinhole and ledge has been beveled or countersunk.

with a proximal slice (Fig. 10-38); and the pinledge with a proximal groove (Fig. 10-39, *A*). The latter two can serve equally well as retainers for an FPD; choosing one over the other depends primarily on tooth configuration and the presence or absence of caries. A tooth with a slight proximal convexity can often be prepared successfully with a proximal slice, whereas one with a small carious lesion often lends itself better to the proximal groove variation. The pinledge preparation with proximal slice is described first.

Design

1. Draw the outline of the proposed preparation onto the tooth (Fig. 10-40). A line is marked along the height of contour of the incisal edge and on the proximal wall to include the area needed for a connector. The lingual chamfer is placed immediately adjacent to the crest of the marginal ridge. The cervical extent of the margin is on the height of contour of the cingulum, but it may be extended farther cervically at a later stage to blend into the proximal aspect of the preparation.

Proximal Reduction

2. Prepare the proximal slice with a tapered diamond. (Disks may be preferred by some operators.) The diamond is either held parallel to the path of withdrawal or given a slight lingual inclination. The primary purpose of this step is to provide sufficient reduction to allow adequate metal in the area for a subsequent connector. The proximal reduction includes the proximal contact area, but care

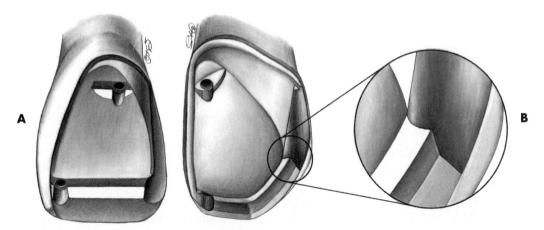

Fig. 10-39. **A,** Modified pinledge preparation with a proximal groove. The path of withdrawal of this groove is compatible with the preparation as well as with the pinholes. **B,** A similar preparation on a maxillary canine. Note two similarities with the three-quarter crown: the heavy lingual chamfer and the incisal offset blending into the proximal groove to provide additional bulk for reinforcement.

must be taken not to extend the reduction too far facially, because this will alter the outline form of the tooth. For esthetic reasons, the reduction must not extend onto the labial surface.

Incisal and Lingual Reduction

3. Prepare the incisal bevel with the diamond inclined slightly toward the lingual. It extends just beyond the previously placed pencil line on the crest of the incisal edge, but it must remain within the curvature of the incisal edge to minimize display of metal. Sufficient clearance provides functional contact on metal rather than on the junction between metal and tooth structure. The desired metal thickness is 1 mm, except in the area close to the margin.

4. Perform the lingual reduction with a football- or wheel-shaped diamond after placing reduction grooves as has been described in other anterior preparations. Metal thickness of 1 mm is required in the intercuspal position and throughout excursive movements. The reduction follows the lingual marginal ridge and continues its chamfer configuration cervically until it runs into the proximal reduction. To facilitate subsequent stages of the preparation, care must be taken to maintain as much tooth structure as possible in the incisal third.

5. Smooth the incisal and lingual reduction with fine-grit diamonds and stones before preparing the ledges and pinholes.

Ledges and Indentations.
Two ledges are prepared across the reduced lingual surface. They will provide room for sufficient bulk of metal to ensure rigidity. The restoration would otherwise not be very strong because it would consist of only a thin sheet of metal.

The ledges are prepared parallel to the incisal edge of the tooth as viewed from the lingual and parallel to one another as viewed from the incisal. In selected areas they will be widened to provide indentations of sufficient size to accommodate the pinholes. The determination of the incisocervical location of the ledges depends on the configuration of the pulp and the available bulk of tooth structure (Fig. 10-41). Usually the incisal ledge is prepared 2

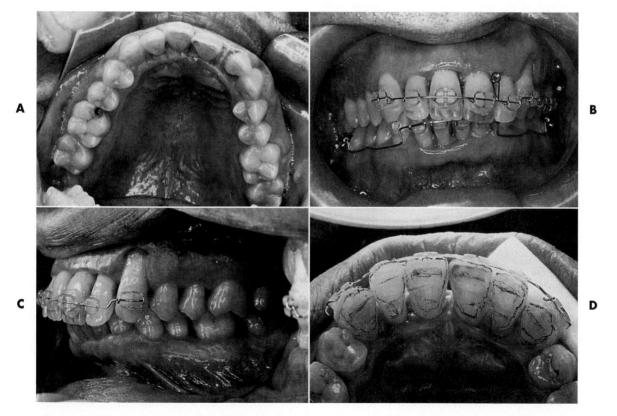

Fig. 10-40. **A,** Although periodontally compromised and malpositioned, these six caries-free anterior teeth are excellent for pinledge preparations. **B,** Orthodontic repositioning of the teeth. **C,** Stabilization after the repositioning. **D,** Outline of the proposed preparations drawn on the teeth.

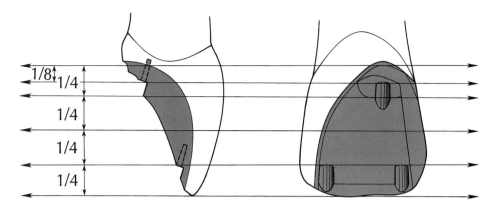

Fig. 10-41. Proximal lingual view of the location of ledges relative to the height of the crown. The incisal ledge is placed so its floor is one fourth of the preparation's height from the incisal edge. The cervical ledge is placed so its floor bisects the cervical fourth. Note that the path of insertion is parallel to the incisal two thirds of the labial wall. Adequate offset of the cervical pinhole either mesially or distally is needed to prevent pulpal exposure.

to 2.5 mm cervical to the incisal edge, or one fourth of the total height of the preparation from the incisal edge. The cervical ledge is placed on the crest of the cingulum at the center of the cervical one fourth of the preparation.

6. Prepare two ledges with a cylindrical carbide bur. The recommended minimum width for the ledge is 0.7 mm. Drawing the proposed location of the ledges on the lingual surface of the tooth is helpful. The design of the ledges must be compatible with the path of withdrawal of the restoration, which is parallel to the incisal two thirds of the labial surface of the tooth.

7. Make indentations in the left and right sides of the incisal ledge and slightly off center in the cervical ledge to prevent subsequent pulp exposure when the pinholes are placed. These incisal indentations will be as widely spaced as possible to retain as much dentin as possible between the pinholes and the pulp. Because the completed pinhole must be surrounded by sound dentin, it is not possible to place holes in the extreme corners because of the tooth's morphology. However, every effort should be made to prepare the indentations so that the pinholes will be surrounded by dentin and away from the pulp. This is particularly important for younger patients. The relationship between recommended pinhole locations and the pulp is illustrated in Fig. 10-42. Generally this means that the indentations are just within the mesial and distal marginal ridges, about 1.5 mm inside the external tooth contour (Fig. 10-43). The same carbide bur can be used to prepare the inden-

tations. When completed, the configuration of the indentations should resemble a half cylinder. Again, their orientation is parallel to the selected path of withdrawal and their floor should be smooth and continuous with the floor of the ledges. When combined, they should provide a flat area 1 to 1.2 mm wide buccolingually.

Pinhole Preparation

8. Sink pilot channels with either a small, round bur or a small twist drill. The shallow indentations will prevent skating of the selected bur. The depth of the completed pinhole should be at least 2 mm but can be as much as 3 mm when the placement and orientation of the pilot channels are satisfactory.

9. Enlarge and deepen the pilot channels with a tapered carbide bur when their placement and orientation are satisfactory. At this stage, any small corrections in orientation can be made. Less experienced operators may spend a great deal of time attempting to determine the correct alignment of the bur. However, it should be remembered that the design and location of the pinholes have already been determined by the placement of the ledges and indentations, so the only remaining concern should be verification of the position of the rotary instrument and attainment of the minimum depth of the pinholes. Some operators find it helpful to place a second bur in a prepared pinhole to help transfer the path of withdrawal, although precautions must be taken to prevent its being swallowed or inhaled. Preparing multiple

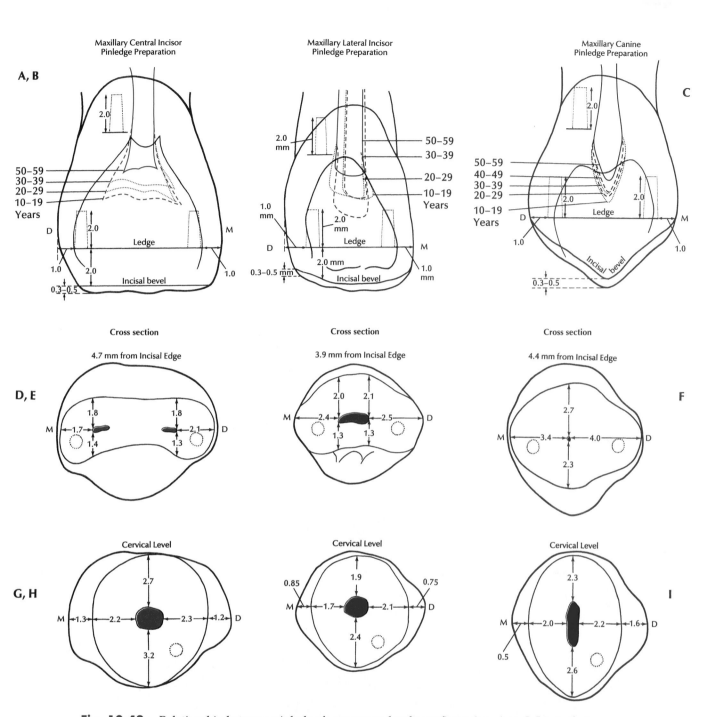

Fig. 10-42. Relationship between pinhole placement and pulp configuration. **A** to **C,** Lingual view. **D** to **F,** Cross section through incisal pinholes. **G** to **I,** Cross section through cervical pinholes. Dotted lines show the mean pulp chamber size of various age groups.
(Data from Ghashi Y: Shikagakuho 68:726, 1968.)

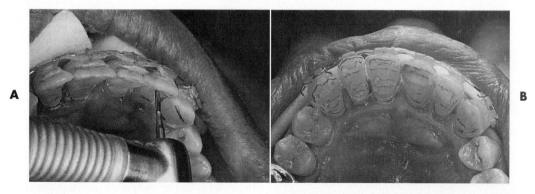

Fig. 10-43. **A,** Proposed location of the ledges marked on the teeth with a pencil. Note the orientation of the carbide relative to the long axis of the tooth. **B,** Ledge preparation completed on one side. Pilot holes for some pinholes have been placed.

pinholes a little at a time may also be helpful, moving from one to the next and gradually deepening each. This will permit alignment verification as the pinholes are prepared.

10. Bevel the junction between pinhole and indentation with a round bur slightly larger than the largest diameter of the pinhole (Fig. 10-44). (The required interproximal clearance is illustrated in Fig. 10-45.)

11. Inspect all surfaces of the preparation for smoothness and evaluate the margin. Correct any area that requires more distinct delineation (Fig. 10-46).

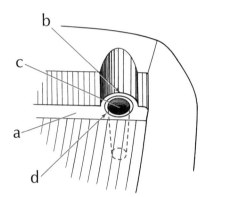
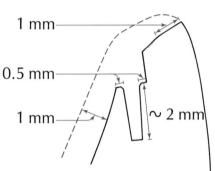

Fig. 10-44. Note the relation among the ledge, the indentation, and the pinhole. Recommended dimensions are given in the buccolingual cross section on the right. *a*, Ledge; *b*, indentation; *c*, pinhole; *d*, countersink.

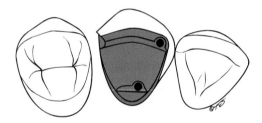

Fig. 10-45. Modified pinledge preparation with a proximal groove. Adequate interproximal clearance has resulted from the proximal flare.

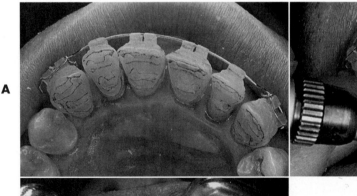
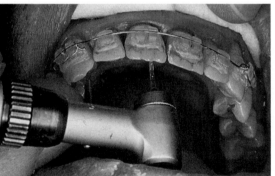
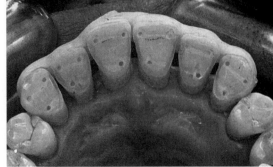

Fig. 10-46. **A,** Ledges and indentations prepared. **B,** Pinhole preparation with low-speed handpiece. **C,** The completed pinledge preparations. Utility wax has been placed over the brackets for impression making.

INLAYS AND ONLAYS

INDICATIONS

An inlay can be used instead of amalgam for patients with a low caries rate who require a small Class II restoration in a tooth with ample supporting dentin. It is among the least complicated cast restorations to make and can be very durable when it is carefully done. An onlay allows the damaged occlusal surface to be restored with a casting in the most conservative manner. It should be considered in the restoration of a severely worn dentition when the teeth are otherwise minimally damaged or for the replacement of an MOD amalgam restoration when sufficient tooth structure remains for retention and resistance form.

CONTRAINDICATIONS

Since these restorations rely on intracoronal (wedging) retention, inlays and onlays are contraindicated unless there is sufficient bulk to provide resistance and retention form. MOD inlays may increase the risk of cusp fracture and are generally not recommended. Extensive onlays, required where caries or existing restorations extend beyond the facial or lingual line angles, are contraindicated unless pins are used to supplement retention and resistance.

ADVANTAGES

Cast inlays and onlays can prove to be extremely long-lived restorations because of the excellent mechanical properties of the gold alloy. Low creep and corrosion mean that if inlay or onlay margins are accurately cast and finished, they will not deteriorate. The lack of corrosion may be an esthetic advantage. Gold will not lead to the tooth discoloration sometimes associated with dental amalgam. Unlike an inlay or amalgam, an onlay can support cusps, reducing the risk of tooth fracture.

DISADVANTAGES

In the restoration of a small carious lesion, an inlay is not very conservative of tooth structure. This is because additional tooth removal is necessary after minimal proximal extension to achieve a cavity preparation without undercuts and to permit access for impression making. This extension may lead to additional display of metal and gingival encroachment, which is undesirable for periodontal health. Since they do not encircle the tooth, inlays rely on the bulk of the buccal and lingual cusps for resistance and retention form. There is concern that high occlusal force will lead to cusp fracture due to wedging from the inlay.

PREPARATION

Armamentarium (Fig. 10-47). Carbide burs are usually used for inlay or onlay preparations, but diamonds can be substituted if preferred:

- Tapered carbide burs
- Round carbide burs
- Cylindrical carbide burs
- Finishing stones
- Mirror
- Explorer and periodontal probe
- Chisels
- Hatchet
- Gingival margin trimmers
- Excavators
- High- and low-speed handpieces
- Articulating film

CLASS II INLAY PREPARATION (FIG. 10-48)

Occlusal Analysis

1. Carefully assess the occlusal contact relationship and mark it with articulating film. The margins of the restoration should not be too close (<1.0 mm) to a centric contact; otherwise, there will be damaging stresses at the gold-enamel junction.
2. Apply rubber dam. Because good visibility and moisture control are essential during tooth preparation and caries excavation, the use of a rubber dam is strongly recommended.

Outline Form

3. Penetrate the central groove just to the depth of the dentin (typically about 1.8 mm) with a small, round or tapered carbide bur held in the path of withdrawal of the inlay. Generally this will be perpendicular to an imaginary line connecting the buccal and lingual cusps, not necessarily perpendicular to the occlusal plane. For example, on mandibular premolars it will be angled toward the lingual.

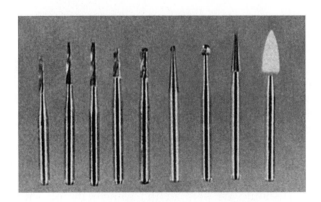

Fig. 10-47. Armamentarium for inlays and onlays.

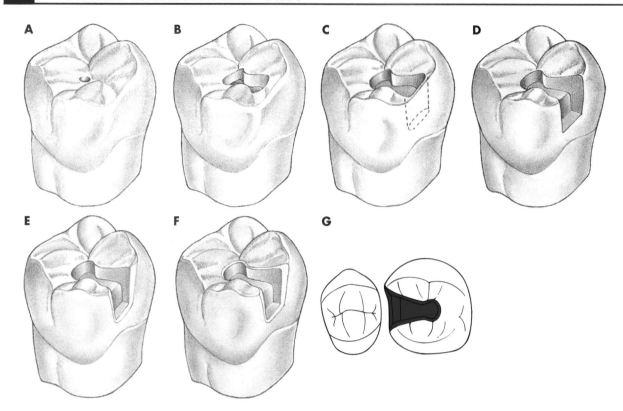

Fig. 10-48. The MO inlay preparation. **A,** Depth hole extending just into the dentin. **B,** An occlusal outline is prepared following the central groove. **C,** The outline is extended proximally and then gingivally, undermining the marginal ridge and removing caries. **D,** Unsupported enamel is removed, and the walls of the proximal box are defined. This is easily accomplished with hand instruments. **E,** Proximogingival bevels can be placed with tapered or flame-shaped carbides and hand instruments. **F,** An occlusal bevel or chamfer complete the preparation. **G,** Occlusal view of the completed preparation.

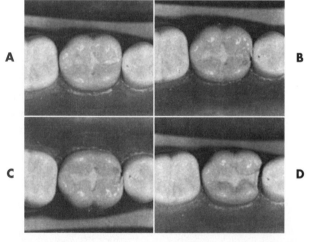

Fig. 10-49. Preparation of a mandibular molar tooth for an MO inlay. **A,** Occlusal outline. **B,** Proximal box initiated. **C,** Proximal box extended to remove contact. **D,** Completed preparation.
(Courtesy Dr. H. Bowman.)

4. Extend the occlusal outline through the central groove with the tapered carbide. The bur should be held in the same path of withdrawal and kept at the same depth—just into dentin. The buccolingual extension should be as conservative as possible to preserve the bulk of the buccal and lingual cusps. Resistance to proximal displacement is achieved with a small occlusal dovetail or pinhole. The outline should avoid the occlusal contacts.

5. Extend the outline proximally, undermining the marginal ridge, and stop it at the height of contour of the ridge (Fig. 10-49, *A*).

6. Advance the bur cervically to the carious lesion and then lingually and buccally, taking care to hold it in the precise path of withdrawal. There should be a thin layer of enamel remaining between the side of the bur and the adjacent tooth (Fig. 10-49, *B*). This will prevent accidental damage. The bur should move parallel to the original unprepared proximal surface, creating a convex axial wall in the box. The opposing buccal and lingual walls contribute significantly to retention, so great care must be taken not to tilt the bur during this step. It should be held in the path of withdrawal throughout. The width of the gingival floor of the box should be about

1.0 mm (mesiodistally). Correct cervical, lingual, and buccal extension at this stage is just beyond the proximal contact area. The completed inlay will require a minimum of 0.6 mm of proximal clearance to allow an impression to be made, but some of this will be achieved with the proximal flares and gingival bevels. Sharp line angles between the occlusal outline and proximal box are rounded at this time (Fig. 10-49, C).

Caries Excavation

7. Identify and remove any caries not eliminated by the proximal box preparation, using an excavator or a round bur in the low-speed handpiece.
8. Place a cement base to restore the excavated tissue in the axial wall and/or pulpal floor. If necessary, the preparation can be extended buccally or lingually. NOTE: an inlay is not a suitable restoration for extensive caries, and carrying it beyond the line angles will lead to a significant loss of retention and resistance form.

Axiogingival Groove and Bevel Placement

9. Prepare a small, well-defined groove at the junction of axial and gingival walls at the base of the proximal box to enhance resistance form and prevent distortion of the wax pattern during manipulation. It is easily placed with a gingival margin trimmer held in contact with the axial wall to prevent creating an undercut.
10. Place a 45-degree gingival margin bevel with a thin, tapered carbide or fine-grit diamond. Correct orientation is achieved by holding the instrument parallel to the gingival one third of the proximal surface of the adjacent tooth. The bur should not be tilted buccally or lingually to the path of withdrawal; otherwise, an undercut will be created at the corners of the box (a commonly seen fault in inlay preparations).
11. Prepare proximal bevels on the buccal and lingual walls with the tapered bur oriented in the path of withdrawal. There should be a smooth transition between the proximal and gingival bevels.
12. Place an occlusal bevel to improve marginal fit and allow finishing of the restoration. When the cuspal anatomy is steep, a conventional straight bevel will create too little gold near the margin for strength and durability. A hollow-ground bevel or chamfer is

normally preferred and can be conveniently placed with a round bur or stone.
13. As a final step, smooth the preparation where necessary, paying particular attention to the margin (Fig. 10-49, D).

MOD Onlay Preparation (Fig. 10-50)

The occlusal outline and proximal boxes of an onlay preparation are similar to those of an inlay. The additional steps are the occlusal reduction and a functional (centric) cusp ledge.

Outline Form

1. Prepare the occlusal outline with a tapered carbide bur just beyond the enamel-dentin junction (approximately 1.8 mm deep) and extend it through the central groove, incorporating any deep buccal or lingual grooves. Existing amalgam restorations are removed as part of this step.
2. Extend the outline both mesially and distally to the height of contour of the marginal ridge. As with an inlay, the boxes with an MOD onlay are prepared by advancing the bur gingivally and then buccally and lingually, always holding it in the precise path of withdrawal of the preparation. By ensuring that there is a thin section of proximal enamel remaining as the bur advances, damage to the adjacent tooth will be prevented (Fig. 10-51, A). Correct gingival, buccal, and lingual extension of the preparation normally depends on the contact area with the adjacent tooth. A minimum clearance of 0.6 mm is needed for impression making. Sometimes existing restorations or caries require a box to be extended beyond optimal. However, if a box requires extension beyond the transitional line angle, the preparation will have little resistance form, and an alternative restoration such as a complete crown should be considered. Preparing the boxes is a key step when fabricating an onlay. The tapered bur should be held precisely in the planned path of withdrawal throughout. Tilting, often caused by trying to advance the bur too quickly, is commonly done and is difficult to correct.
3. Round sharp line angles between the occlusal outline and proximal boxes.

Caries Excavation

4. Remove any remaining caries using an excavator or a round bur in the low-speed handpiece.
5. Place a cement base to restore the excavated tissue. Good judgment is needed to ensure

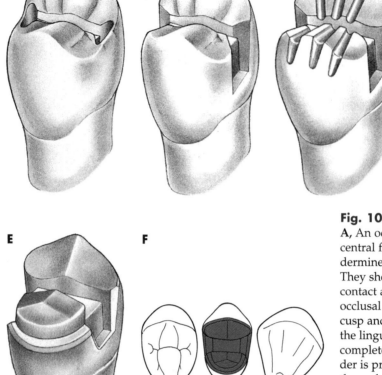

Fig. 10-50. The MOD onlay preparation. **A,** An occlusal outline is prepared to follow the central fossa, and the marginal ridges are undermined. **B,** The proximal boxes are refined. They should extend just beyond the proximal contact area. **C,** Depth grooves are placed for occlusal reduction—0.8 mm on the noncentric cusp and 1.3 mm on the centric cusp. **D,** Note the lingual functional cusp bevel as part of the completed occlusal reduction. A lingual shoulder is prepared, approximately at the level of the occlusal isthmus. **E,** Continuous bevel completes the preparation. The bevel on the lingual shoulder makes a smooth transition into the proximal bevel of the box. A small contrabevel is placed on the buccal cavosurface margin. **F,** Occlusal view of the completed preparation.

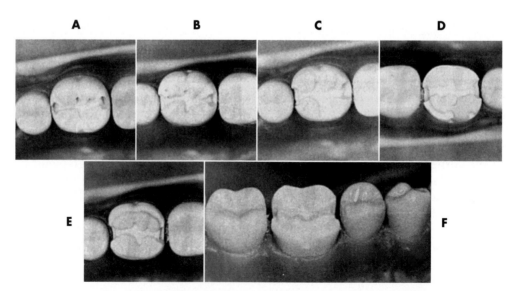

Fig. 10-51. Preparation of a mandibular molar tooth for an MOD onlay. **A,** Preparation outline. **B,** Proximal boxes extended to remove contacts. **C,** Occlusal reduction grooves. **D,** Centric cusp ledge placed for distal half. **E** and **F,** Completed preparation. *(Courtesy Dr. H. Bowman.)*

that adequate sound dentin is present on the axial walls to provide retention and resistance.

Occlusal Reduction

6. Place depth grooves on the centric (functional) cusps. To give additional clearance at the cusp tip, the bur must be oriented more horizontally than the intended restoration cusp. The grooves should be 1.3 mm deep, allowing 0.2 mm for smoothing.

7. Place 0.8 mm grooves on the noncentric cusps. On noncentric cusps, the bur is oriented parallel to the cuspal inclines. As with all depth grooves, it is assumed that the tooth is in good occlusal relation before preparation. If it is not, a vacuum-formed matrix made from the diagnostic waxing procedure is recommended as a guide.

8. Connect the grooves to form the occlusal reduction, maintaining the general contour of the original anatomy.

9. Prepare a 1.0-mm centric cusp ledge with the cylindrical carbide bur (Fig. 10-51, D). This will give the restoration bulk in a high-stress area, preventing deformation during function. The ledge should be placed about 1 mm apical to the opposing centric contacts. It extends into the proximal boxes but should not be positioned too far apically; otherwise, the resistance form from the boxes will be lost.

10. Round any sharp line angles, particularly at the junction of the ledge and occlusal surface.

11. Check for adequate occlusal reduction by having the patient close into soft wax and measuring with a thickness gauge.

Margin Placement

12. Establish a smooth, continuous bevel on all margins. The gingival bevel is placed, as for an inlay, with the thin carbide or diamond held at 45 degrees to the path of withdrawal, or approximately parallel to the adjacent tooth contour. This will blend smoothly with the buccal and lingual bevels, which have been prepared with the bur held in the path of withdrawal.

13. Bevel the noncentric and centric cusps. Where additional bulk at the margin is needed, a chamfer should be substituted for the straight bevel. This can be placed with a round-tipped diamond.

14. Complete the preparation by rechecking the occlusal clearance in all excursions and assessing for smoothness (Fig. 10-51, E and F).

Study Questions

1. What are the indications and contraindications for partial veneer crowns?
2. What are the advantages and disadvantages of partial veneer crowns?
3. What is the recommended armamentarium and in what sequence should a maxillary premolar be prepared for a partial veneer crown?
4. What are the minimal criteria for each step described above?
5. What are the indications and contraindications for inlay/onlay restorations?
6. What are the advantages and disadvantages for inlay/onlay restorations?
7. What is the recommended armamentarium and in what sequence should a mandibular molar be prepared for an inlay/onlay restoration?
8. What are the minimal criteria for each step described above? Why?

SUMMARY CHART

Indications	Contraindications	Advantages	Disadvantages
Sturdy clinical crown of average length or longer	Short teeth	Conservative of tooth structure	Less retentive than complete cast crown
Intact buccal surface not in need of contour modification and well-supported by sound tooth structure	High caries index	Easy access to margins	Limited adjustment of path of withdrawal
	Extensive destruction	Less gingival involvement than with complete cast crown	Some display of metal
No conflict between axial relationship of tooth and proposed path of withdrawal of FPD	Poor alignment		
	Bulbous teeth	Easy escape of cement and good seating	
	Thin teeth	Verification of seating simple	
		Electric vitality test feasible	

SUMMARY CHART

Indications	Contraindications	Advantages	Disadvantages
Sturdy clinical crown of average length or longer	Short teeth	Conservation of tooth structure	Less retentive than complete cast crown
Intact labial surface that is not in need of contour modification and that is supported by sound tooth structure	Nonvital teeth	Easy access to margins for finishing (dentist) and cleaning (patient)	Limited adjustment of path of insertion
	High caries index		Some display of metal
	Extensive destruction	Less gingival involvement than with complete cast crown	Not indicated on nonvital teeth
No discrepancy between axial relationship of tooth and proposed path of withdrawal of FPD	Poor alignment with path of withdrawal of FPD		
	Cervical caries	Easy escape of cement and good seating	
	Bulbous teeth	Easy verification of complete seating	
	Thin teeth	Electric vitality test feasible	

PARTIAL VENEER CROWN PREPARATION, POSTERIOR TEETH

Preparation Steps	Recommended Armamentarium	Criteria
Depth grooves for occlusal reduction	Tapered carbide fissure bur or tapered round-tipped diamond	0.8 mm on noncentric cusps 1.3 mm on centric cusps
Occlusal reduction	Round-tipped diamond	Clearance of 1 mm on noncentric cusps, 1.5 mm on centric cusps
Depth grooves for axial reduction	Round-tipped diamond	Chamfer depth of 0.5 mm (no more than half the width of diamond)
Axial reduction	Round-tipped diamond	Axial reduction parallel to long axis of tooth
Chamfer finishing	Large, round-tipped diamond	Smooth and continuous to minimize marginal length and facilitate finishing; distinct resistance to vertical displacement by periodontal probe
Proximal groove	Tapered carbide fissure bur	Distinct resistance to lingual displacement by probe; parallel to path of withdrawal of restoration; 90-degree angle between prepared axial wall and buccal or lingual aspect of groove
Buccal and occlusal bevel (maxillae), chamfer (mandible)	Round-tipped diamond	Maxillary teeth: bevel extends just beyond cusp tip but remains within curvature of cusp tip Mandibular teeth: minimum of 1 mm of cast gold in area of centric stops
Finishing	Large, round-tipped diamond or carbide	All sharp internal line angles (except grooves) rounded to smooth transitions

PARTIAL VENEER CROWN PREPARATION, ANTERIOR TEETH

Preparation Steps	Recommended Armamentarium	Criteria
Depth grooves for lingual reduction	Round-tipped diamond	Should allow for 1 mm of clearance
Lingual reduction	Football-shaped diamond	Should have 1 mm of clearance
Incisal bevel	Round-tipped diamond	Allows for metal thickness ≥ 0.7 mm
Depth grooves for axial reduction	Round-tipped diamond	Allows for 0.5 mm of metal thickness at margin
Axial reduction	Round-tipped diamond	Extends into interproximal about 0.4 mm lingual of contact area; parallel to incisal two thirds of labial surface
Retention form (proximal grooves and lingual pinhole)	Tapered carbide fissure bur and half-round bur	Grooves parallel to incisal two thirds of labial surface; should resist lingual displacement; pinhole should be between 2 and 3 mm deep Lingual wall of groove meets proximoaxial wall at angle of 90 degrees
Finishing and flare	Fine-grit, tapered diamonds (large and small) or carbide	All surfaces smooth; buccal wall of groove flared to break proximal contact; resulting cavosurface angle is 90 degrees; no unsupported enamel remaining

SUMMARY CHART

Indications	Contraindications	Advantages	Disadvantages
Undamaged anterior teeth in caries-free mouth	Large pulps	Minimal tooth reduction	Less retentive than complete coverage
Alteration of lingual contour of maxillary anterior teeth or alteration of occlusion	Thin teeth	Minimal margin length	Alignment can prove difficult
Anterior splinting	Nonvital teeth	Minimum gingival involvement	Technically demanding
	Carious involvement	Optimum access for margin finishing and hygiene	Not usable on nonvital teeth
	Problems with proposed path of withdrawal of FPD	Adequate retention	

SUMMARY CHART

Indications	Contraindications	Advantages	Disadvantages
Small carious lesion in otherwise sound tooth	High caries index	Superior material properties	Less conservative than amalgam
Adequate dentinal support	Poor plaque control	Longevity	May display metal
Low caries rate	Small teeth	No discoloration from corrosion	Gingival extension beyond ideal
Patient's request for gold instead of amalgam or composite resin	Adolescents	Least complex cast restoration	"Wedge" retention
	MODs		
	Poor dentinal support requiring a wide preparation		

SUMMARY CHART

Indications	Contraindications	Advantages	Disadvantages
Worn or carious teeth with intact buccal and lingual cusps	High caries index	Support of cusps	Lacks retention
MOD amalgam requiring replacement	Poor plaque control	High strength	Less conservation than amalgam
Low caries rate	Short clinical crown or extruded teeth	Longevity	May display metal
Patient's request for gold instead of amalgam	Lesions extending beyond transitional line angles		Gingival extension beyond ideal

PINLEDGE PREPARATION

Preparation Steps	Recommended Armamentarium	Criteria
Reduction of marginal ridge and contact area adjacent to edentulous space	Round-tipped, tapered diamond	Should provide space for adequate bulk of metal in area of connector
Lingual reduction	Football-shaped diamond	Should provide for clearance of at least 0.7 mm
Ledges	Straight carbide fissure bur	Ledges must be parallel to one another when viewed from lingual and from incisal; maximum width 1 mm
Indentations	Straight carbide fissure bur	Indentation should provide at least 0.5 mm of space for metal reinforcement around opening of pinhole
Pilot channels and pinholes	Tapered carbide bur	Pinholes must be between 2 and 3 mm deep; minimal width of ledge around pinholes is 0.5 mm
Finishing	Finishing stones or carbides	All surfaces must be as smooth as possible (obtain with fine-grit rotary instruments) to facilitate removal of this delicate wax pattern from die

CLASS II INLAY PREPARATION

Preparation Steps	Recommended Armamentarium	Criteria
Occlusal outline	Tapered carbide	Includes central groove, avoids centric contacts, includes dovetail or pinhole for resistance; approx. 1.8 mm deep
Proximal box	Tapered carbide	Follows curvature of original tooth surface
Caries removal	Excavator or round bur	Tissue replaced with base
Axiogingival groove	Gingival margin trimmer	Detectable with explorer tip (0.2 mm deep)
Gingival and proximal bevels	Thin, tapered carbide or diamond	45 degrees; approximately 0.8 mm wide
Occlusal bevel	Round carbide or stone	Hollow ground, avoid centric contacts.

MOD ONLAY PREPARATION

Preparation Steps	Recommended Armamentarium	Criteria
Occlusal outline	Tapered carbide	Includes central, buccal, and lingual grooves; about 1.8 mm deep
Proximal boxes	Tapered carbide	Follows curvature of original tooth surface
Caries removal	Excavator or round bur	Tissue replaced with base / Adequate dentin for resistance and retention
Occlusal reduction	Tapered carbide	Following anatomic contours / 1.5-mm centric cusp; 1.0-mm noncentric cusp
Centric cusp ledge	Tapered carbide	About 1.0 mm wide (before beveling) / About 1.0 mm apical to centric contact
Gingival and proximal bevels	Thin, tapered carbide	45 degrees; about 0.8 mm wide

CHAPTER ELEVEN

TOOTH PREPARATION FOR ALL-CERAMIC RESTORATIONS

All-ceramic inlays, onlays, veneers, and crowns are some of the most esthetically pleasing prosthodontic restorations. Because there is no metal to block light transmission, they can resemble natural tooth structure better in terms of color and translucency than any other restorative option. Their chief disadvantage is their susceptibility to fracture, although this is lessened by use of the resin-bonded technique.

The restorations may be fabricated in several ways. The technique (first developed over 100 years ago) originally called for a platinum foil matrix to be intimately adapted to a die. This supported the porcelain during firing and prevented distortion. The foil was removed before cementation of the restoration.

Today, popular fabrication processes for the restorations include hot-pressing and slip-casting. These options are discussed in Chapter 25.

COMPLETE CERAMIC CROWNS

Complete ceramic crowns should have relatively even thickness circumferentially. For the hot-pressed ceramic crown (IPS Empress* or Optimal†) (Fig. 11-1) usually about 1 to 1.5 mm is needed to

---

*Ivoclar-AG: Schaan, Liechtenstein.
†Jeneric/Pentron, Inc: Wallingford, Conn.

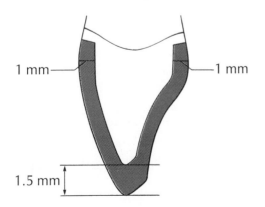

1 mm ——

—— 1 mm

1.5 mm

Fig. 11-1. Recommended reduction for the all-ceramic crown.

create an esthetically pleasing restoration. Incisally, a greater ceramic thickness may be required.

Only minor differences in tooth preparation design exist among the restorations fabricated with the various techniques. Therefore, the hot-pressed crown preparation is described in detail, and the necessary variations are discussed when pertinent.

ADVANTAGES

The advantages of a complete ceramic crown include its superior esthetics, its excellent translucency (similar to that of natural tooth structure), and its generally good tissue response. Lack of reinforcement by a metal substructure permits slightly more conservative reduction of the facial surface than is possible with the metal-ceramic crown, although the lingual surface needs additional reduction for strength. The appearance of the completed restoration can be influenced and modified by selecting different colors of luting agent. However, changing cement color under restorations that rely on an opaque core for strength, such as the slip cast alumina core system (InCeram*), will be ineffective.

DISADVANTAGES

The disadvantages of a complete ceramic crown include reduced strength of the restoration because of the absence of a reinforcing metal substructure. Because of the need for a shoulder-type margin circumferentially, significant tooth reduction is necessary on the proximal and lingual aspects. Porcelain brittleness, when combined with the lack of a reinforcing substructure, requires the incorporation of a circumferential support with a shoulder. Thus, by comparison, the proximal and lingual reductions are less conservative than those needed for a metal-ceramic crown.

Difficulties may be associated with obtaining a well-fitting margin when certain techniques are used. The "unforgiving" nature of porcelain, if an

---

*Vita Zahnfabrik: Bad Säckingen, Germany.

inadequate tooth preparation goes uncorrected, can result in fracture.

Proper preparation design is critical to ensuring mechanical success. A 90-degree cavosurface angle is needed to prevent unfavorable distribution of stresses and to minimize the risk of fracture (Fig. 11-2). The preparation should provide support for the porcelain along its entire incisal edge. Thus a severely damaged tooth (Fig. 11-3) should not be restored with a ceramic crown.

All-ceramic restorations are not effective as retainers for a fixed partial denture, although the strongest of the slip-cast materials (In-Ceram zirconia) and the higher-strength pressed systems (IPS Empress 2) may be suitable for anterior applications. The brittle nature of porcelain requires that connectors of large, cross-sectional dimension (a minimum of 4 × 4 mm is recommended) be incorporated in the FPD design. Typically this leads to impingement on the interdental papilla by the connector, with increased potential for periodontal failure.

Wear has been observed on the functional surfaces of natural teeth that oppose porcelain restorations. This also applies to teeth opposed by metal-ceramic restorations, especially the mandibular incisors, which can exhibit significant wear over time (see Fig 17-1).

INDICATIONS

The complete ceramic crown is indicated in areas with a high esthetic requirement where a more conservative restoration would be inadequate (Fig. 11-4). Usually such a tooth has proximal and/or facial caries that can no longer be effectively restored with composite resin. The tooth should be relatively intact with sufficient coronal structure to support the restoration, particularly in the incisal area, where it is important not to exceed a maximum porcelain thickness of 2 mm; otherwise, brittle failure of the material will occur.

Because of the relative weakness of the restoration, the occlusal load should be favorably distributed (Fig. 11-5). Generally this means that centric contact must be in an area where the porcelain is

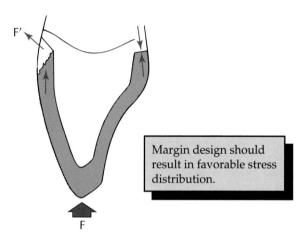

Margin design should result in favorable stress distribution.

Fig. 11-2. A sloping shoulder is not recommended for the all-ceramic crown. It does not support the porcelain. Incisal loading will lead to tensile stresses near the margin.

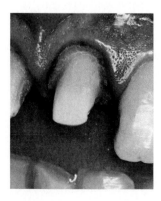

Fig. 11-3. Removal of an existing anterior crown. Defects in this tooth make it unsuitable for an all-ceramic crown.

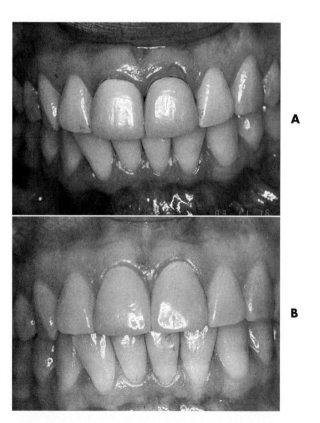

Fig. 11-4. **A,** Inadequately fitting all-ceramic crowns have led to recurrent caries and gingival recession around these central incisors. The patient, a professional model, had a high esthetic requirement. **B,** The gingival defect was corrected by minor periodontal recontouring, the teeth were reprepared, and new all-ceramic crowns were provided.

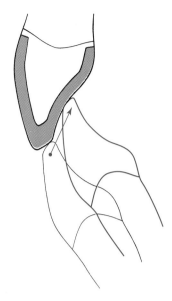

Fig. 11-5. The occlusion on an all-ceramic crown is critical for avoiding fracture. Centric contacts are best confined to the middle third of the lingual surface. Anterior guidance should be smooth and consistent with contact on the adjacent teeth. Leaving the restoration out of contact is not recommended. Future eruption may lead to protrusive interferences, precipitating fracture.

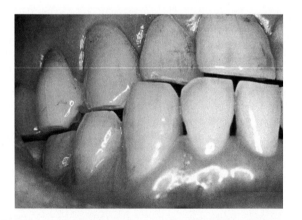

Fig. 11-6. Unfavorable occlusal loading such as this edge-to-edge relationship on the lateral incisor is a contraindication to the all-ceramic crown, particularly in view of the parafunctional activity of this patient.

supported by tooth structure (e.g., in the middle third of the lingual wall).

CONTRAINDICATIONS

The ceramic crown is contraindicated when a more conservative restoration can be used. Rarely are they recommended for molar teeth. The increased occlusal load and the reduced esthetic demand make metal-ceramics the treatment of choice. If occlusal loading is unfavorable (Fig. 11-6) or if it is not possible to provide adequate support or an even shoulder width of at least 1 mm circumferentially, a metal-ceramic restoration should be considered instead.

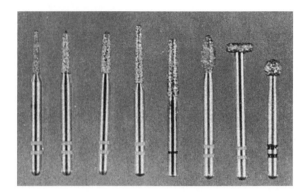

Fig. 11-7. Armamentarium for an all-ceramic crown preparation.

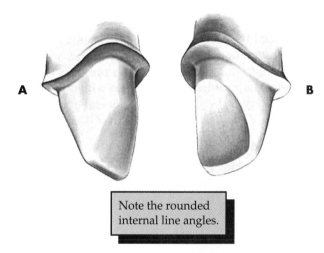

Note the rounded internal line angles.

Fig. 11-8. All-ceramic crown preparation. **A,** Labial view. **B,** Lingual view. To prevent stress concentrations in the ceramic, all internal line angles should be rounded. The shoulder should be as smooth as possible to facilitate the technical aspects of fabrication.

PREPARATION

Armamentarium (Fig. 11-7). The instruments needed for preparing a ceramic crown include the following:
- Narrow, round-tipped, tapered diamonds, regular and coarse grit (0.8 mm)
- Square-tipped, tapered diamond, regular grit (1.0 mm)
- Football-shaped diamond
- Finishing stones and carbides
- Mirror
- Periodontal probe
- Explorer
- Chisels and hatchets
- High- and low-speed handpieces

Step-by-Step Procedure (Fig. 11-8). The preparation sequence for a ceramic crown is similar to that for a metal-ceramic crown; the principal difference is the need for a 1-mm-wide chamfer circumferentially (Fig. 11-9).

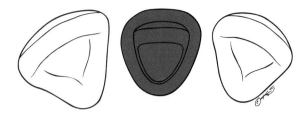

Fig. 11-9. Note the uniform chamfer width of 1 mm on this all-ceramic crown preparation.

Incisal (Occlusal) Reduction. The completed reduction of the incisal edge should provide 1.5 to 2 mm of clearance for porcelain in all excursive movements of the mandible. This will permit fabrication of a cosmetically pleasing restoration with adequate strength. If the restoration is used for posterior teeth (rare), 1.5 to 2 mm of clearance is needed on all cusps.

1. Place three depth grooves in the incisal edge, initially keeping them approximately 1.3 mm deep to allow for additional loss of tooth structure during finishing. The grooves are oriented perpendicular to the long axis of the opposing tooth to provide adequate support for the porcelain crown.
2. Complete the incisal reduction, reducing half the surface at a time, and verify its adequacy upon completion.

Facial Reduction

3. After placing depth grooves, reduce the facial or buccal surface and verify that adequate clearance exists for 1 mm of porcelain thickness. One depth groove is placed in the middle of the facial wall, and one each in the mesiofacial and distofacial transitional line angles. The reduction is then performed with a cervical component parallel to the proposed path of withdrawal and an incisal component parallel to the original contour of the tooth. The depth of these grooves should be approximately 0.8 mm to allow finishing. The reduction is performed on half of the facial surface at a time.
4. Do the bulk reduction with the round-tipped tapered diamond (which will result in a heavy chamfer margin). Be sure to maintain copious irrigation throughout.

Lingual Reduction

5. Use the football-shaped diamond for lingual reduction after placing depth grooves approximately 0.8 mm deep. The lingual reduction is done like the other anterior tooth preparations (see Chapters 9 and 10) until a clearance of 1 mm in all mandibular excur-

sive movements has been obtained. Adequate space must exist for the porcelain in all load-bearing areas.

6. After the selected path of withdrawal has been transferred from the cervical wall of the facial preparation, place a depth groove in the middle of the cingulum wall.
7. Repeat the shoulder preparation, this time from the center of the cingulum wall into the proximal, until the lingual shoulder meets the facial shoulder. This margin should follow the free gingival crest and should not extend too far subgingivally.

Chamfer Preparation. For subgingival margins, displace the tissue with cord before proceeding with the chamfer preparation. The ultimate objective is to direct stresses optimally in the completed porcelain restoration. This is accomplished when the chamfer or rounded shoulder margin completely supports the crown; then any forces exerted on the crown will be in a direction parallel to its path of withdrawal. A sloping shoulder will result in unfavorable loading of the porcelain, with a greater likelihood of tensile failure. A 90-degree cavosurface angle is optimal. Care must be taken, however, that no residual unsupported enamel is overlooked, because it might chip off.

The completed chamfer should be 1 mm wide, smooth, continuous, and free of any irregularities.

Finishing

8. Finish the prepared surfaces to a final smoothness as described for the other tooth preparations. Be sure to round any remaining sharp line angles to prevent a wedging action, which can cause fracture.
9. Perform any additional margin refinement as needed, using either the diamond or a carbide rotary instrument of choice.

■ CERAMIC INLAYS AND ONLAYS

For patients demanding esthetic restorations, ceramic inlays and onlays provide a durable alternative to posterior composite resins. The procedure consists of bonding the ceramic restoration to the prepared tooth with an acid-etch technique. The bonding mechanism relies on acid etching of the enamel and the use of composite resin, as seen in the resin-retained FPD technique (see Chapter 26). Bonding to porcelain is achieved by etching with hydrofluoric acid and the use of a silane coupling agent (materials are identical to those marketed as porcelain repair kits). A similar restoration uses indirectly fabricated composite resin instead of the ceramic inlays.

INDICATIONS

A ceramic inlay can be used instead of amalgam or a gold inlay for patients with a low caries rate requiring a Class II restoration and wishing to restore the tooth to its original appearance. It is the most conservative ceramic restoration and enables most of the remaining enamel to be preserved.

CONTRAINDICATIONS

Because these restorations are time consuming and expensive, they are contraindicated in patients with poor oral hygiene or active caries. Because of their brittle nature, ceramics may be contraindicated in patients with excessive occlusal loading, such as bruxers.

ADVANTAGES

Ceramic inlays and onlays can be extremely esthetic restorations. The restoration wear associated with posterior composite restorations is not a problem with the ceramics. Marginal leakage associated with polymerization shrinkage and high thermal coefficient of expansion of the resin is reduced, because the luting layer is very thin.

DISADVANTAGES

Accurate occlusion can be difficult to achieve with ceramic inlays and onlays. Because they are fragile, intraoral occlusal adjustment is impractical before they are bonded to place. Therefore, any areas of adjustment need careful finishing and polishing, which is a time-consuming procedure. Rough porcelain is extremely abrasive of the opposing enamel. Castable glass-ceramics (see Chapter 25) are less abrasive than the traditional feldspathic porcelain. Wear of the composite resin-luting agent can be a problem, leading to marginal gaps. These will eventually allow chipping or recurrent caries. Accuracy is important with these restorations, because accurately fitting restorations (marginal gaps less than 100 μm) have been shown to reduce this problem significantly. Finishing of the margins can be difficult in the less accessible interproximal areas. Resin flash or overhangs are difficult to detect and can initiate periodontal disease.

Bonded ceramic inlays are a relatively new concept, and long-term clinical performance is hard to judge. The patient should always be made aware that unforeseen problems may surface over time when a newer procedure is used.

PREPARATION (FIG 11-10)

Armamentarium (Fig 11-11). As for metal inlays, carbide burs are used in the preparation, but diamonds may be substituted:

- Tapered carbide burs
- Round carbide burs
- Cylindrical carbide burs
- Finishing stones
- Mirror
- Explorer and periodontal probe
- Chisels

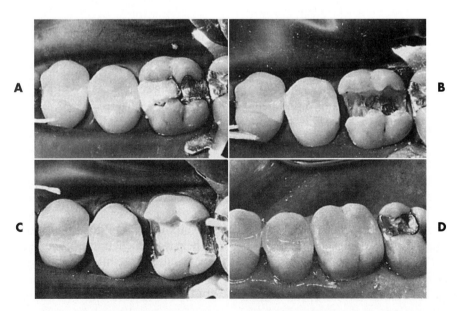

Fig. 11-10. Maxillary first molar preparation for an MOD ceramic inlay. **A,** Defective restoration. **B,** The restoration and caries removed. **C,** Unsupported enamel removed and glass ionomer base placed. **D,** The completed ceramic restoration. *(Courtesy Dr. R. Seghi.)*

- Gingival margin trimmers
- Excavators
- High- and low-speed handpieces
- Articulating film

Step-by-Step Procedure. Rubber dam isolation is recommended for visibility and moisture control. Before applying the dam, mark and assess the occlusal contact relationship with articulating film. To avoid chipping or wear of the luting resin, the margins of the restoration should not be at a centric contact.

Outline Form

1. Prepare the outline form. This will generally be governed by the existing restorations and caries and is broadly similar to that for conventional metal inlays and onlays (see Chapter 10). Because of the resin bonding, axial wall undercuts can sometimes be blocked out with resin-modified glass ionomer cement, preserving additional enamel for adhesion. However, undermined or weakened enamel should always be removed. The central groove reduction (typically about 1.8 mm) follows the anatomy of the unprepared tooth rather than a monoplane. This will provide additional bulk for the ceramic. The outline should avoid occlusal contacts. Areas to be onlayed need 1.5 mm of clearance in all excursions to prevent ceramic fracture.

2. Extend the box to allow a minimum of 0.6 mm of proximal clearance for impression making. The margin should be kept supragingival, which will make isolation during the critical luting procedure easier and will improve access for finishing. If necessary, electrosurgery or crown lengthening (p. 150) can be done. The width of the gingival floor of the box should be approximately 1.0 mm.

3. Round all internal line angles. Sharp angles lead to stress concentrations and increase the likelihood of voids during the luting procedure.

Caries Excavation

4. Remove any caries not included in the outline form preparation with an excavator or a round bur in the low-speed handpiece.

5. Place a resin-modified glass ionomer cement base to restore the excavated tissue in the gingival wall.

Margin Design

6. Use a 90-degree butt joint for ceramic inlay margins. Bevels are contraindicated because bulk is needed to prevent fracture. A distinct heavy chamfer is recommended for ceramic onlay margins.

Finishing

7. Refine the margins with finishing burs and hand instruments, trimming back any glass ionomer base. Smooth, distinct margins are essential to an accurately fitting ceramic restoration.

Occlusal Clearance (for Onlays)

8. Check this after the rubber dam is removed. A 1.5-mm clearance is needed to prevent fracture in all excursions. This can be easily evaluated by measuring the thickness of the resin provisional restoration with a dial caliper.

PORCELAIN LAMINATE VENEERS

Laminate veneering (Fig. 11-12) is a conservative method of restoring the appearance of discolored,

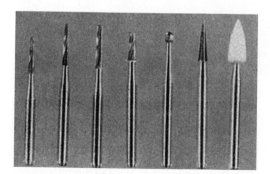

Fig. 11-11. Armamentarium for the porcelain laminate veneer preparation.

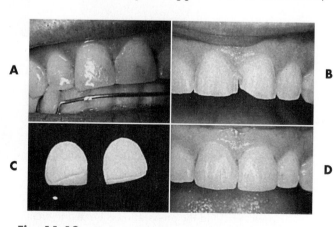

Fig. 11-12. Esthetic facial veneers. **A,** Discolored maxillary central incisors. **B,** Prepared for porcelain veneers. **C,** The laminates etched before bonding. **D,** Restorations in place.
(Courtesy Dr. C. Zmick.)

pitted, or fractured anterior teeth. It consists of bonding thin ceramic laminates onto the labial surfaces of affected teeth. The bonding procedure is the same as that for ceramic inlays.

ADVANTAGES AND INDICATIONS

The main advantage of facial veneers is that they are conservative of tooth structure. Typically only about 0.5 mm of facial reduction is needed. Since this is confined to the enamel layer, local anesthesia is not usually required. The main disadvantage of the procedure relates to difficulty in obtaining restorations that are not excessively contoured. This is almost inevitable in the gingival area if enamel is left for bonding. Currently, little has been reported about the effect of the restorations on long-term gingival health and whether or how often they will need replacement over a patient's lifetime.

Esthetic veneers should always be considered as a conservative alternative to cemented crowns. In many practices they have largely replaced metal-ceramic crowns for the treatment of multiple discolored but otherwise sound teeth.

PREPARATION

Armamentarium. The instruments needed for preparing a porcelain laminate veneer include the following:

- 1-mm round bur or 0.5-mm depth cutter
- Narrow, round-tipped, tapered diamonds, regular and coarse grit (0.8 mm)
- Finishing strip
- Finishing stones
- Mirror
- Periodontal probe
- Explorer

Step-by-Step Procedure (Fig. 11-13). The gingival third and proximal line angles are often overcontoured with these restorations. Therefore, maximum reduction should be achieved with minimum penetration into the dentin.

1. Make a series of depth holes with a round bur to help avoid penetrating abnormally thin enamel. The required amount of reduction will depend somewhat on the extent of discoloration. A minimum of 0.5 mm is usu-

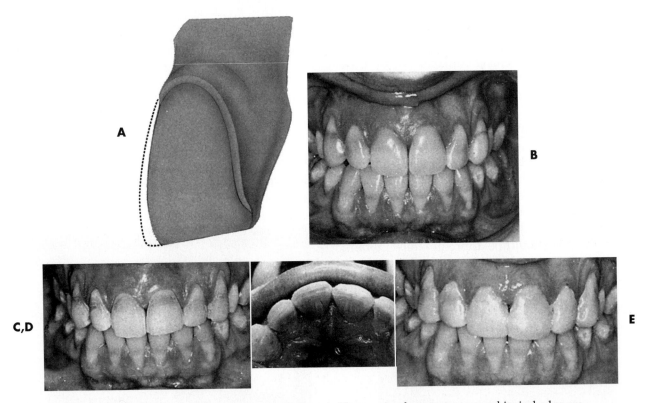

Fig. 11-13. Porcelain facial veneer preparation. **A,** The proximal contact areas and incisal edge are preserved, and the preparation is limited to enamel. Normally a reduction depth of about 0.5 mm is recommended, but making a series of depth holes with a round bur will guard against penetrating thin enamel. **B,** Tetracycline-stained teeth. Composite resin veneers were placed earlier but failed to mask the discoloration satisfactorily. Six maxillary porcelain labial veneers will be provided. **C and D,** Completed tooth preparations. **E,** Provisionals made directly with composite resin, which are retained by etching small areas of enamel (see Chapter 15).

ally adequate. The reduction should follow the anatomic contours of the tooth.

2. Place the "long chamfer" margin (Fig. 11-14). This design has an obtuse cavosurface angle, which exposes the enamel prism ends at the margin for better etching. The margin should closely follow the gingival crest so that all discolored enamel will be veneered without undue encroachment on the gingival sulcus.

3. Wherever possible, place the preparation margin labial to the proximal contact area to preserve it in enamel. However, slight clearance for separating the working cast and for accessing the proximal margins for finishing and polishing is essential. A diamond finishing strip helps create the necessary clearance. Sometimes the proximal margins are extended lingually to include existing restorations. This can necessitate considerable tooth

reduction to avoid creating an undercut. Some authorities advocate placing the ceramic margin on composite rather than extending the preparation to enamel, but this is not recommended. Extensive existing restorations are a contraindication for porcelain laminate veneers.

4. If possible, do not reduce the incisal edge (Fig. 11-15); this helps support the porcelain and makes chipping less likely. If the incisal edge length is to be increased, the preparation should extend to the lingual. Care is needed to avoid undercuts with this modification. Visualizing the path of insertion of the restoration is important, because an undercut will prevent placement of the veneer.

5. To prevent areas of stress concentration in the porcelain, be sure that all prepared surfaces are rounded (see Fig. 11-13, *C, D*).

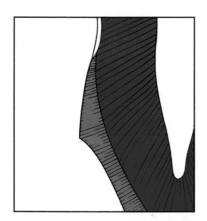

Fig. 11-14. The recommended margin ("long chamfer") for facial veneers has an obtuse cavosurface angle so the ends of the enamel prisms will be exposed for differential etching.

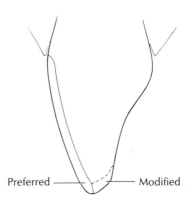

Fig. 11-15. The preferred design for porcelain laminate veneers maintains part of the incisal edge in enamel. If the edge is to be lengthened, a modified preparation with lingual extension will be needed (*dotted line*).

Study Questions

1. What are the indications and contraindications for all-ceramic crowns and porcelain laminate veneers?
2. What are the advantages and disadvantages for all-ceramic crowns and porcelain laminate veneers?
3. What is the recommended armamentarium, and in what sequence should a maxillary central incisor be prepared for an all-ceramic crown and porcelain laminate veneer?
4. What are the minimal criteria for each step described above? Why?
5. Discuss the advantages, disadvantages, indications, and contraindications for ceramic inlays and onlays.
6. What is the recommended armamentarium, and in what sequence should a mandibular molar be prepared for a ceramic inlay and onlay?
7. What are the minimal criteria for each step described above? Why?

SUMMARY CHART

Indications	Contraindications	Advantages	Disadvantages
High esthetic requirement	When superior strength is warranted and metal-ceramic crown is more appropriate	Esthetically unsurpassed	Reduced strength compared to metal-ceramic crown
Considerable proximal caries	High caries index	Good tissue response even for subgingival margins	Proper preparation extremely critical
Incisal edge reasonably intact	Insufficient coronal tooth structure for support	Slightly more conservative of facial wall than metal ceramic	Among least conservative preparations
Endodontically treated teeth with post-and-cores	Thin teeth faciolingually		Brittle nature of material
Favorable distribution of occlusal load	Unfavorable distribution of occlusal load		Can be used as single restoration only
	Bruxism		

SUMMARY CHART

Indications	Contraindications	Advantages	Disadvantages
Demand for esthetics	High caries index	Superior esthetics	Abrasive of opposing tooth
Low caries rate	Poor plaque control	Conservative	Occlusion difficult to adjust
Intact buccal and lingual enamel	Bruxism	Durable	Wear of luting agent
			Expensive
			Long-term success rate unknown

SUMMARY CHART

Indications	Contraindications	Advantages	Disadvantages
Discolored or damaged anterior teeth	High caries index	Superior esthetics	Increased tooth contour
	Poor plaque control	Wear and stain resistant	Expensive
	Extensive existing restorations		
	Bruxism		

ALL-CERAMIC CROWN PREPARATION

Preparation Steps	Recommended Armamentarium	Criteria
Depth grooves for incisal reduction	Tapered diamond	Approximately 1.3 mm deep to allow for additional reduction during finishing; perpendicular to long axis of opposing tooth
Incisal reduction	Tapered diamond	Clearance of 1.5 mm; check excursions
Depth grooves for facial reduction	Tapered diamond	Depth of 0.8 mm needed for additional reduction during finishing
Facial reduction	Tapered diamond	Reduction of 1.2 mm needed; two planes, as for metal-ceramic crown preparation
Depth grooves and lingual reduction	Tapered and football-shaped diamonds	Initial depth 0.8 mm; recreate concave configuration; do not maintain any convex configurations (stress)
Depth grooves for cingulum reduction	Tapered diamond	Parallel to cervical aspect of facial preparation; 1 mm of reduction; shoulder follows free gingival margin
Lingual shoulder preparation	Square-tipped diamond	Rounded shoulder 1 mm wide; minimize "peaks and valleys"; 90-degree cavosurface angle
Finishing	Fine-grit diamond or carbide	All surfaces smooth and continuous; no unsupported enamel; 90-degree cavosurface angle

CERAMIC INLAY AND ONLAY PREPARATION

Preparation Steps	Recommended Armamentarium	Criteria
Outline	Tapered carbide	Includes existing restorations and caries; about 1.8 mm deep; small undercuts tolerated
Proximal box	Tapered carbide	Gingival floor 1 mm wide Clearance for impression 0.6 mm
Caries removal	Excavator or round bur	Block out undercuts with glass ionomer
Margins	Finishing burs Hand instruments	90-degree butt joint Heavy chamfer for onlays
Occlusal clearance	Round-tipped diamond	Clearance in all excursions of 1.5 mm
Finishing	Finishing burs Fine-grit diamonds	Rounded internal angles Smooth margins

PORCELAIN LAMINATE VENEERS

Preparation Steps	Recommended Armamentarium	Criteria
Depth cuts	1-mm round bur or 0.5-mm depth cutter	A series of depth cuts to determine dentin exposure
Facial reduction	Round-tipped diamond	Follows curvature of original tooth surface
Proximal reduction	Round-tipped diamond	Extended to gingival crest, leaving contact area intact
Incisal and lingual reduction	Round-tipped diamond	None unless incisal margin is extended to lingual to allow lengthening
Margins	Round-tipped diamond	Long chamfer
Finishing	Fine-grit diamonds, carbides, or finishing stones	No sharp internal margins

RESTORATION OF THE ENDODONTICALLY TREATED TOOTH

KEY TERMS

canal configuration
embedment depth
ferrule
multipiece post-and-cores
post-and-core
post configuration
post removal

post type
prefabricated posts
root diameter
stress distribution
surface texture
tooth length

An endodontically treated tooth should have a good prognosis. It can resume full function and serve satisfactorily as an abutment for a fixed or removable partial denture. However, special techniques are needed to restore such a tooth. Usually a considerable amount of tooth structure has been lost because of caries, endodontic treatment, and the placement of previous restorations. The loss of tooth structure makes retention of subsequent restorations more problematic and increases the likelihood of fracture during functional loading.

Two factors influence the choice of technique: the type of tooth (whether it is an incisor, canine, premolar, or molar) and the amount of remaining coronal tooth structure. The latter is probably the most important indicator when determining the prognosis.

Different clinical techniques have been proposed to solve these problems, and opinions vary about the most appropriate one. Recent experimental data have improved our understanding of the difficulties inherent in restoring an endodontically treated tooth. This chapter offers a rational and practical approach to the challenge.

TREATMENT PLANNING

Extensive caries or periodontal disease may make removal of a tooth more sensible than endodontically treating it, although a severely damaged tooth occasionally can be restored after orthodontic repositioning or **root** resection (Fig. 12-1). This should be done if its loss will significantly jeopardize the pa-

tient's occlusal function or the total treatment plan, particularly if dental implants are not an option. When the decision is made to treat the tooth endodontically, consideration must have been given to its subsequent restoration. Before restoration, existing endodontically treated teeth need to be assessed carefully for the following[1]:

- Good apical seal
- No sensitivity to pressure
- No exudate
- No fistula
- No apical sensitivity
- No active inflammation

Inadequate root fillings should be retreated. If doubt remains, the tooth should be observed until there is definite evidence of success or failure.

If the coronal structures are largely intact and loading is favorable as on anterior teeth that are farther removed from the fulcrum, a simple filling can be placed in the access cavity (Fig. 12-2, *A*). However, if a substantial amount of coronal structure is missing, a cast **post-and-core** is indicated instead (Fig. 12-2, *B*). Molars are often restored with amalgam or a combination of one or more cemented posts and amalgam or composite resin (Fig. 12-2, *C* and *D*).

Although one-piece post-crowns were once made, such prostheses are of historical interest only. Superior results can now be obtained with a two-step technique (Fig. 12-3) consisting of a post-and-core foundation and a separate crown. Most often a metal post is used, which provides the necessary retention for the core. This replaces any lost coronal tooth structure of the tooth preparation. The shape of the residual coronal tooth structure, combined with the core, should result in an ideal shape for the preparation (Fig. 12-4).

Prefabricated metal, carbon fiber, ceramic, and glass fiber posts are available. These last two options provide esthetic alternatives to metal posts.[2,3] They are used in conjunction with a plastic material such as composite resin, amalgam, or glass ionomer.

With the two-step approach of fabricating a separate crown over a cast post-and-core, achieving a

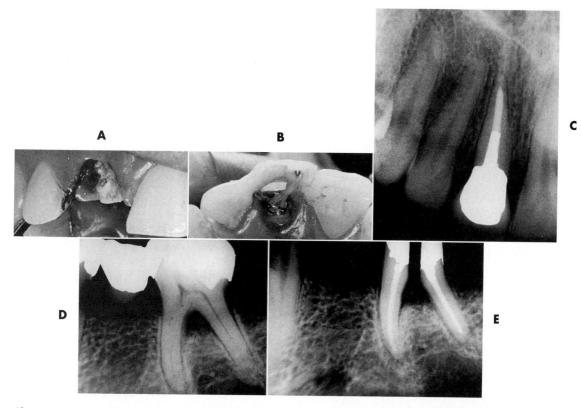

Fig. 12-1.   **A** to **C,** A severely damaged tooth can sometimes be retained after orthodontic extrusion (see Chapter 6). **D** and **E,** Plaque control around periodontally compromised teeth may be improved after hemisectioning (see Chapter 5).
(*D and E courtesy Dr. H. Kahn.*)

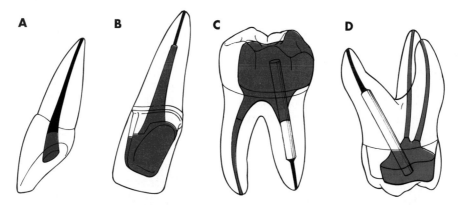

Fig. 12-2.   **A,** An anterior tooth with intact clinical crown can be predictably restored with a composite restoration in the access cavity. **B,** When most coronal tissue is missing, a cast post-and-core is indicated to obtain optimal tooth preparation form. **C,** In mandibular molars an amalgam foundation is supported by a cemented prefabricated post in the distal canal. **D,** In maxillary molars the palatal canal is most often used.

satisfactory marginal fit is easier because the expansion rate of the two castings can be controlled individually. A cast post-and-core needs to be slightly smaller than the canal to achieve optimal internal seating, whereas the crown needs to be slightly larger to achieve optimal seating (see Chapter 7). The two-step approach further permits fabrication of a replacement crown, if necessary, without the

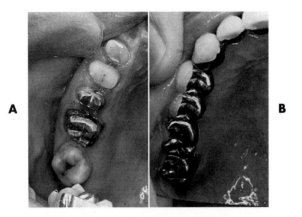

Fig. 12-3. **A,** The first molar and second premolar have been restored with post-and-cores. Note the margins, optimally located on sound tooth structure, cervical to the castings. **B,** Extracoronal restorations in place.

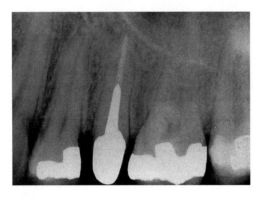

Fig. 12-4. The second premolar has been restored with a cast post-and-core, before a metal-ceramic crown. *(Courtesy Dr. R. Webber.)*

need for **post removal**. Finally, a different path of placement than the one selected for the post-and-core may be selected for the crown. This is often helpful when the tooth is restored to serve as an abutment for a fixed partial denture (FPD).

CLINICAL FAILURE

Morphologic and functional differences between anterior teeth and posterior teeth require that they be treated differently after endodontic therapy, mainly because different loading considerations apply.

One retrospective analysis[4] involving 638 patients evaluated 788 post-and-cores: 456 custom cast post-and-cores and 332 foundations with ParaPosts. Four to five years after cementation, reported failure rates in males were significantly higher than in females, and failure rates above age 60 were three times as high as failure rates for younger patients. Maxillary failure rates (15%) were three times as high as mandibular failure rates (5%), and more prevalent in lateral incisors, canines, and premolars than central

incisors and molars. Failure rate under fixed partial dentures was significantly lower than under single crowns. The latter may be due to load reduction resulting from bracing by the FPD. No correlation was apparent between failure and reduced marginal height of the encasing bone. Custom cast post-and-cores exhibited slightly higher failure rates than amalgam foundations. This observation was also made by Sorensen and Martinoff.[5] However, Torbjörner et al[4] suggest that custom cast post-and-cores tend to be used more often in teeth that already have considerably weakened root structure. Thus, regardless of the technique selected for subsequent restoration, the teeth themselves are already more prone to failure. Distal cantilevers appear to contribute to post-and-core failure in endodontically treated abutment teeth that support the cantilever.

Most of the failures just discussed are influenced by load. In general, as loading increases, failure rates appear to increase concomitantly. Failure loads have been shown to increase as the load angle approaches parallelism to the long axes of the teeth.[6] This suggests that failure will occur more readily under lateral loading. When planning the restoration of endodontically treated teeth, the practitioner's prognosis must consider the strength of the remaining tooth structure weighed carefully against the load to which the restored tooth will be subjected.

CONSIDERATIONS FOR ANTERIOR TEETH

Endodontically treated anterior teeth do not always need complete coverage by placing a complete crown, except when plastic restorative materials have limited prognosis (e.g., if the tooth has large proximal composite restorations and unsupported tooth structure). Many otherwise intact teeth function satisfactorily with a composite resin restoration.

Although commonly believed, it has not been demonstrated experimentally that endodontically treated teeth are weaker or more brittle than vital teeth. Their moisture content, however, may be reduced.[7] Laboratory testing[8] has actually revealed a similar resistance to fracture between untreated and endodontically treated anterior teeth. Nevertheless, clinical fracture does occur, and attempts have been made to strengthen the tooth by removing part of the root canal filling and replacing it with a metal post. In reality, placement of a post requires the removal of additional tooth structure (Box 12-1), which is likely to weaken the tooth.

Cementing a post in an endodontically treated tooth is a fairly common clinical procedure despite the paucity of data to support its success. In fact, a laboratory study[9] and two **stress** analyses[10,11] have

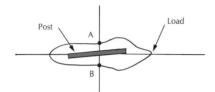

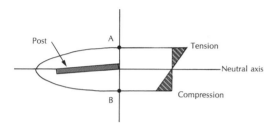

Fig. 12-5. Experimental stress distributions in an endodontically treated tooth with a cemented post. When the tooth is loaded, the lingual surface is in tension, and the facial surface is in compression. The centrally located cemented post lies in the neutral axis (i.e., not in tension or compression).
(Redrawn from Guzy GE, Nicholls JI: J Prosthet Dent 42:39, 1979.)

> It takes some practice to estimate remaining wall thickness after preparation for the future extracoronal restoration.

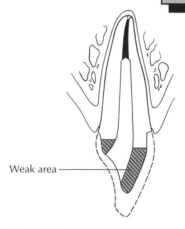

Fig. 12-6. Cross section through a central incisor. The dotted line indicates the original tooth contour before preparation for a metal-ceramic restoration. Even with minimum reduction for the extracoronal restoration, note the weakened facial wall, which would not be able to support a prosthesis successfully. The sharp lingual wall complicates pattern fabrication.

DISADVANTAGES TO THE ROUTINE USE OF A CEMENTED POST   BOX **12-1**

- Placing the post requires an additional operative procedure.
- Preparing a tooth to accommodate the post removes additional tooth structure.
- It may be difficult to restore the tooth later, when a complete crown is needed, because the cemented post may have failed to provide adequate retention for the core material.
- The post can complicate or prevent future endodontic retreatment if this becomes necessary.

---

determined that no significant reinforcement results. This might be explained by the hypothesis that, when the tooth is loaded, stresses are greatest at the facial and lingual surfaces of the root and an internal post, being only minimally stressed, does not help prevent fracture (Fig. 12-5). Other studies, however, contradict this assumption.[8,12] Cemented posts may further limit or complicate endodontic retreatment options if these are necessary. In addition, if coronal destruction occurs, post removal may be necessary to provide adequate support for a future core.

For these reasons, a metal post is not recommended in anterior teeth that do not require complete coverage restorations. This view is supported by a retrospective study[13] that did not show any improvement in prognosis for endodontically treated

anterior teeth restored with a post. In another study, post placement did not influence the position or angle of radicular fracture.[14]

Discoloration in the absence of significant tooth loss may be more effectively treated by bleaching[15] than by the placement of a complete crown, although not all stained teeth can be bleached successfully. Resorption can be an unfortunate side effect of nonvital bleaching.[16] However, when loss of coronal tooth structure is extensive or the tooth will be serving as an FPD or RPD abutment, a complete crown becomes mandatory. Retention and support then must be derived from within the canal because a limited amount of coronal dentin remains once the reduction for complete coverage has been completed. Coupled with the loss of internal tooth structure necessary for endodontic treatment, the remaining walls become thin and fragile (Fig. 12-6), often requiring their reduction in height.

CONSIDERATIONS FOR POSTERIOR TEETH

Endodontically treated posterior teeth are subject to greater loading than anterior teeth because of their closer proximity to the transverse horizontal axis. This, combined with their morphologic characteristics (having cusps that can be wedged apart), makes them more susceptible to fracture. Careful occlusal adjustment will reduce potentially damaging lateral

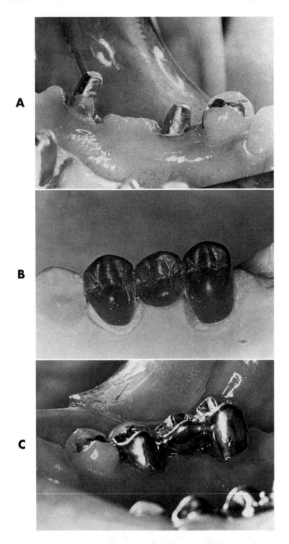

Fig. 12-7. **A,** Mandibular premolar and hemisected molar restored with cast post-and-cores. **B,** Waxed three-unit FPD. **C,** The FPD cemented in place. *(Courtesy Dr. F. Hsu.)*

forces during excursive movements. Nevertheless, endodontically treated posterior tooth should receive cuspal coverage to prevent biting forces from causing fracture. Possible exceptions are mandibular premolars and first molars with intact marginal ridges and conservative access cavities not subjected to excessive occlusal forces (i.e., posterior disclusion in conjunction with normal muscle activity).

Complete coverage is recommended on teeth with a high risk of fracture. This is especially true for maxillary premolars, because complete coverage gives the best protection against fracture, since the tooth is completely encircled by the restoration. However, considerable tooth reduction is required, particularly when a metal-ceramic restoration is to be used. When significant coronal tooth loss has occurred, a cast post-and-core (Fig. 12-7) or an amalgam foundation restoration is needed.

◨ PRINCIPLES OF TOOTH PREPARATION

Many of the principles of tooth preparation discussed in Chapter 7 apply equally to the preparation of endodontically treated teeth, although certain additional concepts must be understood to avoid failure.

CONSERVATION OF TOOTH STRUCTURE

Preparation of the Canal (Fig. 12-8). When creating post space, great care must be used to remove only minimal tooth structure from the canal. Excessive enlargement can perforate or weaken the root, which then may split during cementation of the post or subsequent function. The thickness of the remaining dentin is the prime variable in fracture resistance of the root. Experimental impact testing of teeth with cemented posts of different diameters[7] showed that teeth with a thicker (1.8 mm) post fractured more easily than those with a thinner (1.3 mm) one.

Photoelastic stress analysis also has shown that internal stresses are reduced with thinner posts. Conversely, the root can be compared to a ring. The strength of a ring is proportional to the difference between the fourth powers of its internal and external radii. This implies that the strength of a prepared root comes from its periphery, not from its interior, so a post of reasonable size should not weaken the root significantly.[17] Nevertheless, it is difficult to enlarge a root canal uniformly and to judge with accuracy how much tooth structure has been removed and how thick the remaining dentin is. Most roots are narrower mesiodistally than faciolingually and often have proximal concavities that cannot be seen on a standard periapical radiograph. Experimentally, most root fractures originate from these concavities because the remaining dentin thickness is minimal.[18] Therefore the root canal should be enlarged only enough to enable the post to fit accurately yet passively while ensuring strength and retention. Along the length of the post space, enlargement seldom needs to exceed what would have been accomplished with one or two additional file sizes beyond the largest size used for endodontic treatment. Because of the more coronal position of the post space, a much larger file must be used to accomplish this (Fig. 12-9).

Preparation of Coronal Tissue. Endodontically treated teeth often have lost much coronal tooth structure as a result of caries, of previously placed restorations, or in preparation of the endodontic access cavity. However, if a cast core is to be used, further reduction is needed to accommodate a complete crown and to remove undercuts from the

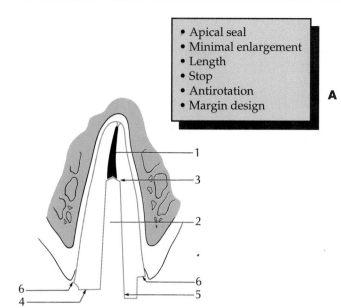

- Apical seal
- Minimal enlargement
- Length
- Stop
- Antirotation
- Margin design

Fig. 12-8. Faciolingual cross section through a maxillary central incisor prepared for a post-and-core. Six features of successful design are identified: *1*, Adequate apical seal; *2*, minimum canal enlargement (no undercuts remaining); *3*, adequate post length; *4*, positive horizontal stop (to minimize wedging); *5*, vertical wall to prevent rotation (similar to a box); *6*, extension of the final restoration margin onto sound tooth structure.

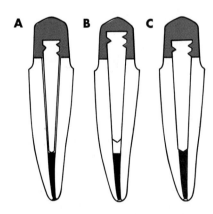

Fig. 12-9. Use of a prefabricated post entails enlarging the canal one or two file sizes to obtain a good fit at a predetermined depth. **A,** Incorrect; the prefabricated post is too narrow. **B,** Incorrect; the prefabricated post does not extend to the apical seal. **C,** Correct; the prefabricated post is fitted by enlarging the canal slightly.

chamber and internal walls. This may leave very little coronal dentin. Every effort should be made to save as much of the coronal tooth structure as possible, because this helps reduce stress concentrations at the gingival margin.[19] The amount of remaining tooth structure is probably the single most important predictor of clinical success. If more than 2 mm of coronal tooth structure remains, the post design probably has a limited role in the fracture re-

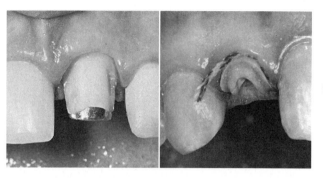

Fig. 12-10. **A,** It is preferable to maintain as much coronal tooth structure as possible, provided it is sound and of reasonable strength. **B,** Extensive caries has resulted in the loss of all coronal tooth structure. This is less desirable than the situation in **A,** because greater forces are transmitted to the root.

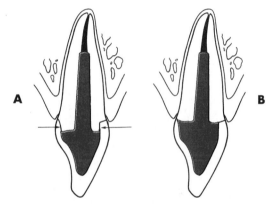

Fig. 12-11. Extending a preparation apically creates a ferrule and helps prevents fracture of an endodontically treated tooth during function. **A,** Prepared with a ferrule *(arrows)*. **B,** Prepared without a ferrule.

sistance of the restored tooth.[20,21] The once common clinical practice of routine coronal reduction to the gingival level before post-and-core fabrication is outmoded and should be avoided (Fig. 12-10). Extension of the axial wall of the crown apical to the missing tooth structure provides what is known as a *ferrule* (Fig. 12-11) and is thought to help bind the remaining tooth structure together, preventing root fracture during function.[22-24] Although there is evidence that preserving as much coronal tooth structure as possible will enhance prognosis, it is less clear whether the prognosis will improve by creating a **ferrule** in an extensively damaged tooth by surgical crown-lengthening. In this latter circumstance, although the crown-lengthening allows a ferrule, it also leads to a much less favorable crown-to-root ratio and therefore increased leverage on the root during function (Fig. 12-12). One recent laboratory study showed that creating a ferrule through

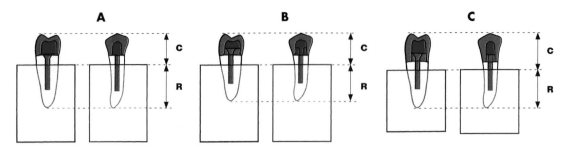

Fig. 12-12. Effect of apical preparation on crown-to-root ratio. **A,** Schematic of extensively damaged premolar tooth. Apical extension of the gingival margin would encroach on the biologic width (p. 150). This preparation has no ferrule. **B,** Creating a ferrule with orthodontic extrusion (see Fig. 6-21) reduces root length *(R)* while crown length *(C)* remains unchanged. **C,** Surgical crown lengthening also reduces root length *(R)* but increases crown length *(C)*. This results in a much less favorable crown-to-root ratio, which may not in fact strengthen the restoration.
(Courtesy Dr. A.G. Gegauff. From Gegauff AG: J Dent Res 78:223, 1999 [abstract].)

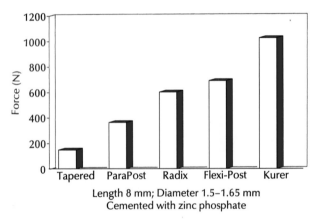

Fig. 12-13. Comparison of forces needed to remove different prefabricated post systems.
(Redrawn from Standlee JP, Caputo AA: J Prosthet Dent 68:436,1992.)

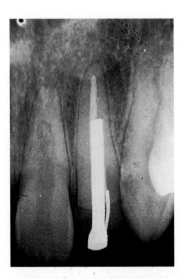

Fig. 12-14. The use of a parallel-sided post in a tapered canal requires considerable enlargement of the post space, which can weaken the root significantly.
(Courtesy Dr. R. Webber.)

crown lengthening resulted in a weaker, rather than a stronger, restored tooth.[25] Creating a ferrule with orthodontic extrusion may be preferred as, although the root is effectively shortened, the crown is not lengthened (see Fig. 12-12, *B*).

RETENTION FORM

Anterior Teeth. Dislodgment of a post-retained anterior crown is frequently seen clinically and results from inadequate retention form of the prepared root. Post retention is affected by the preparation geometry, post length, diameter, **surface texture,** and by the luting agent.

Preparation Geometry. Some canals, particularly in maxillary central incisors, have a nearly circular cross section (see Table 12-3). These can be prepared with a twist drill or reamer to provide a cavity with parallel walls or minimal taper, allowing the use of a preformed post of corresponding size and configuration. Conversely, canals with elliptical cross sections must be prepared with a restricted amount of taper (usually 6 to 8 degrees) to ensure adequate retention while eliminating undesired undercuts. This is analogous to an extracoronal preparation (see Chapter 7). With extracoronal preparations, retention increases rapidly as vertical wall taper is reduced (see Chapter 7). Although retention can be further increased by using a threaded post, which screws into dentin, this procedure is not recommended because of residual stress in the dentin. If the procedure is used, however, threaded posts must be "backed off" to ensure passivity; otherwise, the root will fracture.

Laboratory testing[26-28] has confirmed that parallel-sided posts are more retentive than tapered posts and that threaded posts are the most retentive (Fig. 12-13). However, these comparisons are relevant

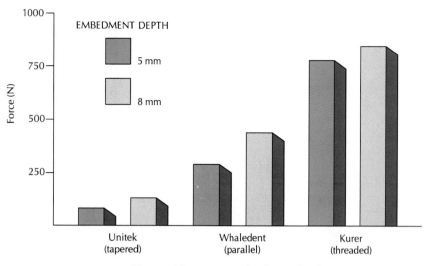

Fig. 12-15. Effect of the depth of embedding a post on its retentive capacity. *(Data from Standlee JP et al: J Prosthet Dent 39:401, 1978.)*

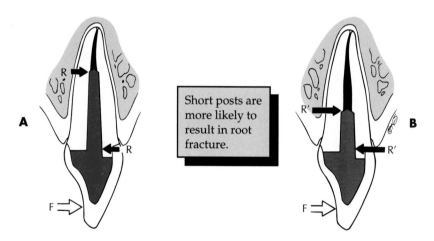

Fig. 12-16. Faciolingual longitudinal sections through a maxillary central incisor. **A,** With a post of the correct length, a force *(F)* applied near the incisal edge of the crown will generate a resultant couple *(R)*. **B,** When the post is too short, this couple will be greater *(R')*, leading to the increased possibility of root fracture.

only if the post fits the root canal properly, because retention is proportional to the total surface area.

Circular parallel post systems are only effective in the most apical portion of the post space because the majority of prepared post spaces demonstrate considerable flare in the occlusal half. Similarly, when the root canal is elliptical, a parallel-sided post will not be effective unless the canal is considerably enlarged, which would significantly weaken the root unnecessarily (Fig. 12-14).

Post Length. Studies[26,28,29] have shown that as post length increases, so does retention. However, the relationship is not necessarily linear (Fig. 12-15). A post that is too short will fail (Fig. 12-16), whereas one that is too long may damage the seal of the root

canal fill or risk root perforation if the apical third is curved or tapered (Fig. 12-17). Absolute guidelines for optimal post length are difficult to define. Ideally, the post should be as long as possible without jeopardizing the apical seal or the strength or integrity of the remaining root structure. Most endodontic texts advocate maintaining a 5-mm apical seal. However, if a post is shorter than the coronal height of the clinical crown of the tooth, the prognosis is considered unfavorable, because stress is distributed over a smaller surface area, thereby increasing the probability of radicular fracture. A short root and a tall clinical crown present the clinician with the dilemma of having to compromise the mechanics, the apical seal, or both. Under such circumstances, an apical seal of 3 mm is considered acceptable.

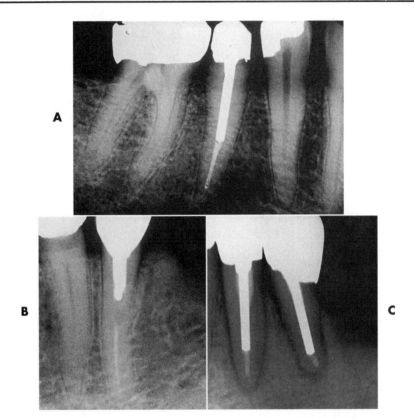

Fig. 12-17. **A,** Correct post length. **B,** The post is too short; the consequences are inadequate retention and increased risk of root fracture. **C,** The post is too long, jeopardizing the apical seal.

Post Diameter. Increasing the post diameter in an attempt to increase retention is not recommended because it may unnecessarily weaken the remaining root. Although one group of investigators[30] reported that increasing the post diameter increased retention, other groups do not confirm this.[26,27] Empirical evidence suggests that the overall prognosis is good when post diameter does not exceed one third of the cross-sectional diameter of the root.

Post Surface Texture. A serrated or roughened post is more retentive than a smooth one,[27] and controlled grooving of the post and root canal[31] (Fig. 12-18) considerably increases the retention of a tapered post.

Luting Agent. When considering traditional cements, the choice of luting agent seems to have little effect on post retention[32,33] or the fracture resistance of dentin.[34] However, adhesive resin luting agents (see Chapter 31) have the potential to improve the performance of post-and-core restorations; laboratory studies have shown improved retention.[35,36] Resin cements may be indicated if a post becomes dislodged. Resin cements are affected by eugenol-containing root canal sealers, which should

be removed by irrigation with ethanol or etching with 37% phosphoric acid if the adhesive is to be effective.[37] Zinc phosphate and glass ionomer have similar retentive properties—polycarboxylate and composite resin have slightly less.[38] Some resin and glass ionomer cements have demonstrated significantly higher retention in comparison to hybrid cements.[39] Although the choice of luting agent may become more important if the post has a poor fit within the canal,[40] a post-and-core should be remade if any rotation or wobble is present.

Posterior Teeth (Fig. 12-19). Relatively long posts with a circular cross section provide good retention and support in anterior teeth but should be avoided in posterior teeth, which often have curved roots and elliptical or ribbon-shaped canals. For these teeth, retention is better provided by two or more relatively short posts in the divergent canals.

When amalgam is used as the core material, it can be condensed either around cemented metal posts or directly into short, prepared post spaces. If more than 3 to 4 mm of coronal tooth structure remains, use of the root canals for retention is not necessary, and this avoids the chance of perforation.[41] Using the canals for retention can provide good results,[42] although the strength of the tooth once a complete

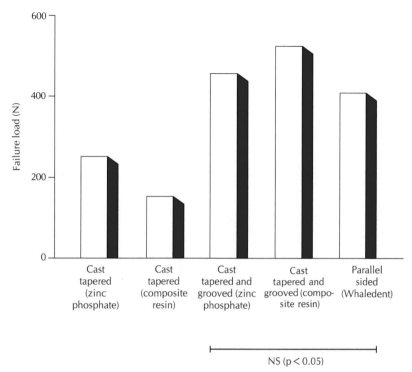

NS (p < 0.05)

Fig. 12-18.   Effect of horizontal grooving on the retention of tapered posts. *NS,* Not significant. *(Modified slightly from Wood WW: J Prosthet Dent 49:504, 1983.)*

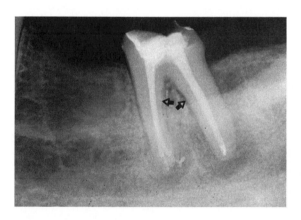

Fig. 12-19.   When preparing posterior teeth for intra-coronal retention, the practitioner must be careful to avoid perforation, especially on the distal surface of mesial roots and the mesial surface of distal roots, where residual tooth structure is normally thinnest *(arrows).*

crown has been provided is not dramatically influenced by differences in technique.

Mandibular premolars and molars with a reasonable amount of remaining coronal tooth structure, when coupled with a circumferential cervical band of tooth structure with restricted taper of about 2 mm, can often be restored with amalgam directly condensed into the chamber. Core buildups in molars with one or more missing cusps will benefit from one or more cemented posts around which the amalgam can be condensed. The posts provide the

additional retention, which was compromised because of the missing tooth structure. In mandibular molars, the larger distal canal is recommended for post placement. In maxillary molars, the palatal canal is used (see Fig.12-2, *C* and *D*).

Although it is possible to restore a molar with three or more missing cusps with multiple posts and amalgam, the tooth's overall importance must be assessed. If retaining the tooth is critical, a cast core can be used (made in sections that have different paths of withdrawal) (Fig. 12-20). An alternative preparation method for a posterior tooth is selecting the canals that are widest (normally the palatal of maxillary molars and the distal of mandibular molars) for the major post and then preparing short auxiliary post spaces in the other canals with the same path of withdrawal (Fig. 12-21).

RESISTANCE FORM

Stress Distribution.   One of the functions of a post-and-core is to improve resistance to laterally directed forces by distributing them over as large an area as possible. However, excessive internal preparation of the root weakens it, and the possibility of failure increases. The post design should distribute stresses as evenly as possible. The incidence of radicular fracture increases with the use of threaded posts, and threaded flexible posts do not appear to reduce stress concentrations during function.

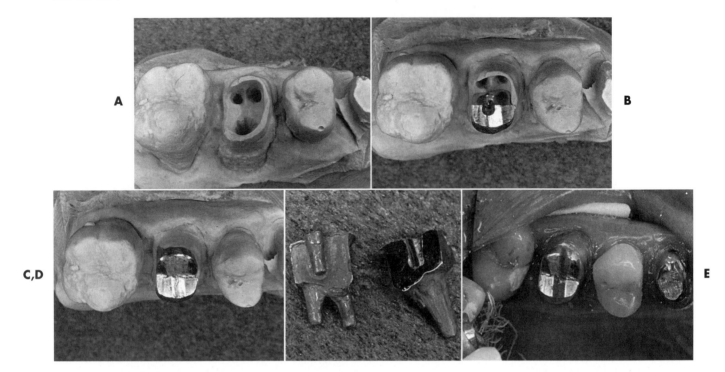

Fig. 12-20. Cast cores for posterior teeth can be made in interlocking sections, with each section having its own path of withdrawal.

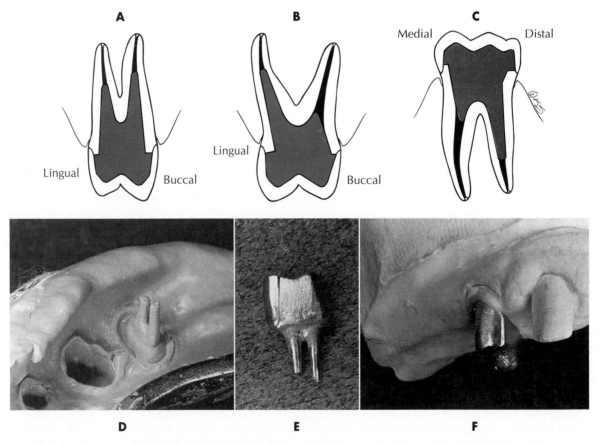

Fig. 12-21. Single-piece castings can be made by selecting the larger-diameter canal and extending a second post for a limited distance into the smaller canal. **A,** A maxillary first premolar. **B,** A maxillary first molar. **C,** A mandibular first molar. **D** to **F,** Post-and-core provided for a maxillary first premolar by the indirect technique.

The influence of post design on **stress distribution** has been tested using photoelastic materials,[18,29,43-45] strain gauges,[46,47] and finite element analysis.[48,49] From these laboratory studies, the following conclusions have been drawn:

1. The greatest stress concentrations are found at the shoulder, particularly interproximally, and at the apex. Dentin should be conserved in these areas if possible.
2. Stresses are reduced as post length increases.
3. Parallel-sided posts may distribute stress more evenly than tapered posts, which may have a wedging effect. However, parallel posts generate high stresses at the apex.
4. Sharp angles should be avoided because they produce high stresses during loading.
5. High stress can be generated during insertion, particularly with smooth, parallel-sided posts that have no vent for cement escape.
6. Threaded posts can produce high stress concentrations during insertion and loading, but they have been shown to distribute stress evenly if the posts are backed off a half-turn and when the head contact area is of sufficient size.[35]
7. The cement layer results in a more even stress distribution to the root with less stress concentrations.

Rotational Resistance (Fig. 12-22). It is important that a post with a circular cross section does not rotate during function. This should not present a problem in areas where sufficient coronal tooth structure remains, because rotation is usually prevented by a vertical coronal wall. In areas where coronal dentin has been completely lost, a small groove placed in the canal can serve as an antirota-

tional element. The groove is normally located where the root is bulkiest, usually on the lingual aspect. Alternatively, rotation can be prevented by an auxiliary pin in the root face. Rotation of a threaded post can also be prevented[28] by preparing a small cavity (half in the post, half in the root) and condensing amalgam into it after the post is cemented.

PROCEDURES

Tooth preparation for endodontically treated teeth can be considered a three-stage operation:

1. Removal of the root canal filling material to the appropriate depth
2. Enlargement of the canal
3. Preparation of the coronal tooth structure

REMOVAL OF THE ENDODONTIC FILLING MATERIAL

The root canal system should first be completely obturated; space should then be made for a post, thus ensuring that lateral canals are sealed. A post cannot be placed if the canal is filled with a full-length silver point, so these must be removed and the tooth retreated with gutta-percha.

There are two commonly used methods to remove gutta-percha (Fig. 12-23): one uses a warmed endodontic plugger, and the other uses a rotary instrument, which is sometimes used in conjunction with chemical agents. Although it is more time consuming, the warmed endodontic plugger is preferred because it eliminates the possibility that the rotary instrument will inadvertently damage the dentin. If it is more convenient, the gutta-percha can be removed with a warmed condenser immediately after obturation (although not with a rotary instrument). This will not disturb the apical seal.[50,51] This method offers the additional advantage of allowing the operator to work in an area where the root canal anatomy is still familiar.

1. Before removing gutta-percha, calculate the appropriate length of the post. It should be adequate for retention and resistance but not long enough to weaken the apical seal. As a guide, make the post length *equal to the height of the anatomic crown* (or two-thirds the length of the root), but *leave 5 mm of apical gutta-percha*. On short teeth, it will not be possible to meet both these restrictions, and a compromise must be made. An absolute minimum of 3 mm of apical fill is needed. If this cannot be achieved without having a very short post, the tooth's prognosis is seriously impaired.
2. Avoid the apical 5 mm if possible. Curvatures and lateral canals may be found in this segment. Average values for crown and root length are given in Table 12-1. If the working length of the root canal is known, the length

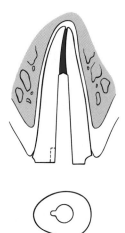

Fig. 12-22. Rotational resistance in an extensively damaged tooth can be obtained by preparing a small groove in the root canal. This must be in the path of placement of the post-and-core.

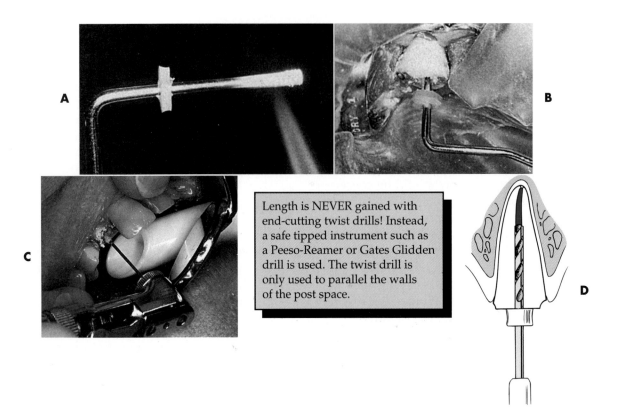

Fig. 12-23. Gutta-percha can be removed from the canal with a heated endodontic plugger (**A** and **B**), a non–end-cutting bur (**C**) (e.g., a Gates Glidden drill), or a ParaPost drill (**D**) (with a rubber stop to ensure accuracy of the preparation depth).
(*A and B courtesy Dr. D.A. Miller.*)

Length is NEVER gained with end-cutting twist drills! Instead, a safe tipped instrument such as a Peeso-Reamer or Gates Glidden drill is used. The twist drill is only used to parallel the walls of the post space.

Average Crown and Root Lengths (mm) (n = 50 for each tooth)				TABLE 12-1
	Mean Crown Length*	Mean Root Length*	Two Thirds Root Length	Root Length (to 4 mm from apex)
MAXILLARY TEETH				
Central incisor	10.8 ± 0.7	12.5 ± 1.6	8.3	8.5
Lateral incisor	9.7 ± 0.9	13.1 ± 1.4	8.7	9.1
Canine	10.2 ± 0.8	15.8 ± 2.1	10.5	11.8
First premolar	8.6 ± 0.8	12.7 ± 1.7	8.5	8.7
Second premolar	7.5 ± 0.6	13.5 ± 1.4	9.0	9.5
First molar	7.4 ± 0.5	MF 12.5 ± 1.2	8.3	8.5
		DF 12.0 ± 1.3	8.0	8.0
		L 13.2 ± 1.4	8.8	9.2
Second molar	7.4 ± 0.5	MF 12.8 ± 1.5	8.5	8.8
		DF 12.0 ± 1.4	8.0	8.0
		L 13.4 ± 1.3	8.9	9.4
MANDIBULAR TEETH				
Central incisor	9.1 ± 0.5	12.4 ± 1.4	8.3	8.4
Lateral incisor	9.4 ± 0.7	13.0 ± 1.5	8.7	9.0
Canine	10.9 ± 0.9	14.3 ± 1.4	9.5	10.3
First premolar	8.7 ± 0.7	13.4 ± 1.3	8.9	9.4
Second premolar	7.8 ± 0.6	13.6 ± 1.7	9.1	9.6
First molar	7.4 ± 0.5	M 13.5 ± 1.3	9.0	9.5
		D 13.4 ± 1.3	8.9	9.4
Second molar	7.5 ± 0.5	M 13.4 ± 1.2	8.9	9.4
		D 13.3 ± 1.3	8.9	9.3

MF, Mesiofacial M, Mesial
DF, Distofacial D, Distal
L, Lingual.

Data from Shillingburg HT et al: *Calif Dent Assoc J* 10:43, 1982.
*SD listed after mean length.

of the post space can be easily determined. Therefore, the incisal or occlusal reference point must not be lost as a result of premature removal of coronal tooth structure.

3. To prevent aspiration of an endodontic instrument, apply a rubber dam before preparing the post space.

4. Select an endodontic condenser large enough to hold heat well but not so large that it binds against the canal walls.

5. Mark it at the appropriate length (normally endodontic working length minus 5 mm), heat it, and place it in the canal to soften the gutta-percha.

6. If the gutta-percha is old and has lost its thermoplasticity, use a rotary instrument, making sure that it follows the gutta-percha and does not engage dentin (this will cause a root perforation). For this reason, high-speed instruments and conventional burs are contraindicated. Special post preparation instruments are available (Fig. 12-24). Peeso-Reamers and Gates Glidden drills are often used for this purpose. These are considered "safe-tip" instruments because they are not end-cutting burs. The friction generated between the fill and the tip of these burs softens the gutta-percha, allowing the rotary instrument to track the canal with reasonable predictability. One study comparing rotary instruments[52] concluded that the Gates Glidden drill conformed to the original canal more consistently than the ParaPost drill, which is an end-cutting instrument. The latter is a twist drill and should only be used to parallel the walls of the post space. Considerable heat can be generated when using these rotary instruments, especially during the ParaPost preparation stage.[53]

NOTE: End-cutting instruments should *never* be used to gain length because root perforation will result!

7. If using a rotary instrument, choose it to be slightly narrower than the canal.

8. Make sure the instrument follows the center of the gutta-percha and does not cut dentin. Often, only a part of the root canal fill needs to be removed with a rotary instrument, and the remainder can be removed with the heated condenser. A rotary instrument should not be used immediately after obturation, because it may disturb the apical seal.[54]

9. When the gutta-percha has been removed to the appropriate depth, shape the canal as needed.

This can be accomplished by using an endodontic hand instrument or a low-speed drill. This procedure removes undercuts and prepares the canal to receive an appropriately sized post without excessively enlarging the canal. Files are a conservative approach to shaping the canal walls and permit simultaneous removal of any small residual undercuts in the chamber. If a parallel-shaped post is desired, a low-speed twist drill set to the same length as the most recently used Peeso-Reamer can be used.

The post should be no more than one third the diameter of the root,[1,55] with the root and walls at least 1 mm thick. Obviously, when deciding on appropriate post diameters, a knowledge of average root dimensions is important. These have been calculated[56] and are presented in Table 12-2. Knowledge of root canal cross section also is significant in post selection. **Prefabricated posts** are circular in cross section, but many root canals are elliptical, which makes uniform reduction with a drill impossible. A summary of canal shapes is presented in Table 12-3.

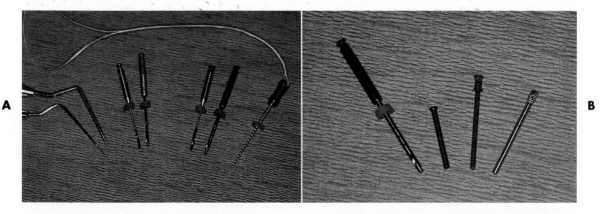

Fig. 12-24. Commonly used instruments for gutta-percha removal and canal enlargement. **A,** Endodontic pluggers, two sizes of Peeso-Reamers with corresponding twist drills and endodontic file. Note attached floss as a safety precaution. **B,** The ParaPost twist drill corresponds in size to an aluminum post used to fabricate provisionals, a plastic post for patterns, and a stainless-steel or titanium post. *(Courtesy Dr. J.A. Nelson.)*

Average Root Diameters and Recommended Post Sizes (mm)* — TABLE 12-2

	CEJ	Furcation†	Midpoint	Diameter 4 mm from Apex‡	Recommended Post Diameter
MAXILLARY TEETH					
Central incisor	MD 6.3 ± 0.5	—	5.2 ± 0.5	3.8 ± 0.4	1.7
	FL 6.4 ± 0.4	—	5.8 ± 0.4	4.3 ± 0.4	
Lateral incisor	MD 4.9 ± 0.5	—	4.0 ± 0.5	3.2 ± 0.5	1.3
	FL 5.7 ± 0.5	—	5.4 ± 0.5	4.2 ± 0.4	
Canine	MD 5.4 ± 0.5	—	4.4 ± 0.5	3.3 ± 0.5	1.5
	FL 7.7 ± 0.6	—	7.2 ± 0.6	4.8 ± 0.6	
First premolar	MD 4.1 ± 0.3	Facial MD —	3.6 ± 0.4	2.6 ± 0.4	0.9
	FL 8.1 ± 0.7	FL —	3.4 ± 0.4	2.4 ± 0.4	
		Lingual MD —	3.3 ± 0.3	2.5 ± 0.4	0.9
		Fl —	3.3 ± 0.4	2.4 ± 0.5	
Second premolar	MD 4.9 ± 0.3	—	3.8 ± 0.4	3.2 ± 0.6	1.1
	FL 7.9 ± 0.5	—	7.0 ± 0.7	5.0 ± 0.7	
First molar	MD 7.7 ± 0.4	Mesio- MD 3.4 ± 0.3	3.1 ± 0.3	2.9 ± 0.4	1.1
	FL 10.5 ± 0.5	Facial FL 6.8 ± 0.5	5.8 ± 0.7	4.8 ± 0.7	
		Disto- MD 3.1 ± 0.2	2.8 ± 0.3	2.6 ± 0.4	1.1
		Facial FL 5.0 ± 0.4	4.4 ± 0.5	3.8 ± 0.5	
		Lingual MD 5.7 ± 0.5	5.0 ± 0.5	4.4 ± 0.5	1.3
		FL 4.3 ± 0.4	3.7 ± 0.4	3.3 ± 0.4	
Second molar	MD 7.3 ± 0.4	Mesio- MD 3.4 ± 0.3	3.1 ± 0.3	2.7 ± 0.4	1.1
	FL 10.4 ± 0.6	Facial FL 6.6 ± 0.5	5.6 ± 0.7	4.5 ± 0.7	
		Disto- MD 3.1 ± 0.4	2.8 ± 0.3	24 ± 0.4	0.9
		Facial FL 4.3 ± 0.4	3.8 ± 0.4	3.2 ± 0.4	
		Lingual MD 4.9 ± 0.5	4.2 ± 0.5	3.6 ± 0.5	1.3
		FL 4.5 ± 0.4	3.9 ± 0.4	3.1 ± 0.4	
MANDIBULAR TEETH					
Central incisor	MD 3.3 ± 0.3	—	2.7 ± 0.3	2.1 ± 0.2	0.7
	FL 5.5 ± 0.5		5.6 ± 0.4	4.3 ± 0.6	
Lateral incisor	MD 3.6 ± 0.3	—	2.7 ± 0.4	2.0 ± 0.2	0.7
	FL 5.9 ± 0.4		5.7 ± 0.5	4.3 ± 0.5	
Canine	MD 5.2 ± 0.6	—	4.0 ± 0.5	3.2 ± 0.7	1.5
	FL 7.8 ± 0.8		7.3 ± 0.6	5.0 ± 0.5	
First premolar	MD 5.1 ± 0.4	—	4.0 ± 0.4	3.2 ± 0.4	1.3
	FL 6.6 ± 0.4		6.0 ± 0.5	4.3 ± 0.5	
Second premolar	MD 5.3 ± 0.3	—	4.3 ± 0.3	3.5 ± 0.5	1.3
	FL 7.0 ± 0.5		6.0 ± 0.6	4.4 ± 0.5	
First molar	MD 8.9 ± 0.6	Mesio- MD 3.7 ± 0.2	3.2 ± 0.3	2.8 ± 0.3	1.1
	FL 8.3 ± 0.6	Facial FL 3.4 ± 0.3	3.1 ± 0.3	2.8 ± 0.4	
		Mesio- MD 3.4 ± 0.3	2.9 ± 0.3	2.5 ± 0.3	0.9
		Lingual FL 3.5 ± 0.4	3.2 ± 0.3	2.7 ± 0.4	
		Distal MD 3.5 ± 0.4	2.8 ± 0.4	2.7 ± 0.4	1.1
		FL 7.6 ± 0.8	6.6 ± 1.2	5.4 ± 0.8	
Second molar	MD 9.3 ± 0.7	Mesio- MD 3.6 ± 0.3	3.1 ± 0.3	2.6 ± 0.3	0.9
	FL 8.3 ± 0.7	Facial FL 3.2 ± 0.3	2.8 ± 0.3	2.4 ± 0.4	
		Mesio- MD 3.6 ± 0.4	3.0 ± 0.4	2.5 ± 0.4	0.9
		Lingual FL 3.2 ± 0.5	2.8 ± 0.4	2.3 ± 0.4	
		Distal MD 4.1 ± 0.4	3.5 ± 0.4	3.0 ± 0.4	1.1
		FL 6.8 ± 0.8	5.9 ± 0.9	4.7 ± 0.7	

Data from Shillingburg HT et al: *Calif Dent Assoc J* 10:43, 1982.

*N = 50 for each tooth.

†Furcation distance from the CEJ: maxillary first molar, 4.1 mm; maxillary second molar, 3.2 mm; mandibular first molar, 3.1 mm; mandibular second molar, 3.3 mm.

‡Because of greater root length, the mean distance from the apex on maxillary canine measurements is 5.1 mm.

ENLARGEMENT OF THE CANAL

Before enlargement of the canal, the type of post system to be used for fabrication of the post-and-core must be chosen.

The advantages and disadvantages of different **post types** are summarized in Table 12-4. Because no system has universal application, being familiar with more than one technique is a significant

Root Canal Configurations — TABLE 12-3

Circular	Elliptical Buccolingual	Elliptical Mesiodistal
Maxillary central incisor	Maxillary lateral incisor Maxillary canine Mandibular incisors Mandibular canine	
Maxillary first premolar (two roots)	Maxillary first premolar (single root) Mandibular first premolar	
Mandibular second premolar	Maxillary second premolar	
Maxillary molars (distobuccal roots)	Maxillary molars (mesiobuccal roots) Mandibular molars (mesial and distal roots)	Maxillary molars (palatal roots)

From Weine FS: *Endodontic therapy,* ed 4, St Louis, 1989, Mosby, pp 225–269.

Available Post-and-Core Systems — TABLE 12-4

	Advantages	Disadvantages	Recommended Use	Precautions
Amalgam	Conservative of tooth structure Straightforward technique	Low tensile strength Corrosion with base metal	Molars with adequate coronal tooth structure	Not recommended in teeth under lateral load (anteriors)
Glass ionomer	Conservative of tooth structure Straightforward technique	Difficult condensation Low strength	Teeth with minimum tooth structure missing	Not recommended in teeth under lateral load
Composite resin	Conservative of tooth structure Straightforward technique	Low strength Continued polymerization Microleakage	Teeth with minimum tooth structure missing	Not recommended in teeth under lateral load
Custom cast post-and-core	High strength Better fit than prefabricated	Less stiff than wrought Time consuming, complex procedure	Elliptical or flared canals	Care to remove nodules before try-in
Wire post and cast core	High strength High stiffness	Corrosion of base metal Pt-Au-Pd wire expensive	Small circular canals	Care to avoid perforation during preparation
Tapered prefabricated post	Conservative of tooth structure High strength and stiffness	Less retentive than parallel-sided or threaded systems	Small circular canals	Not recommended for excessively flared canals
Parallel-sided prefabricated post	High strength Good retention Comprehensive system	Precious-metal post expensive Corrosion of stainless-steel Less conservative of tooth structure	Small circular canals	Care during preparation
Threaded post	High retention	Stresses generated in canal may lead to fracture Not conservative of coronal and radicular tooth structure	Only when maximum retention is essential	Care to avoid fracture during seating
Carbon fiber post	Dentin bonding Easy removal	Low strength Microleakage Black color	Minimal missing tooth structure Uncertain endodontic prognosis	Not recommended for teeth under lateral load
Zirconia ceramic posts	Esthetics High stiffness	Uncertain clinical performance	High esthetic demand	
Woven fiber posts	Esthetics Dentin bonding	Low strength Uncertain clinical performance	High esthetic demand	Not recommended for teeth under lateral load

advantage. A wide range of prefabricated posts are available. They come in many shapes and sizes (Table 12-5 and Figs. 12-25 and 12-26). The diameters of nine popular prefabricated posts are given in Table 12-6. Parallel-sided prefabricated posts are recommended for conservatively prepared root canals in teeth with roots of circular cross section. Excessively flared canals (e.g., those found in young persons or in individuals after retreatment of an endodontic failure) are most effectively managed with a custom post. However, situations should be evaluated on an individual basis.

Text continued on p. 297

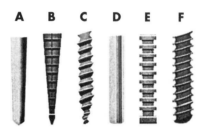

Fig. 12-25. Classification of prefabricated posts. **A,** Tapered, smooth-sided posts. **B,** Tapered, serrated posts. **C,** Tapered, threaded posts. **D,** Parallel, smooth-sided posts. **E,** Parallel, serrated posts. **F,** Parallel, threaded posts.
(Redrawn from Shillingburg HT, Kessler JC: Restoration of the endodontically treated tooth, Chicago, 1982, Quintessence Publishing.)

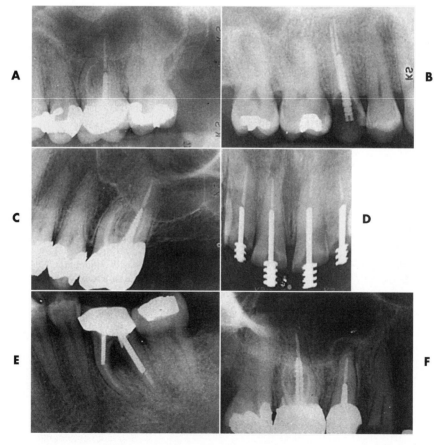

Fig. 12-26. Radiographs of the six categories of endodontic posts. **A,** KG Endowel, tapered and smooth sided. **B,** Unimetric, tapered and serrated. **C,** Dentatus, tapered and threaded. **D,** CTH Beta, parallel sided and smooth. **E,** ParaPost (two sizes), parallel sided and serrated. **F,** Flexi-Post (in the right maxillary first molar), parallel sided and threaded (note the split shank).
(A courtesy Dr. D.A. Miller and Dr. H.W. Zuckerman; B courtesy Dr. I.A. Roseman; C courtesy Dr. F.S. Weine and Dr. S. Strauss; D courtesy Dr. J.F. Tardera; E courtesy Dr. J.L. Wingo; F courtesy Dr. L.R. Farsakian.)

TABLE 12-5 Currently Available Prefabricated Posts*

Example†	Product (Vendor)	Composition‡	Shank Characteristics	Diameter (mm)§
TAPERED SMOOTH POSTS				
	C-I Post (Parkell Products)	PB, SS	Flat tip	1.3 & 1.6
	ER Casting Post (Brasseler USA)	PB	Flat tip	1.1 to 1.7
	ER Cerapost (Brasseler USA)	ZrO₂	Blunt tip	1.1 to 1.7
	ER Post System (Brasseler USA)	Ti alloy	Blunt tip	1.1 to 1.7
	ER PCR Post (Brasseler USA)	Ti alloy	Blunt tip	1.1 to 1.7
	Cytco (Dentsply Maillefer)	Ti alloy	Blunt tip, 3 coronal threads	0.9 & 1.2
	Filpost (Filhol Dental USA)	Ti	Blunt tip	1.3 & 1.6
	Plastic Impression Pin (Union Broach)	PB	Blunt tip	1.4 & 1.7
	Colorama (Metalor Dental USA)	PB	Blunt tip	1.3 to 2.0
	Endodontic Post (Sterngold)	PB	Blunt tip	1.7 & 1.8
	Luscent Anchors (Dentatus USA)	Fiberglass-resin	Blunt tip	1.1 to 1.6
	Stress-Free Post (Denovo)	SS	Blunt tip, ISO‖ sizes: 50 to 130	0.7 to 1.5
	Endowel (Star Dental)	PB	Pointed tip, ISO‖ sizes: 80 to 140	1.0 to 1.6
	UM C-POST (Bisco)	Carbon fiber-resin	Pointed tip, ISO‖ sizes: 100, 120, 140	1.2 to 1.6
	PD Sprues (R Chige)	PB, SS	Pointed tip	1.1 to 2.1
TAPERED SERRATED POSTS				
	Unimetric (Dentsply Maillefer)	Ti alloy	Knurled	1.6 to 1.8
	PD Solid & Hollow Post (R Chige)	SS	Knurled	1.1 to 2.1

*Posts are categorized by their radiographic silhouette from the apical 8 mm of the shank.
†Posts are not photographed to scale.
‡Composition key: *Au,* Gold; *Brass,* alloy of copper and zinc (brass posts are gold plated); Carbon fibers bound by epoxy-resin matrix; *Cu,* copper; *Ni,* nickel; *PB,* plastic burnout; *Pd,* palladium; *SS,* stainless steel; *Ti,* titanium (*Ti* indicates approximately 99% pure titanium; *Ti alloy* indicates a content of approximately 90% titanium); *ZrO₂,* zirconium dioxide.
§Shank diameter includes the threads of relevant posts; diameters of tapered posts are taken 8 mm from the apical tip.
‖ISO indicates that the post corresponds to standardized file sizes (set by the International Standards Organization).

Continued

TABLE 12-5 Currently Available Prefabricated Posts—cont'd

Example[†]	Product (Vendor)	Composition[‡]	Shank Characteristics	Diameter (mm)[§]
	TAPERED SERRATED POSTS—cont'd			
	NuBond (Ellman International)	SS	Knurled	0.9 to 2.0
	Davis Crown Post (Union Broach)	SS	Deeply grooved	1.8 to 2.0
	Luminex (Dentatus USA)	PB	Deeply grooved	1.1 to 1.8
	TAPERED THREADED POSTS			
	Ancorex (E C Moore)	Ti	Tightly threaded	1.1 to 1.8
	Ancorextra (E C Moore)	Ti	Tightly threaded	1.1 to 1.8
	Dentatus Classic Post (Dentatus USA)	Ti, SS, Brass	Tightly threaded	1.1 to 1.8
	Tapered Obturation Post (Union Broach)	SS	Tightly threaded	1.2 to 1.6
	Ventra-Post (Ellman International)	SS	Sparsely threaded	1.4
	PARALLEL-SIDED SMOOTH POSTS			
	C-Post (Bisco)	Carbon fiber-resin	Dual size shank, tapered apical end	1.4 to 2.1
	Aestheti-Post (Bisco)	Carbon fiber-resin	Dual size shank, tapered apical end	1.4 to 2.1
	IntegraPost System (Premier)	Ti alloy	Vertical serrations, flat tip	0.9 to 1.5
	CTH Beta Post (CTH)	SS	Vertical grooves, flat tip	1.1 to 1.6
	CTH R Series (CTH)	SS	Vertical grooves, flat tip	1.1 to 1.6
	ProPost (Dentsply Tulsa Dental)	SS	Smooth, tapered apical end	0.8 to 1.4
	Vario Cast Passive Post (Brasseler USA)	PB	Smooth, blunt tip	1.2 to 1.6
	PARALLEL-SIDED SERRATED POSTS			
	ParaPost (Coltène/Whaledent)	Ti alloy, PB, SS	Fine serrations, flat tip	0.9 to 1.8
	ParaPost XP (Coltène/Whaledent)	Ti alloy, PB, SS	Diamond-shaped grooves, flat tip	0.9 to 1.8
	Unity (Coltène/Whaledent)	Ti alloy, PB	Diamond-shaped grooves, flat tip	0.9 to 1.8

Currently Available Prefabricated Posts—cont'd

TABLE 12-5

Example†	Product (Vendor)	Composition‡	Shank Characteristics	Diameter (mm)§
	ParaPost XH (Coltène/Whaledent)	Ti alloy	Diamond-shaped-grooves, flat tip	0.9 to 1.8
	ParaPost Plus (Coltène/Whaledent)	Ti alloy, SS	Serrated ledges, flat tip	0.9 to 1.8
	FibreKor Post System (Jeneric/Pentron)	Glass fiber-resin	Serrated ledges, flat tip	1.0 to 1.5
	ExactaCast (Essential Dental Systems)	PB	Wide grooves, flat tip	0.7 to 1.5
	Vario Passive Post (Brasseler USA)	Ti alloy	Wide grooves, flat tip	1.2 to 1.6
	Vario PCR Passive Post (Brasseler USA)	Ti alloy	Wide grooves, flat tip	1.2 to 1.6
	Vlock Passive Post (Brasseler USA)	Ti alloy	Wide grooves, flat tip	1.2 to 1.6
	Micropost (Danville Engineering)	Ti alloy	Fine grooves, flat tip	0.8 to 1.6
	SB Post (J Morita USA)	SS	Fine grooves, tapered tip	0.8 to 1.6
	Versadowel-A Series (Western Dental)	SS	Fine grooves, tapered tip	0.8 to 1.3
	Versadowel-M Series (Western Dental)	SS	Fine grooves, tapered tip	0.8 to 1.3
	Versadowel-U Series (Western Dental)	SS	Fine grooves, tapered tip	0.8 to 1.3
	AccessPost (Essential Dental Systems)	SS	Spiraling groove, flat tip	0.8 to 1.6
	AccessPost Overdenture (Essential Dental Systems)	SS	Spiraling groove, flat tip	1.1 to 1.6
	ERA Direct Overdenture (Sterngold)	SS	Fine serrations, flat tip	1.4 & 1.7
	PARALLEL-SIDED THREADED POSTS			
	Compo-Post (Henry Schein)	Brass	Tightly threaded, pointed tip	1.1 to 1.8
	Golden Screw Post (EC Moore)	Brass	Tightly threaded, pointed tip	1.1 to 1.8
	Titanium Screw Post (EC Moore)	Ti	Tightly threaded, pointed tip	1.1 to 1.8
	Boston Post (Roydent Dental Products)	Ti	Tightly threaded, pointed tip	1.0 to 1.6
	Obturation Post (Union Broach)	SS	Tightly threaded, pointed tip	1.3

Continued

TABLE 12-5

Currently Available Prefabricated Posts—*cont'd*

PARALLEL-SIDED THREADED POSTS—cont'd

Example†	Product (Vendor)	Composition‡	Shank Characteristics	Diameter (mm)§
	K4 Ready Core Anchor (Teledyne Water Pik)	SS	Tightly threaded, flat tip	1.6 to 2.0
	K4 Universal Anchor (Teledyne Water Pik)	SS	Tightly threaded, flat tip	1.5 to 2.0
	K4 Custom Core Anchor (Teledyne Water Pik)	SS	Tightly threaded, flat tip	1.7 to 2.0
	K4 Denture Anchor (Teledyne Water Pik)	SS	Tightly threaded, flat tip	1.8 to 2.0
	Sure-Grip (R Chige)	SS	Sparsely threaded, blunt tip	0.9 to 1.9
	Vlock Active Post (Brasseler USA)	Ti alloy	Sparsely threaded, blunt tip	1.3 to 1.8
	Vario Active Post (Brasseler USA)	Ti alloy	Sparsely threaded, blunt tip	1.3 to 1.8
	Vario ELO Active Post (Brasseler USA)	Ti alloy	Sparsely threaded, flat tip	1.3 to 1.8
	Radix-Ankor (Dentsply Maillefer)	Ti alloy	Sparsely threaded, flat tip	1.2 to 1.6
	ParaPost XT (Coltène/Whaledent)	Ti alloy	Sparsely threaded, grooves, flat tip	0.9 to 1.5
	Flexi-Post (Essential Dental Systems)	Ti alloy, SS	Sparsely threaded, split shank	1.0 to 1.9
	Flexi-Flange (Essential Dental Systems)	Ti alloy, SS	Sparsely threaded, split shank	1.1 to 1.9
	Flexi-Overdenture (Essential Dental Systems)	Ti alloy, SS	Sparsely threaded, split shank	1.4 to 1.9

Post	0.80	0.90	0.95	1.00	1.05	1.15	1.20	1.25	1.35	1.40	1.45	1.50	1.60	1.65	1.75	1.80	1.85	1.90	2.00
Diameters of 8 Commonly Used Prefabricated Posts (mm) — TABLE **12-6**																			
Boston*		X					X					X							
Dentatus*			X		X		X			X		X		X					
Flexi-Post*		X		X						X				X				X	
Stress-free post size 70	†	‡																	
Ky Universal Anchor										X		X	X				X		X
ParaPost		X		X				X			X				X				
Radix*					X		X					X	X						
Vlock Passive Post					X		X					X							

*Diameter includes threads.
†5 mm from tip.
‡10 mm from tip.

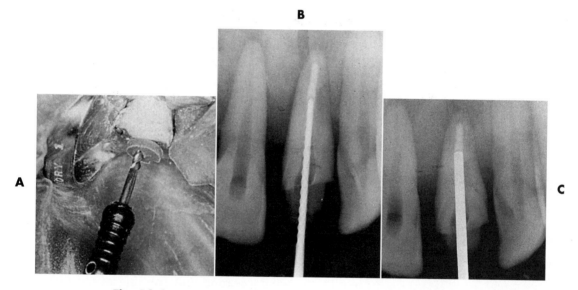

Fig. 12-27. Enlargement of the root canal for a prefabricated post.

Prefabricated Posts (Fig. 12-27)

1. Enlarge the canal one or two sizes with a drill, endodontic file, or reamer that matches the configuration of the post (see Fig. 12-27, *A* and *B*). When using rotary instruments, alternate between the Peeso-Reamers and twist drills that correspond in size. In the case of a threaded post, the appropriate drill is followed by a tap that prethreads the internal wall of the post space. Parallel-sided posts are more retentive and distribute stresses better than tapered posts, but they do not conform well to the shape of a canal that has been flared to facilitate condensation of gutta-percha. In this situation, it may not be possible to enlarge the canal sufficiently to provide adequate retention for the post; in that case, a tapered custom-made post is preferred.

2. Use a prefabricated post (see Fig. 12-27, *C*) that matches standard endodontic instruments. A tapered post will conform better to the canal than a parallel-sided post and requires less removal of dentin to achieve an adequate fit. However, it will be slightly less retentive and will cause greater stress concentrations, although retention may be improved by controlled grooving.[31]

3. Be especially careful not to remove more dentin at the apical extent of the post space than is necessary (see Figs. 12-14 and 12-27).

NOTE: If careful measurement techniques have been followed, radiographs are not normally required to verify the post space preparation.

Most of the time a preformed parallel-sided post will fit only in the most apical portion of the canal. Modified posts are available with tapered ends, and these conform better to the shape of the canal although they have slightly less retention than parallel-sided posts do, particularly the shorter ones.[29] In the absence of a vertical stop on sound tooth structure, such posts can also create an undesirable wedging effect.

Custom-made Posts (Fig. 12-28)

1. Use custom-made posts in canals that have a noncircular cross section or extreme taper. Enlarging canals to conform to a preformed post may lead to perforation. Often very little preparation will be needed for a custom-made post. However, undercuts within the canal must be removed, and some additional shaping usually is necessary.

2. Be most careful on molars to avoid root perforation. In mandibular molars the distal wall of the mesial root is particularly susceptible. In maxillary molars the curvature of the mesiobuccal root makes mesial or distal perforation more likely[57] (Fig. 12-29).

PREPARATION OF THE CORONAL TOOTH STRUCTURE

After the post space has been prepared, the coronal tooth structure is reduced for the extracoronal

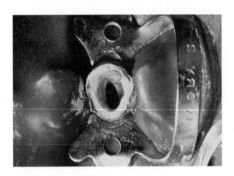

Fig. 12-28. Custom-made posts are indicated for teeth with root canals whose cross section is not circular or is extremely tapered. Further enlargement of the root canal is often not necessary on these teeth.

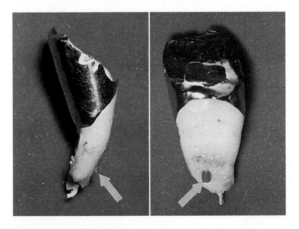

Fig. 12-29. Distal root curvature contributed to this mesial perforation *(arrow)* of a mandibular molar and necessitated removal of the distal root segment. *(Courtesy Dr. J. Davila.)*

restoration. Anterior teeth requiring a post-and-core are most effectively restored with a metal-ceramic crown (see Chapters 9 and 24).

1. Ignore any missing tooth structure (from previous restorative procedures, caries, fracture, or endodontic access) and prepare the remaining tooth as though it were undamaged (i.e., if a porcelain labial margin restoration is planned, a facial shoulder and lingual chamfer are placed).

2. Be sure that the facial structure of the tooth is adequately reduced for good esthetics.

3. Remove all internal and external undercuts that will prevent withdrawal of the pattern.

4. Remove any unsupported tooth structure, but preserve as much of the crown as possible. Because tooth structure has been removed internally and externally, the remaining walls often are thin and weakened. Defining absolute measurements for the dimensions of the residual coronal walls is difficult, but ideally they should be at least 1 mm wide. Wall height is reduced proportionally to the remaining wall thickness because tall, thin walls have a tendency to fracture when the provisional restoration is removed and during try-in and seating of the casting.

5. In addition, be sure that part of the remaining coronal tissue is prepared perpendicular to the post (see step 4 in Fig. 12-8), because this will create a positive stop to prevent overseating and splitting of the tooth. Similarly, rotation of the post must be prevented by preparing a flat surface parallel to the post (see step 5 in Fig. 12-8). If insufficient tooth structure for this feature remains, an antirotation groove should be placed in the canal (see Fig. 12-22).

6. Complete the preparation by eliminating sharp angles and establishing a smooth finish line.

POST FABRICATION

Prefabricated Posts. Technique simplicity is one advantage of using prefabricated posts. A post is selected to match the dimensions of the canal, and only minimum adjustment is needed for seating it to the full depth of the post space. The coronal half of the post may have an inadequate fit because the root canal has been flared. This can be corrected by adding material when the core is made.

Available Materials (see Table 12-5). Prefabricated parallel-sided posts are made of platinum-gold-palladium (Pt-Au-Pd or PGP), nickel-chromium

(Ni-Cr), cobalt-chromium (Co-Cr), or stainless steel clasp wire. Serrated posts come in stainless steel, titanium, or nonoxidizing noble alloy. Tapered posts are available in Au-Pt, Ni-Cr, and titanium alloys. All these posts have a high modulus of elasticity and an elongated grain structure, which contribute to their more suitable physical properties as compared to cast posts. Essentially, they are more rigid.

Failure of posts cast in Type III gold when loaded at a 45-degree angle has been attributed to bending.[58] Although posts cast in stiffer (Type IV) gold or Ni-Cr alloys can be expected to resist bending better, prefabricated posts should possess even more desirable physical properties, although their properties can deteriorate when a core is cast to a wrought post.[59]

Carbon-fiber posts have increased in popularity during recent years.* These posts consist of bundles of stretched aligned carbon fibers embedded in an epoxy matrix. The resulting post is strong but has significantly lower stiffness and strength when compared to ceramic and metal posts.[60] Preliminary retrospective study of this system appears promising[61] (Fig 12-30). However, a laboratory study comparing teeth restored with carbon fiber posts and composite-resin foundations and teeth restored with custom post-and-cores cast in Type III alloy showed significantly higher fracture thresholds for the cast post-and-cores.[62] One advantage of a carbon fiber post is the ease of its removal for retreatment. The preferred technique involves drilling apically. The very strong carbon fibers prevent the drill from tracking laterally, avoiding penetration of the dentin. Therefore, if concern exists about the long-term prognosis of an endodontically treated tooth, a carbon fiber post should be considered. The chief disadvantage of a carbon fiber post is its black appearance, which presents an esthetic problem (as can metal posts).

Manufacturers have developed high-strength ceramic[63,64] (zirconia) posts† (Fig. 12-31) and ceramic composite‡ (Fig 12-32) and woven fiber (e.g., polyethylene) posts,§ all of which have excellent esthetic properties (see also Chapters 25 and 27). Ceramic is very strong and rigid; woven fiber is less strong and more flexible.[65] Because the systems are relatively new, judging how well the foundations will per-

form in clinical practice is difficult, but they should be considered where esthetic demands are high.

Corrosion Resistance. Several reports[66-68] have linked root fracture to corrosion of base metal prefabricated post-and-core systems. One study,[63] reporting on 468 teeth with vertical or oblique root fracture, attributed 72% of these failures to electrolytic action of dissimilar metals used for the post and the core (reaction occurring between tin in the amalgam core and stainless steel, German silver, or brass in the post). The authors suggested that volume changes produced by corrosion products split the root. Although possible fracture mechanisms have been suggested,[64,65] these studies are confusing cause with effect: The corrosion may have occurred subsequent to root fracture rather than causing it.

Further study is needed to answer the question conclusively. However, in the meantime, avoiding the use of potentially corrodible dissimilar metals for post, core, and crown is recommended.

Custom-made Posts. A custom-made post can be cast from a direct pattern fabricated in the patient's mouth, or an indirect pattern can be fabricated in the dental laboratory. A direct technique using autopolymerizing or light-polymerized resin is recommended for single canals, whereas an indirect procedure is more appropriate for multiple canals.

Direct Procedure
1. Lightly lubricate the canal and notch a loose-fitting plastic dowel (Fig. 12-33, *A*). It should extend to the full depth of the prepared canal.
2. Use the bead-brush technique (Fig. 12-33, *B*) to add resin to the dowel (Fig. 12-33, *C*) and seat it in the prepared canal. This should be done in two steps: Add resin only to the canal orifice first. An alternative is to mix some resin and roll it into a thin cylinder. This is introduced into the canal and pushed to place with the **monomer**-moistened plastic dowel.
3. Do not allow the resin to harden fully within the canal. Loosen and reseat it several times while it is still rubbery.
4. Once the resin has polymerized, remove the pattern (Fig. 12-33, *D*).
5. Form the apical part of the post by adding additional resin and reseating and removing the post, taking care not to lock it in the canal.
6. Identify any undercuts that can be trimmed away carefully with a scalpel.

The post pattern is complete when it can be inserted and removed easily without binding in the

*C-Posts, Bisco: Chicago.
†CosmoPost, Ivoclar: Amhurst, N.Y.
‡Æstheti-Post, Bisco: Chicago.
§FibreKor, Jeneric/Pentron Inc.: Wallingford, Conn.
Luscent Anchor, Dentatus: New York.

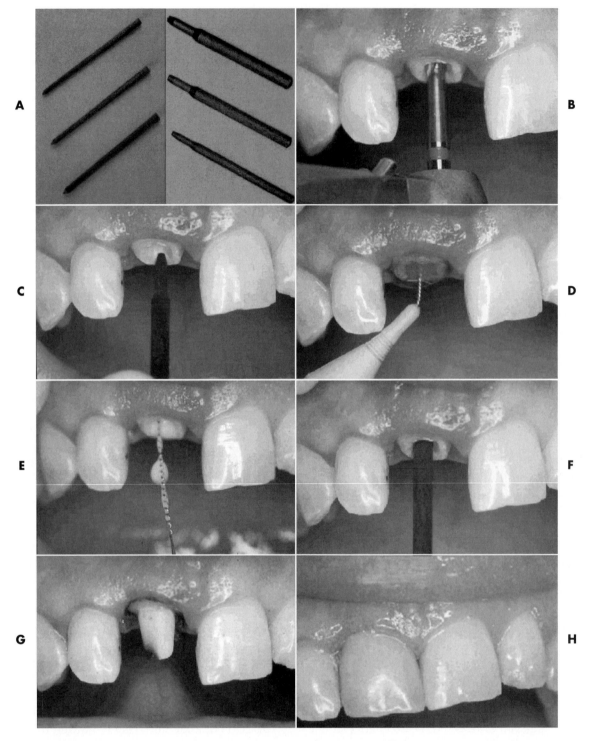

Fig. 12-30. Carbon fiber posts. **A,** The C-Post system is available in various sizes and configurations. **B,** Gutta-percha is removed with hot instruments or a Gates Glidden drill. The canal is prepared sequentially with the drills provided by the manufacturer. **C,** The post is seated in the canal and shortened with a diamond rotary instrument or disk. Wire cutters should *never* be used to cut carbon fiber composites, because they crush and weaken the composite structure. **D,** The canal is prepared by etching and priming according to the manufacturer's recommendations. Then the post is prepared by airborne particle abrasion. **E,** The luting resin is introduced into the canal with a lentulo spiral. **F,** The post is seated and the core built up with the recommended core resin. **G,** The preparation is finalized. **H,** The completed restoration. *(Courtesy Bisco, Inc.)*

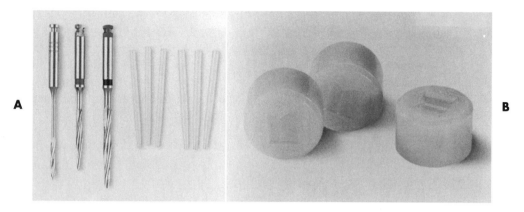

Fig. 12-31.   **A,** Zirconia posts, such as the CosmoPost, shown with the corresponding rotary instruments, are esthetic and strong. **B,** Special pressable ceramics are available to form the core (composite resin can also be used). (See also Fig. 25-19.)
(Courtesy Ivoclar North America.)

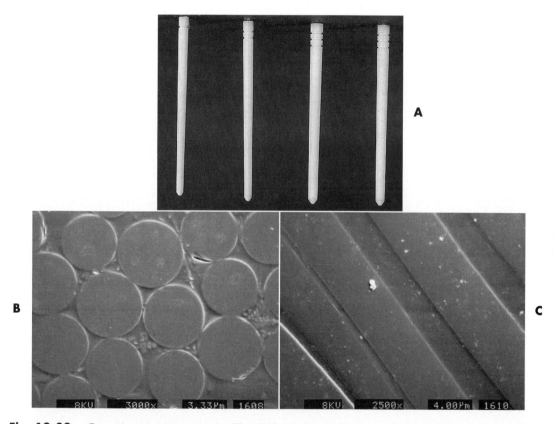

Fig. 12-32.   Ceramic composite post. **A,** The Æstheti-plus post system uses ceramic fibers in a resin matrix. **B,** Cross-sectional and **C,** longitudinal sections of the fiber composite.
(A courtesy Bisco, Inc.; B and C courtesy Dr. J. Wang.)

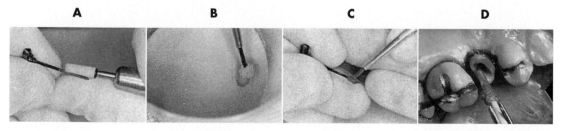

Fig. 12-33.   Fabrication of an acrylic resin pattern for a custom-made post.
(Courtesy Dr. R. Webber.)

canal. Once the pattern has been made, additional resin or light-polymerized resin* is added for the core.

Pattern Fabrication with Thermoplastic Post (Fig. 12-34)

1. Fit the plastic rod to the prepared post space. Trim the rod until the bevel area is approximately 1.5 to 2 mm occlusal to the finish line for the core.
2. Lubricate the canal with a periodontal probe and petroleum jelly.
3. Heat the thermoplastic resin over a flame until the material turns clear or heat the resin in a low-temperature glue gun†.
4. Apply a small amount of the heated resin to the apical end of the rod to cover two thirds of the anticipated length of the post pattern.
5. Fully insert the rod into the prepared post space. Lift after 5 to 10 seconds and reseat. Inspect the post pattern for completeness and remove any projections that result from undercuts in the canal with a scalpel blade.

---

*LX Gel, Dentatus: New York; Palavit G LC, Heraeus Kulzer, Inc.: South Bend, Indiana.

†Thermogrip, Black and Decker, Inc: Hunt Valley, Md.

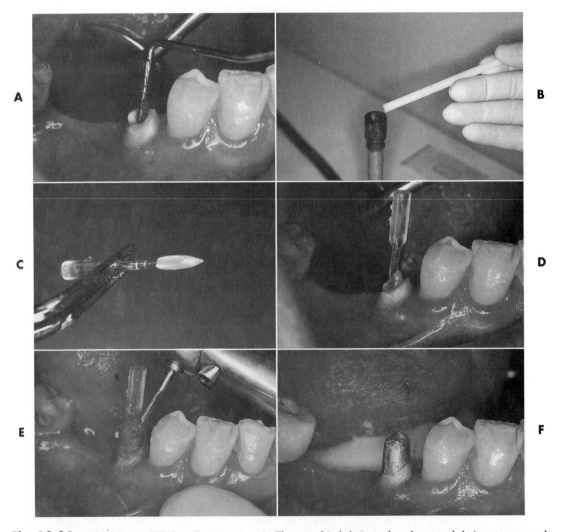

Fig. 12-34. The Merritt EZ Cast Post system. **A,** The canal is lubricated and excess lubricant removed with paper points. The post was previously trimmed until its beveled portion protrudes about 1.5 to 2 mm above the tooth preparation. **B,** A stick of the thermoplastic material is heated. **C,** The plastic rod is covered for about two thirds of the anticipated post length. **D,** The coated post is inserted and can be removed in 5 to 10 seconds. **E,** After any protrusions have been removed, the core is built from autopolymerizing resin and trimmed to ideal tooth preparation form. **F,** The completed custom post-and-core. *(From Rosenstiel SF et al: J Prosthet Dent 77:209, 1997.)*

6. For the direct technique, fabricate the core with conventional autopolymerizing resin using the brush-bead technique or syringe a light polymerized pattern resin (an easier technique).

7. If the indirect technique is preferred, pick up the pattern with an elastomeric impression material, which can be poured in the conventional manner. Soak the cast in warm water to help release the pattern. Reseat the post pattern and wax the core.

8. Invest and cast the post-and-core. Phosphate-bonded investment is recommended because of its higher strength.

Indirect Procedure (Fig. 12-35). Any elastomeric material will make an accurate impression of the root canal if a wire reinforcement is placed to prevent distortion.

1. Cut pieces of orthodontic wire to length and shape them like the letter J (Fig. 12-35, *A*).

2. Verify the fit of the wire in each canal. It should fit loosely and extend to the full depth of the post space. If the fit is too tight, the impression material will strip away from the wire when the impression is removed.

3. Coat the wire with tray adhesive. If subgingival margins are present, tissue displacement may be helpful. Lubricate the canals to facilitate removal of the impression without distortion (die lubricant is suitable).

4. Using a lentulo spiral, fill the canals with elastomeric impression material. Before loading the impression syringe, verify that the lentulo will spiral material in an apical direction (clockwise). Pick up a small amount of material with the largest lentulo spiral that fits into the post space. Insert the lentulo with the handpiece set at low rotational speed to slowly carry material into the apical portion of the post space. Then increase handpiece speed and slowly withdraw the lentulo from the post space. This technique prevents the impression material from being dragged out. Repeat until the post space is filled.

All of the elastomeric impression materials require some form of reinforcement when making a post space impression.

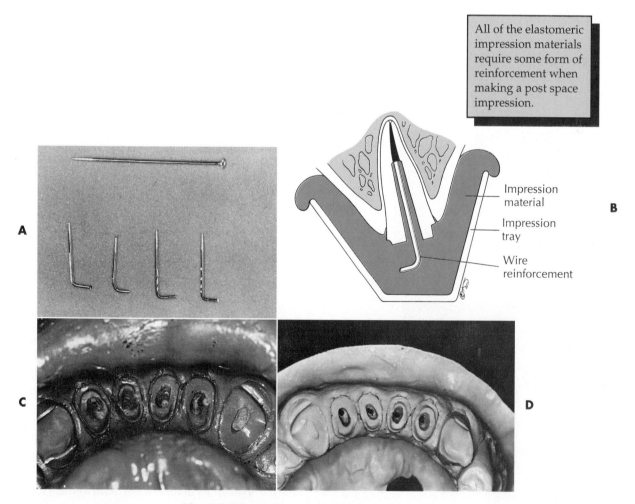

Impression material

Impression tray

Wire reinforcement

Fig. 12-35. Indirect procedure for post-and-cores.

5. Seat the wire reinforcement to the full depth of each post space, syringe in more impression material around the prepared teeth, and insert the impression tray (see Fig. 12-35, *B*).

6. Remove the impression (see Fig. 12-35, *C*), evaluate it, and pour the working cast (see Fig. 12-35, *D*) as usual (see Chapter 17).

NOTE: Access for waxing is generally adequate without placement of dowel pins or sectioning of the cast.

7. In the laboratory, roughen a loose-fitting plastic post (a plastic toothpick is suitable) and, using the impression as a guide, make sure that it extends into the entire depth of the canal.

8. Apply a thin coat of sticky wax to the plastic post and, after lubricating the stone cast, add soft inlay wax in increments (Fig. 12-36). Start from the most apical and make sure that the post is correctly oriented as it is seated to adapt the wax. When this post pattern has been fabricated, the wax core can be added and shaped.

9. Use the impression to evaluate whether the wax pattern is completely adapted to the post space.

CORE FABRICATION

The core of a post-and-core restoration replaces missing coronal tooth structure and thereby forms

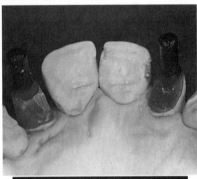

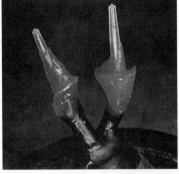

Fig. 12-36. Post-and-core patterns made by adding wax to prefabricated plastic posts.

the shape of the tooth preparation. It can be shaped in resin or wax and added to the post pattern before the assembly is cast in metal. This prevents possible failure at the post-core interface. The core can also be cast onto most prefabricated post systems (although there is then some concern that the casting process may unfavorably affect the physical properties of wrought metal posts). A third alternative is to make the core from a plastic restorative material such as amalgam, glass ionomer, or composite resin.

Plastic Filling Materials. The advantages of amalgam, glass ionomer, or resin[58,69,70] include the following:

1. Maximum tooth structure can be conserved because undercuts do not need to be removed.

2. Treatment requires one less patient visit.

3. There are fewer laboratory procedures.

4. Testing generally shows good resistance to fatigue testing[71] and good strength characteristics,[72] possibly because of the good adaptation to tooth structure. However, these plastic restorative materials, especially the glass ionomers, have lower tensile strength than do cast metals.

Disadvantages include the following:

1. Long-term success may be affected by corrosion of amalgam cores, the low strength of glass ionomer,[73] or the continued polymerization[74] and high thermal expansion coefficients of composite resin cores.

2. Microleakage with temperature fluctuations (thermocycling) is greater under composite resin and amalgam cores than under conventional crown preparations[75] (however, the extent of leakage under cast cores has yet to be determined).

3. Difficulty may be encountered with certain operative procedures such as rubber dam or matrix application (particularly on badly damaged teeth).

Amalgam cores are suitable for restoring posterior teeth, particularly when some coronal structure remains. The procedure described by Nayyar et al,[42] with amalgam also used for the posts, is conservative of tooth structure. The cores are placed during the same appointment as the root canal obturation, because then the teeth are still isolated by the rubber dam, the root canal morphology is still fresh in the practitioner's mind, and the cores can serve as a support for the provisional restoration (Fig. 12-37).

Step-by-Step Procedure for Amalgam (see also Chapter 6).

1. Apply the rubber dam and remove gutta-percha from the pulp chamber as well as 2 to 4 mm into each root canal if less than 4 mm of coronal height remains. Use a warmed endodontic instrument.

2. Remove any existing restoration, undermined enamel, or carious or weakened dentin. Establish the cavity form using conventional principles of resistance and retention form. Even if cusps are missing, pins are not normally required because adequate retention can be gained by extending the amalgam into the root canals.

3. If you suspect that the floor of the pulp chamber is thin, protect it from condensing pressures with a cement base.

4. Fit a matrix band. Where lack of tooth structure makes the application of a conventional matrix system difficult, an orthodontic or annealed copper band may be used.

5. Condense the first increments of amalgam (select a material with high early strength) into the root canals with an endodontic plugger.

6. Fill the pulp chamber and coronal cavity in the conventional manner.

7. Carve the alloy to shape. The impression can be made immediately. Alternatively, the amalgam can be built up to anatomic contour and later prepared for a com-plete crown. Under these circumstances, avoid forces that would fracture the tooth or newly placed restoration.

Cast Metal. Cast metal cores have the following advantages:

1. They can be cast directly onto a prefabricated post, providing a restoration with good strength characteristics.

2. Conventional high-noble, metal-content alloys can be used.

3. An indirect procedure can be used, making restoration of posterior teeth easier.

Direct Procedure for Single-rooted Teeth

Direct patterns can be formed by combining a prefabricated post with **autopolymerizing resin**. Alternatively, a thermoplastic material can be used to create a post pattern,[76] and the core portion can be developed in either autopolymerizing resin, light polymerized resin, or wax.

Pattern Fabrication with Autopolymerizing Resin (Fig. 12-38)

1. Use a prefabricated metal or custom acrylic resin post.

2. Add resin by the "bead" technique, dipping a small brush in monomer and then into

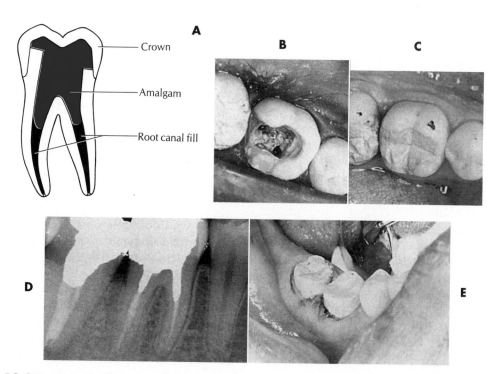

Fig. 12-37. Retention for an amalgam core can be obtained from the root canal system, preserving as much tooth structure as possible.
(*B to D courtesy Dr. M. Padilla.*)

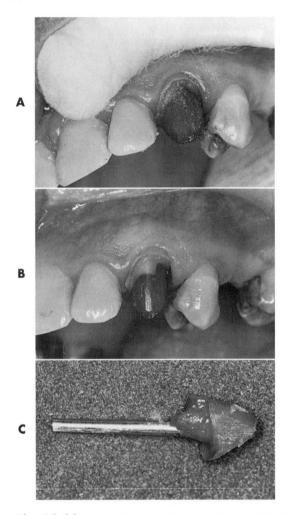

Fig. 12-38. Direct pattern for a single-rooted tooth.

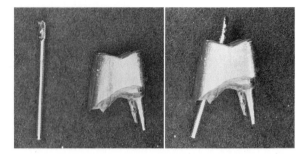

Fig. 12-39. A direct post-and-core for posterior teeth can be made by cementing a prefabricated post through a casting. Here the two buccal canals had a common path of withdrawal and could be incorporated into the core casting. More typically, only one canal has a fixed post, and the others are cemented through the core.

The procedure is simple, as long as smooth parallel-sided or tapered posts are used.

1. Fit prefabricated posts into the prepared canals. One post is roughened; the others are left smooth and lubricated. All posts should extend beyond the eventual preparation.
2. Build up the core with autopolymerizing resin, using the bead technique.
3. Shape the core to final form with carbide finishing burs.
4. Grip the smooth, lubricated posts with forceps and remove them.
5. Remove, invest, and cast the core with the roughened single post. When this has been done, the holes for the auxiliary posts can be refined with the appropriate twist drill.
6. After verifying the fit at try-in, cement the core and auxiliary posts to place.

Indirect Pattern for Posterior Teeth (Fig. 12-40)

1. Wax the custom-made posts as described previously.
2. Build part of the core around the first post.
3. Remove any undercuts adjacent to other post holes and cast the first section.
4. Wax additional sections and cast them.

Using dovetails to interlock the sections makes the procedure more complicated and is probably of limited benefit, especially because the final buildup is held together by the fixed cast restoration.

PROVISIONAL RESTORATIONS (see Chapter 15)

To prevent drifting of opposing or adjacent teeth, an endodontically treated tooth requires a proper provisional restoration immediately following completion of endodontics (Fig. 12-41). Of particular importance are good proximal contacts to prevent

polymer and applying it to the post. Some experts recommend light-cured resin to facilitate this step.[77]

3. Slightly overbuild the core and let it polymerize fully (Fig. 12-38, *A*).
4. Shape the core with carbide finishing burs or paper disks (Fig. 12-38, *B*). Use water spray to prevent overheating of the acrylic resin. Correct any small defects with wax.
5. Remove the pattern (Fig. 12-38, *C*); sprue and invest it immediately.

Direct Pattern for Multirooted Teeth (Fig. 12-39)

A direct pattern can be used for multirooted posterior teeth, although limited access may make the indirect approach easier. A single-piece core with auxiliary posts is used, as opposed to the multisection core recommended for indirect posterior cast post-and-cores. The core is cast directly onto the post of one canal. (The other canals already have prefabricated posts that pass through holes in the core.)

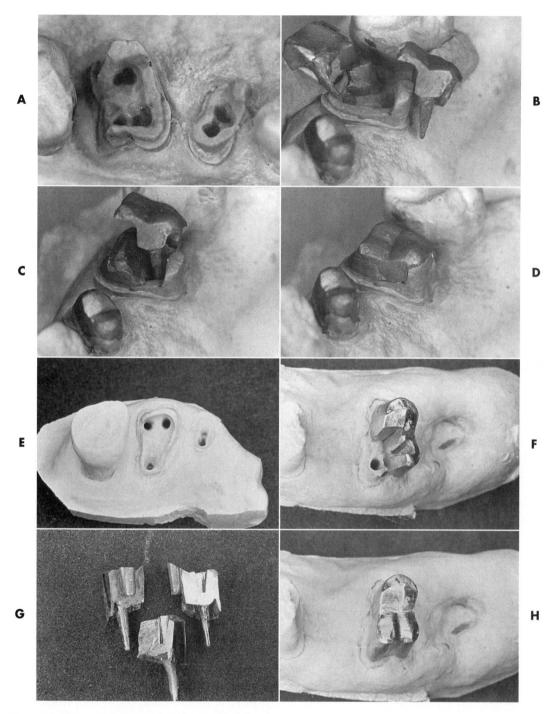

Fig. 12-40. **A to D, Multipiece post-and-cores** can be made by the indirect technique, waxing each section to ensure that no undercuts are created. **E to H,** Alternatively, interlocking sections can be made, but this complicates the laboratory phase.

tooth migration leading to unwanted root proximity. If a cast post-and-core is made, an additional provisional restoration is needed while the post-and-core is being fabricated. This can be retained by fitting a wire (e.g., a paper clip or orthodontic wire) into the prepared canal. The restoration is then conveniently fabricated with autopolymerizing resin by the direct technique.

INVESTING AND CASTING

A cast post-and-core should fit somewhat loosely in the canal. A tight fit may cause root fracture. The casting should be slightly undersized, which can be accomplished by restricting expansion of the investment (i.e., by omitting the usual ring liner or casting at a lower mold temperature [see Chapter 22]). An accelerated casting technique may facilitate the

It is not essential that the reline material extend all the way down the post space. By engaging the apical portion of the post space, the wire will enhance resistance of the provisional.

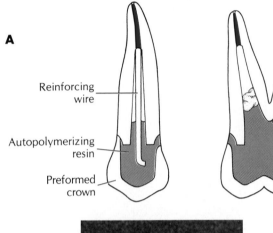

A

Reinforcing wire

Autopolymerizing resin

Preformed crown

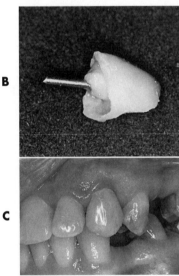

B

C

Fig. 12-41. Provisional restorations made for endodontically treated teeth by lining a polycarbonate crown with autopolymerizing resin. The post is made of metal wire (orthodontic wire or a paper clip, [see Chapter 15]).
(*A from Taylor GN, Land MF: In Clark JW, editor:* Clinical dentistry, *New York, 1985, Harper & Row.*)

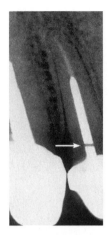

Fig. 12-42. Fractured post. (*Courtesy Dr. D. Francisco.*)

EVALUATION

The practitioner must be particularly careful that casting defects do not interfere with seating of the post; otherwise, root fracture will result. Post-and-cores should be inserted with gentle pressure. However, the marginal fit of a cast foundation is not as critical as that of other cast restorations, because the margins will be covered by the final casting. Air-abrading the surface to a matte-type finish may help detect interferences at try-in (Fig. 12-43).

The shape of the foundation is evaluated and adjusted as necessary. No adjustments should be made immediately after cementation because vibration from the bur could fracture the setting cement and cause premature failure.

CEMENTATION

The luting agent must fill all dead space within the root canal system (Fig. 12-44). Voids may be a cause of periodontal inflammation via the lateral canals. A rotary (lentulo) paste filler or cement tube (Fig. 12-45) is used to fill the canal with cement. The post-and-core is inserted gently to reduce hydrostatic pressure, which could cause root fracture. If a parallel-sided post is being used, a groove should be placed along the side of the post to allow excess cement to escape.

REMOVAL OF EXISTING POSTS

Occasionally an existing post-and-core must be removed (e.g., for retreatment of a failed root canal filling). Patients must understand in advance that post removal is a risky process and occasionally results in radicular fracture. If sufficient length of post is exposed coronally, the post can be retrieved with thin-beaked forceps. Vibrating the post first with an ultrasonic scaler will weaken brittle cement and facilitate removal. A thin scaler tip or

laboratory phase.[78] The casting alloy should have suitable physical properties. Extra-hard partial denture gold (ADA Type IV) or nickel chromium alloys have high moduli of elasticity and are suitable for cast posts. A sound casting technique is essential because any undetected porosity could lead to a weakened casting that might fail in function (Fig. 12-42).

Casting a core onto a prefabricated post avoids problems of porosity, but the preheating temperature of the investment mold should be restricted if recrystallization of the wrought post[79] is to be avoided.

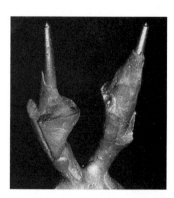

Fig. 12-43. The fitting surface of the casting must be carefully evaluated. Any nodules could lead to root fracture if undetected.

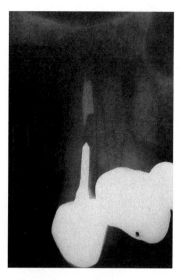

Fig. 12-44. Residual voids after cementation can cause inflammation.
(Courtesy Dr. D. Francisco.)

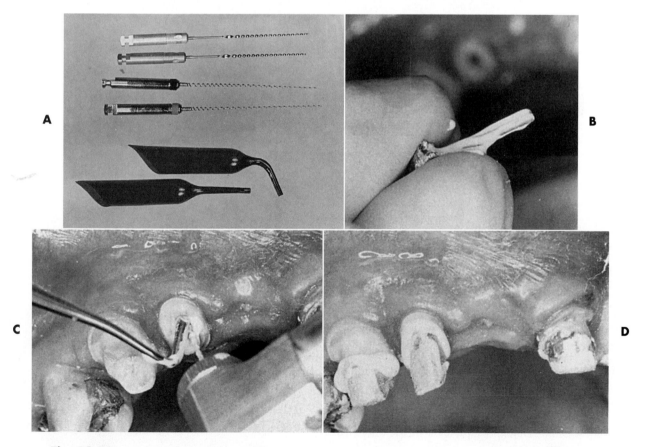

Fig. 12-45. **A,** Lentulo rotary paste fillers or a cement tube are used to fill the post space completely. **B,** The post is first coated with cement. **C,** The canal is filled with cement. **D,** To avoid the risk of fracture, the post-and-core is very gently seated. A small cement line is not usually significant, because dissolution is prevented by the presence of the definitive restoration.
*(**B** to **D** courtesy Dr. M. Padilla.)*

special post removal tip is recommended (Fig. 12-46). Although histologic examination with animal models shows no harmful effect in the periodontal tissues,[80] ultrasonic removal is slower than other methods and may result in an increased number of canal and intradentin cracks.[81] Alternatively, a post puller can be used.[82] This device consists of a vise to grip the post and legs that bear on the root face. A screw activates the vise and extracts the post.

A post that has fractured within the root canal cannot be removed with a post puller or forceps. The post can be drilled out, but great care is needed to avoid perforation. The technique is best limited to relatively short fractured posts (Fig. 12-47).

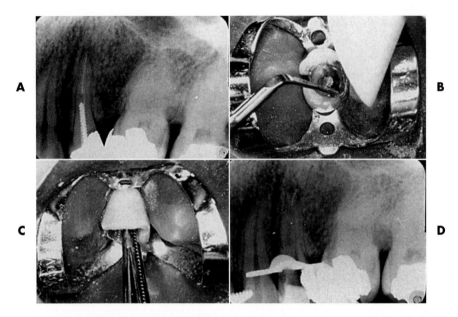

Fig. 12-46. Post removal by ultrasonic device. **A,** Preoperative radiograph of the left maxillary first premolar with a parallel-sided threaded post that had to be removed for endodontic retreatment. **B,** After the coronal portion of the post has been well isolated, the tip of the ultrasonic device is placed against it, and energy is applied to disrupt the cement interface. Note the suction tip, which removes water spray used with the ultrasonic handpiece. **C,** After a time, the post becomes loose within the canal and can be retrieved by forceps. **D,** Radiograph of the premolar after post removal. *(Courtesy Dr. L. L. Lazare.)*

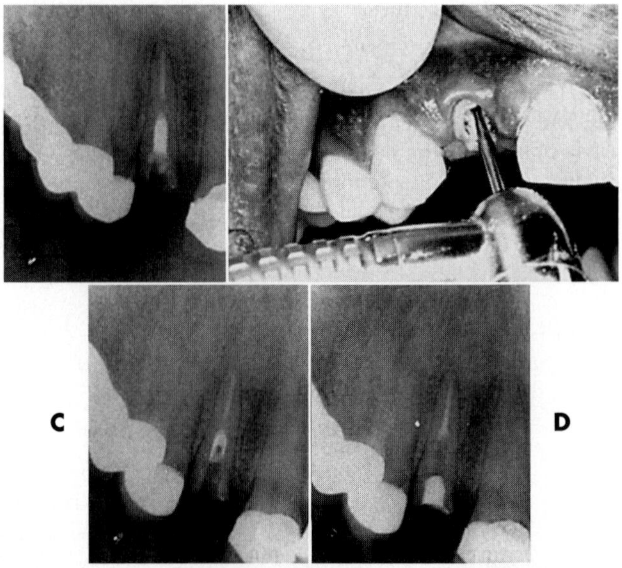

Fig. 12-47. Post removal by high-speed bur. **A,** Preoperative radiograph of the right maxillary lateral incisor, in which both the crown and part of a post have been fractured off. A portion of the Kurer-type, parallel-sided, threaded post remains within the canal. **B,** Because of the large diameter of the post and its position within the canal, a high-speed handpiece was chosen to drill it out. **C,** Radiograph to verify the correct orientation of the bur's progress inside the canal. With this method of post removal, the operator must be extremely careful not to let the high-speed bur contact the canal wall, which would seriously compromise tooth structure. **D,** Radiograph of the incisor after post removal and retreatment. *(Courtesy Dr. D. A. Miller.)*

Another means of handling an embedded fractured post (described by Masserann[83] in 1966) uses special hollow end-cutting tubes (or trephines) to prepare a thin trench around the post (Fig. 12-48). This technique has shown success.[84] Retrieval can be facilitated by using an adhesive to attach a hollow tube extractor[85] or by using a threaded extractor[86] (Fig. 12-49).

SUMMARY

Although the restoration of endodontically treated teeth has been rationalized considerably by recent laboratory research data, information from controlled long-term clinical trials is still necessary and difficult to obtain. Different clinical procedures have been advocated, many of which are successful if properly used. Where the crown is preserved, an *anterior* tooth can be safely restored with a plastic filling. To prevent fracture of *posterior* teeth, cast restorations providing cuspal coverage are recommended.

Preserving as much tooth structure as possible is important, particularly within the root canal, where the amount of remaining dentin may be difficult to assess.

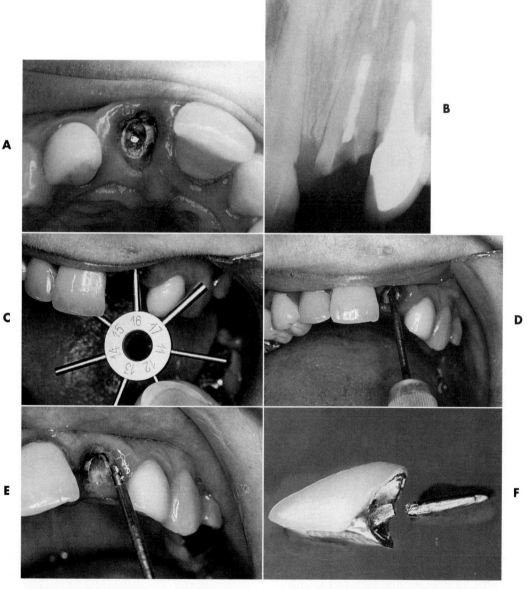

Fig. 12-48.   Masserann technique for the removal of fractured posts. **A** and **B,** Maxillary incisor with a post that has fractured inside the canal. **C,** The diameter of the post is gauged with a sizing tool. **D,** The selected trephine is carefully rotated counterclockwise to create a narrow channel around the post. **E,** When the instrument has removed sufficient material, the post is recovered. **F,** The fractured crown and post after removal.

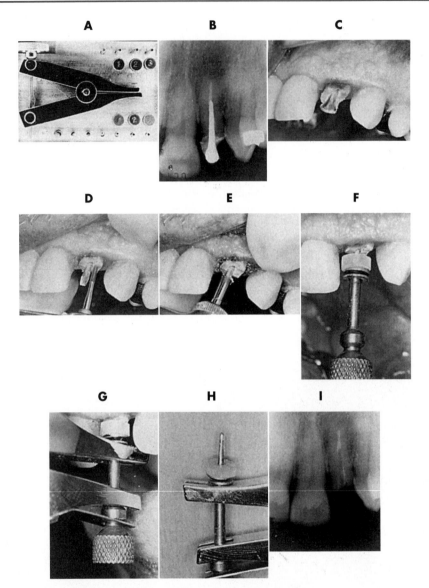

Fig. 12-49. Post removal by extractor. **A,** The Thomas (Gonon) post-removing system. It includes pliers, trephine burs, mandrels, and washers. **B,** Preoperative radiograph of the left maxillary lateral incisor with a post. **C,** Note the flared shape of the post in this preoperative view and the height of the surrounding tooth structure. **D,** A high-speed bur is used to free the post from coronal tooth structure and parallel its sides. (NOTE: An ultrasonic device may be used at this point to disturb the cement interface.) **E,** A trephine bur machines the post to the correct diameter and places threads for the mandrel. **F,** The mandrel is threaded onto the post with special washers, which distribute the forces from the extractor evenly over the tooth. **G,** The beaks of the pliers are fitted onto the mandrel; the knob of the pliers is then rotated, which separates the beaks, and the post is extruded from the tooth. H, The removed post, still attached to the mandrel and pliers. I, Radiograph of the lateral incisor after post removal. *(Courtesy Dr. D. A. Miller.)*

A post-and-core is used to provide retention and support for a cast restoration. It should be of adequate length for good stress distribution but not so long as to jeopardize the apical seal. The safest method to create post space is to use a warmed endodontic plugger to remove the gutta-percha. Anterior teeth, particularly those with flared or elliptical canals, should be built up with a custom cast post-and-core, although prefabricated posts can be used successfully too. Esthetic post materials should be considered if a dark post would ruin an esthetic restoration. Amalgam can be used satisfactorily on posterior teeth, although a casting may be preferred if much coronal tooth structure is missing.

Study Questions

1. What must be determined to ensure that an endodontically treated tooth is ready for subsequent restorative treatment?
2. What six features must be incorporated in the tooth preparation for a cast post-and-core?
3. Discuss five variables that have an impact on retention form for cast post-and-cores.
4. Discuss four different post-and-core systems, their advantages and disadvantages, and typical indications and precautions.
5. Which canal configurations are circular? Which are elliptical?
6. Describe recommended step-by-step procedures for the following:
   1. Custom-made direct procedure post-and-core pattern fabrication for a maxillary second premolar.
   2. Amalgam post-and-core on a mandibular molar.
7. How is a provisional restoration fabricated for a mandibular second premolar that has been prepared for a cast post-and-core?

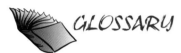 GLOSSARY

anatomic crown: the portion of a natural tooth that extends coronal from the cementoenamel junction—called also *anatomical crown.*

apex: *n, pl* **apexes:** or **apices:** (1601) *1:* the uppermost point; the vertex; *2:* in dentistry, the anatomic end of a tooth root.

autopolymerizing resin: a resin whose polymerization is initiated by a chemical activator.

avulsion: *n* (1622): a forcible separation or detachment, as in a tearing away of a body part surgically or accidentally.

dowel: *n* (13c): a post, usually made of metal that is fitted into a prepared root canal of a natural tooth. When combined with an artificial crown or core, it provides retention and resistance for the restoration.

elastic: *adj* (1653): susceptible to being stretched, compressed, or distorted and then tending to resume the original shape.

elastic modulus: the stiffness or flexibility of a material within the elastic range. Within the elastic range, the material deforms in direct proportion of the stress applied as represented by Hooke's law.

endoscope: *n* (1861): a flexible or rigid thin tube used for examining the interior of a structure.

exposure: *n* (1606) *1:* the act of laying open, as a surgical or dental exposure *2:* in radiology, a measure of the roentgen rays or gamma radiation at a certain place based on its ability to cause ionization. The unit of exposure is the roentgen, called also exposure dose.

ferrule: *n* (15c) *1:* a metal band or ring used to fit the root or crown of a tooth *2:* any short tube or bushing for making a tight joint.

monomer: *n* (1914): a chemical compound that can undergo polymerization; any molecule that can be bound to a similar molecule to form a polymer.

polymerization: *n* (1872): the forming of a compound by the joining together of molecules of small molecular weights into a compound of large molecular weight.

post-core: see dowel.

resin: *n* (14c) *1:* any of various solid or semisolid amorphous natural organic substances that usually are transparent or translucent and brown to yellow; usually formed in plant secretions; are soluble in organic solvents but not water; are used chiefly in varnishes, inks, plastics, and medicine; and are found in many dental impression materials *2:* a broad term used to describe natural or synthetic substances that form plastic materials after polymerization. They are named according to their chemical composition, physical structure, and means for activation of polymerization.

root: *n* (bef. 12c): the portion of the tooth apical to the cementoenamel junction that is normally covered by cementum and is attached to the periodontal ligament and hence to the supporting bone.

stress: *n* (14c): force per unit area; a force exerted on one body that presses on, pulls on, pushes against, or tends to invest or compress another body; the deformation caused in a body by such a force; an internal force that resists an externally applied load or force. It is normally defined in terms of mechanical stress, which is the force divided by the perpendicular cross sectional area over which the force is applied.

wax pattern: a wax form that is the positive likeness of an object to be fabricated.

REFERENCES

1. Johnson JK et al: Evaluation and restoration of endodontically treated posterior teeth, *J Am Dent Assoc* 93:597, 1976.

2. Kakehashi Y et al: A new all-ceramic post and core system: clinical, technical, and in vitro results, *Int J Periodont Restor Dent* 18:586, 1998.

3. Blitz N: Adaptation of a fiber-reinforced restorative system to the rehabilitation of endodontically treated teeth, *Pract Periodont Aesthet Dent* 10:191, 1998.

4. Torbjörner A et al: Survival rate and failure characteristics for two post designs, *J Prosthet Dent* 73:439, 1995.

5. Sorensen JA, Martinoff JT: Clinically significant factors in dowel design, *J Prosthet Dent* 52:28, 1984.

6. Loney RW, Moulding MB, Ritsco RG: The effect of load angulation on fracture resistance of teeth restored with cast post and cores and crowns, *Int J Prosthodont* 8:247, 1995.

7. Helfer AR et al: Determination of the moisture content of vital and pulpless teeth, *Oral Surg* 34:661, 1972.

8. Trabert KC et al: Tooth fracture: a comparison of endodontic and restorative treatments, *J Endodont* 4:341, 1978.

9. Guzy GE, Nicholls JI: In vitro comparison of intact endodontically treated teeth with and without endo-post reinforcement, *J Prosthet Dent* 42:39, 1979.

10. Hunter AJ et al: Effects of post placement on endodontically treated teeth, *J Prosthet Dent* 62:166, 1989.

11. Ko CC et al: Effects of posts on dentin stress distribution in pulpless teeth, *J Prosthet Dent* 68:421, 1992.

12. Kantor ME, Pines MS: A comparative study of restorative techniques for pulpless teeth, *J Prosthet Dent* 38:405, 1977.

13. Sorensen JA, Martinoff JT: Intracoronal reinforcement and coronal coverage: a study of endodontically treated teeth, *J Prosthet Dent* 51:780, 1984.

14. Lu YC: A comparative study of fracture resistance of pulpless teeth, *Chin Dent J* 6:26, 1987.

15. Warren MA et al: In vitro comparison of bleaching agents on the crowns and roots of discolored teeth, *J Endodont* 16:463, 1990.

16. Madison S, Walton R: Cervical root resorption following bleaching of endodontically treated teeth, *J Endodont* 16:570, 1990.

17. McKerracher PW: Rational restoration of endodontically treated teeth. I. Principles, techniques, and materials, *Aust Dent J* 26:205, 1981.

18. Felton DA et al: Threaded endodontic dowels: effect of post design on incidence of root fracture, *J Prosthet Dent* 65:179, 1991.

19. Henry PJ: Photoelastic analysis of post core restorations, *Aust Dent J* 22:157, 1977.

20. Assif DF et al: Photoelastic analysis of stress transfer by endodontically treated teeth to the supporting structure using different restorative techniques, *J Prosthet Dent* 61:535, 1989.

21. Milot P, Stein RS: Root fracture in endodontically treated teeth related to post selection and crown design, *J Prosthet Dent* 68:428, 1992.

22. Sorensen JA, Engelman MJ: Ferrule design and fracture resistance of endodontically treated teeth, *J Prosthet Dent* 63: 529, 1990.

23. Libman WJ, Nicholls JI: Load fatigue of teeth restored with cast posts and cores and complete crowns, *Int J Prosthodont* 8:155, 1995.

24. Isidor F et al: The influence of post length and crown ferrule length on the resistance to cyclic loading of bovine teeth with prefabricated titanium posts, *Int J Prosthodont* 12:78, 1999.

25. Gegauff AG: Change in strength from creating a ferrule via crown-lengthening, *J Dent Res* 78:223, 1999 (abstract).

26. Standlee JP et al: Retention of endodontic dowels: effects of cement, dowel length, diameter, and design, *J Prosthet Dent* 39:401, 1978.

27. Ruemping DR et al: Retention of dowels subjected to tensile and torsional forces, *J Prosthet Dent* 41:159, 1979.

28. Kurer HG et al: Factors influencing the retention of dowels, *J Prosthet Dent* 38:515, 1977.

29. Cooney JP et al: Retention and stress distribution of tapered-end endodontic posts, *J Prosthet Dent* 55:540, 1986.

30. Krupp JD et al: Dowel retention with glass-ionomer cement, *J Prosthet Dent* 41:163, 1979.

31. Wood WW: Retention of posts in teeth with non-vital pulps, *J Prosthet Dent* 49:504, 1983.

32. Hanson EC, Caputo AA: Cementing mediums and retentive characteristics of dowels, *J Prosthet Dent* 32:551, 1974.

33. Chapman KW et al: Retention of prefabricated posts by cements and resins, *J Prosthet Dent* 54:649, 1985.

34. Driessen CH et al: The effect of bonded and nonbonded posts on the fracture resistance of dentin, *J Dent Assoc S Afr* 52:393, 1997.

35. Mendoza DB, Eakle WS: Retention of posts cemented with various dentinal bonding cements, *J Prosthet Dent* 72:591, 1994.

36. O'Keefe KL et al: In vitro bond strength of silica-coated metal posts in roots of teeth, *Int J Prosthod* 5:373, 1992.

37. Tjan AH, Nemetz H: Effect of eugenol-containing endodontic sealer on retention of prefabri-

cated posts luted with adhesive composite resin cement, *Quintessence Int* 23:839, 1992.

38. Radke RA et al: Retention of cast endodontic posts: comparison of cementing agents, *J Prosthet Dent* 59:318, 1988.

39. Love RM, Purton DG: Retention of posts with resin, glass ionomer and hybrid cements, *J Dent* 26:599, 1998.

40. Assif D et al: Retention of endodontic posts with a composite resin luting agent: effect of cement thickness, *Quintessence Int* 19:643, 1988.

41. Kane JJ et al: Fracture resistance of amalgam coronal-radicular restorations, *J Prosthet Dent* 63:607, 1990.

42. Nayyar A et al: An amalgam coronal-radicular dowel and core technique for endodontically treated posterior teeth, *J Prosthet Dent* 43:511, 1980.

43. Mentink AG et al: Qualitative assessment of stress distribution during insertion of endodontic posts in photoelastic material, *J Dent* 26:125, 1998.

44. Standlee JP et al: The retentive and stress-distributing properties of a threaded endodontic dowel, *J Prosthet Dent* 44:398, 1980.

45. Thorsteinsson TS et al: Stress analysis of four prefabricated posts, *J Prosthet Dent* 67:30, 1992.

46. Dérand T: The principal stress distribution in a root with a loaded post in model experiments, *J Dent Res* 56:1463, 1977.

47. Leary JM et al: Load transfer of posts and cores to roots through cements, *J Prosthet Dent* 62:298, 1989.

48. Peters MCRB et al: Stress analysis of a tooth restored with a post and core, *J Dent Res* 62:760, 1983.

49. Yaman SD, Alacam T, Yaman Y: Analysis of stress distribution in a maxillary central incisor subjected to various post and core applications, *J Endodont* 24:107, 1998.

50. Schnell FJ: Effect of immediate dowel space preparation on the apical seal of endodontically filled teeth, *Oral Surg* 45:470, 1978.

51. Bourgeois RS, Lemon RR: Dowel space preparation and apical leakage, *J Endodont* 7:66, 1981.

52. Gegauff AG et al: A comparative study of post preparation diameters and deviations using ParaPost and Gates-Glidden drills, *J Endodont* 14:377, 1988.

53. Hussey Dl et al: Thermographic assessment of heat generated on the root surface during post space preparation, *Int Endodont J* 30:187, 1997.

54. Dickey DJ et al: Effect of post space preparation on apical seal using solvent techniques and Peeso reamers, *J Endodont* 8:351, 1982.

55. Caputo AA, Standlee JP: Pins and posts: why, when, and how, *Dent Clin North Am* 20:299, 1976.

56. Shillingburg HT et al: Root dimensions and dowel size, *Calif Dent Assoc J* 10(10):43, 1982.

57. Abou-Rass M et al: Preparation of space for posting: effect on thickness of canal walls and incidence of perforation in molars, *J Am Dent Assoc* 104:834, 1982.

58. Perez Moll JF et al: Cast gold post and core and pin-retained composite resin bases: a comparative study in strength, *J Prosthet Dent* 40:642, 1978.

59. Phillips RW: *Skinner's science of dental materials,* ed 9, Philadelphia, 1991, WB Saunders, p 550.

60. Asmussen E, Peutzfeldt A, Heitmann T: Stiffness, elastic limit, and strength of newer types of endodontic posts, *J Dent* 27:275, 1999.

61. Frederiksson M et al: A retrospective study of 236 patients with teeth restored by carbon fiber epoxy resin posts, *J Prosthet Dent* 80:151,1998.

62. Martinez-Insua A et al: Comparison of the fracture resistances of pulpless teeth restored with a cast post and core or carbon-fiber post with a composite core, *J Prosthet Dent* 80:527, 1998.

63. Kakehashi Y et al: A new all-ceramic post and core system: clinical, technical, and in vitro results, *Int J Periodont Restor Dent* 18:586, 1998.

64. Ahmad I: Zirconium oxide post and core system for the restoration of an endodontically treated incisor, *Pract Periodont Aesthet Dent* 11:197, 1999.

65. Sirimai S et al: An in vitro study of the fracture resistance and the incidence of vertical root fracture of pulpless teeth restored with six post-and-core systems, *J Prosthet Dent* 81: 262, 1999.

66. Rud J, Omnell KA: Root fractures due to corrosion: diagnostic aspects, *Scand J Dent Res* 78:397, 1970.

67. Angmar-Manansson B et al: Root fracture due to corrosion. I. Metallurgical aspects, *Odontol Rev* 20:245, 1969.

68. Silness J et al: Distribution of corrosion products in teeth restored with metal crowns retained by stainless steel posts, *Acta Odontol Scand* 37:317, 1979.

69. Chan RW, Bryant RW: Post-core foundations for endodontically treated posterior teeth, *J Prosthet Dent* 48:401, 1982.

70. Lovdahl PE, Nicholls JI: Pin-retained amalgam cores vs. cast-gold dowel-cores, *J Prosthet Dent* 38:507, 1977.

71. Reagan SE et al: Effects of cyclic loading on selected post-and-core systems, *Quintessence Int* 30: 61, 1999.

72. Foley J, Saunders E, Saunders WP: Strength of core build-up materials in endodontically treated teeth, *Am J Dent* 10:166, 1997.

73. Kovarik RE et al: Fatigue life of three core materials under simulated chewing conditions, *J Prosthet Dent* 68:584, 1992.

74. Oliva RA, Lowe JA: Dimensional stability of composite used as a core material, *J Prosthet Dent* 56:554, 1986.

75. Larson TD, Jensen JR: Microleakage of composite resin and amalgam core material under complete cast crowns, *J Prosthet Dent* 44:40, 1980.

76. Rosenstiel SF et al: Custom-cast post fabrication with a thermoplastic material, *J Prosthet Dent* 77:209, 1997.

77. Waldmeier MD, Grasso JE: Light-cured resin for post patterns, *J Prosthet Dent* 68:412, 1992.

78. Campagni WV, Majchrowicz M: An accelerated technique for the casting of post and core restorations, *J Prosthet Dent* 66:155, 1991.

79. Brunell G: Casting and microstructure of post and core at different mold temperatures, *Acta Odontol Scand* 40:241, 1982.

80. Yoshida T et al: An experimental study of the removal of cemented dowel-retained cast cores by ultrasonic vibration, *J Endodont* 23:239, 1997.

81. Altshul JH et al: Comparison of dentinal crack incidence and of post removal time resulting from post removal by ultrasonic or mechanical force, *J Endodont* 23:683, 1997.

82. Warren SR, Gutmann JL: Simplified method for removing intraradicular posts, *J Prosthet Dent* 42:353, 1979.

83. Masserann J: The extraction of posts broken deeply in the roots, *Actual Odontostomatol* 75:329, 1966.

84. Williams VD, Bjorndal AM: The Masserann technique for the removal of fractured posts in endodontically treated teeth, *J Prosthet Dent* 49:46, 1983.

85. Gettleman BH et al: Removal of canal obstructions with the Endo Extractor, *J Endodont* 17:608, 1991.

86. Machtou P et al: Post removal prior to retreatment, *J Endodont* 15:552, 1989.

CHAPTER THIRTEEN

IMPLANT-SUPPORTED FIXED PROSTHESES

Edwin A. McGlumphy

KEY TERMS

cover screw
dental implant
fixed abutment
healing abutment
healing cap
hybrid prosthesis
implant abutment types
implant analog
implant angulation

implant body
implant placement
implant prosthodontics
implant substructure
implant surgery
osseointegration
peri-implantitis
transosteal dental implant

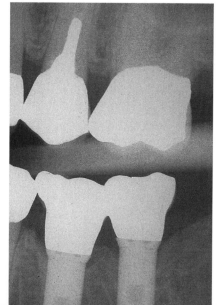

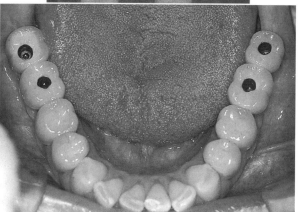

Fig. 13-1. **A**, Radiograph of two-unit fixed partial denture supported by two dental implants. **B**, Clinical example of bilateral two-unit fixed partial dentures.

Today the continued high rate of success achieved with osseointegrated **dental implants** allows a greater number of patients to enjoy the benefits of fixed rather than removable restorations.[1-3] The main indications for implant restorations in the partially edentulous patient are the free-end distal extension where no posterior abutment is available (Fig. 13-1) and the long edentulous span. In both these situations, the conventional dental treatment plan would include a removable partial denture. However, with the advent of implant abutments, the patient can benefit from fixed restorations. Additionally, in the short edentulous span, the single implant is a popular option (Fig. 13-2).

■ IMPLANT TYPES

There are three major subgroups of dental implants: subperiosteal, transosteal, and endosteal (Fig. 13-3). The first two, subperiosteal and transosteal, are designed primarily to anchor dentures in the completely edentulous patient and thus fall outside the scope of this chapter. The third, endosteal implants, are surgically placed within alveolar or basal bone and are most commonly used for the treatment of partially edentulous patients, either singly or in multiples. They can be further subdivided by shape into blade form (plateform) and root form (cylindrical). Blades are wedge shaped or rectangular in cross section and are generally 2.5 mm wide, 8 to 15

mm deep, and 15 to 30 mm long. Root forms are 3 to 6 mm in diameter and 8 to 20 mm long, often with external threads (Fig. 13-4). Endosteal implants are also categorized as one stage or two stage. The one-stage implant is designed to be placed in the bone and to immediately project through mucosa

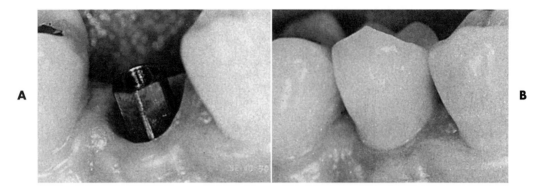

Fig. 13-2. **A,** Single-tooth implant abutment tightened to place. **B,** Implant crown replacing a single missing tooth (cement retained).

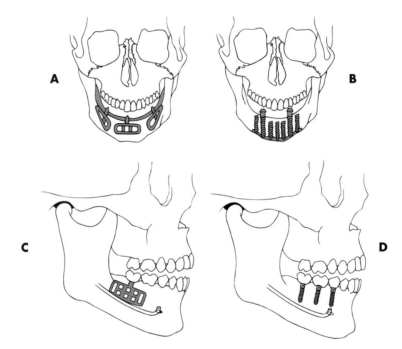

Fig. 13-3. The three major subgroups of dental implants. **A,** Subperiosteal. **B,** Transosteal. **C** and **D,** Endosteal. Endosteal implants can be further subdivided into plate form **(C)** and root form **(D).**

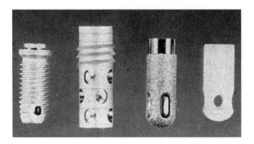

Fig. 13-4. Common types of root-form implants. Left to right: titanium screw, titanium alloy hollow basket, titanium plasma-sprayed cylinder, hydroxyapatite-coated cylinder.

into the oral cavity. The two-stage implant requires two surgical procedures. First, the implant is placed in bone to the level of the cortical plate and the oral mucosa is sutured over it; this is left for a prescribed healing period (usually 3 months in the mandible and 6 to 9 months in the maxilla), depending on the quality of bone. Then, in a second surgery, the mucosa is reflected from the superior surface of the implant, and an extension collar or abutment that projects into the oral cavity is fastened to the implant. Some authors have suggested shortening the time before implant loading, but the long-term consequences of this are unknown.[4,5]

PLATE IMPLANTS (BLADES)

Blades were the first dental implant to experience reasonable success in a large number of patients. All the original studies on blades used one-stage systems, but the success rates were considerably lower than those of current root-form implants. It has been suggested[6] that many of the problems of blade implants can be traced to the high temperature at which the bone sites were prepared and the routine immediate loading of this type of implant. Both these practices have been linked to the fibrous encapsulation that occurred with many of the original blade implants. Consequently, submergible titanium blades are now available, and more recent blade studies[7] have reported success rates above 80% for 5 years. However, the drawbacks to blade implants remain—difficulty of preparing precision slots for blade placement compared to placing holes accurately for root-form implants and the disastrously large circumferential area of the jaw that can be affected when a blade fails.

ROOT-FORM IMPLANTS (CYLINDERS)

Cylindrical root-form dental implants are considered to be state-of-the-art implant dentistry. Advantages include adaptability to multiple intraoral locations, uniformly precise implant-site preparation, and comparatively low adverse consequences similar to that experienced when a tooth is lost. Most root forms are made of titanium or titanium alloy with or without hydroxyapatite coating, materials that are perceived to have the highest biofunctionality. Both threaded and nonthreaded designs are available and are quite popular. Today many of the titanium implants are grit blasted or acid etched to roughen the surface and increase the area for bone contact.

The NIH consensus conference[1] in 1988 reported that root-form implants already constituted 78% of the implant market. This trend is credited to the Brånemark system, which set the precedent for surgical techniques and restorative procedures that result in predictably successful implants. Two of the most important additions from the Swedish research team, led by P.I. Brånemark, were atraumatic **implant placement** and delayed implant loading. These factors contributed to a remarkably increased degree of implant predictability. The original Brånemark success rate of 91% in the mandible over 15 years[2] has become the benchmark by which other implant systems are judged.[8] Many of the other root-form implant systems are also believed to have reached or exceeded this high level of long-term success.

TREATMENT PLANNING FOR THE IMPLANT PATIENT

Implant success reported from major research institutions is quite high. However, meticulous attention to the procedures of patient selection, diagnosis, and treatment planning is required to duplicate this suc-

cess. Indications for dental implant treatment in the partially edentulous patient are provided in Box 13-1.

A combined surgical and restorative treatment plan must be devised for prospective implant patients. Feasible nonimplant alternatives should be included in the overall treatment discussions. Patients need to be evaluated preoperatively and assessed as to whether they will be able to tolerate the procedure. The predictable risks and expected benefits should be weighed for each person. Although the placement of dental implants does entail some risks, they are relatively minor. Absolute contraindications, based on immediate surgical and anesthetic risks, are limited to individuals who are acutely ill, individuals with uncontrolled metabolic disease, and pregnant women (contraindications that apply to virtually all elective surgical procedures).

Local and systemic contraindications that threaten long-term implant retention must also be evaluated. Implants may be contraindicated in patients with abnormal bone metabolism, poor oral hygiene, and previous radiation to the implant site. Most potential implant placement patients became edentulous or partially edentulous from caries and periodontal disease resulting from poor oral hygiene. Suspicion that inadequate hygiene will continue is a relative contraindication to implant placement. Patients must be motivated and educated in oral hygiene techniques as part of their preparation for implants. Some individuals, such as those suffering from paralysis of the arms, debilitating arthritis, cerebral palsy, and severe mental retardation, may not be able to improve their hygiene. Implants are contraindicated in these patients unless adequate oral hygiene will be provided by caregivers. A summary of contraindications to implant placement is presented in Box 13-2.

CLINICAL EVALUATION

Evaluation of the planned implant site begins with a thorough clinical examination. This examination will determine whether there is adequate bone and

---

INDICATIONS FOR IMPLANT PLACEMENT IN THE PARTIALLY EDENTULOUS PATIENT BOX **13-1**

1. Inability to wear a removable partial or complete denture
2. Need for long-span fixed partial denture with questionable prognosis
3. Unfavorable number and location of potential natural tooth abutments
4. Single tooth loss that would necessitate preparation of minimally restored teeth for fixed prosthesis

will identify anatomic structures that could interfere with ideal implant placement. Visual inspection and palpation allow the detection of flabby excess tissue, bony ridges, and sharp underlying osseous formations and undercuts that would limit implant insertion. However, clinical inspection alone may not be adequate if there is thick overlying soft tissue that is dense, immobile, and fibrous.

RADIOGRAPHIC EVALUATION

Radiographic evaluation is also necessary. The best initial film is the panoramic view. However, there can be variations in magnification (5% to 35%); a small radiopaque reference object should therefore be placed near the proposed implant placement site during the exposure (Fig. 13-5). Measurement of this image on the actual radiograph will enable the practitioner to correct for any magnification error (Fig. 13-6). A ball bearing placed in wax on a denture baseplate or in poly(vinyl siloxane) impression putty works well. Some new panoramic radiography machines have standardized enlargement ratios, which makes correction markers less necessary.

The widths of the posterior mandible and maxilla are determined primarily by clinical examination. Bone width not revealed on a panoramic film can be evaluated in the anterior maxilla and mandible with a cephalometric film (Fig. 13-7). The location of the inferior alveolar canal and maxillary sinus can be determined by specialized CT scans, although high radiation exposure and considerable expense may limit their routine use.

DIAGNOSTIC CASTS

Accurately mounted diagnostic casts (see Chapter 2) are essential for treatment planning. They are used to study the remaining dentition, evaluate the residual bone, and analyze maxillomandibular relationships. They can be helpful to the surgeon for fixture placement. A diagnostic waxing is done on the cast or on a duplicate. Proposed fixture installation sites are checked for proper alignment, direction, location, and relation to the remaining dentition. The waxing helps determine the most esthetic placement of the

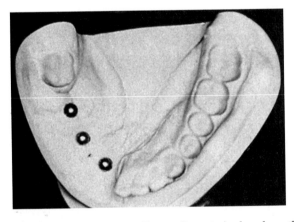

Fig. 13-5. Ball bearings (5-mm diameter) placed on the diagnostic cast at the proposed implant site.

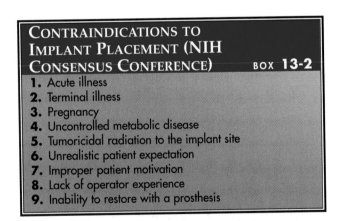

> **CONTRAINDICATIONS TO IMPLANT PLACEMENT (NIH CONSENSUS CONFERENCE)**   BOX **13-2**
> 1. Acute illness
> 2. Terminal illness
> 3. Pregnancy
> 4. Uncontrolled metabolic disease
> 5. Tumoricidal radiation to the implant site
> 6. Unrealistic patient expectation
> 7. Improper patient motivation
> 8. Lack of operator experience
> 9. Inability to restore with a prosthesis

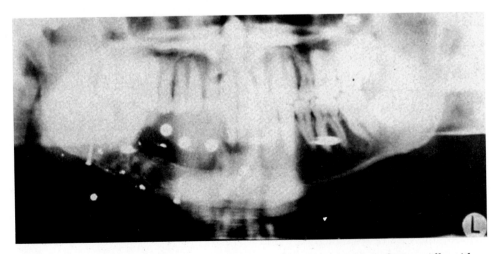

Fig. 13-6. A panoramic radiograph exposed with the ball bearings positioned intraorally with a wax or resin baseplate.

teeth to be restored and the potential for functional speech disturbances. After adjustments and the diagnostic waxing are completed, a resin template can be made from the cast to guide the surgeon during implant placement (Fig. 13-8). Diagnostic waxings and surgical templates are essential when planning implants as part of a full-mouth reconstruction or when restoring the anterior esthetic zone (Fig. 13-9).

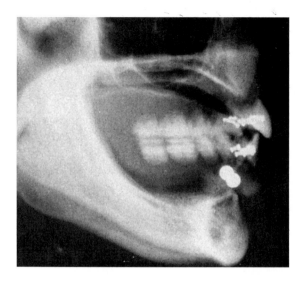

Fig. 13-7. The lateral cephalometric radiograph can indicate bone width in the anterior midline.

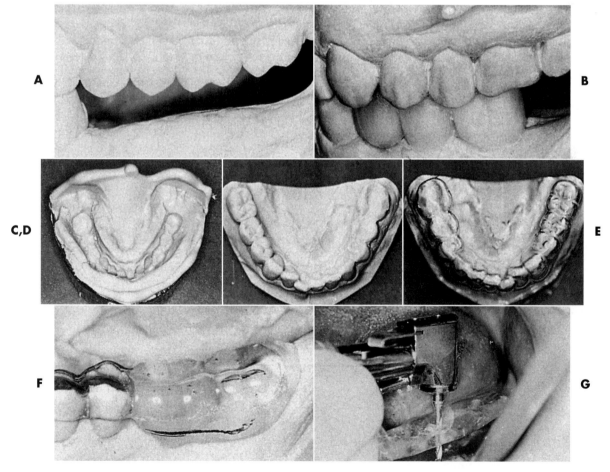

Fig. 13-8. **A,** Mounted diagnostic casts show an edentulous ridge and the interarch distance. **B,** Diagnostic waxing of a three-unit fixed prosthesis to replace the posterior teeth. **C,** To fabricate the surgical template, an alginate impression is made of the diagnostic waxing. **D,** An impression is poured to make a stone cast of the diagnostic waxing. **E,** A 1.5-mm vacuum-formed matrix is adapted to the stone cast. **F,** The matrix is trimmed from the duplicate cast and returned to the partially edentulous cast. The hollow matrix area is filled with autopolymerizing clear resin. The resin can be trimmed and holes drilled to guide the surgeon during implant site preparation **(G).**

BONE SOUNDING

When the results of clinical and radiographic examinations are equivocal and additional information is needed, sounding of the bone with a probe may be attempted. Under local anesthesia, a needle or sharp caliper is pushed through the tissue until it contacts bone. This can help judge soft tissue thickness at the planned implant sites.

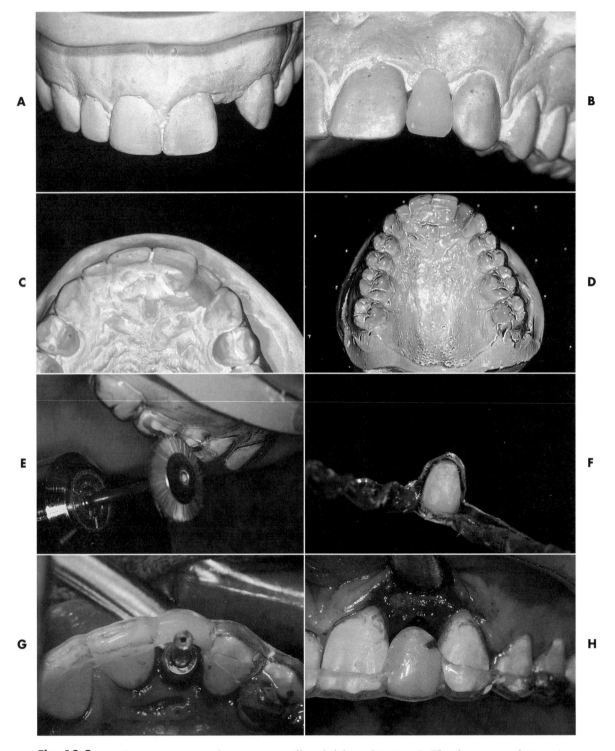

Fig. 13-9.   A, Diagnostic cast with missing maxillary left lateral incisor. **B,** The denture tooth is positioned for optimum esthetics. **C,** The denture tooth is trimmed from the lingual side until it is 2 mm thick. **D,** If the tooth is held in position with light-cured composite, a vacuum matrix can be performed directly without duplicating the cast. **E,** The matrix can be trimmed to the height of contour with a stiff bristle brush. **F,** The denture tooth can be glued back into the matrix. **G** and **H,** The surgeon can use this template to guide both horizontal and vertical positioning.

PRINCIPLES OF IMPLANT LOCATION

ANATOMIC LIMITATIONS

To maximize the chance of success, the implant should be placed entirely within bone and away from significant anatomic structures (e.g., the inferior alveolar canal). Ideally, 10 mm of vertical bone dimension and 6 mm of horizontal should be available for implant placement. These dimensions will prevent encroachment on anatomic structures and allow 1.0 mm of bone on both the lingual and the facial aspect of the implant. There should also be adequate space between adjacent implants. The minimum recommended distance varies slightly among implant systems but is generally accepted as 3.0 mm (Fig. 13-10). This space is needed to ensure bone viability between the implants and to allow adequate oral hygiene once the restorative dentistry is complete. Specific limitations due to anatomic variations among different areas of the jaws also must be considered. These include implant length, diameter, proximity to adjacent structures, and time required for integration.

The anterior maxilla, posterior maxilla, anterior mandible, and posterior mandible each require special considerations in placing implants. Some common guidelines include staying 2.0 mm above the superior aspect of the inferior alveolar canal, 5.0 mm anterior to the mental foramen, and 1.0 mm from the periodontal ligament of adjacent natural teeth.

After tooth loss, resorption of the ridge follows a pattern that results in crestal bone thinning and a change in angulation of the residual ridge. These sequelae most often cause problems in the anterior mandible and maxilla. The irregular anatomy of the residual ridge may lead to problems with achieving ideal **implant angulation** or adequate bone thickness along the labial aspect of the implant. Techniques for the management of these problems during surgery will be discussed, but they must be anticipated in the preoperative phase.

Anterior Maxilla. The anterior maxilla must be evaluated for proximity to the nasal cavity. A minimum of 1.0 mm of bone should remain between the apex of the implant and the nasal vestibule. Due to resorption of the anterior maxilla, the incisive foramen may be located near the residual ridge, especially in patients whose edentulous maxilla has been allowed to function against a natural mandibular anterior dentition. Anterior maxillary implants should be located slightly off midline, on either side of the incisive foramen.

Posterior Maxilla. Implant placement in the posterior maxilla poses two specific concerns:

First, the bone of the posterior maxilla is less dense than that of the posterior mandible. It has larger marrow spaces and a thinner cortex, which can affect treatment planning, since increased time must be allowed for integration of the implants and additional implants may be needed. A minimum of 6 months is usually needed for adequate integration of implants placed in the maxilla. In addition, one implant for every tooth that is being replaced is normally recommended, especially in the posterior maxilla.

The second concern is that the maxillary sinus is close to the edentulous ridge in the posterior maxilla. Frequently, because of the resorption of bone and increased pneumatization of the sinus, only a few millimeters of bone remain between the ridge and the sinus (Fig. 13-11, A). In treatment planning for implants in the posterior maxilla, the surgeon should leave 1.0 mm of bone between the floor of the sinus and the implant so the implant can be anchored apically into cortical bone of the sinus floor. Adequate bone height for implant stability can usually be found between the nasal cavity and the maxillary sinus. If there is not adequate bone for implant placement and support, bony augmentation through the sinus should be considered (Fig. 13-11).

Anterior Mandible. With respect to anatomic limitations, the anterior mandible is usually the most straightforward area for treatment planning. It usually has adequate height and width for implant

Implants should be placed at least 3 mm apart and 1 mm from adjacent teeth.

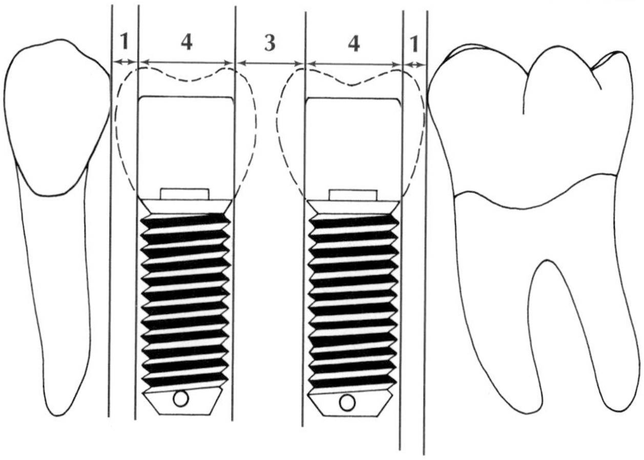

Fig. 13-10. Recommended minimum distances (in millimeters) between implants and between implants and natural teeth.

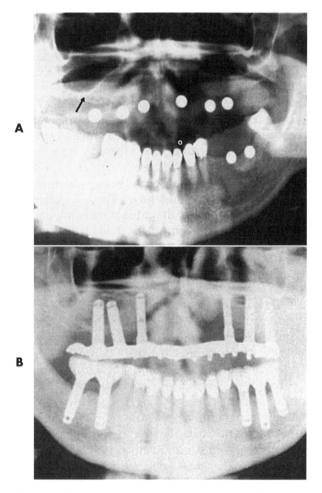

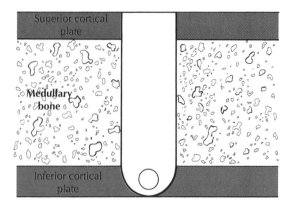

Fig. 13-12. Whenever possible, implants should engage two cortical plates of bone.

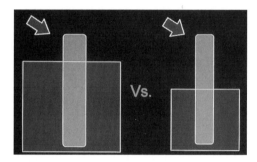

Fig. 13-13. Shorter implants usually have two problems: (1) less bone contact and (2) longer crowns, which increase the forces acting on the implant.

Fig. 13-11. **A,** The arrow denotes thin maxillary bone inferior to the sinus, which would be inadequate for implant placement without additional grafting procedures. **B,** The patient, successfully treated with dental implants after graft placement.

placement, and the bone quality is normally excellent, which makes it require the least amount of time for integration. Some success with immediate loading of implants in the anterior mandible has even been reported.

When possible, an implant in the anterior mandible should be placed through the entire cancellous bone so the apex of the implant will engage the cortex of the inferior mandibular border (Fig. 13-12). In the premolar area, care must be taken that the implant does not impinge on the inferior dental nerve. Since this nerve courses as much as 3.0 mm anterior to the mental foramen before turning posteriorly and superiorly to exit at the foramen, an implant should be at least 5.0 mm anterior to the foramen.

Posterior Mandible. The posterior mandible poses some limitations on implant placement. The inferior alveolar nerve traverses the mandibular body in this region, and treatment planning must allow for a 2.0-mm margin from the apex of the im-

plant to the superior aspect of the inferior alveolar canal. This is an important guideline: disregarding it can cause damage to the nerve and numbness of the lower lip. If adequate length is not present for even the shortest implant, nerve repositioning, onlay grafting, or a conventional nonimplant-borne prosthesis must be considered.

Implants placed in the posterior mandible are usually shorter, do not engage cortical bone inferiorly, and must support increased biomechanical occlusal forces once they are loaded due to their location in the posterior area. Consequently, allowing slightly more time for integration may be beneficial. In additional, if short implants (8 to 10 mm) are used, "overengineering" and placing more implants than usual to withstand the occlusal load is recommended. Short implants are often necessary because of bone resorption, thus increasing the crown-to-implant ratio when the normal plane of occlusion is reestablished (Fig. 13-13).

The width of the residual ridge must be carefully evaluated in the posterior mandible. Attachments of the mylohyoid muscle maintain it along the superior aspect of the ridge, and a deep (lingual) depression exists immediately below it. This area should

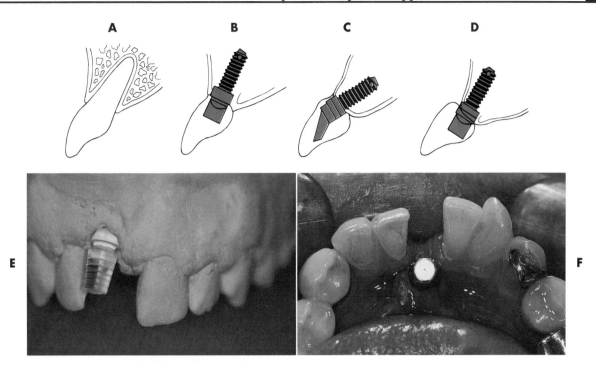

Fig. 13-14. Implant placement and angulation dictate the screw emergence position and crown contours. Esthetics and access for hygiene can be greatly affected. **A,** The natural tooth. **B,** Ideal implant location with acceptable crown contours and lingual screw emergence. **C** and **D,** Less ideal implant location. **E,** Laboratory example of an implant placed too far apically and facially. **F,** Clinical example of an implant placed too far lingually.

be palpated at the time of evaluation and examined at surgery:

RESTORATIVE CONSIDERATIONS

Implant Placement. Implant placement is critically important to the design of the restoration. Thus the treatment-planning aspects of implant placement must begin with a restorative dentistry consultation. Implant placement dictates the appearance, contour, and long-term function of the prosthesis. To prevent damage, staying at least 1.0 mm away from the adjacent natural tooth is essential, but staying as close to the natural tooth as possible is also important, so acceptable contours can be created by the restorative dentist. For proper access during oral hygiene procedures, a minimum of 3.0 mm should be left between implants. In addition, implants must not encroach on the embrasure spaces or be angled so that screw access is necessary through the facial surfaces of the completed restoration (Fig. 13-14).

To minimize harmful lateral forces, the long axis of the implant should be positioned in the central fossae of the restoration. This dictates placing the implant accurately in all three planes of space. Superoinferior placement is important to ensure the optimal emergence profile of the restoration. Ideally, the superior surface of the implant should be 2.0 to 3.0 mm directly inferior to the emergence po-

sition of the planned restoration, particularly when the restoration is to be located in the anterior esthetic zone (see Fig. 13-15).

Implant and Restoration Size. The choice of implant and its superior-inferior placement location are modified by the diameter of the intended restoration and can be adjusted for different sizes of teeth.

For example, the typical root diameter of a maxillary central incisor is 8.0 mm; the average implant diameter is 4.0 mm. Therefore, a distance of 2.0 to 3.0 mm is needed to make the transition gradually from 4.0 to 8.0 mm. If this is done over too short a distance, the restoration will be overcontoured or look unnatural. By contrast, many mandibular centrals and laterals are smaller than 4.0 mm at the cementoenamel junction. Therefore, an esthetic restoration on a 4.0-mm implant is impossible. Smaller-diameter implants (about 3.0 mm) have been developed to allow esthetic restoration in these areas. It is also possible to use a larger implant (5.0 to 6.0 mm) for molar restorations with adequate bone (Fig. 13-16).

Restoration size must always be considered during the treatment-planning stage so that a properly sized implant will be placed in the ideal location.

Accurate implant depth is critical to a successful result.

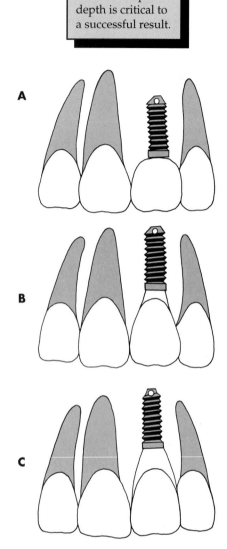

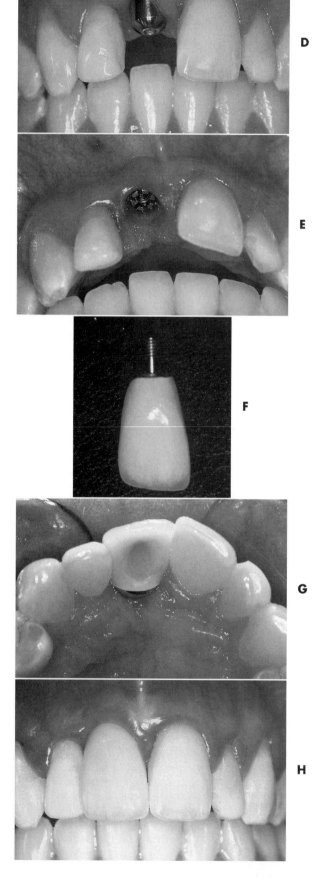

Fig. 13-15. Superior or inferior positioning may affect crown contours and pocket depth. **A,** The implant is not placed deep enough. This creates a short, overcontoured crown. **B,** Placement 2 to 3 mm apical to the tooth emergence position is ideal. **C,** Placing the implant 4 mm apical to the crown contours may create an excessively deep gingival sulcus. **D** to **H,** Clinical example of a properly positioned implant, both facially and apically, resulting in good esthetics.

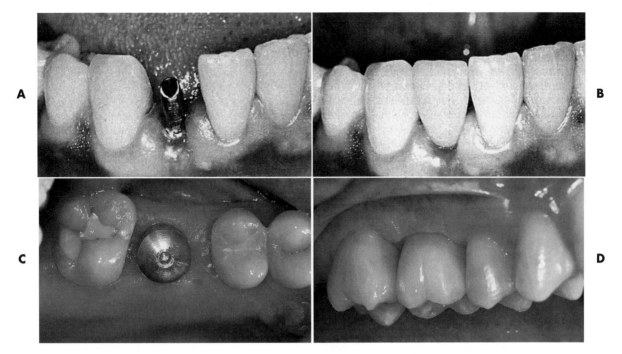

Fig. 13-16. **A,** Small-diameter implant and abutment positioned to restore a mandibular lateral incisor. The **fixed abutment** can be custom prepared and narrowed to allow restoration of a small-diameter tooth. **B,** Completed implant restoration of the mandibular lateral incisor. **C,** Wide-diameter (5.0 mm) implant in position to replace maxillary first molar. **D,** Completed implant restoration of the maxillary first molar.

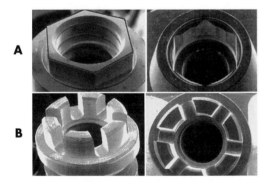

Fig. 13-17. **A,** Scanning electron micrograph (SEM) of the standard external hexagon on an implant and corresponding abutment. **B,** SEM of six finger projections from an implant (known as a *spline interface*).

Single Tooth Implant. Treatment planning for the single tooth restoration, particularly in the anterior esthetic zone, is one of the most challenging problems faced by the implant restorative dentist. Placement of the implant for both esthetics and biomechanical loading (to minimize screw loosening) is especially critical. In addition, at the treatment-planning stage, the decision to place an implant with an antirotational feature built into the system (e.g., a spline or a hexagon) is essential (Fig. 13-17).

SURGICAL GUIDE

The coordination of surgical and prosthetic procedures through proper treatment planning is one of the more critical factors in obtaining ideal esthetic results for the implant restoration. A surgical guide template is extremely useful for anterior implants because slight variations in angulation can significantly affect the appearance of the final restoration. Construction of the surgical guide template has become a requirement in those patients in whom it is necessary to optimize fixed replacement and ensure correct emergence profiles. Surgical templates can also be beneficial in areas where esthetics is less important. The objectives for using a surgical template in partially edentulous patients are as follows: (1) delineate the embrasures, (2) locate the implant within the restoration contour, (3) align implants with the long axis of the completed restoration, and (4) identify the level of the CEJ or tooth emergence from the soft tissue.

A clear resin facial veneer template is recommended for anterior implant placement to allow the surgeon access to the osseous receptor site and an unimpeded view of the frontal and sagittal angulations as the site is being prepared. This type of template is fabricated from a diagnostic waxing or denture tooth arrangement on a mounted cast. The waxing is duplicated with alginate or poly(vinyl siloxane) and poured in quick-setting stone. Then 1.5 mm (0.060 inch) of vacuum-formed matrix material is adapted to the replicated cast. For accurate orientation, the vacuum-formed matrix should be trimmed to extend over the full facial surface of the teeth being restored and about a third of the facial surface of the remaining dentition. This template is removed from the duplicate cast and returned to the original cast. A 2-mm thickness of autopolymerizing resin is added to the lingual surface to compensate for the space occupied by the porcelain on the implant restoration (Fig. 13-18). (The total thickness, including an additional millimeter from the vacuum-formed matrix, will be about 3.0 mm.) The surgeon must stay as close as possible to this guide during implant placement, which will allow maximum flexibility in selecting an implant site without violating the facial surface or forcing screw access holes to be located inappropriately in the facial restoration. Following this guide will enable the surgeon to place a fixture in the best location with minimum

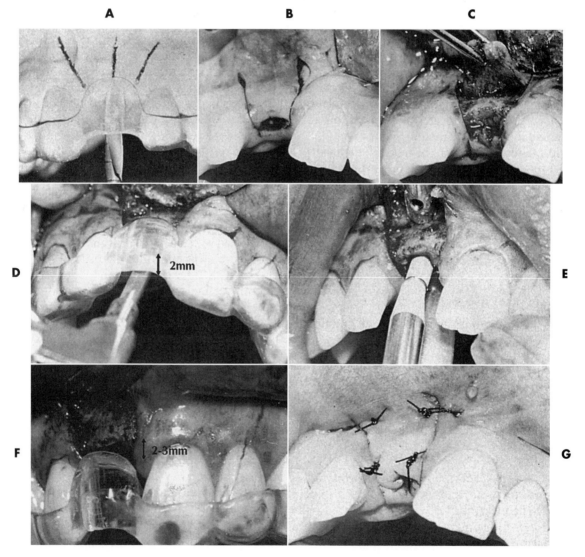

Fig. 13-18. Anterior surgical guide template fabrication. **A,** The apical extent of the template is not removed, which allows the superior-inferior orientation of implant placement to be determined. **B,** Full-thickness flap incisions are made, preserving the interdental papilla. **C,** A tissue flap is reflected to expose bone for preparation of the implant site. **D,** Resin (2.0 mm) has been added to the lingual aspect of the matrix; the rest of the lingual area was left open so the surgeon can choose the best available bone. The site should be prepared as close to the template as possible. **E,** The implant is tapped into position at an angle that allows optimum esthetics and access for hygiene. **F,** The implant is positioned 2.0 to 3.0 mm apical to the desired emergence position of the final restoration. **G,** The surgical site is sutured. A 6-month healing time will be allowed.
(Courtesy Dr. J.A. Holloway.)

undesirable sagittal angulation. If a cement-retained restoration is desired, the orientation of the implant can be slightly more facial.

Although the use of a guide is most necessary in the maxillary anterior region, where bony dimensions are sometimes surprising and often unfavorable, the guide may also be useful in posterior areas with wide edentulous ridges. However, a different type of guide or template is fabricated in this area. Holes are drilled through the resin into the underlying cast and are paralleled with a milling machine or dental surveyor. Such templates even more accurately locate the placement of an implant and direct the inclination of its long axis.

Surgical templates also can be fabricated for a maxillary edentulous arch that is to be restored with a fixed prosthesis. Such templates are described later in the chapter, but the same preoperative planning and interspecialty cooperation are as important here as was just described.

IMPLANT SURGERY

Peter E. Larsen

Implant surgery can be performed in an ambulatory setting under local anesthesia. However, it requires more time than other surgical procedures, so conscious sedation may be preferred. Although placing an implant is less traumatic than extracting a tooth, patients expect it to be more traumatic. Preoperative education and conscious sedation should lessen the anxiety.

For a complete description of the surgical procedures involved in implant placement, refer to one of the current standard texts.[9,10]

Surgical Access

Several types of incision can be used to gain access to the residual ridge for implant placement. The incision chosen should allow retraction of the soft tissue for unimpeded implant placement and should preserve attached tissue esthetics and quantity.

When the quantity of attached tissue is adequate and the underlying bone is expected to be of sufficient width, a simple crestal incision is recommended. However, closure must be performed carefully, because the implant lies directly beneath. In the posterior mandible, an incision may be placed toward the buccal aspect of the ridge to allow the flap to be retracted by a suture. This may be a disadvantage, however, because the incision line is then immediately over the area where the bone may be thinnest, and a dehiscence can occur during surgery. An incision slightly to the palatal side is particularly effective in the maxillary anterior zone.

After the bone is exposed, the surgical template is positioned, and a periodontal probe is used to make a preliminary assessment of the potential implant site. The residual ridge may have areas that are uneven or with sharp ridges. These areas should be smoothed before implant placement.

Implant Placement

Placement procedures for all implant systems require atraumatic preparation of the recipient site. Thermal injury to bone is minimized by using a low-speed, high-torque handpiece, along with copious irrigation. The irrigation is either externally or internally applied and directed through channels in the drill. Manufacturer recommendations relating to the type of irrigation and speed of the drilling equipment should be followed. Threaded implants often require final thread preparation in the bone at very low speeds.

The implant recipient site is prepared with a series of gradually enlarged burs. All implant systems have an initial small-diameter drill used to mark the implant site. The implant site is located using the surgical template, which may also assist in directing angulation of the implant. The center of the implant recipient site is marked with the initial drill, and a pilot hole is prepared. A paralleling pin is then placed in the preparation to check alignment and angulation.

At this point, a final determination is made regarding the adequacy of the recipient site for implant placement. Although implant placement is a surgical procedure, it is influenced by critical restorative parameters. The stent communicates the range of acceptable implant positions and angulations. At this step, if it is apparent that supporting bone will not allow proper positioning of the implant, further osseous augmentation may be necessary, either simultaneously with implant placement, or as a separate procedure with implant placement delayed until proper osseous support is available.

After the desired depth and diameter of the recipient site are achieved, the implant is placed. For titanium implants, an uncontaminated surface oxide layer is required for **osseointegration.** Hydroxyapatite-coated implants are also sensitive to contamination.

Nonthreaded implants are positioned in the recipient site and gently tapped into place with a mallet and seating instrument. Threaded implants are screwed into place, which also requires cutting the screw threads in the recipient site. Self-tapping implants are available for use in the maxilla, where the bone is soft enough to make prethreading unnecessary. After all implants are placed, tension-free closure prevents wound dehiscence.

POSTOPERATIVE EVALUATION

A radiograph should be taken postoperatively to evaluate the position of the implant in relation to adjacent structures (e.g., the sinus and the inferior alveolar canal) and other implants. Any significant problems noticed at this time should be corrected.

Patients are given mild analgesics and 0.12% chlorhexidine gluconate rinses for 2 weeks after surgery to keep bacterial populations to a minimum during healing. Weekly evaluations are recommended until soft tissue healing is complete (2 to 3 weeks). If possible, complete or removable partial dentures should not be worn for 1 week after surgery. The resin over the implant can then be reduced by 2.0 or 3.0 mm and replaced with a soft liner, so that the denture can be worn without injuring the healing implant site.

IMPLANT UNCOVERING

If a two-stage system is used, implant uncovering is performed after complete implant fixture integration has been achieved. The time interval for integration to occur varies and depends on the particular site and patient. Longer times may be required if the bone quality and surgery were less than ideal or if the bone-to-implant interface was questionable at the time of placement. In general, recommended integration times are 6 months in the maxilla, 3 months in the anterior mandible, and 4 months in the posterior mandible.

The goals of surgical uncovering are to accurately attach the abutment to the implant, to preserve attached tissue, and to recontour tissue as necessary. These goals may be accomplished with any of these three techniques: the tissue punch, crestal incision, or flap repositioning.

After the implant is exposed, the implant abutment is placed. There are two approaches for this procedure. The first approach is to place the same abutment as will be used in the restoration. The second approach is to place a temporary **healing cap** that will remain until the tissue heals and will then be replaced by the abutment during the surgical treatment procedures.

When the abutment is placed, the superstructure must be completely seated on the **implant body** without gaps or intervening tissue. In systems with antirotational facets in the implant (see Fig. 13-17), these features must be aligned to allow complete seating of the abutment. The superstructure–implant body interface should be evaluated radiographically immediately after the uncovering. If a gap is present, the superstructure must be repositioned.

• • •

IMPLANT RESTORATIONS

Osseointegrated implants are generally designed to support screw- or cement-retained implant restorations. These implant systems offer many advantages over conventional dental restorations and one-stage implants (Box 13-3).

Fabrication of screw-retained implant restorations requires a number of components unique to implant dentistry. For less experienced clinicians, the large number of parts included within one system might create problems. This section describes in generic terms the component parts typically needed to restore an osseointegrated implant. There are many implant systems, and although all the major components are available for each system, many differ slightly in specific design and materials. The basic steps for implant restoration fabrication are described in Figure 13-19.

CLINICAL IMPLANT COMPONENTS

Terms used to describe similar implant components vary widely among manufacturing companies. A list of terms used in this book and a partial list of alternative terms are described in Box 13-4.

Implant Body. The implant body is the component placed within the bone during first-stage surgery. It may be a threaded or nonthreaded root form and is normally made of either titanium or titanium alloy of varying surface roughnesses, with or without a hydroxyapatite coating (Fig. 13-20). Although some controversy exists regarding the optimum shape and surface coating for an implant in different parts of the mouth, the significant factors for success are precise placement, atraumatic surgery, unloaded healing, and passive restoration.

ADVANTAGES OF OSSEOINTEGRATED IMPLANTS   BOX 13-3

1. Surgical
   a. Documented success rate
   b. In-office procedure
   c. Adaptable to multiple intraoral locations
   d. Precise implant site preparation
   e. Reversibility in the event of implant failure
2. Prosthetic
   a. Multiple restorative options
   b. Versatility of second-stage components
      • Angle correction
      • Esthetics
      • Crown contours
      • Screw- or cement-retained options
   c. Retrievability in the event of prosthodontic failure

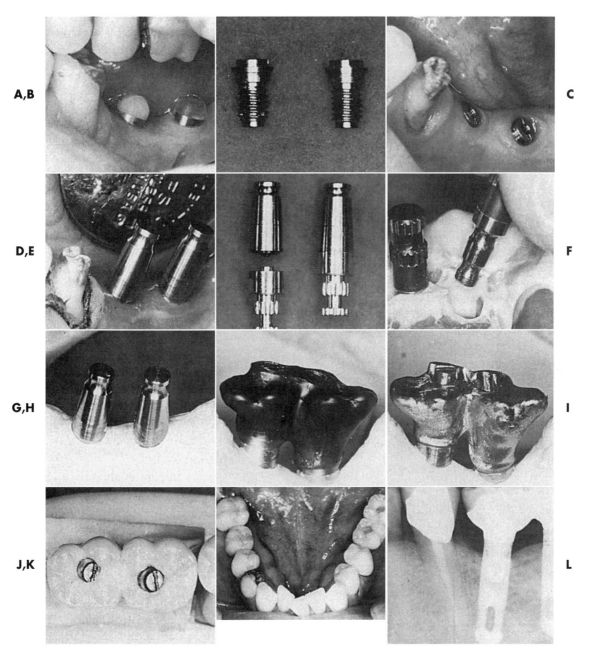

Fig. 13-19. **A,** Healing caps in place 2 weeks after second-stage surgery. A two-unit implant prosthesis will be fabricated distal to the conventional crown on the mandibular second premolar. **B,** Two abutments are selected to thread into the implants when the healing caps are removed. **C,** The abutments are placed intraorally, and the premolar is prepared for a conventional crown. **D,** The impression posts are tightened onto the abutments, and a displacement cord is placed only around the conventional preparation. **E,** After an impression is made, the impression posts are removed from the mouth and attached to the laboratory analogs. **F,** Impression posts and analogs are relocated in the impression before pouring. **G,** The impression posts locate the analogs in the same position on the cast as the abutments are in the mouth. **H,** Impression posts removed from the analogs. Waxing sleeves are attached, and a full-contour waxing is completed and cut back. **I,** The unit is then cast, incorporating the waxing sleeves in the prosthesis, and is fitted back on the cast. **J,** Porcelain is applied to the prosthesis, which is secured by retaining screws countersunk below the occlusal surface. **K,** The completed prosthesis replaces the mandibular first and second molars. Composite resin covers the screw access holes. The prosthesis is not joined to the conventional crown on the mandibular second premolar. **L,** Radiograph of the completed restorations.

IMPLANT TERMINOLOGY

BOX **13-4**

TEXT TERM	ALSO KNOWN AS	FUNCTION
Implant body (see Fig. 13–20)	Implant fixture screw Cylinder	Portion of the implant system within the bone
Cover screw (see Fig. 13–21)	Sealing screw Healing screw First stage cover screw	Seals the occlusal surface of the implant during osseointegration
Healing abutment (see Fig. 13–22)	Temporary gingival cuff Healing collar Implant healing cap	A cover, attached to the implant, that is used to maintain the opening through the tissue until the restoration is completed
Healing cap (see Fig. 13–22, B)	Temporary screw Comfort cap Abutment healing cap	A cover that is attached to the top of a transmucosal abutment, protecting the internal threads and interface surfaces of the abutment
Standard abutment (see Fig. 13–23 A)	Transmucosal abutment Tissue extension Permucosal extension	An intermediate component placed between the implant and metal framework/restoration, providing support and retention for a fixed-removable restoration. Excellent for bar overdentures
Tapered abutment (see Fig. 13–23, B)	Conical abutment Transmucosal abutment Tissue extension Permucosal abutment	An intermediate component placed between the implant and restoration, providing support and retention for a fixed-removable restoration. The abutment is cone shaped for maximum esthetics. Excellent for screw-retained fixed prostheses.
Hex driver (see Fig. 13–32, C)	Hex tool Screw driver	Used for placing and removing all hex screws (i.e., abutment fastening screws), impression post-retaining screws, and healing abutments. Available in two lengths: Short (19 mm - for posterior) and long (24 mm - for anterior); and three hex sizes: 0.048", 0.050", and 0.062"
Abutment driver or seating tool	Name of each driver/tool is specific based on its use	Used to seat the abutment directly onto the implant
Impression post (see Fig. 13–32, A, B, D)	Impression coping Impression pin Transfer pin Transfer post	Component used during the impression procedure to transfer the position of the implant to the cast
Laboratory analog (see Fig. 13–32, G)	Implant fixed analog Abutment analog Implant body analog Fixture replica	Replicates the implant for use in the cast
Temporary abutment sleeve (see Fig. 13-49, H)	Temporary cylinder Temporary coping Provisional abutment	Provides support and retention for acrylic temporary/provisional restorations. May also be used for occlusal rim and wax set-up try-in procedures for overdentures.
Fixed abutment (see Fig. 13–23, B, C)	Straight abutment Coping abutment Abutment post Crown and bridge abutment (slang)	An abutment used for a cement retained restoration (Also available in 15° and 25° angles)
Plastic sleeve (see Fig. 13–36)	Plastic sheath Waxing sleeve Plastic coping Castable abutment Castable coping	A castable plastic pattern used to form an abutment during the laboratory waxing procedure
Gold cylinder (see Fig. 13–37) (waxing sleeve)	Gold sleeve Gold coping	A premachined abutment that is waxed and cast to. It interfaces directly onto the transmucosal abutment.
Prosthesis-retaining screw Fastening screw (see Fig. 13–40)	Gold screw Coping screw Fastening screw	Screw used to secure a screw-retained metal (bar) framework or restoration to transmucosal abutments (i.e., conical or standard abutments)

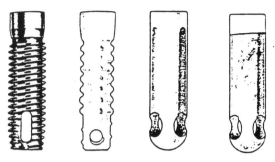

Fig. 13-20. Four main categories of osseointegrated implants. *Left to right:* titanium screw, hydroxyapatite-coated screw, hydroxyapatite-coated cylinder, titanium plasma-sprayed cylinder.

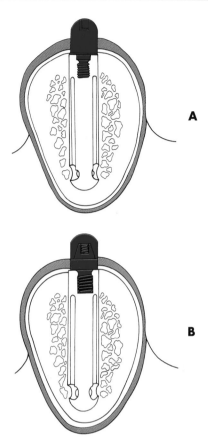

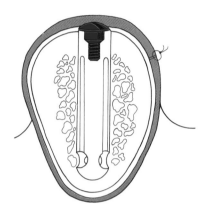

Fig. 13-21. Cover screw in place during the initial implant-healing phase. Soft tissue is sutured over the implant. A removable prosthesis can be worn over this area during healing.

Fig. 13-22. Two types of healing abutments. Both allow for soft tissue healing after second-stage surgery. **A,** This type screws into the implant. **B,** This type screws into the abutment. It is more commonly referred to as a healing cap.

All contemporary dental implants have an internally threaded portion that can accept second-stage screw placements. These implants also may incorporate an antirotational feature within the design of the fixture body. If it is incorporated, the antirotational feature may be either internal or external.

Implant bodies can also be classified as *one stage* or *two stage*. One-stage implants project through the soft tissue immediately after Stage I surgery. Two-stage implants are typically covered with soft tissue at this point. When a tall **cover screw** or healing cap is placed on a two-stage implant to project it through the tissue at the time of placement, this is referred to as "using a two-stage implant with a one-stage protocol."

Cover Screw. During the healing phase following first-stage surgery, a screw is normally placed in the superior aspect of the fixture. It is usually low in profile to facilitate the suturing of soft tissue in the two-stage implant or to minimize loading in the one-stage implant (Fig. 13-21). At second-stage surgery, it is removed and replaced by subsequent components. In some systems the screw is made slightly

larger than the diameter of the implant, which facilitates abutment placement by ensuring that bone does not grow over the edge of the implant. The implant surgeon should always be sure that the sealing screw is completely seated after stage-one surgery to prevent bone from growing between the screw and the implant. If this occurs, removing the bone may damage the superior surface of the implant and affect the fit of subsequent components.

Healing Abutment. Healing abutments are dome-shaped screws placed after second-stage surgery and before insertion of the prosthesis. They range in length from 2 to 10 mm and project through the soft tissue into the oral cavity. They may screw directly into the fixture or, in some systems, onto the abutment immediately after second-stage surgery. Those that screw onto the abutment are commonly referred to as *healing caps* (Fig. 13-22). Both healing abutments are made of titanium or titanium alloy. In areas where esthetics is paramount, healing should be sufficiently completed around a healing cap to stabilize the gingival margin. At this time, abutments of appropriate length are selected to ensure that the metal-porcelain interface of the restoration will be located subgingivally. In areas where tissue esthetics is not critical, adequate healing for impressions usually takes 2 weeks. In esthetic zones, 3 to 5 weeks may be required before abutment selection. In addition, knowing the length of the healing cap can expedite abutment selection.

Abutments. Abutments are the component of the implant system that screw directly into the implant. They will eventually support the prosthesis in screw-retained restorations, since they accept the retaining screw of the prosthesis. For cement-retained restorations, they may be shaped like a conventional crown preparation. Abutments take many forms (Fig. 13-23). Their walls are usually smooth, polished, and straight-sided titanium or titanium alloy. Their length ranges from 1 to 10 mm. In nonesthetic areas, 1 to 2 mm of titanium should be allowed to penetrate the soft tissue to maximize the patient's ability to clean the prosthesis (Fig. 13-24). In esthetic areas, an abutment can be selected to allow porcelain to be carried subgingivally for optimum esthetics (Fig. 13-25).

In implant systems that incorporate an antirotational feature, the abutment must have two components that move independently of each other—one engages the antirotational feature, and the other secures the abutment within the fixture (Fig. 13-26).

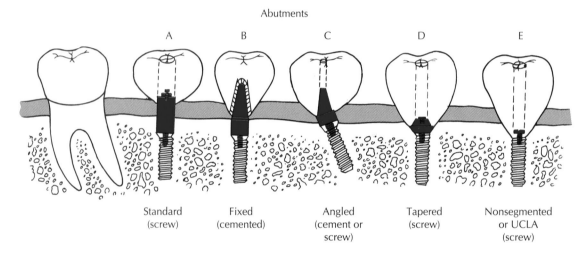

Fig. 13-23. Types of abutments *(left to right):* **A,** Standard. Length can be selected to make the margin subgingival or supergingival. **B,** Fixed. This abutment is much like a conventional post-and-core. It is screwed into the implants, has a prepared finish line, and receives a cemented restoration. **C,** Angled. This type is available when implant angles must be corrected for esthetic or biomechanical reasons. **D,** Tapered. This type can be used to make the transition to restoration more gradual in larger teeth. **E,** Nonsegmented, or direct. This type is used in areas of limited interarch distance or areas where esthetics is important. The restoration can be built directly on the implant, so there is no intervening abutment. This direct restoration technique has been called the *UCLA abutment.*
(Modified from Peterson et al: Contemporary oral surgery, *ed 3, St Louis, 1998, Mosby.)*

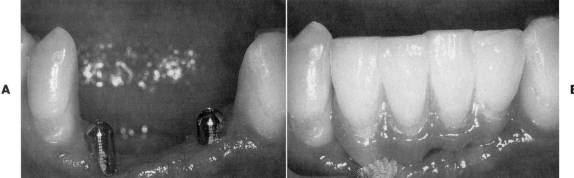

Fig. 13-24. **A,** Healing abutments projecting through the soft tissue. **B,** Implant restorations supported by standard abutments that allow easy access for oral hygiene.

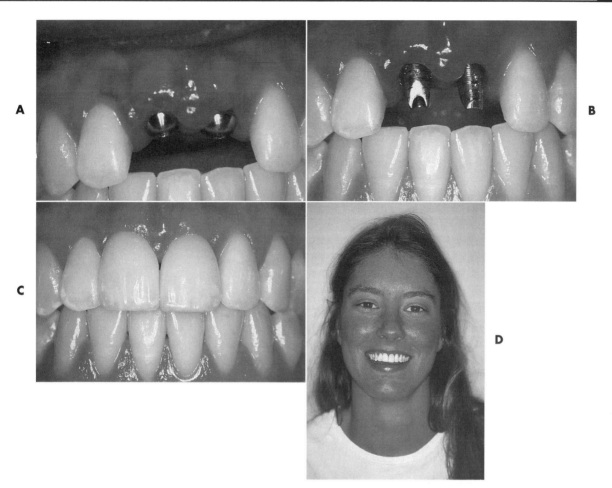

Fig. 13-25. **A,** Healing abutments projecting through the tissue for implant restoration of maxillary central incisors. **B,** Fixed abutments selected with margins 1 to 2 mm subgingival. **C,** Completed, cemented restorations. **D,** Overall esthetic result.

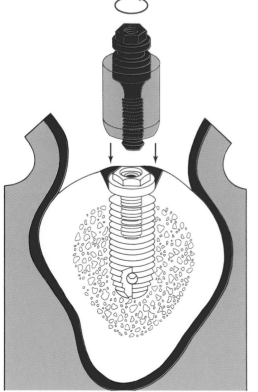

Fig. 13-26. When an antirotational feature is to be engaged by the abutment, one component of the abutment (the sleeve) must fit the hexagon whereas the other (the screw) independently tightens the components together.

Angled abutments use a similar technique to correct divergently placed implants (Figs. 13-27 and 13-28). Some systems have recently included tapered or wide-base abutments, which allow teeth with larger cross-sectional diameters to be restored with more physiologic contours. The nonsegmented implant crown (UCLA) bypasses the abutment portion by using a sleeve waxed directly to the implant. Using nonsegmented implant crowns may be necessary when soft tissue thickness is less than 2 mm. All-ceramic components designed to be tightened directly to the implant also have been introduced (Fig. 13-29).

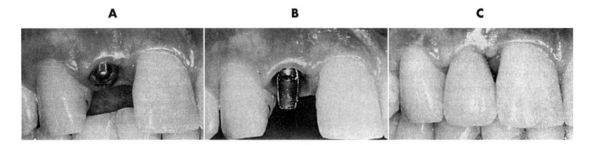

Fig. 13-27. **A,** This implant in the maxillary lateral incisor position is angled too far facially to restore with a straight abutment. **B,** An abutment angled 15 degrees with subgingival margins is screwed to place. **C,** The completed crown cemented onto the angled abutment. A provisional luting agent can be used to maintain retrievability, although choosing a suitable material that retains the restoration adequately but can still be removed is not always easy.

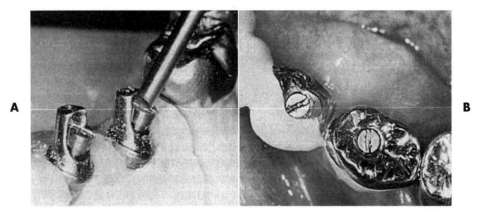

Fig. 13-28. **A,** Severely angled implants require 25-degree angled abutments. **B,** Completed restoration on 25-degree angled abutments with retaining screws redirected toward the occlusal surface.

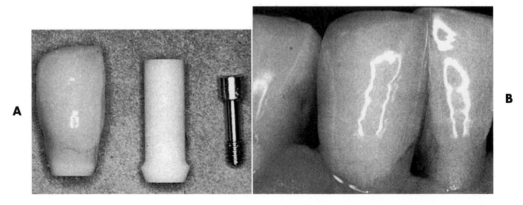

Fig. 13-29. **A,** An all-ceramic abutment designed to fit directly against the implant is compatible with aluminous dental porcelain. **B,** A screw-retained, all-ceramic restoration can be used on larger teeth and has excellent esthetics.
(Courtesy Drs. A. Ingber and V. Prestipino.)

The choice of abutment size will depend on the vertical distance between the fixture base and opposing dentition, the existing sulcular depth, and the esthetic requirements in the area being restored. For acceptable appearance, fixtures in the posterior maxilla or mandible may require margin termination at or below the gingival crest. An anterior maxillary crown may require 2 to 3 mm of subgingival porcelain at the facial gingival margin to create the proper emergence profile and appearance. Framework fit should be checked on multiple unit restorations if abutment margins are no more than 1 mm subgingivally. Periodontal probing of the sulcus after the healing cap is removed will reveal the space

available for subgingival extension and can be performed at the time of abutment placement or following a period of tissue healing around a provisional restoration. When these measurements have been made, the correct abutment is attached to the implant. The abutment length can have a dramatic effect on restoration contours (Fig. 13-30).

Impression Posts. Impression posts facilitate transfer of the intraoral location of the implant or abutment to a similar position on the laboratory cast. They may screw into the implant or onto the abutment and are customarily subdivided into fixture types or abutment types (Fig. 13-31).

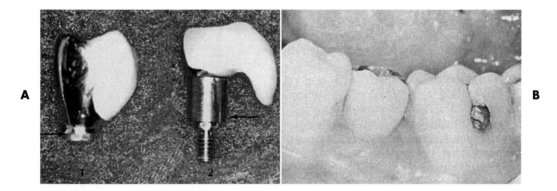

Fig. 13-30. **A,** Two crowns fabricated for the same lingually tipped mandibular implant. The arrows denote the connection to the implant body for both units. Crown 2 is fabricated on a 4-mm abutment. Crown 1 is connected directly to the implant body, allowing the creation of more physiologic contours. **B,** One-year follow-up of crown 1. The soft tissue response is excellent despite a poorly placed implant.

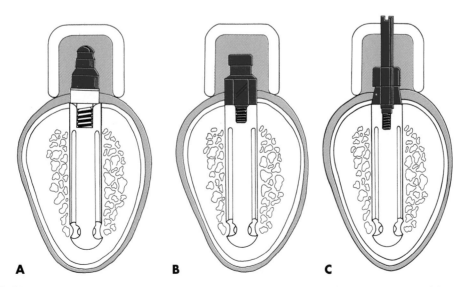

Fig. 13-31. Types of impression posts. **A,** A one-piece (screws onto abutment) is used if the abutment does not need to be changed on the laboratory cast. **B,** A one-piece (transfer) is attached directly to the fixture if the abutment does need to be changed on the cast (it should have a flat side if angle correction will be necessary). **C,** A two-piece (pick-up), used to orient the antirotational feature or to make impressions of very divergent implants.

With the transfer impression post in place, an impression is made intraorally. Both of these can be further subdivided into transfer types (indirect) and pick-up (direct) types after radiographs are taken to confirm complete engagement. Heavier-body impression materials (e.g., poly[vinyl siloxane] and polyether) are usually recommended, although any conventional impression material can be used. When the impression is removed from the mouth, the impression post remains in place on the implant abutment or on the fixture. It is then removed from the mouth and joined to the laboratory analog before being transferred to the impression in the proper orientation. If the clinician anticipates that the implant angulation will have to be corrected on the laboratory cast, a flat-sided impression post that goes directly into the fixture or implant should be used (Fig. 13-32). The flat side of the post will accurately orient the location of the implant and position the threads and the antirotational feature. When an angled abutment is placed or screwed into the implant, it must be oriented in the same position as the prosthesis was fabricated in the laboratory. Completely symmetric impression posts are contraindi-

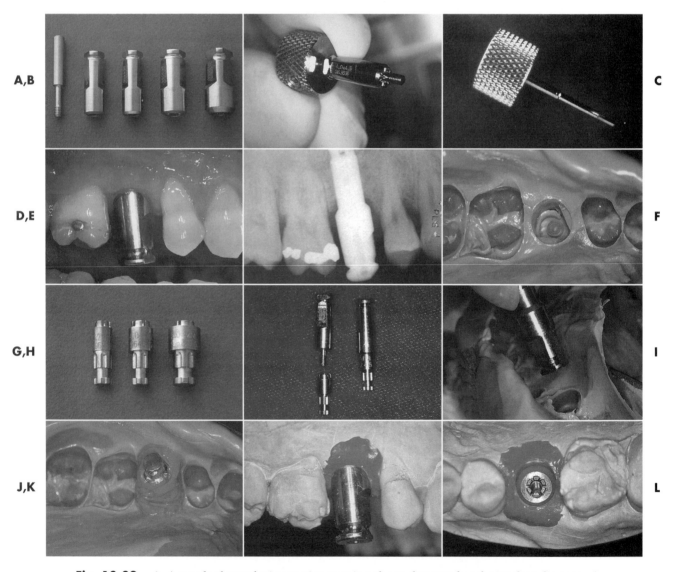

Fig. 13-32.   **A,** A standard transfer impression post is a sleeve that matches the implant diameter. A screw penetrates through its center. **B,** The screw can be placed through the impression post sleeve and carried to the mouth with the standard hex driver **(C). D,** Impression post seated into the implant. **E,** Radiograph confirming complete seating. **F,** Complete impression, clearly showing flat sides. **G,** Laboratory analog corresponding to the size of the implant. **H,** Impression post removed from the mouth and attached to a laboratory analog. **I,** Impression post/analog complex inserted into the impression with flat sides properly oriented. **J,** Polyether impression material injected around the complex before pouring. **K** and **L,** Impression post orients the laboratory analog to cast as the implant body is positioned in the mouth.

cated if angle correction may be necessary. If the clinician decides to transfer the orientation of an antirotational feature from the mouth to the laboratory model, the two-piece pick-up (direct) impression technique should be used. This technique requires a two-piece impression post with a removable guide pin that screws directly into the abutment or onto the fixture. It uses a square coping with a long guide pin and usually an open-top tray. The impression coping is designed with square side walls to prevent rotation in the impression material. An open-top impression tray allows access to the guide pin for unscrewing after the material has set so that the copings can be picked up within the impression when removed from the mouth (Fig. 13-33). When implants are oriented at significantly divergent angles, the pick-up technique is generally considered to be the more accurate of the two procedures. The transfer technique is more convenient and sometimes mandatory when space is limited and screwdriver access would be limited. Before an implant impression is taken, a radiograph should be made

to ensure that the components are properly assembled. This requirement is especially important when an antirotational feature is involved.

Laboratory Analogs. Laboratory analogs are made to represent exactly the top of the implant fixture or the abutment in the laboratory cast. Therefore, they can be classified as fixture analogs and abutment analogs (Fig. 13-34). Both types screw directly into the impression post after it has been removed from the mouth, and the joined components are returned to the impression before pouring. The final impression should be poured in either dental stone or die stone. The gingival tissues can be reproduced by injecting an elastomer (e.g., Permadyne*) to represent soft tissue around the laboratory analog before pouring. This will facilitate removal of the impression post from the stone cast and the placement of subsequent abutments without breaking the stone and losing the reference point of the soft tissue (Fig. 13-35).

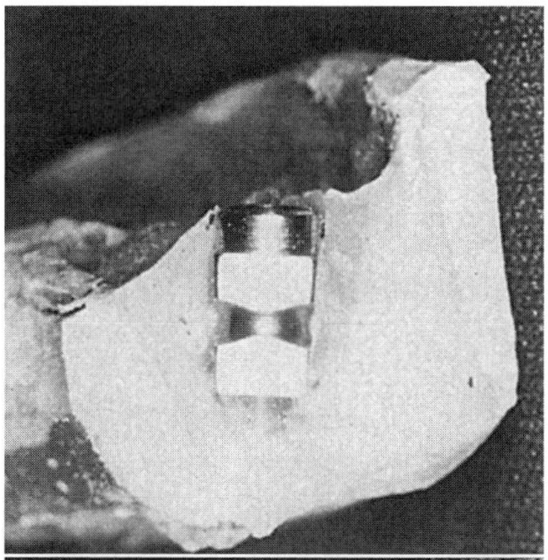

Abutment analogs are generally attached to an implant impression post. Implant body impression posts are normally attached to implant body analogs. The advantage of using the implant body analog is that the abutments can be changed in the laboratory. Also, if a flat-sided impression post has been used to orient the threads or the hexagon of the implant body analog properly, the decision to correct the implant angulation can be deferred until the laboratory stage. If the clinician is confident that the appropriate abutment has been selected, using the abutment impression post and abutment analog can simplify the procedure. If a supragingival

*ESPE-North America: Norristown, Pa.

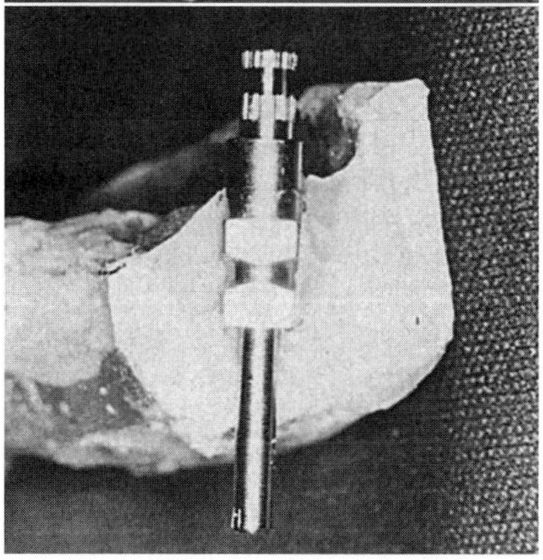

Fig. 13-33. A, Cross-sectional view of the two-piece impression post, which remains within the impression material. B, The impression screw passes through the coping to attach the laboratory analog.

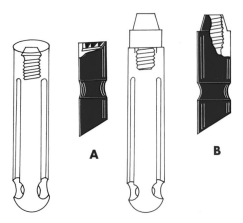

Fig. 13-34. Laboratory analogs. These represent either implants or abutments. A duplicates the top of the implant. B duplicates the top of the abutment.

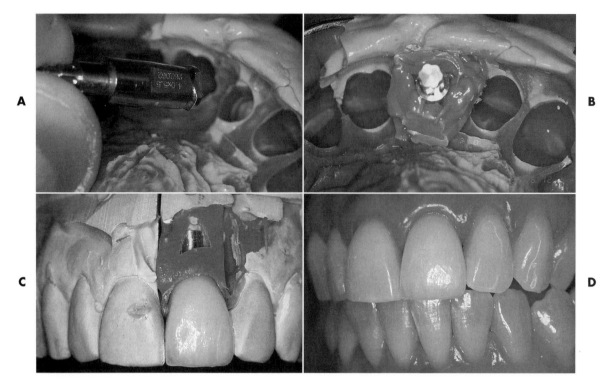

Fig. 13-35. **A** and **B,** Polyether impression material injected around a laboratory analog before the impression is poured. The gingival material should not cover any retention features of the analog. **C,** The impression material reproduces the patient's soft tissue contours adjacent to the implant. The impression post may be removed and other components inserted without losing the associated anatomic landmarks. **D,** Completed restoration.
(Courtesy Dr. C. Pechous.)

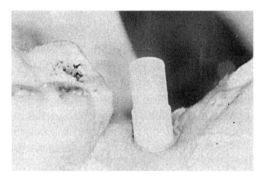

Fig. 13-36. Plastic waxing sleeve tightened to a laboratory analog.

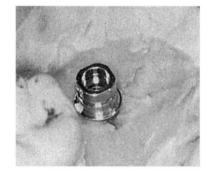

Fig. 13-37. Gold cylinder tightened to a laboratory analog.

abutment margin has been selected, a soft tissue cast will not be necessary.

Waxing Sleeves. Waxing sleeves are attached to the abutment by the relating screw on the laboratory model. They will eventually become part of the prosthesis. In nonsegmented implant crowns, they are attached directly to the implant body analog in the cast.

Commonly referred to as *UCLA abutments,* they may be plastic patterns that will be burned out and cast as part of the restoration framework (Fig. 13-36), precious metal that will be incorporated in

the framework when it is cast to the precious alloy cylinder, or a combination of each (Fig. 13-37). Using a metal waxing sleeve ensures that two machined surfaces will always be in contact. The cast surface of the plastic waxing sleeve may be retooled before it is returned to the fixture.

Waxing sleeves are available in several vertical dimensions. Tall ones can be shortened to conform to the requirements of the occlusal plane. Today, most waxing sleeves are a combination of gold alloy and plastic (Fig. 13-38). This combination allows the machined fit of the alloy at the implant, with the cost advantage of plastic at the waxing surface.

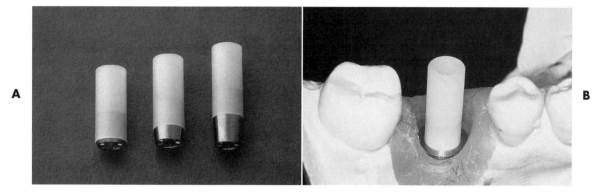

Fig. 13-38. **A,** Waxing sleeves with gold alloy base and plastic extension. **B,** On the laboratory cast, the technician can wax to the plastic extension. The wax and plastic will be burned out, and the new alloy will be "cast to" the original alloy base.

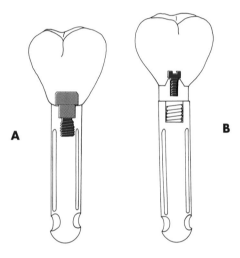

Fig. 13-39. Two types of prosthesis-retaining screws. **A,** Nonsegmented crown retained to implant. **B,** Crown retained on abutment.

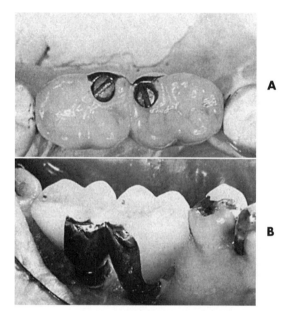

Fig. 13-40. **A,** Prosthesis-retaining screws countersunk below the occlusal surface of the restoration. **B,** Composite resin placed in screw access holes after the retaining screws are tightened.

Prosthesis-retaining Screws. Prosthesis-retaining screws penetrate the fixed restoration and secure it to the abutment (Fig. 13-39). They are tightened with a screwdriver and attach nonsegmented crowns to the body of the implant. They generally are made of titanium, titanium alloy, or gold alloy and may be long (which allows them to penetrate the total length of the implant crown) or short (which requires countersinking them into the occlusal surface of the restoration). Screws that are countersunk must be covered by an initial layer of resilient material (e.g., gutta-percha, cotton, or silicone). A subsequent seal of composite resin is placed over the resilient plug (Fig. 13-40).

IMPLANT RESTORATIVE OPTIONS

Distal-extension Implant Restoration. Implant support offers major advantages in the treatment of partially edentulous patients in whom no terminal abutment is available. In this situation, the conventional dental treatment plan would include a re-

movable partial denture. However, with the implant alternative, patients can avoid the discomfort and inconvenience of a removable prosthesis.

There are two distal-extension restorative options. One option is to place an implant distal to the most posterior natural abutment and fabricate a fixed prosthesis connecting the implant with the natural tooth. However, there are problems associated with implants connected to natural teeth (see p. 356). The other option is to place two or more implants posterior to the most distal natural tooth and fabricate a completely implant-supported restoration (Fig. 13-41). If the crown-to-implant ratio is favorable, two implants to support a three-unit fixed partial denture may be considered. If implants are short and crowns are long, one implant to replace

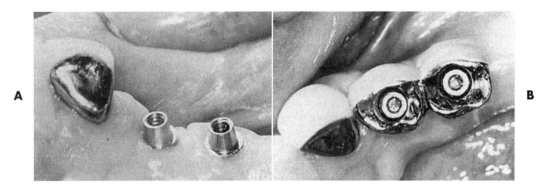

Fig. 13-41. **A,** Two implants placed distal to the mandibular canine. **B,** The completed restoration is not connected to the natural tooth.

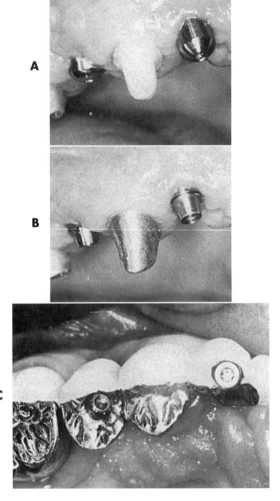

Fig. 13-42. **A,** Natural tooth prepared between two implants. **B,** Telescopic coping permanently cemented onto the natural tooth. **C,** Prosthesis placed with screw retention on the implants and temporary cement retention on the telescopic coping.

each missing tooth is highly recommended. If doubt remains, more implants are used when heavier forces are expected (e.g., the posterior part of the mouth in patients with evidence of parafunctional activity). Fewer implants are used when lighter forces are expected (e.g., those opposing a complete denture or those supporting a prosthesis in the anterior part of the mouth).

Long Edentulous Span Restoration. Similar options can be used when treating a long edentulous span. The clinician may choose to have multiple implants placed between the remaining natural teeth and to fabricate a fully implant-supported restoration. As an alternative, one or two implants can be placed in the long edentulous span and the final restoration connected to natural teeth. When it is necessary to connect implants and the natural teeth, protecting the teeth with telescopic copings is recommended (Fig. 13-42). In this manner, prosthesis retrievability can be maintained. In addition, some long edentulous spans require the reconstruction of soft and hard tissue as well as teeth. In these instances, using resin teeth processed to a metal substructure rather than a conventional metal-ceramic restoration is recommended. Soft tissue esthetics can be more easily and accurately mimicked with heat-processed resin and large defects (Fig. 13-43). This type of restoration has been called a *hybrid* because it combines the principles of conventional fixed and removable prosthodontics. For smaller defects, pink porcelain can be used to compensate for missing soft tissue (see Fig. 13-24, *B*).

Single-tooth Implant Restoration. The use of single implants in restoring missing teeth is an attractive option for the patient and the dentist. However, it requires careful implant placement and precise control of all prosthetic components. Single-tooth restorations supported by implants may be indicated in the following situations:
1. An otherwise intact dentition
2. A dentition with spaces that would be more difficult to treat with conventional fixed prosthodontics

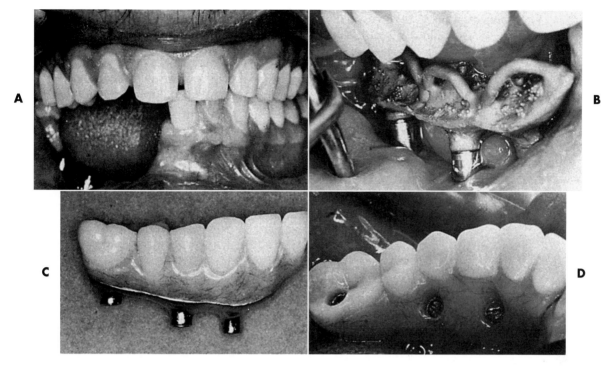

Fig. 13-43. **A,** Large mandibular defect created by a shotgun wound. **B,** Metal substructure of a hybrid prosthesis tried onto three implants in this defect. **C,** Denture resin can more effectively recreate the soft tissue color and contours in the completed restoration than dental porcelain. **D,** Hybrid restoration restoring the defect.

3. Distally missing teeth when cantilevers or removable partial dentures are not indicated
4. A prosthesis that needs to closely mimic the missing natural tooth

The requirements for single-tooth implant crowns are as follows:

1. Esthetics
2. Antirotation—to avoid prosthetic component loosening
3. Simplicity—to minimize the amount of components used
4. Accessibility—to maintain optimum oral health
5. Variability—to allow the clinician to control the height, diameter, and angulation of the implant restoration

Several systems have been developed to comply with these demands. Common indications include congenitally missing maxillary lateral incisors (Fig. 13-44) and teeth in which endodontic treatment was unsuccessful (Fig. 13-45). Screw loosening has most commonly been associated with the terminally positioned single molar implant crown (Fig. 13-46).

Matching the soft tissue contours of adjacent natural teeth remains the most difficult challenge for completing the anterior single-tooth restoration. These contours can be reliably created with provisional restorations. One technique, which combines soft tissue contouring and provisional placement, is

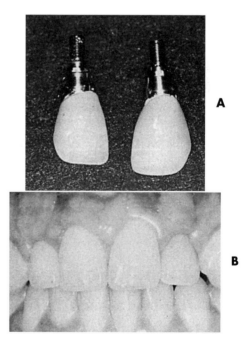

Fig. 13-44. **A,** Lateral incisor crowns attached to implant abutments. **B,** Single tooth implant crowns replacing the maxillary lateral incisors.

shown in Figure 13-47. When the tissue has matured around the provisional restoration, a final impression can be taken to complete the definitive restoration (Fig. 13-48). Impressions can also be made at

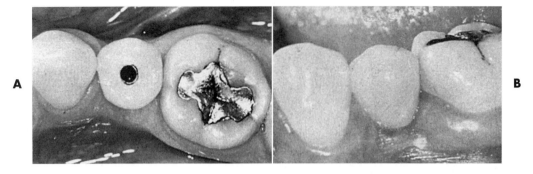

Fig. 13-45. **A,** Occlusal view of a single tooth implant crown replacing a fractured mandibular premolar. **B,** Buccal view of a single-tooth implant crown replacing a mandibular premolar.

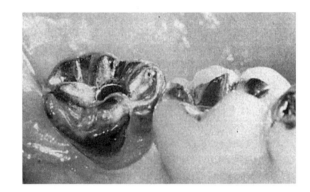

Fig. 13-46. Screw loosening is most commonly associated with single-tooth molar implant crowns.

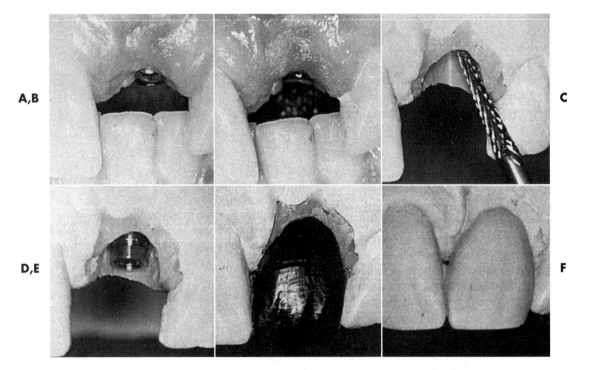

Fig. 13-47. **A,** Soft tissue healing 2 weeks after second-stage surgery and placement of a healing cap. **B,** The healing cap removed. Note that the interdental papilla has been preserved. An impression post may be placed, and an implant master cast prepared. **C,** Soft tissue cast prepared with a laboratory bur to create the ideal soft tissue architecture. **D,** A gold waxing sleeve attached to the laboratory analog retains the provisional restoration. **E,** A full-contour wax pattern can be used to fabricate the provisional. **F,** Duplicate cast of the full-contour wax pattern.

Continued

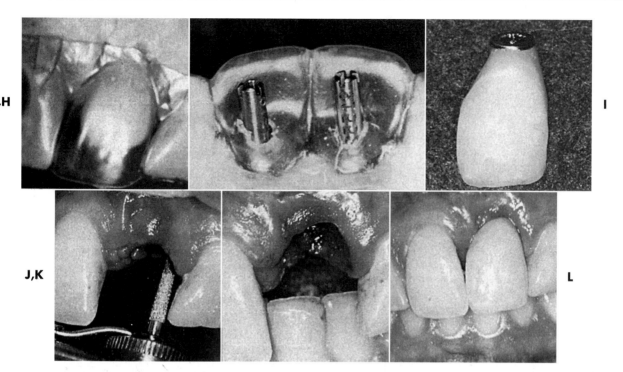

Fig. 13-47, cont'd. **G,** An acrylic template is adapted to the duplicate cast and returned to the master cast. **H,** Waxing posts to create a screw access hole in the provisional restoration. **I,** A provisional implant restoration is fabricated by one of the techniques described in Chapter 15. **J,** The soft tissue is contoured to accept a provisional restoration. A diamond curettage bur can be used when sufficient attached tissue is present. **K,** Soft tissue contouring improves esthetics, minimizes pocket depths, and allows more physiologic restoration contours. **L,** The provisional restoration. Soft tissue is allowed to heal for 4 to 6 weeks before the final impression is made.

the time of Stage I surgery so that a provisional can be delivered at Stage II to facilitate more ideal soft tissue contours (Fig. 13-49). The best soft tissue esthetics are still generally achieved when interdental papillae are present before the surgery. If soft tissue contours are deficient before surgery, the patient should expect some compromise in the final soft tissue result.

Fixed Restoration in the Completely Edentulous Arch. For completely edentulous patients who require nonremovable restorations, there are two implant options: a **hybrid prosthesis** and a fixed metal-ceramic rehabilitation (Figs. 13-50 to 13-52).

The hybrid prosthesis is a cast alloy framework with processed denture resin and teeth. It requires a minimum of five implants in the mandible and six in the maxilla. One major determining factor for selecting this option is the amount of bone and soft tissue lost. For patients who have had moderate bone loss, the prosthesis restores both bone and soft tissue contours.

The metal-ceramic rehabilitation also requires five implants in the mandible and six in the maxilla. It can be made esthetically pleasing only if minimal

bone loss has occurred and is best suited for patients who have recently lost their natural teeth (within 5 years). For patients with severe bone loss, there is probably only one option: a removable restoration (Fig. 13-53).

The main advantage of a completely fixed restoration, whether it is hybrid or metal-ceramic, is that it is completely retained by the patient at all times. Therefore, patients experience the psychologic benefit of having a restoration that closely resembles their original natural teeth. In addition, movement within the system is minimized, and the components tend to wear out less quickly. Because the prosthesis is screw retained, the dentist can remove it, allowing access for cleaning and repairs. A potential disadvantage is that the implants must be precisely placed, especially in the maxillary anterior esthetic zone. Implants placed in embrasure spaces can lead to disastrous esthetic results and can impede access for hygiene. With a hybrid prosthesis, the clinician must decide between leaving enough space for hygiene access and minimizing space for optimum esthetics. Some patients may be concerned by the amount of metal shown in a hybrid prosthesis. However, from a conversational distance,

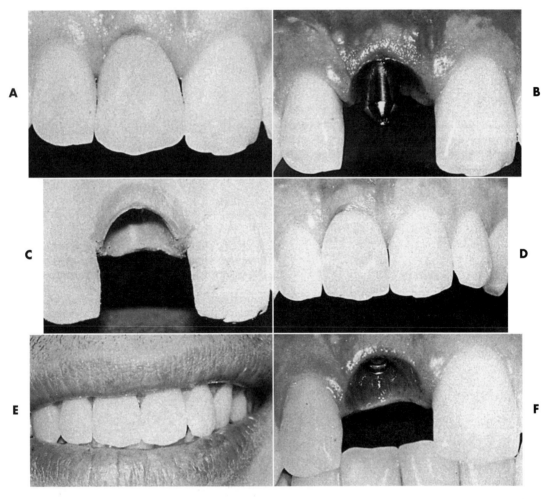

Fig. 13-48.   **A,** Soft tissue around a maxillary implant provisional restoration after 6 weeks of healing. **B,** New soft tissue contours compared to the healing abutment previously in place. **C,** Final impression made and a master cast fabricated. The new soft tissue contours are reproduced. **D,** Implant crown placed on the maxillary right central incisor. **E,** Preservation of the interdental papilla is important for patients with medium to high smile lines. **F,** One-year follow-up showing that the patient has maintained healthy soft tissue contours.
(Courtesy Dr. J. Holloway.)

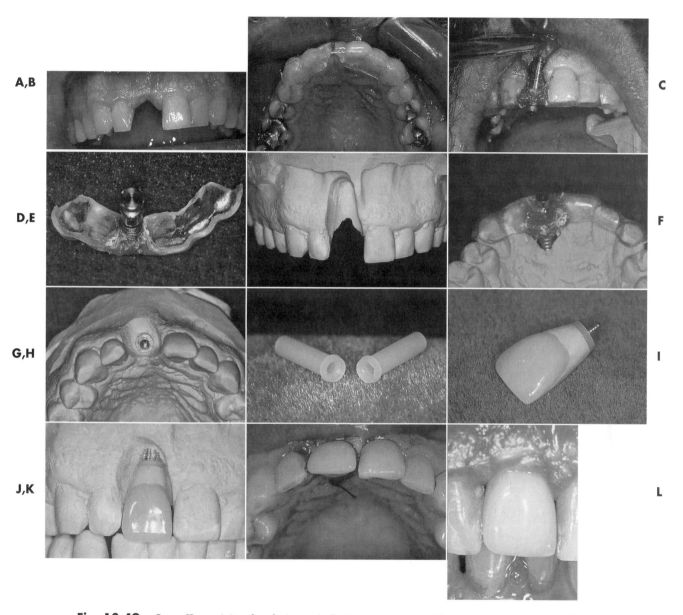

Fig. 13-49. Stage II provisional technique. **A,** Patient missing maxillary right central incisor. **B,** Surgical template in position. **C,** Once the screw-shaped implant is in place, the fixture mount is luted to the surgical template with resin before it is unscrewed from the mouth. **D,** Analog attached to the fixture mount. **E,** Diagnostic stone cast prepared to position analog. **F,** Template placed back on diagnostic cast. **G,** Dental stone is flowed around the analog. The position of the analog is identical to the position of the implant in the mouth. **H to L,** A plastic sleeve is used for the fabrication of a provisional restoration that can be delivered at Stage II surgery.

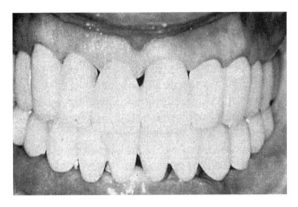

Fig. 13-50. A metal-ceramic implant restoration may be indicated if adequate bone and soft tissue contours are available.

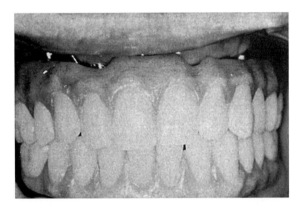

Fig. 13-51. Hybrid restorations are the treatment of choice for edentulous patients with moderate bone resorption.

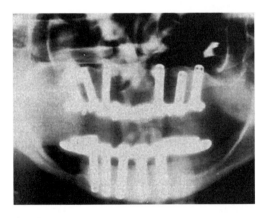

Fig. 13-52. Radiograph showing fixed restorations supported by six implants in the maxilla and five in the mandible.

Treatment-planning implant options for edentulous patients depend on bone resorption.

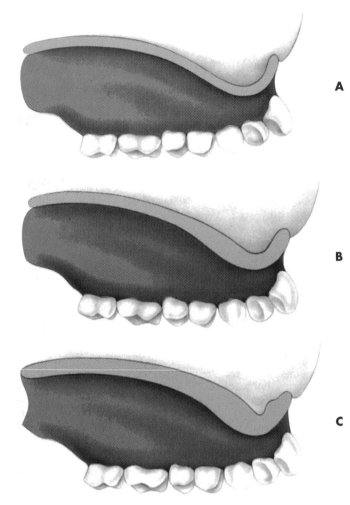

Fig. 13-53. The amount of bone resorption dictates the treatment options for an edentulous patient. **A,** Minimal resorption may allow metal-ceramic restorations. **B,** Moderate resorption may necessitate resin-to-metal (hybrid) restorations. **C,** Severe resorption will require only implant-supported overdentures for optimum esthetic results.

a properly made prosthesis will be hardly noticeable. Esthetic and phonetic problems in the maxillary arch can often be avoided by not placing implants near the midline and restoring the incisor teeth with pontics. This approach to implant placement improves the restorative outcome considerably (Fig. 13-54).

CEMENT-RETAINED VERSUS SCREW-RETAINED IMPLANT CROWNS

Cemented implant crowns can be luted to a screw-retained abutment. Zinc phosphate, glass ionomer, and composite resin cements have all been suggested for this purpose. However, retrievability of the implant restoration is ordinarily not considered when a permanent cement is used. The provisional cements have been recommended because they allow restoration retrieval. However, unpre-

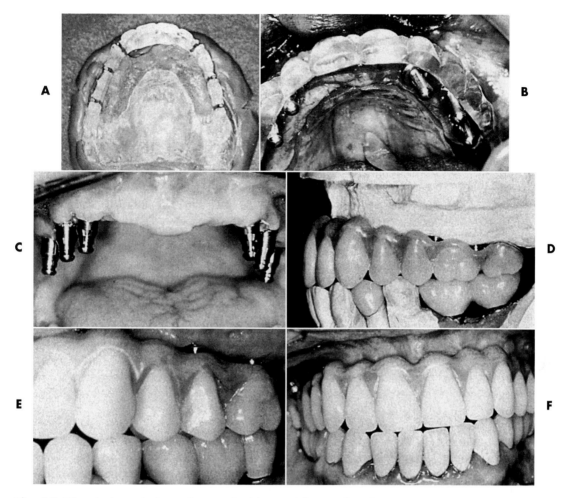

Fig. 13-54. **A,** A surgical template can be fabricated for an edentulous patient by duplicating the existing denture in clear resin. **B,** The lingual aspect of the template is removed, leaving the most facial 2 mm of resin intact. The surgeon will have access to the bone, but it will be confined to the arch form. **C,** The ideal positions for maxillary implants are the canine, second premolar, and second molar areas. Cross arch implant parallelism is also important. **D,** Access for hygiene must be allowed around implant abutments. **E,** If implants are located posterior to the canine, access for hygiene can be created without compromising esthetics or phonetics. **F,** Reasonable esthetics and phonetics can be accomplished with a hybrid restoration if modified ridge-lap pontics are used in the maxillary central and lateral incisor positions.

dictability of the temporary luting agents can lead to a difficult retrieval or premature displacement.[11]

Simplicity and, in some systems, economy are the major advantages of cement-retained restorations. In addition, cementing allows minor angle corrections to compensate for discrepancies between the implant inclination and the facial crown contour (Fig. 13-55). Resistance to rotation is particularly critical with cemented prosthetics, and the abutment should then incorporate an antirotational feature. Very small teeth are most easily replaced with cement-retained implant crowns (Fig. 13-56).

One misconception about cement-retained crowns is that they are simpler and have fewer screw-loosening episodes. They actually require more chair time and have the same propensity to

loosen. They are, however, more esthetically pleasing and less expensive.

The screw-retained implant crown is fastened either to the abutment or directly to the implant. The main advantage of this restoration is its retrievability. Retrievability allows for crown removal, which can facilitate soft tissue evaluation, calculus debridement, and any other necessary modifications. In addition, future treatment considerations can be made more easily and are less costly if the implant restoration is retrievable. However, in screw-retained restorations, the access hole must be through the occlusal table of posterior teeth or the lingual surface of anterior teeth. Forces can then be directed in the long axis of the implant, and optimum esthetics is more easily achieved. This

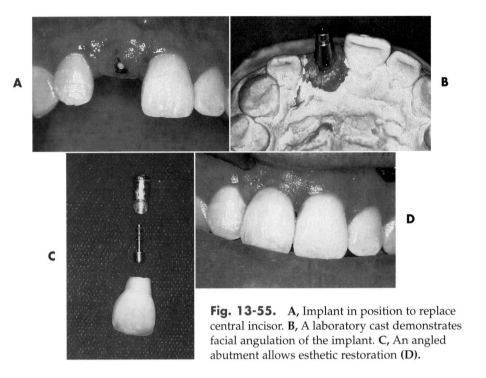

Fig. 13-55. **A,** Implant in position to replace central incisor. **B,** A laboratory cast demonstrates facial angulation of the implant. **C,** An angled abutment allows esthetic restoration **(D).**

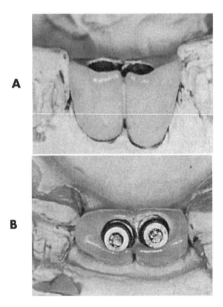

Fig. 13-56. **A,** Very small teeth are difficult to restore esthetically with screw-retained restorations. **B,** Occlusal view of screw-retained mandibular central incisors. Note the discrepancy in incisal edge widths caused by the screw access holes.

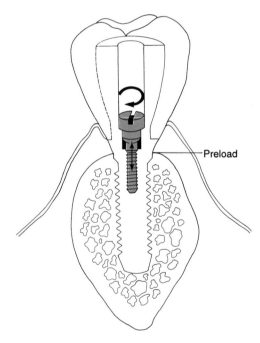

Fig. 13-57. Torque on the screw develops a preload (clamping force) between the implant and the crown.

requirement dictates an ideal surgical location, which is not always possible because of anatomic limitations. The primary disadvantage of a screw-retained implant restoration is that the screw may loosen during function. Many techniques for retaining screw connection have been reported. The direct mechanical interlock or antirotational feature appears to be the most effective.

If the screw is sufficiently tightened into the implant crown to seat it, a clamping load or preload is developed between the implant and the crown (Fig. 13-57). If this clamping force is greater than the forces trying to separate the joint between implant and crown, the screw will not loosen. An implant screw should be tightened with sufficient force to seat the crown, but not so much as to affect the

Screw loosening can
be a problem with
implant prostheses.

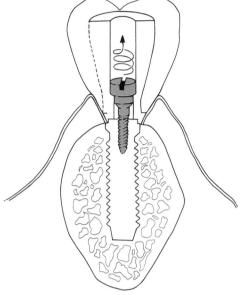

Fig. 13-58. The screw will loosen only if the joint-separating force is greater than the clamping force.

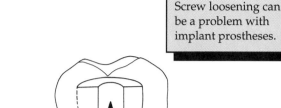

> **LOOSE IMPLANT SCREWS**   BOX **13-5**
> CHECK:
> **1.** Excessive occlusal contacts not in the long axis of the implant
> **2.** Excessive cantilever contacts
> **3.** Excessive lateral contacts
> **4.** Excessive interproximal contacts
> **5.** Inadequately tightened screws

bone-implant interface. Torque wrenches are available to achieve this. In addition, lateral forces (which tend to separate the joint) should be eliminated or reduced (Fig. 13-58 and Box 13-5.)

BIOMECHANICAL FACTORS AFFECTING LONG-TERM IMPLANT SUCCESS

OCCLUSION (BOX 13-6)

Bone resorption around dental implants can be caused by premature loading or repeated overloading. Vertical or angular bone loss is usually characteristic of bone resorption caused by occlusal trauma. When pressure from traumatic occlusion is concentrated, bone resorption occurs by osteoclastic activity. In the natural dentition, bone remodeling typically occurs once the severe stress concentration

> **IMPLANT OCCLUSION**   BOX **13-6**
> **1.** Direct forces in long axis of the implant.
> **2.** Minimize lateral forces on the implant.
> **3.** Place lateral forces when necessary as far anterior in the arch as possible.
> **4.** When it is impossible to minimize or move lateral forces anteriorly, distribute them over as many teeth and implants as possible.

is reduced or eliminated. However, in the osseointegrated implant system, after bone resorbs, it usually does not reform. Because dental implants most effectively resist forces directed primarily in their long axis, lateral forces on implants should be minimized.

Lateral forces in the posterior part of the mouth are greater and more destructive than lateral forces in the anterior part of the mouth. When they cannot be completely eliminated from the implant prosthesis, efforts should be made to distribute them equally over as many teeth as possible.

Implant restorations should be designed to minimize damaging forces at the implant-bone interface, with particular attention to the occlusion. Flatter inclines can be developed on implant cusps, creating more vertical resultant forces and a shorter moment arm (Fig. 13-59). Whenever possible, a cusp-fossa relationship should be established in the intercuspal position with no eccentric occlusal contacts (see Chapter 18). The maxillary single-tooth restoration is vulnerable to screw loosening due to occlusal contacts, which usually produce an inclined resultant force with increased torque on the retaining screw. Optimum implant orientation will effectively reduce these forces.

In general, the location and inclination of force should be seriously considered in the restorative phase of implant treatment. Divergent implant placement increases the moment arm through which force is transmitted to the bone-implant interface; this could exceed the threshold for bone resorption. Interchangeable components to alter implant angles have been produced by implant body manufacturers. However, it has been shown[12] that increasing abutment angles also produces increased stresses at the bone-implant interface. Angled abutments may solve immediate esthetic or contour problems while masking potential long-term consequences created by an implant placement that is poorly planned or dictated by the patient's anatomy.

Inadequate implant distribution may also lead to excessive cantilevers or forces that could potentiate overloading of implant bodies. Whenever possible, dental implants should be joined so that forces may be more equally distributed over multiple implants.

A carefully designed occlusion is critical to implant success.

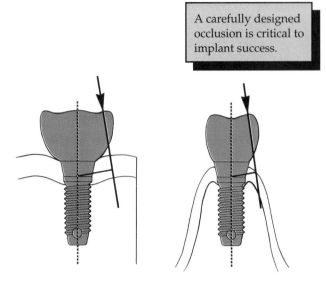

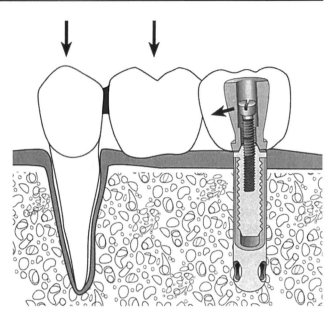

Fig. 13-59. Sharper cusp inclines and wider occlusal tables increase the resultant force on implant components.

Fig. 13-60. When a single implant is attached to a natural tooth, biting forces on the natural tooth and pontic cause stress to be concentrated at the superior portion of the implant.

Ideally, one implant for every tooth to be restored should be placed. This number is particularly important when shorter implants are placed in poorer-quality bone. When implants longer than 13 mm can be placed in dense bone, two for every three teeth being replaced are acceptable. Full arch restorations should not be considered on less than six implants in the maxilla and five in the mandible. Implant cantilevers should be kept as short as possible. However, cantilevering considerable distances off five well-integrated fixtures in the anterior mandible is possible. Quite often, cantilevering to the first molar is possible. Equations based on the distribution and length of fixtures have been proposed.[13]

CONNECTING IMPLANTS TO NATURAL TEETH

It has been suggested[14] that connecting a single osseointegrated implant to one natural tooth with a fixed partial denture can create excessive forces because of the relative immobility of the osseointegrated implant compared to the functional mobility of a natural tooth. During function, the tooth moves within the limits of its periodontal ligament, which can create stress at the neck of the implant up to two times the implied load on the prosthesis (Fig. 13-60). Potential problems with this type of restoration include (1) breakdown of the osseointegration, (2) cement failure on the natural abutment, (3) screw or abutment loosening, and (4) failure of the implant prosthetic component. This situation is encountered clinically when the most posterior abutment is lost in the dental arch and a fixed prosthesis is needed to connect a single implant to the natural tooth. If possible, a totally implant-supported fixed partial den-

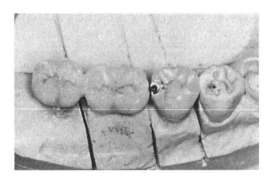

Fig. 13-61. A semi-precision attachment may compensate for vertical displacement forces in the tooth and an implant-supported fixed prosthesis. It does not compensate for forces in the buccolingual direction. *(Courtesy Dr. G. Seal.)*

ture with two or more implants should be provided. However, anatomic limitations of the maxillary sinus or the mandibular canal often limit restorative efforts directed at a single fixture site.

When connecting an implant to a natural tooth is necessary, multiple implant or natural tooth abutments should be used. A semi-precision attachment (keyway) in the prosthesis between the implant and the natural tooth may solve potential problems[14] (Fig. 13-61). However, under most circumstances, when a load is applied to the pontic, the additional movement at the attachment actually increases the cantilever effect on the implant abutment. In practice, the only advantage of a semi-precision attachment may be that it allows a screw-retained implant abutment crown to be removed for periodic evaluation.

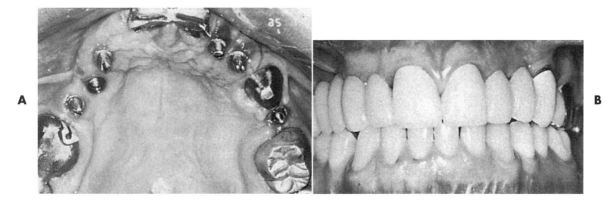

Fig. 13-62. **A,** Metal try-in for maxillary rehabilitation using implant abutments and a telescopic coping on the maxillary left premolar. **B,** Prosthesis screw retained on implants with temporary luting agent over the telescopic coping.

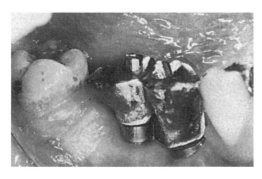

Fig. 13-63. Metal framework fit should be evaluated with only a single retaining screw in place.

When circumstances dictate using a natural tooth abutment, a telescopic coping should be considered. This is permanently cemented to the natural tooth and can prevent decay if loosening occurs. Provisional cement is used to attach the prosthesis to the coping. If it leaches out of the implant crown, the natural tooth will still be protected (Fig. 13-62).

IMPLANT AND FRAMEWORK FIT

Pathogenic forces can be placed on an implant if the framework does not fit passively. When all the prosthesis-retaining screws are tightened, gaps between the abutment and a poorly fitting framework will close, giving the appearance of an acceptable fit. However, significant compressive forces are placed on the interfacial bone, which can lead to implant failure. The fit of all implant frameworks should be checked with only one screw in place. No visible amounts of space or any amounts of movement with finger pressure should be discernible on any of the other implant abutments (Fig. 13-63). If a non-passively fitting framework is identified, it should be sectioned and soldered and then reassessed for passive fit. A relation record should also be made.

SHOCK-ABSORBING ELEMENTS

Because there is no movement between the bone and an osseointegrated implant, incorporating some type of shock-absorbing layer to reduce occlusal impact forces may be necessary. One theory claims that such forces may exceed the threshold necessary for bone resorption to occur. This shock absorber could be specially designed into the implant system, or the occlusal surface of the restoration might be constructed of acrylic resin to accomplish the same effect. These recommendations are based on theoretical calculations rather than on clinical data, and the need for shock-absorbing elements remains a controversial subject in implant dentistry.

MAINTENANCE

The goal of implant maintenance is to eradicate microbial populations affecting the prosthesis. Although dental implants may be more resistant than natural teeth to the effects of bacterial plaque, this has yet to be definitively proved. Until more research is available, proper and timely home care measures for prolonging the lifetime of an implant are most effective. Clinicians must ensure that the patient receives thorough instruction in maintenance techniques, including an initial session with the clinician. This should be reinforced by a training session with the dental hygienist during a recall visit. Recall visits should be scheduled at least every 3 months during the first year. The patient's oral hygiene should be evaluated and documented at a recall visit; reinstruction should be provided when necessary. Sulcular debridement must be perfomed with plastic or wooden scalers, since conventional instruments will scratch the titanium. Implant abutments may be polished using rubber cups with a low-abrasive polishing paste or tin oxide.

At each recall appointment, implant mobility should be evaluated; any bleeding after probing should be examined. Framework fit and occlusion also must be checked. Attention to both biologic and biomechanical factors is important to the long-term success of dental implants.

COMPLICATIONS

BONE LOSS

The primary complication with dental implant therapy is bone loss around the implant (Fig. 13-64). Any loss exceeding 0.2 mm per year is cause for concern. Multiple factors are associated with implant bone loss:

1. Inappropriate size and shape of the implant
2. Inadequate number of implants or implant positioning
3. Poor quality or inadequate amount of available bone
4. Initial instability of the implant
5. Compromised healing phase
6. Inadequate fit of the prosthesis
7. Improper design of the prosthesis (e.g., excessive cantilever, poor access for hygiene)
8. Excessive occlusal forces
9. Deficient fit of abutment components (i.e., gaps that allow bacterial colonization)
10. Inadequate oral hygiene
11. Systemic influence (e.g., tobacco use, diabetes)

The restorative dentist should pay particular attention to the fit of the prosthesis, the access for hygiene, and the presence of excessive occlusal forces. If bone loss reaches 25% to 30%, revision surgery should be considered.

PROSTHETIC FAILURE

Additional implant prosthetic complications include fracture of the implant components or the prosthesis. Fracture of implant components is usually attributed to fatigue from biomechanical overload (Fig. 13-65). Failure of the implant prosthesis is usually traceable to less than ideal laboratory procedures or prosthesis design (Figs. 13-66 and 13-67).

SUMMARY

Implant-supported prostheses, using cylindrical osseointegrated fixtures placed by a two-stage surgical technique, should be considered in the treatment of any partially edentulous patient. They are a reliable solution to many situations that are difficult to treat by conventional measures: the patient who

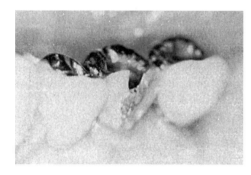

Fig. 13-65. Fractured abutment screw on a tooth and implant-supported prosthesis.

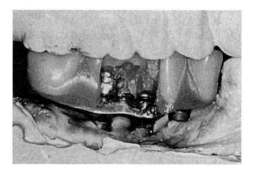

Fig. 13-66. Porcelain fracture on an implant prosthesis with inadequate metal support.

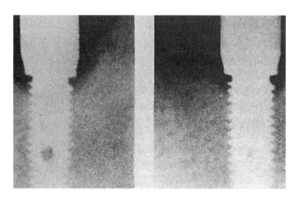

Fig. 13-64. To monitor cimplant bone loss, radiographs should be evaluated once a year.

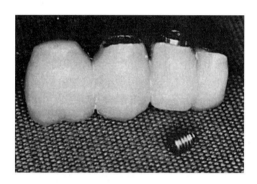

Fig. 13-67. Resin fracture on a hybrid prosthesis. The prosthesis can be retrieved easily for repair.

cannot wear removable appliances, the patient with a long edentulous span or other circumstance (e.g., short roots) that diminishes the prognosis for an FPD, and the patient with a single missing tooth but sound adjacent teeth.

Success with implant prosthodontics requires the same attention to detail and careful planning as conventional fixed prosthodontics. Often a team approach is recommended, with a surgeon placing the implant and a restorative dentist designing the prosthesis. The critical stage is optimum placement of the implant(s). The surgeon's main concern is that it be well within the available bone and away from vital structures (e.g., the inferior dental canal). The restorative dentist's main concern is that the positioning and angulation of each fixture allow optimum occlusion, esthetics, and tissue health as well as minimum stresses at the implant-bone interface. Information obtained from a clinical examination, radiographs, and a diagnostic waxing on articulated casts is crucial to planning. Surgery is guided by a template made from the diagnostic waxing.

Depending on the implant site, a two-stage surgical technique requires 3 to 6 months for bone to heal against the implant. In a second surgery, the implant is uncovered and implant abutments are screwed into place. Subsequently, a screw-retained prosthesis is fabricated to restore function and appearance.

Several implant systems are available, each with a variety of components for restorative management (e.g., an antirotational feature incorporated in an implant for single tooth replacement).

Problems unique to implant prosthodontics include screw loosening and bone loss from premature loading or repeated overloading. Occlusal considerations, prosthesis fit, plaque control, and follow-up care are all primary concerns to the professionals who deal with implants and conventionally supported prostheses.

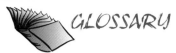

GLOSSARY

dental implant: a prosthetic device of alloplastic material implanted into the oral tissues beneath the mucosal or/and periosteal layer, and/or within the bone to provide retention and support for a fixed or removable prosthesis; a substance that is placed into or/and upon the jaw bone to support a fixed or removable prosthesis—*usage:* although dental implants may be classified by their silhouette or geometrical form (i.e., fin, screw, cylinder, blade, basket, rootform, etc.) generally, dental implants are classified based on their anchorage component as it relates to the alveolar bone that provides support and stability. Thus, there are *eposteal dental implants, endosteal dental implants,* and *transosteal dental implants.* Some dental implants possess both eposteal and endosteal components (by design or subsequent anchorage change); the decision as to what anchorage system provides the most support at initial placement determines which category is used to best describe the dental implant.

endosteal dental implant: a device placed into the alveolar and/or basal bone of the mandible or maxilla and transecting only one cortical plate. The endosteal dental implant is composed of an anchorage component, the *dental implant body,* which, ideally, is within the bone, and a retentive component(s), the *dental implant abutment,* which connects to the implant body, passes through the oral mucosa, and serves to support and/or retain the prosthesis. Such an abutment may be for interim or definitive application—*usage: interim abutment, definitive abutment.* Descriptions of the implant body that use silhouette or geometric forms, such as cylinder, blade, basket, or endodontic, may be used as adjectives to enhance understanding of the geometry of any endosteal dental implant. *Interim or definitive abutments* may be composed of one or more *elements.* The abutment elements usually are

Study Questions

1. Discuss the history and scientific basis for osseointegration.
2. Discuss the indications and contraindications for implant-supported fixed partial dentures.
3. When treatment-planning the replacement of a congenitally missing lateral incisor with an implant restoration, describe the necessary minimum bone dimensions vertically, horizontally, and between roots. Also describe the guidelines used to position the implant in the appropriate anteroposterior and superoinferior location.
4. Describe the technique used to replicate the intraoral location of an implant on the laboratory cast.
5. List and describe the various types of abutments used for implant restorations. When is each type recommended? Why?
6. Describe some common problems with implant restorations and recommend methods to manage them.

described by means of their geometric form, i.e., screw, coping, cylinder, lug.

hybrid prosthesis: *slang:* a nonspecific term for any prosthesis that does not follow conventional design. Frequently it is used to describe a prosthesis that is composed of different materials, types of denture teeth (porcelain, plastic, composite), variable acrylic denture resins, differing metals, etc. It may refer to a fixed partial denture or any removable prosthesis.

¹implant: *v* (1890): to graft or insert a material such as an alloplastic substance, an encapsulated drug, or tissue into the body of a recipient.

²implant: *n* (1809): any object or material, such as an alloplastic substance or other tissue, which is partially or completely inserted or grafted into the body for therapeutic, diagnostic, prosthetic, or experimental purposes.

implant abutment: the portion of a dental implant that serves to support and/or retain any prosthesis— *usage:* frequently dental implant abutments, especially those used with endosteal dental implants, are changed to alter abutment design or use before a definitive prosthesis is fabricated. Such a preliminary abutment is termed an *interim abutment.* The abutment chosen to support the definitive prosthesis is termed a *definitive abutment.*

implant body: the portion of a dental implant that provides support for the abutment(s) through adaptation upon (eposteal), within (endosteal), or through (transosteal) the alveolar bone—usage: eposteal dental implants alveolar bone support system has, heretofore, been termed the *implant frame, implant framework, or implant substructure;* however, this is an integral component of that dental implant and is not subservient to any other component.

implant prosthodontics: the phase of prosthodontics concerning the replacement of missing teeth and/or associated structures by restorations that are attached to dental implants.

implant substructure: the metal framework of a eposteal dental implant that is embedded beneath the soft tissues, in contact with the bone, and stabilized by means of endosteal screws. The periosteal tissues retain the framework to the bone. The framework supports the prosthesis, frequently by means of abutments and other superstructure components.

implant surgery: (1993): the phase of implant dentistry concerning the selection, planning, and placement of the implant body and abutment.

implantology *obs:* a term historically conceived as the study or science of placing and restoring dental implants.

osseous: *adj* (1707): bony.

osseous integration: (1993) *1:* the apparent direct attachment or connection of osseous tissue to an inert, alloplastic material without intervening connective tissue *2:* the process and resultant apparent direct connection of an exogeous material's surface and the host bone tissues, without intervening fibrous connective tissue present *3:* the interface between alloplastic materials and living tissue.

peri-implantitis: in periodontics, a term used to describe inflammation around a dental implant, usually its abutment.

transosteal dental implant: *1:* a dental implant that penetrates both cortical plates and passes through the full thickness of the alveolar bone *2:* a dental implant composed of a metal plate with retentive pins to hold it against the inferior border of the mandible that supports transosteal pins that penetrate through the full thickness of the mandible and pass into the mouth in the parasymphyseal region— called also *staple bone plant, mandibular staple implant, transmandibular implant.*

REFERENCES

1. NIH Consensus Development Conference: Statement on dental implants, *J Dent Educ* 52:824, 1988.

2. Adell R et al: A 15-year study of osseointegrated implants in the treatment of the edentulous jaw, *Int J Oral Surg* 10:387, 1981.

3. Kent J et al: Biointegrated hydroxylapatite-coated dental implants: 5-year clinical observations, *J Am Dent Assoc* 121:138, 1990.

4. Lazzara RJ et al: A prospective multicenter study evaluating loading of osseotite implants two months after placement: one-year results, *J Esthet Dent* 10:280, 1998.

5. Buser D et al: Removal torque values of titanium implants in the maxillofacial of miniature pigs, *Int J Oral Maxillofac Implant* 13:611, 1998.

6. Smithloff M, Fritz ME: Use of blade implants in a selected population of partially edentulous patients, *J Periodontol* 53:413, 1982.

7. Kapur KK: VA cooperative dental implant study: comparisons between fixed partial dentures supported by blade-vent implants and removable partial dentures. II. Comparisons of success rates and periodontal health between two treatment modalities, *J Prosthet Dent* 62:685, 1989.

8. Smith D, Zarb GA: Criteria for success for osseointegrated endosseous implants, *J Prosthet Dent* 62:567, 1989.

9. McGlumphy EA, Larsen PE: Contemporary implant dentistry. In Peterson LJ et al, editors: *Contemporary oral and maxillofacial surgery,* ed 3, St Louis, 1998, Mosby.

10. Hobo S et al, editors: *Osseointegrated and occlusal rehabilitation,* Tokyo, 1990, Quintessence Publishing.

11. Chiche GI, Pinault A: Considerations for fabrication of implant-supported posterior restorations, *Int J Prosthod* 4:37, 1991.

12. Clelland N, Gilat A: The effect of abutment angulation on the stress transfer for an implant, *J Prosthod* 1:24, 1992.

13. Takayama H: Biomechanical considerations on osseointegrated implants. In Hobo S et al, editors: *Osseointegrated and occlusal rehabilitation*, Tokyo, 1990, Quintessence Publishing.

14. Sullivan D: Prosthetic considerations for the utilization of osseointegrated fixtures in the partially edentulous arch, *Int J Oral Maxillofac Implants* 1:39, 1986.

CHAPTER FOURTEEN

TISSUE MANAGEMENT AND IMPRESSION MAKING

KEY TERMS

accelerator
custom impression tray
dimensional stability
elastomer
hydrocolloid
impression
impression material

ischemia
monomer
polyether
polysulfide
reversible hydrocolloid
tissue displacement

Because it is neither possible nor desirable to make patterns for fixed prostheses directly in the mouth, an **impression,** or negative likeness of the teeth and surrounding structures, is necessary to obtain a cast. This cast is then used to make a restoration in the laboratory. To obtain the cast, an elastic **impression material** is placed in a tray that is inserted into the patient's mouth. When the material has set, it is removed from the mouth. A suitable dental stone is then poured into the "negative" impression, and a positive likeness or working cast is obtained.

An acceptable impression must be an exact record of all aspects of the prepared tooth. This means it must include sufficient unprepared tooth structure immediately adjacent to the margins for the dentist and laboratory technician to identify the contour of the tooth and all prepared surfaces. The contour of the unprepared tooth structure cervical to the preparation margin is critical information that must be available when the restoration is fabricated in the dental laboratory. If the impression does not reproduce this critical area where tooth and future restoration meet, fabricating the restoration with proper contours is not possible (barring some lucky guesswork).

All teeth in the arch and the soft tissues immediately surrounding the tooth preparation must be reproduced in the impression. They will allow the cast to be accurately articulated and will contribute to proper contouring of the planned restoration. Particular attention is given to reproducing the lingual surfaces of anterior teeth because they influence anterior guidance, which determines the occlusal mor-

phology of the posterior teeth (see Chapter 4). The impression must be free of air bubbles, tears, thin spots, and other imperfections that might produce inaccuracies.

The patient's mouth is a challenging environment in which to make an accurate impression. Moisture control is probably one of the most important aspects of successful impression making. Except for the **polyethers**, all elastomeric impression materials are hydrophobic[1] (i.e., they do not tolerate or displace moisture). Any moisture will result in voids. Consequently, saliva flow into the area must be reduced and diverted to obtain the necessary dry field of operation.

When the preparation margins extend subgingivally, the adjacent gingival tissues must be displaced laterally to allow access and to provide adequate thickness of the impression material. This may require enlarging the gingival sulcus through mechanical, chemical, or surgical means and must be done without jeopardizing periodontal health. Improper manipulation of impression material and **tissue displacement** can lead to permanent soft tissue damage.

PREREQUISITES

TISSUE HEALTH

After the teeth are prepared and a provisional restoration has been made (see Chapter 15), the health of the surrounding soft tissues must be reevaluated. Careful preparation will result in minimal tissue damage; however, if a subgingival margin is needed, some tissue trauma in the sulcular area may be unavoidable. The effects of this trauma can be transient as long as the patient receives a properly made provisional restoration and maintains adequate oral hygiene. However, if the provisional is poorly contoured, not polished, or has defective margins, plaque retention will lead to a localized inflammatory response. The combination of such tissue trauma in the presence of preexisting periodontal disease can produce disastrous results.

Periodontal disease must be treated and resolved before fixed prostheses are placed.

On occasion, a defective restoration will contribute to the inflammatory sulcular response. If this is the case, a properly adapted and well-contoured polished provisional must be fabricated and cemented on the prepared teeth; the focus must shift from the teeth to the soft tissues, which must be re-turned to a state of optimum health before impression making is even considered.

SALIVA CONTROL

Depending on the location of the preparations in the dental arch, several techniques can be used to create the necessary dry field of operation (Fig. 14-1). In areas where only supragingival margins are present,

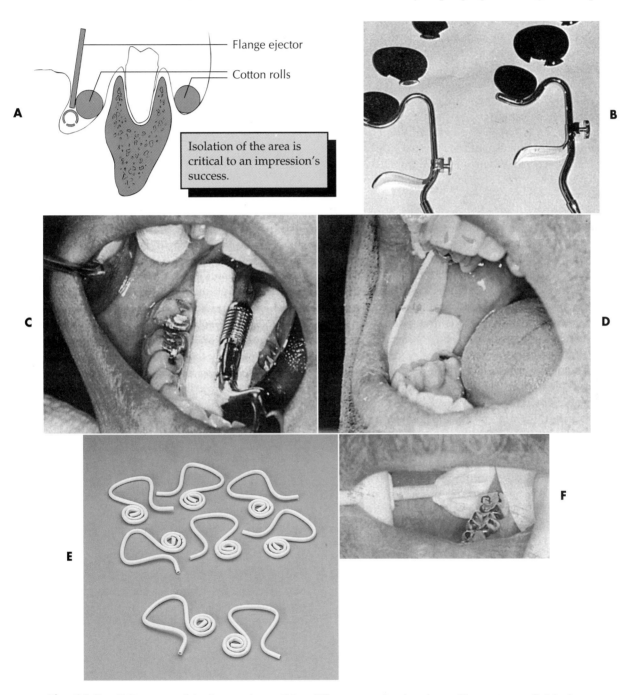

Fig. 14-1. Saliva control for impression making. When correctly placed, maxillary cotton rolls block salivary flow from the parotid gland. **A,** The evacuator removes saliva from the floor of the mouth, keeping the prepared tooth dry while the flange displaces the tongue medially. **B,** Svedopter and Speejector saliva evacuators. **C,** Placement of the Svedopter with cotton rolls. **D,** An absorbent card. **E,** The disposable Hygoformic aspirator system. **F,** Denta Pops aspirator system.
(E courtesy Sullivan-Schein Dental.)

moisture control with a rubber dam is probably the most appropriate method. However, in most instances a rubber dam cannot be used, and absorbent cotton rolls must be placed at the source of the saliva; an evacuator must be placed where the saliva pools. In the maxillary arch, placing a single cotton roll in the vestibule immediately buccal to the preparation and a saliva evacuator in the opposing lingual sulcus is usually sufficient. When working on a maxillary second or third molar, multiple cotton rolls must sometimes be placed immediately buccal to the preparation and slightly anterior to block off the parotid duct, which opens just anterior to the maxillary first molar. If a maxillary roll does not stay in position but slips down, it can be retained with a finger or the mouth mirror. When making a mandibular impression, placing additional cotton rolls to block off the sublingual and submandibular salivary ducts is usually necessary. Rolls on the buccal and lingual sides of the prepared teeth will help with soft tissue retraction—the cotton on the buccal side displaces the cheek laterally, and the cotton on the lingual side displaces the tongue medially. One or two cotton rolls placed vertically between the horizontally placed cotton rolls in the buccal vestibules will help maintain the latter in position.

An alternative to multiple cotton rolls is placement of one long roll "horseshoe fashion" in the maxillary and mandibular mucobuccal folds. However, when part of the cotton is saturated, the entire roll must be replaced. The use of moisture-absorbing cards (see Fig. 14-1, D) is another method for controlling saliva flow. These cards are pressed-paper wafers covered with a reflective foil on one side. The paper side is placed against the dried buccal tissue and adheres to it. In addition, two cotton rolls should be placed in the maxillary and mandibular vestibules to control saliva and displace the cheek laterally.

The tongue can be a problem when working in the mandibular arch. Saliva evacuators may help eliminate excess flow, but most of these are displaced easily by a "probing" tongue. If lingually placed cotton rolls continually become dislodged or, in conjunction with a conventional saliva evacuator, fail to control moisture adequately, a flanged-type evacuator (e.g., the Svedopter* or the Speejector†) should be considered (see Fig. 14-1, B). To avoid the risk of soft tissue trauma, this device must be placed carefully. A cotton roll between the blade and the

mylohyoid ridge of the alveolar process will minimize intraoral patient discomfort. Simultaneously, if properly positioned, this type of device will provide a "stop" that prevents the flange from being displaced farther buccally, allowing excellent lingual access to mandibular posterior teeth. Care must be taken not to tighten the chin clamp excessively, because considerable discomfort can result from pressure to the floor of the mouth. A disposable saliva ejector designed to displace the tongue may also be effective (see Fig 14-1, E and F).

In addition to the pain control normally needed during tissue displacement, local anesthesia may help considerably with saliva control during impression making. Nerve impulses from the periodontal ligament form part of the mechanism that regulates saliva flow; when these are blocked by the anesthetic, saliva production is considerably reduced.

When saliva control is especially difficult, a medication with antisialagogic action may be considered. Dry mouth is a side effect of certain anticholinergics[2,3] (drugs that inhibit parasympathetic innervation and thereby reduce secretions, including saliva). This group of drugs includes atropine, dicyclomine, and methantheline. Anticholinergics should be prescribed with caution in older adults and should not be used in any patient with heart disease. They are also contraindicated in individuals with glaucoma, because they can cause permanent blindness. The incidence of undiagnosed glaucoma in the general population is high, and some physicians recommend that all patients be evaluated ophthalmologically before anticholinergics are used.

Clonidine,[4] an antihypertensive drug, has successfully reduced salivary output. It is considered safer than anticholinergics and has no specified contraindications. However, it should be used cautiously in patients who take hypertension medication. In a clinical trial,[5] 0.2 mg of clonidine reduced salivary flow as effectively as 50 mg of methantheline.

DISPLACEMENT OF GINGIVAL TISSUES

Tissue displacement is commonly needed to obtain adequate access to the prepared tooth to expose all necessary surfaces, both prepared and not prepared. This is most effectively achieved by placement of a displacement cord (generally impregnated with a chemical agent). Sometimes gingival tissue is excised with a scalpel or with electrosurgery.

Displacement Cord. Some enlargement of the gingival sulcus can be obtained by placing a nonimpregnated cord and leaving it in place for a sufficient length of time. The cord is pushed into the sulcus and

---

*EC Moore Co.: Dearborn, Mich.

†Pulpdent Corporation of America: Brookline, Mass.

mechanically stretches the circumferential periodontal fibers. Placement is often easier if a braided (e.g., Gingibraid)* or a knitted (e.g., Ultrapak†) cord is used. However, larger sizes of braided cord should be avoided because they have a tendency to "double up" and can become too thick for atraumatic intrasulcular placement. In areas where very narrow sulci preclude placement of the smaller sizes of twisted or braided cord, wool-like cords that can be flattened are preferable for initial displacement of tissue.

Better sulcus enlargement can be achieved with a chemically impregnated cord or by dipping the cord in an astringent (e.g., Hemodent‡). These materials contain aluminum or iron salts and cause a transient **ischemia**, shrinking the gingival tissue. Even so, the sulcus closes quickly (less than 30 seconds) after the cord is removed; therefore, the impression must be taken immediately.[6] In addition, medicaments help control seepage of gingival fluid. Aluminum chloride ($AlCl_3$) and ferric sulfate ($Fe_2(SO_4)_3$) are suitable because they cause minimal tissue damage. As an alternative, a sympathomimetic amine-containing eye wash§ or nasal decongestant‖ have been shown to be effective.[7]

Many of the chemicals used for their astringent effect are stable only at narrow ranges of low pH levels. Table 14-1 shows the mean pH of some commonly used materials. The low pH levels have raised concern about the effect of acidic solutions on tooth structure and, perhaps more importantly, on the smear layer.[8,9] Figure 14-2 represents scanning electron micrographs of dentin after various durations of exposure to a commonly used ferric sulfate

---

*Van R Dental Products, Inc.: Los Angeles, Calif.
†Ultradent Products, Inc.: Salt Lake City, Utah.
‡ESPE-Premier: Norristown, Pa.
§Visine (tetrahydrozoline HCl, 0.05%).
‖Afrin (oxymetazoline, 0.05%).

solution. Contact between the astringent and the prepared tooth surfaces must be minimized if the smear layer is to be maintained. A nonacidic hemostatic agent can be used as an alternative.

Several displacement cords preimpregnated with epinephrine are available commercially. Epinephrine should be used with caution, because it may cause a tachycardia,[10] particularly if it is placed on lacerated tissue. Dosage control is also a potential problem. In a recent study,[11] clinicians were unable to detect any advantages of using gingival retraction cords that were impregnated with epinephrine.

Step-by-step Procedure
1. Isolate the prepared teeth with cotton rolls, place saliva evacuators as required, and dry the field with air.
2. Cut a length of cord sufficient to encircle the tooth (Fig. 14-3, A and B). Do not overdesiccate the tooth, because this may lead to postoperative sensitivity.
3. Dip the cord in astringent solution and squeeze out the excess with a gauze square. An impregnated cord can be placed dry but should be moistened in situ to prevent the thin sulcular epithelium from sticking to it and tearing when it is removed.
4. If a nonbraided cord is used, twist it tightly for easier placement.
5. Loop the cord around the tooth and gently push it into the sulcus with a suitable instrument (Fig. 14-3, C).

It is best to start in the interproximal area (Fig. 14-3, D), because the cord can be more easily placed here than facially or lingually. The instrument should be angled toward the tooth so the cord is pushed directly into the area. It should also be angled slightly toward any cord already packed; otherwise, that portion might be displaced. A second instrument (Fig. 14-3, E) may aid placement.

Acidity of Commonly Used Hemostatic Agents   TABLE 14-1

Agent	Manufacturer	Active Ingredient	Vehicle	Mean pH
Astringedent	Ultradent	15.5% $Fe_2(SO_4)_3$	Aqueous	0.7
Gingi-Aid	Gingi-Pak	Buffered 25% $AlCl_3$	Aqueous	1.9
Styptin	Van R	20% $AlCl_3$	Glycol	1.3
Hemodent	Premier	21.3% $AlCl_3$-6-hydrate	Glycol (aqueous)	1.2
Hemogin-L	Van R	$AlCl_3$	Aqueous	0.9
Orostat 8%	Gingi-Pak	8% Racemic epinephrine HCl	Aqueous	2.0
VicoStat	Ultradent	20% $Fe_2(SO_4)_3$	Aqueous	1.6
Aluminum chloride 25%	USP	25% $AlCl_3$	Aqueous	1.1
Stasis	Gingi-Pak	Basic $Fe_2(SO_4)_3$		0.8
For comparison: Ketac Dentin Etching Liquid				1.7

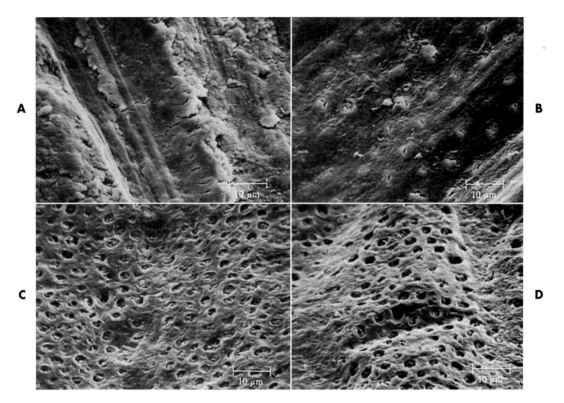

Fig. 14-2. Disturbance of the dentinal smear layer after contact with hemostatic agents. **A,** Dentin surface prepared with a high-speed, fine-grit diamond. **B,** After exposure to 15.5% $Fe_2(SO_4)_3$ solution for 30 seconds. The smear layer is largely removed, but many dentinal tubules are still occluded. **C,** After 2 minutes of exposure. Now the smear layer is totally removed, although the peritubular dentin appears to be largely intact. **D,** After 5 minutes of exposure. Now the dentin is etched, and the peritubular dentin has been removed.
(From Land MF et al: J Prosthet Dent *72:4, 1994.)*

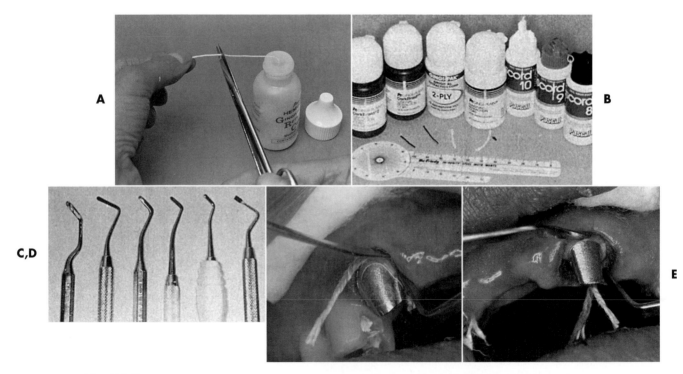

Fig. 14-3. **A,** Cutting a section of cord of adequate length to surround the tooth. **B,** From *left to right:* twisted cord, braided cord, wool-like cord in various sizes. **C,** Most cord-packing instruments have a slightly rounded tip with serrations to hold the cord while positioning it intrasulcularly. **D,** Initial proximal cord placement. **E,** An additional instrument prevents the cord from dislodging.

NOTE: Tissue displacement must be done gently but with sufficient firmness to place the cord just apical to the margin. Overpacking should be avoided because it could cause tearing of the gingival attachment, leading to irreversible recession. Repeated use of displacement cord in the sulcus also should be avoided, since this can cause gingival recession.

Evaluation

Difficulty with tissue displacement is often the result of gingival inflammation. The inflamed and swollen tissue bleeds easily, preventing access by the impression material.

Initial assessment of cord placement can be a useful indicator of the amount of displacement accomplished. When looking at the tooth preparation from the occlusal aspect, one should be able to see the preparation margin circumferentially and the uninterrupted cord, with no soft tissue folded over it, in contact with the tooth. If there is any doubt, assessing displacement by removing the cord is a good idea. The entire preparation margin should be clearly visible and will remain directly accessible for about a minute.

Typically, if the result is acceptable, a second cord is quickly inserted to maintain the displacement while the impression material is mixed. If the sulcus enlargement is not favorable, the tissue health should be reassessed, particularly if adequate displacement cannot be obtained by repeating the previous steps.

Sometimes a double cord is helpful. First, a thin cord is placed and trimmed so that its ends do not overlap. A second, larger cord is then placed in the normal manner and removed. The thin, first cord remains during impression making. When using this technique, the clinician should be careful not to damage the epithelial attachment.

On many occasions it is better to delay impression making and concentrate on how to improve tissue health (e.g., by reassessing the quality of the provisional restoration and reinforcing oral hygiene instructions) rather than attempting impression making under adverse conditions. Minor hemorrhaging can sometimes be controlled with an astringent* or by infiltrating a local anesthetic directly into the adjacent gingival papillae.

Electrosurgery.   An electrosurgery unit[12-15] (Fig. 14-4, *A*) may be used for minor tissue removal before impression making. In one technique,[16] the inner epithelial lining of the gingival sulcus is removed, thus improving access for a subgingival crown margin (Fig. 14-4, *B* and *C*) and effectively controlling postsurgical hemorrhage[17] (provided the tissues are not inflamed). Unfortunately, there is the potential for gingival tissue recession after treatment.[18]

An electrosurgery unit works by passage of a high-frequency current (1 to 4 million Hz†) through the tissue from a large electrode to a small one. At the small electrode, the current induces rapid localized polarity changes that cause cell breakdown

---

*ViscoStat or Astringedent (15.5% ferric sulfate) used with the Dento-Infusor tips according to the recommendations of Ultradent Products, Inc., has been effective.
†1 hertz = 1 cycle/second.

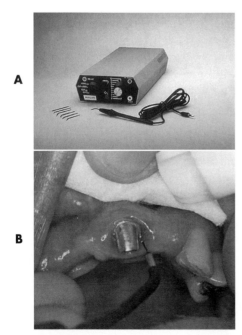

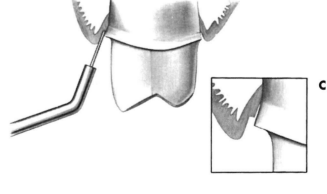

Fig. 14-4.   **A,** An electrosurgery unit. **B** and **C,** Procedure for enlarging the gingival sulcus. *(A courtesy Macan Engineering Co.)*

("cutting"). For restorative procedures, an unmodulated alternating current is recommended, because it will minimize damage to deeper tissues.[13]

The following facts should be considered before attempting electrosurgery:

1. It is contraindicated on or near patients with any electronic medical device (e.g., a cardiac pacemaker, TENS unit, insulin pump)[19] or patients with delayed healing as a result of debilitating disease or radiation therapy.
2. It is not suitable on thin attached gingivae (e.g., the labial tissue of maxillary canines).
3. It should not be used with metal instruments, because contact could cause electric shock. (Plastic mirrors and evacuation tubes are available.)
4. Profound soft tissue anesthesia is mandatory.
5. A thin wire electrode is best for sulcular enlargement. Gingival contouring is usually performed with a loop electrode.
6. The instrument should be set to unmodulated alternating current mode.
7. The electrode should be passed rapidly through the tissue with a single light stroke and kept moving at all times.
8. If the tip drags, the instrument is at too low a setting and the current should be increased.
9. If sparking is visible in the tissue, the instrument is at too high a setting and the current should be decreased.
10. A cutting stroke should not be repeated within 5 seconds.
11. The electrode must remain free of tissue fragments.
12. The electrode must not touch any metallic restoration. Contact lasting just 0.4 second has been shown to lead to irreversible pulpal damage in dogs.[20]
13. The sulcus should be swabbed with hydrogen peroxide before the displacement cord is placed.

MATERIALS SCIENCE

James L. Sandrik
ELASTIC IMPRESSION MATERIALS

There is an extensive variety of materials for making a precision negative mold of soft and hard tissues. In order of their historical development, they consist of the following:

1. **Reversible hydrocolloid**
2. **Polysulfide** polymer
3. Condensation silicone
4. Polyether
5. Addition silicone

Irreversible hydrocolloid is not sufficiently accurate for cast restorations. Each material has advantages and disadvantages, and none is entirely free of shortcomings. However, they all share one important characteristic: when handled correctly, they can produce casts of sufficient accuracy[21] and surface detail[22] for the fabrication of clinically acceptable fixed prostheses.

Nevertheless, there are reasons for selecting one material over another: If it becomes necessary to store the impression before a cast will be made, the polyethers and addition silicones are preferable because they exhibit sufficient long-term **dimensional stability**; the other materials, particularly the reversible hydrocolloids, must be poured immediately. If the impression will be poured in epoxy or will be electroplated (see Chapter 17), reversible hydrocolloid should not be selected because it is compatible only with die stone.

The advantages and disadvantages of the elastic impression materials are summarized in Table 14-2.

Reversible Hydrocolloid (Fig. 14-5).   Reversible hydrocolloid (also called *agar hydrocolloid* or simply *hydrocolloid*) was originally derived as a natural product of kelp. However, the material currently available is considerably different.

If poured immediately, reversible hydrocolloid produces casts of excellent dimensional accuracy and acceptable surface detail. At elevated temperatures, it changes from a gel to a sol. This change is reversible—i.e., as the material cools, the viscous fluid sol is converted to an elastic gel. Agar changes from gel to sol at 99° C (210° F) but remains a sol as low as 50° C (122° F), forming a gel only slightly above body temperature. These unique characteristics are very favorable for its use as an impression material.

Reversible hydrocolloid is supplied in a range of viscosities. Generally a heavy-bodied tray material is used with a less viscous syringe material. The required temperature changes are effected with a special conditioning unit and water-cooled impression trays.

Reversible hydrocolloid's lack of dimensional stability is due primarily to the ease with which water can be released from or absorbed by the material (syneresis and imbibition). The accuracy of a reversible hydrocolloid impression is improved if the material has as much bulk as possible (low surface area/volume ratio). This contrasts with the elastomeric impression materials, whose accuracy is improved by minimizing bulk (e.g., polysulfide and condensation silicone), because stresses produced during removal are reduced.[23] Therefore, an additional advantage of reversible hydrocolloid is that a **custom impression tray** is not required.

Available Elastic Impression Materials

TABLE 14-2

	Advantages	Disadvantages	Recommended Uses	Precautions
Irreversible hydrocolloid	Rapid set Straightforward technique Low cost	Poor accuracy and surface detail	Diagnostic casts Not suitable for working casts	Pour immediately
Reversible hydrocolloid	Hydrophilic Long working time Low material cost No custom tray required	Low tear resistance Low stability Equipment needed	Multiple preparations Problems with moisture	Pour immediately Use only with stone
Polysulfide polymer	High tear strength Easier to pour than other elastomers	Messy Unpleasant odor Long setting time Stability only fair	Most impressions	Pour within 1 hr; allow 10 min to set
Addition silicone	Dimensional stability Pleasant to use Short setting time Automix available	Hydrophobic Poor wetting Some materials release H_2 Hydrophilic formulations imbibe moisture	Most impressions	Delay pour of some materials Care to avoid bubbles when pouring
Condensation silicone	Pleasant to use Short setting time	Hydrophobic Poor wetting Low stability	Most impressions	Pour immediately Care to avoid bubbles when pouring
Polyether	Dimensional stability Accuracy Short setting time Automix available	Set material very stiff Imbibition Short working time	Most impressions	Care not to break teeth when separating cast

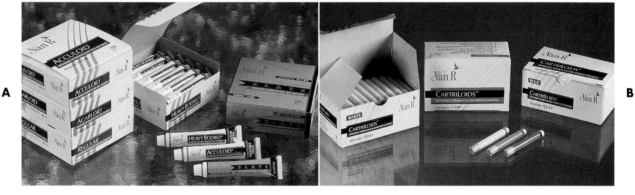

A   B

Fig. 14-5. Reversible hydrocolloid impression material. **A,** Tray material. **B,** Syringe material. *(Courtesy Sullivan-Schein Dental.)*

Polysulfide Polymer (Fig. 14-6). The polysulfides, commonly (though erroneously) known as *rubber bases*,* were introduced in the early to middle 1950s. They were received enthusiastically by dentists because they had better dimensional stability and tear strength than hydrocolloid. Nevertheless, they should be poured as soon as possible after impression making; delays of more than an hour result in clinically significant dimensional change.[19]

There is a slight contraction of polysulfide during polymerization, but the effects can be minimized with a custom impression tray to reduce the bulk of the material.[24] Generally a double-mix technique is used with a heavy-bodied tray material and a less viscous syringe material. These polymerize simultaneously, forming a chemical bond of adequate strength.[25]

The high tear resistance[26,27] and enhanced elastic properties of polysulfide facilitate impression making in sulcular areas and pinholes, and it has improved dimensional stability over hydrocolloid (inferior to polyether and addition silicone). Although it is the least expensive **elastomer**, it is not well-liked by patients because of its unpleasant sulfide odor and long setting time in the mouth (about 10

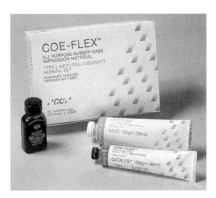

Fig. 14-6. Polysulfide polymer.
(Courtesy Sullivan-Schein Dental.)

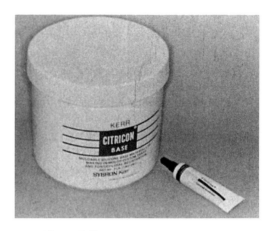

Fig. 14-7. Condensation silicone.

minutes). Furthermore, high humidity and temperature dramatically reduce its working time,[28] which may be so short that polymerization begins before it is inserted in the mouth, resulting in severe distortion). Although air conditioning is common in dental operatories, temperatures near 25° C (77° F) with humidity in excess of 60% can create problems.

Most polysulfide materials are polymerized with the aid of lead peroxides, which explains this material's typical brown color. The unpolymerized product is sticky and should be handled carefully, because it stains clothing permanently. Alternatives to lead are available; copper hydroxide is the most common. $Cu(OH)_2$-polymerized polysulfide is light green and shares many of the characteristics of the PbO_2-polymerized material (except for a reduced setting time).

Condensation Silicone (Fig. 14-7). Some of polysulfide's disadvantages have been overcome by condensation silicone, which is essentially odorless and can be pigmented to virtually any shade. Unfortunately, its dimensional stability is less than that of polysulfide but greater than that of reversible hydrocolloid. An additional advantage of this silicone is its relatively short setting time in the mouth (about 6 to 8 minutes). As a result, patients tend to prefer condensation silicone over polysulfide. In addition, condensation silicone is also less affected by high operating room temperatures and humidity.[23]

Silicone's main disadvantage is its poor wetting characteristics, which stems from its being extremely hydrophobic (for this reason, it is used in commercial sprays that protect automobile electrical systems from moisture). In this context, the prepared teeth and gingival sulci must be completely free of moisture to make possible a defect-free impression. Pouring without trapping air bubbles is also more difficult than with other impression materials, and a surfactant may be needed. Silicone impression material is available in a variety of viscosities. One technique involves a heavily filled

putty material that is used to customize a stock impression tray in the mouth, generally with a polyethylene spacer. The spacer allows room for a thin wash of light-bodied material, which makes the impression. The technique requires considerable care in seating, however, to prevent strain in the set putty. If this happens, the impression will rebound when removed from the mouth, resulting in dies that are too small.[29] Care is also needed to avoid contaminating the putty surface with saliva, which will prevent the wash impression from adhering properly.[30]

Silicone and polysulfide have a dimensional instability that results from their mode of polymerization. They are both condensation polymers, which as a by-product of their polymerization reactions, give off alcohol and water, respectively. As a result, evaporation from the set material causes dimensional contraction in both.

Polyether (Fig. 14-8). Polyether impression material, developed in Germany in the mid-1960s, has a polymerization mechanism unlike those of the other elastomers. No volatile by-product is formed, which results in excellent dimensional stability. In addition, its polymerization shrinkage[31] is unusually low compared with most room temperature–cured polymer systems. However, its thermal expansion[32] is greater than that of polysulfide.

With the high dimensional stability of polyether, accurate casts can be produced when the material is poured more than a day after the impression has been made. This is especially useful when pouring the impression immediately is impossible or inconvenient. Another advantage of polyether is its short setting time in the mouth (about 5 minutes, which is less than half the time required for polysulfide). For these reasons, polyether is used by many practitioners.

However, polyether has certain disadvantages. The stiffness of the set material is one such disad-

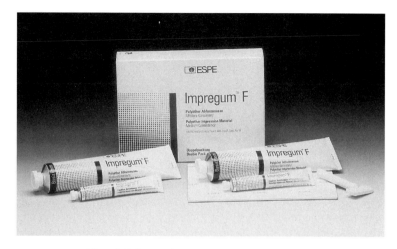

Fig. 14-8. Polyether impression material. *(Courtesy Sullivan-Schein Dental.)*

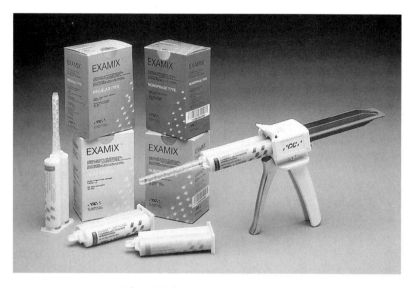

Fig. 14-9. Addition silicone. *(Courtesy Sullivan-Schein Dental.)*

vantage, which causes problems when separating a stone cast from the impression. Thin and single teeth, in particular, are liable to break unless the practitioner uses great care. Polyether is stable only if stored dry, because it will absorb moisture and undergo significant dimensional change. Polyether's relatively short working time may limit the number of prepared teeth that can be reliably captured in a single impression. Isolated cases of allergic hypersensitivity[33] to polyether elastomer have been reported (manifested as sudden onset of burning, itching, and general oral discomfort). Therefore, the allergic patient's record should carry a warning against polyether's future use, and an alternative elastomer should be chosen. Recent improvements in these materials have reportedly reduced this problem.

Addition Silicone (Fig. 14-9). Addition silicone was introduced as a dental impression material in

the 1970s. Also known as *poly(vinyl siloxane)* (*polysiloxane* is the generic chemical expression for silicone resins), it is similar in many respects to condensation silicone, except that it has much greater dimensional stability[34] (equivalent to polyether polymer), and its working time is more affected by temperature.[22] The set material is less rigid than polyether but stiffer than polysulfide. As with the other materials previously described, adverse soft-tissue responses have been reported.[35] One disadvantage of this material is the setting inhibition caused by some brands of latex gloves.[36] The problem is most apparent if a hand-mixed putty is used, but problems can occur if the tissues are touched with gloved hands immediately before impression placement. If the putty system is used, gloves that do not interfere with setting should be selected.[37] Like condensation silicone, addition silicones are hydrophobic. Some formulations contain surfactants, which gives them hydrophilic properties,[38] imparting wettability similar to polyethers.[39] However, these products also expand like polyether when in contact with moisture.[40] Addition silicone is generally used as a two-viscosity system, although monophase formulations are also available. It is easier to trap bubbles when using the monophase.[41]

Manufacturer recommendations should be followed when a cast is being poured, and pouring should be delayed with some of the earlier products. If this is not done, a generalized porosity of the cast surface caused by gas from the impression material will develop. Newer products contain "scavengers" that prevent the escape of gas at the polymer-cast interface. Addition silicone that contains scavenger material can be poured immediately.

• • •

CUSTOM TRAY FABRICATION

A custom tray improves the accuracy[42] of an elastomeric impression by limiting the volume of the material, thus reducing two sources of error: stresses during removal and thermal contraction. Although reducing the bulk of an elastomeric impression material increases its accuracy, the opposite is true for reversible hydrocolloid impressions. In hydrocolloid impressions, dimensional change is due to water loss (or gain) from the surface of the impression. A bulky hydrocolloid impression has a lower surface area/volume ratio and is therefore less subject to dimensional change.

Generally a custom tray is made from autopolymerizing acrylic resin (Fig. 14-10), although thermoplastic or photopolymerized resins are sometimes

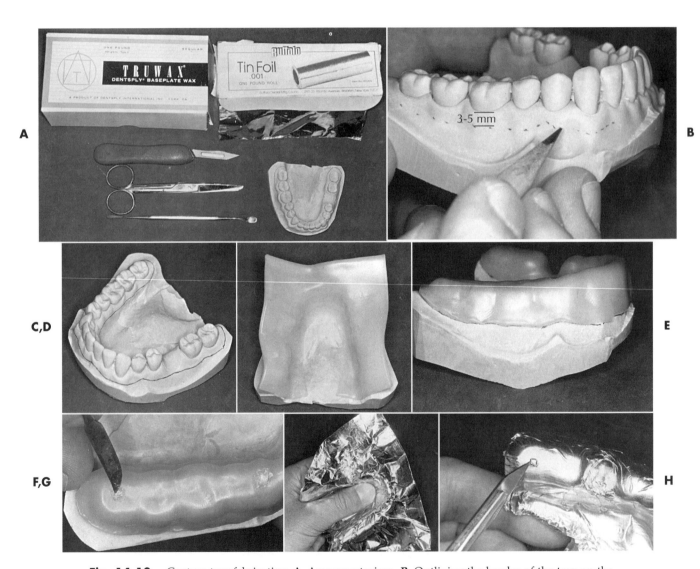

Fig. 14-10. Custom tray fabrication. **A,** Armamentarium. **B,** Outlining the border of the tray on the diagnostic cast. **C,** The tray should extend 3 to 5 mm from the gingival margin and about 3 mm beyond the most distal tooth. **D,** Softened baseplate wax is adapted to form a spacer. Typically two thicknesses will provide the recommended 2 to 3 mm of space. **E,** Spacer is trimmed to the pencil line. **F,** Wax is removed to form the tray stops. **G,** Covered with tinfoil. **H,** The foil is adapted to the stops.

Continued

used. Thermoplastic materials can be softened in a waterbath and adapted either manually or with a vacuum former with a heating element (Figs. 14-11 and 14-12). The accuracy of impressions made with a thermoplastic tray material or light-polymerized materials is comparable to that made with an autopolymerized resin.[43,44] Light-polymerized materials are convenient because a storage period is not needed for the completion of polymerization[45] (Fig. 14-13). In addition, the resin is less susceptible to distortion in moisture, making the impression suitable for the electroformed die technique (see Chapter 17). With the appropriate adhesive, it produces a better bond to the impression material.[46]

With any system, tray rigidity is important, because even slight flexing of the tray will lead to a distorted impression. This is particularly frustrating because the errors are usually undetectable until the practitioner attempts to seat the restoration. For this reason, thin, disposable plastic trays are unacceptable.[47] Resin thicknesses of 2 to 3 mm are needed for adequate rigidity. Clearance between the tray and the teeth should also be 2 to 3 mm; however, greater clearance is necessary for the more rigid polyether materials.

Armamentarium (see Fig. 14-10, *A*)
- Baseplate wax

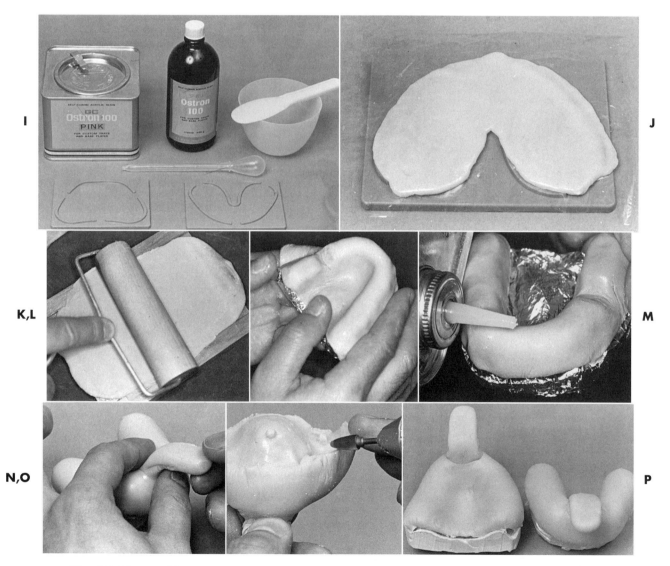

Fig. 14-10, cont'd. **I,** Custom tray resin. **J,** While it is still doughy, the resin is molded to a horseshoe shape (semicircle for maxillary trays). **K,** Wooden slab and roller used in an alternative method. **L,** The resin is gently adapted to the cast, and the excess is trimmed. **M** and **N,** Resin is moistened with monomer to attach the handle. **O,** When the resin has cured, the periphery is shaped with an acrylic-trimming bur. **P,** Maxillary and mandibular custom trays.

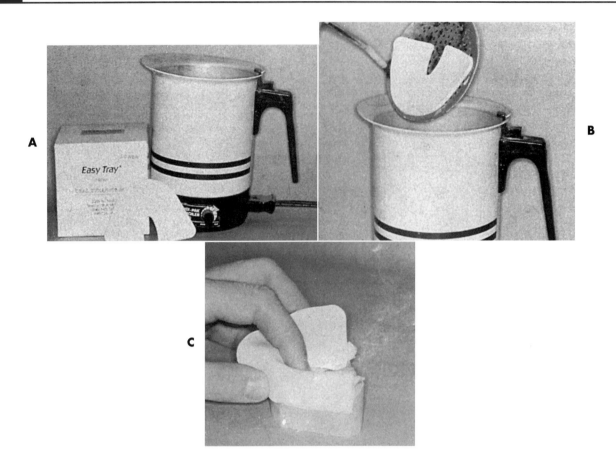

Fig. 14-11.   Thermoplastic custom tray material. **A** and **B,** The material is softened in hot water. **C,** The material has been adapted to the spaced cast.

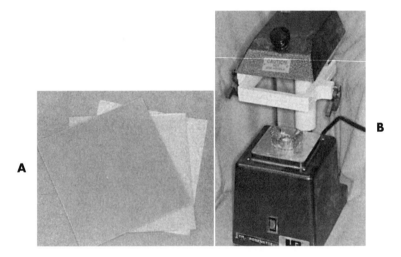

Fig. 14-12.   Vacuum-formed custom tray material. **A,** The thermoplastic sheets are much thicker and more rigid than those used for making provisional restorations (see Chapter 15), but the same equipment is used **(B).**

- 0.025 mm (0.001 in) tinfoil
- Scalpel
- Scissors
- Waxing instrument

Step-by-step Procedure (see Fig. 14-10, *B* to *P*)
1.   Using a pencil, mark the border of the tray on the diagnostic cast (see Fig. 14-10, *B*) approximately 5 mm apically to the crest of the free

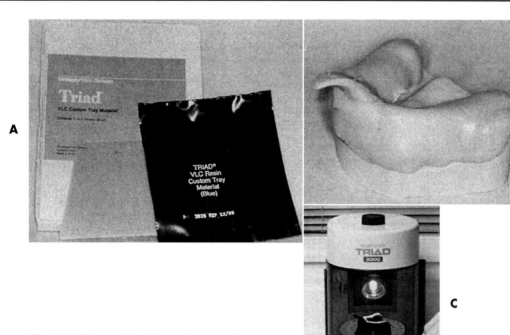

Fig. 14-13. Visible light-polymerized custom tray material. **A** and **B,** The material is removed from the packet and adapted to the spaced cast. **C,** The assembly is placed on the turntable of a special curing unit and exposed to intense light.

gingiva. Allow for muscle and frenum attachments (see Fig. 14-10, *C*). Maxillary trays do not always necessitate covering the entire palate, although this may be desirable if a removable appliance is planned after completion of the fixed prostheses. Under no circumstances should the posterior border extend farther than the demarcation between hard and soft palates.

2. Adapt a wax or other suitable spacer to the diagnostic cast (see Fig. 14-10, *D*). Two layers of baseplate wax will result in a combined thickness of approximately 2.5 mm (the sheets should be measured with a thickness gauge, because wax thicknesses vary).

3. Soften the wax by carefully heating it over a Bunsen burner or in hot water. Overheating may melt it and produce an undesirable thin spot. Only light pressure should be applied.

4. After the second sheet of wax has been applied, trim it back (see Fig. 14-10, *E*) until the pencil line is just visible. An alternative technique involves repeated dipping of the cast in molten wax. The cast is thoroughly wetted and then dipped three or four times to obtain a sufficient and uniform wax thickness (about 2 or 3 mm). This creates the space needed for the impression material. Three stops are needed in the tray to maintain even

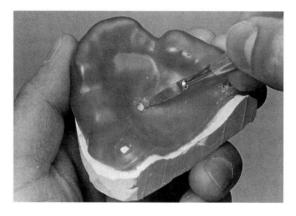

Fig. 14-14. If necessary, a tray stop can be placed on the hard palate.

space for the impression material in the oral cavity. These are placed on noncentric cusps of teeth that are not to be prepared (buccal cusps of the maxillary, lingual cusps of the mandibular). If all teeth are involved, a larger soft tissue stop (Fig. 14-14) can be placed on the crest of the alveolar ridge or in the center of the hard palate. Stops are made (Fig. 14-15) by removing wax at an angle of 45 degrees to the occlusal surfaces of three teeth that have a tripodal arrangement in the arch. This will lend stability to the tray, and the 45-degree slope will help center the tray during insertion.

5. Apply a layer of tinfoil over the wax (which may melt from the polymerization heat of the material) to prevent it from contaminating the inside of the tray.

6. Mix autopolymerizing acrylic resin (see Fig. 14-10, *I*) according to the manufacturer's recommendations. The use of vinyl gloves is recommended to prevent the development of sensitivity to the monomer.

7. After the resin is mixed, set it aside until it is doughy (with the consistency of putty). A template (see Fig. 14-10, *J*) or a wooden slab and roller (see Fig. 14-10, *K*) may help obtain a consistent thickness, although with practice the resin can be thinned out accurately by hand. Care must be taken not to stretch the material when manipulating it; thin areas in the resin may lead to a flexible tray and produce distortions.

8. Gently adapt the resin to the cast (see Fig. 14-10, *L*). A handle made from the excess resin can be attached at this time. If working time is unavailable, it can also be attached later with a separate second mix of acrylic resin (see Fig. 14-10, *M* and *N*). Buccal ridges, which are helpful with impression removal, can also be added (Fig. 14-16).

9. After the material has polymerized, remove it from the cast and trim it with an acrylic-trimming bur (see Fig. 14-10, *O*) where the indentation made by the wax

ledge is visible. All rough edges should be rounded to prevent soft tissue trauma.

10. If necessary, fill defects in the stops with additional resin, wetting the set tray material with monomer to ensure a good bond. To prevent the material from lifting up, some pressure should be maintained during this phase.

Evaluation

The completed custom tray (see Fig. 14-10, *P*) needs to be rigid, with a consistent thickness of 2 to 3 mm. It should extend about 3 to 5 mm cervical to the gingival margins and should be shaped to allow muscle attachments. It should be stable on the cast with stops that can maintain an impression thickness of 2 or 3 mm. The tray must be smooth, with no sharp edges. Finally, the handle should be sturdy and shaped to fit between the patient's lips (Fig. 14-17).

To avoid distortion from continued polymerization of the resin,[48] the tray should be made at least 9 hours before its use. When a tray is needed more urgently, it can be placed in boiling water for 5 minutes and allowed to cool to room temperature. A light-polymerized tray can also be made (see Fig. 14-13).

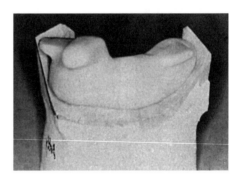

Fig. 14-16. Buccal ridges can be provided to facilitate removal of the impression.
(Courtesy Dr. H. Lin.)

> Once it is fully seated on its stops, a custom tray should be stable.

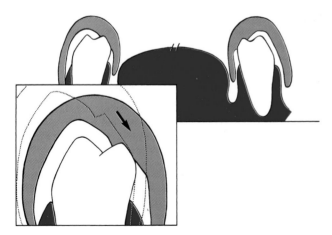

Fig. 14-15. Cross section through a mandibular custom tray. Stops have been placed on the noncentric cusps so that distortion will not interfere with the intercuspal relationship. The 45-degree slope helps to center the tray. Space exists for the impression material.

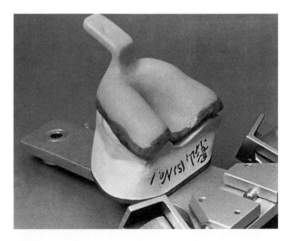

Fig. 14-17. A custom tray should be smooth and well finished. This will enhance patient acceptance.

◪ IMPRESSION MAKING

ELASTOMERIC MATERIALS

NOTE: When performing the following steps, an assistant is essential, unless the automix technique is used.

Step-by-step Procedure
Heavy Body–Light Body Combination

1. Try the custom tray in the mouth to verify its fit. Correct as needed.
2. Apply tray adhesive to extend a few millimeters onto the external surface of the tray (Fig. 14-18, *A*).

3. Isolate the abutment teeth and place gingival displacement cord in the sulcus.
4. On separate pads (one for the tray and one for the syringe material), disperse equal amounts of base and **accelerator** (Fig. 14-18, *B* and *C*).

NOTE: When mixing polysulfide polymers, pick up the brown catalyst first (Fig. 14-18, *D*) rather than the white base material, because the base will stick to the spatula and make it virtually impossible to incorporate all the catalyst.

5. Blend the two pastes thoroughly (Fig. 14-18, *E*). Initially, the spatula is kept somewhat vertical

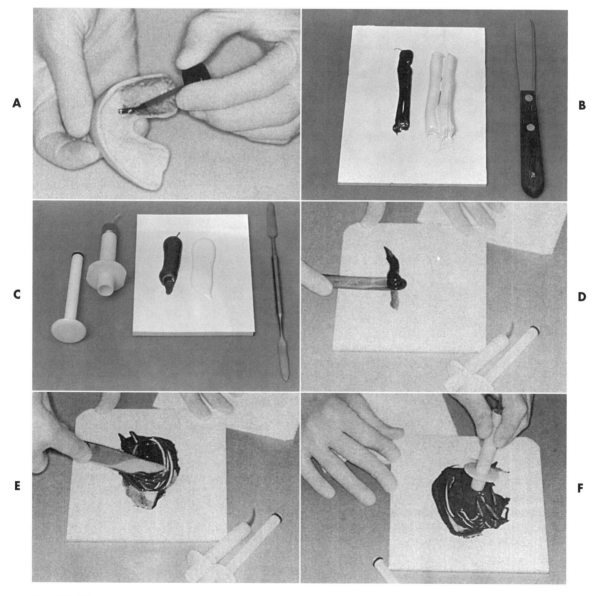

Fig. 14-18. Elastomeric impression making (polysulfide polymer). **A,** Adhesive applied to the tray. Sufficient time is allowed for drying. **B,** Heavy-bodied tray material. **C,** Light-bodied syringe material. **D,** The brown catalyst is picked up first. **E,** The light-bodied (white) material is thoroughly spatulated. **F,** Impression syringe being loaded.

Continued

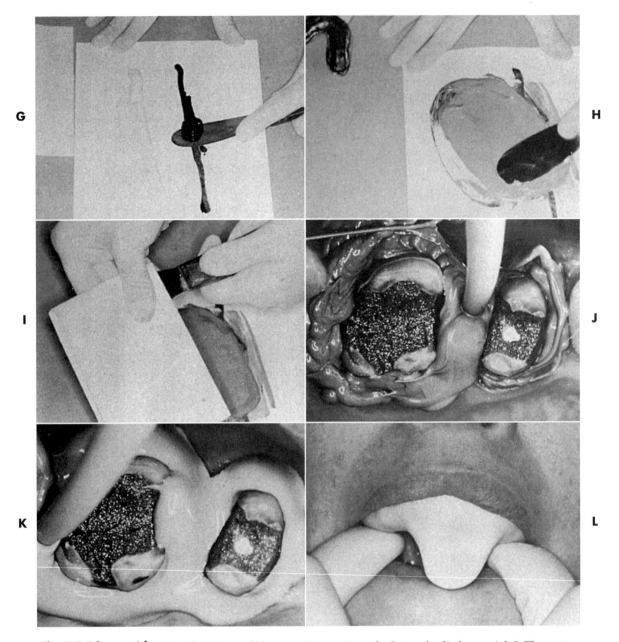

Fig. 14-18, cont'd.   **G** and **H,** Meanwhile, an assistant mixes the heavy-bodied material. **I,** The spatula is wiped to prevent unmixed material from being incorporated into the impression. **J** and **K,** Displacement cord is removed, and the impression material is syringed into the sulcus, around the prepared teeth, and into the grooves of the occlusal surfaces. **L,** The impression tray is filled with heavy-bodied material and seated.

during mixing, which is changed gradually to a more horizontal position as the two pastes become better incorporated. At this time, the spatula is wiped on a clean paper towel. Mixing continues for another 10 seconds to ensure that the material is homogeneous.

6. Load the syringe. This can be done by holding the barrel vertically and pushing it through the mix and then angling and sliding it sideways over the mixing pad. The syringe

can also be loaded from the other end (Fig. 14-18, *F*) by picking up the mixing sheet, forming a funnel, and expressing the material into the breech of the syringe.

NOTE: Concurrently with steps 5 through 9, have the assistant mix the heavy-bodied material in a similar manner as the light-bodied material (Fig. 14-18, *G* to *I*) and load the tray.

7. Remove the displacement cord and gently dry the preparation with compressed air.

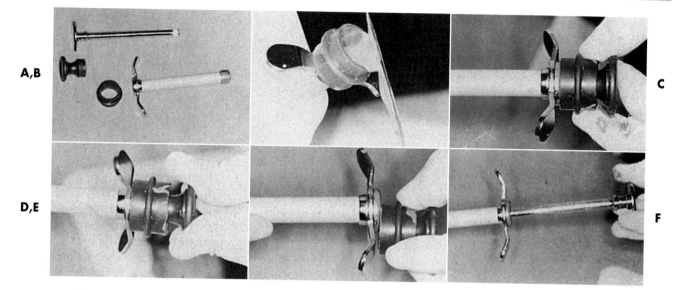

Fig. 14-19. **A,** A syringe-loading system is useful, especially for the single-mix technique. **B,** The mixed impression material is placed in a plastic sleeve attached to the rear of an impression syringe. **C and D,** It is forced into the barrel with a plastic piston. **E,** The piston-sleeve unit is removed, and the impression syringe barrel is inserted **(F).**

8. Place the tip of the syringe nozzle so that it touches the margin and inject the material slowly (Fig. 14-18, *J*). The tip should be inserted into the most distal embrasure first. This will prevent the material from flowing down over the preparation and trapping air bubbles. The tip is moved so that it follows the material rather than travelling ahead of it. When all the margins and axial surfaces have been covered, the material is air-blown into a thin layer. This improves the accuracy of the impression because the light-bodied material has greater polymerization shrinkage than the tray material.

9. Syringe along any edentulous spaces, lingual concavities of the anterior teeth (which are important for guidance), and occlusal surfaces of the posterior teeth (which are important for obtaining an accurate articulation) (Fig. 14-18, *K*).

10. Seat the tray (Fig. 14-18, *L*). It must remain immobile while the material undergoes polymerization (6 to 12 minutes, depending on the material). Otherwise, strains will form in the elastomer, which can cause distortion of the impression when it is removed. The manufacturer's recommendations for maximum working time and minimum setting time should be followed. It is difficult to judge clinically when elastomers start to develop elasticity.[49] Any delay in seating the tray will result in a distorted impression. It is

tempting to remove the impression too soon, since the patient may find it uncomfortable. However, premature impression removal is a common cause of distorted impressions. Because setting times vary from batch to batch, allowing the impression to set longer than what the manufacturer recommends is a wise precaution.

Single-mix Technique (Fig. 14-19). The same steps are performed for the single-mix technique as for the heavy body–light body technique; however, as the name indicates, only one mix is used to load the syringe and fill the tray. Most single-mix materials tend to produce a more viscous combination with a slightly shorter working time. (An alternate technique for loading the syringe is shown in Figure 14-19.)

Automix Technique (Fig. 14-20). Most manufacturers offer impression material in prepackaged cartridges with a disposable mixing tip attached. The cartridge is inserted in a caulking gunlike device, and the base and catalyst are extruded into the mixing tip, where mixing occurs as they progress to the end of the tube. The homogeneously incorporated material can be directly placed on the prepared tooth and impression tray. One of this system's advantages is the elimination of hand mixing on pads; the elimination of this variable has been shown to produce fewer voids in the impression.[50] Following the manufacturer's directions and bleeding the cartridge before inserting the tip are crucial.

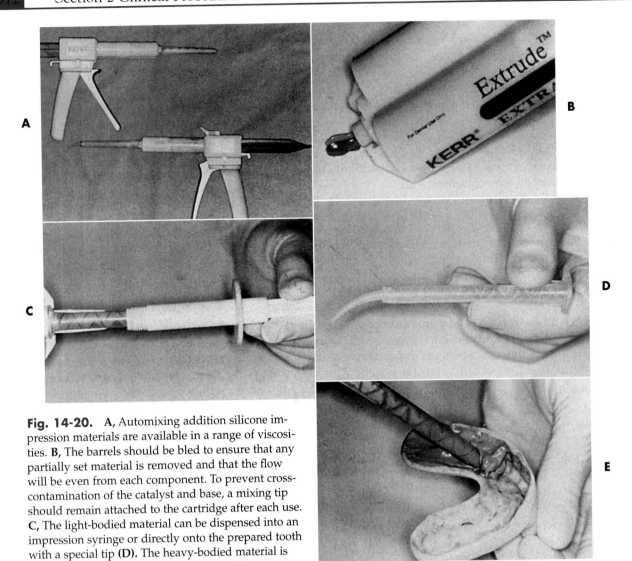

Fig. 14-20. **A,** Automixing addition silicone impression materials are available in a range of viscosities. **B,** The barrels should be bled to ensure that any partially set material is removed and that the flow will be even from each component. To prevent cross-contamination of the catalyst and base, a mixing tip should remain attached to the cartridge after each use. **C,** The light-bodied material can be dispensed into an impression syringe or directly onto the prepared tooth with a special tip **(D).** The heavy-bodied material is dispensed into the adhesive-coated tray **(E).**

Automixing is not available for the polysulfide polymers because these materials are too sticky for proper combination.

Machine Mixing Technique (Fig. 14-21). An alternative method for improving impression mixing is to use a machine mixer.* This system is convenient and produces void-free impressions.

Evaluation (Fig. 14-22)

The impression must be inspected for accuracy when it is removed. (Magnification is helpful.) If bubbles or voids appear in the margin, the impression must be discarded. An intact, uninterrupted cuff of impression material should be present beyond every margin. Streaks of base or catalyst material indicate

improper mixing and may render an impression useless. If the impression passes all these tests, it can then be disinfected (see p. 376) and poured to obtain a die and working cast (see Chapter 17).

REVERSIBLE HYDROCOLLOID

Reversible hydrocolloid impression material requires a special conditioning unit (Fig. 14-23), which is made up of three thermostatically controlled water baths:

1. A liquefaction bath (100° C [212° F]) for the heavy-bodied tray material and the light-bodied syringe material
2. A storage bath (about 65° C [150° F]) for maintaining liquefied materials until needed
3. A tempering bath (about 40° C [105° F]) for reducing the temperature of the heavy-bodied tray material enough to avoid tissue damage.

*Pentamix, ESPE America, Inc: Norristown, Pa.

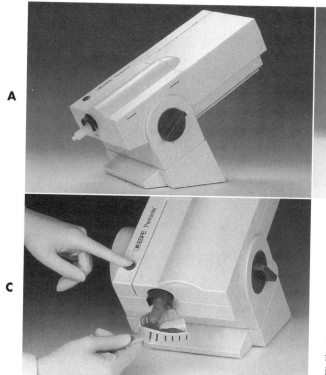

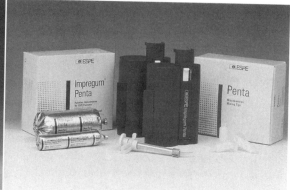

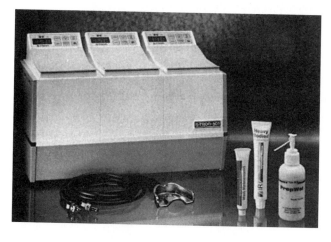

Fig. 14-21. Machine mixing system. **A,** Pentamix machine. **B,** Polyether impression material. **C,** Loading an impression tray.
(Courtesy ESPE America, Inc.)

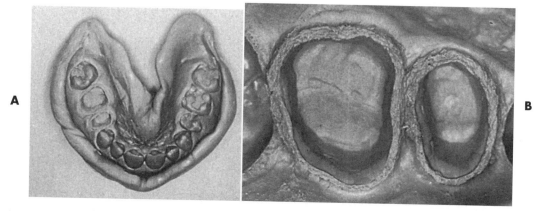

Fig. 14-22. **A,** The impression is removed and evaluated after the recommended setting time. **B,** There should be an uninterrupted cuff of material around each preparation margin.

Fig. 14-23. Hydrocolloid conditioning equipment consists of three thermostatically controlled water baths: boiling, storage, and tempering.
(Courtesy Van R Dental Products, Inc.)

Step-by-step Procedure

1. Select the correct size of water-cooled impression tray. For maximum accuracy, use as large a size as can be comfortably accommodated by the patient.
2. Place small modeling compound or prefabricated stops (tripod fashion) in the tray to prevent overseating.
3. For adequate access, displace the gingival tissues as previously described.
4. Fill the impression tray with heavy-bodied material from the storage bath wash hydro-colloid (Fig. 14-24, *A*). Squeeze some onto the tray material (Fig. 14-24, *B*) and submerge the tray in a tempering bath (Fig. 14-24, *C*). Load the syringe and replace it in the storage tank.
5. Carefully remove the cord from the sulcus, flood the sulcus with warm water (Fig. 14-24, *D*) (some techniques omit this step), and inject the light-bodied impression material as for polysulfide polymer. Then cover the entire surface of the prepared tooth.
6. Remove the impression tray from the tempering tank, wipe off the surface layer with a

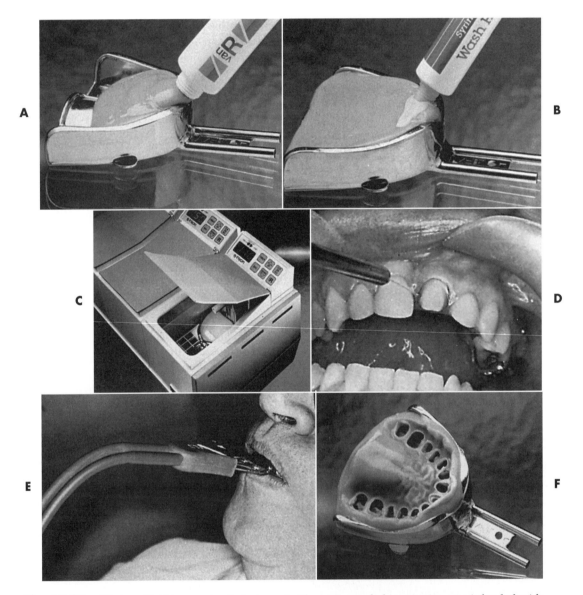

Fig. 14-24. Hydrocolloid impression technique. **A,** The water-cooled impression tray is loaded with heavy-bodied material. **B,** The wash hydrocolloid is squeezed onto the tray material in the area of the preparations. **C,** The filled tray is placed in a tempering bath for the recommended 7 minutes. **D,** The entire arch is flooded with water or a surfactant. **E,** The tray is seated, and water-cooling tubes are connected. **F,** The completed impression. Light-bodied material should have been displaced by the tray material. *(Courtesy Van R Dental Products, Inc.)*

gauze square, and place it in the patient's mouth. After seating, cold water is circulated through the tray until the impression material is completely set (Fig. 14-24, *E*). This usually takes 5 or 6 minutes.

7. Hold the tray firmly in the patient's mouth while the impression material is setting.

8. Remove the tray with a rapid motion, wash it with cold water, disinfect it (see Table 14-3), immerse it in potassium sulfate solution (if the manufacturer recommends this), and evaluate it for accuracy.

9. After the impression is judged to be acceptable, pour immediately in Type IV or V stone.

Evaluation (Fig. 14-24, *F*)

A reversible hydrocolloid impression is evaluated in the same manner as polysulfide polymer. However, the translucency of the material may make small imperfections difficult to detect. If doubt exists, it may be expedient to make a new impression, because this does not require additional tissue displacement and can be easily accomplished.

SPECIAL CONSIDERATIONS

Certain modifications of the basic **impression technique** are sometimes needed, particularly for making impressions with additional retention features such as pinholes and post space.

Pin-retained Restorations (Fig. 14-25). Elastomeric impression materials are strong enough to reproduce a pinhole without tearing. However, to avoid bubbles, they must be introduced carefully into the pinhole with a lentulo or cement tube. With reversible hydrocolloid, a special nylon bristle must be used for the impression.

Step-by-step Procedure

1. Apply a separating medium (e.g., die lubricant) to the pinholes and isolate and displace the tissue in the conventional manner.

2. After mixing the light-bodied impression material, set aside a small amount for placement into the pinholes.

Cement Tube

3. Fill the tube and squeeze a small amount of material into each pinhole. Make sure that no air is trapped in the base of the pinhole (insert an explorer into the material, remove, and repeat the application).

Lentulo

4. Be sure that the slow-speed handpiece is rotating clockwise before picking up a small quantity of impression material.

5. Spiral the material into the pinholes, rotating slowly while moving the lentulo along the side of the pinhole.

6. Increase the speed of the lentulo while backing it out (to prevent the material from being pulled out).

Prefabricated Plastic Pin

7. When making a reversible hydrocolloid impression of a pin-retained restoration, use elastomer bristles to register the pin holes. The bristles can be modified as necessary with a sharp scalpel to eliminate any inaccuracy relating to fit. Their lengths should be adjusted so that they do not contact the impression tray. (A bristle should extend 2 mm above the opening of the pinhole.)

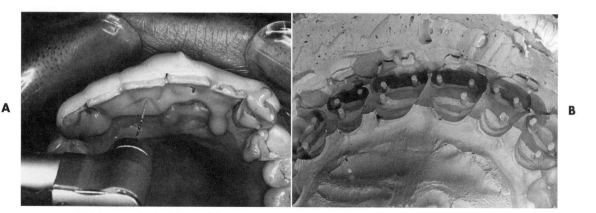

Fig. 14-25. Elastomeric impression for pin-retained restorations. **A,** A lentulo fills each pinhole; then material is syringed around the prepared teeth in the normal way, and the tray is seated. **B,** The completed impression.

8. Apply a separating medium to the pinhole before placing the bristle and completing the impression.

Post-and-cores. Elastomeric materials can be successfully used to make impressions of the post space when endodontically treated teeth are being restored. The procedure involves reinforcing the impression with a plastic pin or suitable wire (e.g., orthodontic wire) as described in Chapter 12.

DISINFECTION

When they are removed from the patient's mouth, it must be assumed that all impression materials have been in contact with body fluids. They should be disinfected according to the recommended procedures for the material being used. After being removed from the patient's mouth, the impression is immediately rinsed with tap water and dried with an air syringe. Suitable chemicals should be used, such as glutaraldehyde solutions or iodophor sprays. Table 14-3 shows the most commonly recommended techniques for the materials discussed in this section. Some are perfectly acceptable for one material but unsuitable for others. Because of its tendency to distort and absorb moisture, polyether or "hydrophilic" addition silicone impression materials should be sprayed and stored in a plastic bag rather than submerged and soaked in a glutaraldehyde solution. Disinfection is an essential step for preventing cross-infection and exposure of laboratory personnel. If it is performed properly, disinfection will not affect the accuracy or surface reproduction of the elastomer.[51, 52]

EVALUATION

After disinfection, the completed impression (Fig. 14-26) is inspected carefully before the working cast is made. An elastomeric impression should be dried before it is evaluated. The following points are then considered:

1. Has the material been properly mixed? An impression that contains visible streaks of base or catalyst material should be rejected.
2. Is there an area where the custom tray shows through? This must be identified and its potential impact on the quality of the impression assessed. A common error is rotation and the resulting inaccurate seating of the tray. This can result in the tray contacting several teeth and an uneven thickness of impression material. Normally this will occur only at the tray stops, but when it touches a critical area, the impression must be discarded and a new one made. However, if a thin spot is not near the prepared teeth, it can sometimes be allowed to remain.
3. Are there any voids, folds, or creases? These should have been avoided by careful technique; however, the impression may still be acceptable when a small defect occurs in a noncritical area (e.g., away from the margin of a prepared tooth). Careful judgment must be exercised.
4. Is there an even, uninterrupted extension of impression material beyond the margins of the prepared teeth? This is essential if restorations with well-fitting margins and correct contours are to be made.
5. Has the impression material separated from the tray? This is a common cause of distorted impressions and results from improper application and/or inadequate drying of the adhesive.

Recommended Disinfection Method by Impression Material   TABLE 14-3

Disinfection Solution	Irreversible* Hydrocolloid	Reversible* Hydrocolloid	Polysulfide	Silicones	Polyether†
Glutaraldehyde 2% (10-minute soak time)	Not recommended	Not recommended	Yes	Yes	No
Iodophors (1:213 dilution)	Yes	Yes	Yes	Yes	No
Chlorine compounds (1:10 dilution of commercial bleach)	Yes	Yes	Yes	Yes	Yes
Complex phenolics	Not recommended	Limited data	Yes	Yes	No
Phenolic glutaraldehydes	Not recommended	Yes	Yes	Yes	No

Modified from Merchant VA: *CDA J* 20:10, 31, 1992.

*Immersion time should be minimized. Dip in glutaraldehyde, rinse in sterile water, dip again, and delay pouring for 10 minutes while maintaining a humid environment. Alternatively, spray with sodium hypochlorite, rinse, and respray with a similar 10-minute delay before pouring.

†Note: Imbibition distortion results from prolonged immersion. 1:10 hypochlorite or chlorine dioxide: spray, rinse, repeat, spray again, and delay pouring for approximately 10 minutes.

SUMMARY

An impression or negative likeness of the teeth and surrounding structures is used to obtain a cast, on which the planned restoration is fabricated. A good impression is an exact negative replica of each prepared tooth and must include all of the prepared surfaces and an adequate amount of unprepared tooth structure adjacent to the margin.

Healthy soft tissues and the control of saliva flow are essential for a successful impression. However, caution must be exercised to prevent injury to the gingiva. Cotton rolls, cards, and saliva evacuators are needed for adequate moisture control. During the impression procedure, using a local anesthetic to minimize discomfort and to reduce saliva flow is recommended.

Both mechanical-chemical and surgical methods for enlargement of the gingival sulcus can be used to obtain access to subgingival margins of prepared teeth. However, a narrow cord impregnated with a mild astringent (e.g., $AlCl_3$) is recommended. To protect the smear layer, excessive contact between hemostatic agents and cut tooth structure should be avoided.

A custom acrylic resin tray should be used when making an impression with any of the elastomeric materials. All impression materials should be rinsed, dried, and disinfected when removed from the mouth. Impressions made with polysulfide polymer should be poured within 1 hour. Impressions made with polyether or addition silicone have high dimensional stability and can be stored considerably longer before pouring. When making pin-retained restorations, a cement tube, lentulo, or nylon bristle is needed for an accurate impression of the pinholes or post spaces. In this technique and others, a good impression is critical for an accurately fitting restoration.

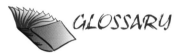 *GLOSSARY*

accelerator: *n* (1611) *1:* a substance that speeds a chemical reaction *2:* in physiology, a nerve, muscle, or substance that quickens movement or response

agar: *n* (1889): a complex sulfated polymer of galactose units, extracted from Gelidium cartilagineum, Gracilaria confervoides, and related red algae. It is a mucilaginous substance that melts at approximately 100°C and solidifies into a gel at approximately 40°C. It is not digested by most bacteria and is used as a gel in dental impression materials and solid culture media for microorganisms.

autopolymer: *n:* a material that polymerizes by chemical reaction without external heat, as a result of the addition of an activator and a catalyst—**autopolymerization** *vb*

catalyst: *n* (1902): a substance that accelerates a chemical reaction without affecting the properties of the materials involved

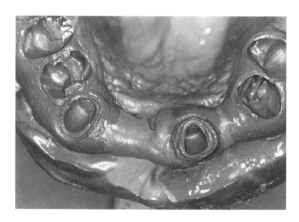

Fig. 14-26. The completed impression. Careful technique will ensure a complete cuff of impression material beyond the margin and will greatly facilitate trimming of the die and contouring of the wax pattern.

Study Questions

1. Discuss the prerequisites to successful and predictable impression making with elastomeric impression materials.
2. Discuss three ways to ensure access to prepared tooth structure for impression making. What are the respective indications and contraindications?
3. Name three classes of impression materials for fixed prosthodontics, and discuss their advantages and disadvantages. Illustrate their indicated use with three clinical scenarios.
4. Describe 10 considerations before implementing electrosurgery.
5. What are the requirements for a successful custom impression tray?
6. Disinfection techniques vary among materials. Select three classes of impression material and illustrate how the respective disinfection techniques change for each.

custom tray: an individualized impression tray made from a cast recovered from a preliminary impression. It is used in making a final impression

dimensional stability: the ability of a material to retain its size and form

elastomer: *n* (ca. 1934): a polymer whose glass transition temperature is below its service temperature (usually room temperature). These materials are characterized by low stiffness and extremely large elastic strains—**elastomeric** *adj*

final impression: the impression that represents the completion of the registration of the surface or object

gingival displacement: the deflection of the marginal gingiva away from a tooth

hydrocolloid: *n* (1916): a colloid system in which water is the dispersion medium; those materials described as a colloid sol with water that are used in dentistry as elastic impression materials

impression: *n:* a negative likeness or copy in reverse of the surface of an object; an imprint of the teeth and adjacent structures for use in dentistry

impression material: any substance or combination of substances used for making an impression or negative reproduction

impression technique: *obs:* a method and manner used in making a negative likeness (GPT-4)

impression tray: *1:* a receptacle into which suitable impression material is placed to make a negative likeness *2:* a device that is used to carry, confine, and control impression material while making an impression

ischemia: *n* (ca. 1860): local and temporary deficiency of blood, chiefly resulting from the contraction of a blood vessel

master impression: the negative likeness made for the purpose of fabricating a prosthesis

monomer: *n* (1914): a chemical compound that can undergo polymerization; any molecule that can be bound to a similar molecule to form a polymer

polyether: *adj:* an elastomeric impression material of ethylene oxide and tetra-hydrofuron copolymers that polymerizes under the influence of an aromatic ester

polysulfide: *n* (1849): an elastomeric impression material of polysulfide polymer (mercaptan) that cross-links under the influence of oxidizing agents such as lead perioxide

polyvinylsiloxane: *n:* an addition reaction silicone elastomeric impression material of silicone polymers having terminal vinyl groups that cross-link with silanes on activation by a platinum or palladium salt catalyst

reversible hydrocolloid: colloidal gels in which the gelation is brought about by cooling and can be returned to the sol condition when the temperature is sufficiently increased

tissue displacement: the change in the form or position of tissues as a result of pressure

tissue reaction: the response of tissues to an altered condition

REFERENCES

1. McCormick JT et al: Wettability of elastomeric impression materials: effect of selected surfactants, *Int J Prosthod* 2:413, 1989.

2. Council on Dental Therapeutics, American Dental Association: *Accepted dental therapeutics,* ed 38, Chicago, 1979, The Association, p. 247.

3. Sherman CR, Sherman BR: Atropine sulfate: a current review of a useful agent for controlling salivation during dental procedures, *Gen Dent* 47:56, 1999.

4. Findlay D, Lawrence JR: An alternative method of assessing changes in salivary flow: comparison of the effects of clonidine and tiamenidine (HOE 440), *Eur J Clin Pharmacol* 14:231, 1978.

5. Wilson EL et al: Effects of methantheline bromide and clonidine hydrochloride on salivary secretion, *J Prosthet Dent* 52:663, 1984.

6. Laufer BZ et al: The closure of the gingival crevice following gingival retraction for impression making, *J Oral Rehabil* 24:629, 1997.

7. Bowles WH et al: Evaluation of new gingival retraction agents, *J Dent Res* 70:1447, 1991.

8. Land MF et al: Disturbance of the dentinal smear layer by acidic hemostatic agents, *J Prosthet Dent* 72:4, 1994.

9. Land MF et al: Smear layer instability caused by hemostatic agents, *J Prosthet Dent* 76:477, 1996.

10. Pelzner RB et al: Human blood pressure and pulse rate response to racemic epinephrine retraction cord, *J Prosthet Dent* 39:287, 1978.

11. Jokstad A: Clinical trial of gingival retraction cords, *J Prosthet Dent* 81:258, 1999.

12. Harris HS: *Electrosurgery in dental practice,* Philadelphia, 1976, JB Lippincott.

13. Gnanasekhar JD, al-Duwairi YS: Electrosurgery in dentistry, *Quintessence Int* 29:649, 1998.

14. Louca C, Davies B: Electrosurgery in restorative dentistry. I. Theory, *Dent Update* 19:319, 1992.

15. Louca C, Davies B: Electrosurgery in restorative dentistry. II. Clinical applications, *Dent Update* 19:364, 1992.

16. Podshadley AG, Lundeen HC: Electrosurgical procedures in crown and bridge restorations, *J Am Dent Assoc* 77:1321, 1968.

17. Maness WL et al: Histologic evaluation of electrosurgery with varying frequency and waveform, *J Prosthet Dent* 40:304, 1978.

18. DeVitre R, Galburt RB, Maness WJ: Biometric comparison of bur and electrosurgical retraction methods, *J Prosthet Dent* 53:179, 1985.

19. Walter C: Dental treatment of patients with cardiac pacemaker implants, *Quintessence Int* 8:57, 1975.

20. Krejci RF et al: Effects of electrosurgery on dog pulps under cervical metallic restorations, *Oral Surg* 54:575, 1982.

21. Tjan AH et al: Clinically oriented evaluation of the accuracy of commonly used impression materials, *J Prosthet Dent* 56:4, 1986.

22. Setz J et al: Profilometric studies on the surface reproduction of dental impression materials, *Dtsch Zahnarztl Z* 44:587, 1989.

23. Luebke RJ et al: The effect of delayed and second pours on elastomeric impression material accuracy, *J Prosthet Dent* 41:517, 1979.

24. Eames WB et al: Elastomeric impression materials: effect of bulk on accuracy, *J Prosthet Dent* 41:304, 1979.

25. Cullen DR, Sandrik JL: Tensile strength of elastomeric impression materials, adhesive and cohesive bonding, *J Prosthet Dent* 62:142, 1989.

26. Herfort TW et al: Tear strength of elastomeric impression materials, *J Prosthet Dent* 39:59, 1978.

27. Hondrum SO: Tear and energy properties of three impression materials, *Int J Prosthodont* 7:517, 1994.

28. Harcourt JK: A review of modern impression materials, *Aust Dent J* 23:178, 1978.

29. Fusayama T et al: Accuracy of the laminated single impression technique with silicone materials, *J Prosthet Dent* 32:270, 1974.

30. Tjan AH: Effect of contaminants on the adhesion of light-bodied silicones to putty silicones in putty-wash impression technique, *J Prosthet Dent* 59:562, 1988.

31. Henry PJ, Harnist DJR: Dimensional stability and accuracy of rubber impression materials, *Aust Dent J* 19:162, 1974.

32. Mansfield MA, Wilson HJ: Elastomeric impression materials: a method of measuring dimensional stability, *Br Dent J* 139:267, 1975.

33. Nally FF, Storrs J: Hypersensitivity to a dental impression material: a case report, *Br Dent J* 134:244, 1973.

34. Lacy AM et al: Time-dependent accuracy of elastomer impression materials. II. Polyether, polysulfides, and polyvinylsiloxane, *J Prosthet Dent* 45:329, 1981.

35. Sivers JE, Johnson GK: Adverse soft tissue response to impression procedures: report of a case, *J Am Dent Assoc* 116:58, 1988.

36. Reitz CD, Clark NP: The setting of vinyl polysiloxane and condensation silicone putties when mixed with gloved hands, *J Am Dent Assoc* 116:371, 1988.

37. Matis BA et al: The effect of the use of dental gloves on mixing vinyl polysiloxane putties, *J Prosthodont* 6:189, 1997.

38. Boening KW et al: Clinical significance of surface activation of silicone impression materials, *J Dent* 26:447, 1998.

39. Pratten DH, Craig RG: Wettability of a hydrophilic addition silicone impression material, *J Prosthet Dent* 61:197, 1989.

40. Oda Y et al: Evaluation of dimensional stability of elastomeric impression materials during disinfection, *Bull Tokyo Dent Coll* 36:1, 1995.

41. Millar BJ et al: In vitro study of the number of surface defects in monophase and two-phase addition silicone impressions, *J Prosthet Dent* 80:32, 1998.

42. Millstein P et al: Determining the accuracy of stock and custom tray impression/casts, *J Oral Rehabil* 25:645, 1998.

43. Gordon GE et al: The effect of tray selection on the accuracy of elastomeric impression materials, *J Prosthet Dent* 63:12, 1990.

44. Martinez LJ, von Fraunhofer JA: The effects of custom tray material on the accuracy of master casts, *J Prosthodont* 7:106, 1998.

45. Wirz J et al: Light-polymerized materials for custom impression trays, *Int J Prosthod* 3:64, 1990.

46. Bindra B, Heath JR: Adhesion of elastomeric impression materials to trays, *J Oral Rehabil* 24:63, 1997.

47. Burton JF et al: The effects of disposable and custom-made impression trays on the accuracy of impressions, *J Dent* 17:121, 1989.

48. Pagniano RP et al: Linear dimensional change of acrylic resins used in the fabrication of custom trays, *J Prosthet Dent* 47:279, 1982.

49. McCabe JF, Carrick TE: Rheological properties of elastomers during setting, *J Dent Res* 68:1218, 1989.

50. Chong YH et al: The effect of mixing method on void formation in elastomeric impression materials, *Int J Prosthod* 2:323, 1989.

51. Drennon DG et al: The accuracy and efficacy of disinfection by spray atomization on elastomeric impressions, *J Prosthet Dent* 62:468, 1989.

52. Drennon DG, Johnson GH: The effect of immersion disinfection of elastomeric impressions on the surface detail reproduction of improved gypsum casts, *J Prosthet Dent* 63:233, 1990.

CHAPTER • FIFTEEN

PROVISIONAL RESTORATIONS

Anthony G. Gegauff

Julie A. Holloway

KEY TERMS

acrylic resin
autopolymerizing resin
exotherm
external surface form (ESF)

poly(methylmethacrylate)
poly(R' methacrylate)
provisional luting agent
tissue surface form (TSF)

Provisional crowns or fixed partial dentures are essential to prosthodontic therapy. The word *provisional* means established for the time being, pending a permanent arrangement. Even though a definitive restoration may be placed as quickly as 2 weeks after tooth preparation, the provisional restoration must satisfy important needs of the patient and dentist. Unfortunately, *temporary* usually connotes laxity, and this may imply that requirements pertaining to the more permanent condition are ignored. If this connotation becomes a philosophy governing the provisional phase of treatment, the dentist will needlessly be reducing clinical efficiency and treatment quality. Experience has repeatedly shown that the time and effort expended in fulfilling the requisites of provisional restorations are well spent.

Because of unforeseen events (e.g., laboratory delays or patient unavailability), a provisional restoration may have to function for an extended period. On the other hand, a delay in placing the definitive restoration may be deliberate (e.g., because the etiologic factors of a temporomandibular disorder or periodontal disease must be corrected). Whatever the intended length of time of treatment, a provisional will have to be adequate to maintain patient health. Thus it should not be casually fabricated on the basis of expected short-term use.

Provisional procedures also must be efficiently performed, because they are done while the patient is in the operatory and during the same appointment that the teeth are prepared. Costly chairside time should be used efficiently with the practitioner producing an acceptable restoration. Failure to do so will result in the eventual loss of more time than was initially thought saved. For example, an inadequate restoration may lead to unnecessary repairs or to the need to treat gingival inflammation and remake the impression. Such problems can be avoided if one thoroughly understands what is required of the provisional and makes the effort to meet these requirements.

■ REQUIREMENTS

An optimum provisional restoration must satisfy many interrelated factors, which can be classified as biologic, mechanical, and esthetic (Fig. 15-1).

BIOLOGIC REQUIREMENTS

Pulp Protection. A provisional restoration must seal and insulate the prepared tooth surface from the oral environment to prevent sensitivity and further irritation to the pulp. Because of the sec-

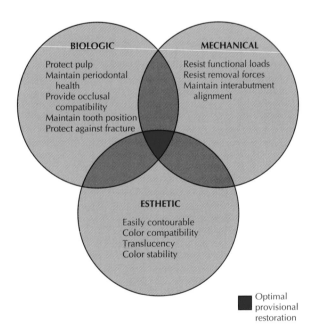

Fig. 15-1. Factors to be considered in making a provisional restoration. The dark red area represents the optimum, in which biologic, mechanical, and esthetic requirements are adequately met.

tioning of dentinal tubules, a certain degree of pulp trauma is inevitable during tooth preparation (Fig. 15-2).

When healthy, each tubule contains the cytoplasmic process of a cell body (the odontoblast), whose nucleus is in the pulp cavity. Unless the environment around the exposed dentin is carefully controlled, adverse pulp effects can be expected.[1] In addition, the pulp health of a tooth requiring a cast restoration is likely to be compromised before and after preparation (Table 15-1). In severe situations, leakage can cause irreversible pulpitis and the resulting need for root canal treatment.[2]

Periodontal Health. To facilitate plaque removal, a provisional restoration must have good marginal fit, proper contour, and a smooth surface.

This is particularly important when the crown margin will be placed apical to the free gingival margin.[3] If the provisional restoration is inadequate and plaque control is impaired, gingival health will deteriorate.[4]

The maintenance of good gingival health is always desirable, but it has special practical significance when fixed prosthodontics is undertaken. Inflamed or hemorrhagic gingival tissues make subsequent procedures (e.g., impression making and cementation) very difficult. The longer the provisional restoration must serve, the more significant become any deficiencies in its fit and contour (Fig. 15-3). When gingival tissue is impinged upon, ischemia is likely. This can be detected initially as tissue blanching. If it is not corrected, a localized inflammation or necrosis will develop.

Occlusal Compatibility and Tooth Position. The provisional restoration should establish or maintain proper contacts with adjacent and opposing teeth (Fig. 15-4). Inadequate contacts allow supraeruption and horizontal movement.

Supraeruption is detected at try-in when the definitive restoration makes premature contact. Correcting this in the operatory is possible, but the effort is time consuming and often leads to a restoration with poor occlusal form and function. Horizontal movement results in excessive or deficient proximal contacts. The former requires tedious chairside adjustment; the latter involves a laboratory procedure to add metal or ceramic to the deficient site. This often results in a compromised

Factors Contributing to Pulp Death	TABLE 15-1
Past	Present (During Fixed Prosthodontic Therapy)
Caries	Preparation trauma
Operative dentistry	Microbial exposure
Bruxism	Desiccation
Periodontal surgery	Chemical exposure
Prosthodontic therapy	Thermal exposure

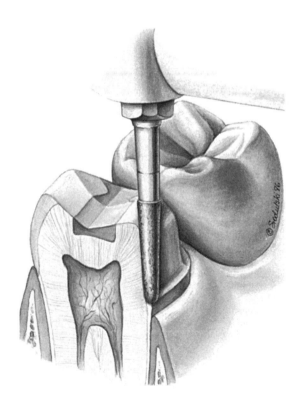

Fig. 15-2. Pulp trauma and exposure of the dentinal tubules from tooth preparation.

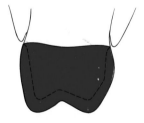 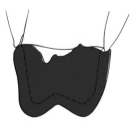

Rough margins around provisionals will jeopardize subsequent procedures.

Fig. 15-3. A provisional restoration should have good marginal fit, proper contour, and a smooth surface finish. **A,** The properly contoured provisional. Smoothly continuous with the external surface of the tooth. **B,** Overcontouring. Irregular transition from the restoration to the root surface and inadequate marginal adaptation. These factors contribute to plaque accumulation and an unhealthy periodontium.

If a provisional does not ensure positional stability, tooth movement can occur, and additional treatment will be necessary.

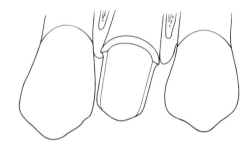

Fig. 15-4. Proper occlusal and proximal contacts promote patient comfort and maintain tooth position.

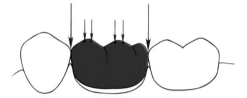

Fig. 15-5. A missing proximal contact allows tooth migration. The resulting root proximity may require surgical or orthodontic correction for impression making (see Fig. 6-26).

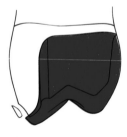

Fig. 15-6. The provisional restoration must protect the tooth. Fracture of a tooth after the impression phase delays treatment and jeopardizes restorability.

proximal contour. This, along with root proximity (Fig. 15-5), impairs oral hygiene measures.

Prevention of Enamel Fracture (Fig. 15-6). The provisional restoration should protect crown preparation margins. This is particularly true with partial-coverage designs in which the margin of the preparation is close to the occlusal surface of the tooth and could be damaged during chewing. Even a small chip of enamel will make the definitive restoration unsatisfactory and necessitate a time-consuming remake.

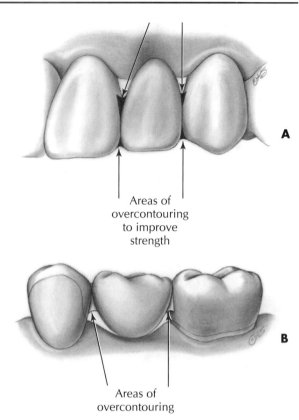

Areas of overcontouring to improve strength

Areas of overcontouring

Fig. 15-7. The connectors of a provisional fixed partial denture are often purposely overcontoured. **A,** In the anterior region, the degree of overcontouring is substantially limited by esthetic requirements. **B,** In the posterior region, esthetics is less restrictive, but overcontouring still must not jeopardize maintenance of periodontal health.

MECHANICAL REQUIREMENTS

Function. The greatest stresses in a provisional restoration are likely to occur during chewing. Unless the patient avoids contacting the prosthesis when eating, internal stresses will be similar to those occurring in the definitive restoration. The strength of **poly (methyl methacrylate)** resin is about one-twentieth that of metal-ceramic alloys,[5] making fracture of the provisional restoration much more likely. Fracture is not usually a problem with a complete crown as long as the tooth has been adequately reduced. Breakage occurs more frequently with partial-coverage restorations and fixed partial dentures. Partial-coverage restorations are inherently weaker because they do not completely encircle the tooth.

An FPD must function as a beam in which substantial occlusal forces are transmitted to the abutments. This creates high stresses in the connectors,[6] which are often the site of failure. To reduce the risk of failure, connector size must be increased in the provisional compared to the definitive restoration (Fig. 15-7). Greater strength is achieved by reducing

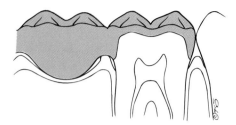

Fig. 15-8. In this mesiodistal section, an overcontoured connector crowds the gingiva. Pressure ischemia and poor access for plaque removal promote gingivitis.

INDICATIONS FOR HIGH-STRENGTH PROVISIONAL RESTORATIONS BOX 15-1
- A long-span posterior FPD
- Prolonged treatment time
- Patient unable to avoid excessive forces on the prosthesis
- Above-average masticatory muscle strength
- History of frequent breakage

---

the depth and sharpness of the embrasures. This increases the cross-sectional area of the connector while reducing the stress concentration associated with sharp internal line angles. The biologic and sometimes the esthetic requirements place limits on just how much larger connectors can be made. To avoid jeopardizing periodontal health, they should not be overcontoured near the gingiva (Fig. 15-8). Good access for plaque control must have high priority.

In some instances high-strength provisionals (e.g., cast metal, fiber reinforced or heat-processed resin) can spare the practitioner and the patient inconvenience, lost time, and the expense of remaking a restoration (Box 15-1).

Displacement. To avoid irritation to the pulp and tooth movement, a displaced provisional must be recemented promptly. An additional office visit is usually required, resulting in considerable inconvenience to the patient and the dentist. Displacement is best prevented through proper tooth preparation and a provisional with a closely adapted internal surface. Excessive space between the restoration and the tooth places greater demands on the luting agent, which has lower strength than regular cement and thus cannot tolerate the added force. For this and for biologic reasons, unlined **preformed crowns** should be avoided.

Removal for Reuse. Provisional restorations often need to be reused and therefore should not be damaged when removed from the teeth. In most in-

stances, if the cement is sufficiently weak and the provisional has been well fabricated, it will not break when removed.

ESTHETIC REQUIREMENTS

The appearance of a provisional restoration is particularly important for incisors, canines, and sometimes premolars. Although it may not be possible to duplicate exactly the appearance of an unrestored natural tooth, tooth contour, color, translucency, and texture are essential attributes. When conditions require it, esthetic enhancement procedures are available to create personalized details; however, because these are not routinely called for, they are addressed on p. 413, following the discussion of cementation and repair.

The degree to which a material matches the color of adjacent teeth initially is an essential requirement of prosthodontics. However, color stability can govern the selection of materials when a long period of service is anticipated, because some resins discolor after several months in the mouth.[7] The propensity for discoloration due to stain accumulation[8] or secondary to home bleaching procedures[9] differs according to resin composition (see Table 15-3, *F*).

The provisional is often used as a guide to achieving optimum esthetics in the definitive restoration. In complete denture prosthodontics, it is customary to have a wax try-in so the patient can respond to the dentist's esthetic interpretation before the denture is processed. Many dentists consider this essential because of the frequency of patient requests for changes and the ease with which such changes can be made. When fixed prosthodontics is being performed in the anterior oral cavity, it greatly influences appearance; the patient should be given an opportunity to voice an opinion. Beauty and personal appearance are highly subjective and difficult to communicate verbally, and a facsimile prosthesis can play a vital role in the patient's consideration of esthetics and the impact that the prosthesis will have on self-image. Obtaining the opinions of others whose judgment is valued is also important. An accurate provisional is a practical way of obtaining specific feedback for the design of a definitive restoration. Verbal descriptions are often too vague and frequently cause overcorrections, which are difficult to reverse in the definitive restoration. The provisional is shaped and modified until its appearance is mutually acceptable to the dentist and the patient. When this is achieved, an impression is made of the provisional (Fig. 15-9) and a cast is poured. This cast accompanies the fixed prosthodontic working cast to the laboratory, where the contours are duplicated. This process is

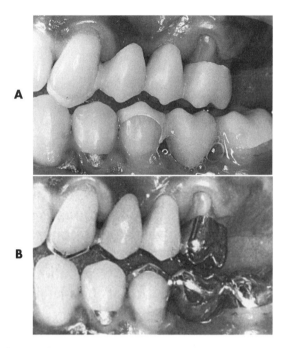

Fig. 15-9. **A,** This provisional FPD established anterior guidance and pontic form before work on the definitive restoration was begun. (Note the facial cavosurface margin of the mandibular second premolar covered by the provisional to protect it from damage.) **B,** The definitive restoration closely matches its predecessor in form and function.

more efficient when it begins with diagnostic waxing procedures. Involving the patient in decision-making results in greater patient satisfaction.

▣ MATERIALS AND PROCEDURES

Many procedures using a wide variety of materials are available to make satisfactory provisional restorations (Fig. 15-10). As new materials are introduced, associated techniques are reported, creating even more variety. Particularly helpful is the fact that all the procedures have in common the formation of a mold cavity into which a plastic material is poured or packed. Furthermore, the mold cavity is created by two correlated parts: one forms the external contour of the crown or fixed partial denture, and the other forms the prepared tooth surfaces and (when present) the edentulous ridge contact area. The terms *external surface form (ESF)* and *tissue surface form (TSF)* are suggested for these mold parts. This terminology will be used in the ensuing discussions.

EXTERNAL SURFACE FORM

There are two general categories of external surface forms: custom and preformed.

Custom. A custom ESF is a negative reproduction of either the patient's teeth before preparation or a modified diagnostic cast. It may be obtained directly with any impression material. Impressions made in a quadrant tray with irreversible hydrocolloid or silicone rubber are convenient. The higher cost of silicone rubber may be offset by its ability to be retained for possible reuse at any future appointment. Accurate reseating of the ESF is easier, and the mold cavity produces better results if thin areas of impression material (as may be found interproximally or around the gingival margin) are trimmed away (Fig. 15-11). Moldable putty materials are popular because they can be used without a tray and can be easily trimmed to minimum size with a sharp knife. In addition, their flexibility facilitates subsequent removal of the polymerized resin (Fig. 15-12).

A custom ESF can be produced from thermoplastic sheets, which are heated and adapted to a stone cast with vacuum or air pressure while the material is still pliable (Fig. 15-13). This produces a transparent form with thin walls, which makes it advantageous in the direct technique because of its minimum interference with the occlusion. It is filled with resin, placed in the mouth, and fully seated as the patient closes into maximum intercuspation. Little additional effort is required to adjust the occlusal contacts. The thinness of the material may also be a disadvantage in the direct technique, however. The material is a poor dissipater of the heat released during resin polymerization,[10] so care must be taken to remove it from the mouth before injury can occur. A thermoplastic ESF has other uses in fixed prosthodontic treatment, in both the clinical and the laboratory phase; for example, it can help evaluate the adequacy of tooth reduction[11,12] (Fig. 15-14).

Transparent sheets are available in cellulose acetate or polypropylene and come in various sizes and thicknesses; a 125 × 125 mm sheet of 0.5 mm thickness is recommended for provisional restorations. Polypropylene is preferred because it produces better surface detail and is more tear resistant. Better tear resistance makes initial removal from the forming cast less tedious and enables the ESF to be used more than once.

Although thermoplastic sheets have a number of advantages, a wide variety of other materials and methods can be used successfully. For example, some practitioners favor baseplate wax because it is convenient and economical (see Fig. 15-10, *B*).

Preformed. A variety of preformed "crowns" is available commercially. On their own, they rarely sat-

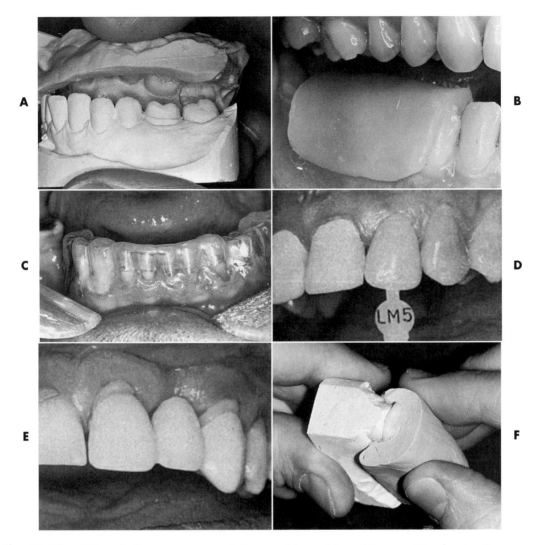

Fig. 15-10. Although there are many variations, molds used in making provisional restorations consist of an external surface form (ESF) and a tissue surface form (TSF). Direct techniques use the patient's mouth directly as the TSF. **A,** Indirect technique: ESF, An alginate impression; TSF, a quick-set plaster cast. **B,** Direct technique: ESF, A baseplate wax impression; TSF, the patient. **C,** Direct technique: ESF, A vacuum-formed acetate sheet; TSF, the patient. **D,** Direct technique: ESF, A polycarbonate preformed shell; TSF, the patient. **E,** Indirect-direct technique: ESF, A custom preformed three-unit FPD shell (nos. 9 to 11) made indirectly; TSF, the patient. **F,** Indirect technique: ESF, A silicone putty impression; TSF, a quick-set plaster cast.

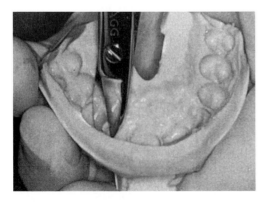

Fig. 15-11. Shortening proximal projections of the impression material facilitates complete reseating of the ESF. Note that excess impression material palatally and facially has been trimmed away with a sharp knife for this reason. The anterior sextant tray shown was selected because it adequately captures the teeth adjacent to the proposed provisional restoration.

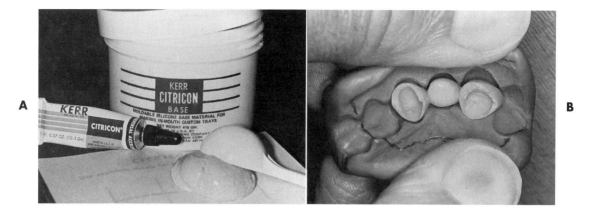

Fig. 15-12. **A,** One of the flexible silicone putties suitable for making external surface forms. **B,** The putty form has been spread apart. Note the completed resin provisional in place, to demonstrate the degree of putty flexibility.

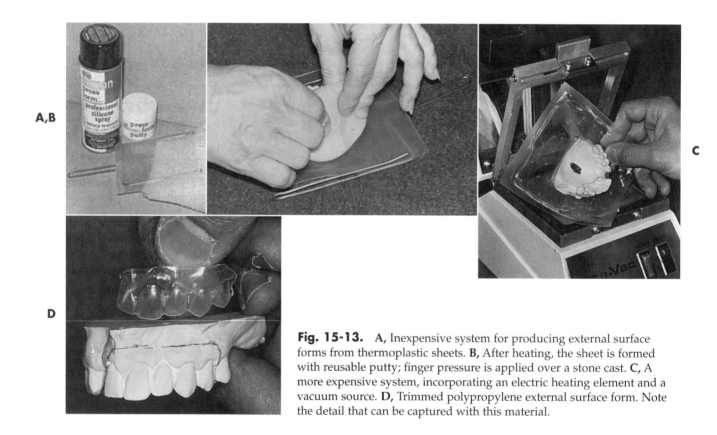

Fig. 15-13. **A,** Inexpensive system for producing external surface forms from thermoplastic sheets. **B,** After heating, the sheet is formed with reusable putty; finger pressure is applied over a stone cast. **C,** A more expensive system, incorporating an electric heating element and a vacuum source. **D,** Trimmed polypropylene external surface form. Note the detail that can be captured with this material.

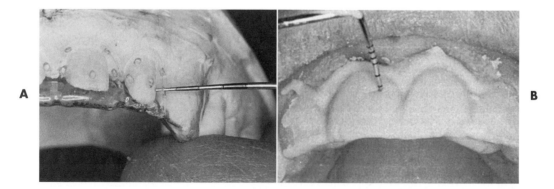

Fig. 15-14. **A,** The thinness and transparency of these ESFs allow their use directly as tooth-reduction guides both in and out of the mouth. **B,** Tooth reduction may be assessed by using the ESF to mold alginate over the prepared tooth. When the alginate is set, the ESF is removed, and a periodontal probe is pushed through the alginate for measurements at desired locations.

isfy the requirements of a provisional restoration, but they can be thought of as ESFs rather than as finished restorations and therefore must be lined with **autopolymerizing resin.** Most crown forms need some modification (e.g., internal relief, axial recontouring, occlusal adjustment) in addition to the lining procedure (Fig. 15-15). When extensive modification is required, a custom ESF is superior because it is less time consuming. Preformed crowns are generally limited to single restorations, since using them as pontics for fixed partial dentures is not feasible.

Materials from which preformed ESFs are made (Fig. 15-16) include polycarbonate, cellulose acetate, aluminum, tin-silver, and nickel-chromium. These are available in a variety of tooth types and sizes (Table 15-2).

Polycarbonate. Polycarbonate (Fig. 15-17) has the most natural appearance of all the preformed materials. When properly selected and modified, its appearance rivals a well-executed porcelain restoration and is a very color-stable resin. Although it is available in only one shade, this can be modified to a limited extent by the shade of the lining resin. Polycarbonate ESFs are supplied in incisor, canine, and premolar tooth types.

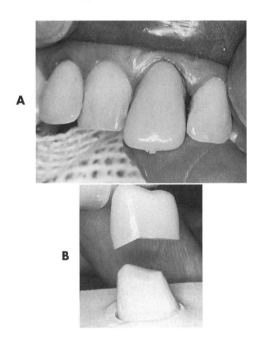

Fig. 15-15. **A,** The time required to modify this particular preformed crown outweighs the advantages it might provide. If a custom external surface form were available, it would be more efficient and more economical. **B,** The excessively tapered internal lingual wall of this preformed crown requires grinding to accommodate a properly prepared tooth. (The stone cast in the lower portion of the illustration duplicates the internal surface of the preformed crown.)

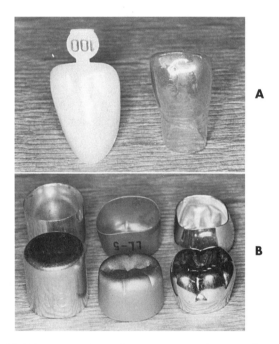

Fig. 15-16. **A,** Preformed anterior crown forms: polycarbonate *(left)* and cellulose acetate *(right)*. **B,** Preformed posterior crown forms: aluminum shell *(left)*, aluminum anatomic *(center)*, and tin-silver anatomic *(right)*.

Preformed Crowns					Sizes in Each Mold	TABLE **15-2** Approximate Cost
	Area of Use*					
	I	C	P	M		($/unit)
RESIN						
Cellulose acetate	X	X	X	X	5	0.95
Polycarbonate	X	X	X		6	0.85
METAL						
Aluminum			X	X	20	0.05
Aluminum (anatomic)			X	X	6	1.50
Tin-silver (anatomic)			X	X	10	1.50
Nickel-chromium (anatomic)	X†	X†	X	X	6	2.50

*Incisor, canine, premolar, molar.
†Primary teeth

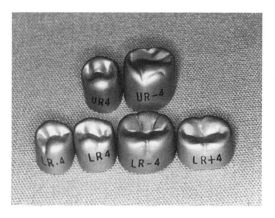

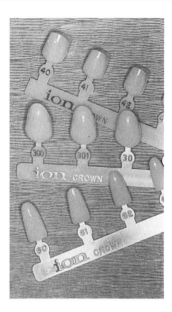

Fig. 15-17. Polycarbonate crowns. Available in maxillary and mandibular incisor, canine, and premolar shapes.

Fig. 15-18. Aluminum anatomic crowns. Available in a variety of sizes and shapes. The manufacturer has produced two maxillary and four mandibular shapes for the left and right side of the mouth, each in six sizes.

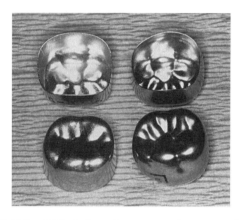

Fig. 15-19. Nickel-chromium anatomic crowns. Available also in an array of sizes and shapes, including ones for the primary teeth, with straight and contoured axial surfaces.

Cellulose Acetate. Cellulose acetate is a thin (0.2 to 0.3 mm) transparent material available in all tooth types and a range of sizes (see Fig. 15-16, *A*). Shades are entirely dependent on the autopolymerizing resin. The resin does not chemically or mechanically bond to the inside surface of the shell, so after polymerization the shell is peeled off and discarded to prevent staining at the interface. However, removing the shell requires the addition of resin to reestablish proximal contacts.

Aluminum and Tin-silver (Fig. 15-18). Aluminum and tin-silver are suitable for posterior teeth. The most elaborate crown forms have anatomically shaped occlusal and axial surfaces. The most basic and least expensive forms are merely cylindrical shells resembling a tin can (see Fig. 15-16, *B*).

Nonanatomic cylindrical shells are inexpensive but require modification to achieve acceptable occlusal and axial surfaces. Using crowns that have been preformed as individual maxillary and mandibular posterior teeth is more efficient. Care must also be taken to avoid fracturing the delicate cavosurface margin of the tooth preparation when fitting a metal crown form. This risk is greater if adaptation is carried out directly by having the patient forcefully occlude on the crown shell. The edge of the shell can engage the margin and fracture it under biting pressure. An even greater risk occurs when the crown has a constricted cervical contour. Tin-silver crowns are deliberately designed this way (see Fig. 15-16, *B*). This highly ductile alloy allows the crown cervix to be stretched to fit the tooth closely. Direct stretching on the tooth is practical only where featheredge margins are used. For other margin designs, cervical enlargement should be performed indirectly on a swaging block, which are supplied with the crown kit.

Nickel-chromium (Fig. 15-19). Nickel-chromium shells are used primarily for children with extensively damaged primary teeth. In that application they are not lined with resin but are trimmed, adapted with contouring pliers, and luted with a high-strength cement. They may be applied to secondary teeth but are more suitable for primary teeth. Nickel-chromium alloy is very hard and therefore can be used for longer-term provisional restorations.

TISSUE SURFACE FORM

There are two primary categories of tissue surface forms: indirect and direct. A third category, indirect-

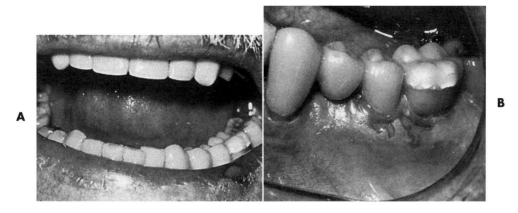

Fig. 15-20. Labial **(A)** and gingival **(B)** ulcerations subsequent to brief poly(methyl methacrylate) monomer exposure.

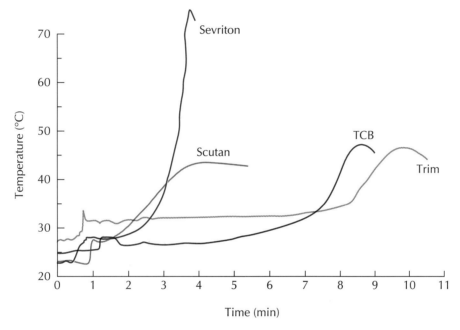

Fig. 15-21. Heat generated during resin polymerization. Under nonclinical experimental conditions, the temperature increases are severe. Sevriton, a poly(methyl methacrylate) resin, produced significantly higher temperatures than the others represented. This is useful information when selecting intraoral resins. However, under clinical conditions, the differences may be insignificant. *(Redrawn from Braden M et al:* Br Dent J *141:269, 1976.)*

direct, results from the sequential application of these two forms.

Indirect Procedure. An impression is made of the prepared teeth and ridge tissue and is poured in quick-setting gypsum or poly(vinyl siloxane).[13] The provisionals are fabricated outside the mouth. This technique has the following advantages over direct procedures:

1. There is no contact of free monomer with the prepared tooth or gingiva, which might cause tissue damage[14] and an allergic reaction or sensitization.[15-18] One group of investigators[19] reported a 20% incidence of allergic sensitivity in

subjects previously exposed to a monomer patch test. The risk of sensitization in patients who are not allergic to monomer increases with the frequency of exposure. In allergic patients, an exposure to even small amounts of monomer usually causes painful ulceration and stomatitis (Fig. 15-20).

2. The procedure avoids subjecting a prepared tooth to the heat created from polymerizing resin. The **exotherm** charted in Figure 15-21 indicates temperature increases with time for several materials under similar experimental conditions. Clinical simulation experiments[20,21] have shown peak temperature increases of

approximately 10° C in the pulp chambers of prepared teeth upon which direct provisional restorations had been made. That amount of temperature elevation is capable of causing irreversible pulp damage.[22] The simulation experiments also indicate that an increase in temperature depends directly on the type and volume of resin present. Therefore, a directly made restoration with a large pontic is more likely to cause injury than one for a single crown (especially if the tooth is prepared conservatively). These studies also demonstrate that the heat-conducting properties of the ESFs significantly influence the maximum temperature reached. However, it is important to note that peak temperatures were not reached until 7 to 9 minutes had elapsed[21] (Fig. 15-22). For this reason, and also because it must be drawn through the undercuts of adjacent proximal tooth surfaces, the resin should be removed at the rubbery stage of polymerization, which typically occurs 2 to 3 minutes after insertion in the mouth. In Figure 15-22, the temperature increase is negligible at 3 minutes, suggesting that thermal injury is easily avoidable.

3. The marginal fit of provisional restorations that have been polymerized undisturbed on stone casts is significantly better than that of provisionals that have been removed from the mouth before becoming rigid.[23,24] This is because (a) the stone restricts resin shrinkage during polymerization and (b) separating the resin from the tooth causes distortion. Directly made long-span or multi-abutment FPDs are likely to have unacceptable marginal discrepancies caused by shrinkage and distortion.

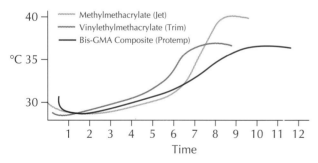

Fig. 15-22. These exotherms (time in minutes) are derived from a simulated clinical procedure for making a single crown using silicone putty as the ESF. A thermocouple probe in the pulp chamber of an extracted tooth was used to measure temperature changes. Initial readings reflect the cooling effect of room-temperature resin mixtures. For all three classes of resins tested, the temperatures did not exceed 35° C until more than 6 minutes had elapsed. *(Redrawn from Tjan AHL et al: J Prosthet Dent 62:622, 1989.)*

4. When a dimensionally stable elastomer impression is made to form the TSF,[13] it can be retained for possible reuse with the ESF. This allows replacement restorations to be made without having the patient present. For example, if a patient calls to report a lost interim FPD, a replacement can be made at the dentist's convenience before the patient arrives. This minimizes disruption of the office schedule and earns the patient's appreciation. It is not known whether using an elastomer TSF results in margins that fit as well as those obtained with a gypsum TSF. The elastomer may not resist polymerization shrinkage as effectively as the gypsum.

5. This technique gives the patient a chance to rest and lets the dentist perform other tasks, provided an assistant is trained to carry out the laboratory procedures.

Direct Procedure. The patient's prepared teeth and gingival tissues (in the case of an FPD) directly provide the tissue surface form, so the intermediate steps of the indirect technique are eliminated. This is convenient when assistant training and office laboratory facilities are inadequate for efficiently producing an indirect restoration. However, the direct technique has significant disadvantages: potential tissue trauma from the polymerizing resin and inherently poorer marginal fit. Therefore, the routine use of directly formed provisional restorations is not recommended when indirect techniques are feasible.

Indirect-direct Procedure. In this technique, the indirect component produces a "custom-made-preformed ESF" similar to a preformed polycarbonate crown. In most cases the practitioner uses a custom ESF with an underprepared diagnostic cast as the TSF. The resulting mold forms a shell that is lined with additional resin after tooth preparation (using the patient for the TSF). This last step is the direct component of the procedure. Another method of creating the shell eliminates the need for an indirect TSF. It is accomplished by painting monomer liquid into the ESF and carefully sprinkling or blowing resin powder on it. The thickness of the resin shell is difficult to control with this technique, however, and may result in time-consuming corrective grinding.

The indirect-direct approach offers these advantages:

1. Chairside time is reduced. Most of the procedures are completed before the patient's visit.
2. Less heat is generated in the mouth. The volume of resin used during lining is comparatively small.

3. Contact between the resin monomer and soft tissues is minimized compared to the direct procedure. Because pontic ridge areas do not normally require lining, there is a reduced risk of allergic reaction.

However, even with the diagnostic cast method, adjustments are frequently needed to seat the shell completely on the prepared tooth. This is the primary disadvantage of the indirect-direct procedure.

PROVISIONAL RESTORATIVE MATERIALS

While in a fluid state, the provisional restorative materials fill the cavity formed by the external and tissue surface forms; they then solidify, producing a rigid restoration.

Ideal Properties.   An ideal provisional material has the following characteristics:
- Convenient handling—adequate working time, easy moldability, rapid setting time
- Biocompatibility—nontoxic, nonallergenic, nonexothermic
- Dimensional stability during solidification
- Ease of contouring and polishing
- Adequate strength and abrasion resistance

- Good appearance—translucent, color controllable, color stable
- Good patient acceptance—nonirritating, odorless
- Ease of adding to or repairing
- Chemical compatibility with provisional luting agents

Currently Available Materials (Fig. 15-23).   The ideal provisional material has not yet been developed. A major problem still to be solved is dimensional change during solidification. These materials shrink during polymerization, which causes marginal discrepancy,[23-25] especially when the direct technique is used (Fig. 15-24). In addition, the resins currently used are exothermic and not entirely biocompatible.

The materials can be divided into four resin groups:

Poly(methyl methacrylate)

Poly(R′ methacrylate)*

---

*The *R′* represents an alkyl group larger than methyl (e.g., ethyl or isobutyl).

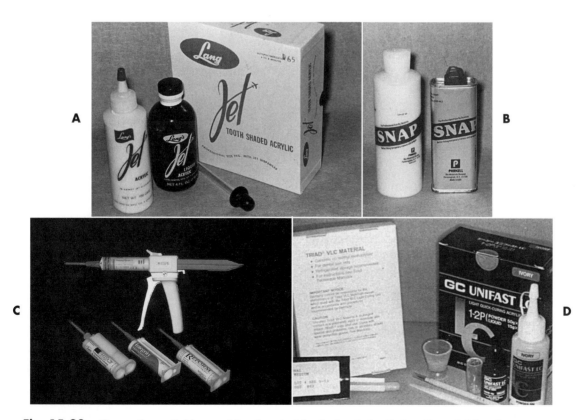

Fig. 15-23.   Currently available provisional materials: **A,** A poly(methyl methacrylate) resin. **B,** A poly(R′ methacrylate) resin. **C,** Microfilled composite resins using an automixing delivery system. **D,** Light-cured resins: a microfilled urethane-dimethacrylate (*left*) and a light-cured poly(ethyl methacrylate).

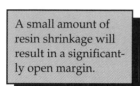

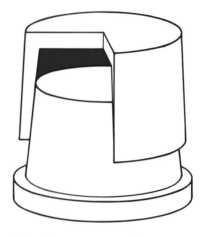

A small amount of resin shrinkage will result in a significantly open margin.

Fig. 15-24. With ideal axial wall convergence, a 2% reduction in crown diameter results in a comparatively high marginal discrepancy.

Ranked Characteristics of Representative Provisional Restoration Resins   TABLE 15-3

Material/Characteristic	A	B	C	D	E	F	G	H	I	J	K	L	M	N
Jet (PMMA)	2*	2‡	3	1‖	1‡	3‡	1†	2	1	1	2#	1	3	1
Duralay (PMMA)	1‡	-	3	-	-	-	1	2	1	1	-	1	3	1
Trim (PR'MA)	2‡	1‡	2	3‖	-	3‡	2‡	3	1	1	3#	1	2	1
Snap (PR'MA)	2‡	2‡	2	-	-	2‡	2	3	1	1	-	1	2	1
Protemp Garant (Bis-GMA comp.)	1*	1	1	2	2	1	2‡	3	2	2	1#	2	1	2
Unifast LC (light-cured, PR'MA)	2*	2§	3	-	-	2¶	2	1	3	1	-	2	3	2
Triad (light-cured, Ureth. DMA comp.)	2†	3‡	1	1	1‡	1‡	3‡	1	3	3	-	3	1	3

1, Most desirable
2, Less desirable
3, Least desirable
A, Marginal adaptation (indirect)
B, Temperature release during reaction
C, Toxicity/allergenicity
D, Strength (fracture toughness)
E, Repair strength (% original)
F, Color stability (UV light)
G, Ease of trimming and contouring
H, Working time
I, Setting time

J, Flowability for mold filling
K, Contaminated by free eugenol
L, Special equipment needed
M, Odor
N, Unit volume cost
*Tjan AHL et al: *J Prosthet Dent* 77:482, 1997.
†Kounijan HJ, Holmes JB: *J Prosthet Dent* 63:639, 1990.
‡Moore BK et al: *Int J Prosthod* 2:173, 1989.
§Castelnouvo J et al: *J Prosthet Dent* 78:441, 1997.
‖Gegauff AG, Pryor HG: *J Prosthet Dent* 58:23, 1987.
¶Doray PG et al: *J Prosthod* 6:183, 1997.
#Gegauff AG, Rosenstiel SF: *Quintessence Int* 18:841, 1987.

Microfilled composite
Light-cured

The properties of these resins are compared in Table 15-3. Overall performances are similar, with no resin being superior in all categories. A material should be chosen according to the specific requirements or conditions of the particular treatment. For example, materials with the least toxicity and least polymerization shrinkage should be chosen for a direct technique. When a long-span prosthesis is being fabricated, high strength is an important selection criterion.

■ MATERIALS SCIENCE

William M. Johnston

The material used for fabrication of a provisional restoration consists of pigments, monomers, filler, and an initiator, which combine to form an esthetic restorative substance. The pigments are incorporated by the manufacturer, so the set material will resemble a natural tooth structure as much as possible, with a variety of shades available. Although the other ingredients have a role in the handling, setting, and final properties of the provisional, the primary monomer determines many of the material's important characteristics. The monomer's ability to convert to a polymer allows the material (after it has been formed as desired) to set into a solid that is durable enough to withstand the oral environment for the necessary interim period.

Depending on the brand, the most commonly used monomers are methyl methacrylate, ethyl methacrylate, isobutyl methacrylate, bis-GMA, and urethane dimethacrylate. Each of these monomers, whether used whole or in combinations, may be converted to a polymer by free-radical polymerization, although the conversion process is never perfectly complete.

FREE-RADICAL POLYMERIZATION

The polymerization process invokes chemical, mechanical, dimensional, and thermal changes that affect the success of these materials in dentistry. Since monomers may be unpleasant or even harmful biologically, the chemical conversion of a monomer to a biologically inert polymer is desirable. Also, if the polymerization process is prematurely terminated or not properly initiated, the resulting restoration may not have adequate mechanical properties and will likely fail. However, because the density of the polymer is inherently and often substantially greater than that of the monomer, a dimensional contraction occurs during polymerization. The polymerization reaction is exothermic, which causes the material to become hot before it loses its fluidity. As a result, an additional contraction occurs when the restoration cools. If a direct technique is being used, the heat of reaction can cause irreversible damage to nearby pulpal tissues, which may already have been thermally insulted during cavity preparation (see p. 389).

Initiation. Free-radical polymerization begins with the formation of a free radical (a process called *activation*) and the subsequent combination of this free radical with a monomer. Free radicals are formed by the decomposition of a chemical (the initiator). The method of decomposition depends on the nature of the initiator. Possible initiators include benzoyl peroxide and camphoroquinone.

Benzoyl peroxide decomposes to free radicals at approximately 50° C or higher in a process called *thermal activation*. Excessive temperatures should be avoided during the early stages of thermal activation, because some monomers vaporize at temperatures near 100° C, with subsequent formation of porosity in the resultant polymer. Thermal activation results in greater contraction on cooling than with other activation methods and is therefore usually avoided for provisional restorations.

Benzoyl peroxide also decomposes to free radicals when catalyzed by a tertiary amine; this process is called *chemical activation*. Chemical activation occurs when the activator, initiator, and monomer are mixed together, so these materials are usually supplied separately—the monomer and activator are in one container, and the initiator and filler are in another. To prevent voids, proper mixing is essential. Since chemical activation requires intimate contact between the chemical activator and the initiator, it is not as efficient as thermal activation. Inefficient activation of the initiator results in more residual monomer and less color stability of the restoration, since unreacted benzoyl peroxide can cause color changes. However, since benzoyl peroxide is decomposed by both thermal and chemical activation, increased temperature can enhance its decomposition in a chemically cured system and will not increase contraction if the restoration initially undergoes chemical setting. Heating a recently set restoration in 100° C water will promote greater polymerization efficiency and remove any unconverted monomer, which might cause a sensitivity reaction in a patient susceptible to monomer irritation.

Camphoroquinone decomposes to free radicals in the presence of both an aliphatic amine and blue light energy; this process is called *visible-light activation*. Light-activated materials have two advantages: (1) the ingredients can be mixed by the manufacturer with little porosity, and (2) working time is virtually unlimited because no setting occurs if the material is kept in a dark environment. A limitation of this method is the depth to which visible light can penetrate (less for darker materials). Whenever possible, the activation illumination should be directed toward the center of the restoration from all surfaces. For darker materials, the exposure time should be longer.

Propagation. When it has begun, the polymerization process continues by including more monomer molecules in the growing molecular chain. The material must not be disturbed, because defects can be easily incorporated if the material is jostled during this phase. During propagation, the following occurs:

1. The setting material undergoes an increase in density, causing contraction.
2. The exothermic heat of reaction may cause a substantial increase in temperature, with subsequent increased contraction.
3. Other physical properties (e.g., rigidity, strength, and resistance to dissolution) increase.

Termination. Due to the randomness of position of the growing chains, some of them may combine and terminate the growth process. This type of termination cannot be avoided, although it is better to have termination only after polymerization of all the monomer has occurred. Termination may also result from the reaction with eugenol, hydroquinone, or oxygen, so contact with these substances must be avoided, or at least minimized, when possible.

PROPERTIES ASSOCIATED WITH THE MONOMER

The various monomers exhibit different initial and setting characteristics and result in polymers with significantly different properties (i.e., viscosity before setting, exothermic heat of reaction, dimensional change on setting, and strength). In general, the exothermic heat of reaction on setting and the physical strength of the set mass is inversely proportional to the size of the monomer molecule. Properties of available materials are presented in Table 15-3.

Filler. Although the primary properties of a provisional restorative material are determined by the monomer(s) involved, a decrease in the less desirable setting and mechanical properties is accomplished mainly with the filler. An increase in filler content reduces the relative amounts of exothermic heat and contraction while increasing the strength of the set material. However, too much filler can lead to insufficient handling characteristics before setting, and this will impede mixing and shaping and will introduce porosity in the set restoration. For light-activated systems, the amount of filler is determined by the manufacturer; for other systems, incorporating as much filler as possible without interfering in the handling or manipulation characteristics of the material is preferred.

• • •

PROCEDURES

To minimize duplication, a basic clinical and laboratory armamentarium are listed here once; they can be referred to throughout the chapter as needed. As each new procedure is discussed, only items necessary to augment the basic armamentarium will be listed.

Clinical Armamentarium (Fig. 15-25)
- Gloves
- Face mask
- Protective eyewear
- Mouth mirror
- Explorer
- Periodontal probe
- Saliva evacuator

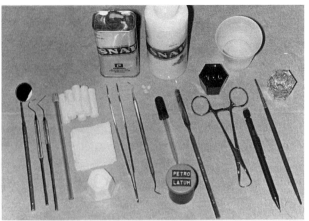

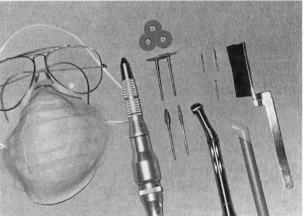

Fig. 15-25. Basic clinical armamentarium.

- Cotton rolls
- Gauze squares
- Gingival displacement cord
- Astringent solution
- Cotton-roll pliers
- Plastic filling instrument
- Cotton pellets
- Petrolatum
- Autopolymerizing resin
- Dropper
- Three dappen dishes
- Cement spatula
- Backhaus towel clamp forceps
- Soft lead pencil
- Straight, slow-speed handpiece
- Carborundum disks with mandrels, SHP
- Fine garnet paper disks (7/8-inch diameter) with mandrels, SHP
- Tungsten carbide burs, SHP
- High-speed handpiece with air-water supply
- Round bur (no. 4), FG
- Tungsten carbide 12-fluted finishing bur, FG (e.g., 7803)
- High-volume evacuation
- Articulating ribbon and holder
- Camel hair brush (no. 0)
- Cup of warm water

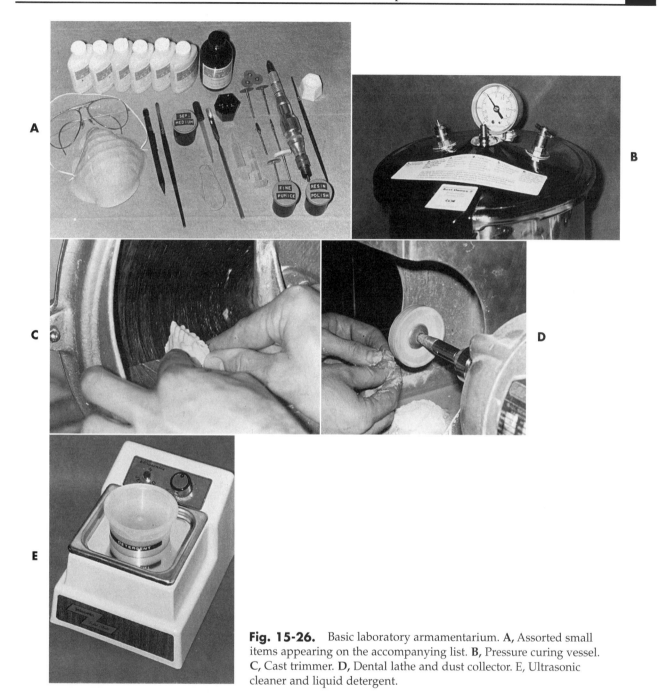

Fig. 15-26. Basic laboratory armamentarium. **A,** Assorted small items appearing on the accompanying list. **B,** Pressure curing vessel. **C,** Cast trimmer. **D,** Dental lathe and dust collector. E, Ultrasonic cleaner and liquid detergent.

Laboratory Armamentarium (Fig. 15-26)
- Protective eyewear
- Face mask (for respiratory protection)
- Soft lead pencil
- Camel hair brushes (nos. 4 and 6)
- Gypsum-resin separating medium
- Autopolymerizing resin
- Dropper
- Two dappen dishes
- Cement spatula
- Polypropylene syringe
- Rubber bands
- Pressure vessel

- Cast trimmer
- Straight, slow-speed handpiece
- Carborundum disks with mandrels, SHP
- Fine garnet paper disks (⅞-inch diameter) with mandrels, SHP
- Tungsten carbide burs, SHP
- Dental lathe
- Muslin wheels
- Robinson bristle brushes
- Felt wheels (1-inch diameter) with mandrels
- Fine pumice
- Resin-polishing compound
- Ultrasonic cleaner with detergent solution

Custom Indirect Provisional Fixed Partial Dentures

The custom indirect procedure is probably the best overall technique for FPDs and should provide the most predictable results with the least risk to patient health.

Additions to Clinical Armamentarium

- Shade guide
- Irreversible hydrocolloid impression material
- Rubber bowl
- Impression tray
- Mixing spatula

Step-by-step Procedure

1. After shade selection and tooth preparation, obtain an impression tray for an irreversible hydrocolloid impression. A sextant impression is adequate only if it extends one tooth beyond the abutments, so the external surface form will index accurately with the cast (TSF).
2. Displace the gingiva if necessary to expose the cavosurface margins (Fig. 15-27).
3. Make an irreversible hydrocolloid impression. Other clinical procedures (e.g., making the definitive impression) can be performed while the assistant is pouring the cast.

Additions to Laboratory Armamentarium

- Accelerated-setting plaster
- Rubber bowl
- Spatula
- Vibrator
- External surface form

Step-by-step Procedure

Plaster setting can be accelerated by shaking dry powder with the water before mixing (1 teaspoon of powder/30 ml).[26] A commercially available quick-setting plaster may also be used.

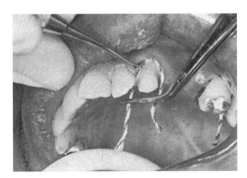

Fig. 15-27. Subgingival margins often require tissue displacement before an adequate impression can be made. Alginate in a disposable tray produces an economical and satisfactory impression. After treatment for infection control, the impression is cast in quick-set plaster to create the TSF.

1. Pour the quick-setting stone or plaster into the irreversible hydrocolloid impression and allow it to set for 8 minutes.
2. Remove the cast and trim it to provide proper indexing with the external surface form. The external surface form is normally made from a diagnostic waxing of the proposed restoration. Make sure the two forms fit together passively and completely.
3. Paint the cast uniformly with separating medium (Fig. 15-28). Avoid leaving unpainted "islands" on the cast, especially at the cavosurface margin areas. Drying can be accelerated by a gentle air stream. Do not forcefully blow the medium from the surface of the cast. When the cast is thoroughly dry, mark the cavosurface margins of the preparations with a soft lead pencil to serve later as a guide for trimming. This is optional and should not be done where the margins are highly visible.
4. Mix autopolymerizing resin (methyl methacrylate is a good choice) and load it into a polypropylene syringe. The orifice of the syringe tip should be about 2 or 3 mm in diameter.
5. Fill the external surface form methodically with the syringe, starting at one end of the restoration space and working to the other.

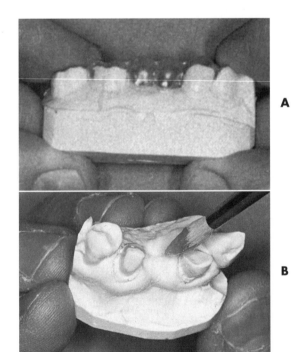

Fig. 15-28. **A,** After trimming, the indirect TSF is mated with the ESF to verify accurate passive indexing. **B,** When this is accomplished, the forms are separated, and the TSF is completely coated with a resin-gypsum separating medium (brushed on).

To avoid trapping air, keep the syringe tip in constant contact with the resin. The mold should not be overfilled; the resin should just reach the level of the gingiva (Fig. 15-29).

6. Seat the tissue surface form into the filled external surface form (Fig. 15-30). They can be lightly held together by rubber bands. The assembly is then placed in warm water (40° C/100° F) in a pressure vessel, and air is applied at about 0.15 MPa (20 psi). Pressure curing will reduce resin porosity.
7. Remove the assembly after 5 minutes.
8. Separate the external surface form from the cured resin restoration, which usually re-

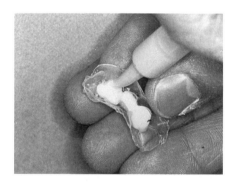

Fig. 15-29. A polymer syringe with a widened orifice (2-mm diameter) is useful for filling the ESF. To avoid entrapping air, it is best to begin at one end and progress slowly to the other, keeping the syringe tip in contact with the expressed resin.

mains in contact with the tissue surface form (Fig. 15-31). The bulk of the stone can be removed on a cast trimmer and with a Carborundum disk (Fig. 15-32). If the margins were marked with lead, dielike remnants of the tissue surface form should be retained as a guide for correct trimming. However, the tissue surface form often separates completely from the resin during handling. This is an advantage, because it eliminates any further effort to remove the stone. Even if the margins were marked, it would probably be better to discard the stone and carefully mark the resin margins with a fine-point graphite pencil. This should not be postponed, because the margins are more difficult to identify accurately after trimming begins.

9. Eliminate resin flash with an acrylic-trimming bur and a fine-grit garnet paper disk.
10. Contour the pontic areas according to proper pontic design procedures (Fig. 15-33). (See Chapter 19.)
11. Finish the restoration with wet pumice. Do not neglect the gingival surface of the pontic. If this area is not accessible, use a Robinson brush on a straight handpiece.
12. Check for and remove any resin blebs or remnants of stone on the internal surfaces of the restoration.

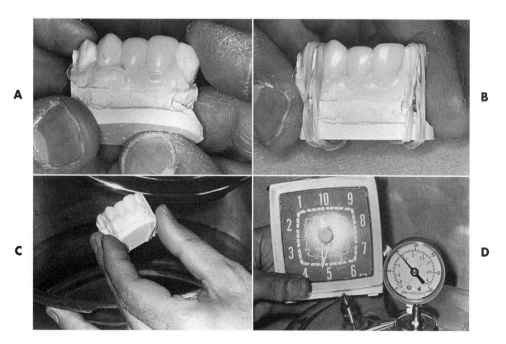

Fig. 15-30. **A,** The resin-filled external surface form placed on the tissue surface form. **B,** Rubber bands around the mold assembly and located over adjacent unprepared teeth. This will avoid distorting the external surface form. **C,** The assembly is placed into a pressure vessel filled with warm water. **D,** The resin cures for 5 minutes under 0.15-MPa (20-psi) pressure.

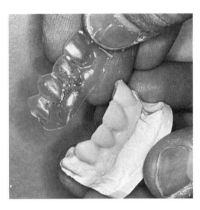

Fig. 15-31. External surface form removed.

13. Using proper infection-control procedures, clean the restoration in preparation for clinical try-in.

Evaluation. The provisional FPD should be evaluated in the patient's mouth for proximal contacts, contour, surface defects, marginal fit, and occlusion. Deficient proximal contacts, imperfections in contour, or surface defects can be corrected by adding resin, using the bead-brush technique (Figs. 15-34 and 15-68).

Unacceptable marginal fit can be corrected in the same manner as custom indirect-direct fixed partial dentures (p. 401, steps 3 to 9), as long as the patient

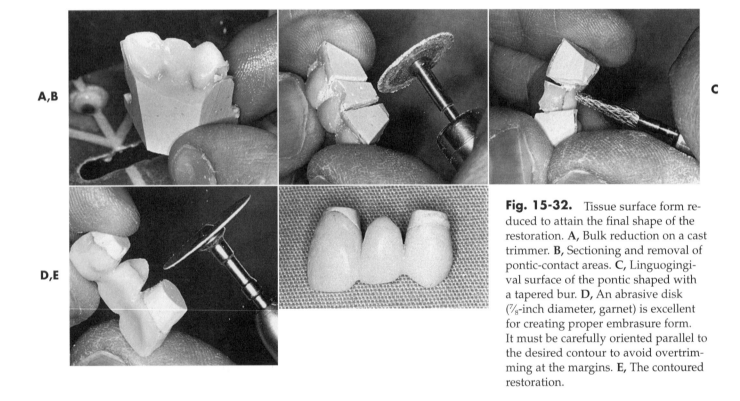

A,B

C

D,E

Fig. 15-32. Tissue surface form reduced to attain the final shape of the restoration. **A,** Bulk reduction on a cast trimmer. **B,** Sectioning and removal of pontic-contact areas. **C,** Linguogingival surface of the pontic shaped with a tapered bur. **D,** An abrasive disk (⅞-inch diameter, garnet) is excellent for creating proper embrasure form. It must be carefully oriented parallel to the desired contour to avoid overtrimming at the margins. **E,** The contoured restoration.

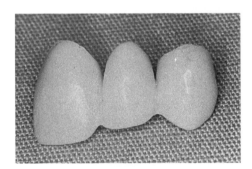

Fig. 15-33. The restoration before try-in.

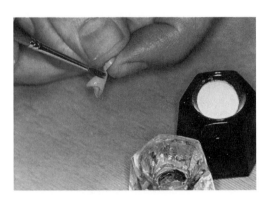

Fig. 15-34. Proximal contact added by the bead-brush technique. When the resin reaches the doughy stage, the restoration is set on the prepared tooth to form the contact.

has no history of a monomer allergy. If occlusal correction is needed, the restoration is marked with articulating ribbon and adjusted with a 12-fluted tungsten carbide finishing bur rotating at high speed. Copious air-water spray is used to prevent the resin from melting (Fig. 15-35). Adequate intraoral evacuation and eye protection are essential.

14. After practicing appropriate infection-control procedures, return to the laboratory for final wet pumice finishing and dry polishing with a resin-polishing compound. If access to the gingival surfaces of the pontics is restricted, a ¾-inch diameter felt wheel can be used for polishing.

CUSTOM INDIRECT-DIRECT PROVISIONAL FIXED PARTIAL DENTURES

The custom indirect-direct procedure may be a good compromise when laboratory support is not immediately available and chair time must be minimized.

Additions to Laboratory Armamentarium
(Fig. 15-36)
- Diagnostic tissue surface form (duplicate of conservatively prepared diagnostic cast)

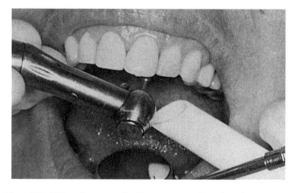

Fig. 15-35. Intraoral adjustment of occlusal contacts.

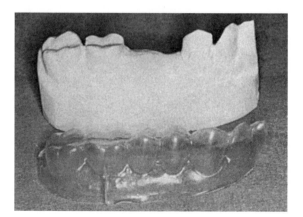

Fig. 15-36. Additions to the basic laboratory armamentarium for the indirect-direct procedure: the diagnostic tissue surface form and the polypropylene external surface form.

- External surface form (vacuum-formed polypropylene sheet)
- Original diagnostically prepared cast mounted on an articulator
- Articulating ribbon

Step-by-step Procedure
1. Prepare the abutment teeth on accurately mounted diagnostic casts (Fig. 15-37). The diagnostic preparation should be more conservative than the eventual tooth preparation and should have supragingival margins. These preparations are often helpful for treatment planning (see Chapter 3).
2. Make an irreversible hydrocolloid impression of the diagnostic preparations to duplicate them in stone (Fig. 15-38).
3. Coat the stone tissue surface form with separating medium.
4. Perform a diagnostic waxing procedure on the articulated casts. This step is also often recommended in the treatment-planning phase. The external surface form is made from the diagnostically waxed cast. If a thermoplastic sheet is used, it should be molded over a stone duplicate of the cast rather than directly on the wax (which will melt if contacted by the heated sheet) (Fig. 15-39).
5. Make sure the external and tissue surface forms fit together accurately (Fig. 15-40).

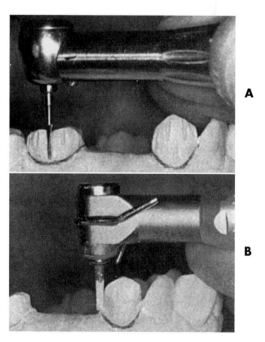

A

B

Fig. 15-37. Preparations involved in making the articulator-mounted diagnostic cast. **A,** Conservative depth-orientation grooves. **B,** Placement of supragingival cavosurface margins.

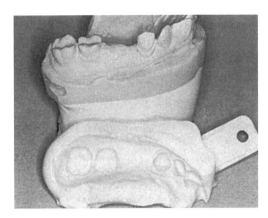

Fig. 15-38. The prepared cast is duplicated with an alginate impression. This creates the indirect tissue surface form. Quick-set plaster is used.

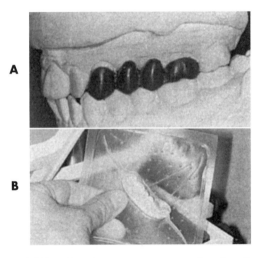

Fig. 15-39. Creating a custom external surface form from a diagnostic waxing. **A,** The diagnostically waxed articulated casts. Patterns should satisfy biologic, mechanical, and esthetic requirements. **B,** If a thermoplastic ESF is desired, the completed waxing must be duplicated in stone.

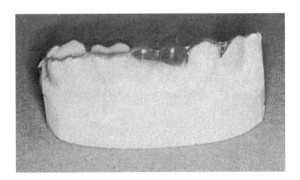

Fig. 15-40. Proper relationship between the ESF and the TSF. If it is necessary to remove any cast artifacts to correct the relationship, this should be done before the separating medium is applied.

6. Syringe the resin into the external surface form and complete the provisional restoration as described in the preceding section (see Figs. 15-29 to 15-33).

7. If the wax has been removed from the diagnostic cast (after duplication), seat the completed provisional (custom-preformed ESF) on it and refine the occlusion with the articulator. If this cannot be done, more time will be required for adjustment.

8. Finish and clean the preformed ESF for try-in, which will follow tooth preparation (Fig. 15-41).

Addition to Clinical Armamentarium
• Custom-preformed ESF

Step-by-step Procedure
1. Prepare the patient's teeth in the usual manner.

2. Try-in the preformed ESF (Fig. 15-42). If it is not compatible with the occlusion (i.e., it does not seat completely) and the teeth have been

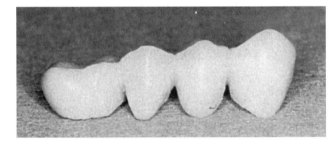

Fig. 15-41. The completed custom-preformed ESF. This is the end product of the indirect component of the indirect-direct technique.

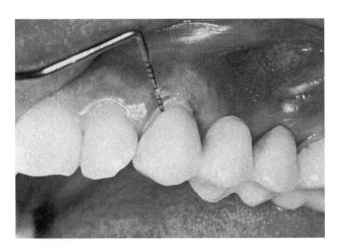

Fig. 15-42. The custom-preformed ESF fully seated over the prepared teeth. Note the marginal discrepancy on each abutment. The tip of the periodontal probe easily fits into the space, which will be filled by a direct lining procedure.

reduced adequately, the internal surface of the ESF should be relieved until the occlusion is acceptable. If necessary, reduce the teeth further; the ESF should then be reevaluated and adjusted. The adjustment process can be tedious, particularly if the preliminary steps were not performed carefully enough. This is the indirect-direct procedure's primary disadvantage. The remaining steps outline the (direct) procedure for lining, which is necessary for internal and marginal adaptation (Fig. 15-43). Because of their relatively low potential for tissue trauma, resins in the poly(-R' methacrylate) group are recommended for direct procedures.

3. Apply a uniform coat of petrolatum on the prepared abutment teeth, gingival tissues, and external surfaces of the ESF.

4. Make a vent hole with a round bur through the occlusal (or lingual) surface of each abutment retainer.

5. Fill the retainers with resin, and after it loses its surface sheen, seat the restoration. The quantity of excess resin expressed around the margin can be controlled by placing fingertips over the vent holes in a manner similar to playing a flute. When a small amount of excess resin appears around the entire periphery of the margin, the fingertip is lifted, allowing trapped air and remaining excess resin to escape. Resin on the occlusal surface can be wiped away immediately, eliminating the need to grind it off after it sets.

6. When the rubbery stage of polymerization is reached (about 2 minutes in the mouth), engage the facial and lingual surfaces of an abutment retainer with the Backhaus forceps and rock the provisional buccolingually to loosen it. Move to the other retainer and rock it in a similar manner. When the FPD is loosened at both ends, remove it from the mouth. The forceps tines make small indentations in the resin, but this is not usually a concern for posterior units. The defects can be smoothed later during the finishing procedures.

7. Place the provisional in warm water (37° C) to hasten polymerization.

8. After 3 to 5 minutes, mark the margins with a sharp pencil and eliminate the excess resin. The bulk can be removed with an **acrylic resin–trimming bur** or Carborundum disk (Fig. 15-44). A fine-grit garnet paper disk completes axial shaping. Accurate trimming to the margins can be simplified by holding the disk parallel to the desired final contour. A paper-thin extension remaining beyond the marked margin indicates that the contour is correct and the cavosurface margin is fully covered. Often this flash can be easily peeled away from the margin with the fingers (Fig. 15-45).

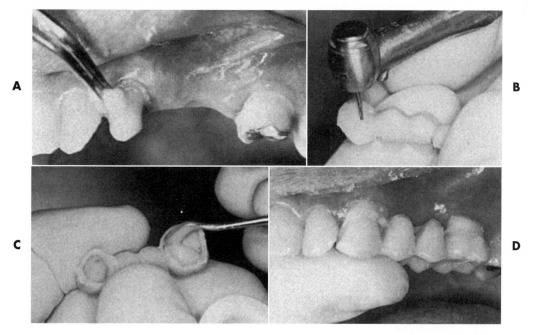

Fig. 15-43. Lining the custom-preformed external surface form. This is the direct component of the indirect-direct technique. **A,** Oral tissues are protected with petrolatum. **B,** Vent holes help to eliminate trapped air. **C,** Abutment retainers filled with lining resin. **D,** The restoration completely seated. (The amount of resin at the margins is controlled by covering or uncovering the vent holes.)

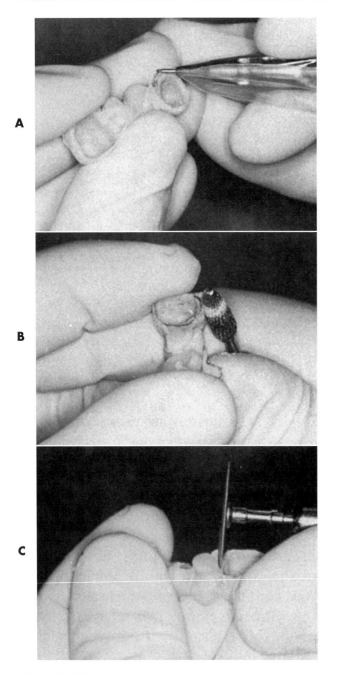

Fig. 15-44. Removal of excess after the lining resin hardens. **A,** Margins are marked with a sharp soft lead pencil. **B,** Gross resin excess is quickly removed. (Margins must be avoided.) **C,** The final axial contours, connectors, and marginal fit are perfected with an abrasive disk rotating toward the margin to prevent debris from obscuring the pencil line. Note the orientation of the disk, parallel to the desired final contour.

9. Confirm the marginal fit and occlusion, refinish and polish where necessary, and cement the restoration (Fig. 15-46).

CUSTOM SINGLE-UNIT PROVISIONAL RESTORATIONS

Complete Crown. Single-unit complete crowns or splinted crowns may be made directly or indi-

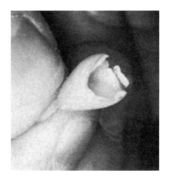

Fig. 15-45. Flash at the margin of a restoration whose axial surface was contoured with proper disk orientation.

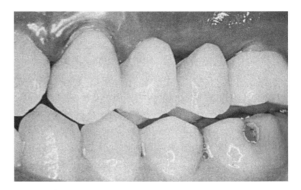

Fig. 15-46. Occlusal contacts of the completed restoration are checked and adjusted before polishing.

rectly by following the basic procedures described for fixed partial dentures. Because pontics are not involved, creating an external surface form is simpler. Diagnostic procedures are not required unless extensive coronal changes are planned. For example, extensive changes are usually required when increasing the vertical dimension of occlusion. If diagnostic procedures are not needed, an alginate impression of the crown or crowns before tooth preparation should be adequate. The impression can serve directly as the ESF or indirectly when a cast has been poured in another impression material.

Onlay and Partial Veneer Crown. The technique for making onlay and partial veneer provisionals is similar to that for custom single crowns. However, the provisionals are more easily distorted during handling because of the conservative tooth preparations that interrupt the continuity of the axial walls. The direct method therefore demands extra care when separating the resin from the tooth. Significantly better results can be expected with the indirect procedure.

Two other points deserve mention. When trimming the polymerized resin to the margin, leaving excess resin at the occlusal cavosurface margin (see

Fig. 15-9) is recommended. This will help prevent fracture of enamel, which is likely to result from the lower strength of resin compared to metal. Second, if lining is needed, an occlusal vent hole is not necessary, because the shape of these restorations provides an adequate escape for trapped air and excess resin.

Inlay. Inlays are small and difficult to handle, especially during trimming. Making interim restorations requires a number of modifications.

Additions to Clinical Armamentarium
- Tofflemire retainer/matrix band
- Wedges
- Amalgam condenser
- Spoon excavator
- Scalpel handle and blade (no. 15)

Step-by-step Procedure
1. For a two- or three-surface inlay, apply the matrix band and wedges in the same manner as condensing a Class II amalgam restoration. The wedges should be placed with firm pressure so that proximal contact is reestablished when the band is removed. The band must seal all aspects of the proximal cavosurface margins.
2. Using petrolatum on a small cotton pellet, lightly coat all sides of the cavity preparation and the matrix band.
3. Make a handle to remove the resin by placing one end of a 2- to 3-cm length of unwaxed dental floss in the preparation cavity.
4. Mix a small amount of poly-R′ methacrylate. When it can be kneaded like bread dough, mold a small cone of it on the end of an amalgam condenser.
5. Lightly condense the resin into the cavity, being careful not to force it past the matrix into an undercut. Immediately remove as much occlusal excess as possible with a sharp spoon excavator.
6. Monitor the polymerization by light probing with a hand instrument. When the resin reaches the late rubbery stage, remove it by tugging the floss handle with cotton roll forceps along the path of withdrawal (Fig. 15-47).
7. Place the resin in a cup of warm water (37° C) for 5 minutes.
8. Mark the margins with a sharp pencil and trim away any flash.
9. Return the cured resin to the cavity preparation and adjust the occlusion using marking film and a slow-speed handpiece. (Take extreme

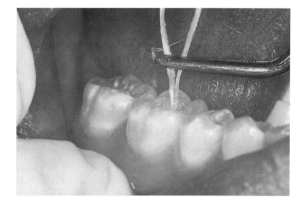

Fig. 15-47. A floss handle facilitates removal of an inlay resin provisional during the late rubbery stage.

care to avoid removing tooth structure if the definitive impression has already been made.) Leave the floss handle in place as long as it does not interfere with occlusal adjustments.

10. Remove the adjusted provisional with the floss handle and put it aside where it may be found easily after impression making for the definitive inlay.
11. Clean and dry the cavity preparation and place a thin coat of provisional cement on the cavity walls. Immediately insert the provisional restoration.
12. When the cement is set, remove the excess with an explorer and a spoon excavator. Carefully cut off the floss handle with the scalpel blade.

Laminate Veneers
Additions to Clinical Armamentarium
- Composite resin shade guide
- Light-cured composite resin
- Hand-held curing light
- Phosphoric acid etchant gel
- Light-cured unfilled resin bonding agent

Step-by-step Procedure
1. Select the most appropriate resin shade or combination of shades before preparing the tooth.
2. When tooth preparation is complete, apply a thin coat of petrolatum to the prepared tooth surface.
3. Using a plastic instrument wetted with alcohol, form the preselected shade of light-cured resin to the desired contour on the lubricated tooth.

NOTE: If the material is difficult to control, placement and curing may be accomplished in stages.

Another option is forming the veneers indirectly by creating a TSF and an ESF, as was recommended for the fixed partial denture provisional restoration. The indirect method may be more efficient if multiple veneers are being made.

4. Light-cure the resin and remove it from the tooth surface.

5. Thoroughly clean the petrolatum from the prepared tooth enamel and internal surface of the veneer if necessary. Apply the etchant gel to three 1-mm diameter areas to form an equilateral triangle (two corners at the mesioincisal and distoincisal line angles and the third centered more cervically). Allow the etchant to remain for 20 seconds, rinse completely with water, and dry.

6. Place a small amount of the unfilled bonding agent on the three etched areas. Immediately place the veneer on the tooth, hold it in place, and light-cure for 10 seconds. Remove any excess bonding agent, then cure for 60 seconds.

7. At the patient's return visit, remove the veneers with a spoon excavator.

MASS-PRODUCED ESF PROVISIONAL CROWNS

Under most circumstances, a custom external surface form will produce the best results in the shortest time. However, there are times when a custom ESF is not available (e.g., a first-visit emergency in which a crown is missing and must be replaced). If by coincidence a crown form closely matches the size and shape of the desired provisional, the mass-produced form is more convenient than initiating custom procedures (generating a diagnostic cast and waxing the missing crown contours). Such coincidences are not routine and should not be relied upon. Regardless of the situation, mass-produced provisional crowns should be thought of as ESFs; they need to be lined with resin to meet the basic requirements of a provisional restoration.

POLYCARBONATE CROWN FORMS

Polycarbonate crown forms are useful for provisional restorations on single anterior teeth and premolars.

Additions to Clinical Armamentarium
- Assorted polycarbonate crowns
- Boley gauge or dividers
- Green stone, SHP

Step-by-step Procedure
1. Measure the mesiodistal width of the crown space with dividers (some crown kits provide a selection guide) and select a shell with the same or slightly larger width (Fig. 15-48).

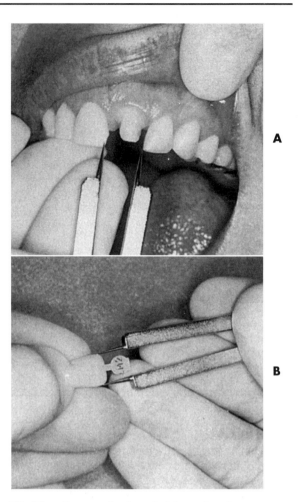

Fig. 15-48. Crown selection. **A,** Measuring the mesiodistal width of the space with dividers. **B,** Appropriate crown size for the measured space.

2. Mark the crown height (from the incisal edge) with a pencil (Fig. 15-49). Use this measurement as a guide to trimming the shell so it matches the approximate curvature of the prepared cavosurface margin. A green stone should be used for this trimming.

3. Try the shell on the prepared tooth (Fig. 15-50), being especially careful that the incisal edge and labial surface of the shell align properly with those of the adjacent teeth. The internal surface of the shell will often need reduction to achieve this match. Since it is usually better to adjust it after lining, the occlusion should be ignored for now. When the shell can be properly positioned without forceful gingival contact, it is ready to be lined with resin.

4. Apply a uniformly thin coat of petrolatum to the prepared teeth and adjacent gingivae (Fig. 15-51). This will prevent direct contact of the monomer with these tissues and will reduce the risk of injury.

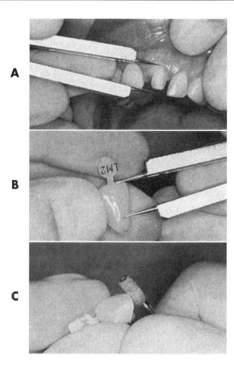

Fig. 15-49. Crown length adjustment. **A,** Incisocervical height required for the completed restoration. **B,** Measurement transferred to the crown. **C,** Cervical portion of the crown adjusted to duplicate the curvature of the cavosurface margin.

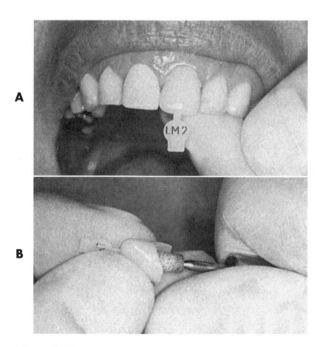

Fig. 15-50. **A,** The cervical portion of the crown is trimmed until the length and axial inclination are correct. **B,** If necessary, internal surfaces are adjusted for proper orientation of the crown.

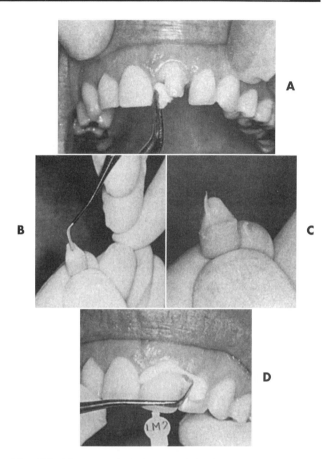

Fig. 15-51. Lining the adjusted shell. **A,** Protection with petrolatum. The shell is filled with resin **(B)** and seated **(C),** when the resin does not slump after a peak is formed with the tip of an explorer. **D,** Excess resin is immediately removed after the crown has been positioned.

5. Mix the autopolymerizing resin and fill the shell (poly[R' methacrylate] is recommended). When the surface just loses its gloss or the resin forms a peak without slumping, place the shell over the tooth and align the incisal and labial surfaces with those of the adjacent teeth.

6. Immediately eliminate any marginal excess. If polymerization is too far advanced, the doughy resin will pull away from the margin and require later repair.

7. When the rubbery stage of polymerization is reached (after about 2 minutes), rock the crown faciolingually to loosen and remove it. The Backhaus forceps should be kept within easy reach in case there is difficulty separating the crown from the tooth. However, because it makes small indentations in the crown surface, the forceps should be used only when needed on anterior units.

8. Place the crown in warm water (37° C) (Fig. 15-52).

9. When the resin has fully set (about 5 minutes), mark the margins with a sharp pencil. The axial surfaces can be shaped, and flash eliminated, with SHP carbide burs or abrasive disks.

A **B** **C**

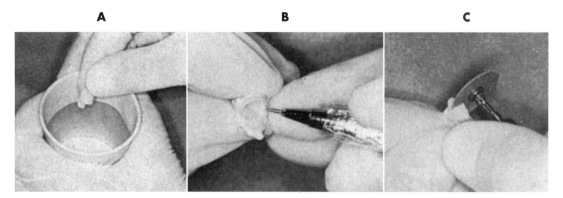

Fig. 15-52. **A,** When the resin has reached the rubbery stage, the crown is removed and placed in warm water (37° C). Hot water must not be used, because it will increase resin shrinkage. However, warm water is not recommended for poly(methyl methacrylate) resin, because excessive shrinkage will make the marginal fit unacceptable. **B,** After about 5 minutes in warm water, the resin should be rigid enough for marking the margins. **C,** Initial removal of the excess lining resin is accomplished with a coarse garnet disk.

A **B** **C**

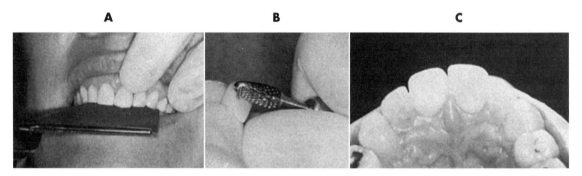

Fig. 15-53. **A,** A considerable amount of lingual reduction may be required. If it is only minor, it can be done intraorally. **B,** To increase efficiency and to facilitate patient comfort, any bulk reduction should be done extraorally. **C,** Finalized lingual contour that promotes gingival health and allows access for oral hygiene. Note the more natural contour of the left central incisor compared to that of the provisional crown on the right central.

A **B** **C**

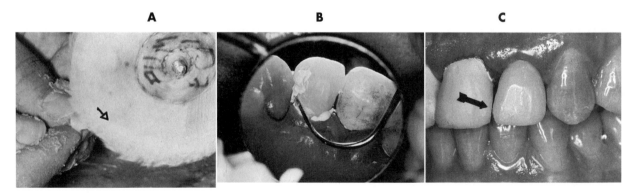

Fig. 15-54. **A,** A rag wheel and pumice are used before polishing with compound. Note the parallel orientation of the wheel to the crown's axial surface at the point of contact *(arrow)*. The crown should be positioned so the wheel rotates from the surface toward the margin. **B,** An explorer and dental floss are used to carefully remove all excess cement. **C,** Overpolishing results in a deficient mesial contact *(arrow)*. The bead-brush technique is recommended for correcting a small inadequacy.

10. Try on the newly lined crown and adjust the lingual surface to the desired occlusion and contour (Fig. 15-53).
11. Polish and cement the restoration (Fig. 15-54).

ALUMINUM CROWN FORMS

Aluminum shells are useful for restoring single posterior teeth, where their unnatural appearance is not a disadvantage.

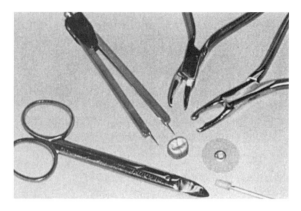

Fig. 15-55. Additions to the basic clinical armamentarium.

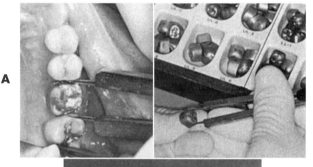

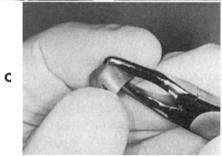

Fig. 15-56. Aluminum crown selection and modification. **A,** Mesiodistal dimension of the space. **B,** Appropriate crown size, nearest this measurement. **C,** Contouring pliers to make small size modifications. This is frequently unnecessary.

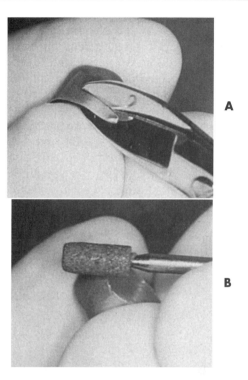

Fig. 15-57. **A,** Cervical portion of the crown trimmed to proper length. **B,** Smoothing the cut edge to prevent gingival injury.

Additions to Clinical Armamentarium
(Fig. 15-55)
* Assorted aluminum crowns
* Dividers
* Crown-and-collar scissors
* Contouring pliers
* Cylindrical green stone, SHP
* Coarse garnet paper disk (⅞-inch diameter)

Step-by-step Procedure
1. Measure the mesiodistal width of the crown space with dividers and select an appropriate shell type with a width as close as possible to that measured. A slightly larger or smaller shell can be deformed with contouring pliers to achieve the proper fit (Fig. 15-56).

2. Measure the occlusocervical height and trim the shell with crown-and-collar scissors so that it extends about 1 mm apical to the cavosurface margin (Fig. 15-57). Sharp burrs left by the scissors should be smoothed or rounded with the green stone.
3. Place the trimmed shell over the prepared tooth and gradually apply seating pressure while observing the gingiva. Trim the margins further wherever the gingiva blanches. The shell margin should not engage the prepared tooth margin.
4. Repeat the try-in and trim as necessary.
5. Instruct the patient to close with moderate force. The soft aluminum should deform until normal intercuspation is reached (Fig. 15-58).
6. Apply petrolatum to the prepared tooth and adjacent gingival tissues; mix poly (R′ methacrylate) resin and fill the shell.
7. When the resin surface becomes matte, place the shell over the tooth and guide it to a slightly supraclusal position. Instruct the patient to close (Fig. 15-59).
8. To avoid pulling the resin away from the cavosurface margin, immediately remove the marginal excess.
9. When the rubbery stage of polymerization is reached (about 2 minutes in the mouth), engage the crown with the Backhaus forceps to

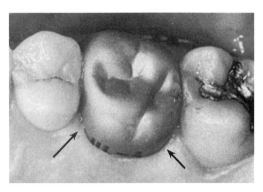

Fig. 15-58. The patient is instructed to bite on the shell after the length has been adjusted. Note the occlusal indentation and gingival blanching *(arrows)*. Additional shortening should be done where the blanching occurs.

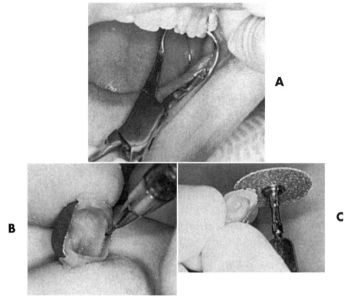

Fig. 15-60. **A,** Backhaus forceps provides definite purchase of the shell for controlled removal. **B,** After 5 minutes in warm water, the margin is marked with a pencil. A coarse garnet disk is recommended for initial contouring of the axial surfaces. This usually requires partially removing the aluminum shell. After the overcontoured aluminum has been ground away, a fine garnet disk is used to finalize the axial contours (including the marginal areas). Again, disk orientation is important to establishing a straight emergence profile and well-adapted margins.

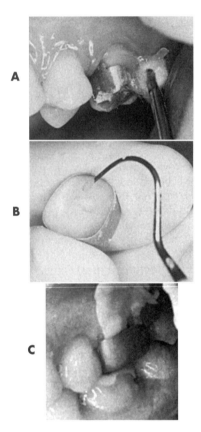

Fig. 15-59. **A,** Protection with petrolatum. **B,** The adjusted shell is filled with lining resin and seated just short of its final position after the resin has lost its sheen. **C,** The final position is determined by the patient's closing into maximum intercuspation. Excess resin is immediately removed.

just penetrate the aluminum shell (Fig. 15-60). Loosen and remove the crown by rocking it buccolingually or by using the thumb and index finger of the other hand to apply occlusally directed force under the tines.

The small buccal and lingual holes created in the surface of the aluminum will not usually be a problem and can be ignored until the patient returns; at that time, they may be used to remove the crown again.

10. Place the shell in a cup of warm water (37° C).
11. After about 5 minutes, mark the margins and trim away any excess. To establish periodontally healthy axial contours, the aluminum shell frequently is ground away in certain areas (Fig. 15-61).
12. Replace the crown and adjust the occlusion as deemed necessary. If either proximal surface lacks contact, resin can be added to correct the deficiency. Metal must be ground away in the contact area to provide a resin-to-resin bond (Fig. 15-62).
13. Polish, clean, and cement the restoration.

POST-AND-CORE PROVISIONAL RESTORATIONS

Intraradicular retention and support are often obtained from a cast metal post-and-core (see Chapter 12). A provisional restoration will be needed while the casting is being made.

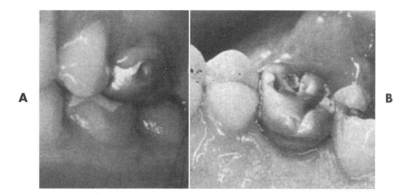

Fig. 15-61. **A,** Proper contouring of the axial walls exposes lining resin in the cervical area. Note the indentations in the shell from the Backhaus forceps. **B,** Final occlusal adjustment will remove the anodized gold finish, but this is of no concern.

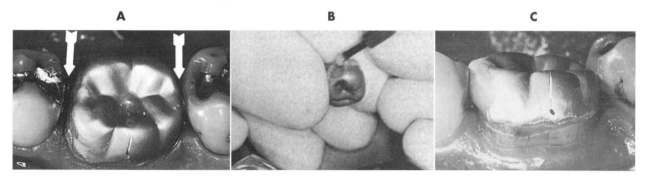

Fig. 15-62. Adding proximal contacts to aluminum crowns. **A,** Contacts are absent in this lined crown *(arrows).* **B,** The metal in the contact area is ground away to expose the underlying resin. The bead-brush technique is then used for correcting the deficiency. **C,** Crown after resin addition to the mesial surface. To improve the gingival embrasure form, further contouring with a disk is recommended.

Additions to Clinical Armamentarium
- Wire
- Wire-cutting pliers
- Cylindrical green stone, SHP
- Wire-bending pliers
- Paper points

Step-by-step Procedure
1. Place a piece of wire (e.g., a straightened paper clip) in the post space. To avoid root fracture, it must extend passively to the end of the post space. If binding occurs, a mounted stone can be used to taper the wire.
2. Mark the wire with a pencil at the mouth of the post space. Then, at a point slightly occlusal to this mark, use the pliers to make a 180-degree bend in the wire (Fig. 15-63).
3. Lubricate the tooth and surrounding soft tissues with petrolatum. Paper points are convenient for lubricating the post space.
4. Fill the ESF with provisional resin (polyR' methacrylate is recommended).

5. When the resin loses its surface gloss, place the wire in the post space and seat the ESF over it (Fig. 15-64).

NOTE: Precautions should be taken to protect the patient from swallowing or aspirating the wire.

6. Remove the ESF while the resin is still rubbery (about 2 to 2½ minutes). The stage of polymerization should be monitored. If the resin is allowed to become rigid and lock into the undercut surfaces within the post preparation, removing it and the wire will be time consuming and will risk the tooth's restorability. Usually the provisional will remain in the ESF, which can be placed in warm water to hasten polymerization. The wire must not be disturbed while the resin is soft. If the provisional remains on the tooth, it should be loosened and reseated several times and then removed before the resin has fully polymerized.
7. Mark the margins with a pencil, and trim and contour the restoration with disks or SHP carbide burs.

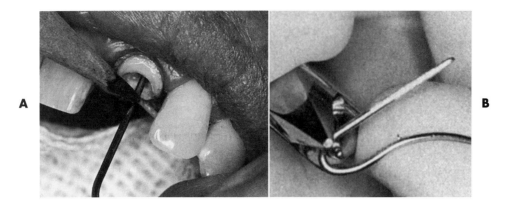

Fig. 15-63. Provisional post preparation. **A,** The wire is marked so that the bend will be made at the correct level. When in position, the wire must not interfere with the external surface form. **B,** A 180-degree or greater bend in the wire to resist displacement in the lining resin.

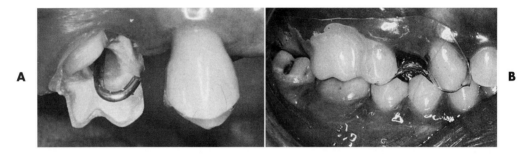

Fig. 15-64. **A,** Wire in the post space just before placement of the filled external surface form. A gauze throat pack is recommended to protect the patient from aspirating or swallowing the wire. **B,** Filled ESF seated.

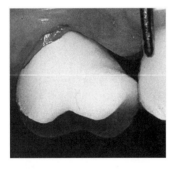

Fig. 15-65. The completed provisional post and crown restoration. Note the unusual mesial contour (which is the result of a mesiobuccal root amputation).

8. Try-in the restoration and adjust as necessary.
9. Polish, clean, and cement the restoration (Fig. 15-65).

CEMENTATION

The primary function of the provisional luting agent is to provide a seal, preventing marginal leakage and pulp irritation. The luting agent should not be relied upon to resist occlusal forces, because it is purposely formulated to have low strength. Unintentional displacement of a provisional restoration is frequently caused by a nonretentive tooth preparation or excessive cement space rather than the choice of luting agent.

Ideal Properties.   Desirable characteristics of a provisional luting agent are as follows:
• Ability to seal against leakage of oral fluid
• Strength consistent with intentional removal
• Low solubility
• Blandness or obtundency
• Chemical compatibility with the provisional polymer
• Convenience of dispensing and mixing
• Ease of eliminating excess
• Adequate working time and short setting time
• Compatibility with the definitive luting agent

Available Materials (Fig. 15-66).   Of the presently available materials, zinc oxide–eugenol cements appear to be the most satisfactory. Zinc phosphate, zinc polycarboxylate, and glass ionomer cements are not recommended because their comparatively high strength makes intentional removal difficult. High-strength cements frequently damage the restoration or even the tooth when removal is at-

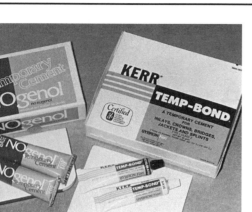

Fig. 15-66. A noneugenol and a eugenol provisional luting agent.

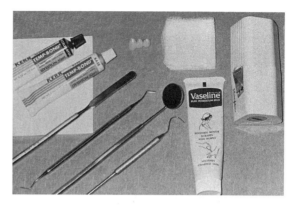

Fig. 15-67. Provisional restoration luting armamentarium.

tempted. Weaker ZOE cements allow easy removal, which enables reuse of the restoration. In addition to its acceptable sealing properties, ZOE also has an obtundent effect on the pulp.[27] Unfortunately, *free* eugenol acts as a plasticizer of methacrylate resins. It has been shown to reduce surface hardness[28] and presumably strength. New resin applied over polymerized resin previously in contact with free eugenol results in softening[29] of the added resin, making linings or repairs unsuccessful. The R' methacrylates are severely affected by free eugenol. Methyl methacrylates are affected moderately, and the composites are only slightly softened. These adverse effects have prompted the marketing of provisional luting agents without eugenol. However, several studies have shown that the mere presence of eugenol in a cement is not enough to cause adverse effects. Unreacted or free eugenol must also be present to cause problems. Therefore, when using products that contain eugenol, one must be sure that the correct proportions are blended. It is still unclear whether free eugenol is necessary to elicit pulpal desensitization.

Temporary cements that contain eugenol are also a concern when resin luting agents will be used to cement the definitive restoration. One study demonstrated that both residual ZOE- and noneugenol-containing temporary cements reduced the tensile bond strength of resin luting agents.[30] In practice, all traces of temporary cement should be thoroughly removed to maximize adhesion. Air abrasion with aluminum oxide will effectively remove residual ZOE cement residue, but alcohol and organic solvents will not.[31] Similarly, cleansing with pumice will leave a ZOE residue mixed with pumice, which can inhibit bonding.[32] Etching with 37% phosphoric acid after cleaning with pumice may be an alternative means of ZOE removal when

a resin luting agent is planned.[33] The retention of cast crowns cemented with zinc phosphate cement or resin-modified glass ionomer or composite resin cores exposed to ZOE does not appear to be affected.

In situations when the tooth preparation lacks retention, when a span is great or long-term use is anticipated, or when parafunction exists, using a higher-strength cement may be desirable. A good compromise would be reinforced zinc oxide-eugenol; another might be eugenol-free zinc oxide, which has slightly greater strength than cements containing eugenol.[34] Conversely, sometimes minimum strength is desired, as with temporary placement of the definitive restoration. (Its removal may be needed to refire the porcelain.) Petrolatum can be mixed with equal parts of the provisional cement base and catalyst to reduce the cement's strength by more than half.

Armamentarium (Fig. 15-67)
- Provisional luting agent
- Mixing pad
- Cement spatula
- Plastic filling instrument
- Petrolatum
- Mirror and explorer
- Dental floss

Step-by-step Procedure (Fig. 15-68)
Most provisional luting agents are supplied as a two-part system.
1. To facilitate removal of excess cement, lubricate the polished external surfaces of the restoration with petrolatum (see Fig. 15-68, *A*).
2. Mix the two pastes together rapidly and apply a small quantity just occlusal to the cavosurface margin (see Fig. 15-68, *B*). A marginal

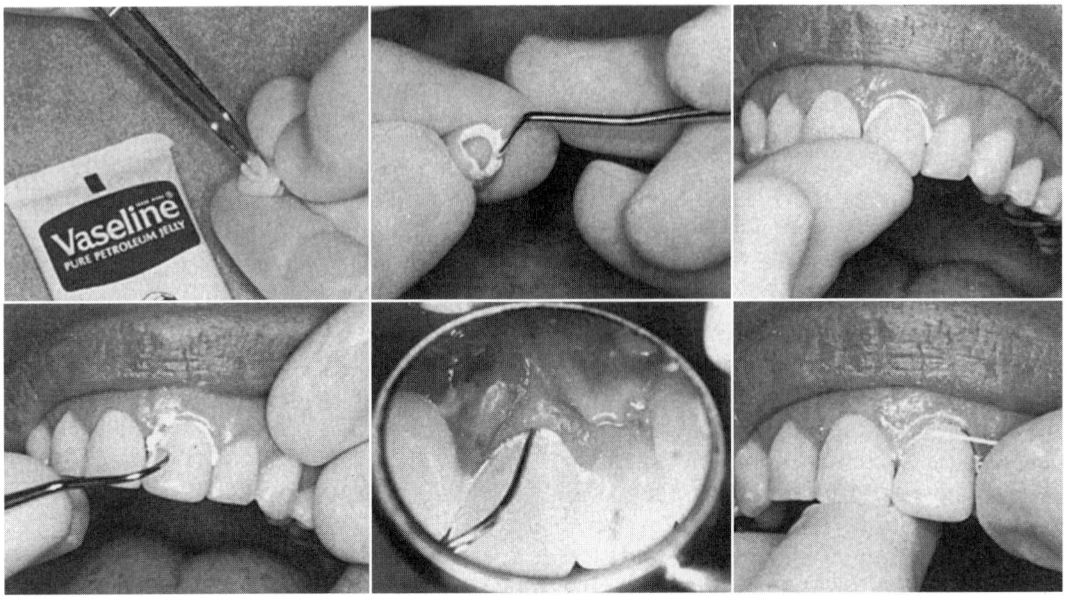

Fig. 15-68. Luting procedure. **A,** The external surface is lightly coated with petrolatum to aid removal of the set cement. **B,** Careful placement of the cement will seal the margins and reduce the cleanup effort. **C,** The restoration is seated with firm finger pressure, or (for posterior restorations) the patient may occlude on a cotton roll. **D** and **E,** An explorer is used to remove excess and to probe the sulcus gently for remnants. **F,** The proximal contact areas and sulcus are cleaned with dental floss, followed by copious irrigation with the air-water syringe.

bead of cement forms the required seal against oral fluids. Filling the crown or abutment retainers should be avoided, because it prolongs cleanup and increases the risk of leaving debris in the sulcus.

3. Seat the restoration and allow the cement to set (see Fig. 15-68, *C*).
4. Carefully remove excess with an explorer and dental floss (see Fig. 15-68, *D* to *F*).

NOTE: Cement remnants left in the sulcus irritate the gingiva and may cause severe periodontal inflammation with possible bone loss. Therefore, the sulcus must be carefully checked and irrigated with the air-water syringe.

Removal, Recementation, and Repair

The provisional restoration is removed when the patient returns for placement of the definitive restoration or for continued preparation. Fracture of the prepared tooth or foundation must be avoided. This risk can be minimized if removal forces are directed parallel to the long axis of the preparation. The Backhaus or a hemostatic forceps is effective for obtaining sound purchase on a single unit (Fig. 15-69). A slight buccolingual rocking motion will help break the cement seal.

Damage can occur when a fixed partial denture is being removed. If one abutment retainer suddenly breaks loose, the other can be subjected to severe

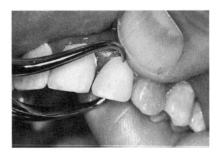

Fig. 15-69. Backhaus towel clamp forceps provide positive purchase on provisional restorations. For maximum control, occlusal finger pressure is applied directly to the tines.

flexure stresses when the FPD acts as a lever arm. Care must be exercised to remove the prosthesis along the path of withdrawal. Looping dental floss under the connector at each end of the FPD is sometimes helpful.

Armamentarium

- Backhaus towel clamp or hemostatic forceps
- Spoon excavator
- Ultrasonic cleaner with cement-remover solution

Step-by-step Procedure

1. If the provisional restoration is going to be recemented, clean out the bulk of the cement with a spoon excavator.

A   **B**   **C**

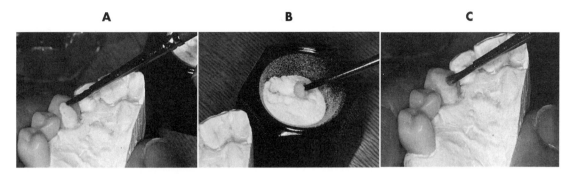

Fig. 15-70. Bead-brush technique for repairs. **A,** Monomer liquid is painted on the surface of the thoroughly cleaned restoration to which resin will be added. The brush is dipped in monomer and briefly touched to the powder, forming a small bead on the tip. **C,** The bead is touched to the repair site, and the brush handle is rolled to deposit it. Bead placement continues in this manner until the desired contour is achieved. To prevent excessive porosity, the unset resin should be painted lightly with monomer until it is hard.

2. Place the provisional in a cement-dissolving solution and set this in the ultrasonic cleaner.
3. Line the provisional with a fresh mix of resin if necessary (e.g., if the tooth preparation has been modified). The internal surface is relieved slightly and painted with monomer to ensure good bonding of the new lining.

A fractured or damaged provisional can be easily repaired with resin added directly by using the bead-brush technique (Fig. 15-70).

ESTHETIC ENHANCEMENT

Contour, color, translucency, and texture are the key elements of coronal appearance. Contour and color are fundamental and more important than the other two elements. The indirect FPD procedure just described includes methods for controlling contour and color. Diagnostic waxing provides the ultimate control of contour. Using a shade guide before tooth preparation gives the operator some control of color. If contour and color are well controlled, most provisional restorations will have a very acceptable, and even excellent, appearance. However, skill and attention to detail are required if this to be routinely achieved. Although it is listed third, translucency can be a significant appearance element for patients with unabraded teeth. Texture, the least important element of appearance, usually can be controlled easily.

Color. Although some resin manufacturers use only general color descriptions (e.g., light, medium, dark) for their products, most cross-reference their colors to popular shade guides for porcelain or denture teeth. However, even when cross-referenced, manufacturer and material differences make shade matching inaccurate. More effective control of color

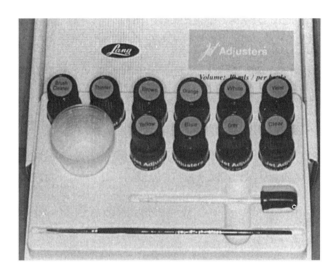

Fig. 15-71. This provisional stain kit contains violet, blue, yellow, orange, brown, white, and gray paint-on colorants to create custom effects and a clear material used to form a glazed, translucent surface. The liquids are designed to dry quickly, which requires that they be kept covered until immediately before use. A thinner and brush cleaner are provided.

can be accomplished with a custom shade guide. This can be easily made by casting the resins into an elastomeric putty mold of an extracted incisor crown. A wider selection of shades can be created by combining two or more existing hues in known proportions. Resin coloring tints are also an option.

Custom color effects that simulate intrinsic and extrinsic stains, cracks, or hypocalcification of adjacent teeth may be added to provisional restorations with paint-on stain kits (Fig. 15-71). These should be applied quickly, avoiding overmanipulation, which causes streaking and surface roughness. Under ideal conditions, the surface should have a glazed appearance similar to porcelain. Thickening of stains as a result of the evaporation of solvent is a common problem that hampers manipulation. Poor resistance to abrasion is another problem with paint-on colorants. Loss of the pigments in high-abrasion areas produces an unattractive mottled effect.

Translucency. Coronal translucency is determined by the type and amount of enamel present. At the incisal edge of an unworn anterior tooth where there is no dentin in the light path, a blue or gray hue often appears, which results from the dark oral cavity. This effect is most pronounced with enamel that scatters very little light due to the absence of pigments or opacifying mineralization (e.g., fluorosis). Although less obvious, the translucent appearance of enamel is observable over the entire incisal or occlusal third of the crown. Therefore, when it is visible in adjacent teeth or when a more realistic appearance is desired, translucency can be simulated in the provisional. The procedure requires two resins—one colored to match the body and one to match the enamel of the tooth. Some manufacturers produce enamel or incisal shades that may be used without modification. When these are not available or when variation is needed, clear resin powder may be mixed with a smaller fraction of the "body" powder to produce the desired translucency.

Two procedures can be used to create a translucent effect. In the first, which is more difficult to control, the enamel color resin is carefully bead-brushed onto the occlusal or incisal surface of the ESF and tapered to end at the middle or cervical third. The resin's tendency to flow where it is not wanted can be controlled by the orientation of the ESF with respect to gravity and by manipulation with the brush tip. When the desired distribution of enamel color resin is achieved, a disposable syringe is loaded with body color resin and the ESF is immediately filled, avoiding disruption of the enamel color resin. The TSF is then positioned in the ESF, and normal procedures are followed. The result is a more natural-appearing provisional restoration with translucency in the incisal or occlusal portion that closely matches the existing dentition (Fig. 15-72).

In the second procedure, the enamel color resin is allowed to polymerize on the ESF without adding body color resin or the TSF. The rigid enamel veneer is removed from the ESF and trimmed to occupy only the space intended for enamel. Checking that the ESF and TSF can be mated without interference from the in-place veneer is important. With the veneer in place, monomer liquid is painted on it, and the body color resin is added. The TSF is then in-

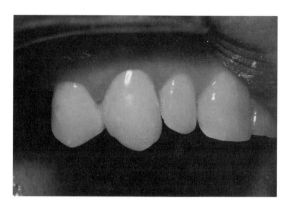

Fig. 15-72. The layering of translucent resin and dentin-shaded resin allow a more realistic appearance of the premolar and canine provisionals. They serve as RPD abutments and are splinted together to help resist dislodgment by the RPD clasp assembly.

serted, and standard procedures are followed for the remainder of the restoration. The timing for this procedure is less critical than for the first and may be better suited to practitioners with less experience. A disadvantage is that sometimes there is an obvious demarcation between the enamel and the body resins.

Texture. Texture effects require only a small amount of time, but in some cases they contribute significantly to the overall appearance of the provisional. These effects are most important for maxillary anterior teeth adjacent to teeth with well-defined lobes, imbrication lines, or developmental defects.

Developmental lobes are most effectively simulated in wax during the final stage of the diagnostic waxing. To produce a natural effect, it is critical to avoid making grooves that are straight or sharp-edged or have uniform cross sections. Instead, grooves should be created with a gentle crescent shape, with softening of the edges and slight varying of the cross section by burnishing with the largest-diameter waxing wire. If a polypropylene sheet is used to form the ESF, these subtle details can be reproduced in the resin.

Placement of developmental defects is most effectively accomplished in the resin just before pumice and rag wheel finishing. Depending on their size and definition, these features may be created with a sharp-edged, inverted-cone green stone rotating parallel to the occlusal plane and touched briefly to the resin. Often the defects are most noticeable in the cervical third of the tooth, but an adjacent tooth is the best guide for determining their distribution.

Imbrication lines may be simulated with a coarse diamond rotary instrument rotating slowly and moved across the facial surface from proximal to proximal. This will reduce the surface reflectance of the resin after it is finished and polished. However, as with all texture effects, overfinishing will obliterate these lines. Care must be taken to monitor the finishing by rinsing pumice from the surface and drying it. A completely smooth and highly polished provisional may be excellent for plaque control but will not be esthetically compatible with the adjacent teeth. The patient should be asked which of these two factors is more important.

SUMMARY

Although provisional restorations are usually intended for short-term use and then discarded, they can be made to provide pleasing esthetics, adequate support, and good protection for teeth while maintaining periodontal health. They may be fabricated in the dental office from any of several commercially available materials and a number of practical methods. The success of fixed prosthodontics often depends on the care with which the provisional is designed and fabricated.

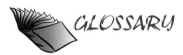 GLOSSARY

acrylic resin: *1:* pertaining to polymers of acrylic acid, meth-acrylic acid, or acrylonitril; for example, acrylic fibers or acrylic resins *2:* any of a group of thermoplastic resins made by polymerizing esters of acrylic or methylmethacrylate acids

autopolymer: *n:* a material that polymerizes by chemical reaction without external heat, as a result of the addition of an activator and a catalyst—**autopolymerization** *vb*

autopolymerizing resin: a resin whose polymerization initiated by a chemical activator

bench set: a stage of resin processing that allows a chemical reaction to occur under the conditions present in the ambient environment; also used to describe the continuing polymerization of impression materials beyond the manufacturer's stated set time

methyl methacrylate resin: a transparent, thermoplastic acrylic resin that is used in dentistry by mixing liquid methyl methacrylate monomer with the polymer powder. The resultant mixture forms a pliable plastic termed a dough, which is packed into a mold before to initiation of polymerization

photoactive: *adj:* reacting chemically to visible light or ultraviolet radiation—**photoactivation**

pumice: *n 1:* a type of volcanic glass used as an abrasive. It is prepared in various grits and used for finishing and polishing *2:* a polishing agent, in powdered form, used for natural teeth and fixed and removable restorations

resin: *n 1:* any of various solid or semisolid amorphous natural organic substances that usually are transparent or translucent and brown to yellow; usually formed in plant secretions; are soluble in organic solvents but not water; are used chiefly in varnishes, inks, plastics, and medicine; and are found in many dental impression materials *2:* a broad term used to describe natural or synthetic substances that form plastic materials after polymerization. They are named according to their chemical composition, physical structure, and means for activation of polymerization

resin crown: a resin restoration that restores a clinical crown without a metal substructure

thermoplastic: *adj* (1883): a characteristic or property of a material that allows it to be softened by the application of heat and return to the hardened state on cooling—**thermoplasticity** *n*

Study Questions

1. What are the ideal properties of a provisional restorative material? What are the ideal properties of the optimal provisional luting agent?
2. List at least five requirements of a successful provisional restoration.
3. Explain why these factors are critical to clinical success. What would occur if they were not appropriately performed or obtained?
4. Select three techniques for fabricating a provisional restoration for a single tooth. Identify the factors involved when a certain technique is selected for an indication or tooth.
5. What are the currently available materials for fabrication of provisional restorations? What are their respective material properties, advantages, and disadvantages?
6. Explain the basic chemistry involved in resin polymerization.
7. What factors should be considered when deciding between a direct, indirect, or indirect-direct fabrication technique for provisional fixed partial dentures?

REFERENCES

1. Seltzer S, Bender IB: *The dental pulp: biologic considerations in dental procedures*, ed 3, Philadelphia, 1984, JB Lippincott, p 191.

2. Seltzer S, Bender IB: op cit, pp 267-272.

3. Larato DC: The effect of crown margin extension on gingival inflammation, *J S Calif Dent Assoc* 37:476, 1969.

4. Waerhaug J: Tissue reactions around artificial crowns, *J Periodontol* 24:172, 1953.

5. Anusavice KJ: *Phillips' science of dental materials*, ed 10, Philadelphia, 1996, WB Saunders, pp. 285, 431.

6. El-Ebrashi MK et al: Experimental stress analysis of dental restorations. VII. Structural design and stress analysis of fixed partial dentures, *J Prosthet Dent* 23:177, 1970.

7. Koumjian JH et al: Color stability of provisional materials in vivo, *J Prosthet Dent* 65:740, 1991.

8. Scotti R et al: The in vitro color stability of acrylic resins for provisional restorations, *Int J Prosthod* 10:164, 1997.

9. Robinson FG et al: Effect of 10 percent carbamide peroxide on color of provisional restoration materials, *J Am Dent Assoc* 128:727, 1997.

10. Castelnuovo J et al: Temperature rise in pulpal chamber during fabrication of provisional resinous crowns, *J Prosthet Dent* 78:441, 1997.

11. Preston JD: A systematic approach to the control of esthetic form, *J Prosthet Dent* 35:393, 1976.

12. Moskowitz ME et al: Using irreversible hydrocolloid to evaluate preparations and fabricate temporary immediate provisional restorations, *J Prosthet Dent* 51:330, 1984.

13. Roberts DB: Flexible casts used in making indirect interim restorations, *J Prosthet Dent* 68:372, 1992.

14. Hensten-Pettersen A, Helgeland K: Sensitivity of different human cell lines in the biologic evaluation of dental resin-based restorative materials, *Scand J Dent Res* 89:102, 1981.

15. Munksgaard EC: Toxicology versus allergy in restorative dentistry, *Adv Dent Res* 6:17, 1992.

16. Dahl BL: Tissue hypersensitivity to dental materials, *J Oral Rehabil* 5:117, 1978.

17. Weaver RE, Goebel WM: Reactions to acrylic resin dental prostheses, *J Prosthet Dent* 43:138, 1980.

18. Giunta J, Zablotsky N: Allergic stomatitis caused by self-polymerizing resin, *Oral Surg* 41:631, 1976.

19. Spealman CR et al: Monomeric methyl methacrylate: studies on toxicity, *Industrial Med* 14:292, 1945.

20. Moulding MB, Teplitsky PE: Intrapulpal temperature during direct fabrication of provisional restorations, *Int J Prosthod* 3:299, 1990.

21. Tjan AHL et al: Temperature rise in the pulp chamber during fabrication of provisional crowns, *J Prosthet Dent* 62:622, 1989.

22. Zach L, Cohen G: Pulpal response to externally applied heat, *Oral Surg* 19:515, 1965.

23. Crispin BJ et al: The marginal accuracy of treatment restorations: a comparative analysis, *J Prosthet Dent* 44:283, 1980.

24. Monday JJL, Blais D: Marginal adaptation of provisional acrylic resin crowns, *J Prosthet Dent* 54:194, 1985.

25. Robinson FB, Hovijitra S: Marginal fit of direct temporary crowns, *J Prosthet Dent* 47:390, 1982.

26. Von Fraunhofer JA, Spiers RR: Accelerated setting of dental stone, *J Prosthet Dent* 49:859, 1983.

27. Pashley EL et al: The sealing properties of temporary filling materials, *J Prosthet Dent* 60:292, 1988.

28. Rosenstiel SF, Gegauff AG: Effect of provisional cementing agents on provisional resins, *J Prosthet Dent* 59:29, 1988.

29. Gegauff AG, Rosenstiel SF: Effect of provisional luting agents on provisional resin additions, *Quintessence Int* 18:841, 1987.

30. Terata R et al: Characterization of enamel and dentin surfaces after removal of temporary cement—effect of temporary cement on tensile bond strength of resin luting cement, *Dent Mater J* 13:148, 1994.

31. Stark H: Does temporary cementing have an effect on the bond strength of definitively cemented crowns? *Dtsch Zahnartzl Z* 46:774, 1991.

32. Mojon P, Hawbolt EB, MacEntee MI: A comparison of two methods for removing zinc oxide-eugenol provisional cement, *Int J Prosthodont* 5:78, 1992.

33. Schwartz R, Davis R, Mayhew R: Effect of a ZOE temporary cement on the bond strength of a resin luting cement, *Am J Dent* 3:28, 1990.

34. Olin PS et al: Retentive strength of six temporary dental cements, *Quintessence Int* 21:197, 1990.

LABORATORY PROCEDURES

COMMUNICATING WITH THE DENTAL LABORATORY

KEY TERMS

certified dental technician (CDT)   margin design
infection control   work authorization

To make a high-quality fixed prosthesis, all members of the dental team must understand what they can reasonably expect from each other. A mutual

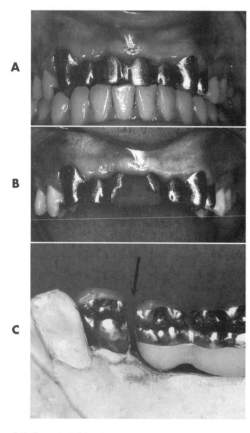

Fig. 16-1. **A,** This six-unit anterior metal-ceramic framework did not seat. After sectioning between the incisors, the adaptation of the individual components was satisfactory. Note the (correct) narrow width of the soldering gap. **B,** The two segments indexed with autopolymerizing resin for subsequent soldering. **C,** The dentist sectioned this FPD incorrectly: the soldering gap is much too wide *(arrow),* and distortion during soldering will almost certainly result. A remake of at least one of the FPD components is indicated.

knowledge of individual limitations is also critical. The dentist who does not understand and appreciate the challenges faced by the technician is at a serious disadvantage when prescribing and delegating laboratory procedures (Fig. 16-1). Critical to the development of sound clinical judgment is a thorough understanding of technical procedures and their rationale, which will be described in the chapters of this section.

DENTAL TECHNOLOGY CERTIFICATION

The National Organization of Dental Laboratories is committed to upholding and advancing the commercial dental laboratory industry. They emphasize the following information[1]:

In 46 states there are no laws to set minimum qualifications for performance of dental technology or the operation of a dental laboratory. Technicians and laboratories that become certified do so as evidence of their commitment to maintaining professional standards in dental technology. The standards and requirements for certification do not vary across state lines. A **certified dental technician (CDT)** tested in New England must demonstrate the same competencies as a CDT tested on the Pacific coast.

Whenever and wherever the credibility and responsibility of a dental technician or laboratory is measured, the objective third-party certificate credential is the reliable hallmark of competence. Certification is endorsed by dental organizations, encouraged by military services, and acknowledged by third-party payers and courts of law.

The first CDTs were tested in 1958. Today the National Board for Certification (NBC) tests more than 1700 technicians annually. In 1978 the current standards for laboratory certification were adopted; today there are more than 500 certified dental laboratories. To qualify for certification, technicians must have a 2-year dental technology degree (or the equivalent) and must pass written and practical examinations. To maintain certification, they must document at least 10 hours of continuing education annually, including study of **infection control.** The requirements for a certified dental laboratory include certification (CDT) of its supervisory technicians; professional standards of health, safety, and maintenance in the laboratory facility; and conscientious training and practice in infection control techniques. Certification must be renewed annually.*

MUTUAL RESPONSIBILITIES

Good communication is the key to a dental team's technical success.[2,3] This requires a close working relationship between the dentist and laboratory technician. Anticipating satisfactory results is absolutely unrealistic if the dentist does not have a reasonable amount of experience with, and a thorough understanding of, dental laboratory procedures. Active participation is paramount, and clinicians who take the time to develop an in-depth understanding of laboratory work make better clinical decisions because of their understanding of applicable technical and materials science limitations. Only then can a dentist select the best compromise between technical restrictions on the one hand and biologic factors and esthetic needs on the other. Similarly, if the technician does not appreciate and respect the clinical rationale of the treating dentist, the results will be less than satisfactory (Fig. 16-2). The dentist can earn this respect by being prepared to meet personal responsibilities and by actively participating in the technical decision-making process.

A survey[4] of fixed prosthodontic laboratories revealed that dentists delegate a significant proportion of this responsibility. The technicians surveyed were often dissatisfied with the quality of work received; complaints included insufficient informa-

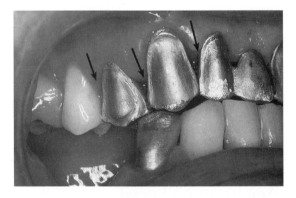

Fig. 16-2. It is often difficult for the technician to appreciate soft tissue contours and embrasure form. These substructures were not cut back sufficiently interproximally (*arrows*).

*Reproduced by permission of National Organization of Dental Laboratories.

tion about the **work authorization,** deficient impressions, and inadequate records. This survey highlighted significant problems in dentist-technician communication. In other studies and opinions concerning dentist-technician interaction, whether written by dentists or technicians, the authors emphasized that improvement is achievable only by improving communication.[5]

The American Dental Association (ADA) has issued guidelines to improve the relationship between dentist and technicians.[6] They are reprinted here:

Working relationships between dentists and dental laboratories: The current high standard of prosthetic dental care is directly related to, and remains dependent upon, mutual respect within the dental team for the abilities and contributions of each member. The following guidelines are designed to foster good relations between dental laboratories, dental laboratory technicians and the dental profession.

The dentist, being duly licensed, should:

(1) Provide the laboratory with signed written instructions detailing the work which is to be performed and prescribing the appropriate materials to be used;

(2) Provide the laboratory with accurate impressions, casts, interocclusal records or mountings;

(3) Identify the margins, postdam, borders, relief and/or prosthetic design on all submitted cases;

(4) Furnish a shade description, photograph, drawing or shade button that most closely achieves the desired results;

(5) Provide a verbal or written approval for the laboratory to proceed with the fabrication of the prosthesis or approve modifications, if notified by the laboratory that a submitted case may have questionable areas or unclear instructions and submit written approval to the laboratory after the item in question has been clarified;

(6) Retain a copy of the written instructions for a period of time as may be required by law;

(7) Follow appropriate laboratory infection control protocol as outlined in the ADA's infection control guidelines.

The dental laboratory should:

(1) Produce dental prostheses following the written instructions provided by the dentist and using the impressions, casts, interocclusal records or mountings as submitted;

(2) Review the case with the prescribing dentist for clarification if a question arises;

(3) Match the shade as described in the original instructions, within the limitations of the materials available for use;

(4) Notify the dentist immediately if it is determined that work on the case cannot proceed;

(5) Fabricate the prostheses in a timely manner;

(6) Inform the dentist of the materials used in the fabrication of the case;

(7) Follow appropriate laboratory infection control protocol as outlined in the ADA's infection control guidelines.*

RESPONSIBILITIES OF THE DENTIST

The dentist has the overall responsibility for the treatment rendered. Delegating many procedures to auxiliary personnel is possible if all the necessary information is provided to enable them to deliver high-quality service. However, errors such as insufficient tooth reduction, uncertainty about the location of tooth preparation margins, improper interocclusal records and articulations, and ambiguity in communicating the desired shades for esthetic restorations to the technician hamper this responsibility.

INFECTION CONTROL

The U.S. Department of Health and Human Services[7] and the ADA[8] have issued guidelines about the disinfection and handling of impressions and other material transferred from the dental office to the dental laboratory. Applicable guidelines are detailed in Chapter 14. Strict adherence to infection control guidelines

---

*Reproduced by permission of The American Dental Association.

cannot be overemphasized, because the potential for infection of dental laboratory personnel exists. In a 1990 sample,[9] 67% of all materials sent from dental offices to dental laboratories were contaminated.

TOOTH PREPARATION

An organized approach to tooth preparation has been discussed in Chapters 7 to 12, which provide the criteria for minimally necessary clearances for the various restorations.

Inadequate tooth reduction in the cervical third for a metal-ceramic restoration is a common error. Obviously, on long clinical crowns of vital teeth (e.g., after periodontal surgery) it will not always be possible to reduce the desired 1.2 to 1.5 mm without pulp exposure. Nevertheless, it is generally impossible, even for an experienced ceramist, to achieve superior esthetic results if the tooth is underprepared.[10] Inexperienced technicians tend to resolve the problem by overcontouring (Fig. 16-3), but this usually leads to the initiation or recurrence of periodontal disease. Esthetic difficulties like this should be discussed during the treatment planning phase. Communication regarding any deviation from "ideal" criteria is essential and can prevent misunderstanding, frustration, and ultimate failure.

PREPARATION MARGINS

Margins should be easily discernible and accessible on the casts submitted to the technician. The saying "If you can't see it, you can't wax it" describes the

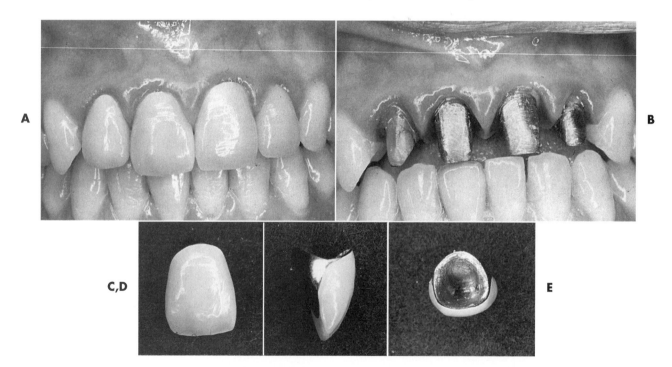

Fig. 16-3. Restoration failure resulting from excessive axial contours. **A,** Recently placed metal-ceramic crowns have contributed to gingival inflammation. **B,** The crowns removed. **C** and **D,** Excessive contour. **E,** The fault is readily appreciated from a gingival view.   *Continued*

situation well. (The requirements for dies are listed in Chapter 17.)

The dentist should outline the margins on the dies[11] (Fig. 16-4). However, in practice, few dentists do this.[12] If the teeth are properly prepared and the impression is accurate, the margins should be obvious, which makes this step unnecessary. When doubt exists, the dentist's knowledge of the extent of the preparation should resolve any uncertainty.

Dentists must understand the importance of **margin design.** For instance, it is unrealistic to request a collarless restoration on a shoulder-bevel type of margin or an all-ceramic crown restoration on a tooth with a narrow chamfer finish line (Figs. 16-5 and 16-6).

Although an experienced technician will probably bring any unrealistic demands to the attention of the dentist, some well-meaning technicians may attempt to meet a request that is doomed to failure from the beginning. To quote one excellent dentist, "When you discover an error has occurred, STOP. Don't proceed. Return to the step where the error occurred and correct it. Attempting to blunder on without correcting it properly will only compound and complicate the error."

ARTICULATION

Proper articulation of opposing casts is the responsibility of the dentist. Often it is advisable to schedule a separate appointment with the patient for verification of the articulation. This is particularly critical as the complexity of treatment increases (Fig. 16-7). An apparently slight discrepancy may require a remake or hours of

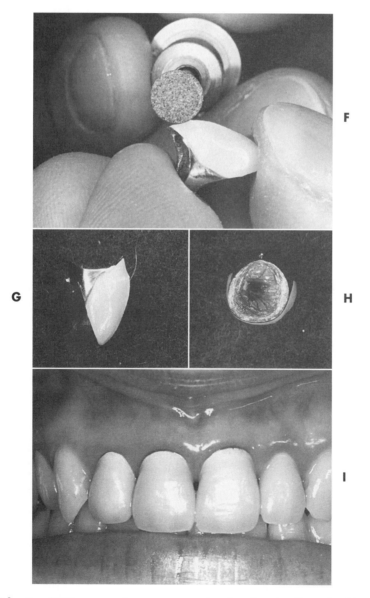

Fig. 16-3, cont'd. F to H, The restorations recontoured and reglazed. I, Tissue health quickly improves when the recontoured restorations are temporarily recemented. Replacements were later made for esthetic reasons.

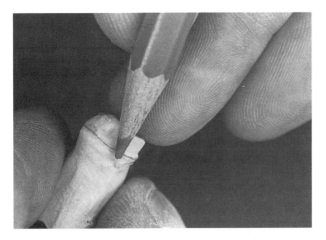

Fig. 16-4. Marking the preparation margin with a colored pencil. The line must be clearly visible but of minimal thickness.

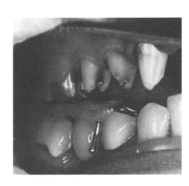

Fig. 16-5. The expectations of the dentist are not realistic. These cervically under-reduced preparations are unsuitable for the metal-ceramic restorations requested. Also, buccolingual resistance is compromised by the excessive taper.

Fig 16-6. Three types of esthetic restorations. The restoration with the metal collar can be fabricated on a shoulder or shoulder-bevel margin. The porcelain labial margin metal-ceramic crown can be fabricated on a shoulder margin; the all-ceramic crown requires a slightly rounded internal angle. The last two require margins that are "glasslike" in smoothness.

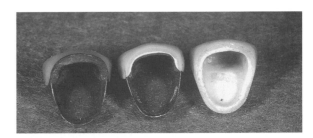

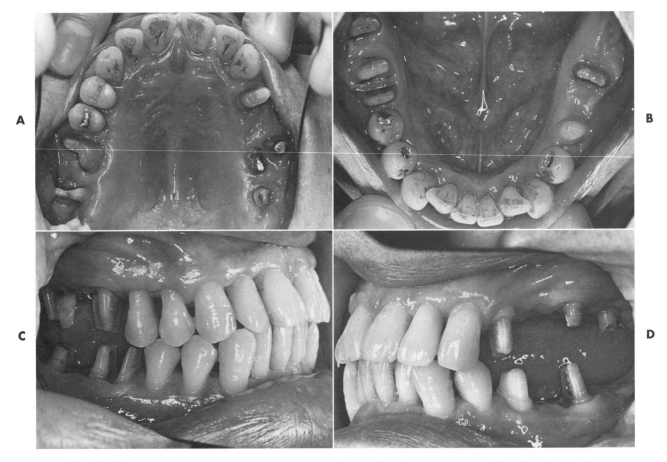

Fig. 16-7. A to D, In the presence of compromised periodontal support, optimal loading is critical to enhance the prognosis. Accurate occlusion is essential to successful restoration of this periodontally compromised patient for whom multiple hemisections, root resections, and amputations have been performed. Extensive communication with the technician is necessary.

Continued

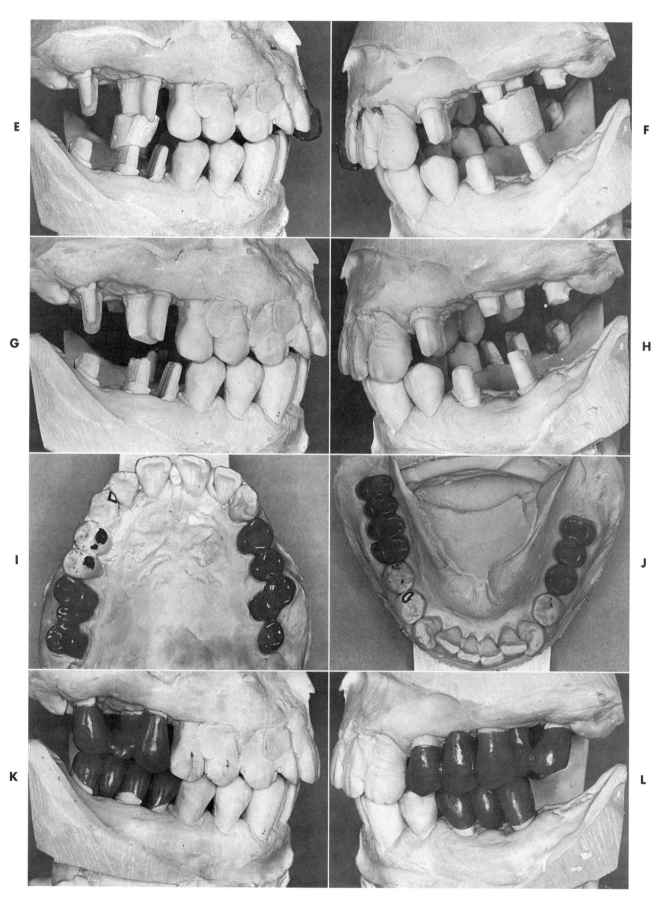

Fig. 16-7, cont'd. **E** to **H,** The occlusal relationship is transferred to the articulator with small impression plaster indices and a Lucia jig made from autopolymerizing resin (see Chapter 2). **I** to **L,** Wax patterns are designed to combine occlusal function with maximum access for oral hygiene. Note the buccolingual reduction in width of the occlusal table **(I)** and the emergence profile on the maxillary molars **(K** and **L).**

Continued

Fig. 16-7, cont'd.   M and N, Restorations on the working cast. O to S, Restorations in place. Note that occlusal rests have already been incorporated in the fixed prostheses in the mandibular arch **(S)** to prepare for possible future failure (see Chapter 32). **T** and **U,** Note that embrasure design allows proper cleaning.

corrective grinding and a compromised result. With careful planning, verification of the articulation can be done efficiently and will result in peace of mind.

WORK AUTHORIZATION

In addition to certain general information that is required by law, a work authorization form (Fig. 16-8) should include the following:

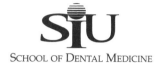

SCHOOL OF DENTAL MEDICINE

**DENTAL LABORATORY
WORK AUTHORIZATION**

School of Dental Medicine, 2800 College Avenue, Alton, IL 62002-4700

Student _____   Rec. by SDM Lab _____ Units Rec. _____
Patient _____   F. P. Sec. Head Begin _____
Patient # _____   Technician _____
Lab _____   F.P. Sec. Head Complete _____
                                    Received by Student _____
Date Due _____   (Name & Date for each of the above)

SHADE GUIDE

INDICATE CHARACTERIZATIONS

PONTIC DESIGN (circle)

MODIFIED-RIDGE LAP   CONICAL   HYGIENIC

MAXILLARY

MANDIBULAR

Tooth #	Rest. Type	Metal	Guide	Shade Incisal	Shade Gingival	Margin 0.3 mm metal	Margin Porc. Shoulder	Contacts Metal	Contacts Porcelain	Articulator Settings R / L
										Cond. Guid.
										Inc. Guid.
										ISS
										PSS

Porcelain Shades

Articulator Number

R℞

Dental License No. _____   Signature _____   D.M.D.
                                                                                    D.D.S.

Office Use Only   Business Office Paid

Wax [ ]   Bridge Units [ ]
Cast [ ]
Porc. [ ]   Crown Units [ ]
Sold. [ ]

EML 11/89   White–Lab. Credit Voucher / Yellow–Lab. Record Copy / Pink–File Copy   1810-23   rev. 4/99

Fig. 16-8. Work authorization form.

1. General description of the restoration to be made
2. Material specification (e.g., ADA Type IV gold)
3. Desired occlusal scheme
4. Connector design for FPDs
5. Pontic design, including the material specification for tissue contact
6. Substructure design for metal-ceramic restorations
7. Information regarding the shade selection for esthetic restorations
8. Proposed RPD design (if applicable)
9. Date of the next scheduled patient appointment and the stage of completion required by then

The dentist must be familiar with the materials the technician prefers to use for certain procedures. Specifying those materials can save both time and effort. The technician should also respect the selection when the dentist requests a specific material. Written instructions should be explicit.[13]

Communication improves if the technician and dentist discuss a particular choice rather than a bald statement written on the work authorization form. It may be inconvenient for the technician to comply with a request, so its importance should be discussed.

Occlusion. The work authorization form should designate the location of the occlusal contacts. It must be specified whether they are to be on metal or porcelain. In theory, the two most desirable occlusal schemes are cusp-fossa and cusp-marginal ridge. Assuming that these will be attained in every case is unrealistic, however, because they can only be accomplished consistently when the opposing teeth are reasonably close to ideal relative positions (Angle Class I—see Chapter 1). Compromises often must be made, especially when teeth are being restored to conform to an existing dentition. For example, when a mandibular molar is in a buccolingual end-to-end posterior relationship with its antagonist, a decision must be made whether to restore the tooth in a cross-bite relationship or whether the tooth preparation should be modified (additional reduction of the buccal functional cusp bevel) to accommodate a more conventional occlusal relationship. As an alternative, restoring the opposing tooth may need to be considered.

If the dentist has performed a diagnostic tooth preparation and waxing (see Chapter 2), it is possible to prescribe the desired occlusal relationship with good accuracy. Occasionally, when a single crown is to be made, an existing malocclusion may be accepted. This can limit the need for more extensive treatment, although it makes sense only if the opposing teeth will not need a restoration in the near future.

Connectors. The work authorization form should specify which connectors are to be cast, which are to be preceramic soldered, and which are to be postceramic soldered. The sequence of the planned procedures should be indicated and discussed when necessary or when clarity can be enhanced. If nonrigid connectors are requested, the desired type of connector and path of placement should be specified.

Pontic and Substructure Design. Pontic design is discussed in Chapter 20. A simple checklist on the work authorization form should suffice if the dentist and technician have agreed on applicable expectations and requirements.[13,14]

The design of metal substructures for metal-ceramic restorations is somewhat controversial. Many technicians believe that it is not necessary to first create the contours of the completed restoration in wax and then cut back the veneering area. We disagree, and present our reasoning in Chapter 19 (Fig 16-9). The authorization should specify whether the anatomic contour wax patterns are to be returned for evaluation and possible modification. The more complex the restorative effort, the more critical a careful evaluation becomes at this stage. Long-term success is the goal, and inadequate framework design is a relatively common cause of failure for which the dentist will bear the responsibility (although often blaming the ceramist).

Shade Selection. With the prevalence of metal-ceramic restorations, dentists and technicians have become acutely aware of the difficulty involved in communicating shade selection. A thorough understanding of the principles of color science (presented in Chapter 23) and the use of internal and surface colorants (discussed in Chapters 24 and 30) is essential to both parties.

Many dentists and technicians have found a diagram of the tooth that allows specifications of multiple shades helpful (Fig. 16-10).[15] The diagram should be large enough to designate a cervical shade, an incisal shade, and any applicable individual characterization. Diagrams on most preprinted laboratory prescription forms do not provide adequate space (see Fig. 16-8), so other space must be available. A separate entry regarding the value or brightness can be helpful. When selecting a shade, the dentist should use a guide that corresponds to the ceramic system used by the technician. On occasion, it may not be possible to obtain a match with a simple shade guide (e.g., the Vita Lumin vacuum system). In those cases an alternative guide or a shade distribution chart (outlined in Chapter 23)

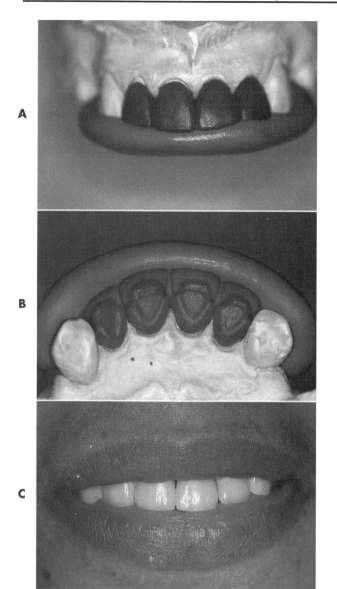

Fig. 16-9. Full contour waxing **(A)** and cutback **(B)** with the use of incisal **(A)** and facial **(B)** vinyl polysiloxane indexes leads to predictable success when esthetics are paramount **(C)**.

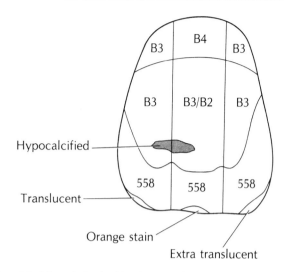

Fig. 16-10. A shade distribution chart must be adequate in size to permit inclusion of enough detail. Subtle differences observed in cervical shades are identified, as are surface details such as hypocalcification, incisal translucency, and stains.

tomized tab is sent to the dental laboratory. The ceramist then has an actual reference and can compare the work and make the required modifications, thus ensuring predictable success.

If esthetic requirements are extensive or difficult to communicate through the means described above, involving dental laboratory personnel in the shade selection process may be helpful. The ADA takes the position that when a dentist requests the assistance of a dental laboratory technician in the shade selection process, this does not constitute the practice of dentistry by the technician, provided the activity is undertaken in consultation with the dentist and that it complies with the dentist's written instructions.

Such assistance is most appropriately provided in the dentist's office.[5]

Additional Information. Additional information will often help the technician considerably. Reference to diagnostic waxing can communicate specific information about desired tooth length and form or a desired occlusal arrangement. A custom anterior guide table (see Chapter 2) provides specific information to follow as anterior guidance is established in maxillary and/or mandibular anterior crowns. Casts of provisional restorations are invaluable to the technician when he or she is asked to fabricate fixed partial dentures with a high esthetic requirement. They provide information about midlines, incisal edge position, and coronal form and are the most practical way of accurately conveying information to the laboratory (Fig. 16-11). The diagnostic waxing enables the dentist to explore all the treatment

should be used. The dentist must have excellent color perception skills and should be able to precisely transfer those onto a written prescription that includes a large, detailed diagram that allows the ceramist to accurately reproduce the shade observed and described by the clinician. Close communication and cooperation are obviously necessary, and a trial porcelain firing may be needed.

A practical alternative to written color communication is the use of light-cured, resin-based staining kits to custom-stain a shade-tab. The closest matching shade-tab is selected and modified using stains mixed with liquid resin. Once the desired match has been obtained, the resin is light-cured, and the cus-

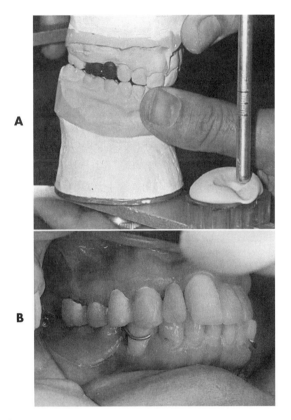

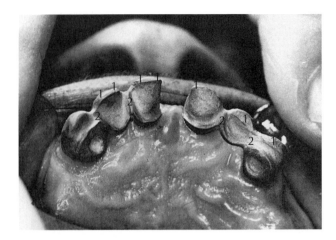

Fig. 16-12. Substructure try-in. At this stage the location of the porcelain-metal junction is assessed. Errors here include the following: (1) rounding is needed on the veneering surface (see Chapter 19) and (2), the closed cervical embrasures need to be enlarged by reducing the size of the connectors and correction of the interproximal emergence profile to minimize periodontal problems.

Fig. 16-11. **A,** Diagnostic casts, guide table, and waxing provide additional information for the technician. **B,** Carefully adjusted provisional restorations can be duplicated in an irreversible hydrocolloid impression and replicated in the definitive prosthesis by the technician.

alternatives before choosing a course of therapy. A resin provisional can be fabricated and adjusted intraorally as necessary for optimum appearance and function. Color photographs can be especially helpful in conveying essential additional information.

APPROPRIATE CHECKS

In any new working relationship between a dentist and a technician, every step of initial treatments in laboratory procedures should be reviewed in detail. Only then can teamwork develop over time. As the dentist and technician become familiar with each other's preferences, several steps may then be combined.

The initial review may include the wax patterns for corrective shaping of occlusal and axial contours of retainers and pontics. When treating patients with fixed partial dentures and metal-ceramic crowns, the dentist must decide whether the restorations should be completed through porcelain application in the laboratory or whether a preliminary metal substructure try-in appointment is needed. We recommend that a try-in of the metal

substructure for metal-ceramic restorations be routinely done. As an example, the technician may not have adequate information to evaluate how far the veneering area should be extended into the cervical embrasures, and this can be readily determined by the dentist during try-in (Fig. 16-12). When soldering FPDs, often it is best to index the component parts directly in the mouth rather than rely on the accuracy of the working cast. A try-in appointment can facilitate making small corrections of discrepancies that could later become significant errors. Similarly, it may be advantageous to plan a try-in appointment for final contouring, texturing, and staining of a metal-ceramic restoration in the bisque bake, before glazing. It takes time and effort to perform these clinical procedures (see Chapter 30), but patients will recognize and appreciate the improved results.

The use of checklists by both clinician and technician can be helpful.[16] For instance, before an impression leaves the dental office, the dentist and auxiliary personnel can use a standard protocol to confirm that finish lines are distinct; no blood or saliva is present in impressions and disinfection protocols were followed; no voids, tears, defects, or areas where the tray was seated; nor has contact occurred between occlusal surfaces and the tray, creating thin spots that can lead to articulation errors. For casts, die trimming, the absence of undercuts, retention form, adequacy of reduction for facial porcelain and porcelain margins, and occlusal clearance need to be confirmed.

Where retainers for RPDs are involved, the prescription and cast are checked to ensure availability of all pertinent information relative to the path of insertion of the RPD, guideplanes, rest seats, and the desired heights of contour.

SUMMARY

The key to high-quality fixed prosthodontics lies in good communication between the dentist and the technician. All too often each lives in a vacuum—the dentist forgets how a straightforward step such as rounding line angles can expedite the fabrication of a restoration or the technician is unaware of the difficulties of a particular clinical phase (e.g., impression making or a remount procedure).

Through mutual respect and a coordinated effort, each can contribute to the delivery of patient care and at the same time keep failures to a minimum.

The most common problems seen by the dentist at try-in are poor marginal adaptation, poor occlusion, poor axial contour (specifically overcontouring of the cervical third of the tooth), and haphazard pontic and substructure design. The most common problems encountered by the technician are inadequate tooth reduction, "mystery margins," improper articulation, and vagueness in color communication.

The use of certain ancillary devices (e.g., diagnostic waxing and casts of provisional restorations) will help both dentist and technician deliver more effective treatment to the prosthodontic patient.

The student and practitioner involved in fixed prosthodontic treatment must acquire an in-depth understanding of the laboratory procedures described in the following chapters in this section. Often such understanding is most rapidly developed by personal involvement in the technical aspects of clinical dentistry. Over time, this will lead to significantly improved interaction with dental technicians, resulting in improved clinical decision making and more predictable and successful fixed prostheses.

REFERENCES

1. http://nadl.org/html/essential_facts.html
2. Small BW: Laboratory communication for esthetic success, *Gen Dent* Nov-Dec 566, 1998.
3. Gleghorn T: Improving communication with the laboratory when fabricating porcelain veneers, *J Am Dent Assoc* 128:1571, 1997.
4. Aquilino SA, Taylor TD: Prosthodontic laboratory and curriculum survey. III. Fixed prosthodontic laboratory survey, *J Prosthet Dent* 52:879, 1984.
5. Landesman HM: Proc. of Pros. 21. Clinical practice: professional affairs, *J Prosthet Dent* 64:252, 1990.
6. American Dental Association: *Current policies, 1954-1991*, pp 64-65.
7. U.S. Department of Health and Human Services, Public Health Service: Recommended infection control practices for dentistry, *MMWR* 35:237, 1986.
8. JADA Reports: Infection control recommendations for the dental office and the dental laboratory, *J Am Dent Assoc* 116:241, 1988.
9. Powell GL et al: The presence and identification of organisms transmitted to dental laboratories, *J Prosthet Dent* 64:235, 1990.
10. Jorgenson MW, Goodkind RJ: Spectrophotometric study of five porcelain shades relative to dimensions of color, porcelain thickness, and repeated firings, *J Prosthet Dent* 42:96, 1979.
11. Leeper SH: Dentist and laboratory: a "love-hate" relationship, *Dent Clin North Am* 23:87, 1979.
12. Olin PS et al: Current prosthodontic practice: a dental laboratory survey, *J Prosthet Dent* 61:742, 1989.
13. Drago CJ: Clinical and laboratory parameters in fixed prosthodontic treatment, *J Prosthet Dent* 76:233, 1996.

Study Questions

1. Discuss the guidelines issued by the American Dental Association relative to working relationships between dentists and dental laboratories. What are specific responsibilities of the dentist? What are the responsibilities of the dental technician?
2. What is a CDT? What are requirements for certification?
3. Write a series of complete and comprehensive prescriptions for the various stages of laboratory fabrication of an anterior metal-ceramic FPD from tooth #8 to #11 (two pontics), to be fabricated in two segments and soldered after clinical evaluation and before porcelain application. List the various materials and models to be submitted with each prescription.
4. What is the purpose of submitting an anterior custom acrylic guide table to the dental laboratory? When would this be advisable?

14. Deyton G: Communications checksheet will ease relations with laboratories, *Mo Dent J* 74(5):32, 1994.

15. Pensler AV: Shade selection: problems and solutions, *Compendium* 19:387, 1998.

16. Maxson BB: Quality assurance for the laboratory aspects of prosthodontic treatment, *J Prosthodont* 6:204, 1997.

CHAPTER SEVENTEEN

WORKING CASTS AND DIES

KEY TERMS

blockout	epoxy resin
cyanoacrylate	gypsum products
dental cast	master cast
dental stone	mounting
die trimming	multiple pour technique
dowel pin	split-cast procedure
electroplated die	stone die
electroplating	vacuum mixing

Because direct fabrication of patterns for extracoronal restorations in the mouth is inconvenient, difficult, time consuming, and virtually impossible, practically all wax patterns are made in the laboratory with the indirect technique. This technique requires an accurate reproduction of the prepared tooth, the surrounding soft tissues, and the adjacent and opposing teeth. A cast-and-die system captures the necessary information so that it can be transferred to the laboratory.

The working (or master) cast is the replica of the prepared teeth, ridge areas, and other parts of the dental arch. The die is the positive reproduction of the prepared tooth and consists of a suitable hard substance of sufficient accuracy (usually an improved stone, resin, or metal) (Fig. 17-1).

The accuracy of a cast and die is a function of the completeness and accuracy of the impression. *The cast cannot contain more information than the impression from which it was made.*

This chapter describes the requirements of a cast-and-die system and correlates these with the available materials. The procedures are generally straightforward, but the steps must be followed carefully if the intended prosthesis is to be successful.

PREREQUISITES

The cast that will be used to make the fixed restoration must meet certain requirements. It must reproduce all details captured in the impression and should be free of defects. Depending on their location, however, minor imperfections may be

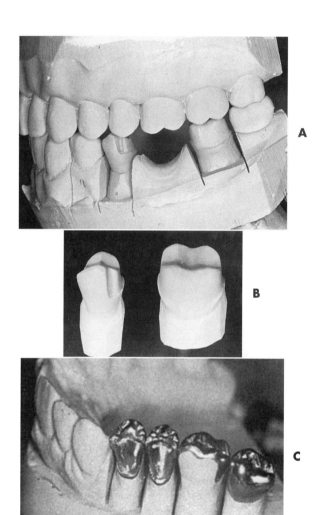

Fig. 17-1. Removable die system. **A,** Working cast. **B,** The individual dies. **C,** Epoxy die. (*C courtesy Dr. J. H. Bailey.*)

acceptable (Fig. 17-2). The cast must meet certain requirements:

1. It must reproduce both prepared and unprepared tooth surfaces.
2. The unprepared teeth immediately adjacent to the preparation must be free of voids.
3. All surfaces of any teeth involved in anterior guidance and the occlusal surfaces of all

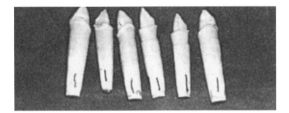

Fig. 17-2. Individual dies.

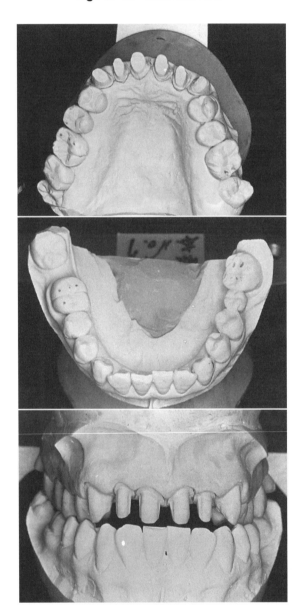

Fig. 17-3. Defect-free occlusal surfaces are essential to permit precise articulation.

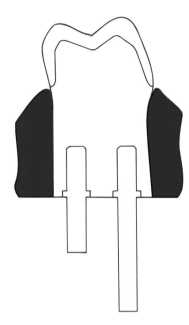

Fig. 17-4. To facilitate trimming, the impression should extend beyond the preparation margin. A properly trimmed die must have the same cervical contour as the tooth. (The red area indicates the parts of the die to be removed during trimming.)

1. It must reproduce the prepared tooth exactly.
2. All surfaces must be accurately duplicated, and no bubbles or voids can be accepted.
3. The remaining unprepared tooth structure immediately cervical to the finish line should be easily discernible on the die, ideally with 0.5 to 1 mm visible (enough must be present to help the technician establish the correct cervical contour of the restoration) (Fig. 17-4).
4. Adequate access to the margin is imperative.

MATERIALS SCIENCE

James L. Sandrik
GYPSUM

The two critical characteristics of cast-and-die materials, dimensional accuracy and resistance to abrasion while the wax pattern is being formed, are adequately achieved with gypsum. This material is inexpensive, easy to use, and produces consistent results. Manufactured in enormous quantities for industrial use, it can easily be modified for dental use.

Dental **gypsum products** are available in five forms (ADA Types I to V)—defined as impression plaster; model plaster; **dental stone;** high-strength dental stone; and high-strength, high-expansion stone. The gypsum components are identical chemically. The setting reaction is due to the hydration of calcium sulfate hemihydrate:

unprepared teeth must allow for precise articulation of the opposing casts (Fig. 17-3).
4. All relevant soft tissues should be reproduced in the working cast, including all edentulous spaces and residual ridge contours that will be involved in the fixed prosthesis.

The die for the fixed restoration also must meet certain requirements:

$$CaSO_4 \cdot \tfrac{1}{2} H_2O + 1\tfrac{1}{2} H_2O \rightarrow CaSO_4 \cdot 2H_2O$$

The hemihydrate is manufactured by heating the dihydrate under controlled conditions to drive off some of the water of crystallization (a process called *calcination*). The differences between the various types of dental gypsum are attributable to calcination. The improved physical properties of die stone over dental stone and plaster result from the fact that less water is needed to obtain a sufficiently fluid mix.*

Hand mixing of gypsum products is easy, but results are better when the mixing is done mechanically in a vacuum. Porosity is reduced, with a concomitant increase in strength, after only 15 seconds of mechanical mixing. Newly poured casts should be left undisturbed for at least 30 minutes; superior results are achieved at 1 hour, although these times may vary among brands.

Surface detail reproduction is acceptable with Type IV and Type V gypsum products. The materials are capable of reproducing a 20-μm-wide line as prescribed by ADA specification No. 19.[1] However, not all brands of die stone are compatible with all brands of impression material,[2,3] and if poor surface detail reproduction is experienced, an alternative product should be selected.

With some techniques (e.g., when preparing a cast for duplication), it is necessary to soak the set gypsum in water. However, although it appears to be insoluble, the gypsum slowly dissolves, ruining the surface detail of the cast. If soaking is required, it should be done in water saturated with plaster slurry, and only enough to achieve the desired degree of wetting.

Gypsum's greatest disadvantage is its relatively poor resistance to abrasion. Attempts to overcome this have included the use of so-called "gypsum hardeners." Although these materials (e.g., colloidal silica) have relatively little effect on the hardness of the stone, they improve abrasion resistance (some by as much as 100%).[4] Their use is accompanied by a slight increase in setting expansion, but it is probably not clinically significant. An alternative approach[5] is to impregnate the surface of the die with a low-viscosity resin such as **cyanoacrylate.** As mentioned earlier, abrasion resistance is the physical property most improved by this technique. Care

is needed when selecting and applying the resin so that the resin film will have no significant thickness.[6] Experts continue their efforts to improve the properties of die stone. One approach is to apply additives used in industrial applications (e.g., concrete manufacture) to dental gypsum products.[7] Another is the use of a gum arabic, calcium hydroxide mixture.[8] Resin-strengthened gypsum products such as ResinRock,* with high strength and low expansion,[9] are also popular and are particularly suitable for implant casts (see Chapter 13).

Additional, even stronger, die materials are also available. These include resin and **electroplated dies.**

RESIN

Resins are used as a die material to overcome the low strength and abrasion resistance of die stone. Most available resin die materials are **epoxy resins,** but polyurethane is also used. Epoxy resin is well known as a household and industrial adhesive. It can be cured at room temperature without expensive or complicated equipment, and it yields a form that is reasonably stable dimensionally. Its abrasion resistance is many times greater than that of gypsum products. However, it is more expensive than gypsum, and it undergoes some shrinkage during polymerization.

Epoxy resins suitable for fabrication of precision dies are available, although there is a great deal of variability among brands.[10] The amount of shrinkage upon polymerization is approximately equal to the expansion with gypsum. Polymerization shrinkage is less of a problem with newer formulations[11] and polyurethane resin.[12] When used with polyvinyl siloxane, contemporary resin systems produce complete arch casts with similar dimensional accuracy to traditional die stone.[13] In general, detail reproduction is better[14]; however, prostheses fabricated on resin dies will fit more tightly than those made on gypsum.[15]

Certain impression materials (i.e., polysulfide and hydrocolloid) are not compatible with resin. However, good results are achieved with silicone and polyether.

ELECTROPLATED DIES

Besides resin, **electroplating** can be used to overcome the poor abrasion resistance of gypsum. This technique[16] has been in use for many years and involves the deposition of a coat of pure silver or copper on the impression. The areas to be plated are first coated with finely powdered silver or graphite

---

*Thus 100 g of plaster requires 45 to 50 ml of water, 100 g of dental stone requires 30 to 35 ml, and 100 g of die stone requires 20 to 25 ml, depending on the particular brand. Theoretically, the stoichiometric amount of water needed for the setting reaction is 18.6 ml. Only die stone has suitable physical properties for making cast restorations. However, its properties are totally dependent on accurate measurement of the water/powder ratio.

---

*Whip Mix: Louisville, Ky.

to make them conduct electricity, and the impression is then placed in an electroplating bath. A layer of pure metal is deposited on the impression and is supported with Type IV stone or resin.

Although electroplating has been in use for some time, several problems remain. Variable degrees of distortion commonly occur, and the technique must be performed slowly; otherwise, distortion in the metal will subsequently stress the impression. The time required to produce a cohesive film of metal (typically 8 hours) is ample for the development of dimensional changes in the impression. However, when done properly, an electroplated die can be as accurate as a stone die,[17,18] although not all impression materials are suitable for plating. Because of their low surface energies, silicone impression materials are difficult to electroplate evenly. However, some brands are easier to plate than others.[19] Polyether impressions, because of their hydrophilic nature, imbibe water and become distorted. They therefore cannot be plated accurately. Polysulfide polymers can be silver plated, but it is much more difficult to copper plate them. The main drawback of silver plating is the use of a cyanide solution, which requires special precautions because of its extreme toxicity.

FLEXIBLE DIE MATERIALS

Flexible die materials are similar to heavy-bodied silicone or polyether impression materials (see Chapter 14) and have been used to make provisional restorations[20,21] or indirect composite resin inlays or onlays[22,23] chairside. The advantages of the flexible material over a stone die include more rapid setting and the ease of removal of the provisional or inlay. When choosing materials for flexible dies, be sure to select a compatible combination of impression and die materials that provides good surface details. One study found the best detail reproduction was obtained when combining Impregum F die material* with Extrude Light impression material.†[24]

SELECTION CRITERIA

Choosing one cast-and-die system over another depends on several factors:

1. The material must allow a dimensionally accurate cast and should be strong and resistant to abrasion.
2. It should be easily sectionable and easy to trim with the routinely available equipment.

3. It should be compatible with the separating agent that will be used so that the wax pattern does not stick.
4. It should reproduce surface detail accurately.
5. It should be available in a color that contrasts with the wax used so that the preparation margin can be seen.
6. It should be easily wettable by the wax. In addition, it must be compatible with the impression material.
7. Finally, the type of restoration needs to be considered, because certain procedures (e.g., some all-ceramic crowns) require the strength of metal or epoxy resin and cannot be as readily fabricated on a weaker stone die.

The advantages and disadvantages of the available materials are summarized in Table 17-1.

AVAILABLE METHODS

Removable Dies. In a removable die system (see Fig. 17-1), the die is an integral component of the **master cast** and can be lifted from the cast to facilitate access. Precise relocation of the die in the master cast is critical to this system's success and is usually accomplished with brass pins or dowels (Fig. 17-5). When a single dowel is used, it should have at least one flat surface to provide resistance against rotation. Alternative methods (e.g., the popular Pindex* system [Fig. 17-6]), use multiple or interlocking dowels to ensure such resistance.

The cast is made in two pours of Type IV or V stone† of contrasting colors: the first forms the teeth, and the second forms the base of the cast. The area to be removed is coated with a separating agent before the second layer is poured. In other areas, undercuts are provided to prevent unwanted separation. The location and orientation of the dowels are critical; if they are improperly placed, the dowels will not allow the die of the prepared teeth to be withdrawn from the cast (Fig. 17-7).

In normal situations, dowels are positioned in the stone before it is set. However, drilling the cast and cementing the pins into the set stone are also possible.[25]

The Pindex system is designed to facilitate this latter technique. All removable die systems depend on careful execution so the die will separate cleanly and return to place accurately. One recent study found similar accuracy with four removable die systems, although the Pindex showed the least hori-

---

*ESPE America, Inc.: Norristown, Pa.
†SDS Kerr: Orange, Calif.

---

*Coltène/Whaledent, Inc: Mahwah, N.J.
†Type V stone, with greater expansion, will require less die spacing (see Chapter 18) to achieve the appropriate space for luting agent.

Die Materials

TABLE 17-1

	Advantages	Disadvantages	Recommended Use	Precautions
ADA Type IV stone	Dimensional accuracy Straightforward technique Low cost Straightforward in-office procedure	Will be damaged if not handled carefully Lower abrasion resistance	Most situations	Accurate proportioning essential Vacuum mix recommended
ADA Type V stone	Straightforward technique Low cost Straightforward in-office procedure Harder than Type IV	Increased expansion	Most situations	Accurate proportioning essential Vacuum mix recommended
Epoxy resin	High strength Good abrasion resistance	Polymerization shrinkage Time-consuming complex procedure	Complete ceramic crowns	Not compatible with polysulfide and hydrocolloid
Electroplating	High strength Good abrasion resistance	Time-consuming Special equipment needed	Complete ceramic crowns	Silver uses toxic cyanide Incompatible with many impression materials

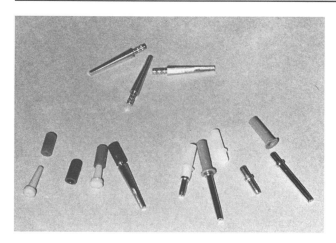

Fig. 17-5. Dowel pins.

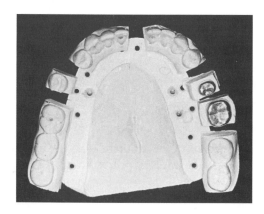

Fig. 17-6. Removable dies made with the Pindex (Whaledent) dowel system (see Fig. 17-20).

zontal movement, and the brass **dowel pins** produced the least occlusogingival reseating discrepancy.[26]

Solid Cast with Individual Die. The solid cast-and-individual die system, also referred to as

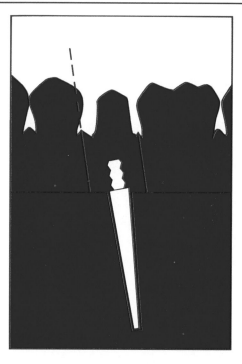

Fig. 17-7. Incorrect alignment of the dowel pin prevents removal of the die. The die will contact the proximal surface of the adjacent tooth *(dotted line).*

the *multiple-pour technique*, has certain advantages over the dowel-removable die system; its primary advantage is its simplicity. It may also be slightly more accurate.[27] When the impression is judged to be satisfactory, it is poured in Type IV or V stone in the area of the preparation(s) only. When set, it is separated. A second pour is then made of the entire arch. (Sometimes the second pour is used for an additional set of individual dies for polishing, and the solid cast is obtained from a third pour.)

The first pour, which is the most accurate, is trimmed into a die with a handle of sufficient length (similar to a tooth root [Fig. 17-8]). The complete arch cast (second pour) is mounted on an articulator. The wax pattern is started on the initial pour (the die) and is then transferred to the articulated cast for refinement of axial contours and occlusal anatomy (see Chapter 18). When completed, this pattern is returned to the die so the margins can be readapted immediately before investing.

An advantage of the solid cast-individual die system is that the working cast requires only minimum trimming. Since the gingival tissues around the prepared teeth are left intact, they can be used as a guide when contouring the restorations. Disadvantages of the solid cast technique include the following:

1. It may be difficult to transfer complex or fragile wax patterns from cast to die.
2. Seating the pattern on the master cast may be problematic because the second pour of

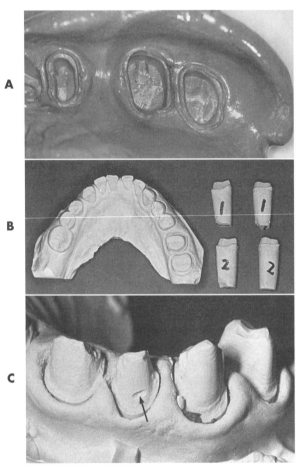

Fig. 17-8. **A,** An accurate impression is essential for successful fixed prostheses. **B,** The first and second pours have been sectioned into individual dies. The third pour will be the master cast. **C,** Small defects *(arrow)* can sometimes be overcome, but they make the laboratory phase much more difficult.

many impression materials is slightly larger than the first; therefore, it may be necessary to relieve the stone slightly to seat the pattern before occlusal evaluation.

3. The technique can be used only with elastomeric impression materials (if reversible hydrocolloid is used, separate impressions are needed for master cast and die).

Alternative Die Systems. The Di-Lok* technique (Fig. 17-9) uses a specially articulated tray for precise reassembly of a sectioned master cast. The impression is poured and the cast trimmed into a horseshoe configuration that fits in the special tray. The tray is filled with a second mix, and the cast is seated. When the stone has set, the tray is disassembled, saw cuts are made on each side of the preparation, and the resulting die is trimmed. The cast and die can be reassembled in the tray, which is then mounted on an articulator. A disadvantage of this system is that the overall size of the tray can make articulation and manipulation awkward and difficult.

The DVA Model System† (Fig. 17-10) and the Zeiser model system‡ (Fig. 17-11) use a precision drill and special baseplates that are aligned and drilled to provide die removal. These systems offer the advantage of allowing for the expansion of stone, which is relieved by the saw cuts.

CHOICE OF WORKING CAST-AND-DIE SYSTEM

The choice of a specific technique relies on operator preference and an assessment of each method's advantages and disadvantages. If they are conducted properly, all the available systems will achieve clinically acceptable accuracy.[28] When establishing a new relationship with a dental technician, it is important to determine which cast-and-die systems are preferred and why the technician has chosen them. Close cooperation between the dentist and technician is a key factor in fixed prosthodontics.

The solid cast technique simplifies cast and die fabrication, but it makes the waxing and porcelain stages more difficult. However, there is no need for special equipment, and the soft tissues immediately adjacent to the preparation are not removed (which facilitates contouring the gingival areas of the restorations). The use of a solid master cast precludes errors caused by incomplete seating of a removable die. In practice, this means that the components of a fixed partial denture can

---

*Di-Equi Dental Products: Wappingers Falls, N.Y.
†DVA Inc.: Corona, Calif.
‡Girrbach Dental GmbH: Pforzheim, Germany.

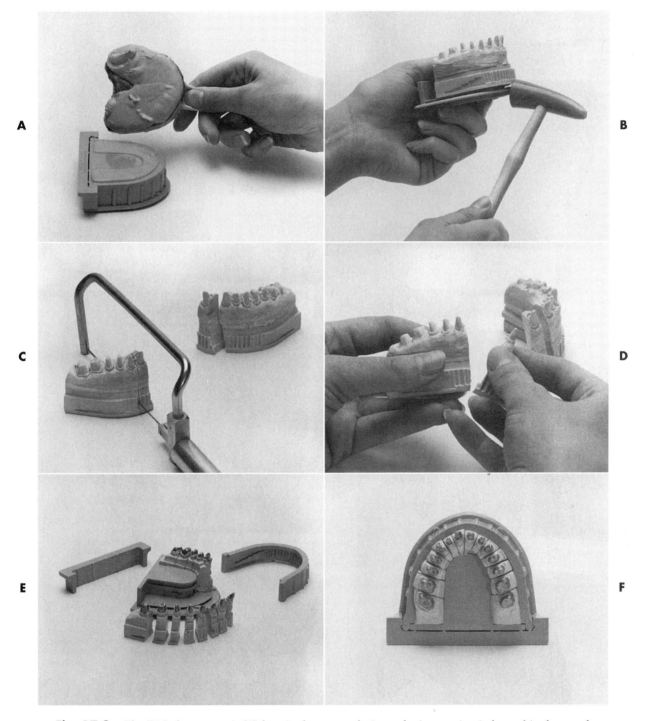

Fig. 17-9. The Di-Lok system. **A,** With a single-pour technique, the impression is formed in the usual way, and the Di-Lok tray is filled. Then the tray is inserted into the impression while the stone is still wet. **B,** After the die stone has fully set, the locking and curved arms of the tray are removed. The cast can then be removed by tapping the anterior pad of the tray base. **C,** The dies are sectioned by sawing three fourths through the stone and are separated **(D)** by breaking the remaining stone base. **E,** Trimmed dies. **F,** Assembled cast ready for articulating.
(Courtesy Di-Equi Dental Products Co.)

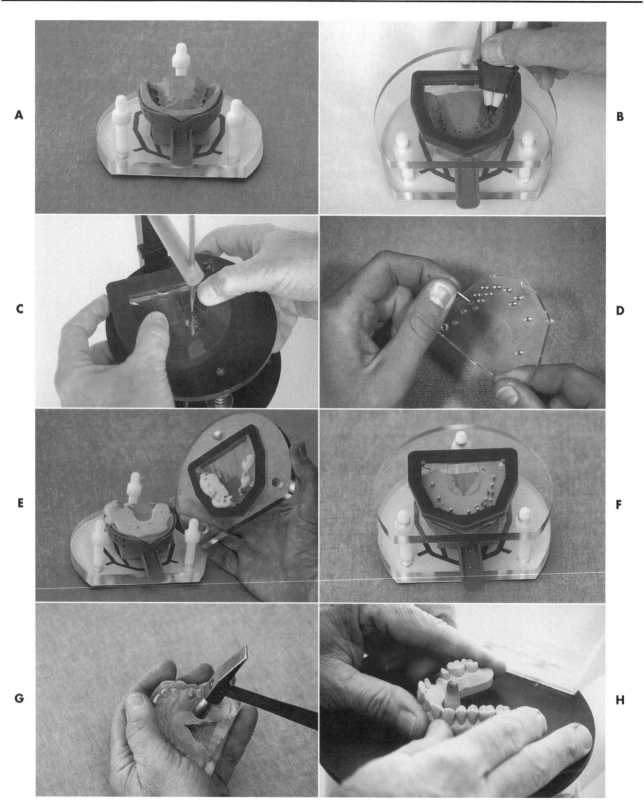

Fig. 17-10. DVA Model System. **A,** Trimmed impression on alignment fixture. **B,** Marking dowel pin locations on clear plate. **C,** Drilling holes for dowel pins as marked. **D,** Inserting dowels in the baseplate. An adhesive is not required. **E,** The impression is poured, stone is placed around dowel pins, and the alignment fixture is replaced over poured impression. **F, G,** Set cast is removed from baseplate and trimmed. **H,** Cast is trimmed.

Continued

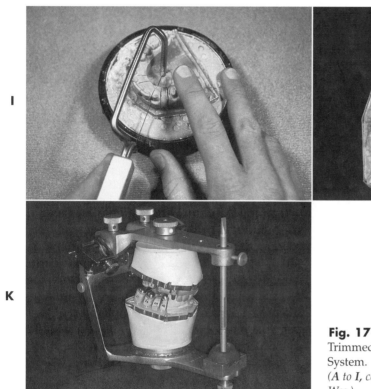

Fig. 17-10, cont'd. I, Cast is sectioned. J and K, Trimmed working casts using the DVA Model System.
(A to I, courtesy DVA, Inc. J and K, courtesy Dr. A.G. Wee.)

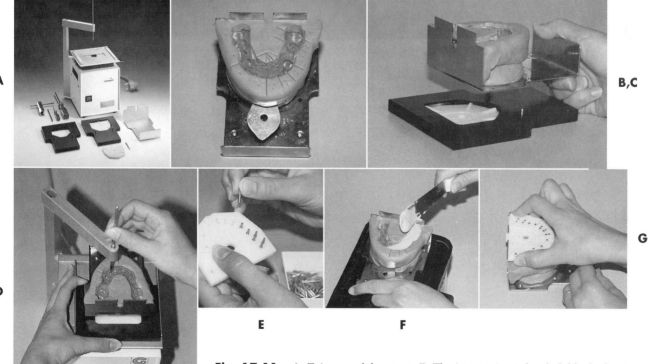

Fig. 17-11. A, Zeiser model system. B, The impression is leveled, blocked out with silcone putty, and positioned over the baseplate. C and D, The pin locations are determined and the pinholes drilled in the base. E, Pins are inserted into the base. F, The impression is poured and the base inverted into the stone (G).   *Continued*

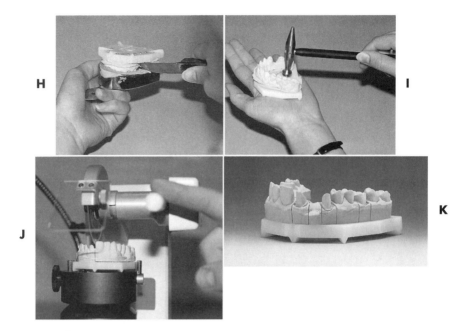

Fig. 17-11, cont'd. **H** and **I,** The cast is separated from the impression when set and then separated from the base. **J,** A precision saw aids sectioning. **K,** The sectioned cast. *(Courtesy Girrbach Dental GmbH.)*

Die Systems				TABLE **17-2**
	Advantages	Disadvantages	Recommended Use	Precautions
Solid cast with individual die	Straightforward procedure No special equipment	Awkward wax and porcelain manipulation	Most situations Can index with confidence from cast	Stone FPD abutment easily broken
Brass dowel pin	Removable die facilitates waxing and porcelain No special equipment	Difficult to master	Most situations	Care needed in cast pouring and dowel placement
Pindex (Whaledent)	Removable die Cast pouring unimpeded	Special equipment needed	Excellent if equipment well maintained	Careful attention to detail
Di-Lok (Di-Equi)	Removable die Cast pouring unimpeded Much less costly than Pindex	Bulky Care needed during reassembly	Awkward to use on some articulators	Care needed when making second pour
DVA Model System (DVA)	Removable die Cast pouring unimpeded Compensates for expansion of cast Single pour	Special equipment needed Quite technique sensitive	Excellent if carefully done	Care needed when seating pins
Zeiser (Girrbach)	Removable die Cast pouring unimpeded Compensates for expansion of cast Single pour	Special equipment needed	Excellent if carefully done	

be indexed from the cast for soldering; on the other hand, it also means that if an FPD is not accurately fabricated, the stone abutment teeth can be easily broken off, which makes subsequent steps more difficult.

The first pour from an elastomeric impression is the most accurate, and readapting the margins of the wax pattern on the first-pour die immediately before the pattern is invested is essential.

A dowel-and-removable die system's main advantage is that it requires less manipulation of the wax pattern, thus reducing the chances of breakage during transfer. In addition, the handling of porcelain restorations is easier, particularly if a porcelain labial margin is used. For these reasons, most technicians believe that the extra steps involved in making a cast with dowels and a removable die are worthwhile.

Nevertheless, the procedures are technically quite difficult. It is not rare to encounter dies that do not seat properly or that have poorly placed dowels. Difficulty also may be encountered in sawing the die out of the cast. Interproximal margins can easily be damaged during this procedure, particularly if clearance between a proximal preparation margin and the adjacent tooth is minimal.

The Pindex system uses a special drilling unit to ensure accurate pin placement. Careful model trimming of the initially poured cast is necessary before drilling the holes for the pins. If done properly, highly accurate and stable removable dies result; however, the cost of the additional equipment must be considered.

The advantages and disadvantages of these cast-and-die systems are summarized in Table 17-2.

TECHNIQUE

The technique for pouring stone dies is similar for most of the popular systems. To avoid repetition, the procedure using single dowel pins is described in detail, with an emphasis on the differences between the solid cast (multiple pour) system and the Pindex system.

Armamentarium (Fig. 17-12)
- Impression
- Small camel hair brush
- Type IV or V stone
- Water
- Surfactant
- Dowel pins ⎫
- Retention devices ⎬ depending on system used
- Orientation aids ⎭
- Vacuum mixer and bowl
- Mixing spatula
- Vibrator
- Petrolatum
- Pencil
- Die saw

After the impression has been removed from the patient's mouth, it is washed under running tap water, blown dry, inspected, and disinfected (see Chapter 14). When it is judged to be satisfactory, it is taken to the laboratory, where the necessary armamentarium should have been prepared for use before impression making. A vacuum mixer (e.g., the Vac-U-Spat*) is strongly recommended. At this time the impression can be sprayed with a surfactant or,

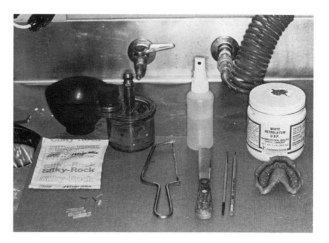

Fig. 17-12.   Armamentarium for pouring dies.

in the case of hydrocolloid, placed in a K_2SO_4 solution (if recommended by the manufacturer).

Step-by-step Procedure
1. If dowels are to be used, position them over the prepared teeth with one of the methods illustrated in Figure 17-13. Their correct location and orientation are important. For example, placing the head of a dowel too deep in the impression may weaken the die; positioning the dowel at an incorrect angle may make die removal impossible. At this stage, some technicians mark the best locations for the dowels in the buccal and lingual sulci or on the palate and place the dowels in the stone after it is poured, because prepositioning the dowels makes pouring more difficult. In addition, the relatively brittle sticky wax commonly used to lute the pins in place can break loose during vibration. If dowels are not prepositioned, the viscosity of the stone should be carefully gauged before dowel placement. If the stone is too runny, the dowels will not remain in place, and a new impression often must be made.
2. Measure the proper proportions of Type IV or V stone and water. To reduce air bubbles in the mix, the water should be placed in the mixing bowl first. The powder is then added and quickly incorporated by hand spatulation. NOTE: The spatula should be wiped clean on the blade of the mechanical mixer rather than on the edge of the mixing bowl, where stone can interfere with the vacuum seal (Fig. 17-14, A to C).

*Whip Mix Corporation: Louisville, Ky.

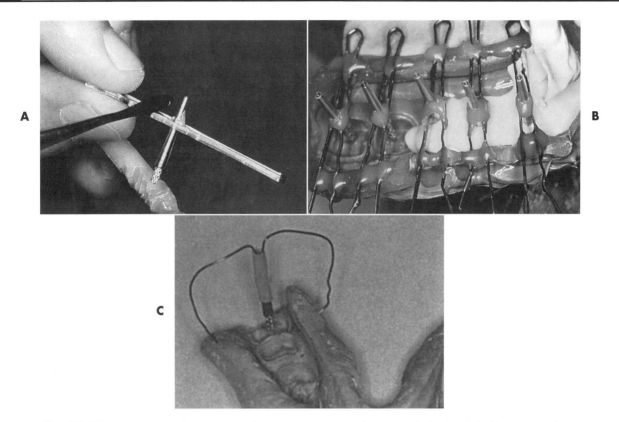

Fig. 17-13. Positioning dowel pins before cast pouring can be accomplished with bobby pins and sticky wax **(A, B)**, or a prefabricated wire-tube aid **(C)**.

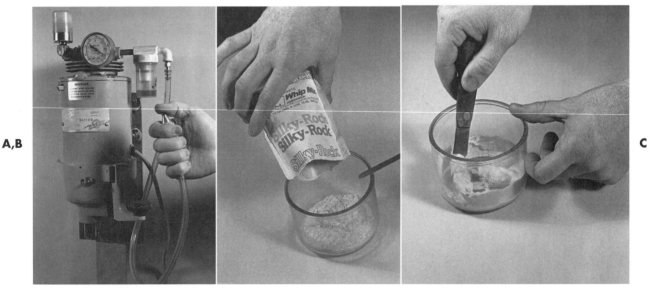

Fig. 17-14. Vacuum mixing ADA Type IV stone. **A,** To verify that the vacuum hose is not blocked and the pump is operating properly, put a thumb over the hose. The vacuum gauge should move from near 0 to about 700 mm (27 inches) Hg. **B,** Add stone to the water in the mixing bowl. **C,** Incorporate the particles by hand.   *Continued*

3. Close the mixing bowl, attach the vacuum hose, and turn on the pump.
4. Insert the drive shaft into the chuck of the mixer and mix the stone for the recommended time. Vibrate the mix to allow the

stone to settle in the bowl. The hose should be pulled out of the bowl before turning the vacuum off; otherwise, stone will sometimes be sucked into the vacuum hose. Whip Mix recommends leaving the mixer on for ap-

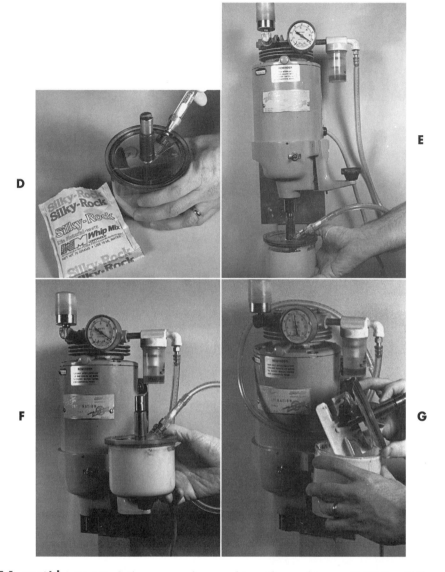

Fig. 17-14, cont'd. **D,** Attach the vacuum hose and turn the machine on. **E,** Wait until the vacuum gauge reaches 700 mm before engaging the drive chuck. Time the mix carefully, because this affects the physical properties of the material. **F,** Vibrate under vacuum. **G,** Remove the hose before turning off the power. This will prevent stone from being drawn into the hose.
(Courtesy Whip Mix Corporation.)

proximately 1 minute after removal of the hose to purge the pump of moisture (Fig. 17-14, *D* to *G*).

5. Blow any excess surfactant out of the impression, pick up a small amount of stone with a suitable brush or instrument, and place it in the most critical area (usually the occlusal aspect of narrow preparations or immediately adjacent to the sulcus area). For small preparations, a thin instrument (e.g., a periodontal probe) may prove helpful with this procedure. Bubbles will be trapped if too much stone is added abruptly or if two sizable masses of stone meet (Fig. 17-15). Therefore, small quantities of stone should be added incrementally in one area, allowing the stone to seek its own path (Fig. 17-16). During pouring, the tray should be held on a vibrator. For easy cleanup, the vibrator table can be covered with a paper towel or plastic bag.

6. Slowly tease the stone into the preparation along the axial walls by tilting the impression and guiding the material with the instrument. Be absolutely sure that the stone flows onto the margins of the preparation without trapping any air bubbles. Bubbles and voids are always a problem when pouring impressions. If the first pour is defective, do not pour a second, because some accuracy is lost. In addition, thin areas of the impression near the

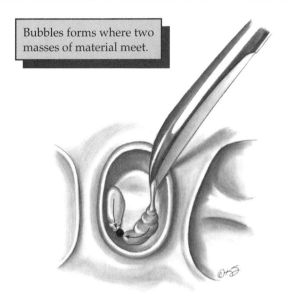

Bubbles forms where two masses of material meet.

Fig. 17-15. Incorrect technique for pouring an impression. An air bubble *(arrows)* will be trapped if two masses of stone are allowed to meet.

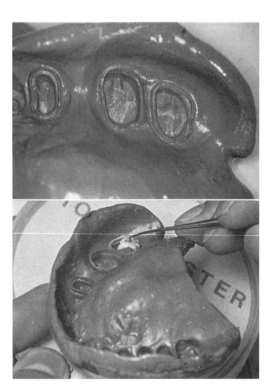

Fig. 17-16. Pouring an impression. To avoid trapping air, start with a very small amount of stone.

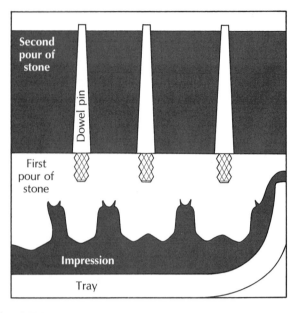

Fig. 17-17. Dowel pins must be carefully positioned so the first pour of stone completely covers the knurled head; otherwise, the parts will not separate cleanly. However, the stone should not extend onto the shaft and reduce stability.

have the lowest contact angle, meaning they are the easiest to pour[29,30]; silicones have the highest contact angle and are the most difficult to pour, although the newer "surface activated" or "hydrophilic" formulations are better.[31] Overall, however, these materials do not seem to greatly facilitate impression making.[32]

7. Place a second amount of stone on top of the first and continue with a third and so forth until the preparation is completely filled. The rest of the impression can then be filled to a height of at least 5 mm beyond the free gingival margins. In areas where individual dowels are used, the head of each dowel must be covered with stone (Fig. 17-17).

SOLID CAST-MULTIPLE POUR SYSTEM

For individual die pours, the stone mass must be built up to a height of approximately 25 mm to obtain a die handle of adequate length. The occlusal surfaces of teeth immediately adjacent to the preparation will be filled with stone, but this is of no concern (Fig. 17-18). When the first pour has set, the cast is separated and repoured. The first pour is then sectioned into individual dies.

---

margin are torn when separating the first pour. For this reason, pouring a bubble-free cast is essential to avoid having to make a new impression. The ease with which an impression can be poured without bubble formation depends on the contact angle that the advancing die stone makes when the impression is wetted. Of the elastomers, polyethers

8. Place retentive devices[33] in areas where there are no dowels so that the two layers of stone will not separate in the wrong place (Fig. 17-19).

9. Allow the stone to set for the recommended time (usually 30 minutes).

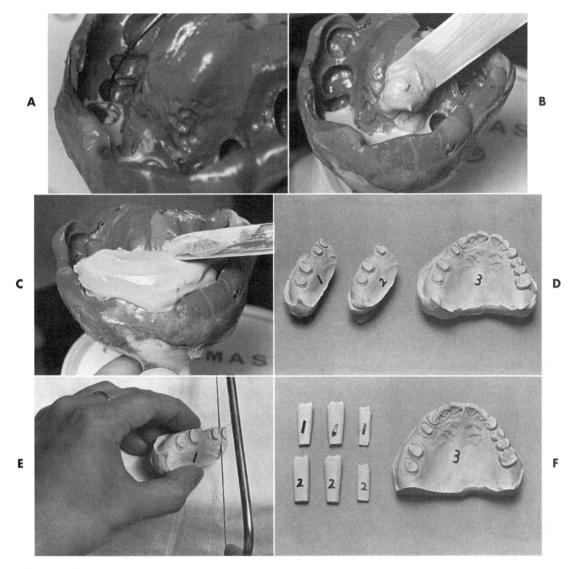

Fig. 17-18. Pouring an impression for individual dies and solid cast (multiple pour system). **A,** Be sure that the critical margin area is covered. **B,** Stone added in the preparation area only. **C,** Sufficient bulk for the die handles. **D,** Pours 1 and 2 (individual dies) and 3 (working cast). **E,** Sectioning the individual dies. **F,** The trimmed dies and working cast before articulation.

10. Inspect the area where separation is required, smooth it as necessary, and coat it with a separating medium (e.g., 10% sodium silicate). Then pour another layer to act as a base and retain the dowels. This second layer should not cover the tips of the dowels. If for some reason the base must be built up more, wax or rubber tubing can be placed on the tip of the dowel to facilitate its retrieval later. Before the base of a mandibular impression is poured, the lingual aspect should be blocked out with a suitable molding material (e.g., Mortite); otherwise, the stone will lock around the tray and hamper removal of the cast from the impression. This is much easier than grinding excess stone away later

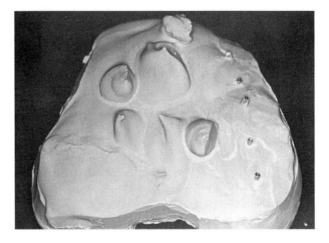

Fig. 17-19. Blobs of stone provide retention in parts of the cast where separation is not desired.

to gain access to the lingual aspect of mandibular preparations (Fig. 17-20). When the cast is separated from the impression, it must be carefully inspected for voids. If any are found in the marginal area of a prepared tooth, the cast is unusable and a new impression must be made. Careful pouring will prevent this. If the cast is satisfactory, it is ready for sectioning and trimming.

11. Trim the buccal and lingual sulcal areas adjacent to the removable sections first so the dies will separate cleanly.

PINDEX* SYSTEM

When the Pindex system is being used, the first pour of stone is removed from the impression once it has set. The base is then ground flat in a plane that must be perpendicular to the intended position of the Pindex pins. The periphery of the cast is trimmed to fit in a special mold. After the cast is dried, the location of the pins is marked and their holes are drilled with a special drill press. The pins are cemented in place with cyanoacrylate resin, special sleeves are positioned over the cemented pins, and the cast is positioned in the second pour that is made in the mold (Fig. 17-21).

Sawing between adjacent prepared teeth is difficult, particularly with small anteriors. If this procedure is not performed carefully, the saw cuts can contact the dowel pin, leading to an unusable die. When the Pindex system is used, removing the part of the first pour that contains the adjacent prepared teeth in one piece before making the critical saw cuts is advantageous. Then the cuts can be carefully marked and started from the base and the tooth side (see Fig. 17-21, M). When sawing from the base, it is important to protect the fragile dies with a soft cloth.

---

*Coltène/Whaledent, Inc: Mahwah, N.J.

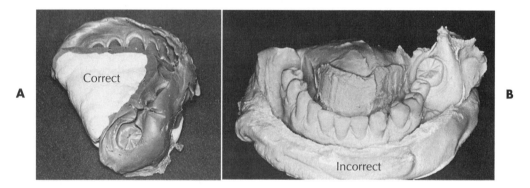

Fig. 17-20. **A,** Use a molding material to block out the lingual aspect before pouring a mandibular impression. **B,** Otherwise, excess stone will have to be ground away to obtain access to the lingual surfaces, which is a tedious process.

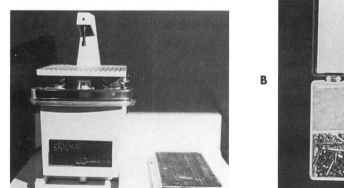
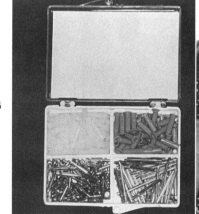
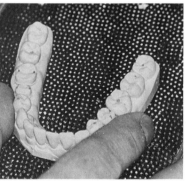

Fig. 17-21. The Pindex system consists of **(A),** a special drill press and **(B),** brass dowels and plastic sleeves. **C,** Pour the impression in stone, separate when set, and trim it to a "horseshoe" shape. The base must be absolutely flat (a trimmer is provided).   *Continued*

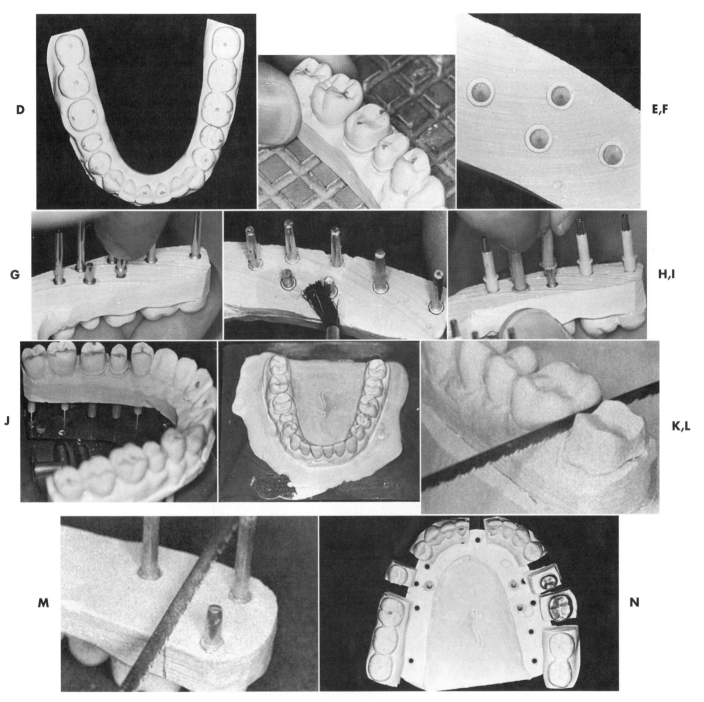

Fig. 17-21, cont'd. **D,** Mark the location of each dowel on the occlusal surface. Two dowels are needed to stabilize each segment. (Alternative single pins are available for small preparations.) **E,** Position the cast on the drill stage; a light indicates the location of the drill. Hold the cast firmly and depress the lever; this activates the drill, which penetrates into the cast. **F,** Each hole should be cleanly drilled; a hand reamer is available if necessary. **G,** Try in the pins and cement them to place. For accessibility, the short locating dowels should be used on the lingual surface. **H,** Coat with petrolatum to ensure clean separation. **I,** Position the plastic sleeves. **J,** Place the assembly in the special mold. **K,** Make the second pour of stone into the mold. **L,** Sawing the dies. **M,** With the Pindex system, removing the first pour and using it as a block and commencing sawing from the base is sometimes helpful. Marking all the saw cuts with a pencil is recommended. **N,** The Pindex cast after sectioning.
(Courtesy Dr. J. O. Bailey.)

12. Mark the position of each saw cut (which should be parallel to the dowel) with a pencil.

13. Carefully insert the saw blade between the preparation and the adjacent tooth; make sure that neither the margin nor the proximal contact is damaged (Fig. 17-22). The cuts must pass completely through the first layer of stone. If this is not done, the die will not separate cleanly. When the saw cuts are made, the dies can be tapped out and are ready for trimming for waxing. (Typical trimmed and untrimmed dies are shown in Figure 17-23.)

All excess stone, with the exception of the critical few millimeters immediately adjacent and cervical to the margin, should be removed with an Arbor band or another cutter in a lathe. The stone that is closer to the margin is removed with a large carbide bur. (Easy access to the margin is mandatory for waxing.) Any residual flash is trimmed away with a sharp scalpel. The margin must not be touched. A binocular microscope is helpful during this step. It is important not to create a ditch apical to the margin, which could lead to poor gingival contour in the completed restoration (Fig. 17-24).

When **die trimming** is completed, the dies are repositioned in the master cast, and their accurate and precise repositioning is verified. The master cast is then mounted on an articulator. NOTE: Trimmed dies must be handled carefully. To minimize potential breakage, they should be secured in a container lined with foam plastic, gauze, or cotton.

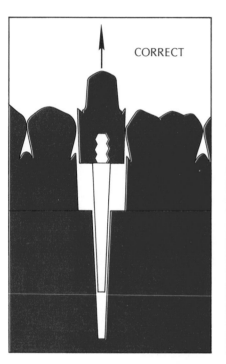

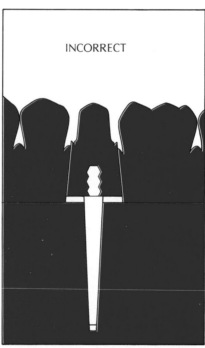

When sectioning the die, the saw cuts should be parallel to each other or should slightly converge (A). Be careful not to create an undercut (B), because the die then will not be readily removable from the cast. Cutting into a pin when sectioning the cast will render it useless, and a new cast will need to be made.

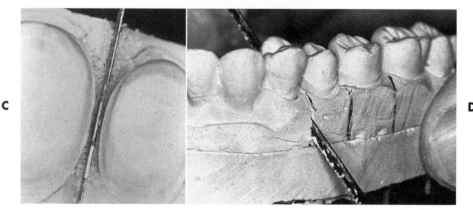

Fig. 17-22. Sectioning removable dies. **A,** The saw cuts should converge slightly toward the dowel; otherwise, **(B)** the die will be locked in by undercuts. **C,** Mark the intended saw cuts in pencil and carefully position the saw blade. It must not touch the prepared tooth. **D,** Saw completely through the first pour. NOTE: Finishing the cut short of the second pour will prevent a clean separation.

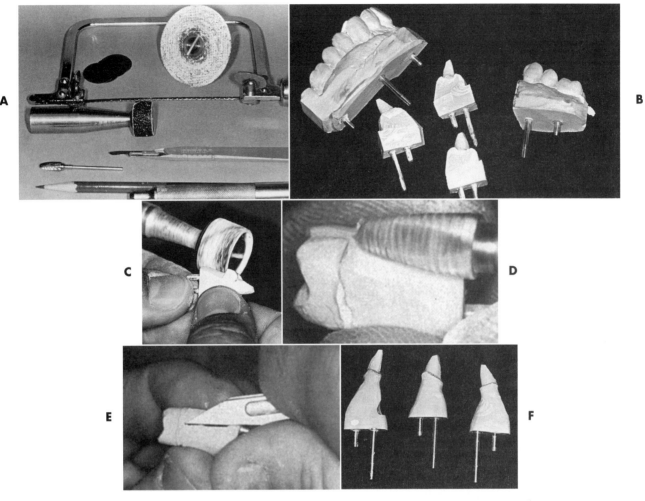

Fig. 17-23. Trimming dies. **A,** Armamentarium. **B,** Sectioned dies. In this instance, the Pindex system has been used. **C,** Bulk trimming is accomplished with an Arbor band on a lathe equipped with efficient dust collection. **D,** An acrylic-trimming bur is used near the margin. **E,** A sharp scalpel is used to trim to final contour, working away from the margin. **F,** The trimmed dies.
(**B, C,** and **F** courtesy Dr. W.V. Campagni.)

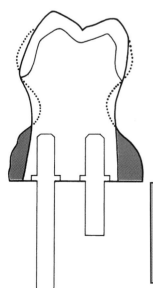

Fig. 17-24. Excessive trimming will lead to a bulky crown, because the trimmed die acts as a guide to gingival contour when the restoration is being waxed.

IMPORTANT! When trimming a die, the original contour of the tooth structure below the margin MUST be preserved. Overtrimming (*dotted line*) will result in overcontoured restorations!

MOUNTING CASTS ON AN ARTICULATOR

The articulation of diagnostic casts is discussed in Chapter 2. The technique for **mounting** a solid working (master) cast is identical. The procedure for attaching a working cast with removable dies to an articulator differs only in that access must be allowed to the area of the base into which the dowels penetrate. This will expedite removal of the dowels (Fig. 17-25).

WORKING CASTS VERSUS DIAGNOSTIC CASTS

The accuracy of the casts and their mounting is even more critical for working casts than for diagnostic casts. Although diagnostic casts can still provide the necessary information, even when mounted slightly inaccurately, working casts must be precisely mounted if lengthy chairside adjustment is to be avoided.

Diagnostic casts are most effectively mounted with a centric relation record (see Chapter 2). This allows the practitioner to visualize the full range of mandibular movement for occlusal diagnosis. The CR record is made at an increased vertical dimension (see Chapter 2). Closing the articulator upon re-

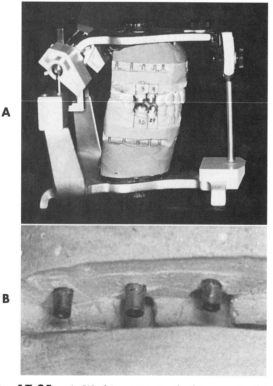

Fig. 17-25. **A,** Working cast attached to an articulator. **B,** To facilitate removal, the mounting should allow access to the end of each dowel.

moval of the record will induce error if an arbitrary facebow is used.[34] There is a slight error even if a kinematic facebow is used.[35] Although such errors are probably not clinically significant with diagnostic casts, they are significant when working casts are involved because the degree of inaccuracy is transferred to restorations fabricated and adjusted on the casts. Whenever possible, working casts should be mounted with a record made at the vertical dimension of occlusion, using maximum intercuspation of unprepared teeth.[36] If this is not possible, a kinematic facebow recording is recommended. Problems associated with mounting casts with a CR record using an arbitrary facebow have been analyzed by Weinberg.[37] He calculated that a 3-mm thick record can create an occlusal discrepancy in the first molar region of 0.2 mm when the arbitrary axis differs from the true hinge axis by 5 mm (a common error).

In addition, an elastomeric (rather than an irreversible hydrocolloid) impression should be made for the opposing cast. The elastomer's improved precision results in a more accurate opposing cast, which reduces the need to adjust the restoration at try-in.

REORGANIZED OCCLUSION

The decision to reorganize a patient's occlusion (e.g., by making CR coincide with MI) is made at the treatment-planning stage (see Chapter 3). Treatment steps may then include occlusal adjustment of the existing dentition by selective reshaping (see Chapter 6) and reorganization of the anterior (incisal) guidance before tooth preparation for definitive cast restorations.

The following question should be asked during treatment planning: Is there any discernible pathology that may have arisen from malocclusion? In the presence of wear facets, widened periodontal ligament spaces, and muscle tenderness, the potential benefits of occlusal adjustment should be weighed. This question must also be asked: Will reorganization of the occlusion benefit the patient? If the answer is yes, occlusal adjustment can be performed (see Chapter 6), after which definitive tooth preparation for fixed prosthodontics should be initiated.

The working casts can then be related at the vertical dimension of occlusion with one of several techniques. Autopolymerizing resin may be used to record the relationship (Fig. 17-26). Alternative materials include impression plaster, zinc oxide-eugenol impression paste on a suitable carrier (e.g., autopolymerizing acrylic resin or gauze), and some

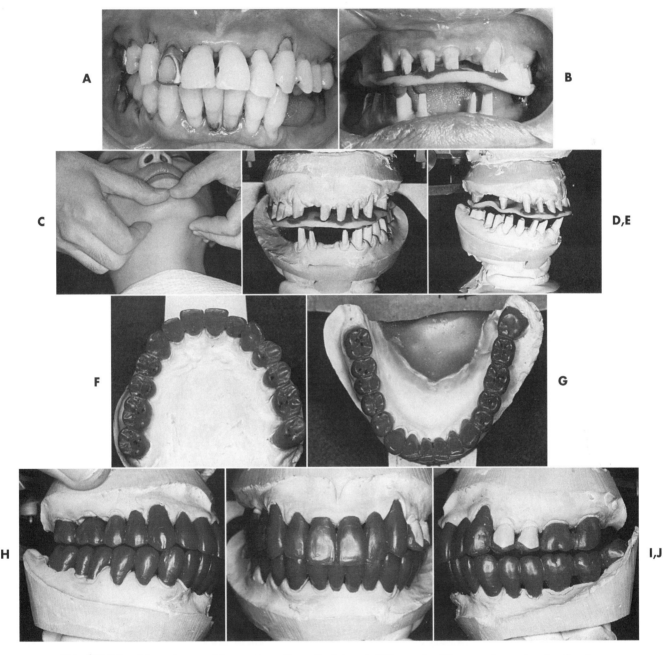

Fig. 17-26. Mounting working casts on the articulator. **A,** When a dentition requires extensive fixed prosthodontic care, accuracy of the articulation is essential to successful treatment. **B,** Recording centric relation at the vertical dimension of occlusion minimizes the error inherent in a facebow transfer. Autopolymerizing acrylic resin was used as the recording medium. **C,** Manipulation of the mandible into centric relation. **D, E,** Working casts articulated with the CR record interposed. **F to J,** Restorations waxed to anatomic contour, with anterior guidance. *Continued*

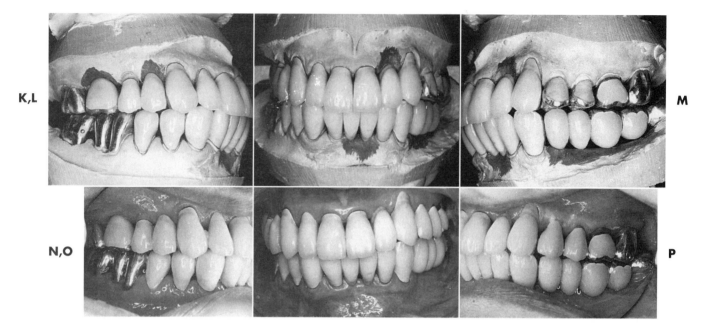

Fig. 17-26, cont'd.   K to M, Metal-ceramic restorations on the working cast. N to P, The completed restorations (see Fig. 32-41).

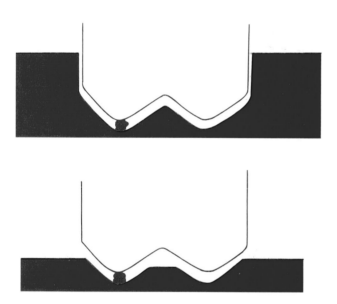

Fig. 17-27.   Trimming the centric relation record. An untrimmed record **(A)** makes assessment of proper cast seating much more difficult than a properly trimmed record **(B)**.

of the stiffer elastomers (polyether or polyvinyl siloxane).

These records are optimal if they include only the cusp tips (Fig. 17-27). If more detail of the grooves is inadvertently captured, it should be carefully trimmed away. Otherwise, the cast will not

seat properly and the restoration will be in supraclusion.

CONFORMATIVE OCCLUSION

On many occasions a cast restoration that conforms to the patient's existing occlusion is made, even if a discrepancy exists between CR and maximum intercuspation position. Typically, if no significant signs of clinical pathology are detected, fabricating simple prostheses in the stable MI position is acceptable. The objective is to maintain rather than reorganize a healthy masticatory apparatus.

When a patient has a symptom-free occlusion and requires relatively few cast restorations (i.e., when only a small part of the dentition needs to be restored), the MI position is the most desirable treatment. Therefore, many patients who need only one or two single crowns (or a small FPD) are best restored to conform with their existing occlusion.

Articulating a working cast for a restoration that is to be waxed conformatively poses certain problems. If the cast is mounted with a CR record (as described for diagnostic casts in Chapter 2), the MI position will not be reproduced accurately enough for precise waxing because it will be in a translated mandibular position. This position cannot be reached with absolute precision on a semi-adjustable articulator. In addition, during closing

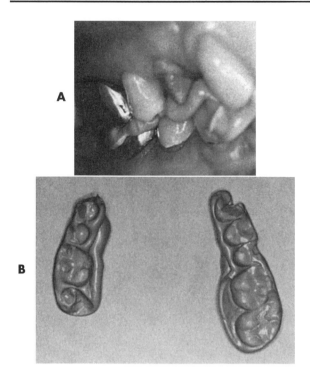

Fig. 17-28. **A,** Conformative interocclusal record made with poly(vinyl siloxane) polymer. **B,** The records before trimming.

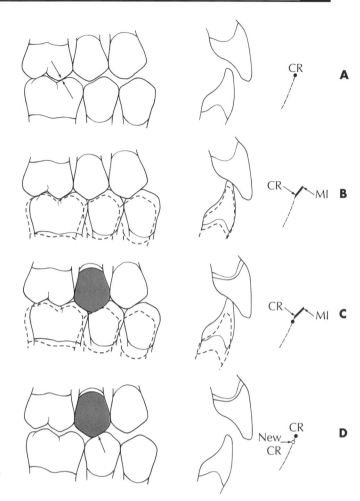

Fig. 17-29. When providing a restoration that conforms to an existing occlusion, it is important to assess both CR and MI carefully. **A,** Before treatment, the CR contact in this patient was on the first molar *(arrows)*. **B,** Preoperative MI. **C,** The new restoration conforms to MI satisfactorily, but notice in **D** that a new CR interference *(arrow)* has been created.

of the instrument, the stone cast can be easily damaged.

Probably the most practical solution is to articulate the working cast in the intercuspal position using a small interocclusal record (e.g., with poly[vinyl siloxane]) interposed between the tooth preparation and the opposing arch in the closed position (Fig. 17-28). At try-in, after the restoration has been fabricated, the patient's CR closure is examined clinically to ascertain that the restoration conforms with the preexisting occlusion. No premature contacts should occur on the new restoration. In CR closure, new occlusal interferences can be introduced on the restoration, and the discrepancy between CR and MI may be effectively increased, leading to new problems (Fig. 17-29). It is then necessary to adjust the restoration to permit the original closing movement of the patient and to provide a smooth transition from the CR to the MI position.

VERIFICATION OF MOUNTING

It is essential to check the accuracy of the articulation before proceeding with the laboratory phase of treatment. For less complex fixed prosthodontics, this can be simply accomplished by comparing the occlusal contacts in the patient's mouth with those made by the casts. (Mylar shim stock or articulating film is suitable.) Occlusal wax (see Chapter 6) is also useful. For more extensive procedures, a second occlusal record is needed that can be compared with the first by using a split-cast mounting technique or a system such as the Vericheck* (see Figs. 2-22; Fig. 17-30).

---

*Teledyne Water Pik: Fort Collins, Colo.

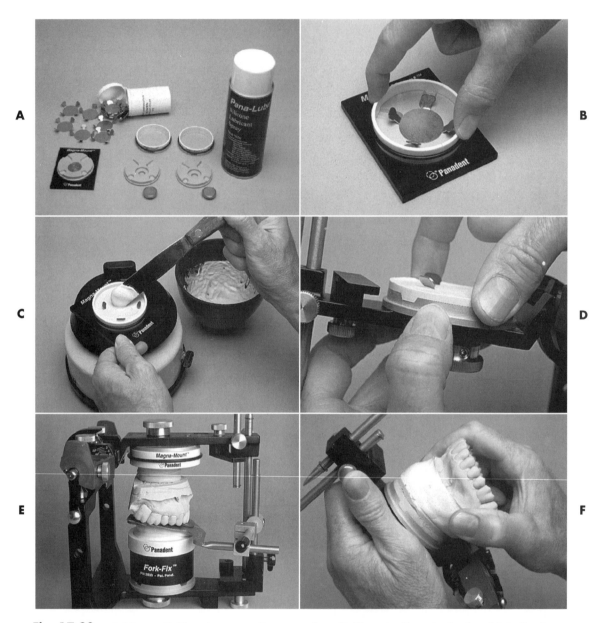

Fig. 17-30. **A,** Magna-Split system mounting procedure. **B,** The retention star is placed into the former and sprayed with silicone. **C,** Mounting stone is poured into the former and allowed to set. **D,** The hardened stone index plate is mated to the semi-permanently attached mounting plate on the articulator. **E,** Mount casts as usual. (Also shown is the Fork-Fix system for supporting the bite fork.) **F,** Mounted casts can be simply removed and replaced by pulling away from the articulator.
(Courtesy Panadent Corp.)

SUMMARY

Accurate working casts and dies are essential to successful cast restorations. There are various materials and techniques that provide an extremely precise reproduction of the prepared teeth. Type IV stone is recommended in most instances, although it requires careful handling to avoid chipping or abrading margins. Epoxy resin and electroplated silver or copper are durable alternatives. The die of the prepared tooth can be made removable by the use of dowels or the more convenient Pindex system. Alternatively, a solid working cast and separate die can be used. Whatever system is chosen, it must articulate precisely with an accurately made opposing cast.

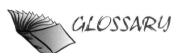

GLOSSARY

block out: *adj 1:* elimination of undesirable undercuts on a cast, *2:* the process of applying wax on another similar temporary substance to undercut portions of a cast so as to leave only those undercuts essential to the planned construction of a prosthesis. A blocked out cast may also include other surface modifications needed relative to the construction of the prosthesis

cyanoacrylate: *n* (20c) a single component, moisture activated, thermoplastic, group of adhesives characterize by rapid polymerization and excellent bond strength

definitive cast: a replica of the tooth surfaces, residual ridge areas, and/or other parts of the dental arch and/or facial structures used to fabricate a dental restoration or prosthesis

dental cast: a positive life size reproduction of a part or parts of the oral cavity

dental stone: the alpha-form of calcium sulfate hemihydrate with physical properties superior to the beta-form (dental plaster). The alpha-form consists of cleavage fragments and crystals in the form of rods or prisms, and is therefore more dense than the beta-form

dowel pin: a metal pin used in stone casts to remove die sections and replace them accurately in the original position

electroplating: *vt* (ca. 1864): the process of covering the surface of an object with a thin coating of metal by means of electrolysis

epoxy resin die: a reproduction formed in epoxy resin

gypsum: *n* (14c) the natural hydrated form of calcium sulfonate, $CaSO_4$ $2H_2O$ gypsum dihydrate

master cast: see definitive cast

mounting: *v* the laboratory procedure of attaching a cast to an articulator or cast relator

plaster: *n* a pastelike composition (usually of water, lime, and sand) that hardens on drying and is used for coating walls, ceilings, and partitions—slang: in dentistry, a colloquial term applied to dental plaster of paris

vacuum mixing: a method of mixing a material such as plaster of paris or casting investment below atmospheric pressure

REFERENCES

1. American Dental Association, Council on Dental Materials and Devices: Specification no. 19 for non-aqueous, elastomeric dental impression materials, *J Am Dent Assoc* 98:733, 1977.
2. Schelb E et al: Compatibility of Type IV dental stone with polysulfide impression materials, *J Prosthodont* 1:32, 1992.
3. Omana HM et al: Compatibility of impressions and die stone material, *Oper Dent* 15:82, 1990.
4. Toreskog S et al: Properties of die materials: a comparative study, *J Prosthet Dent* 16:119, 1966.
5. Fukui H et al: Effectiveness of hardening films on die stone, *J Prosthet Dent* 44:57, 1980.

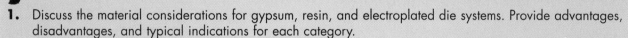

Study Questions

1. Discuss the material considerations for gypsum, resin, and electroplated die systems. Provide advantages, disadvantages, and typical indications for each category.
2. Contrast the advantages, disadvantages, and limitations of the following working cast and dies systems:
   A. Solid cast with individual die
   B. Single brass dowel pin
   C. Pindex
   D. Di-Lok
   E. DVA
3. Discuss the Pindex system in a step-by-step fashion. Identify critical steps and precautions.
4. When articulating working casts, which interocclusal record system results in the most accurate mounting? Why?

6. Campagni WV et al: Measurement of coating agents used for surface protection of stone dies, *J Prosthet Dent* 55:470, 1986.

7. Zakaria MR et al: The effects of a liquid dispersing agent and a microcrystalline additive on the physical properties of type IV gypsum, *J Prosthet Dent* 60:630, 1988.

8. Alsadi S et al: Properties of gypsum with the addition of gum arabic and calcium hydroxide, *J Prosthet Dent* 76:530, 1996.

9. Wee AG et al: Evaluation of the accuracy of solid implant casts, *J Prosthodont* 7:161, 1998.

10. Yaman P, Brandau HE: Comparison of three epoxy die materials, *J Prosthet Dent* 55:328, 1986.

11. Chaffee NR et al: Dimensional accuracy of improved dental stone and epoxy resin die materials. I. Single die, *J Prosthet Dent* 77:131, 1997.

12. Schaffer H et al: Distance alterations of dies in sagittal direction in dependence of the die material, *J Prosthet Dent* 61:684, 1989.

13. Chaffee NR et al: Dimensional accuracy of improved dental stone and epoxy resin die materials. II. Complete arch form, *J Prosthet Dent* 77:235, 1997.

14. Derrien G, Le Menn G: Evaluation of detail reproduction for three die materials by using scanning electron microscopy and two-dimensional profilometry, *J Prosthet Dent* 74:1, 1995.

15. Nomura GT et al: An investigation of epoxy resin dies, *J Prosthet Dent* 44:45, 1980.

16. Stackhouse JA: Electrodeposition in dentistry: a review of the literature, *J Prosthet Dent* 44:259, 1980.

17. Crispin BJ et al: Silver-plated dies. II. Marginal accuracy of cast restorations, *J Prosthet Dent* 51:768, 1984.

18. Cassimaty EM, Walton TR: Effect of three variables on the accuracy and variability of electroplated copper dies, *Int J Prosthodont* 9:547, 1996.

19. Crispin BJ et al: Silver-plated dies. I. Platability of impression materials, *J Prosthet Dent* 51:631, 1984.

20. Nash RW, Rhyne KM: New flexible model technique for fabricating indirect composite inlays and onlays, *Dent Today* 9:26, 1990.

21. Roberts DB: Flexible casts used in making indirect interim restorations, *J Prosthet Dent* 68:372, 1992.

22. Rada RE: In-office fabrication of indirect composite-resin restorations, *Pract Periodont Aesthet Dent* 4:25, 1992.

23. Trushkowsky RD: One-visit composite onlay utilizing a new flexible model material, *Am J Dent* 1:55, 1997.

24. Gerrow JD, Price RB: Comparison of the surface detail reproduction of flexible die material systems, *J Prosthet Dent* 80:485,1998.

25. Smith CD et al: Fabrication of removable stone dies using cemented dowel pins, *J Prosthet Dent* 41:579, 1979.

26. Serrano JG et al: An accuracy evaluation of four removable die systems, *J Prosthet Dent* 80:575, 1998.

27. Aramouni P, Millstein P: A comparison of the accuracy of two removable die systems with intact working casts, *Int J Prosthodont* 6:533, 1993.

28. Covo LM et al: Accuracy and comparative stability of three removable die systems, *J Prosthet Dent* 59:314, 1988.

29. Chong YH et al: Relationship between contact angles of die stone on elastomeric impression materials and voids in stone casts, *Dent Mater* 6:162, 1990.

30. Lepe X et al: Effect of mixing technique on surface characteristics of impression materials, *J Prosthet Dent* 79:495, 1998.

31. Vassilakos N, Fernandes CP: Surface properties of elastomeric impression materials, *J Dent* 21:297, 1993.

32. Boening KW et al: Clinical significance of surface activation of silicone impression materials, *J Dent* 26:447, 1998.

33. Balshi TJ, Mingledorff EB: Matches, clips, needles, or pins, *J Prosthet Dent* 34:467, 1975.

34. Walker PM: Discrepancies between arbitrary and true hinge axes, *J Prosthet Dent* 43:279, 1980.

35. Bowley JF et al: Reliability of a facebow transfer procedure, *J Prosthet Dent* 67:491, 1992.

36. Peregrina A, Reisbick MH: Occlusal accuracy of casts made and articulated differently, *J Prosthet Dent* 63:422, 1990.

37. Weinberg LA: An evaluation of the face-bow mounting, *J Prosthet Dent* 11:32, 1961.

CHAPTER EIGHTEEN

WAX PATTERNS

KEY TERMS

cement space
connector location
curve of Spee
curve of Wilson
cusp-fossa occlusion

cusp-marginal ridge occlusion
emergence profile
lost-wax process
proximal contact location

A large percentage of time and effort spent in fabricating fixed prostheses is devoted to producing a very accurate wax pattern. From this pattern, the finished cast restoration is duplicated by using the **lost-wax process** as part of the indirect procedure.

This technique consists of obtaining an accurate impression of the prepared tooth (Fig. 18-1, *A*) and making a cast from the impression (Fig. 18-1, *B*) on which a wax pattern that resembles the shape of the final restoration is shaped (Fig. 18-1, *C*). A mold is then made around the wax pattern with a refractory investment material (Fig. 18-1, *D*). When the investment has set, the wax is vaporized in an electric furnace. The hollow mold is then filled with molten casting alloy, reproducing every detail of the wax pattern (Fig. 18-1, *E*). The metal casting is retrieved, excess metal is removed, and after polishing, the cast restoration is ready for clinical evaluation (Fig. 18-1, *F*). As

> The lost-wax casting technique dates to the Bronze Age (approximately 3000-3500 BCE), when sand stone molds were used to cast molten metal. Today, the underlying principles remain virtually identical.

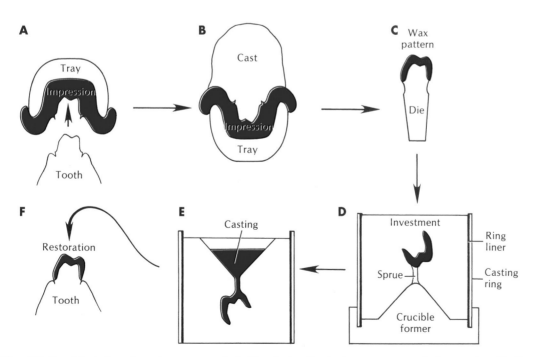

Fig. 18-1. Most dental castings are made indirectly by the lost-wax process. **A,** Impression. **B,** Cast. **C,** Wax pattern on die. **D,** The pattern is attached with sprue to a rubber crucible former and invested. **E,** Casting. **F,** Cemented restoration.

the solidifying metal (casting) cools to room temperature, it shrinks. Dimensional accuracy of the casting is achieved by balancing this shrinkage against precisely controlled expansion of the mold (see Chapter 22). Wax is used to make the patterns because it can be conveniently manipulated and precisely shaped. By heating, it can be completely eliminated from the mold after investing.

The lost-wax technique is widely used in industrial and jewelry manufacturing. The first bronze castings reportedly were made in the third millennium BCE with beeswax and clay refractory materials. Ancient lost-wax castings such as Chinese bronzes, Egyptian deities, and Greek statues have withstood the centuries, yielding information about ancient societies and cultures. The lost-wax method may have been used in Sumeria as early as the Second Early Dynastic Period for figurines and even larger body parts.[1]

In dentistry, *successful results depend on careful handling of the wax*. The practitioner must understand that every defect or void in the wax will appear in the casting. Most defects can be corrected easily in wax, but not in a metal casting. More often than not, compensating for an error in waxing technique is impossible once the metal casting has been formed. Careful evaluation of the pattern, preferably under magnification, is critical to obtaining a good casting.

This chapter approaches the waxing procedure in a logical sequence. As with most aspects of fixed prosthodontics, a successful restoration is possible only if each step is carefully followed and evaluated before moving to the next.

PREREQUISITES

The working die and master cast may require small modifications before waxing is started. Depending on the procedure, the size of the die can be slightly increased by applying a thin layer of painted-on spacer, which helps obtain a slightly larger internal diameter of the restoration.

CORRECTION OF DEFECTS

Even a very small undercut on the die of a tooth preparation will result in an inability to remove the wax pattern. There may be small dimples in the die (resulting from caries removal or loss of a previous restoration) that are undercut relative to the path of placement of the new restoration. Normally such areas are blocked out intraorally with glass ionomer or restored with amalgam or another suitable foundation material as part of the mouth preparation phase (see Chapter 6). Occasionally, however, blocking them out on the working die may be more practical and convenient, as long as the defect does not extend to within 1 mm of the cavity margin. Zinc phosphate cement is a suitable material, but other commercial products (e.g., resin) are available for this purpose (Fig. 18-2).

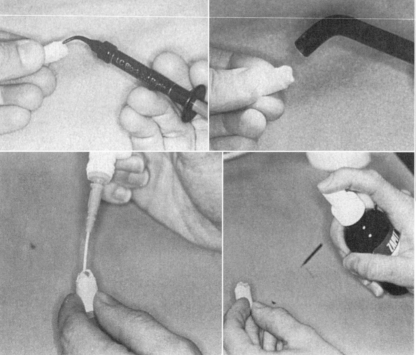
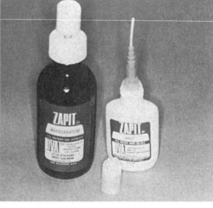

A,B

C

D,E

Fig. 18-2. Blocking out undercuts on a die. **A,** Photopolymerizing resin being applied. **B,** Resin light-cured. **C,** Autopolymerized resin. **D,** Resin is applied. **E,** Monomer spray.

PROVISION OF ADEQUATE CEMENT SPACE

Since the 1920s,[2] practitioners have recognized that a space should exist between the internal surface of the casting and the prepared surface of the tooth everywhere except immediately adjacent to the margin. The space provides room for the luting agent and allows complete seating of the restoration during cementation (see Chapters 7 and 31). At the preparation margin, there should be a band of close adaptation (about 1 mm wide) to prevent dissolution of the luting agent. The ideal dimension[3-5] for the **cement space** has been suggested at 20 to 40 μm for each wall, which implies that a complete crown should have an internal diameter between 40 and 80 μm larger than the diameter of the prepared tooth. By using available techniques in an appropriately standardized manner, such a degree of casting adaptation can routinely be obtained, independent of the geometry of the finish-line.[6,7]

If the cement space is too narrow, the casting will not seat properly during cementation because of hydraulic pressure that develops when the viscous mass of luting agent cannot escape through the narrow gap between crown and preparation as the restoration is seated. Conversely, if the cement space is too wide, the casting will be loose on the tooth, resistance form (see Chapter 7) will be reduced, and the position of the casting will be difficult to maintain accurately during evaluation and occlusal adjustment. In addition, the risk of the crown loosening during function increases considerably, and its longevity is adversely affected. The precise amount of cement space obtained depends on the materials and techniques used in the indirect process, particularly the choice of impression material (see Chapter 14), die material (see Chapter 17), investment (see Chapter 22), and casting alloy (see Chapters 19 and 22 and Fig. 18-1). These factors directly affect the size of the cement space.

Increasing the Cement Space. A number of factors increase the cement space for a complete crown:
1. Thermal and polymerization shrinkage of the impression material (see Chapter 14)
2. Use of a solid cast with individual stone dies (see Chapter 17)
3. Use of an internal (initial) layer of soft wax
4. Use of die spacers
5. Increased expansion of the investment mold (see Chapter 22)
6. Removal of metal from the fitting surface by grinding, airborne-particle abrasion, etching with aqua regia, or electrochemical milling

All factors being equal, the factors just mentioned result in an increased distance between the internal surface of the casting and the surface of the prepared tooth. Although the dentist has little control over the polymerization shrinkage of impression materials, die system selection has a direct influence on the size of the wax pattern. Using a multiple pour system for fabrication of a solid master cast and a separate die will yield a die that is slightly larger with some impression materials, effectively stretching the pattern, which results in a proportionally larger casting. An internal layer of soft wax is subject to slightly more compression by the setting refractory investment material, leading to a looser fit. Spacers enlarge the die by coating the occlusal surface and vertical axial walls with a thin layer of rapidly drying paint. The expansion of the investment mold can be increased by heating the mold to a slightly higher temperature during the wax elimination phase, and metal can be removed from the internal surface of a cast crown through air-abrasion, etching, or milling procedures.

Reduction of the Cement Space. A number of factors reduce the cement space:
1. Use of resin or electroplated dies
2. Use of alloys with a higher melting range
3. Reduced expansion of the investment

Resin and electroplated dies are slightly smaller than stone dies and will therefore result in a smaller casting. As alloys cool over a larger temperature range, the additional shrinkage that takes place will cause the same. If the investment is mixed with an adjusted water/powder ratio resulting in less setting expansion, the size of the resulting casting is again reduced. When problems routinely surface with castings that are either too loose or too tight, any of the previously mentioned variables may be altered, leading to more predictable results.

Problems with fitting castings become apparent at two stages of the indirect procedure: when the casting is tried on the die and when it is cemented. Recognizing problems at each stage and correcting them before proceeding is crucial. Difficulty with seating the casting on the die is generally due to *wax distortion*, the presence of *flash* extending cervical to the preparation margin (excess wax that was not removed before the investing and casting procedure), *improper investment expansion* (underexpansion), or a *casting nodule* (Fig. 18-3). Modification of the investing and casting protocol will solve these problems (see Chapter 22). Consistent problems with castings that do not seat completely when tried on the prepared tooth may be corrected by changing just one variable in the protocol. Although most practitioners

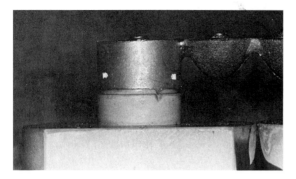

Fig. 18-3. This experimental near-cylindrical casting failed to seat because of inadequate expansion of the investment, not inadequate die spacing.

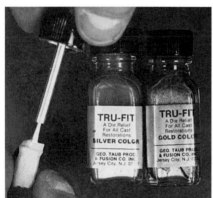

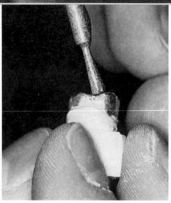

Fig. 18-4. Applying die spacer. Care must be taken to keep the material at least 1 mm from the margin.

advocate the routine use of die spacer, this is just one of many options to influence the size of the resulting cement space.

Die Spacer (Fig. 18-4). This material (similar to model airplane paint[8]) is applied to the die to increase the cement space between axial walls of the prepared tooth and the restoration. It is formulated to maintain constant thickness when painted on the die. However, it should not coat the entire preparation. For adequate marginal adaptation, a band of

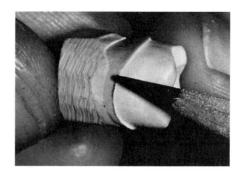

Fig. 18-5. Marking the preparation margin. Note that the side of the colored pencil tip is used to keep line width to a minimum.

about 1 mm must be left unpainted.[9] Thinner is provided to replace the solvent, which tends to evaporate, resulting in an excessive thickness of spacer.

MARKING THE MARGINS

The technician's awareness of the cavosurface margin's location is very important. By marking it with colored pencil, the technician can pinpoint this location (Fig. 18-5). The color should contrast with that of the wax that will be used (e.g., a red pencil can be used for a green wax). An ordinary lead pencil is not recommended, because it can abrade the die, its darker color can interfere with efforts to verify that the wax was properly adapted at the margin, and traces of the graphite (an antiflux) can prevent complete casting of the margins. The marked margins can be coated with low-viscosity cyanoacrylate resin and immediately blown dry. If performed properly, this procedure will add no more than a micrometer[10] to the die. Although removing the excess with acetone is sometimes possible, care must be taken not to create a thick layer of cyanoacrylate, which can result in an unacceptable fit of the final cast restoration. For this reason, higher-viscosity resins should be avoided.

MATERIALS SCIENCE

M.H. Reisbick

Inlay casting wax (the name given all wax used in forming the pattern for cast restorations) is actually composed of several waxes. Paraffin is usually the main constituent (40% to 60%). The remaining balance consists of dammar resin (to reduce flaking) plus carnauba, ceresin, or candelilla wax (to raise the melting temperature), or beeswax. Sometimes a synthetic wax is substituted for the natural material. Dyes are added to provide color contrasts. Exact formulations are trade secrets, but Coleman[11] has published the formula for an experimental compound.

The American National Standards Institute (ANSI) and the American Dental Association (ADA)[12] have categorized waxes into two types:

1. Type I—a medium wax (generally used with the direct technique for making patterns in the oral cavity)
2. Type II—a softer wax (generally used for the indirect fabrication of castings)

Waxes used with direct techniques must not flow appreciably at mouth temperature. Those used with indirect techniques must resist flow at room temperature to maintain their newly shaped forms.

Specifications of the ANSI and ADA govern the important properties of residue, flow, and expansion. Because the mold must burn out cleanly to allow the escape of gases and the complete entry of molten alloy, there can be no residual ash. However, the specifications allow a 0.1% residue, which apparently is effectively negligible. Flow requirements, as previously stated, are necessary to control the stability of the wax once it has reached the temperature at which it is carved, burnished, and polished (37° C [99° F] for direct-type, 25° C [77° F] for indirect-type waxes). In addition, the wax must flow well at typical forming temperatures. Curves of temperature plotted against percentage flow (Fig. 18-6) are furnished by reputable manufacturers and should be consulted when choosing a casting wax. All waxes expand or contract when heated or cooled. Manufacturers' curves of percentage expansion and contraction at various working temperatures (Fig. 18-7) are helpful when considering methods to use in the investing and casting process. For example, a wax that solidifies at a higher temperature will shrink more and will therefore require more compensation to control fit than a wax that solidifies at a lower temperature (a reason for not interchanging Type I and Type II waxes within an established technique). These properties can be adversely affected by repeated heating of the wax, which will drive off the more volatile components.[13] When selecting waxes for optimal casting accuracy, the use of waxes with different properties for the margin and occlusal portions may be necessary.[14] If a casting is to be accurate, the wax pattern must not become significantly distorted. One cause of distortion is that wax has "memory," which means that it exhibits some elasticity unless it is thoroughly liquefied. This problem can be overcome by applying the initial layer of wax in melted increments or drops. As an alternative, the initial coping can be made by dipping the die into thoroughly melted wax.

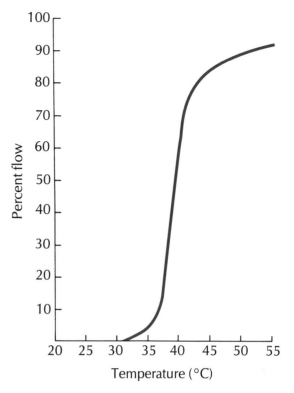

Fig. 18-6. Wax flow curve.

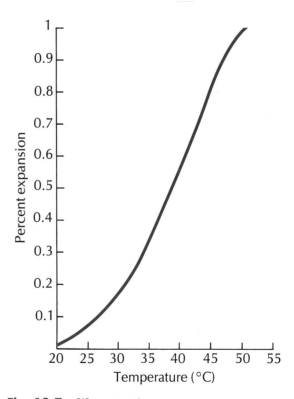

Fig. 18-7. Wax expansion curve.

However, a serious problem exists when the added wax incorporates strain within the pattern as each increment solidifies. This strain tends to be released with time and subsequently distorts the wax pattern. The rate of wax change is temperature dependent, which means that it increases at higher ambient temperatures. Because wax has a relatively high coefficient of thermal expansion and changes dimension subject to air temperature changes, and because the pattern will tend to release its incorporated strain, the margins must be remelted, readapted, and resmoothed immediately before investing. The internal fit of the remelted portion will then be closer to the prepared surface of the tooth than the rest of the casting and therefore may help obtain the necessary space for the luting agent.

• • •

TECHNIQUE

A step-by-step waxing technique is recommended. Each step is evaluated before proceeding to the next, which allows corrections and minimizes extra work. The finished wax patterns should be an accurately shaped anatomic replica of the original teeth. Information needed to shape the restoration correctly is derived from the contours of the unprepared tooth surface, adjacent tooth surfaces, and the opposing occlusal surfaces; however, additional input is needed. This stems from a thorough knowledge of tooth anatomy and the ability to copy three-dimensional structures accurately.

When making a drawing or painting, artists constantly refer to the real-life scene they are trying to reproduce. Similarly, when waxing a restoration, the dentist or technician should refer to a suitable model (e.g., diagnostic casts, unworn extracted teeth, a contralateral tooth) or casts of the unworn natural teeth. It is unwise to copy reproductions of natural teeth (plastic teeth or casts of restored mouths), no matter how skillfully they are made. This would be like an artist trying to render a scene from another artist's painting, rather than from real life.

Evaluating a three-dimensional shape is difficult. The finished wax pattern for a tooth may be too bulbous or too flat. Although it appears "wrong," pinpointing and correcting the exact problem is a skill achieved only after in-depth study of what constitutes "normal" anatomic form. When evaluating occlusal morphology, breaking down the complex surfaces into individual components is helpful. When evaluating axial contours, the practitioner should assess a series of two-dimensional outlines by rotating the wax pattern. These can easily be compared to an appropriate model, and any aberrations can be corrected (Fig. 18-8).

Armamentarium (Fig. 18-9)
- Bunsen burner *(A)*
- Inlay wax *(B)*

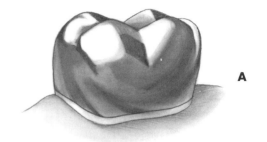

A

View the profile of the pattern while rotating the die against a contrasting background.

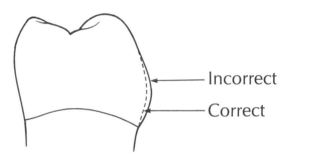

B

Incorrect

Correct

Fig. 18-8. **A,** Incorrect midfacial contour is difficult to determine by looking directly at a three-dimensional object. **B,** It is more easily seen by sequential evaluation of the profile of the pattern as it is rotated.

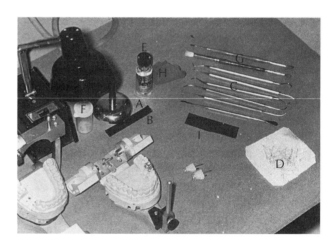

Fig. 18-9. Waxing armamentarium.

- Waxing instruments *(C)*
- Cotton cleaning cloth *(D)*
- Sharp colored pencil (contrasting color to wax)
- Separating liquid *(E)*
- Occlusal indicator powder (zinc stearate* or powdered wax) *(F)*

---

*NOTE: Zinc stearate may present a health hazard if it is inhaled. Powdered wax is a safer alternative.

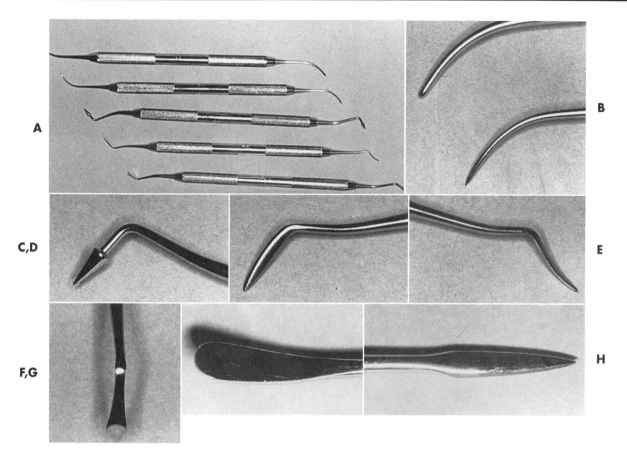

Fig. 18-10. A to F, PKT waxing instruments (**A**, Nos. 1 to 5. **B**, Nos. 1 and 2. **C**, No. 3. **D** and **E**, No. 4. **F**, No. 5) **G** and **H**, The no. 7 waxing spatula.

- Soft toothbrush
- Double-sided brushes (soft/rigid) *(G)*
- Cotton balls
- Fine nylon hose *(H)*
- Shim stock or marking tape *(I)*

Waxing Instruments. Waxing instruments can be categorized by the intent of their design: wax addition, carving, or burnishing. Of the popular PKTs (Fig. 18-10, *A* to *F*) (designed by Dr. Peter K. Thomas specifically for the additive waxing technique), no. 1 and no. 2 are wax addition instruments, no. 3 is a burnisher for refining occlusal anatomy, and nos. 4 and 5 are wax carvers.

Wax is added by heating the instrument in the Bunsen flame, touching it to the wax, and quickly reheating its shank in the flame. Wax flows away from the hottest part of the instrument, so that if the shank is heated, a bead of wax will flow off the tip (Fig. 18-11). However, if the tip is heated, the wax will flow up the shank of the instrument (to the considerable annoyance of inexperienced operators). The PKT no. 1 instrument is used for large increments; the smaller no. 2 is used for lesser additions.

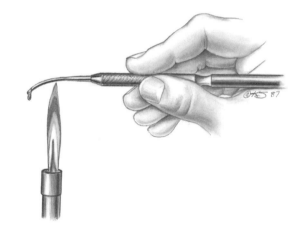

Fig. 18-11. Always heat the shank of the instrument so wax will flow off its tip.

A no. 7 or 7A waxing spatula (see Fig. 18-10, *G* and *H*) is useful for adding large amounts of wax, particularly in forming the initial coping or thimblelike layer of wax that covers all prepared surfaces. Electric waxing instruments (Fig. 18-12) are preferred by some technicians because they allow precise temperature control of the wax, which is important for

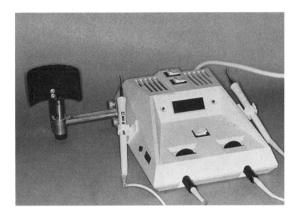

Fig. 18-12. Electric waxing instrument.

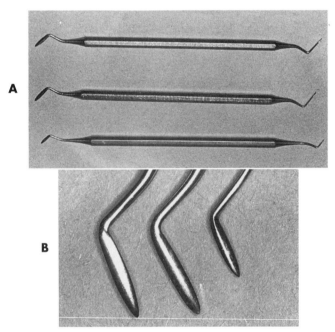

Fig. 18-13. Wax carvers. No. 2 Ward and nos. ½ and 3 Hollenback.

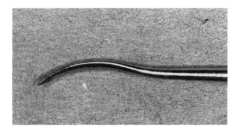

Fig. 18-14. DPT no. 6 wax burnisher.

nishing the occlusal surfaces. The PKT nos. 1 and 2 can be used for burnishing as well as for wax addition. Another popular burnisher is the Darby-Perry trimmer (DPT) no. 6 (Fig. 18-14). For removing wax, burnishing is less effective than carving, but it is probably easier to control and leaves a smoother surface, which can be particularly important when trimming excess wax near the margin. Careless (excessive) carving in this area can result in abrasion of the die, creating a ledge around the finished casting.

POSTERIOR TEETH

The following sequence is recommended for waxing posterior teeth:

1. Internal surface
2. Wax pattern removal and evaluation
3. Proximal surfaces
4. Axial surfaces
5. Occlusal surfaces
6. Margin finishing

Internal Surface. Forming a closely adapted internal surface is the first step in waxing. The wax *must* reproduce all retention features of the restoration.

Step-by-step Procedure

1. Apply die lubricant generously with a clean brush (Fig. 18-15, *A*). Allow it to dry and paint on a second coat (repeat periodically as needed). Waxing should not begin until the lubricant has soaked in completely.
2. Where pinholes have been prepared, fit in plastic pins that match the bur used to sink the hole. Seat the pins in the die and use a heated no. 7 instrument to flatten their tops to provide retention (Fig. 18-15, *B*).
3. Flow wax onto the die from a well-heated, large waxing instrument (Fig. 18-16, *A*), making sure that any previous application is partially remelted. A large instrument will hold sufficient heat to partially remelt previous wax increments and to prevent folds or lines from developing in the fitting surface. Wax-

proper manipulation. Another advantage is that carbon buildup can be kept to a minimum, which easily results from overheating a waxing instrument in a Bunsen flame.

Wax carvers should be kept sharp and should never be heated. In addition to the PKT instruments, the nos. ½ and 3 Hollenback and the no. 2 Ward carvers (Fig. 18-13) are popular. When carving wax, light pressure should be used to obtain the desired smooth surface.

Burnishing is an alternative to carving for obtaining a smooth wax pattern of the desired contour. Burnishing consists of slightly warming a blunt instrument and rubbing the wax. The instrument should not be so hot that it melts the wax surface. The PKT no. 3 instrument is useful for bur-

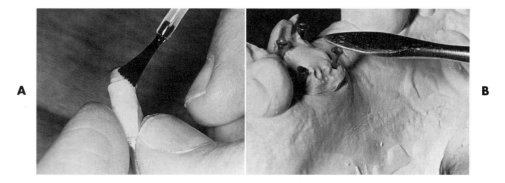

Fig. 18-15. Starting the waxing procedure. **A,** Lubricating the die. **B,** Adapting plastic pins.

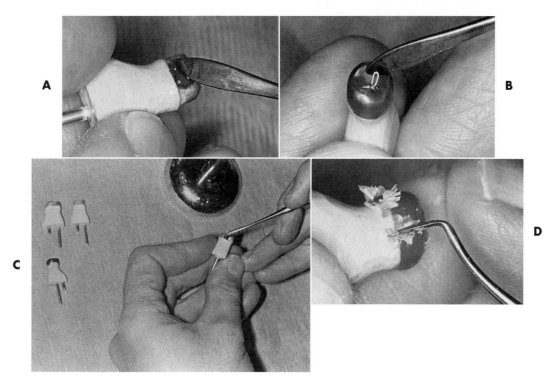

Fig. 18-16. Forming the initial copings. **A,** Use a large instrument to keep the wax sufficiently hot. Ensure that previous applications are remelted as additional wax is added. **B,** Build up adequate bulk for rigidity. **C,** Build up the second coping while allowing the first to cool thoroughly. **D,** Trim the wax very carefully to the margin.

ing will be easier if the instrument is kept clean and only its shank is heated.

4. When applying the initial layer, be sure that the wax is fully molten. If it is not, wax "memory" may cause distortion. Very hot wax flows rapidly over the die. Subsequent waxing of external anatomic details is accomplished with cooler instruments, which allows small additions to be placed accurately. Dipping the lubricated die in a pot of melted wax is an alternative method for making well-adapted internal surfaces (Fig. 18-17). This method is particularly suitable for complete-coverage restorations.

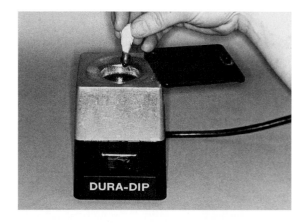

Fig. 18-17. Wax dipping pot.

5. Add sufficient wax with a large instrument to allow the coping to be handled without deformation or breakage (Fig. 18-16, *B*). A large instrument will keep the wax hot more effectively than a small instrument.

6. Give the proximal areas extra bulk to help grip the coping and prevent its distortion when it is removed from the die. The wax should cool between applications (Fig. 18-16, *C*). At this point, no attempt should be made to contour the axial walls.

7. Trim the wax back to the margin (Fig. 18-16, *D*) so the coping can be removed and evaluated. Excess bulk can be removed safely with a carving instrument. When only a thin excess layer remains, trimming is performed most safely with a burnisher. Careless use of a sharp carver at this stage may scratch the fragile margin of the die or chip it. Therefore, a slightly warmed blunt instrument should be used and the margins rubbed with a burnishing action. A carver can be used but requires meticulous technique and great care.

Wax Pattern Removal (Fig. 18-18). The wax should be allowed to cool thoroughly before the coping is removed from the die. A constant light grip is maintained on the pattern by the thumb and forefinger of one hand while pressure is applied against them with the thumb and forefinger of the other hand, which also holds the die (Fig. 18-18, *B*). A small square of washed rubber dam will increase friction between the fingers and the pattern. If the pattern fails to move, there may be excess wax gingival to the margin.

Evaluation (Fig. 18-19). The objective of the first waxing step is a perfectly adapted reproduction of the prepared tooth surfaces. Identifying defects may take some practice. The examiner rotates the pattern under a bright light and looks for shadows formed by folds or creases. A binocular microscope or high-quality magnifying loupe is helpful not only for this step but also throughout the laboratory phase. Ten-power magnification is practical

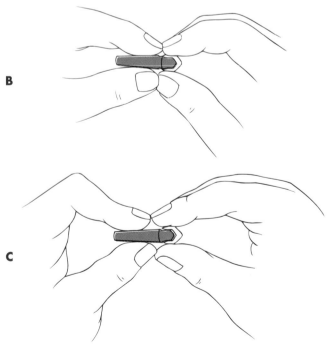

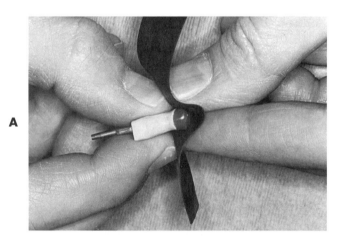

Fig. 18-18. Wax pattern removal. **A,** A sheet of washed rubber dam increases friction and aids removal. **B,** The fingers of the left hand hold the die. The right hand holds the pattern. **C,** The die is pulled from the pattern by bending the fingers of the left hand.

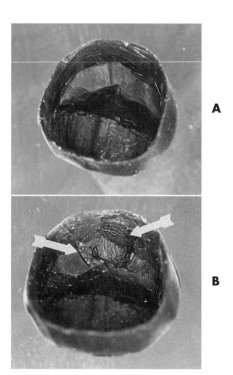

Fig. 18-19. Evaluation. **A,** Well-adapted pattern. **B,** Poor adaptation. Folds and creases *(arrows)* indicate that wax was not hot enough when applied.

and helpful. Using higher power makes maintaining orientation a problem.

Proximal Surfaces (Fig. 18-20). The proximal surfaces of natural teeth are not convex. They tend

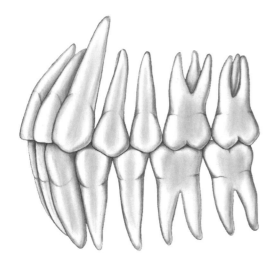

Fig. 18-20. Proximal surfaces gingival to the contact area are normally flat or concave. Note the triangular shape of the posterior embrasures.

to be flat or slightly concave from the contact area to the cementoenamel junction, and any restoration must reproduce this feature. Overcontouring often makes maintaining periodontal health difficult, particularly if drifting of teeth has led to increased root proximity.[15] Excessively concave or undercontoured proximal surfaces also make flossing ineffective and must be avoided.[16]

Contact Areas. The size and location of the contact areas should be established before waxing the remainder of the proximal surfaces. Reference is made to contacts between the contralateral teeth and knowledge of anatomic form.

Abnormally large proximal contact areas make plaque control more difficult and can lead to periodontal disease. Very small (point) contacts may be unstable and cause drifting. Deficient contacts can also lead to food impaction; although this is not a direct cause of chronic periodontal disease, it can be very uncomfortable and painful to the patient.

Most posterior contact areas (Fig. 18-21) are located in the occlusal third of the crown. However, contact between the maxillary first and second

Note how the position of the interproximal contact changes as you progress from anterior to posterior in both the maxillary and mandibular arch.

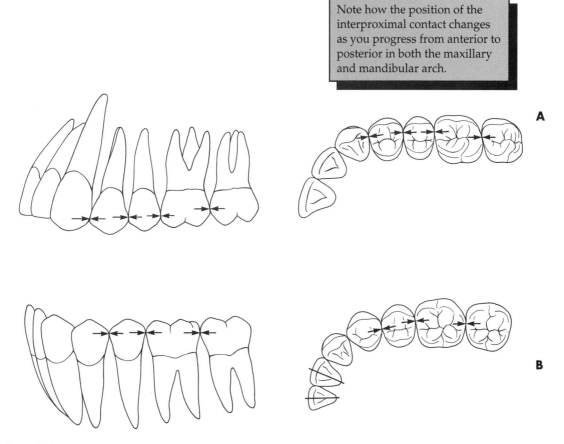

Fig. 18-21. Location of the proximal contact areas. **A,** On maxillary teeth—progressively more occlusal and buccal when progressing anteriorly. **B,** On mandibular posterior teeth—centrally located.

molar occurs in the middle third.[17] The contact areas between mandibular teeth and maxillary molars are generally centrally located. Between maxillary premolars and molars, the contact areas are usually toward the buccal surface (making the lingual embrasure larger than the buccal).

Step-by-step Procedure

1. Replace the wax coping on the lubricated master cast or removable die. When a removable die system is used, extreme care must be taken to ensure that the locating pin and stone surfaces are absolutely free of excess wax or other debris that could prevent complete seating of the die (e.g., small stone particles) (Fig. 18-22).

2. Adjust the coping as necessary to be completely clear of the opposing occlusal surfaces. They will be developed with a wax additive technique later.

3. Add wax to the contact areas until they are the correct size, properly located, and consistent with anatomic form (Fig. 18-23).

4. When this has been accomplished, shape the proximal surfaces gingival to the contacts to the correct contour. A properly trimmed die is of great assistance in accomplishing this. The unprepared tooth structure that was reproduced in the "cuff" of the impression now serves as an effective guide to orienting the waxing instrument properly.

Evaluation. The location of the contact area is checked once again. Where multiple restorations are being made, the proximal embrasure is shaped symmetrically to provide adequate room for the free gingival tissues of adjacent teeth (Fig. 18-24). The proximal surfaces should be flat or slightly concave and should be shaped to eliminate any directional change between the root surface and the finished restoration. The cervical contour of the restoration should be continuous, with the contour of the unprepared tooth structure immediately cervical to the preparation margin.

Axial Surfaces. The buccal and lingual surfaces should be shaped to follow the contours of the adjacent teeth. The location of the height of contour (or survey line for retainers for removable partial dentures) is particularly important. It is generally located in the gingival third of most teeth, although on mandibular molars it is usually in the middle third of the lingual surface.

Restorations are often made too bulky. Natural teeth are rarely more than 1 mm wider at their height of contour than at the CEJ. This should not be exaggerated when recreating a tooth in wax. The tooth surface gingival to its height of contour immediately adjacent to the gingival soft tissues, sometimes called the **emergence profile,**[18] is usually flat or concave. Creation of a convexity in this area or a shelf or ledge[19] makes bacterial plaque removal difficult and has been shown to cause inflammatory and hyperplastic changes in the marginal gingiva. Before dental plaque was identified as the direct etiologic agent in periodontal disease,[20] an excessive axial contour was considered necessary to keep food from entering the gingival sulci.[21] However, there is no evidence to support this concept. Indeed, artificially reduced axial contours (as when a prepared tooth is left unprotected for an extended period)[22] are associated with

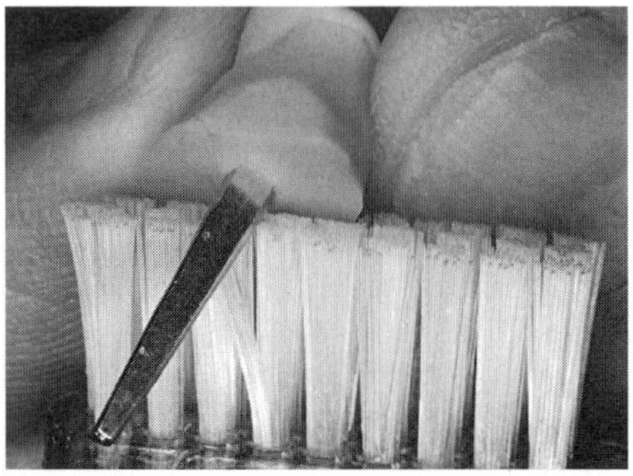

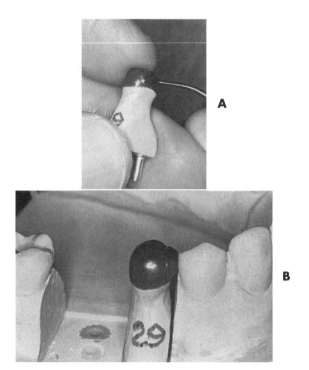

Fig. 18-22. Wax chips that accumulate on the dowel pin or in the sleeve will prevent a die from seating. Periodic cleaning with a brush is recommended.

Fig. 18-23. **A,** Wax is added to the contact area. **B,** The die is seated to establish a correctly located proximal contact.

healthy gingival tissue. Overcontoured axial surfaces result if there has been insufficient axial reduction during tooth preparation. Special care is needed where bone loss has occurred as a result of periodontal disease, particularly when this has exposed the root near the furcation. The axial contour should then be modified to improve access for plaque removal (Fig. 18-25).

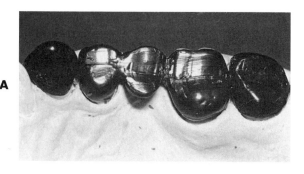

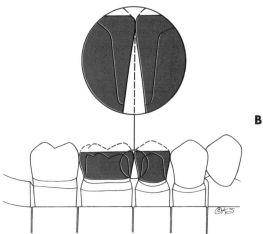

Fig. 18-24.   **A,** From the occlusal view, proper buccal and lingual embrasure form have been established. **B,** The contact areas should be shaped so the gingival embrasures are symmetric.

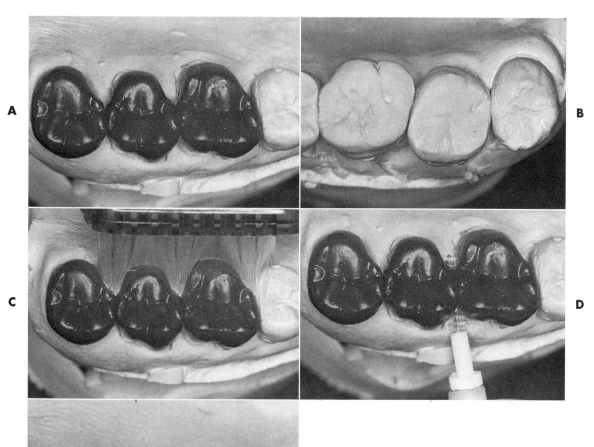

Fig. 18-25.   As the cervical margin is placed near root furcations, the axial contour is modified to improve access for plaque control in patients with extensive bone loss. **A,** Modified wax patterns for a periodontally compromised patient. Note the change in the outline form of the occlusal tables. **B,** Normal axial morphology. **C** to **E,** Modified contour will allow better access for oral hygiene.

Step-by-step Procedure

Axial Contours

1. Establish the location, position, and overall outline of the contour, using the adjacent and contralateral teeth as a guide.
2. Wax the axial surfaces gingivally to form a smooth, flat profile. There should be no change of direction from unprepared tooth structure to the axial restoration contour.
3. Shape the middle third of the axial surface using the adjacent tooth as a guide (Fig. 18-26, *A*).
4. Add wax to join the axial and proximal surfaces and smooth them, paying particular attention to the location and shape of the mesial and distal transitional line angles. A Boley gauge may prove helpful. The line angles should correspond to those on the contralateral teeth if intact (Fig. 18-26, *B*).

Evaluation. The examiner should evaluate the shape of the tooth at its greatest convexity by looking at the wax pattern and comparing it with the shape of the contralateral tooth. Each part of the outline should be carefully scrutinized. If the outline is too square or too round, this can be modified. The buccal and lingual contours and the embrasures should all be assessed. Initially, assessing individual components rather than the entire contour or outline is helpful. Try to relate the shape under evaluation to a "neutral" reference point such as the midsagittal plane when viewing from the occlusal surface. With more experience, the practitioner will find it easier to review multiple forms simultaneously.

Each contact area has four embrasures: gingival, buccal, lingual, and occlusal. All but the occlusal will have been completed by this stage. The embrasures are normally symmetric about a line drawn through the contact area (Fig. 18-27).

Occlusal Surfaces. The cusps and ridges of the occlusal surfaces should be shaped to allow even contact with the opposing teeth while stabilizing the teeth and directing forces along their long axes (see Chapter 4). Noncentric or nonfunctional cusps (buccal of the maxillary teeth, lingual of the mandibular teeth) should overlap vertically and horizontally, preventing accidental biting of the cheek or tongue and keeping food on the occlusal table.

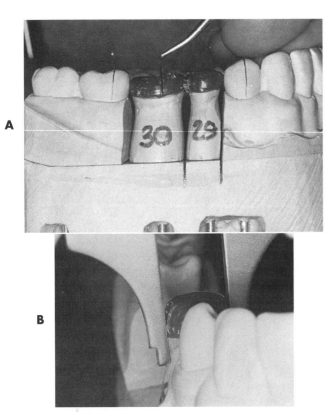

A

B

Fig. 18-26. **A,** Waxing axial contours. **B,** Evaluate the buccolingual dimension with a Boley gauge. This instrument is also helpful in assessing axial shape and height of contour.

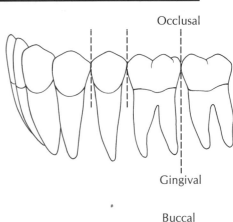

Establishing the correct embrasure form is essential. Only when proper anatomical form is obtained can the patient maintain plaque control.

Occlusal

Gingival

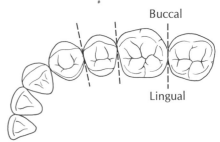

Buccal

Lingual

Fig. 18-27. Symmetry of embrasures.

Point contacts between opposing teeth are preferred to broad, flat occlusal contacts because wear of the restorations will be minimized and mastication of tough or fibrous foods improved. The occlusal surfaces of natural teeth consist of a series of convexities with developmental grooves where the convex ridges meet. The opposing cusps should travel through pathways paralleling these grooves without tooth contact in excursive jaw movements.

The occlusal surfaces can be precisely developed with a wax addition technique similar to the one devised by E.V. Payne[23] that is used in many schools to teach occlusal morphology and function[24-26] (Figs. 18-28 and 18-29).

Occlusal Scheme. Two occlusal schemes are generally recognized and should be understood when planning the restorations: cusp-marginal

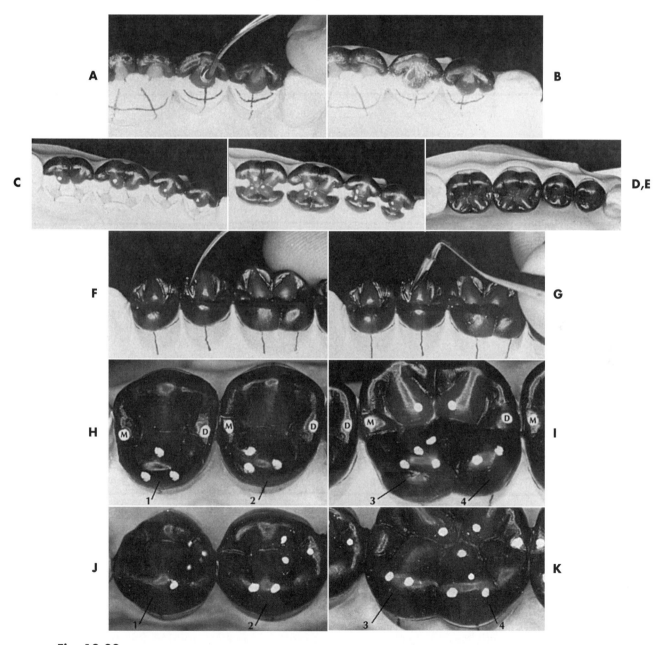

Fig. 18-28. Occlusal waxing using the sequential wax addition technique. **A,** Accurate occlusal contacts are developed by adding small increments of wax and closing the articulator while the addition is still soft. **B,** Powder is used to verify the location and size of the contact. **C,** Cones are used to determine the location of cusp tips. **D** and **E,** The various features of the occlusal surface are developed sequentially in wax. **F** and **G,** Secondary occlusal features can be refined by reflowing the wax and burnishing the fissures. **H** to **K,** Completed waxing with occlusal contacts marked. (For the cusp-marginal ridge scheme, numbers refer to cusp position in Table 18-1.)

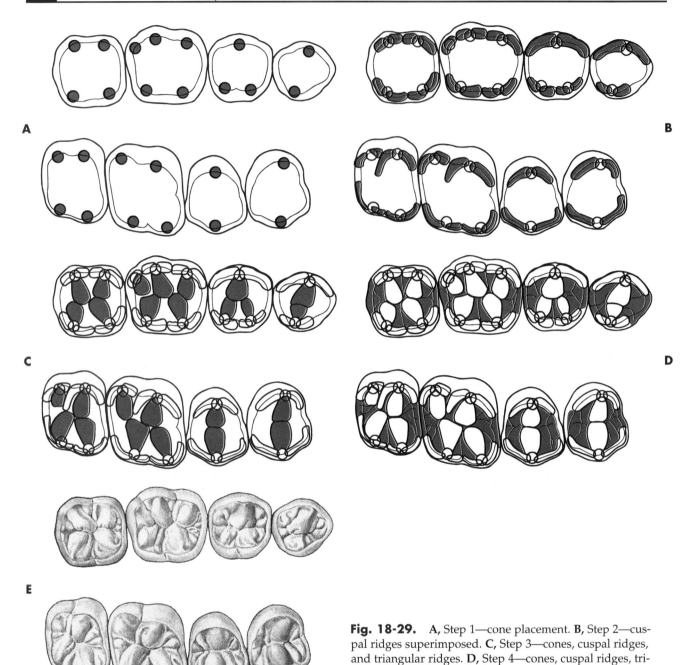

Fig. 18-29. **A,** Step 1—cone placement. **B,** Step 2—cuspal ridges superimposed. **C,** Step 3—cones, cuspal ridges, and triangular ridges. **D,** Step 4—cones, cuspal ridges, triangular ridges, and secondary and marginal ridges. **E,** Step 5—occlusal morphology complete.

ridge and cusp-fossa (see Chapter 4). In the cusp-marginal ridge scheme, the buccal cusps of the mandibular premolars and the mesiobuccal cusps of the mandibular molars contact the embrasures between the maxillary teeth (i.e., they contact two teeth). In the cusp-fossa scheme, these mandibular centric cusps contact farther distally into the mesial fossa of the maxillary tooth and contact only one tooth (Tables 18-1 and 18-2). The lingual (centric) cusps of the maxillary teeth contact the fossae of the mandibular teeth in both schemes.

Most adults with a Class I occlusion and unworn teeth will have a cusp-marginal ridge scheme. In natural dentitions, the cusp-fossa arrangement is found only when a slight Class II malocclusion is present. However, for the following reasons, the cusp-fossa arrangement has been recommended over the cusp-marginal ridge when occlusal reconstruction is undertaken:

1. Food impaction is prevented.
2. Centric relation closure forces are nearer the long axes of the teeth.

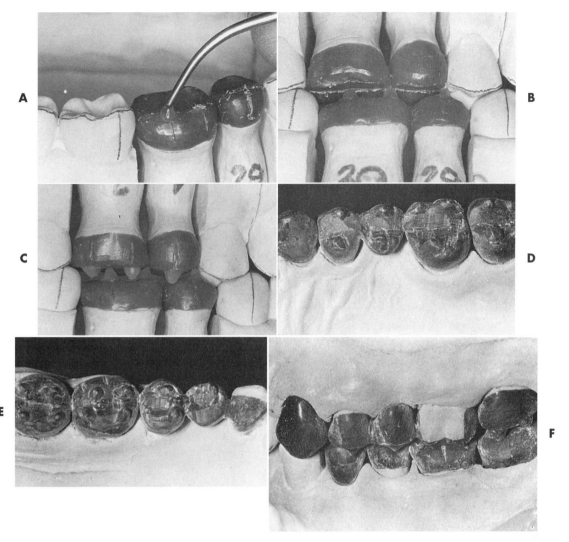

Fig. 18-30. **A,** Adding wax cones to determine cusp height and location. **B,** Marking the central fossae of opposing teeth will help position the centric cusps correctly. **C,** All cones are positioned and tested for interferences in all excursions. **D** to **F,** The wax additive technique is especially useful when multiple restorations are provided.

3. Improved stability results from the tripod contacts for each centric cusp.

When the mesiodistal relationships of opposing teeth favor it, the cusp-fossa scheme is optimal. If these relationships are not present, the coronal contours must be distorted with respect to natural morphology. The cusp-marginal ridge scheme may be a better choice in such cases. However, the decision is not always a clear one. Tooth size and position variations among patients produce a continuum between the optimal cusp-marginal ridge and cusp-fossa schemes. Common sense dictates using the scheme that produces the best overall functional and esthetic result. In many cases, this can be determined only by trial and error. The placement of cones before any other occlusal waxing is often the most efficient way to accomplish this.

Cusp Height and Location (Fig. 18-30)
1. Determine the position and height of the cusps with wax cones. This is done so that necessary modifications can be made rapidly. Add wax cones for each cusp, and mark the central fossae of opposing teeth to help position the cusps correctly.
2. Position the centric or functional cusps (mandibular buccal and maxillary lingual) so they occlude along the buccolingual center of the opposing tooth. The actual cusp tips do not contact the opposing tooth. Greater stability and reduced wear are possible with small points of contact distributed around the cusp tips.
3. Use the mesiodistal location of the cones to determine the type of occlusal scheme to be attempted—cusp-marginal ridge or cusp-

Features of Cusp-Marginal Ridge Scheme: Centric Cusp Articulation (See Fig. 18-31, A.)

TABLE 18-1

Maxilla				
Tooth	Cusp Position	Centric Cusp	Opposing Fossa	Opposing Marginal Ridge (Same Tooth Unless Otherwise Specified)
First premolar	1	L	D	—
Second premolar	2	L	D	—
First molar	3	ML	C	—
	4	DL	—	D and M (second molar)
Second molar	5	ML	C	—
	6	DL	—	D
Mandible				
Tooth	Cusp Position	Centric Cusp	Opposing Fossa	Opposing Marginal Ridge (Same Tooth Unless Otherwise Specified)
First premolar	1	B	—	M
Second premolar	2	B	—	D and M (first premolar)
First molar	3	MB	—	D and M (second premolar)
	4	DB	C	—
Second molar	5	MB	—	D and M (first molar)
	6	DB	C	—

Cusp-Fossa Scheme: Centric Cusp Articulation (See Fig. 18-31, B.)

TABLE 18-2

Maxilla			
Tooth	Cusp Position	Centric Cusp	Opposing Marginal Ridge (Same Tooth)
First premolar	1	L	D
Second premolar	2	L	D
First molar	3	ML	C
	4	DL	D
Second molar	5	ML	C
	6	DL	D
Mandible			
Tooth	Cusp Position	Centric Cusp	Opposing Marginal Ridge (Same Tooth)
First premolar	1	B	M
Second premolar	2	B	M
First molar	3	MB	M
	4	DB	C
	5	D	D
Second molar	6	MB	M
	7	DB	C

L, Lingual; *D*, distal; *M*, mesial; *B*, buccal; *C*, central.
(Courtesy Dr. A. G. Gegauff.)

fossa (see Figs. 18-28, *H* to *K*, Fig. 18-31, and Tables 18-1 and 18-2).

Evaluation (Fig. 18-32). The cones should be positioned so they follow an anteroposterior curve (the **curve of Spee**). The mandibular cusps should become taller farther distally, and the maxillary cusps should become shorter. They should also follow a compensating plane (the **curve of Wilson**) when viewed from the front, with the noncentric (or nonfunctional) cusps slightly shorter than the centric cusps. All eccentric movements should be reproduced on the articulator; if unwanted contact results in protrusive, working, and nonworking excursions, they should be eliminated by either reducing or repositioning the cones. Proper cone height and position are the key to proper occlusal form.

Completion of Axial Contours (Fig. 18-33).

4. Complete the axial contours (marginal ridges and cuspal ridges). Be especially careful not to alter the location or height of the cusps as previously determined with the cones.
5. After each addition of wax, check for occlusal contact by closing the articulator. Do not increase the vertical dimension of occlusion.

Evaluation. At this stage, the buccal, mesial, lingual, and distal surfaces have been completed (see Fig. 18-33, *D* and *E*). When viewed from these perspectives, the wax pattern should appear identical to an intact tooth. When viewed from the buccal perspective, each cusp should have a distinct profile, with the cusp tip highest and a gentle slope down to the marginal ridges. Adjacent marginal ridges should be of the same height. Occlusal contacts in excursive movements must also be evaluated. If there is unwanted contact, grooves can be created in the cuspal ridges to allow the passage of opposing cusps.

Triangular Ridges (see Fig. 18-28, *A*, and Fig. 18-34)

6. Give each cusp a triangular ridge that runs toward the center of the occlusal surface. The apex (or point) of the triangle should be at the

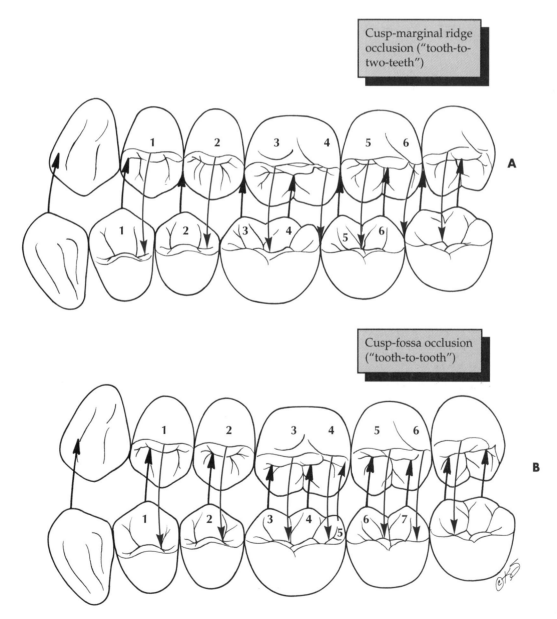

Fig. 18-31. A, Cusp-marginal ridge occlusion. B, Cusp-fossa occlusion. (The numbers refer to Tables 18-1 and 18-2.)

The most critical step in waxing occlusal surfaces is the correct placement of the cusp tips. Use the information provided by adjacent and opposing teeth to determine the optimal position for each cone.

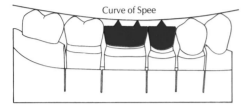

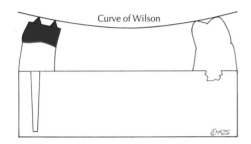

Fig. 18-32. Cones should follow an anteroposterior curve (of Spee) and a lateral curve (of Wilson).

cusp tip, and the base should be in the center of the occlusal surface.

7. Make the bases of the buccal and lingual triangular ridges convex mesiodistally and buccolingually.

8. As each ridge is added, close the articulator. Where the occlusal surface meets an opposing tooth, note the small depression and adjust this to form a convex surface so that pinpoint contact exists.

Evaluation (see Fig. 18-28, *B*, and Fig. 18-35).   The triangular ridges are dusted with zinc stearate or powdered wax. The cusps should still have their correct sharp contour and should not be rounded by improper polishing.

Secondary Ridges (see Fig. 18-28, *F*, and Fig. 18-36)

9. Make two secondary or supplemental ridges adjacent to each triangular ridge. All cusps should have a single triangular ridge and two secondary ridges. The degree of specific delineation between the triangular and secondary ridges varies, depending on the prominence of the cusp within the occlusal table of the tooth that is being waxed.

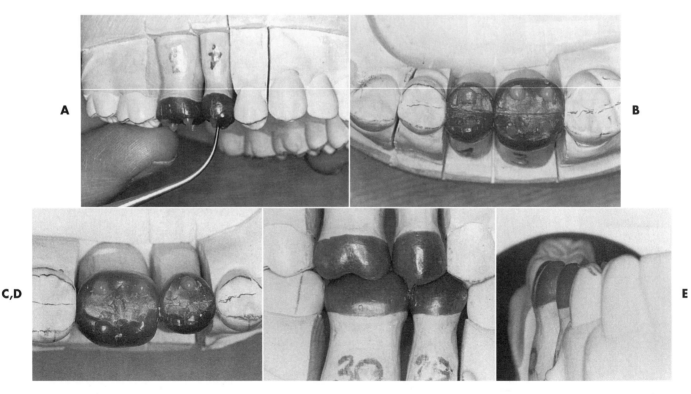

Fig. 18-33.   Completing axial contours. **A** and **B,** Add the maxillary buccal cusp ridges. **C,** Add the mandibular buccal cusp ridges. **D** and **E,** At this stage, the buccal surface is complete and should be evaluated for correct contour.

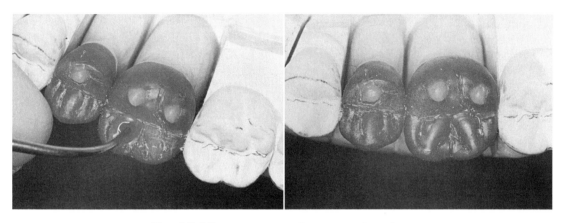

Fig. 18-34. Waxing maxillary triangular ridges.

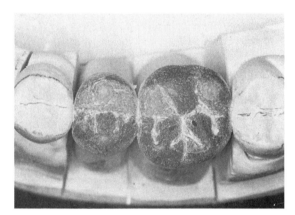

Fig. 18-35. Evaluating occlusal contacts.

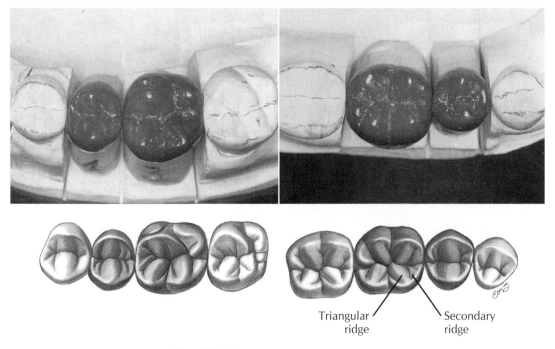

Triangular ridge   Secondary ridge

Fig. 18-36. Adding secondary ridges.

10. Make the secondary ridges convex with grooves where they meet the convexities of the triangular ridges. The most mesial and most distal secondary ridges are often contiguous with the marginal ridges.

Evaluation (Figs. 18-37 and 18-38). If the ridges have been carefully formed, only a small amount of finishing will be needed at this stage. Any pits can be filled with wax and the grooves carefully smoothed (see Fig. 18-28, *G*). Initially, obtaining smooth transitions between the occlusal components may be difficult. Smoothing from the grooves onto the individual occlusal features, rather than back and forth, prevents unnecessary accumulations of wax residue in the grooves.

The occlusal surfaces are redusted with zinc stearate or powdered wax, and the occlusal contacts are checked. If a contact has inadvertently been polished away, it can be quickly re-formed by adding a drop of wax, closing the articulator to verify that contact was restored, and subsequently reflowing and reshaping the occlusal feature to reestablish a convex contour.

Margin Finishing. To optimize the adaptation of the wax pattern (and the cast restoration) to the die, the margins must be reflowed and refinished immediately before investing the wax pattern. The two principal objectives are (1) minimizing dissolution of the luting agent and (2) facilitating plaque control.

If a zone of superior adaptation (i.e., minimum marginal gap width) between the casting and the prepared tooth surface is created, cement dissolution will be reduced.[27] To obtain this superior adaptation, the pattern should be reflowed over a band approximately 1 mm wide, measured from the margin onto the prepared surface (Fig. 18-39).

Plaque control is facilitated by producing cast restorations that exhibit a smooth transition from

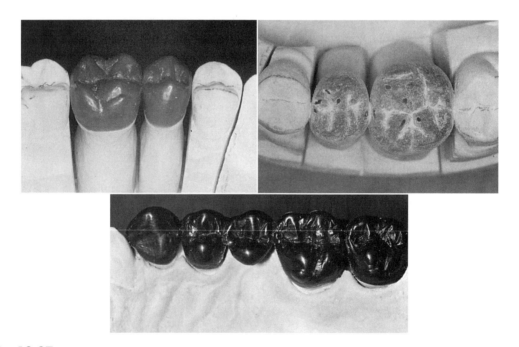

Fig. 18-37. Evaluating the completed wax patterns. *(Courtesy Dr. A.G. Gegauff.)*

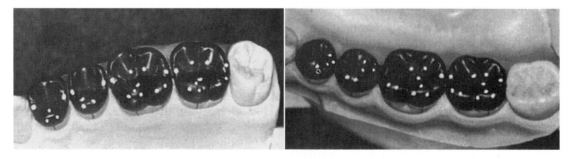

Fig. 18-38. Completed cusp-marginal ridge waxing. The occlusal contacts have been marked.

restoration to tooth without any sudden directional change. In addition, the axial surface of the restoration must be highly polished (see Chapter 29). Because the use of any metal polishing compound or abrasive will result in removal of material, metal finishing procedures should be kept to a minimum near the margin. The best way to prepare for this step is to ensure superior smoothness of the wax pattern when the reflowing process is complete. This should be verified under magnification with loupes or a binocular microscope.

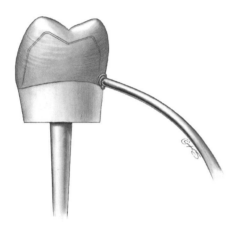

Fig. 18-39. Reflowing the margins. The objective is to create a well-adapted, 1-mm zone to prevent cement dissolution.

Step-by-step Procedure

1. Relubricate the die and reseat the wax pattern (Fig. 18-40, *A*). Because of the time and attention devoted to developing occlusal and axial form, the margins of the pattern are not properly adapted at this stage. A large, well-heated waxing instrument is used to melt completely through the wax.

2. Push the heated instrument through the pattern and completely remelt the marginal 1 to 2 mm (Fig. 18-40, *B*).

3. Draw the instrument along the margin until resistance is felt because the instrument has begun to cool and no longer easily melts the wax.

4. Reheat the instrument and repeat the procedure, always overlapping with the previously melted area to remelt it and to preclude internal folds, voids, and defects. When the entire margin has been reflowed circumferentially, a depression will be seen around the margin as a result of the readaptation.

5. Fill the depression with additional wax (Fig. 18-40, *C*).

6. Trim excess wax from beyond the margin (Fig. 18-40, *D*).

7. Rectify any pits or defects in the axial surfaces and smooth the wax pattern. Wax chips can be removed from the occlusal surface

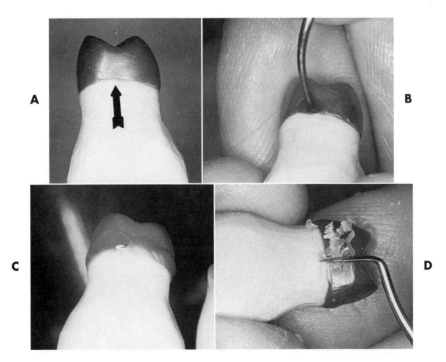

Fig. 18-40. Reflowing margins. **A,** After waxing, a marginal discrepancy is normally apparent *(arrow)*. This must be corrected before investing. **B,** Use a large, well-heated instrument to melt completely through the wax. **C,** Continue around the preparation margin; then add wax to fill the depression. **D,** When the pattern has cooled, carefully trim or burnish the marginal excess.

with a cotton pellet; however, the surface should not be rubbed. Otherwise, the occlusal contacts that were so carefully generated will be destroyed.

The wax pattern is removed from the die without distortion and replaced for final evaluation before investing.

Evaluation. Being thorough at this stage will pay dividends later. Because of the wax pattern's color and glossy surface, small defects can be difficult to identify. If they are not noticed, a later remake may be necessary.

NOTE: Avoid overwaxing. Very little finishing of a cast metal margin is possible without damaging the die. Any flash of wax that extends beyond the finish line *must* be trimmed. Otherwise, it will cause distortion as the pattern is removed or prevent the cast metal restoration from completely seating. A gap between the wax and the die, resulting in an open margin, can be difficult to detect. The die should be oriented so that the observer's line of sight is precisely along the wax-die interface. If the wax is not well adapted, a black shadow line will be visible. This is hard to see in wax but easier to see (but too late) in metal. A binocular microscope or loupe is very helpful for this stage (Fig. 18-41). To

ensure that new debris has not accumulated during the finishing procedures, a final evaluation of the occlusal and axial surfaces is performed. The pattern is now ready for investing. (See Chapter 22.)

Waxing Inlays and Onlays (Fig. 18-42). The sequence of steps for fabricating a wax pattern for an inlay or onlay is similar to that for a complete crown, although the unprepared tooth can often serve as a guide to axial and occlusal contour. Sometimes manipulation of a small inlay can be difficult. One approach is to embed a loop of floss into the pattern for easier removal (Fig. 18-42, *E*).

ANTERIOR TEETH

The approach to waxing anterior teeth is slightly different than the approach to posterior teeth. Anatomic contour waxing is recommended for metal-ceramic restorations, because there is better control over the thickness of porcelain and the smoothness of the metal-ceramic junction. When several anterior teeth are to be restored, a guide to the lingual and labial contours is essential (Fig. 18-43). The contour of the palatal and incisal surfaces significantly influences the articulation. They are most effectively recreated by using a custom an-

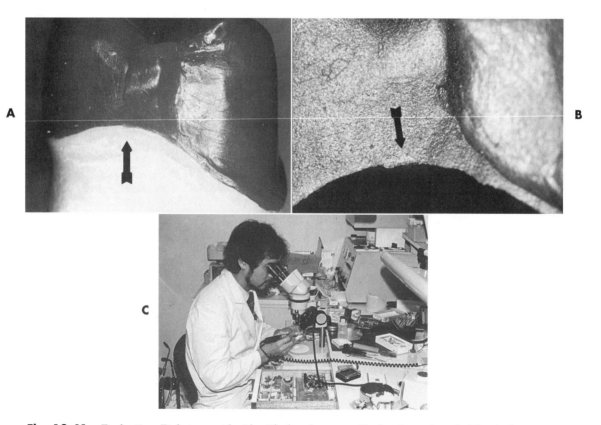

Fig. 18-41. Evaluation. Defects must be identified and corrected before investing. **A,** Marginal excess or flash *(arrow)* is difficult to see in wax but must be carefully removed. **B,** A small defect *(arrow)* is easier to see in the metal but harder to correct. **C,** Magnification is the most practical way to finish margins properly.

terior guidance table (see Chapter 2). This can be made from diagnostic casts (if their initial form was satisfactory) or from a diagnostic waxing or cast made from an impression of provisional restorations. The latter can be used when the provisionals resulted in clinically satisfactory function and appearance. The shape of the anterior teeth will affect the patient's speech, lip support, and appearance. They should be determined carefully and with as many diagnostic aids as necessary.

Lingual and Incisal Surfaces (Fig. 18-44). The position of the incisal edges is determined by the overall arch form of the anterior teeth and the functional occlusal requirements. As with the waxing of posterior occlusal surfaces, cones can be used to initially delineate the approximate position of the incisal edge. Additional wax can then be applied as necessary.

Opposing incisors should contact evenly during protrusive movements but not during lateral excursions. This is achieved by making a concavity in the lingual surface of maxillary incisors. The ability to make this concavity smooth is very important. As a result, the patient is given a smooth envelope of motion, and potential neuromuscular disturbances are

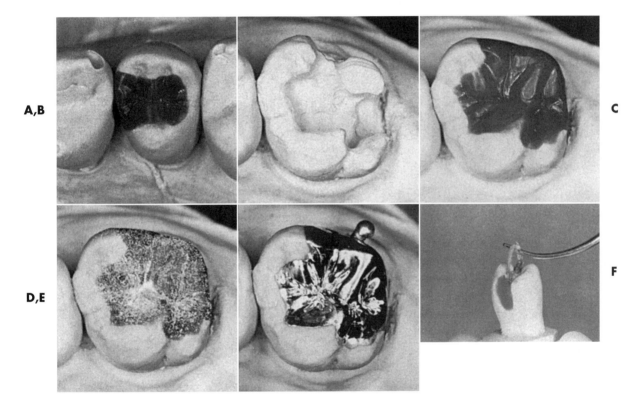

Fig. 18-42. Waxing inlay and onlay restorations. **A,** MO inlay wax pattern. **B** to **E,** DOB onlay wax pattern and casting. **F,** Removal of the inlay wax pattern can be facilitated by embedding a loop of floss.

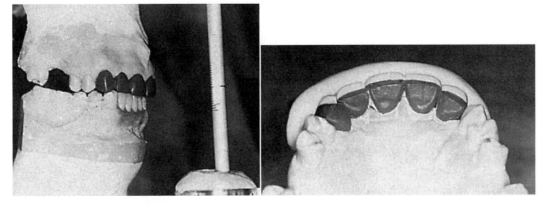

Fig. 18-43. Optimum contours for anterior restorations are developed with the aid of a custom anterior guidance table (see Fig. 19-5).

avoided. In centric closure, anterior teeth ideally should be just out of contact. Mylar shim stock should just "drag" between the patterns. The lingual surfaces of mandibular incisors and canines are noncontacting surfaces. Nevertheless, they should not be overcontoured, but shaped for easy plaque control.

Labial Surfaces (Fig. 18-45). The shape of the labial surfaces, particularly the location of the mesiolabial and distolabial line angles, will determine the appearance of anterior teeth. If the labial surface is too bulbous, plaque control may be difficult, and there may be lingual tilting of the tooth caused by the force exerted by the upper lip. When waxing individual anterior teeth, careful study of the embrasure form of adjacent teeth can be particularly helpful.

WAX CUT-BACK

If a ceramic veneer is to be used, once the final contour of the wax pattern has been completed, the pattern is cut back over an even thickness—usually about 1 mm—to provide room for the porcelain fused

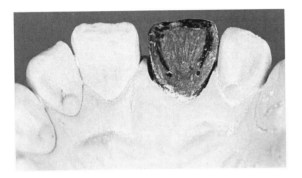

Fig. 18-44. When waxing the lingual surface of an anterior tooth, use the contralateral tooth as a guide.

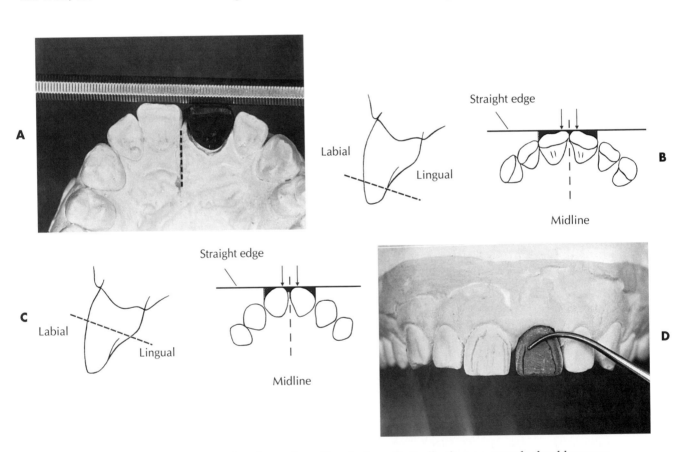

Fig. 18-45. Waxing the labial surfaces of maxillary incisors. Typically, the two centrals should possess mirror symmetry around the midline. **A,** As the waxing progresses, symmetry can be judged by placing a straightedge near the incisal edge and exactly perpendicular to the palatal midline. **B,** The straightedge should contact each central at the same precise distance from the midline (*arrows*). The wax can be easily adjusted if proper contact does not occur. Then the spaces between the straightedge and the wax pattern (*red areas*) are evaluated. The left and right teeth should be mirror images of each other both mesially and distally. **C,** The straightedge is repositioned farther apically, and the analysis is repeated. Note how the form of the embrasures varies at the different locations. **D,** Dusting the wax pattern and marking the mesial and distal line angles. These should correspond to the line angles marked on the contralateral tooth.

onto the cast metal substructure (Fig. 18-46). The design and technique are discussed in Chapter 19.

WAXING CONNECTORS

The connectors that join the separate components of a fixed partial denture or splint are created in wax just before the margins are finalized (Fig. 18-47). Whether the connectors are cast or soldered, they must be shaped in wax so their size, position, and configuration are precisely controlled. Connector size is primarily important from a mechanical perspective. To ensure optimal strength, the connector should be as large as possible. However, from a biologic perspective, connectors should not impinge on the gingival tissues and should be at least 1 mm above the crest of the interproximal soft tissue. Embrasure form below connectors must permit optimal plaque control. The cervical aspect of the connector must be shaped to a smooth archlike configuration. In esthetic areas, (i.e., anterior FPDs) connectors should be hidden behind the esthetic ceramic veneer. Therefore, connectors are often placed slightly lingually when connectors are waxed for anterior prostheses (Fig. 18-48). Connector form and design are discussed in detail in Chapter 28.

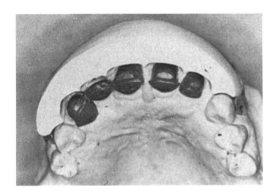

Fig. 18-46.   Wax patterns cut back to provide room for the porcelain. (See Chapter 19.)

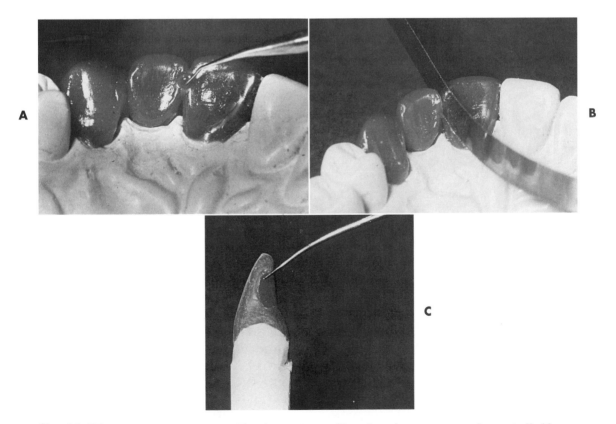

Fig. 18-47.   Waxing connectors. **A,** The shape, size, and location of connectors can be controlled by forming them in wax. **B,** A ribbon saw is then used to section them. **C,** The correct cross-sectional configuration of an anterior connector.

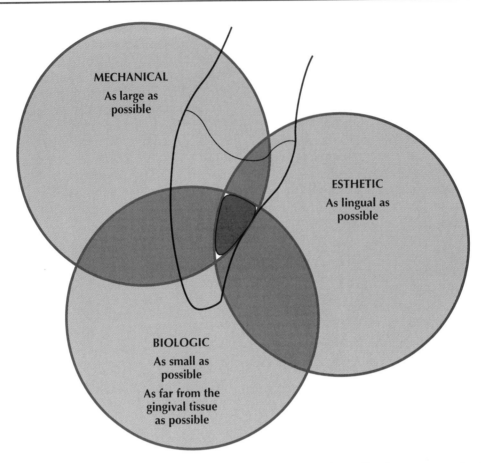

Fig. 18-48. Considerations for anterior connector placement. Mechanically, the connector should be as large as possible for strength. From a biologic perspective, the connector is most effectively placed in the incisal half of the proximal wall. For esthetics, the connector should be placed in the lingual (palatal) half of the proximal wall.

REVIEW OF TECHNIQUE

Figure 18-49 summarizes the steps for waxing to anatomic form.

1. The die is modified as necessary and lubricated (Fig. 18-49, *A*).
2. An initial coping is waxed, forming the internal surface (Fig. 18-49, *B*).
3. The proximal surfaces are developed, with correctly located contact areas (Fig. 18-49, *C*).
4. The axial surfaces are waxed. Overcontouring near the gingival margin must be avoided (Fig. 18-49, *D*).
5. The occlusal surfaces are developed with a wax addition technique, which makes it easier to determine the best location of cusps and occlusal contacts (Fig. 18-49, *E*).
6. The margins are reflowed, and the wax pattern is finished (Fig. 18-49, *F*).

SUMMARY

If the waxing procedure is followed in a sequential order, inexperienced but conscientious operators should have no problem achieving excellent results. With more experience, they can combine and modify some of these steps; however, waxing up teeth "from memory" is not advised. Even the most experienced technician should copy the shape of natural teeth rather than redesign them.

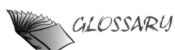 *GLOSSARY*

adaptation: *n* (1610) *1:* the act or process of adapting; the state of being adapted *2:* the act of purposefully adapting two surfaces to provide intimate contact *3:* the progressive adjustive changes in sensitivity that regularly accompany continuous sensory stimulation or lack of stimulation *4:* in dentistry, (a) the degree of fit between a prosthesis and supporting structures, (b) the degree of proximity of a restorative material to a tooth preparation, (c) the adjustment of orthodontic bands to teeth

anteroposterior curve: the anatomic curve established by the occlusal alignment of the teeth, as projected onto the median plane, beginning with

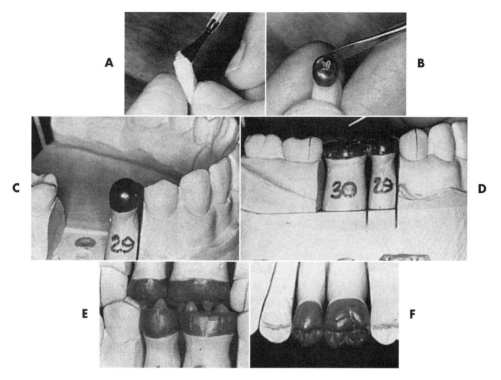

Fig. 18-49. Technique review.

the cusp tip of the mandibular canine and following the buccal cusp tips of the premolar and molar teeth, continuing through the anterior border of the mandibular ramus, ending with the anterior most portion of the mandibular condyle. First described by Ferdinand Graf Spee, German anatomist, in 1890.

Bonwill triangle: [William Gibson Arlington Bonwill, American dentist, 1833-1899]: *eponym* for a 4-inch equilateral triangle bounded by lines connecting the contact points of the mandibular central incisor's in-

cisal edge (or the mid-line of the mandibular residual ridge) to each condyle (usually its mid point) and from one condyle to the other, first described in 1858 while introducing his Anatomical Articulator Bonwill WGA. Scientific articulation of the human teeth as founded on geometrical, mathematical and mechanical laws. Dental Items Int 1899;21: 617-56, 873-80.

casting wax: a composition containing various waxes with desired properties for making wax patterns to be formed into metal castings

centric stop: opposing cuspal/fossae contacts that maintain the occlusal vertical dimension between the opposing arches

compensating curve: *1:* the anteroposterior curvature (in the median plane) and the mediolateral curvature (in the frontal plane) in the alignment of the occluding surfaces and incisal edges of artificial teeth that re used to develop balanced occlusion *2:* the curve introduced in the construction of complete dentures to compensate for the opening influences produced by the condylar and incisal guidances during lateral and protrusive mandibular excursive movements—called also *compensating curvature, compensating curve*

curve of Monson: [George S. Monson, St. Paul Minnesota, U.S. dentist. 1869-1933]: *eponym* for a proposed ideal curve of occlusion in which each cusp and incisal edge touches or conforms to a segment of the surface of a sphere 8 inches in diameter with its center in the region of the glabella
    Monson GS. Occlusion as applied to crown and bridge-work. J Nat Dent Assoc 1920; 7:399-417.
    Monson GS. Some important factors which influence occlusion. J Nat Dent Assoc 1922;9:498-503

curve of occlusion: the average curve established by the incisal edges and occlusal surfaces of the anterior and posterior teeth in either arch

curve of Spee: [Ferdinand Graf Spee, Prosector of Anatomy, Kiel, Germany, 1855-1937]: *eponym* for anteroposterior curve
    Spee FG. Die Verschiebrangsbahn des Unterkiefers am Schadell. Arch Anat Physiol (Leipz) 1890; 16:285-94

curve of Wilson: [George H. Wilson, Cleveland, Ohio, U.S. Dentist, 1855-1922] 1: *eponym* for the mediolateral curve 2: in the theory that occlusion should be spherical, the curvature of the cusps as projected on the frontal plane expressed in both arches; the curve in the lower arch being concave and the one in the upper arch being convex. The curvature in the lower arch is affected by an equal lingual inclination of the right and left molars so that the tip points of the corresponding cross-aligned cusps can be placed into the circumferences of a circle. The transverse cuspal curvature of the upper teeth is affected by the equal buccal inclinations of their long axes
    Wilson GH. A manual of dental prosthetics. Philadelphia: Lea & Febiger, 1911:22-37

cusp angle: the angle made by the average slope of a cusp with the cusp plane measured mesiodistally or buccolingually

cusp height: the perpendicular distance between the tip of a cusp and its base plane

embrasure: *n* (1702) *1:* the space formed when adjacent surfaces flair away from one another *2:* in dentistry, the space defined by surfaces of two adjacent teeth; there are four embrasure spaces associated with each proximal contact area: occlusal/incisal, mesial, distal, and gingival

emergence profile: the contour of a tooth or restoration, such as a crown on a natural tooth or dental implant abutment, as it relates to the adjacent tissues

inlay wax: see Casting Wax

intercuspal contact: the contact between the cusps of opposing teeth

interproximal contact: the area of a tooth that is in close association, connection, or touch with an adjacent tooth in the same arch

oblique ridge: the elevation in the enamel that runs obliquely across the occlusal surface of a maxillary molar

occlusal plane: *1:* the average plane established by the incisal and occlusal surfaces of the teeth. Generally, it is not a plane but represents the planar mean of the curvature of these surfaces *2:* the surface of wax occlusion rims contoured to guide in the arrangement of denture teeth *3:* a flat metallic plate used in arranging denture teeth—comp to Curve of Occlusion

separating medium: *1:* a coating applied to a surface and serving to prevent a second surface from adhering to the first *2:* a material, usually applied on an impression, to facilitate removal of the cast

wax *n:* one of several esters of fatty acids with higher alcohols, usually monohydric alcohols. Dental waxes are combinations of various types of waxes compounded to provide desired physical properties

wax pattern: a wax form that is the positive likeness of an object to be fabricated

waxing *v obs:* the contouring of a wax pattern or the wax base of a trial denture into the desired form (GPT-1)

wax expansion: a method of expanding a wax pattern to compensate for the shrinkage of gold during the casting process

REFERENCES

1. Frankfort H: *The art and architecture of the ancient Orient,* 1956, Penguin p 26 ff.
2. Black GV: The technical procedures in filling teeth. In *Operative dentistry,* vol 2, New York, 1924, Medico Dental Publishing.
3. Cherberg JW, Nicholls JI: Analysis of gold removal by acid etching and electrochemical stripping, *J Prosthet Dent* 42:638, 1979. (Quoting BJ Parkins: *The effect of electropolishing on the unprotected margins of gold castings:* Thesis, Northwestern University, 1969.)
4. Fusayama T et al: Relief of resistance of cement of full cast crowns, *J Prosthet Dent* 14:95, 1964.
5. Eames WB et al: Techniques to improve the seating of castings, *J Am Dent Assoc* 96:432, 1978.

6. Byrne G: Influence of finish-line form on crown cementation, *Int J Prosthod* 5:137, 1992.

7. Syu JZ et al: Influence of finish-line geometry on the fit of crowns, *Int J Prosthod* 1:25, 1993.

8. Campagni WV et al: Measurement of paint-on die spacers used for casting relief, *J Prosthet Dent* 47:606, 1982.

9. Emtiaz S, Goldstein G: Effect of die spacers on precementation space of complete-coverage restorations, *Int J Prosthodont* 10:131, 1997.

10. Fukui H et al: Effectiveness of hardening films on die stone, *J Prosthet Dent* 44:57, 1980.

11. Coleman RL: Physical properties of dental materials, U.S. Bureau of Standards research paper 32, *J Res Natl Bur Stand* 1:867, 1928.

12. Council on Dental Materials, Instruments, and Equipment: Revised ANSI/ADA specification no. 4 for inlay wax, *J Am Dent Assoc* 108:88, 1984.

13. Kotsiomiti E, McCabe JF: Stability of dental waxes following repeated heatings, *J Oral Rehabil* 22:135, 1995.

14. Ito M et al: Effect of selected physical properties of waxes on investments and casting shrinkage, *J Prosthet Dent* 75:211, 1996.

15. Jameson LM, Malone WFP: Crown contours and gingival response, *J Prosthet Dent* 47:620, 1982.

16. Burch JG: Ten rules for developing crown contours in restorations, *Dent Clin North Am* 15:611, 1971.

17. Burch JG, Miller JB: Evaluating crown contours of a wax pattern, *J Prosthet Dent* 30:454, 1973.

18. Stein RS, Kuwata M: A dentist and a dental technologist analyze current ceramo-metal procedures, *Dent Clin North Am* 21:729, 1977.

19. Perel ML: Axial crown contours, *J Prosthet Dent* 25:642, 1971.

20. Löe H et al: Experimental gingivitis in man, *J Periodontol* 36:177, 1965.

21. Wheeler RC: Complete crown form and the periodontium, *J Prosthet Dent* 11:722, 1961.

22. Herlands RE et al: Forms, contours, and extensions of full coverage restorations in occlusal reconstruction, *Dent Clin North Am* 6:147, 1962.

23. Payne EV: Functional occlusal wax-up. In Eissmann HF et al, editors: *Dental laboratory procedures*, vol 2, *Fixed partial dentures*, St Louis, 1980, Mosby.

24. Lundeen HC: *Introduction to occlusal anatomy*, Lexington, Ky, 1969, University of Kentucky Press.

25. Thomas PK: *Syllabus on full-mouth waxing technique for rehabilitation*, San Diego, 1967, Instant Printing Service.

26. Shillingburg HT et al: *Guide to occlusal waxing*, ed 2, Chicago, 1984, Quintessence Publishing.

27. Jacobs MS, Windeler AS: An investigation of dental luting cement solubility as a function of the marginal gap, *J Prosthet Dent* 65:436, 1991.

FRAMEWORK DESIGN AND METAL SELECTION FOR METAL-CERAMIC RESTORATIONS

KEY TERMS

alloy
compressive stress
coping
cut-back
density
ductility
elastic limit

elongation
modulus of elasticity
proportional limit
tensile stress
toughness
yield strength

All patients want a pleasing smile, so esthetics is an essential part of restorative practice, where attention must be given to color, shape, surface texture, and proportion. Because anterior and maxillary posterior teeth are the most visible, they require the greatest attention to esthetic detail.

Tooth-colored restorative materials have evolved from the soluble silicate cements of the past to the composite resin materials and glass ionomer cements of today. Currently metal-ceramic prostheses enjoy wide acceptance and are the most commonly used extracoronal restoration.[1] They combine the superior fit of a casting with the outstanding esthetics of dental porcelain. Because the ceramic veneer is chemically bonded to the metal substructure, this restoration is not subject to the discoloration problems associated with acrylic resin veneer crowns. In addition, the material properties of dental porcelain are able to withstand wear under functional loading better than resin.

The concept of combining a brittle material with an elastic material to arrive at more desirable physical properties has many engineering applications. Dental porcelains (which are, chemically speaking, glasses) resist compressive loading but tend to succumb to **tensile stress**. Therefore, the metal substructure must be designed so that any tensile stresses in the porcelain are minimized.

To avoid fracture, the thickness of a ceramic veneer must not exceed 2 mm; however, a minimum thickness of 1 mm is needed for an esthetically pleasing restoration.

Restorations with porcelain occlusal surfaces must be planned carefully. Although they are esthetically very acceptable, these restorations have disadvantages, especially wear of the opposing enamel. Ideally, an esthetic restoration should wear at approximately the same rate as the enamel it replaces (about 10 μm per year[2]). In addition, the restoration should not increase the wear rate of an opposing enamel surface. Dental porcelain is more abrasive of enamel than other restorative materials (e.g., gold or amalgam[3-7]) and has been implicated in severe occlusal wear, particularly when the porcelain is not glazed or highly polished (Fig. 19-1). This factor should be considered whenever a metal-ceramic restoration is being designed. Less wear on opposing teeth was cited as the most important need for improvement of posterior tooth-colored crowns.[1] In addition, porcelain occlusal coverage leads to restorations with lower strength,[8] and anatomically correct occlusal form with sharp cusps can be difficult to obtain in dental porcelain.

Some technicians may attempt to fabricate a framework by dipping the die into molten wax, obtaining an even thickness. After the excess wax is trimmed away, a gingival collar is added, and the pattern is sprued, invested, and cast. When this is completed, the veneer is then applied. This technique almost always produces an uneven porcelain thickness, with an increased potential for material fracture as a result of the porcelain not being properly supported (Fig. 19-2). If porcelain thickness is not well controlled, appearance will suffer as well, because the shade of the final crown depends on porcelain thickness.[9] For predictable success, the framework must be carefully designed and shaped.

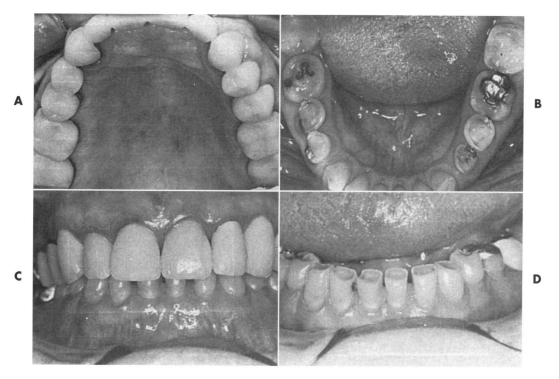

Fig. 19-1. Destructive enamel wear associated with metal-ceramic restorations. *(Courtesy Dr. M. T. Padilla.)*

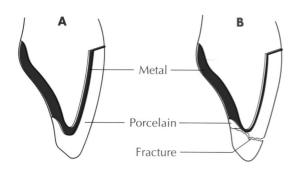

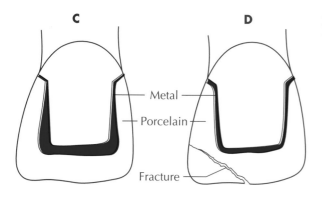

Fig. 19-2. **A** and **C**, Cross section through a metal-ceramic restoration. Ideal porcelain thickness is ensured by waxing to the full anatomic contour and cutting back. **B** and **D**, Incorrect framework design has insufficient support for the incisal porcelain. This can lead to fracture.

PREREQUISITES

The framework design for a fixed prosthesis should be considered during the treatment planning stage (see Chapter 3) and should be evaluated at the diagnostic tooth preparation and waxing stage, par-

ticularly in more complex treatments. A properly designed framework for a metal-ceramic crown or FPD can be achieved routinely only by waxing the restoration to complete anatomic contour first and then cutting back a consistent amount for the veneer. This allows an even thickness of porcelain, proper porcelain-metal interfaces, good connector design, and optimally placed occlusal contacts.

WAXING TO ANATOMIC CONTOUR

The main objective when waxing a framework is a substructure that will support a relatively even thickness of porcelain. Simultaneously, if the retainer is to serve as part of a fixed partial denture (FPD), it must allow for proper connector configuration and location. Furthermore, the restoration must conform to the normal anatomic configuration of the tooth that is being replaced. At the porcelain-metal interface, the ceramic material should be at least 0.5 mm thick. The framework should be shaped to allow for a distinct margin so that the porcelain is not overextended (Fig. 19-3). There should be no abrupt contour change between the metal and the adjacent porcelain.

The most effective way to consistently meet these criteria, with a minimum number of failures, is to develop the final contours of the proposed restoration in wax (Fig. 19-4). Once completed, the area to be veneered can be demarcated and an even thickness of wax removed. If this technique is not followed, one or more of the objectives will almost certainly be missed, and the contours of the framework will not be in harmony with the required ceramic configuration (Fig. 19-5).

OCCLUSAL ANALYSIS

The centric stops of any metal-ceramic restoration can be located on either porcelain or metal. However, they must be at least 1.5 mm away from the junction[10] to prevent porcelain fracture from deformation of the metal (Fig. 19-6). Care is needed to minimize sliding contacts over the porcelain-metal interface. When this is not possible, the framework

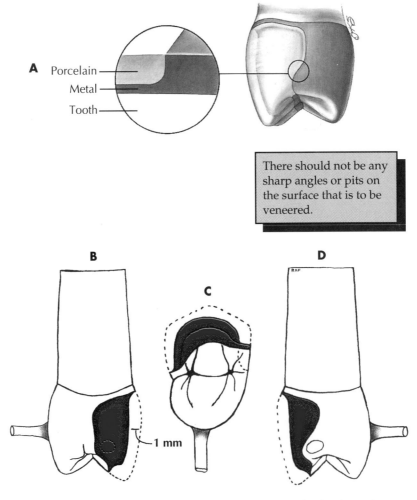

Fig. 19-3. **A,** The metal substructure should have a distinct margin for finishing the veneer. The location of the ceramic-metal interface varies, depending on the material chosen to contact adjacent and opposing teeth. **B,** Cutback for proximal contact in porcelain. **C,** Occlusal contact in metal. **D,** Proximal contact in metal.
(B to D courtesy Dr. R. Froemling.)

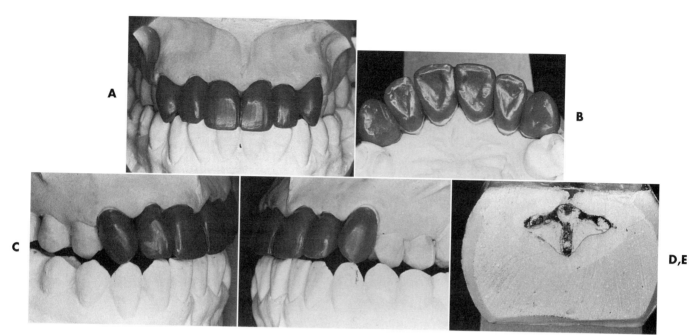

Fig. 19-4. **A** and **B,** Waxing anterior metal-ceramic restorations. **C,** Right lateral excursion. **D,** Left lateral excursion. **E,** The anterior guidance is determined with a custom table fabricated from the diagnostic waxing procedure.

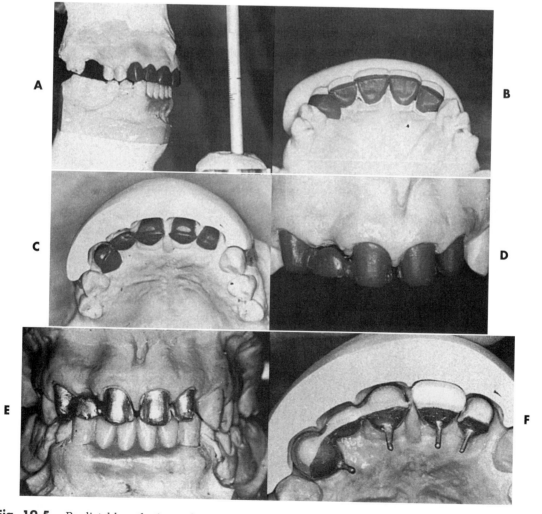

Fig. 19-5. Predictable esthetic result ensured by waxing to anatomical contour. **A,** Anatomic contour wax patterns. **B** and **C,** Incisal and labial indices were used to verify even cut-back. **D,** Completed wax patterns. **E,** Cast substructures. **F,** The labial index is reused during porcelain application. (*Courtesy Dr. M. Chen.*)

Continued

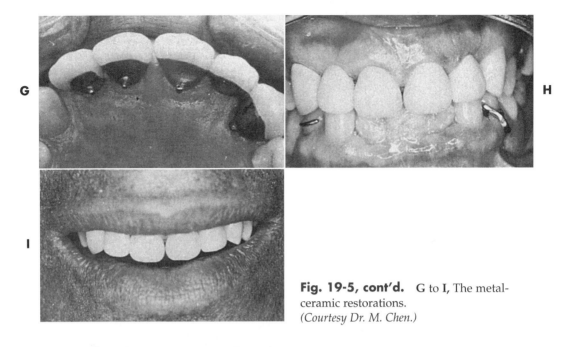

Fig. 19-5, cont'd.   **G** to **I,** The metal-ceramic restorations.
(Courtesy Dr. M. Chen.)

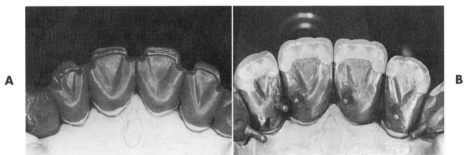

Fig. 19-6.   **A,** The metal-ceramic junction must be carefully placed to avoid areas of high stress near occlusal contacts. **B,** Waxing to the anatomic contour ensures a smooth transition from porcelain to metal.

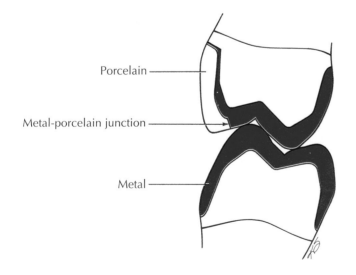

Porcelain

Metal-porcelain junction

Metal

Fig. 19-7.   The metal-ceramic restoration should be designed so that porcelain does not oppose an existing gold restoration. This presents few problems in the maxillary arch because the less visible lingual cusps are in cuspal contact.

must be modified so that the porcelain is well supported in the area of functional contact.

Existing restorations in the opposing arch can influence framework design. Because sliding contact of a porcelain restoration with a cast crown will abrade the gold, the framework design must be modified as necessary. A complete cast crown in the mandibular arch presents little difficulty. It can be opposed by a maxillary restoration with a metal occlusal surface and a facial ceramic veneer only (Fig. 19-7). An exist-

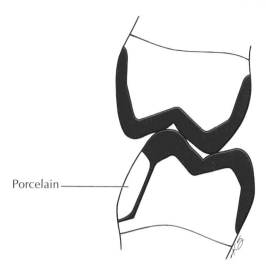

Fig. 19-8. In the mandibular arch, the centric cusps are visible, and only a buccal window of porcelain can be made without contacting an opposing metal crown. Under these circumstances, it must be decided whether the patient should accept an esthetic or functional compromise.

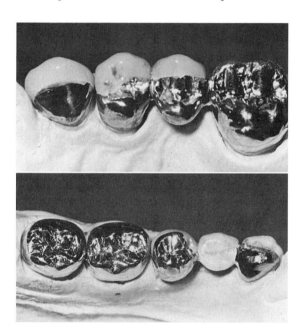

Fig. 19-9. Opposing restorations must be carefully planned so that contacting surfaces will be of the same material (i.e., metal opposing metal, porcelain opposing porcelain).

ing metal crown on a maxillary molar, however, will restrict the design of a mandibular metal-ceramic restoration if metal-to-porcelain contact is to be avoided (Fig. 19-8). Here the facial veneer can no longer be extended to include the buccal cusp tips and associated centric stops without contacting the opposing restoration. A complete cast crown is usually preferred because most patients do not show the facial surfaces of their mandibular posterior teeth. In other situations, particularly on mandibular first premolars, a facial veneer is esthetically essential, and

the design of opposing restorations should allow for it (Fig. 19-9).

CUTTING BACK

The criteria for waxing to anatomic contour have been discussed in Chapter 18. This section deals with cutting back the veneering area.

Armamentarium
- Bunsen burner
- Inlay wax
- Cloth
- Sharp pencil
- Die-wax separating liquid
- Powdered wax
- Waxing instruments
- Nylon hose and silk cloth
- **Cut-back** instrument
- Scalpel
- Discoid carver
- Wax saw
- Waxing brushes

Step-by-step Procedure
Designing the Cut-back. Esthetic and functional needs govern the design of the veneering surface. The ceramic veneer should extend far enough interproximally, particularly in the cervical half of the restoration, to avoid metal display. Wherever possible, the functional occlusal surfaces should be designed in metal, because an accurate occlusion is then easier to achieve (Fig. 19-10). However, esthetic demands may require extension of the porcelain veneer (e.g., on the mesial incline of a mandibular buccal cusp). The extent to which a restoration can be veneered is determined largely by the location of the centric stops.

1. Do not place any proximal contacts on the junction between metal and porcelain. Plaque accumulation there may result in caries of the adjacent tooth. Normally, for good appearance and because it is more easily cleaned, proximal contacts are placed in porcelain. On some posterior teeth, however, where the interproximal area cannot be easily seen, a more conservative preparation may be possible, with the contacts entirely in metal (see Fig. 19-3, *D*).
2. Once the extent of the cut-back area has been determined, use a sharp instrument (e.g., an explorer or scalpel) to mark a line delineating the porcelain interface.
3. Dust the pattern with powdered wax and close the articulator to determine the location of the centric contacts.

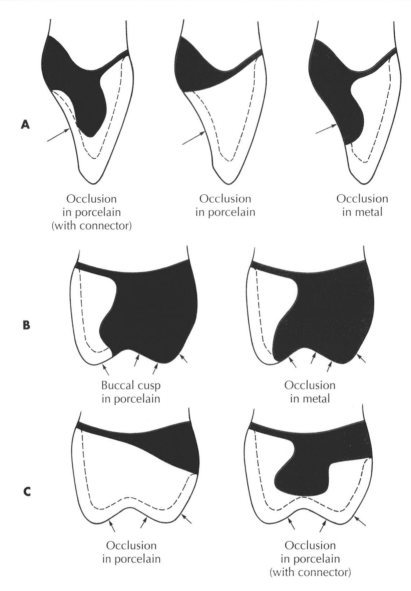

Fig. 19-10. Framework designs for a maxillary incisor **(A)** and a maxillary posterior tooth **(B)**. The cut-back should be designed so the occlusal contacts are 1.5 mm away from the metal-porcelain junction. **C,** Framework designs for porcelain occlusal surfaces.

4. Inspect the design to verify that the proposed junction is far enough away from the contacts (1.5 mm) to prevent distortion of the metal and porcelain fracture.

Troughing the Pattern.   Just as guiding grooves are used to mark the amount of substance to be removed in tooth preparation, depth cuts can be used to standardize the amount of wax to be removed from the veneering area (troughing).

5. Modify an old hand instrument with a separating disk to serve as a depth gauge (Fig. 19-11).* The cutting edge should resemble the

tip of a straight chisel. There should be a shoulder exactly 1 mm from the cutting edge.

6. Make depth cuts around the periphery of the cut-back area perpendicular to the surface of the wax pattern. Depending on the size of the cut-back area, one or more vertical and horizontal cuts can also be made.

7. Remove the islands in between with a scalpel or another carving instrument (Fig. 19-12, *A* to *E*).

Finishing

8. Once the bulk reduction has been completed, smooth the veneering surface of the wax. This will ensure a rounded design and minimize the time spent on metal finishing. Sharp angles on the veneering surface concentrate stresses, which may lead to fracture of the

---

*A suitable instrument is available from Thompson Dental Manufacturing Co.

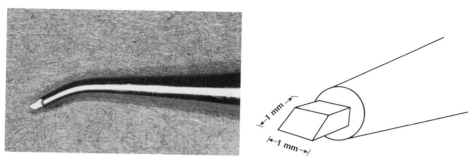

Fig. 19-11. A cut-back instrument can be readily made from a damaged hand instrument.

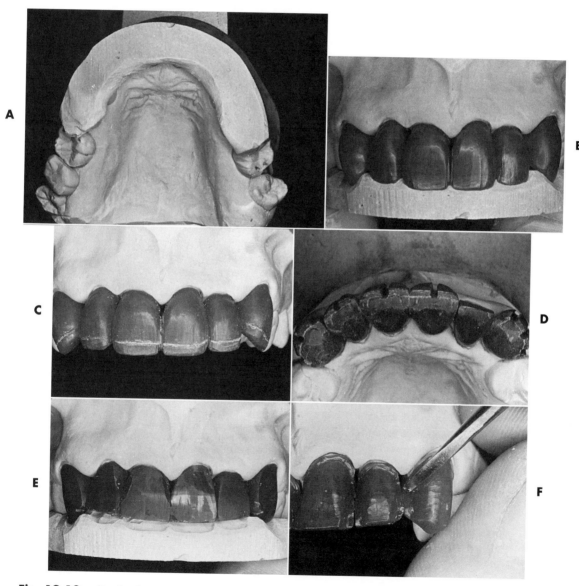

Fig. 19-12. Cut-back procedure. **A** and **B,** For extensive restorations, a matrix or index can be made to facilitate porcelain application. **C,** It is important to follow the incisal contour carefully. **D,** Guiding troughs prepared in the area to be veneered. **E,** Wax is removed from between the troughs. **F,** The porcelain-metal interface is carved to a distinct butt joint.

Continued

restoration.[11] Smoothing is much easier in wax than in metal, although this is not always appreciated initially.

9. Finish the porcelain-metal interface to a 90-degree butt joint (Fig. 19-12, *F* to *J*). Reflowing the margin is essentially the same as for conventional wax patterns (see Chapter 18).

10. Reestablish the collar (obliterated during reflowing) immediately before investing.

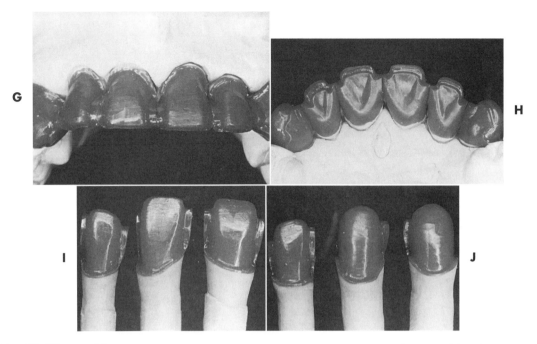

Fig. 19-12, cont'd.   G, Note the correctly shaped proximal. These units will have soldered connectors. **H,** The finished cut-back. **I** and **J,** Patterns before reflowing of the margins.

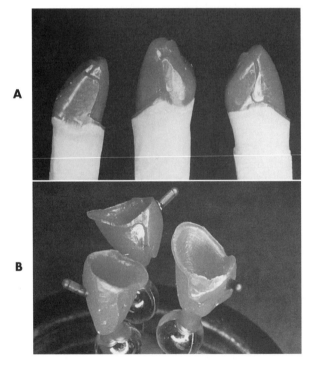

Fig. 19-13.   **A,** Margins reflowed. This will ensure optimum adaptation of the wax pattern in the critical margin area. **B,** Patterns before investing.

Make it slightly thicker (approximately 0.5 mm) to ensure an undistorted complete casting (Fig. 19-13). When waxing for the porcelain labial margin technique (see Chapter 24), some technicians prefer to wax a collar

and cut back the metal; others wax to the collarless shape, but care should be exercised to avoid distorting the fragile pattern.

Connector Design
11.   Establish the connectors in wax as described in Chapters 18 and 28. Properly shaped and positioned connectors are very important. If pre- or post-ceramic application soldering is planned, the patterns are separated with a fine saw.
12.   If only a facial veneer is involved, make the connectors identical to those for a conventional restoration. If the incisal or occlusal aspect is involved in the porcelain veneer, do not displace the connector cervically, because access for oral hygiene will be impeded (Fig. 19-14).

Pontics
13.   Because glazed vacuum-fired porcelain is easy to keep clean, include the tissue-contacting surfaces of pontics in the veneering surface (Fig. 19-15).
14.   To improve handling and stability of the wax pattern, be sure to cut back this area last (see Chapter 20).

Evaluation.   Immediately before investing, the following criteria should have been met:

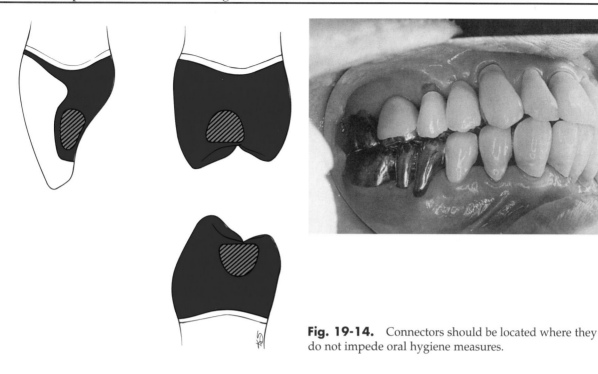

Fig. 19-14. Connectors should be located where they do not impede oral hygiene measures.

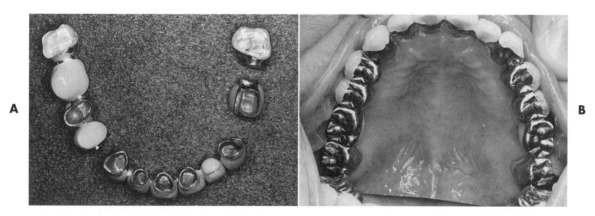

A

B

Fig. 19-15. The tissue contact on the pontics of this extensive fixed prosthesis was established in porcelain.

1. The pattern should conform to normal anatomic form. Centric stops should be located at least 1.5 mm from the porcelain-metal junction.
2. The angle between the veneering surface and the metal framework should be 90 degrees.
3. The internal surface of the veneering area should be smooth and rounded.
4. The collar height should be about 0.5 mm in wax with connectors of adequate size, but it should not impinge on the soft tissue in the interproximal areas.
5. Finally, the pattern should be smooth so that metal-finishing procedures will be minimized.

METAL SELECTION

William A. Brantley

Leon W. Laub

Clinicians and dental laboratories face a potentially bewildering set of choices when selecting **alloys** for metal-ceramic restorations. Both noble metal and base metal casting alloys exist, and there are different alloy types for each of these two major groups. There are advantages and disadvantages for each alloy type, including significant differences in cost. Successful clinical practice depends on the selection of a compatible metal-porcelain combination that will provide predictable results, depending on the particular patient case. Improper selection can cause catastrophic failure (Fig. 19-16). For a better understanding of the different properties provided on the packaging of casting alloys, the meanings and clinical relevance of these properties are discussed next.

DENTAL CONNOTATIONS OF MECHANICAL AND PHYSICAL PROPERTIES FOR CERAMIC ALLOYS

Mechanical properties of major clinical relevance are **modulus of elasticity**, **yield strength** (or **proportional limit**), hardness, and creep or distortion at elevated temperatures. Ultimate tensile strength, **ductility**, and **toughness** should also be reviewed,

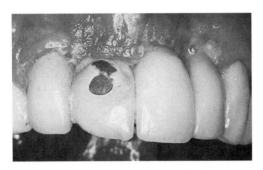

Fig. 19-16. Failure caused by improper material selection.

although these properties have less relevance for metal-ceramic restorations. Except for hardness (and elevated temperature creep or distortion), all these mechanical properties are determined by loading a cast specimen of the alloy to the point of failure in a tension test at room temperature. The physical property of thermal contraction is critically important when choosing an alloy that is compatible with the porcelain selected. From a practical standpoint, the **density** is important to both the economics of alloy selection and the dental laboratory procedure with the casting machine.

Modulus of Elasticity. Figure 19-17 illustrates schematically the tensile stress-strain plot for a ductile casting alloy that undergoes substantial permanent deformation before fracture. This plot consists of two portions: (1) a linear or elastic region that ends at the proportional limit, where the stress is proportional to strain, and (2) a subsequent curved region corresponding to plastic or permanent deformation (that terminates when the test specimen fractures). The modulus of elasticity (called *Young's modulus*) is the slope of the stress-strain plot in the elastic region. The elastic modulus has the same value for tensile and compressive strains, which occur during bending of a prosthesis, where regions on opposite sides of the neutral axis (centerline for a

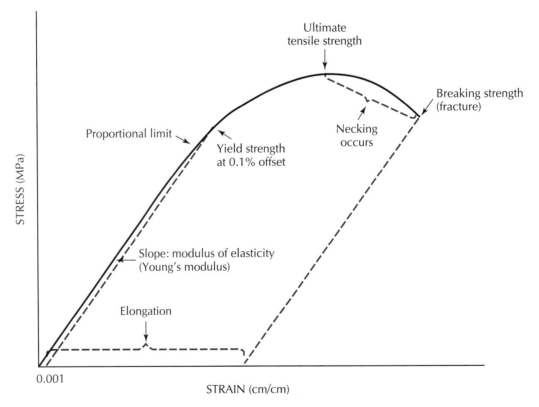

Fig. 19-17. Stress-strain curve.

symmetric cross section) undergo opposite senses of deformation. An alloy with a higher modulus of elasticity has greater stiffness or rigidity for elastic deformation. For the fabrication of a long-span FPD, an alloy with a relatively high modulus of elasticity to reduce the amount of bending deflection under loading is preferred, since excessive flexure can cause fracture of the brittle porcelain (Fig. 19-18). The modulus of elasticity has units of stress/strain and is reported in units of GPa (1 gigapascal [GPa] = 10^9 pascals [Pa] = 145,000 psi [pounds per square inch]). The unit of $1 \text{ Pa} = 1 \text{ N/m}^2$ is much too small to be useful for the elastic modulus of materials.

Proportional Limit and Yield Strength. In standard testing practice, the proportional limit (PL) of an alloy is determined by placing a straight-edge on the stress-strain plot (or performing this operation with computer software) and noting the value at which the plot first deviates from a straight line. The proportional limit is often considered synonymous with the elastic limit, which corresponds to the value of stress at which permanent deformation occurs. However, the value of the elastic limit is highly dependent on the sensitivity of the strain-measuring apparatus. Moreover, precise location of the PL on the stress-strain plot is somewhat problematic. Consequently, dental alloy manufacturers generally report the yield strength (sometimes called *offset yield strength*), which corresponds to the amount of stress for a very small designated amount of permanent deformation, at 0.1% or 0.2% (permanent strains of 0.001 or 0.002, respectively). The units for yield strength (YS) are megapascals (MPa): $1 \text{ MPa} = 10^6 \text{ Pa} = 145 \text{ psi}$. As shown in Figure 19-17, the YS is obtained by constructing a line parallel to the initial straight-line portion of the stress-strain plot, starting with the specified value of offset on the horizontal strain axis and then not-

ing the point of intersection with the curved portion of the plot. Since the 0.2% YS can be substantially higher than the 0.1% YS for a given alloy, depending on the rate of work hardening (slope of the curved portion of the stress-strain plot), manufacturers specify the offset value at which the yield strength was determined on the alloy packaging. The yield strength is often called the *useful strength* of a dental alloy, since stresses due to biting forces should not exceed the YS and result in permanent deformation of the alloy. Although a sufficiently high value of YS is essential for a ceramic alloy, values that are too high will create difficulties when adjusting the casting in the dental laboratory or dental office.

Hardness. The Vickers hardness number (VHN) of dental alloys is generally measured using a symmetric diamond pyramidal indenter, although the Knoop hardness number (KHN), obtained with a different type of diamond indenter having long and short axes, is sometimes reported. Conversion scales available for the two different hardness tests should be used with caution, since such conversions are alloy dependent. Both the Vickers and Knoop tests measure the microhardness, in contrast to the older Brinell and Rockwell tests, which use much larger indenters and measure the macrohardness. When measuring the Vickers hardness of an alloy, an understanding of the microstructure is critical. Use of the standard large indenting load of 1 kg provides information about the overall hardness of the alloy microstructure, whereas light indenting loads (e.g., 10 g) can provide information about the hardness of individual grains, constituents, or phases. The hardness is an important practical property, since very high values of hardness will cause difficulty in the dental laboratory when the casting is ready to be finished. Alloys with hardness values exceeding that of enamel (approximately 350) will cause abrasive wear of opposing teeth.

Elevated-temperature Creep and Distortion. Castings undergo elevated-temperature dimensional changes during the porcelain firing cycles. These changes have many causes, such as bulk creep of the alloy from several metallurgical mechanisms or distortion due to the relief of residual stresses from the casting process and to the alloy oxidation. The latter may be higher for some high-palladium and other alloys that undergo internal and external oxidation with formation of oxide precipitate particles. Measuring the dimensional changes that occur during porcelain bonding is tedious, but concern has been expressed about the clinical fit for castings prepared from certain alloys. Nevertheless,

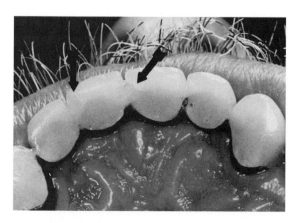

Fig. 19-18. Fracture resulted from flexing of the substructure of this long-span FPD.

in most cases an experienced dental laboratory should be able to vary techniques and obtain successful results.

Ultimate Tensile Strength. The ultimate tensile strength (UTS) (also called *tensile strength* or simply *strength*) is the maximum point on the stress-strain curve (see Fig. 19-17) and represents the greatest value of stress that can be developed in the alloy without fracture. The units for UTS are also MPa. Two types of stress-strain curves are observed for tensile testing of casting alloys. Alloys of high ductility undergo substantial necking between the UTS and the breaking strength, as shown in Figure 19-17. Other alloys of more limited ductility undergo much less necking, and the stress continues to increase after the YS until fracture occurs at the UTS. The tensile strength has minimal practical importance for a ceramic alloy, because the corresponding permanent strain does not occur under clinical conditions for a restoration. Nevertheless, this property is easy to measure, since a strain-gauge extensometer does not need to be attached to the specimen, and manufacturers often quote the tensile strength.

Percentage Elongation. For metals, the ductility, or capability of undergoing permanent tensile deformation, is measured in two ways when the test specimen is loaded to fracture: as percentage **elongation** or as reduction in area. For dental alloy castings, the ductility is measured as the percentage permanent elongation of the starting gauge length, after the two portions of the fractured specimen are placed back together. This is done because the castings typically fracture on inclined planes whose locations are determined by porosity, and a well-defined area for the fracture surface is not available for measurement of the reduction in area. Obtaining precise registration of the two fractured portions and defining the location of the original gauge length are difficult and therefore makes determining the percentage elongation to better than the nearest 1% hard to achieve, although values to the nearest 0.1% have been quoted. In principle, the percentage elongation can be obtained during the stress-strain test if a breakaway extensometer is attached to the specimen. However, extensometers are rarely available in dental materials laboratories. Figure 19-17 exaggerates the more important elastic range of the stress-strain curve, since the values of percentage elongation for casting alloys lie typically within the range of 1% to 10%. When considering the ease of adjustment for cast restorations, remember that both yield strength and elongation are involved.[12] Alloys with high YS will not be hand-burnishable, even if they have a high value of elongation.

Toughness. Historically, toughness, which is the total area under the stress-strain curve, was considered an important property of casting alloys. However, with the focus on stresses that do not exceed the YS, this property no longer receives as much attention. The toughness represents the total energy per unit volume to fracture the alloy and has units of (stress × strain) or MPa. For an alloy that does not work harden greatly and has substantial ductility, toughness is approximately equal to (UTS × elongation). Determining toughness from stress-strain plots is laborious, and manufacturers do not report this property.

Thermal Expansion/Contraction. The linear coefficient of thermal expansion is a critical property for an alloy that is to be bonded to dental porcelain. These coefficients should be closely matched to within about $0.5 \times 10^{-6}/°$ C below the glass transition temperature of the porcelain (approximately 500° to 600° C, depending upon the cooling rate), where the ceramic can no longer undergo viscous flow to relieve thermal incompatibility stresses. The thermal contraction coefficient (α), generally assumed to be the same as for that for thermal expansion, should be slightly higher for the metal so that the ceramic be in a state of beneficial residual **compressive stress** at room temperature. Values typically range from 13.5 to $14.5 \times 10^{-6}/°$ C for metals and 13.0 to $14.0 \times 10^{-6}/°$ C for porcelains.

Density. Density is the ratio of mass to volume; specific gravity is the ratio of the density of a substance to the density of water. Densities for the important types of noble and base metal casting alloys are provided in Table 19-1. The high-gold content alloys have much higher densities than the lower gold-content, palladium-based, and base metal casting alloys. This is due to the much higher density of gold (19.3 g/cm^3), compared to palladium (12.0 g/cm^3), nickel (8.9 g/cm^3) and cobalt (8.8 g/cm^3). These differences in density have two consequences. First, for cast restorations of the same size and configuration, less mass of metal will be required for the lower-density alloy; the difference in the metal cost for a restoration can be substantial when both the unit metal cost and the density difference are considered. Second, there will be additional winding of the spring on the centrifugal casting machine to achieve the needed casting pressure for the lower-density alloys.

TABLE 19-1

Alloys for Porcelain Veneering

High Noble Metal

Brand Name (Manufacturer)	Gold-Platinum-Palladium (Au-Pt-Pd)				Gold-Palladium-Silver (Au-Pd-Ag)				Gold-Palladium (Au-Pd)			
	Jelenko O (Jelenko)	Image 2 (Degussa Ney)	Will-Ceram Y (Williams/ Ivoclar)	Rx CG (Jeneric/ Pentron)	Cameo (Jelenko)	Veritas (Degussa Ney)	Will-Ceram W-2 (Williams/ Ivoclar)	Rx WCG (Jeneric/ Pentron)	Olympia (Jelenko)	Eclipse (Degussa Ney)	Will-Ceram W-3 (Williams/ Ivoclar)	Rx SFC (Jeneric/ Pentron)
Composition (weight %)	Au 87.3 Pt 4.5 Pd 5.9 Ag 1.0	Au 84.5 Pt 6.9 Pd 5.0 Ag 1.0	Au 84.0 Pt 7.1 Pd 5.7 Ag 1.5	Au 87 Pt 6.5 Pd 5 Ag 1	Au 52.5 Pd 27.0 Ag 16.0 In 2.5 Sn 2.0	Au 40.0 Pd 45.0 Ag 5.0	Au 44.8 Pd 40.5 Ag 5.9 In 3.3 Sn 2.2 Ga 1.8	Au 52 Pd 30 Ag 14 In 3	Au 51.5 Pd 38.4 In 8.5 Ga 1.5	Au 52.0 Pd 37.5	Au 48.7 Pd 39.6 In 10.6	Au 52 Pd 38 In 8.5
Yield strength (MPa)	480	670	440	330	450	430	540	550	550	570	500	590
(× 10³ psi)	70	97	64	48	65	62	78	80	80	83	72	85
Modulus of elasticity (GPa)	97	100	81	70	120	120	110	120	120	120	130	140
(× 10⁶ psi)	14	14	12	10	18	17	16	17	18	17	18	20
Tensile strength (MPa)	550	760	490	460	690	760	760	690	790	830	760	830
(× 10³ psi)	80	110	71	67	100	110	110	100	120	120	110	120
Elongation (%)	5	7	10	5	12	40	20	10	20	23	16	18
Hardness: Vickers (VHN)	200	230	170	160	240	230	200	220	260	250	220	220
Density (g/cm³)	18.2	18.0	17.4	18.5	14.1	13.0	13.4	13.8	13.7	13.8	13.8	13.5

Notes:
Alloy composition information was provided by the manufacturers, and small amounts (<1 wt. %) of grain-refining elements (Ru, Ir, and Re) are not shown.
Mechanical properties correspond to the porcelain-fired, heat-treated condition, except for Jeneric/Pentron alloys, which were heated 10 minutes at 950° C and bench cooled (ADA specification no. 38).
Yield strength values correspond to 0.2% offset for Jelenko, Degussa Ney, and Williams/Ivoclar alloys) and to 0.1% offset for Jeneric/Pentron alloys.
Values of mechanical properties have been rounded to two significant figures to reflect the level of accuracy for experimental measurement. Small differences for values in metric and corresponding English units for some alloys with similar values of mechanical properties arise from this rounding procedure and whether the original data from the manufacturer were provided in metric or English units.
Elongation values were determined for 0.5-inch (12.5-mm) or 15-mm gauge length, depending on the manufacturer. Since these values are somewhat approximate, no normalization has been performed.

Austenal Dental Inc., Chicago, Ill.
Degussa Ney, Bloomfield, Conn.
J.F. Jelenko & Co., Armonk, N.Y.
Jeneric/Pentron, Wallingford, Conn.
Williams Division, Ivoclar North America, Amherst, N.Y.

Continued

Alloys for Porcelain Veneering—cont'd

TABLE 19-1

	Noble Metal										
	Palladium-Silver (Pd-Ag)					Palladium-Copper-Gallium (Pd-Cu-Ga)					
Brand Name (Manufacturer)	Jelstar (Jelenko)	Tempo (Degussa Ney)	Will-Ceram W-1 (Williams/ Ivoclar)	Rx Palladent B (Jeneric/ Pentron)	Rx 91 (Jeneric/ Pentron)	Liberty (Jelenko)	Option (Degussa Ney)	Spartan Plus (Williams/ Ivoclar)	Athenium (Williams/ Ivoclar)	Rx Naturelle (Jeneric/ Pentron)	Rx Correct Fit II (Jeneric/ Pentron)
Composition (weight %)	Pd 59.8 Ag 28.0 Sn 6.0 In 6.0	Pd 54.9 Ag 35.0	Pd 53.3 Ag 37.7 Sn 8.5	Pd 60.5 Ag 28 In 6.5 Sn 2.5	Pd 53.5 Ag 37.5 Sn 8.5	Pd 75.9 Cu 10.0 Ga 5.5 Sn 6.0 Au 2.0	Pd 79 Cu 10 Ga 9 Au 2 B < 1	Pd 78.8 Cu 10.0 Ga 9.0 Au 2.0 B 0	Pd 73.8 Cu 14.5 Ga 1.5 In 5.0 Sn 5.0	Pd 79 Cu 10 Ga 9 Au 2	Pd 77 Cu 10 Ga 5 In 6 Au 2
Yield strength (MPa)	440	590	480	550	660	690	900	800	560	900	620
(× 10³ psi)	64	86	70	80	96	100	130	120	81	130	90
Modulus of elasticity (GPa)	120	110	110	92	110	140	94	97	120	110	100
(× 10⁶ psi)	18	16	16	13	16	20	14	14	17	16	14
Tensile strength (MPa)	660	830	650	760	900	970	1200	830	850	1100	970
(× 10³ psi)	95	120	94	110	130	140	170	120	120	160	140
Elongation (%)	18	13	11	10	14	20	23	20	25	16	35
Hardness: Vickers (VHN)	220	240	240	250	240	340	420	310	270	320	260
Density (g/cm³)	10.7	10.8	11.1	10.5	11.0	10.7	10.6	10.7	11.0	10.6	10.5

TABLE 19-1 Alloys for Porcelain Veneering—cont'd

| | Noble Metal | | | | | Predominantly Base Metal | | | | | |
| | Palladium-Gallium (Pd-Ag) | | | | | Nickel-Chromium (Ni-Cr) | | | Cobalt-Chromium (Co-Cr) | | |
Brand Name (Manufacturer)	Legacy (Jelenko)	PTM-88 (Jelenko)	Protocol (Williams/Ivoclar)	LTA (Jeneric/Pentron)	Aspen (Jeneric/Pentron)	Micro-Band NP2 (Austenal)	Rexillium III (Jeneric/Pentron)	Will-Ceram Litecast B (Williams/Ivoclar)	Genesis II (Jelenko)	Neobond II Special (Austenal)	Novarex (Jeneric/Pentron)
Composition (weight %)	Pd 85.2 Ga 10.0 In 1.1 Au 2.0	Pd 86.9 Ga 8.3 Co 4.0	Pd 75.2 Ga 6.0 In 6.0 Au 6.0 Ag 6.5	Pd 80 Ga 6 In 6 Ag 5	Pd 75 Ga 6 In 6 Au 5.5 Ag 6.5 Pt 1	Ni 66.6 Cr 13.0 Ga 7.5 Mo 7.0 Fe 5.0 Si 0.75 Mn 0.15 Be 0	Ni 76 Cr 14 Mo 6 Al 2.5 Be 1.8	Ni 77.4 Cr 12.8 Mo 4.0 Al 3.3 Be 1.8	Co 53.0 Cr 27.0 W 10.0 Ru 3.0 Ga 3.0 Cu 1.0 Nb 1.0 Ta 1.0	Co 52 Cr 28 W 11.5 Ga 2.5 Ru 2.5 Cu 1 Fe 0.87 Nb 0.63 Si 0.5 Ta 0.5	Co 55 Cr 25 W 10
Yield strength											
(MPa)	720	590	500	570	550	260	830	830	520	550	620
($\times 10^3$ psi)	100	85	72	82	80	37	120	120	75	80	90
Modulus of elasticity											
(GPa)	130	120	100	120	130	170	180	190	170	220	220
($\times 10^6$ psi)	19	18	15	17	19	25	26	28	25	32	220
Tensile strength											
(MPa)	970	830	760	900	830	440	1100	1200	760	700	760
($\times 10^3$ psi)	140	120	110	130	120	64	160	170	110	100	110
Elongation (%)	25	25	34	42	21	19	15	12	15	10	7
Hardness: Vickers (VHN)	280	240	240	200	200	170	360	340	350	300	350
Density (g/cm³)	10.9	10.9	11.0	11.2	11	8.6	7.8	7.4	8.8	8.7	8.8

AVAILABLE ALLOY SYSTEMS

The nomenclature for casting alloys usually creates confusion. Classifying noble and base metal casting alloys according to the mechanism for corrosion resistance is the preferred method. The gold-based and palladium-based noble metal casting alloys achieve corrosion resistance because of the inherent nobility of the gold and palladium atoms, which do not form stable oxides at room temperature. In contrast, the base metal casting alloys, where nickel and cobalt are the principal elements, oxidize rapidly to form a passivating chromium oxide surface layer that blocks the diffusion of oxygen and prevents corrosion of the underlying metal.

Historically, terms such as *precious*, *semiprecious*, and *nonprecious* have been used to describe casting alloys. Such precious or semiprecious alloys usually contained a greater quantity of silver, along with more palladium and a reduced gold content. Silver, which is not a noble metal in the oral environment, assumes some noble metal character in the presence of palladium. The terms *precious*, *semiprecious*, and *nonprecious*, which refer to unit metal cost, are much less preferable than the classification of noble and base metals, which refers to the electrochemical character of the alloys.

The major noble metals in dental alloys are gold, platinum, and palladium. The total percentage of these elements is referred to as the *noble metal content of the alloy*. Iridium (much less than 1% by weight) and ruthenium (up to about 1%) are used, respectively, as grain-refining elements in gold-based and palladium-based casting alloys. The original metal-ceramic alloy compositions (e.g., Jelenko "O", shown in Table 19-1) had approximately 98% noble metal content by weight. Rapid increases in the price of gold during the 1970s stimulated the development of lower-gold content (from about 85% to 50% by weight) alloys and base-metal alloys for fixed prosthodontics.[13] During the 1980s, the high-palladium alloys were developed as economic alternatives to the gold-based alloys.[14]*

A classification system[15] developed by the American Dental Association for casting alloys is presented in Table 19-2 and includes alloys for all-metal and metal-ceramic restorations. Because the classification is based solely on noble metal content and ignores other, often critically important, alloying elements, general statements cannot be made about mechanical properties, clinical performance, and biocompatibility, even within each of the three groups in Table 19-2. Hundreds of dental alloys are commercially available, and appropriate testing is necessary to characterize the properties, safety, and efficacy of each. However, when each of these major groups is further subdivided into important alloy types, some accurate generalizations are possible. They are discussed in the following sections.

High Noble Metal Alloys. The high-noble metal content alloys contain a minimum of 60% by weight of noble elements; at least 40% is gold. There are three systems in this class: gold-platinum-palladium, gold-palladium-silver, and gold-palladium (in the historical order of their development). Table 19-1 lists some mechanical properties and the density for representative alloys of each system.

Au-Pt-Pd. As previously noted, these were the first casting alloys formulated to bond with dental porcelain. Because of concern about adverse effects on the color of dental porcelain, copper, which was traditionally used for strengthening the high-gold casting alloys for all-metal restorations, could not be incorporated in the ceramic alloy compositions. Instead, these alloys were strengthened by precipitates of an Fe-Pt intermetallic compound.[16] Porcelain adherence was achieved by incorporating tin and indium in the alloys. During the initial alloy oxidation step for the porcelain firing cycles, these elements (as well as some iron) diffused to the alloy surface and became oxidized. Subsequent chemical bonding was achieved between this oxide layer and the dental porcelain (see Chapter 22). Although these alloys have excellent corrosion resistance, they are susceptible to some dimensional changes during the porcelain firing cycles and are not recommended for multiple-unit FPD restorations.

Au-Pd-Ag. These were the first lower-gold content alternative alloys to be widely used in the 1970s. Platinum was eliminated from the alloy compositions, and the gold content was reduced to about 50%, with corresponding increases in the amounts of

---

*Recently, the price of palladium has greatly increased. In January 1997, palladium was $120 an ounce; by February 2000, this had increased to $800 an ounce. However, by April 2000, the price has decreased to $560 an ounce. Rapid increases in alloy prices can cause many problems for dentists and the dental laboratory industry.

Classification for Dental Casting Alloys	TABLE 19-2
	Noble Metal Content: Au, Pt, PD (Minimum Percentage by Weight)
High-noble metal	60 (greater than 40 gold)
Noble metal	25 (no gold requirement)
Predominantly base metal	Below 25 (no gold requirement)

palladium and silver.[17,18] Some alloy strengthening was achieved by solid solution hardening from the dissimilar atomic sizes of the three major elements (gold, palladium, and silver), which form solutions with each other. Additional solid solution strengthening was hypothesized from tin or indium, which were again incorporated as oxidizable elements to provide porcelain bonding. Further alloy strengthening may occur from precipitates formed by these elements. Although these alloys have excellent mechanical properties and porcelain adherence, green discoloration (resulting from diffusion of silver atoms into the porcelain) has been reported for some alloy-porcelain combinations.[19] Possible reasons for this effect may be the high sodium concentration of the porcelain or the relative sizes of the metal ions in the porcelain. The discolored region can be ground away, but this involves an additional processing step. In addition, silver vapor generated in the porcelain furnace during processing can contaminate the muffle, and periodic purging of the furnace with a carbon block is required. Green discoloration has apparently been eliminated in some porcelain compositions by substituting potassium ions for sodium ions; the larger potassium ions impede the diffusion of silver into the porcelain.

Au-Pd. Gold-palladium alloys that are silver-free were developed during the late 1970s and have become very popular. Alloy strengthening is achieved with a combination of solid solution hardening and microstructural precipitates. The hardness (assumed to be related to strength) of these alloys is independent of heat-treatment temperature within the porcelain-firing range, unlike Au-Pd-Ag alloys.[16] The Au-Pd alloys have excellent mechanical properties, elevated-temperature creep behavior,[20] and porcelain adherence,[21] without the green discoloration associated with Au-Pd-Ag alloys.

Discussion. The data in Table 19-1 show that the Au-Pd and Au-Pd-Ag alloys, when compared to the Au-Pt-Pd alloys, have higher values of yield strength and modulus of elasticity, along with lower density. Consequently, FPD restorations fabricated from alloys in the former two groups will be more resistant to masticatory forces and undergo less bending deflection. They also have the economic advantage of more restorations per unit of alloy cost. Selection of the proper porcelain for Au-Pd-Ag alloys is essential if discoloration problems are to be avoided.

Noble Metal Alloys. The noble-metal alloys have a minimum of 25% by weight of noble metal, with no requirement for gold percentage. There are three alloy systems in this class: palladium-silver, palladium-copper-gallium, and palladium-gallium (in the historical order of their development). Table 19-1 lists some mechanical properties and the density for representative alloys of each system.

Pd-Ag. These alloys, developed in the 1970s, continued the trend by manufacturers of reducing the gold content (to between 0% and 2% by weight), with corresponding increases in the palladium and silver contents.[22] A small percentage of gold in these alloys and the high-palladium alloys has little effect on their properties but may facilitate third-party payments. As previously noted, in the presence of palladium, silver appears to assume noble metal character, which is beneficial for corrosion resistance. Because of their high silver content (30% to 35% by weight), these alloys have been called *semiprecious*, a term that should no longer be used. Compared to the Au-Pd-Ag and Au-Pd alloys, the Pd-Ag alloys have similar values of yield strength and modulus of elasticity and much lower density values. Because of their high silver contents, porcelain greening and furnace contamination can result during fabrication of FPD restorations, unless the porcelain is carefully selected. Nevertheless, these alloys are frequently chosen as a compromise between the more expensive high-noble alloys and the relatively inexpensive base metal alloys.

Pd-Cu-Ga. The Pd-Cu-Ga alloys contain more than 70% by weight of palladium and were developed in the early 1980s as economical alternatives to the gold-based alloys.[12] The melting point of palladium (1555° C) is much higher than that of gold (1064° C); gallium has a melting point of 30° C. The addition of gallium to palladium yields high-palladium alloys that can be fused and cast with the same dental laboratory technology developed for the gold-based casting alloys. Multi-orifice torches are required to fuse the high-palladium alloys, and the use of ceramic crucibles dedicated to individual alloys is recommended.[12] Carbon-containing investments should not be used, because the incorporation of very small amounts of carbon in these alloys degrades the bond strength with porcelain.[23] The Pd-Cu-Ga alloys appear to have castability and casting accuracy comparable to the high noble metal alloys.[24]

Recent measurements[25] of the mechanical properties of some Pd-Cu-Ga alloys have produced values of yield strength, modulus of elasticity, and percentage elongation that differ from values in Table 19-1. This suggests some technique-sensitivity in the fabrication of cast specimens for the tension test. In a recent study, values of yield strength and tensile strength were found to be higher for the Pd-Cu-Ga alloys, compared to Au-Pd-Ag, Au-Pd, and Pd-Ag alloys, while the values for modulus of elasticity and ductility were similar when the same simulated porcelain-firing heat-treatment condition was compared. Although a near-surface eutectic structure was present in Pd-Cu-Ga alloy castings that simulated **copings** for maxillary incisors,[12] this constituent was absent in the 3-mm diameter cast specimens for the tension test.[23] Some Pd-Cu-Ga alloys have hardness values comparable to or exceeding that for tooth enamel, and castings from these alloys may be difficult to finish in the dental laboratory. In addition, chairside adjustments may be difficult for patients. However, substitution of indium for tin yields Pd-Cu-Ga alloys with much lower hardness (VHN approximately 270).[26] All these alloys achieve substantial hardening by solid-solution incorporation of other elements within the palladium crystal structure. The hardest Pd-Cu-Ga alloys (VHN exceeding 300) contain a hard grain boundary phase whose composition is close to that of Pd_5Ga_2.[24] Transmission electron microscopic studies indicate that representative high-palladium alloys have the same bulk ultrastructure.[27] X-ray diffraction analyses have revealed that oxidized Pd-Cu-Ga alloys have complex internal oxidation regions that can contain up to five different oxide phases.[28] Oxides of copper, gallium, tin, indium, and even palladium formed under the conditions present in the porcelain furnace were subsequently detected in the oxidized alloys at room temperature. The results of creep experiments on the Pd-Cu-Ga alloys have been mixed.[18] The creep rates associated with relatively high thermal incompatibility stresses near the glass transition temperature of dental porcelain were high for two Pd-Cu-Ga alloys, whereas these alloys had excellent creep resistance at high temperatures and low stresses simulating the deflection of a long-span FPD due to gravity during processing.

Pd-Ga. The copper-free Pd-Ga alloys were subsequently developed during the 1980s to provide compositions with lower hardness than that of the initial Pd-Cu-Ga formulations. The hard Pd_5Ga_2 phase is absent in these alloys, which are strengthened by solid solution hardening. The alloys have a complex fine precipitate structure at the grain boundaries,[14,29] and their mechanical properties are generally more similar to those of Pd-Ag alloys rather than the Pd-Cu-Ga alloys. Compared to the Pd-Ga alloys, porcelain adherence is superior for the Pd-Cu-Ga alloys.[21] The Pd-Ga-Co alloy[30] in Table 19-1 has a particularly dark oxide that is more difficult to mask with dental porcelain. This alloy has not yet achieved widespread clinical acceptance.

Discussion. A recent study comparing the dimensional changes at various stages of the simu-

lated porcelain firing cycles for copings for metal-ceramic single-unit restorations of selected high-palladium alloys found that most of the selected high-palladium alloys had acceptable high-temperature distortion.[25,31] Because of the considerable price volatility for palladium, the unit metal cost for the Pd-Cu-Ga and Pd-Ga alloys has recently become competitive with the very popular Au-Pd alloys. When the high-palladium alloys were introduced in the 1980s, the unit metal cost was between one-half and one-third of the Au-Pd alloys.[12] Consequently, there has been a trend toward the Au-Pd alloys and the much less expensive Pd-Ag alloys; the latter have comparable density to the high-palladium alloys. However, caution is needed with the Pd-Ag alloys to prevent porcelain with green discoloration. Some biocompatibility concerns have been raised about the high-palladium alloys, particularly in Germany with the Pd-Cu-Ga alloys. Recent review articles[32,33] suggest that there are minimal health hazards associated the high-palladium alloys, although further research in this area is recommended.

Predominantly Base Metal Alloys. Table 19-2 defines these alloys (sometimes termed *nonprecious*) as having less than 25% by weight of noble metal with no requirements for gold. Most of these alloys used for fixed prosthodontics are Ni-Cr alloys, but some Co-Cr alloys have also been formulated for porcelain application.[29,30]

Ni-Cr. Yield strength, hardness, and modulus of elasticity can be greatly affected by small differences in weight percentages of minor elemental components among the compositions of these alloys.[34] Table 19-1 illustrates some of these variations. For example, values of yield strength vary from 260 to 807 MPa, and Vickers hardness varies from 175 to 335. (For comparison, VHN values are 50 to 52, 125 to 127, and 120 to 143 for gold, platinum, and copper, respectively.) Consequently, the selection of a specific brand of Ni-Cr alloy depends on the clinical application. If burnishing or extended finishing of a crown is anticipated, a brand with a relatively low yield strength and hardness should be used.

One benefit of these alloys is their much higher values of modulus of elasticity, compared to the noble metal alloys. Therefore, long-span fixed prostheses fabricated from Ni-Cr alloys will undergo much less flexure than similar prostheses fabricated from noble metal alloys, with less likelihood of fracture of the brittle dental porcelain component. These base metal casting alloys are generally considered more technique-sensitive and difficult to cast that the noble metal casting alloys. However, this assessment may reflect the lack of experience of some dental laboratories with the Ni-Cr alloys. Therefore, the choice of dental laboratory is particularly important when these alloys are selected.

Beryllium. Many Ni-Cr alloy formulations contain up to 2% by weight of beryllium. The major reason for incorporating this element in the alloy is to lower the melting range and to decrease the viscosity of the molten alloy, thereby improving its castability. Beryllium also provides strengthening and affects the thickness of the oxide layer, when the alloy is oxidized for porcelain firing. The latter is an important consideration for base metal casting alloys, which can form much thicker oxide layers than noble metal casting alloys. Fracture through the oxide layer may occur and will cause failure of the base metal-ceramic restoration.

The use of beryllium has created some doubt about the safety of some Ni-Cr alloys. NOTE: When the densities of nickel (8.9 g/cm^3) and chromium (7.2 g/cm^3) are compared to beryllium (1.8 g/cm^3), 2% by weight of beryllium in the alloy composition can be equivalent to nearly 10% beryllium on an atomic basis. Consequently, the atomic proportion of beryllium atoms in these alloy compositions can be relatively large.

Nickel. The U.S. Federal Standard for exposure to metallic nickel and soluble nickel compounds (1 mg/m^3) is much greater than the proposed National Institute for Occupational Safety and Health (NIOSH) recommendation for such exposure (15 μg/m^3 for a 10-hour TWA workday). Occupational exposure of refinery workers to nickel has been associated with lung and nasal cancer. Acute effects of exposure to nickel include skin sensitization that can lead to chronic eczema. Therefore, as a health precaution, an operator should wear a mask and use efficient suction when grinding and finishing a dental nickel-base alloy.

One study reports that 9% of the female population and 0.9% of the male population are sensitive to nickel.[35] This prompts the question: Are such individuals likely to manifest an adverse reaction to dental Ni-Cr alloys? In a 20-patient clinical study[36] to investigate this question, each of 10 controls (who had no known sensitivity to nickel) showed a negative dermal response and a negative intraoral response to a dental Ni-Cr alloy. Among 10 patients with a known sensitivity, 8 showed a positive dermal response to the alloy. When these patients wore an intraoral appliance containing the Ni-Cr alloy, 30% manifested an allergic response within 48 hours.

The ADA has issued a labeling requirement for base metal alloys that contain nickel. It states that such alloys should not be used in individuals with known nickel sensitivity. Another question now arises: Can patients who are not allergic to nickel become sensitive to it from fixed prostheses made with nickel-containing alloys?

A recent investigation[37] found that Ni-Cr alloys not containing beryllium were more resistant than beryllium-containing alloys to in vitro corrosion. The four alloys studied showed lower corrosion rates in cell culture solutions after cold solution sterilization. Although the corrosion products released from the alloys did not alter the cellular morphology and viability of human gingival fibroblasts, reductions in cellular proliferation were observed. The authors concluded that biocompatibility concerns still exist relating to the exposure of local and systemic tissues to elevated levels of corrosion products from the Ni-Cr alloys.

Co-Cr. The potential health problems associated with beryllium- and nickel-containing alloys have led to the development of another alternative base metal alloy system: cobalt-chromium.[38,39] The modulus of elasticity of the Co-Cr system is the highest of any of the ceramic alloy systems discussed so far (see Table 19-1). One alloy, similar in composition and properties to Co-Cr and used for RPD frameworks, has an elongation of 1%. This very low value, combined with its high level of hardness, suggests that finishing restorations made with it may be difficult.

Ti. Titanium-based alloys have been studied since the late 1970s as potential casting alloys.[40] Advantages of titanium-based casting alloys include excellent biocompatibility and corrosion resistance of titanium, which is due to the presence of a thin, adherent, passivating surface layer of TiO$_2$. The low density (4.5 g/cm^3) of titanium, compared to gold or palladium (19.3 and 12.0 g/cm^3, respectively), also results in lighter and potentially less expensive restorations*. Alloys studied have included CP (commercially pure) titanium, Ti-6Al-4V, and a variety of experimental alloys.[40-42] The casting of titanium-based dental alloys poses special problems because of titanium's high melting point (1668° C) and its strong tendency to oxidize and react with other materials.

Special casting machines must be used that provide either a vacuum environment or an argon atmosphere. Both vacuum/argon pressure and centrifugal casting machines have been developed, and both argon-arc melting and induction melting have

---

*However, the laboratory cost of fabricating cast restorations from titanium alloys may be high.

been used to fuse the Ti alloys.[43] Additional studies have discussed the use of face coats on the wax pattern[41] and casting into low-temperature (350° C), phosphate-bonded investments.[44] The effects of the argon gas pressure, permeability of the investment, and mold venting have also been studied.[45-48] Good accuracy for titanium castings on their dies can be achieved with the proper choice of investment.[44] Selecting a dental laboratory experienced in fabricating these castings is essential. Further research is needed to optimize the metallurgical structure and casting technology for titanium alloys, which have a dendritic microstructure[41] resulting from the lack of a suitable grain-refining element. A very hard near-surface region that can exceed 50 μm in thickness is also present on the castings due to reaction of the titanium alloy with the investment and perhaps with the residual atmosphere in the casting machine.[41,44] To overcome the difficulties in casting titanium, a system has been developed that manufactures copings from blocks of pure titanium by machine duplication and spark erosion (Procera*)[49] (Fig. 19-19). Because copings are machined, some error is intro-

*Nobel Biocare: Chicago, Ill.

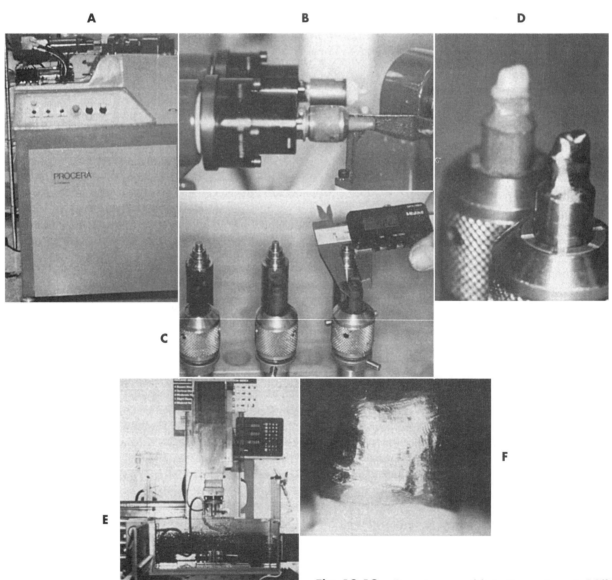

Fig. 19-19. Procera crown fabrication system. **A,** Milling replicator. **B,** Tooth preparation replicated from master die. **C,** Carbon electrodes. **D,** External substructure shape milled out of solid titanium. **E,** Spark erosion unit used to shape the internal surface with the electrodes. **F,** Completed substructure before porcelain application.

duced into the lost wax process. To complete the restoration, an esthetic veneer is applied to the titanium coping. A recent study[50] found no statistically significant differences between the external marginal openings of titanium crowns prepared by electrical discharge machining and cast Au-Pt-Pd crowns.

• • •

REVIEW OF TECHNIQUE

Figure 19-20 summarizes the steps involved in producing wax patterns for metal-ceramic restorations.

1. The restorations are waxed to anatomic contour (Fig. 19-20, *A*).
2. The patterns are troughed to obtain correct porcelain thickness in the completed restoration (Fig. 19-20, *B*).

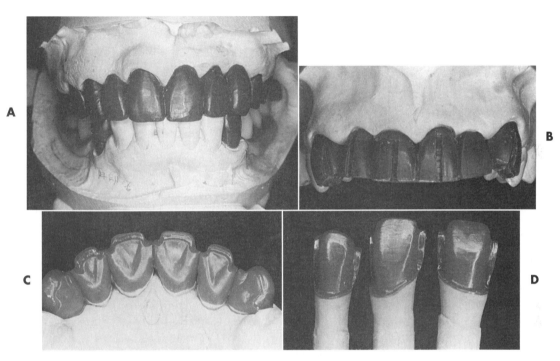

Fig. 19-20. Technique review.

Study Questions

1. Explain all reasons for full-contour waxing before cutting back a wax pattern for a metal-ceramic restoration.
2. Why should the framework of a metal-ceramic crown not be of consistent thickness on the veneering surface?
3. How does one determine the location of the metal-ceramic interface? Interproximally on a maxillary central incisor? Interproximally on a maxillary premolar? Occlusally on a mandibular premolar? Lingually on a maxillary canine?
4. Explain the stress-strain curve. What does it mean when the straight portion of the curve is steeper or more horizontal? What is the importance of a flatter curve versus a more radiused curve? What does it mean if the highest point of the curve is higher or lower? What does the total surface area under the curve signify?
5. Explain the classification of alloy systems for metal-ceramic restorations. Select two categories, and give two examples of alloys in each category. Contrast the physical properties of the alloys chosen, and provide examples of recommended use.
6. Briefly discuss the health hazards that can be associated with the various alloys used in the metal-ceramic technique.

3. The cut-back is completed (Fig. 19-20, C).
4. The margins are finalized before investing (Fig. 19-20, D).

SUMMARY

Framework design for metal-ceramic restorations must be based on an understanding of fundamental material properties. Restorations should be waxed to anatomic contour and then cut back in the area that is to be veneered. This creates an even porcelain thickness, which provides superior mechanical properties in the completed restoration while simultaneously standardizing shade reproduction.

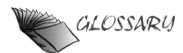 *GLOSSARY*

airborne particle abrasion: the process of altering the surface of a material through the use of abrasive particles propelled by compressed air or other gases.

alloy: *n* (14c) a mixture of two or more metals or metalloids that are mutually soluble in the molten state; distinguished as binary, ternary, quaternary, etc., depending on the number of metals within the mixture. Alloying elements are added to alter the hardness, strength, and toughness of a metallic element, thus obtaining properties not found in the pure metal. Alloys may also be classified on the basis of their behavior when solidified

aluminum oxide: *1:* a metallic oxide constituent of dental porcelain that increases hardness and viscosity *2:* a high-strength ceramic crystal dispersed throughout a glassy phase to increase its strength as in aluminous dental porcelain used to fabricate aluminous porcelain jacket crowns *3:* a finely ground ceramic particle (frequently 50 μm) often used in conjunction with airborne particle abrasion of metal castings before the application of porcelain as with metal ceramic restorations

base metal: any metallic element that does not resist tarnish and corrosion

carat: *n* (15c) a standard of gold fineness. The percentage of gold in an alloy, stated in parts per 24. Pure gold is designated 24 carat

compressive stress: the internal induced force that opposes the shortening of a material in a direction parallel to the direction of the stresses; any induced force per unit area that resists deformation caused by a load that tends to compress or shorten a body

1 coping: *n 1:* a long, enveloping ecclesiastical vestment *2a:* something resembling a cope (as by concealing or covering) *2b:* coping

2 coping: *n* (ca. 1909): a thin covering—usage: see c. impression, transfer c.

degas: *vt;* **degassed:** *pt; pp;* **degassing:** *ppr* (1920) *1:* to remove gas from an object or substance *2:* the name commonly used to denote the first heat cycle (oxidation cycle) in fabrication of a metal ceramic restoration that removes surface impurities from the metallic component and produces surface oxides prior to the application of opaque porcelain

ductility: *n* (14c) the ability of a material to withstand permanent deformation under a tensile load without rupture; ability of a material to be plastically strained in tension. A material is brittle if it does not have appreciable plastic deformation in tension before rupture

elastic limit: the greatest stress to which a material may be subjected and still be capable of returning to its original dimensions when such forces are released

elastic modulus: the stiffness or flexibility of a material within the elastic range. Within the elastic range, the material deforms in direct proportion to the stress applied as represented by Hooke's law

elongation: *n* (14c) *1:* deformation as a result of tensile force application *2:* the degree to which a metal will stretch before breaking *3:* the over eruption of a tooth

fatigue: the breaking or fracturing of a material caused by repeated cyclic or applied loads below the yield limit; usually viewed initially as minute cracks followed by tearing and rupture; termed brittle failure or fracture

Knoop hardness test: [Frederick Knoop, U.S. engineer, U.S. Department of Commerce]: eponym for a surface hardness test using a diamond stylus. It is used for harder materials and is characterized by the diamond or rhomboid shaped indentation. The indentation microhardness test uses a rhombic-based pyramidal diamond indenter. The long diagonal of the resulting indentation is measured to determine the hardness. This test is suitable for most classes of materials including brittle and elastomeric
    Knoop F. Peters CG, Emerson WB. A sensitive pyramidal-diamond tool for indentation measurements. J Res Nat Bur Stand 1939; 12:39-45

malleable: *adj* (14c) capable of being extended or shaped with a hammer or with the pressure of rollers

modulus of elasticity: in metallurgy, the coefficient found by dividing the unit stress, at any point up to the proportional limit, by its corresponding unit of elongation (tension) or strain. A ratio of stress to strain. As the modulus of elasticity rises, the material becomes more rigid

modulus of resilience: the work or energy required to stress a cubic inch of material (in one direction only) from zero up to the proportional limit of the material, measured by the ability of the material to withstand the momentary effect of an impact load while stresses remain within the proportional limit

noble metal: those metal elements that resist oxidation, tarnish, and corrosion during heating, casting, or soldering and when used intraorally; examples include gold and platinum

nonprecious metal: see base metal

proportional limit: that unit of stress beyond which deformation is no longer proportional to the applied load

shearing stress: the internal induced force that opposes the sliding of one plane on an adjacent plane or the force that resists a twisting action

static fatigue: the delayed failure of glass and ceramic materials resulting from stress-enhanced chemical reactions aided by water vapor acting on surface cracks. Analogous to stress corrosion occurring in metals

stress: *n* (14c) force per unit area; a force exerted on one body that presses on, pulls on, pushes against, or tends to invest or compress another body; the deformation caused in a body by such a force; an internal force that resists an externally applied load or force. It is normally defined in terms of mechanical stress, which is the force divided by the perpendicular cross sectional area over which the force is applied

tensile stress: the internal induced force that resists the elongation of a material in a direction parallel to the direction of the stresses

tension: *n* (1533) the state of being stretched, strained, or extended

toughness: *n* the ability of a material to withstand stresses and strains without breaking

ultimate strength: the greatest stress that may be induced in a material at the point of rupture—called also *ultimate tensile strength*

REFERENCES

1. Christensen GJ: The use of porcelain-fused-to-metal restorations in current dental practice: a survey, *J Prosthet Dent* 56:1, 1986.

2. Pintado MR et al: Variation in tooth wear in young adults over a two-year period, *J Prosthet Dent* 77:313, 1997.

3. Monasky GE, Taylor DF: Studies on the wear of porcelain, enamel, and gold, *J Prosthet Dent* 25:299, 1971.

4. Ekfeldt A, Øilo G: Occlusal contact wear of prosthodontic materials, *Acta Odontol Scand* 46:159, 1988.

5. Kelly JR et al: Ceramics in dentistry: historical roots and current perspectives, *J Prosthet Dent* 75:18, 1996.

6. Hacker CH et al: An in vitro investigation of the wear of enamel on porcelain and gold in saliva, *J Prosthet Dent* 75:14, 1996.

7. Ramp MH et al: Evaluation of wear: enamel opposing three ceramic materials and a gold alloy, *J Prosthet Dent* 77:523, 1997.

8. Marker JC et al: The compressive strength of nonprecious versus precious ceramometal restorations with various frame designs, *J Prosthet Dent* 55:560, 1986.

9. Terada Y et al: The influence of different thicknesses of dentin porcelain on the color reflected from thin opaque porcelain fused to metal, *Int J Prosthodont* 2:352, 1989.

10. Craig RG et al: Stress distribution in porcelain-fused-to-gold crowns and preparations constructed with photoelastic plastics, *J Dent Res* 50:1278, 1971.

11. Warpeha WS, Goodkind RJ: Design and technique variables affecting fracture resistance of metal-ceramic restorations, *J Prosthet Dent* 35:291, 1976.

12. Moon PC, Modjeski PJ: The burnishability of dental casting alloys, *J Prosthet Dent* 36:404, 1976.

13. Valega TM, editor: *Alternatives to gold alloys in dentistry*, DHEW Publ. No. (NIH) 77-1227, Washington, DC, 1977.

14. Carr AB, Brantley WA: New high-palladium casting alloys. I. Overview and initial studies, *Int J Prosthodont* 4:265, 1991.

15. American Dental Association Report: Classification system for cast alloys, *J Am Dent Assoc* 109:838, 1984.

16. Fuys A et al: Precipitation hardening in gold-platinum alloys containing small quantities of iron, *J Biomed Mater Res* 7:471, 1973.

17. Civjan S et al: Further studies on gold alloys used in fabrication of porcelain-fused-to-metal restorations, *J Am Dent Assoc* 90:659, 1975.

18. Vermilyea SG et al: Observations on gold-palladium-silver and gold-palladium alloys, *J Prosthet Dent* 44:294, 1980.

19. Moya F et al: Experimental observation of silver and gold penetration into dental ceramic by means of a radiotracer technique, *J Dent Res* 66:1717, 1987.

20. Anusavice KJ et al: Interactive effect of stress and temperature on creep of PFM alloys, *J Dent Res* 64:1094, 1985.

21. Papazoglou E et al: Porcelain adherence to high-palladium alloys, *J Prosthet Dent* 70:386, 1993.

22. Goodacre CJ: Palladium-silver alloys: a review of the literature, *J Prosthet Dent* 62:34, 1989.

23. Herr H, Syverud M: Carbon impurities and properties of some palladium alloys for ceramic veneering, *Dent Mater* 1:106, 1985.

24. Byrne G et al: Casting accuracy of high-palladium alloys, *J Prosthet Dent* 55:297, 1986.

25. Papazoglou E: *On porcelain bonding, oxidation, mechanical properties and high-temperature distortion of high-palladium dental casting alloys*, PhD Dissertation, The Ohio State University, 1999.

26. Wu Q et al: Heat-treatment behavior of high-palladium dental alloys, *Cells Mater* 7:161, 1997.

27. Cai Z et al: Transmission electron microscopic investigation of high-palladium dental casting alloys, *Dent Mater* 13:365, 1997.

28. Brantley WA et al: X-ray diffraction studies of oxidized high-palladium alloys, *Dent Mater* 12:333, 1996.

29. Brantley WA et al: X-ray diffraction studies of as-cast high-palladium alloys, *Dent Mater* 11:154, 1995.

30. Syverud M et al: A new dental Pd-Co alloy for ceramic veneering, *Dent Mater* 3:102, 1987.

31. Papazoglou E et al: High-temperature distortion of high-palladium metal-ceramic crowns, *J Dent Res* 78:484, 1999 (abstract no. 3026).

32. Cai Z et al: On the biocompatibility of high-palladium dental alloys, *Cells Mater* 5:357, 1995.

33. Wataha JC, Hanks CT: Biological effects of palladium and risk of using palladium in dental casting alloys, *J Oral Rehabil* 23:309, 1996.

34. Baran GR: The metallurgy of Ni-Cr alloys for fixed prosthodontics, *J Prosthet Dent* 50:639, 1983.

35. American Dental Association, Council on Dental Materials, Instruments, and Equipment: Biological effects of nickel-containing dental alloys, *J Am Dent Assoc* 104:501, 1982.

36. Moffa JP et al: An evaluation of nonprecious alloys for use with porcelain veneers. II. Industrial safety and biocompatibility, *J Prosthet Dent* 30:432, 1973.

37. Bumgardner JD, Lucas LC: Corrosion and cell culture evaluations of nickel-chromium dental casting alloys, *J Appl Biomater* 5:203, 1994.

38. Vermilyea SG et al: Observations on nickel-free, beryllium-free alloys for fixed prostheses, *J Am Dent Assoc* 106:36, 1983.

39. Barakat MM, Asgar K: Mechanical properties and soldering of some cobalt base metal alloys, *Dent Mater* 2:272, 1986.

40. Waterstrat RM: Comments on casting of Ti-13Cu-4.5Ni alloy. In Valega TM, editor: *Alternatives to gold alloys in dentistry*, DHEW Publ. No. (NIH) 77-1227, Washington, DC, 1977, pp. 224-233.

41. Taira M et al: Studies of Ti alloys for dental castings, *Dent Mater* 5:45, 1989.

42. Hamanaka H et al: Dental casting of titanium and Ni-Ti alloys by a new casting machine, *J Dent Res* 68:1529, 1989.

43. Hamanaka H: Titanium casting – A review of casting machines, *Trans Acad Dent Mater* 6:89, 1993.

44. Takahashi J et al: Casting pure titanium into commercial phosphate-bonded SiO_2 investment molds, *J Dent Res* 69:1800, 1990.

45. Sunnerkrantz PA et al: Effect of casting atmosphere on the quality of Ti-crowns, *Scand J Dent Res* 98:268, 1989.

46. Herr H et al: Mold filling and porosity in casting of titanium, *Dent Mater* 9:15, 1993.

47. Syverud M, Herr H: Mold filling of Ti castings using investments with different gas permeability, *Dent Mater* 11:14, 1995.

48. Watanabe I et al: Effect of pressure difference on the quality of titanium casting, *J Dent Res* 3:736, 1997.

49. Van Roekel NB: Electric discharge machining in dentistry, *Int J Prosthodont* 5:114, 1992.

50. Valderrama S et al: A comparison of the marginal and internal adaptation of titanium and gold-platinum-palladium metal ceramic crowns, *Int J Prosthodont* 8:29, 1995.

CHAPTER TWENTY

PONTIC DESIGN

R. Duane Douglas, contributing author

KEY TERMS

conical pontic
crest
emergence profile
hygienic pontic
modified ridge lap pontic
ovate pontic

residual ridge
residual ridge resorption
ridge augmentation
ridge lap
sanitary pontic

Pontics are the artificial teeth of a fixed partial denture that replace missing natural teeth, restoring function and appearance. They must be compatible with continued oral health and comfort. The edentulous areas where a fixed prosthesis is to be provided may be overlooked during the treatment-planning phase. Unfortunately, any deficiency or potential problem that may arise during the fabrication of a pontic is often identified only after the teeth have been prepared or even when the master cast is ready to be sent to the laboratory. Proper preparation includes a careful analysis of the critical dimensions of the edentulous areas: mesiodistal width, occlusocervical distance, buccolingual diameter, and location of the **residual ridge**. To design a pontic that will meet hygienic requirements and prevent irritation of the residual ridge, particular attention must be given to the form and shape of the gingival surface. Merely replicating the form of the missing tooth or teeth is not enough. The pontic must be carefully designed and fabricated not only to facilitate plaque control of the tissue surface and around the adjacent abutment teeth but also to adjust to the existing occlusal conditions. In addition to these biologic considerations, pontic design must incorporate mechanical principles for strength and longevity as well as esthetic principles for satisfactory appearance of the replacement teeth (Fig. 20-1).

The pontic, as it mechanically unifies the abutment teeth and covers a portion of the residual ridge, assumes a dynamic role as a component of the prosthesis and cannot be considered as a lifeless insert of gold, porcelain, or acrylic.[1]

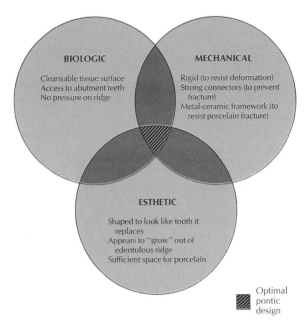

Fig. 20-1. Biologic, mechanical, and esthetic considerations for successful pontic design.

PRETREATMENT ASSESSMENT

Certain procedures will enhance the success of a fixed partial denture (FPD). In the treatment-planning phase, diagnostic casts and waxing procedures may prove especially valuable for determining optimal pontic design (see Chapters 2 and 3).

PONTIC SPACE

One function of an FPD is to prevent tilting or drifting of the adjacent teeth into the edentulous space. If such movement has already occurred, the space available for the pontic may be reduced and its fabrication complicated. At this point, creating an acceptable appearance without orthodontic repositioning of the abutment teeth is often impossible, particularly if esthetics is important. (Modification of abutments with complete-coverage retainers is sometimes feasible.) Careful diagnostic waxing procedures will help determine the most appropriate treatment (see Chapters 2 and 3). Even with a lesser esthetic requirement, as for posterior teeth, overly small pontics are unacceptable because they trap food and are difficult to clean. When orthodontic repositioning is not possible, increasing the proximal contours of adjacent teeth may be better than making an FPD with undersized pontics (Fig. 20-2). If there is no functional or esthetic deficit, the space can be maintained without prosthodontic intervention.

RESIDUAL RIDGE CONTOUR

The edentulous ridge's contour and topography should be carefully evaluated during the treatment-planning phase. An ideally shaped ridge has a smooth, regular surface of attached gingiva, which facilitates maintenance of a plaque-free environment. Its height and width should allow placement of a pontic that appears to emerge from the ridge and mimics the appearance of the neighboring teeth. Facially, it must be free of frenum attachment and of adequate facial height to sustain the appearance of interdental papillae.

Loss of residual ridge contour may lead to unesthetic open gingival embrasures ("black triangles")

(Fig. 20-3, *A*), food impaction (Fig. 20-3, *B*), and percolation of saliva during speech. Siebert[2] has classified residual ridge deformities into three categories (Fig. 20-4):

- Class I defects—faciolingual loss of tissue width with normal ridge height
- Class II defects—loss of ridge height with normal ridge width
- Class III defects—a combination of loss in both dimensions

There is a high incidence (91%) of residual ridge deformity following anterior tooth loss[3]; the majority of these are Class III defects. Because patients with Class II and III defects are frequently dissatisfied with the esthetics of their FPDs,[4] preprosthetic surgery to augment the residual ridge should be carefully considered.

SURGICAL MODIFICATION

Although residual ridge width may be augmented with hard tissue grafts, this is usually not indicated unless the edentulous site is to receive an implant (see Chapter 13).

Class I Defects. Soft tissue procedures have been advocated for improving the width of a Class

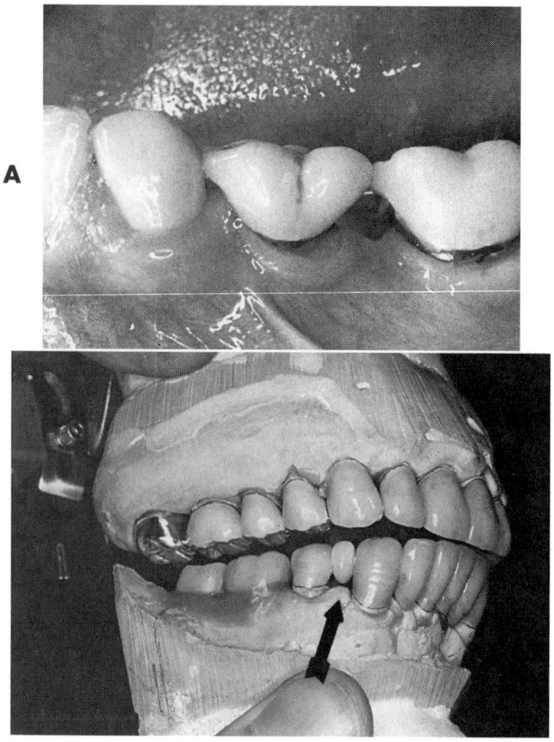

Fig. 20-2. Careful planning is always necessary when deciding how to restore an undersized pontic space where orthodontic treatment is not practical. **A,** In this patient, individual crowns of increased proximal contours were preferred to an FPD with undersized pontics. Excellent plaque control had been demonstrated, and the design provided the optimum occlusal relationship. **B,** Here a small pontic (*arrow*) was preferred to splint an RPD abutment.

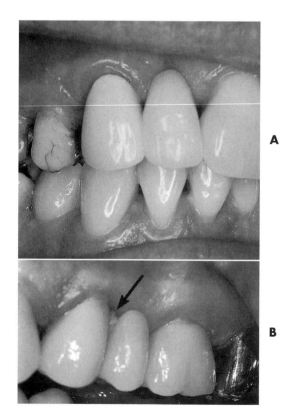

Fig. 20-3. Loss of residual ridge contour leading to unesthetic open gingival embrasures **(A)** and food entrapment (*arrow*) **(B).**

I defect; however, because Class I defects are infrequent and are not esthetically challenging, surgical augmentation of ridge width is uncommon. Paying careful attention to provisional pontic contour will help the operator identify patients who would benefit from surgery. The roll[5] technique uses soft tissue from the lingual side of the edentulous site. The epithelium is removed, and the tissue is thinned and rolled back upon itself, thereby thickening the facial aspect of the residual ridge (Fig. 20-5). Pouches[6] may also be prepared in the facial aspect of the residual ridge, into which subepithelial[7,8] or submucosal[9] grafts harvested from the palate or tuberosity may be inserted (Fig. 20-6).

Class II and III Defects. Unfortunately, few soft tissue surgical techniques can increase the height of a residual ridge with any predictability. The interpositional graft[2,10] is a variation of the pouch technique, in which a wedge-shaped connective tissue graft is inserted into a pouch preparation on the facial aspect of the residual ridge. The epithelial portion of the wedge may be positioned coronally to the surrounding epithelium if an increase of ridge height is desired (Fig. 20-7 *A* and *B*). The onlay graft is designed to gain ridge height[2,11] but also contributes to ridge width, which makes it useful for treating Class III ridge defects. It is a thick "free gingival graft" harvested from partial- or full-thickness palatal donor sites. Since the amount of height augmentation can only be as

thick as the graft, the procedure may have to be repeated several times to reestablish normal residual ridge height. Although the onlay graft has greater potential for increasing ridge height compared to the interpositional graft, its survival is greatly dependent on revascularization, which requires meticulous preparation of the recipient site (Fig. 20-8). Therefore, it is more technique sensitive than the interpositional graft.

GINGIVAL ARCHITECTURE PRESERVATION

Although the degree of **residual ridge resorption** following tooth extraction is unpredictable, resulting deformities are not an inevitable occurrence. Preservation of the alveolar process can be achieved through immediate restorative and periodontal intervention at the time of tooth removal. By conditioning the extraction site and providing a matrix for healing, the pre-extraction gingival architecture (or "socket") can be preserved.

Preparing the abutment teeth before the extraction is the preferred technique. A provisional FPD can be fabricated indirectly, ready for immediate insertion. Because socket preservation is dependent on underlying bone contour, the extraction of the tooth to be replaced should be atraumatic and aimed at preserving the facial plate of bone. The scalloped architecture of interproximal bone forming the extraction site is essential for proper papilla form, as are facial bone levels in the prevention of alveolar collapse. If bone levels are compromised

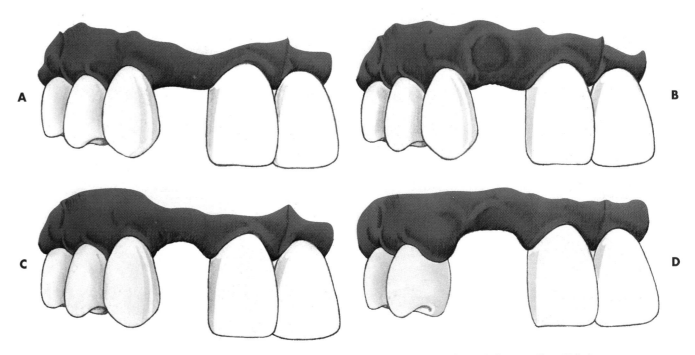

Fig. 20-4. Residual ridge deformities as classified by Siebert.[2] **A, B,** Class I defect. **C,** Class II defect. **D,** Class III defect.

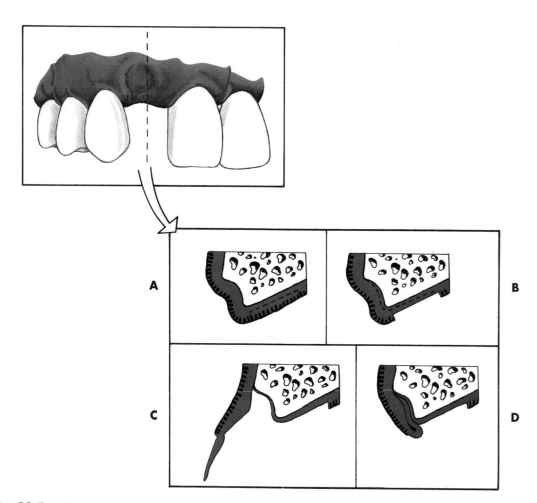

Fig. 20-5. The roll technique for soft tissue ridge augmentation. **A,** Cross section of Class I residual ridge defect before augmentation. **B,** Epithelium removed from palatal surface. **C,** Elevation of flap, creating a pouch on the vestibular surface. **D,** The flap is rolled into the pouch, enhancing ridge width.

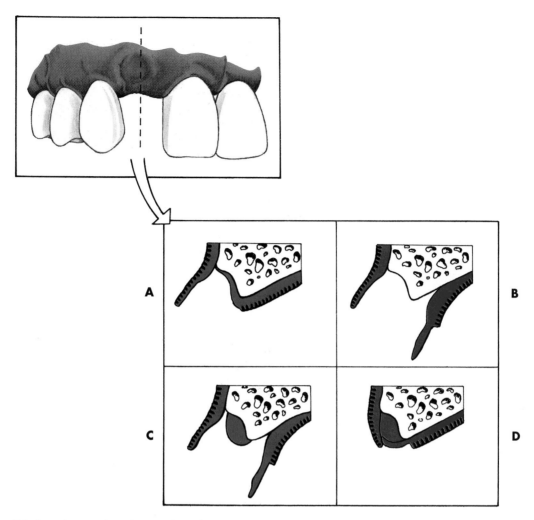

Fig. 20-6. The pouch technique for soft tissue ridge augmentation. **A** and **B,** Split-thickness flap is reflected. **C,** Graft material placed in the pouch increases ridge width. **D,** Flaps sutured in place.

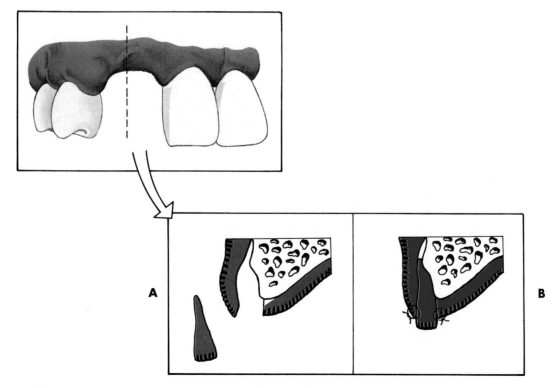

Fig. 20-7. An interpositional graft for augmentation of ridge width and height. **A,** Tissue reflected. **B,** Graft positioned and sutured in place.

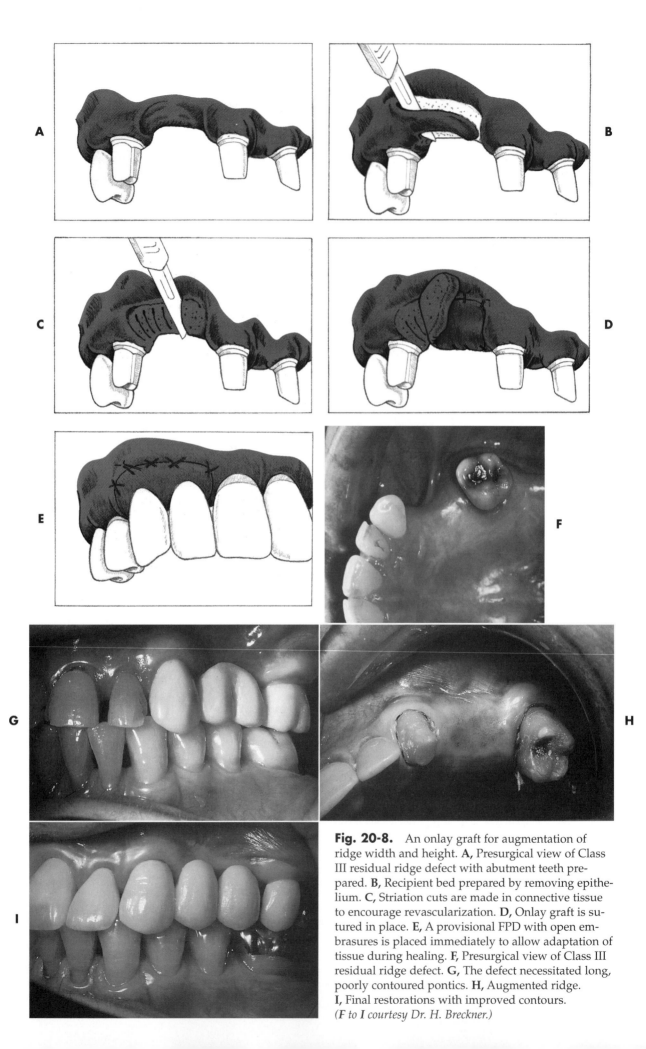

Fig. 20-8. An onlay graft for augmentation of ridge width and height. **A,** Presurgical view of Class III residual ridge defect with abutment teeth prepared. **B,** Recipient bed prepared by removing epithelium. **C,** Striation cuts are made in connective tissue to encourage revascularization. **D,** Onlay graft is sutured in place. **E,** A provisional FPD with open embrasures is placed immediately to allow adaptation of tissue during healing. **F,** Presurgical view of Class III residual ridge defect. **G,** The defect necessitated long, poorly contoured pontics. **H,** Augmented ridge. **I,** Final restorations with improved contours. *(F to I courtesy Dr. H. Breckner.)*

before or during extraction, the sockets can be grafted with an allograft material (hydroxyapatite, tricalcium phosphate, or freeze-dried bone).[12-14]

Immediately after preparation of the extraction site, a carefully shaped provisional FPD is placed (Fig. 20-9, *A* and *B*). The tissue-side of the pontic should be an ovate form, and according to Spear,[15] it should extend approximately 2.5 mm apical to the facial free gingival margin of the extraction socket (Fig. 20-9, *C* and *D*). Because the soft tissues of the socket will begin to collapse immediately after the tooth extraction, the pontic will result in tissue blanching as it supports the papillae and facial/palatal gingiva. The contour of the ovate tissue-side of the pontic is critical and must conform to within 1 mm of the interproximal and facial bone contour to act as a template for healing. Oral hy-

giene in this area is difficult during the initial healing period, so the provisional should be highly polished to minimize plaque retention. After approximately 1 month of healing, oral hygiene access is improved by recontouring the pontic to provide 1 to 1.5 mm of relief from the tissue. When the gingival levels are stable (approximately 6 to 12 months), the final restoration can be fabricated (Fig. 20-9, *E*).

Although maintenance of the residual ridge following extraction is meritorious, socket-preservation techniques are technically challenging and require frequent patient monitoring and conscientious patient hygiene. Even when the procedure is performed meticulously, success is unpredictable because of the variability of patient healing response. Additional surgical augmentation of the ridge may still be necessary for some patients.

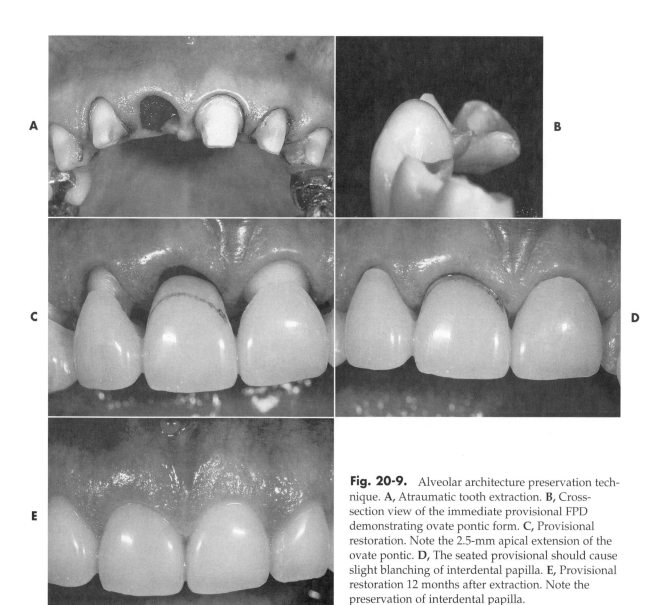

Fig. 20-9. Alveolar architecture preservation technique. **A,** Atraumatic tooth extraction. **B,** Cross-section view of the immediate provisional FPD demonstrating ovate pontic form. **C,** Provisional restoration. Note the 2.5-mm apical extension of the ovate pontic. **D,** The seated provisional should cause slight blanching of interdental papilla. **E,** Provisional restoration 12 months after extraction. Note the preservation of interdental papilla.
(Courtesy Dr. F. Spear and Montage Media.)

PONTIC CLASSIFICATION

Pontic designs are classified into two general groups: those that contact the oral mucosa and those that do not (Box 20-1). There are several classifications within these groups, based on the shape of the gingival side of the pontic. Pontic selection depends primarily on esthetics and oral hygiene. In the anterior region, where esthetics is a concern, the pontic should be well adapted to the tissue to make it appear that it emerges from the gingiva. Conversely, in the posterior regions (mandibular premolar and molar areas), esthetics can be compromised in the interest of designs that are more amenable to oral hygiene. The advantages and disadvantages of the various pontic designs are summarized in Table 20-1.

PONTIC DESIGN CLASSIFICATION BOX 20-1	
A. Mucosal contact	B. No mucosal contact
1. Ridge lap	1. Sanitary (hygienic)
2. Modified ridge lap	2. Modified sanitary
3. Ovate	(hygienic)
4. Conical	

SANITARY OR HYGIENIC PONTIC

As its name implies, the primary design feature of the **sanitary pontic** allows easy cleaning, because its tissue surface remains clear of the residual ridge (Fig. 20-10). This hygienic design permits easier

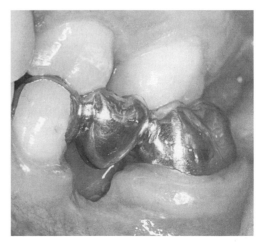

Fig. 20-10. A "hygienic" or "sanitary" pontic replacing a mandibular molar where there has been considerable bone loss.

Pontic Designs

Pontic Design		Recommended Location	Advantages	Disadvantages
Sanitary/hygienic	2 mm	Posterior mandible	Good access for oral hygiene	Poor esthetics
Saddle-ridge-lap		Not recommended	Esthetic	Not amenable to oral hygiene
Conical		Molars without esthetic requirements	Good access for oral hygiene	Poor esthetics
Modified ridge-lap		High esthetic requirement (i.e., anterior teeth and premolars, some maxillary molars)	Good esthetics	Moderately easy to clean
Ovate		Maxillary incisors cuspids and premolars	Superior esthetics Negligible food entrapment Ease of cleaning	Requires surgical preparation

plaque control by allowing gauze strips and other cleaning devices to be passed under the pontic and seesawed in shoe-shine fashion. Its disadvantages include entrapment of food particles, which may lead to tongue habits that may annoy the patient. The **hygienic pontic** is the least "toothlike" design and is therefore reserved for teeth seldom displayed during function (i.e., the mandibular molars).

A modified version of the sanitary pontic has been developed.[16] Its gingival portion is shaped like an archway between the retainers. This geometry permits increased connector size while decreasing the stress concentrated in the pontic and connectors.[17] It is also less susceptible to tissue proliferation that can occur when a pontic is too close to the residual ridge (Fig. 20-11).

SADDLE OR RIDGE LAP PONTIC

The saddle pontic has a concave fitting surface that overlaps the residual ridge buccolingually, simulating the contours and **emergence profile** of the missing tooth on both sides of the residual ridge. How-

ever, saddle or **ridge lap** designs should be avoided because the concave gingival surface of the pontic is not accessible to cleaning with dental floss, which will lead to plaque accumulation (Fig. 20-12). This design deficiency has been shown to result in tissue inflammation[1] (Fig. 20-13).

MODIFIED RIDGE LAP PONTIC

The **modified ridge lap pontic** combines the best features of the hygienic and saddle pontic designs, combining esthetics with easy cleaning. Figs. 20-14 and 20-15 demonstrate how the modified ridge lap design overlaps the residual ridge on the facial (to achieve the appearance of a tooth emerging from the gingiva) but remains clear of the ridge on the lingual. To enable optimal plaque control, the gingival surface must have no depression or hollow. Rather, it should be as convex as possible from mesial to distal (the greater the convexity, the easier the oral hygiene). Tissue contact should resemble a letter T (Fig. 20-16) whose vertical arm ends at the **crest** of the ridge. Facial ridge adaptation is

Indications	Contraindications	Materials
Nonesthetic zones Impaired oral hygiene	Where esthetics is important Minimal vertical dimension	All metal
Not recommended	Not recommended	N/A
Posterior areas where esthetics is of minimal concern	Poor oral hygiene	All-metal Metal-ceramic All-resin
Most areas with esthetic concern	Where minimal esthetic concern exists	Metal-ceramic All-resin
Desire for optimal esthetics High smile line	Unwillingness for surgery	Metal-ceramic All-resin

TABLE 20-1

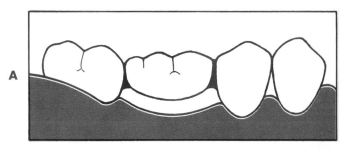
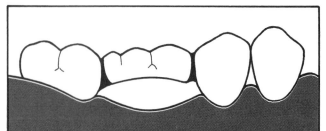

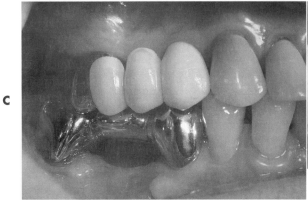
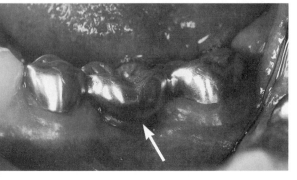

Fig. 20-11. **A,** Sanitary pontic. **B** and **C,** Modified sanitary pontic. **D,** Placement of the pontic, close to the ridge, has resulted in tissue proliferation *(arrow)*.

Fig. 20-12. **A,** Cross-section view of ridge lap pontic. **B,** The tissue surface is inaccessible to cleaning devices.

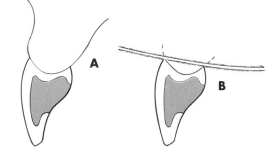

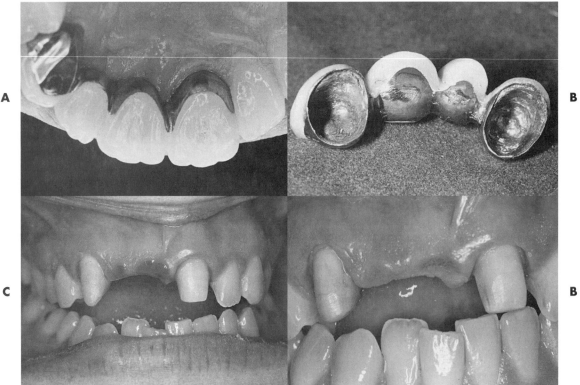

Fig. 20-13. **A** and **B,** FPD with a ridge-lap (concave) gingival surface. **C,** When it was removed, the tissue was found to be ulcerated. **D,** The defective FPD was recontoured and used as a provisional restoration while the definitive restoration was being fabricated. Within 2 weeks the ulceration had re-

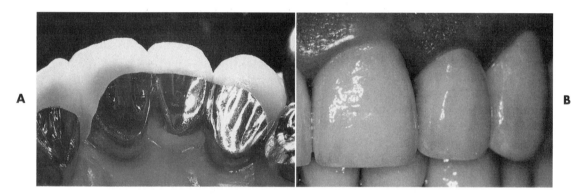

Fig. 20-14. Modified ridge lap pontic. **A,** FPD partially seated. **B,** FPD seated.

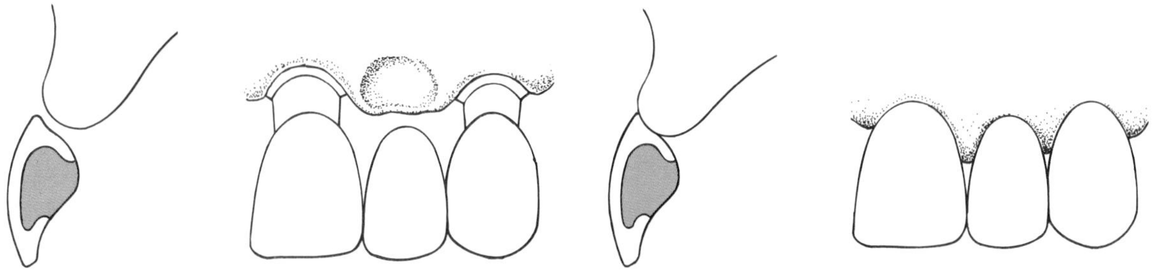

Fig. 20-15. Three-unit FPD replacing the maxillary lateral incisor. **A,** To facilitate plaque control, the lingual surface is made convex. **B,** The facial surface is shaped to simulate the missing tooth.

essential for a natural appearance. Although this design was historically referred to as *ridge-lap*,[18,19] the term *ridge-lap* is now used synonymously with the saddle design. The modified ridge lap design is the most common pontic form used in areas of the mouth that are visible during function (maxillary and mandibular anterior teeth and maxillary premolars and first molars).

Conical Pontic

Often called *egg-shaped, bullet-shaped,* or *heart-shaped,* the **conical pontic** (Fig. 20-17) is easy for the patient to keep clean. It should be made as convex as possible, with only one point of contact at the center of the residual ridge. This design is recommended for the replacement of mandibular posterior teeth where esthetics is a lesser concern. The facial and lingual contours are dependent on the width of the residual ridge; a knife-edged residual ridge will necessitate flatter contours with a narrow tissue contact area. This type of design may be unsuitable for broad residual ridges, because the emergence profile associated with the small tissue contact point may create areas of food entrapment (Fig. 20-18). The sanitary or hygienic pontic is the design of choice in these clinical situations.

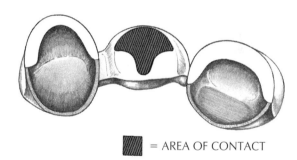

███ = AREA OF CONTACT

Fig. 20-16. Tissue contact of a maxillary FPD should resemble the letter T. This FPD is viewed from the gingival aspect.

Ovate Pontic

The **ovate pontic** is the most esthetically appealing pontic design. Its convex tissue surface resides in a soft tissue depression or hollow in the residual ridge, which makes it appear that a tooth is literally emerging from the gingiva (Fig. 20-19). Careful treatment planning is necessary for successful results. Socket-preservation techniques, which have already been described, should be performed at the time of extraction to create the tissue recess from which the ovate pontic form will emerge. For a preexisting residual ridge, soft tissue surgical augmentation is typically required. When an adequate volume of ridge tissue is established, a socket depression is sculpted into the ridge with surgical diamonds or electrosurgery. In either case, meticulous attention to the contour of the pontic of the provisional restoration is essential when conditioning and shaping the residual ridge that will receive the definitive prosthesis.

The ovate pontic's advantages include its pleasing appearance and its strength. When used successfully with **ridge augmentation**, its emergence from the ridge appears identical to that of a natural

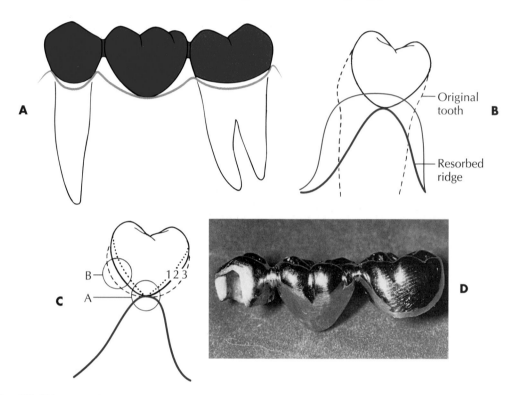

Fig. 20-17. **A** and **B,** A pontic with maximum convexity and single point contact of the tissue surface is the easiest design to keep clean. **C,** Evaluating the contour of three possible pontic shapes (*1, 2,* and *3*). Contour *3* is the most convex in area *B* but is too flat in area *A*. Contour *1* is convex in area *A* but is too flat in area *B*. Contour *2* is the best. **D,** An all-metal FPD with a conical pontic, suitable for replacement of a mandibular molar.

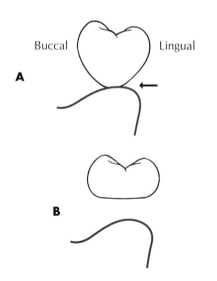

Fig. 20-18. **A,** Conical pontics may create food entrapment on broad residual ridges *(arrow).* **B,** The sanitary pontic form may be a better alternative.

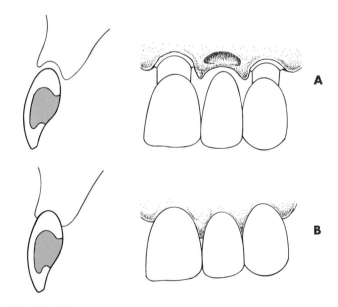

Fig. 20-19. Ovate pontic. **A,** FPD partially seated. **B,** FPD seated.

tooth. In addition, its recessed form is not susceptible to food impaction. The broad convex geometry is stronger than that of the modified ridge lap pontic, because the unsupported, thin porcelain that often exists at the gingivofacial extent of the pontic is eliminated (Fig. 20-20). Because the tissue surface of the pontic is convex in all dimensions, it is accessible to dental floss; however, meticulous oral hygiene is necessary to prevent tissue inflammation resulting from the large area of tissue contact. Other disadvantages include the need for surgical tissue management and the associated cost.

BIOLOGIC CONSIDERATIONS

The biologic principles of pontic design pertain to the maintenance and preservation of the residual ridge, abutment and opposing teeth, and supporting tissues. Factors of specific influence are pontic-ridge contact, amenability to oral hygiene, and the direction of occlusal forces.

RIDGE CONTACT

Pressure-free contact between the pontic and the underlying tissues is indicated to prevent ulceration and inflammation of the soft tissues.[1,20] If any blanching of the soft tissues is observed at try-in, the pressure area should be identified with a disclosing medium (i.e., pressure-indicating paste) and the pontic recontoured until tissue contact is entirely passive. This passive contact should occur exclusively on keratinized attached tissue. When a pontic rests on mucosa, some ulcerations may appear as a result of the normal movement of the mucosa in contact with the pontic (Fig. 20-21). Positive ridge pressure may be due to excessive scraping of the ridge area on the working cast (Fig. 20-22). This was once promoted as a way to improve the appearance of the pontic-ridge relationship. However, because of the ulceration that inevitably results when flossing is not meticulously performed, the concept is not recommended,[1,21,22] unless done as previously described as an ovate pontic.[23,20]

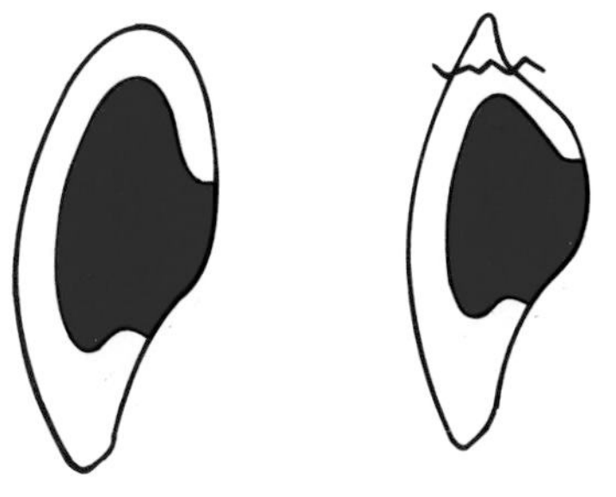

ORAL HYGIENE CONSIDERATIONS

The chief cause of ridge irritation is the toxins released from microbial plaque, which accumulate between the gingival surface of the pontic and the residual ridge, causing tissue inflammation and calculus formation.

Unlike removable partial dentures, FPDs cannot be taken out of the mouth for daily cleaning. Patients must be taught efficient oral hygiene techniques, with particular emphasis on cleaning the gingival surface of the pontic. The shape of the gingival surface, its relation to the ridge, and the materials used in its fabrication will influence ultimate success.

Normally, where tissue contact occurs, the gingival surface of a pontic is inaccessible to the bristles of a toothbrush. Therefore, excellent hygiene habits must be developed by the patient. Devices such as proxy brushes, pipe cleaners, SuperFloss,* and

---

*Oral-B Laboratories: Redwood City, Calif.

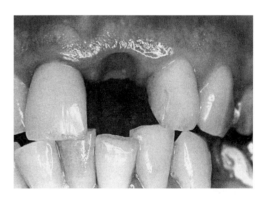

Fig. 20-21. Pressure will inevitably lead to ulceration.

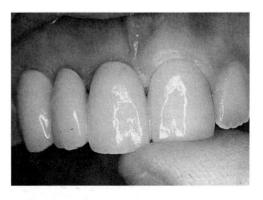

Fig. 20-22. Soft tissue blanching at try-in indicates pressure.

Ovate Modified ridge lap

Fig. 20-20. The ovate pontic design eliminates the potential for unsupported porcelain in the cervical portion of an anterior pontic.

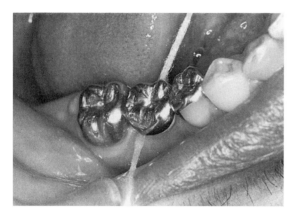

Fig. 20-23. The patient must be instructed how to clean the gingival surface of a pontic with floss.

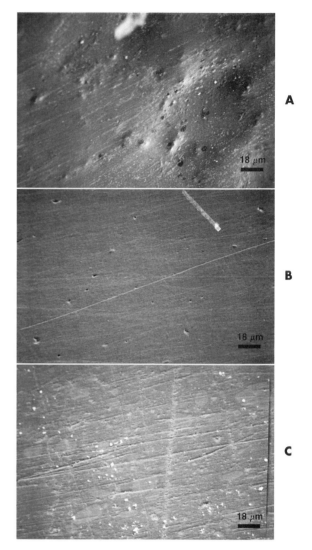

Fig. 20-24. Scanning electron micrographs of glazed porcelain **(A)**, polished gold **(B)**, and polished acrylic resin **(C)**.
(Microscopy by Dr. J.L. Sandrik.)

dental floss with a threader are highly recommended (Fig. 20-23). Gingival embrasures around the pontic should be wide enough to permit oral hygiene aids. However, to prevent food entrapment, they should not be opened excessively. To permit passage of floss over its entire tissue surface, tissue contact between the residual ridge and pontic must be passive.

If the pontic has a depression or concavity in its gingival surface, plaque will accumulate, because the floss cannot clean this area, and tissue irritation[24] will follow. This is usually reversible; when the surface is subsequently modified to eliminate the concavity, inflammation disappears (see Fig. 20-13). Therefore, an accurate description of pontic design should be submitted to the laboratory, and the prosthesis should be checked and corrected if necessary before cementation. Prevention is the best solution for controlling tissue irritation.

PONTIC MATERIAL

Any material chosen to fabricate the pontic should provide good esthetic results where needed; biocompatibility, rigidity, and strength to withstand occlusal forces; and longevity. FPDs should be made as rigid as possible, because any flexure during mastication or parafunction may cause pressure on the gingiva and cause fractures of the veneering material. Occlusal contacts should not fall on the junction between metal and porcelain during centric or eccentric tooth contacts, nor should a metal-ceramic junction occur in contact with the residual ridge on the gingival surface of the pontic.

Investigations into the biocompatibility of materials used to fabricate pontics have centered on two factors: (1) the effect of the materials and (2) the effects of surface adherence. Glazed porcelain is generally considered the most biocompatible of the

available pontic materials,[25-27] and clinical data[21,28] tend to support this opinion, although the critical factor seems to be the material's ability to resist plaque accumulation[29] (rather than the material itself). Well-polished gold is smoother, less prone to corrosion, and less retentive of plaque than an unpolished or porous casting.[30] However, even highly polished surfaces will accumulate plaque if oral hygiene measures are ignored.[31,32]

Although glazed porcelain looks very smooth, when viewed under a microscope, its surface shows many voids and is rougher than either polished gold or acrylic resin[33] (Fig. 20-24). Nevertheless, highly glazed porcelain is easier to clean than other materials. For easier plaque removal and biocompatibility, the tissue surface of the pontic should be

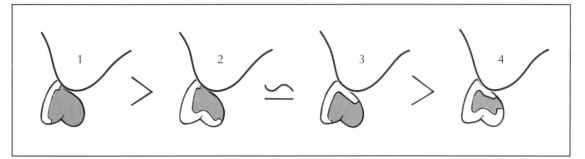

Fig. 20-25. Four pontic designs in descending order of strength based on cross sectional diameter of the metal substructure. When vertical space is minimal, design 4 (porcelain tissue and occlusal coverage) may be contraindicated.

made in glazed porcelain. However, ceramic tissue contact may be contraindicated in edentulous areas where there is minimal distance between the residual ridge and the occlusal table. In these instances, placing ceramic on the tissue side of the pontic may weaken the design of the metal substructure, particularly with porcelain occlusal surface (Fig. 20-25). If gold is placed in tissue contact, it should be highly polished. Regardless of the choice of pontic material, patients can prevent inflammation around the pontic with meticulous oral hygiene.[34]

OCCLUSAL FORCES

Reducing the buccolingual width of the pontic by as much as 30% has been suggested[35,36] as a way to lessen occlusal forces on, and thus the loading of, abutment teeth. This practice continues today, although it has little scientific basis. Critical analysis[37] reveals that forces are lessened only when chewing food of uniform consistency and that a mere 12% increase in chewing efficiency can be expected from a one-third reduction of pontic width. Potentially harmful forces are more likely to be encountered if an FPD is loaded by the accidental biting on a hard object or by parafunctional activities like bruxism rather than by chewing foods of uniform consistency. These forces are not reduced by narrowing the occlusal table.

In fact, narrowing the occlusal table may actually impede or even preclude the development of a harmonious and stable occlusal relationship. Like a malposed tooth, it may cause difficulties in plaque control and may not provide proper cheek support. For these reasons, pontics with normal occlusal widths (at least on the occlusal third) are generally recommended. One exception is if the residual alveolar ridge has collapsed buccolingually. Reducing pontic width may then be desired, thereby lessening the lingual contour and facilitating plaque-control measures.

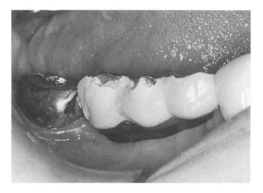

Fig. 20-26. Failure of a long span metal-ceramic FPD subjected to high stress.

🔲 MECHANICAL CONSIDERATIONS

The prognosis of fixed partial denture pontics will be compromised if mechanical principles are not followed closely. Mechanical problems may be caused by improper choice of materials, poor framework design, poor tooth preparation, or poor occlusion. These factors can lead to fracture of the prosthesis or displacement of the retainers. Long-span posterior FPDs are particularly susceptible to mechanical problems. Inevitably, there is significant flexing from high occlusal forces and because the displacement effects increase with the cube of the span length (see p. 71). Therefore, evaluating the likely forces on a pontic and designing accordingly are important. For example, a strong all-metal pontic may be needed in high-stress situations rather than a metal-ceramic pontic (Fig. 20-26), which would be more susceptible to fracture. When metal-ceramic pontics are chosen, extending porcelain onto the occlusal surfaces to achieve better esthetics should also be carefully evaluated. In addition to its potential for fracture, porcelain may abrade the opposing dentition if the occlusal contacts are on enamel or metal.

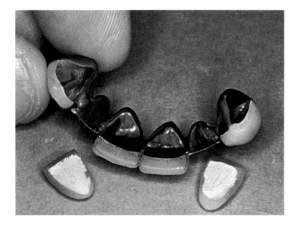

Fig. 20-27. Failure resulting from improper laboratory technique.

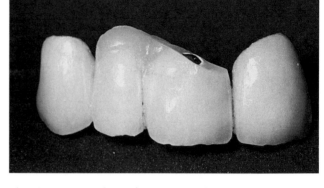

Fig. 20-28. Failure of unsupported gingival porcelain.

AVAILABLE PONTIC MATERIALS

Some fixed partial dentures are fabricated entirely of metal, porcelain, or acrylic resin, but most use a combination of metal and porcelain. Acrylic resin-veneered pontics have had limited acceptance because of their reduced durability (wear and discoloration). The newer indirect composites, based on high inorganic-filled resins and the fiber-reinforced materials (see Chapter 27), have revived interest in composite resin and resin-veneered pontics.

Metal-ceramic Pontics.   Most pontics are fabricated by the metal-ceramic technique. If properly used, this technique is helpful for solving commonly encountered clinical problems. A well-fabricated metal-ceramic pontic is strong, easy to keep clean, and looks natural. However, mechanical failure (Fig. 20-27) can occur and often is attributable to inadequate framework design. The principles of framework design are discussed in Chapter 19, but the following points will be emphasized in this chapter:

1. The framework must provide a uniform veneer of porcelain (approximately 1.2 mm). Excessive thickness of porcelain contributes to inadequate support and predisposes to eventual fracture (Fig. 20-28). This is often true in the cervical portion of an anterior pontic. A reliable technique for ensuring uniform thickness of porcelain is to wax the fixed prosthesis to complete anatomic contour and then accurately cut back the wax to a predetermined depth (Fig. 20-29).
2. The metal surfaces to be veneered must be smooth and free of pits. Surface irregularities will cause incomplete wetting by the porcelain slurry, leading to voids at the porcelain-metal interface that reduce bond strength and increase the possibility of mechanical failure.
3. Sharp angles on the veneering area should be rounded. They produce increased stress concentrations that can cause mechanical failure.
4. The location and design of the external metal-porcelain junction require particular attention. Any deformation of the metal framework at the junction can lead to chipping of the porcelain (Fig. 20-30). For this reason, occlusal centric contacts must be placed at least 1.5 mm away from the junction. Excursive eccentric contacts that might deform the metal-ceramic interface must be watched carefully.

Resin-veneered Pontics.   Historically, acrylic resin-veneered restorations had deficiencies that made them acceptable only as longer-term provisionals. Their resistance to abrasion was lower than enamel or porcelain, and noticeable wear occurred with normal toothbrushing (Fig. 20-31). Furthermore, the relatively high surface area/volume ratio of a thin resin veneer made dimensional change from water absorption and thermal fluctuations (thermocycling) a problem. Because no chemical bond existed between the resin and the metal framework, the resin was retained by mechanical means (e.g., undercuts). Continuous dimensional change of the veneers often caused leakage at the metal-resin interface, with subsequent discoloration of the restoration.

Nevertheless, there are certain advantages to using polymeric materials instead of ceramics: they are easy to manipulate and repair and do not require the high–melting range alloys needed for metal-ceramic techniques. Recently introduced indirect composite resin systems have resolved some

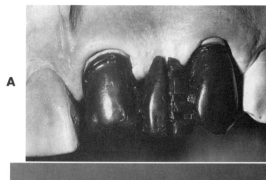

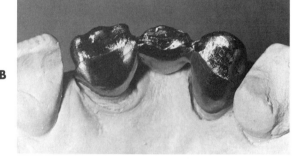

Fig. 20-29. **A,** Waxing to anatomic contour and controlled cut-back are the most reliable approaches to fabricating a satisfactory metal substructure **(B).**

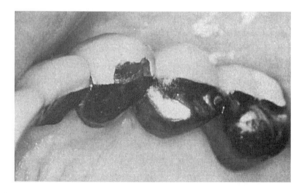

Fig. 20-30. Failure caused by occlusal contact across the metal-ceramic junction.

of the problems inherent in previous indirect resin veneers. These new-generation indirect resins have a higher density of inorganic ceramic filler than traditional direct and indirect composite resins. Most use a post-curing process that results in high flexural strength, minimal polymerization shrinkage, and wear rates comparable to those of tooth enamel.[38] In addition, improvements in the bond between the composite resin and metal[39] may lead to a reappraisal of resin veneers.

Fiber-reinforced Composite Resin Pontics. Composite resins can be used in fixed partial dentures without a metal substructure (see Chapter

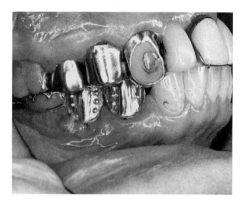

Fig. 20-31. Wear of an acrylic resin-veneered prosthesis.

27). A substructure matrix of impregnated glass or polymer fiber provides structural strength. The physical properties of this system, combined with its excellent marginal adaptation and esthetics, make it a possible metal-free alternative for FPDs, although long-term clinical performance is not yet known.

ESTHETIC CONSIDERATIONS

No matter how well biologic and mechanical principles have been followed during fabrication, the patient will evaluate the result by how it looks, especially when anterior teeth have been replaced. Many esthetic considerations that pertain to single crowns also apply to the pontic (see Chapter 23). Several problems unique to the pontic may be encountered when attempting to achieve a natural appearance.

THE GINGIVAL INTERFACE

An esthetically successful pontic will replicate the form, contours, incisal edge, gingival and incisal embrasures, and color of adjacent teeth. The pontic's simulation of a natural tooth is most often betrayed at the tissue-pontic interface. The greatest challenge here is to compensate for anatomic changes that occur after extraction. Special attention should be paid to the contour of the labial surface as it approaches the pontic-tissue junction to achieve a "natural" appearance. This cannot be accomplished by merely duplicating the facial contour of the missing tooth, because after a tooth is removed, the alveolar bone undergoes resorption and/or remodeling. If the original tooth contour were followed, the pontic would look unnaturally long incisogingivally (Fig. 20-32). To achieve the illusion of a natural tooth, an esthetic pontic must deceive observers into believing they are seeing a natural tooth.

The modified ridge-lap pontic is recommended for most anterior situations; it compensates for lost buccolingual width in the residual ridge by overlapping what remains. Rather than emerging from the crest of the ridge as a natural tooth would, the cervical aspect of the pontic sits in front of the ridge, covering any abnormal ridge morphology resulting from tooth loss. Fortunately, because most teeth are viewed from only two dimensions, this relationship remains undetected. A properly designed, modified ridge-lap provides the required convexity on the tissue side, with smooth and open embrasures on the lingual side for ease of cleaning. This is difficult to accomplish. Clinically, many pontics are seen with less than optimal contour, resulting in an unnatural appearance. This can be avoided with careful preparation at the diagnostic waxing stage (see Chapter 3). Sometimes the ridge tissue must be surgically reshaped to enhance the result.

In normal situations, light falls from above, and an object's shadow is below it. Unexpected lighting or unexpectedly placed shadows (Fig. 20-33) can be confusing to the brain. Because of past experience, the brain "knows" that a tooth grows out of the gingiva, and it therefore "sees" a pontic as a tooth unless telltale shadows suggest otherwise. Special care must be taken when studying where shadows fall around natural teeth, particularly around the gingival margin. If a pontic is poorly adapted to the residual ridge, there will be an unnatural shadow in the cervical area that looks odd and spoils the illu-

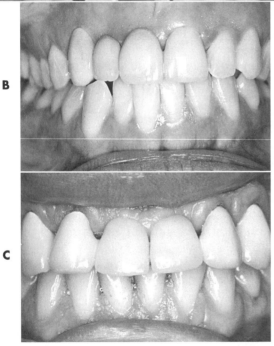

Fig. 20-32. Correct incisogingival height is critical to esthetic pontic design. **A,** Esthetic failure of a four-unit FPD replacing the right central and lateral incisors. The pontics have been shaped to follow the facial contour of the missing teeth, but because of bone loss they look too long. **B,** The replacement FPD. Note that the gingival half of each pontic has been reduced. Esthetics is much improved. **C,** This esthetic failure is the result of excessive reduction. The central incisor pontics look too short.

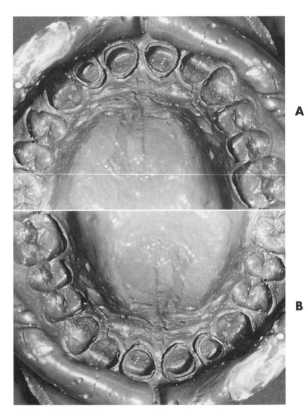

Fig. 20-33. Optical illusion. **A** and **B** are identical except that one image is upside down. Most people make different three-dimensional interpretations of each photograph, interpreting one as a negative impression and the other as a positive cast. (Verify the illusion by turning the book.) The interpretation is based on how shadows fall; in normal situations, objects are seen illuminated from above.

sion of a natural tooth (Fig. 20-34). In additional, recesses occurring at the gingival interface will collect food debris, further betraying the illusion of a natural tooth.

When appearance is of utmost concern, the ovate pontic, used in conjunction with alveolar preservation or soft tissue ridge augmentation, can provide an appearance at the gingival interface that is virtually indistinguishable from a natural tooth. Because it emerges from a soft tissue recess, this pontic is not susceptible to many of the esthetic pitfalls previously described for the modified ridge lap pontic. However, in most cases, the patient must be willing to undergo the additional surgical procedures that an ovate pontic requires.

INCISOGINGIVAL LENGTH

Obtaining a correctly sized pontic simply by duplicating the original tooth is not possible. Ridge resorption will make such a tooth look too long in the cervical region. The height of a tooth is immediately obvious when the patient smiles and shows the gin-

gival margin (Fig. 20-35). An abnormal labiolingual position or cervical contour, however, is not immediately obvious. This fact can be used to produce a pontic of good appearance by recontouring the gingival half of the labial surface (see Fig. 20-35). The observer sees a normal tooth length but is unaware of the abnormal labial contour. The illusion is successful.

Even with moderately severe bone resorption, obtaining a natural appearance by exaggerated contouring of the pontics may still be possible. In areas where tooth loss is accompanied by excessive loss of alveolar bone, however, a pontic of normal length would not touch the ridge at all.

One solution is to shape the pontic to simulate a normal crown and root with emphasis on the cementoenamel junction. The root can be stained to simulate exposed dentin (Fig. 20-36). Another approach is to use pink porcelain to simulate the gingival tissues (Fig. 20-37). However, such pontics then have considerably increased tissue contact and require scrupulous plaque control for long-term

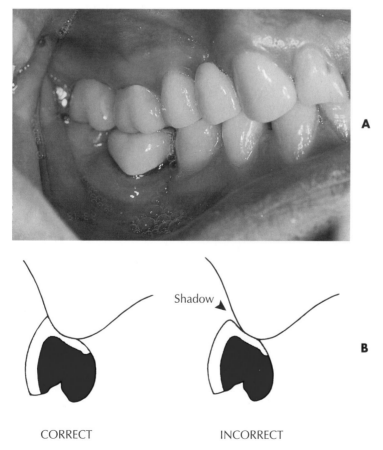

CORRECT   INCORRECT

Fig. 20-34. A pontic should be interpreted as "growing" out of the gingival tissue. The second premolar pontic in the four-unit FPD **(A)** is successful because it is well adapted to the ridge; however, the pontic for the first premolar is evident because of its poor adaptation to the ridge, which creates a shadow. **B,** Shadows around the gingival surface *(arrow)* spoil the esthetic illusion.

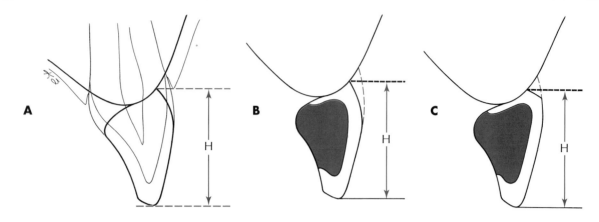

Fig. 20-35. **A,** A pontic should have the same incisogingival height *(H)* as the original tooth. **B,** Correctly contoured pontic. **C,** Incorrect contour. (The dotted lines in **B** and **C** show the original tooth contour.) The shelf at the gingival margin may trap food and create an esthetically unacceptable shadow.

It is often necessary to recontour a substantial portion of the facial surface (**B**) to minimize a shadow or food trap at the cervical of the pontic (**C**).

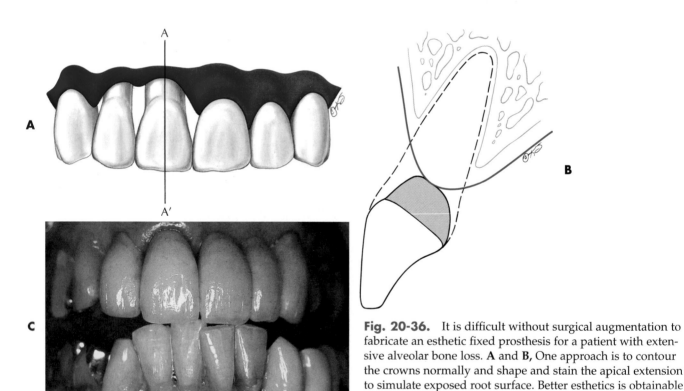

Fig. 20-36. It is difficult without surgical augmentation to fabricate an esthetic fixed prosthesis for a patient with extensive alveolar bone loss. **A** and **B,** One approach is to contour the crowns normally and shape and stain the apical extension to simulate exposed root surface. Better esthetics is obtainable with an RPD (**C**).
*(**A** and **B** redrawn from Blancheri RL: Rev Asoc Dent Mex 8:103, 1950.)*

success. Ridge-augmentation procedures have been successful in correcting areas of limited resorption. When bone loss is severe, the esthetic result obtained with an RPD is often better than with an FPD.

MESIODISTAL WIDTH

Frequently, the space available for a pontic will be greater or smaller than the width of the contralateral tooth. This is usually due to uncontrolled tooth movement that occurred when a tooth was removed and not replaced.

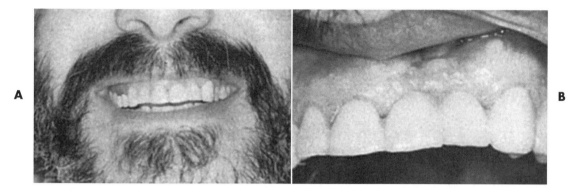

Fig. 20-37. Fixed partial denture replacing maxillary left central and lateral incisors. This patient had lost significant bone from the edentulous ridge. Appearance of the prosthesis was enhanced with the use of pink porcelain between the pontics to simulate gingival tissue. The patient has been able to maintain excellent tissue health through the daily use of SuperFloss.

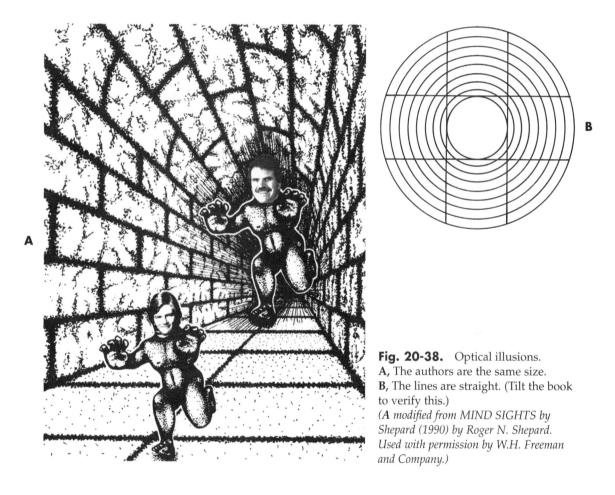

Fig. 20-38. Optical illusions.
A, The authors are the same size.
B, The lines are straight. (Tilt the book to verify this.)
(A modified from MIND SIGHTS by Shepard (1990) by Roger N. Shepard. Used with permission by W.H. Freeman and Company.)

If possible, such a discrepancy should be corrected by orthodontic treatment. If this is not possible, an acceptable appearance may be obtained by incorporating visual perception principles into the pontic design. In the same way that the brain can be confused into misinterpreting the relative sizes of shapes or lines because of an erroneous interpretation of perspective (Fig. 20-38), a pontic of abnormal size may be designed to give the illusion of being a more natural size. The width of an anterior tooth is usually identified by the relative positions of the mesiofacial and distofacial line angles, and the overall shape by the detailed pattern of surface contour and light reflection between these line angles. The features of the contralateral tooth (Fig. 20-39) should be duplicated as precisely as possible in the pontic, and the space discrepancy can be compensated by altering the shape of the proximal areas.

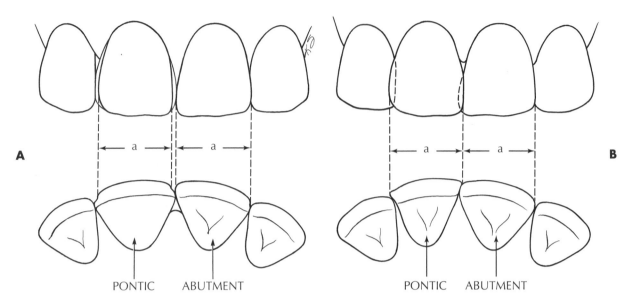

Fig. 20-39. An abnormally sized anterior pontic space can be restored esthetically by matching the location of the line angles and adjusting the interproximal areas. Large **(A)** and small **(B)** pontic spaces. Dimension *a* should be matched in the replacement.
(Redrawn from Blancheri RL: Rev Asoc Dent Mex 8:103, 1950.)

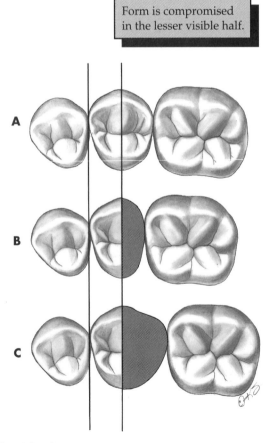

Fig. 20-40. When replacing a posterior tooth **(A)**, duplicate the dimension of the more visible mesial half of the adjacent tooth. Narrow **(B)** and wide **(C)** pontic spaces.
(Redrawn from Blancheri RL: Rev Asoc Dent Mex 8:103, 1950.)

The retainers and the pontics can be proportioned to minimize the discrepancy. (This is another situation in which a diagnostic waxing procedure will help solve a challenging restorative problem.)

Space discrepancy presents less of a problem when posterior teeth are being replaced (Fig. 20-40) because their distal halves are not normally visible from the front. A discrepancy here can be managed by duplicating the visible mesial half of the tooth and adjusting the size of the distal half.

PONTIC FABRICATION

AVAILABLE MATERIALS

Over time, several techniques for pontic fabrication evolved. Prefabricated porcelain facings were very popular for use with conventional gold alloys. As use of the metal-ceramic technique increased during the 1970s, prefabricated facings lost their popularity and essentially disappeared. Although an acceptable substitute, custom-made metal-ceramic facings never gained widespread acceptance. Table 20-2 summarizes the various techniques (Fig. 20-41).

Most pontics are now made with the metal-ceramic technique, which provides the best solution to the biologic, mechanical, and esthetic challenges encountered in pontic design. Their fabrication, however, differs slightly from the fabrication of individual crowns. These differences will be emphasized in the ensuing paragraphs.

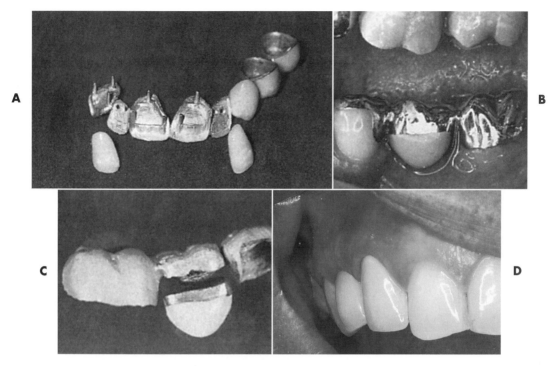

Fig. 20-41. **A,** Eight-unit FPD with porcelain facings. **B** and **C,** This three-unit posterior FPD has been fabricated by postceramic soldering of a metal-ceramic facing to conventional gold. **D,** Metal-ceramic FPD with a modified ridge lap pontic (canine) appears to emerge from the gingiva.

Available Pontic Systems				TABLE 20-2
	Advantages	Disadvantages	Indications	Contraindications

Metal-ceramic	Esthetics
	Biocompatible
		Difficult if an abutment is
		    not metal-ceramic
		Weaker than all-metal
			Most situations	Long spans with
				    high stress

All-metal	Strength
	Straightforward procedure
		Nonesthetic	Mandibular molars,
			    especially under high
			    stress
				Where esthetics is
				    important

Fiber-reinforced
all-resin
	Conservative when used
	    with inlay preparations
	Esthetics
	Ease of repair
		Long-term success
		    unknown
		Limited to short
		    spans
			Areas of high esthetic
			    concern
				Long-span FPDs

Facings	Rarely used—of historical interest only			

METAL-CERAMIC PONTICS

A well-designed metal-ceramic pontic provides easy plaque removal, strength, wear resistance, and esthetics (see Fig. 20-41, *D*). Its fabrication is relatively simple if at least one retainer is also metal-ceramic. The metal framework for the pontic and one or both of its retainers is cast in one piece. This facilitates pontic manipulation during the successive laboratory and clinical phases. In the discus-

sion that follows, it will be assumed that either or both of the retainers are metal-ceramic complete crowns. When this is not the case, an alternate approach is recommended.

Anatomic Contour Waxing. For strength and esthetics, an accurately controlled thickness of porcelain is needed in the finished restoration. To ensure this, a wax pattern is made to the final anatomic contour. This also permits an assessment of connector design adequacy and the relationship between the connectors and the proposed configuration of the ceramic veneer (see Chapter 28).

Armamentarium (Fig. 20-42)
• Bunsen burner
• Inlay wax
• Sticky wax
• Waxing instruments
• Cotton cleaning cloth
• Die-wax separating liquid
• Zinc stearate or powdered wax
• Double-ended brushes
• Cotton balls
• Fine-mesh nylon hose

Step-by-step Procedure
1. Wax the internal, proximal, and axial surfaces of the retainers as described in Chapter 18.
2. Soften the inlay wax, mold it to the approximate desired pontic shape, and adapt it to the ridge. This is the starting point for subsequent modification. Alternatively (and perhaps preferably), an impression may be made of the diagnostic waxing or provisional restoration. Molten wax can then be poured into this to form the initial pontic shape. Prefabricated pontic shapes are also available as a starting point (Fig. 20-43).
3. If a posterior tooth is being replaced, leave the occlusal surface flat because the occlusion is best developed with the wax addition technique outlined in Chapter 18.
4. Lute the pontic to the retainers and, for additional stability, connect its cervical aspect directly to the master cast with sticky wax.

Then wax the pontic to proper axial and occlusal (or incisal) contour (Fig. 20-44).
5. Complete the retainers and contour the proximal and tissue surfaces of the pontic for the desired tissue contact. The pontic is now ready for evaluation before cut-back.

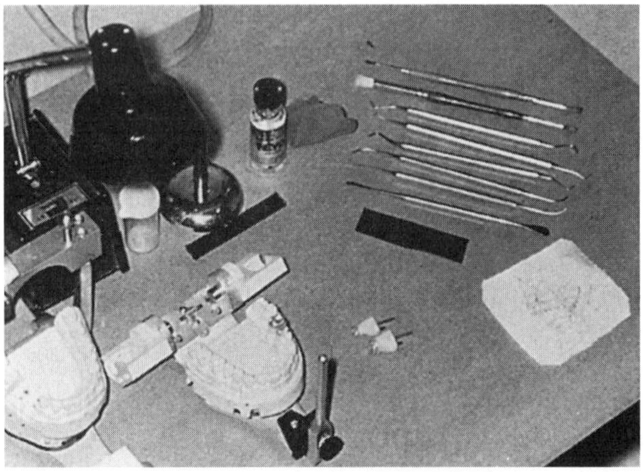

Evaluation (Fig. 20-45). The form of the wax pattern is evaluated and any deficiencies are corrected. Particular attention is given to the connectors,

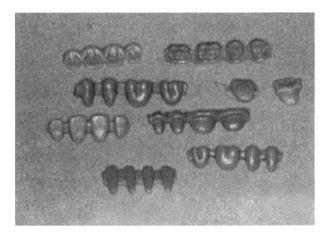

Fig. 20-43. Prefabricated wax pontics.

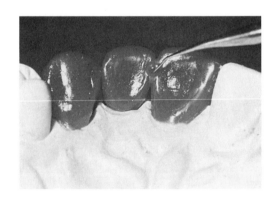

Fig. 20-44. Luting the pontic to the retainers.

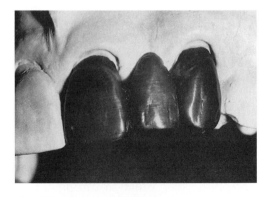

Fig. 20-42. Waxing armamentarium.

Fig. 20-45. Complete contour wax patterns.

which should have the correct shape and size. The connectors provide firm attachment for the pontic so it does not separate from the retainers during the subsequent cut-back procedure.

Cut-back
Armamentarium
- Bunsen burner
- Waxing instruments
- Cut-back instrument
- Scalpel
- Thin ribbon saw blade or sewing thread
- Explorer

Step-by-step Procedure
1. Use a sharp explorer to outline the area that will be veneered with porcelain (Fig. 20-46, *A*). The porcelain-metal junction must be placed sufficiently lingual to ensure good esthetics.
2. Make depth cuts or grooves in the wax pattern (see Chapter 19 and Fig. 20-46, *B*).
3. Complete the cut-back as far as access will allow with the units connected and on the master cast.
4. Section one wax connector with a thin ribbon saw (sewing thread is a suitable alternative) and remove the isolated retainer from the master cast (Fig. 20-46, *C*).
5. Finish the cut-back of this retainer, making sure there is a distinct 90-degree porcelain-metal junction.
6. Reflow and finalize the margins. The pontic is held in position by the other retainer during this procedure.
7. Refine the pontic cut-back where access is improved by removal of the first retainer.
8. Reseat the first retainer, reattach it to the pontic, section the other connector, and repeat the process.

9. Sprue the units and do any final reshaping as needed.
10. Invest and cast in the manner described in Chapter 22.

NOTE: When one connector of a three-unit FPD is to be cast and the other soldered, the cast connector should be sectioned first when the foregoing procedure is followed. The gingival surface of the pontic should be cut back in the metal rather than in the wax, because the tissue contact will help stabilize the pontic. Access is difficult, and it is easy to break the fragile wax connector.

Metal Preparation
Armamentarium
- Separating disk
- Ceramic-bound finishing stones
- Sandpaper disks (nonveneered surfaces only)
- Rubber wheel (nonveneered surfaces only)
- Round carbide bur (no. 6 or 8)
- Airborne abrasion unit (with 25 μm aluminum oxide)

Step-by-step procedure (Fig. 20-47).
1. Recover the castings from the investment and prepare the surfaces to be veneered as described in Chapter 19.
2. Finish the gingival surface of the pontic. Do not overreduce this area.

Evaluation. Less than 1 mm of porcelain thickness is needed on the gingival surface, because once it is cemented, the restoration will be seen from the facial rather than from the gingival. Excessive gingival porcelain is a common fault in pontic framework design and may lead to fracture and poor appearance (see Fig. 20-28).

To facilitate plaque control, the metal-ceramic junction should be located lingually. Then tissue

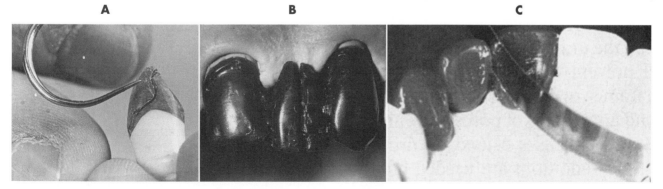

A   **B**   **C**

Fig. 20-46. Cut-back procedure for a three-unit anterior FPD. **A,** Delineating the porcelain-metal junction. **B,** The central incisor has already been cut back, and the pontic has been troughed. The canine is still at anatomic contour. **C,** A ribbon saw is used to section the connector.

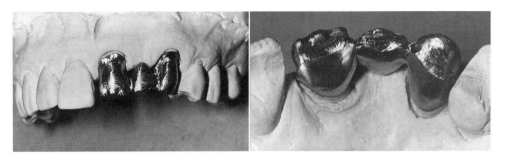

Fig. 20-47. Metal substructure ready for airborne particle abrasion and oxidation.

contact will be on the porcelain and not on metal, which retains plaque more tenaciously.[40]

Porcelain Application. Many of the steps for porcelain application are identical to those in individual crown fabrication (see Chapter 24). There are some features peculiar to pontic fabrication, however, and these will be emphasized.

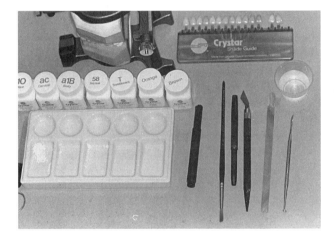

Fig. 20-48. Armamentarium for porcelain application.

Armamentarium (Fig. 20-48)
- Paper napkin
- Glass slab
- Tissues or gauze squares
- Distilled water
- Glass spatula
- Serrated instrument
- Porcelain tweezers or hemostat
- Ceramist's brushes (no. 2, 4, or 6)
- Whipping brush
- Razor blade
- Cyanoacrylate resin
- Colored pencil
- Articulating tape
- Ceramic-bound stones
- Diamond stones
- Diamond disk

Step-by-step Procedure (Fig. 20-49)
1. Prepare the metal and apply opaque as described in Chapter 24.
2. Apply cervical porcelain to the gingival surface of the pontic and seat the castings on the master cast. A small piece of tissue paper adapted to the residual ridge on the cast by moistening with a brush will prevent porcelain powder from sticking to the stone. (Cyanoacrylate resin or special separating agents can be used for the same purpose.)
3. Build up the porcelain (as described in Chapter 24) with the appropriate distribution of cervical, body, and incisal shades. The tissue paper will act as a matrix for the gingival surface of the pontic.

4. When the porcelain has been condensed, section between the units with a thin razor blade. This will prevent the porcelain from pulling away from the framework as a result of firing shrinkage. A second application of porcelain will be needed to correct any deficiencies caused by firing shrinkage. Such additions usually are needed proximally and gingivally on the pontic.
5. Apply a porcelain separating liquid (e.g., Vita Modisol*) to the stone ridge so that the additional gingival porcelain can be lifted directly from the cast as in the fabrication of a porcelain labial margin (see Chapter 24).
6. Mark the desired tissue contact and contour the gingival surface to provide as convex a surface as possible. The pontic is now ready for clinical evaluation and soldering procedures, characterization, glazing, finishing, and polishing (see Chapters 28 to 30).

Evaluation (Fig. 20-50). The porcelain on the tissue surface of the pontic should be as smooth as

---

*Vident: Brea, Calif.

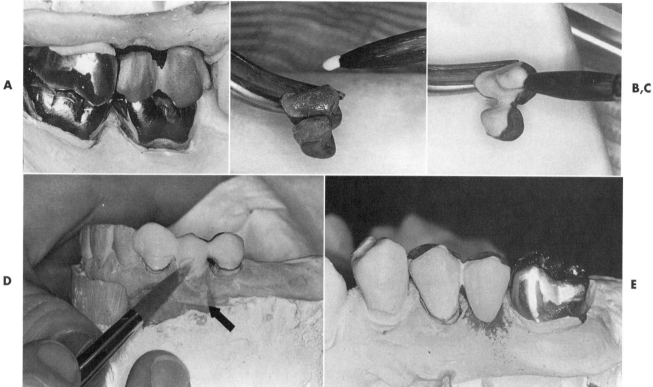

Fig. 20-49. Porcelain application. **A,** Substructure ready for opaquing. **B,** Opaque application. **C,** Body porcelain application. **D,** A piece of moistened tissue paper *(arrow)* on the edentulous ridge. **E,** The porcelain after the first firing.

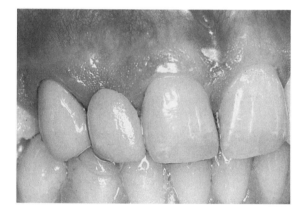

Fig. 20-50. Metal-ceramic pontic replacing a lateral incisor.

possible. Pits and defects will make plaque control difficult and promote calculus formation. The metal framework must be highly polished, with special care directed to the gingival embrasures (where access for plaque removal is more difficult).

ALL-METAL PONTICS

Pontics made from metal (Fig. 20-51) require fewer laboratory steps and are therefore sometimes used for posterior FPDs. However, they have some

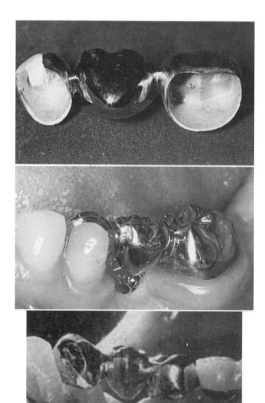

Fig. 20-51. All-metal, three-unit FPDs.

disadvantages (e.g., their appearance). In addition, investing and casting must be done carefully because the mass of metal in the pontic is prone to porosity as the bulk increases. A porous pontic will retain plaque and tarnish and corrode rapidly.

SUMMARY

Designs that allow easy plaque control are especially important to a pontic's long-term success. Minimizing tissue contact by maximizing the convexity of the pontic's gingival surface is essential. Special consideration is also needed to create a design that combines easy maintenance with natural appearance and adequate mechanical strength. When the appropriate design has been selected, it must be accurately conveyed to the dental technician.

There are subtle differences between metal-ceramic pontic fabrication and the fabrication of other types of pontics. Under most circumstances, the metal-ceramic technique is used because it is straightforward and practical. However, it requires careful execution for maximum strength, appearance, and effective plaque control. Alternative procedures may sometimes be helpful, particularly when gold alloys are used for the retainers. Resin-veneered pontics should be restricted to use as longer-term provisional restorations, and all-metal pontics may be the restoration of choice in nonesthetic situations, particularly where forces are high.

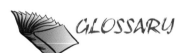 GLOSSARY

center of the ridge: the faciolingual or buccolingual mid-line of the residual ridge.

clinical crown: the portion of a tooth that extends from the occlusal table or incisal edge to the free gingival margin.

crest: *n* (14c): a ridge or prominence on a part of a body; in dentistry, the most coronal portion of the alveolar process.

emergence profile: the contour of a tooth or restoration, such as a crown on a natural tooth or dental implant abutment, as it relates to the adjacent tissues.

hygienic pontic: a pontic that is easier to clean because it has a domed or bullet shaped cervical form and does not overlap the edentulous ridge.

modified ridge lap: a ridge lap surface of a pontic that is adapted to only the facial or buccal aspect of the residual ridge.

pontic: *n:* an artificial tooth on a fixed partial denture that replaces a missing natural tooth, restores its functions, and usually fills the space previously filled by the natural crown.

residual ridge: the portion of the residual bone and its soft tissue covering that remains after the removal of teeth.

residual ridge crest: the most coronal portion of the residual ridge

residual ridge resorption: a term used for the diminishing quantity and quality of the residual ridge after teeth are removed.

Ortman HR. Factors of bond resorption of the residual ridge. J Prosthet Dent 1962; 12:429-40.

Atwood DA. Some clinical factors related to rate of resorption of residual ridges. J Prosthet Dent 1962;12:441-50

ridge augmentation: any procedure designed to enlarge or increase the size, extent, or quality of deformed residual ridge.

ridge crest: the highest continuous surface of the residual ridge not necessarily coincident with the center of the ridge.

Study Questions

1. Outline and discuss a logical classification of pontics.
2. How does pontic design change as a function of location in the dental arch?
3. What are the materials available for pontic fabrication? What are their respective advantages and disadvantages, indications, and contraindications?
4. Discuss the factors that govern the shaping of the facial and lingual surfaces of a modified ridge lap pontic.
5. What common clinical problems might be encountered if a pontic is improperly shaped or fabricated?
6. Discuss the various techniques for soft tissue augmentation and the residual ridge defects they are designed to resolve.
7. What factors should be considered when selecting the pontic material that will be in contact with the residual ridge?

ridge lap: the surface of an artificial tooth that has been shaped to accommodate the residual ridge. The tissue surface of a ridge lap design is concave and envelops both the buccal and lingual surfaces of the residual ridge.

REFERENCES

1. Stein RS: Pontic-residual ridge relationship: a research report, *J Prosthet Dent* 16:251, 1966.

2. Siebert JS: Reconstruction of deformed, partially edentulous ridges, using full thickness onlay grafts. I. Technique and wound healing, *Compend Contin Educ Dent* 4:437, 1983.

3. Abrams H, Kopczyk RA, Kaplan AL: Incidence of anterior ridge deformities in partially edentulous patients, *J Prosthet Dent* 57:191, 1987.

4. Hawkins CH et al: Ridge contour related to esthetics and function, *J Prosthet Dent* 66:165, 1991

5. Abrams L: Augmentation of the deformed residual edentulous ridge for fixed prosthesis, *Compend Contin Educ Dent* 1:205, 1980.

6. Garber DA, Rosenberg ES: The edentulous ridge in fixed prosthodontics, *Compend Contin Educ Dent* 2:212, 1981.

7. Langer B, Calagna L: The subepithelial connective tissue graft, *J Prosthet Dent* 44:363, 1980.

8. Smidt A, Goldstein M: Augmentation of a deformed residual ridge for the replacement of a missing maxillary central incisor, *Pract Periodont Aesthet Dent* 11:229, 1999.

9. Kaldahl WB et al: Achieving an esthetic appearance with a fixed prosthesis by submucosal grafts, *J Am Dent Assoc* 104:449, 1982.

10. Meltzer JA: Edentulous area tissue graft correction of an esthetic defect: a case report, *J Periodontol* 50:320, 1979.

11. McHenry K, Smutko GE, McMullen JA: Reconstructing the topography of the mandibular ridge with gingival autografts, *J Am Dent Assoc* 104:478, 1982.

12. Nemcovsky CE, Vidal S: Alveolar ridge preservation following extraction of maxillary anterior teeth. Report on 23 consecutive cases, *J Periodontol* 67:390, 1996.

13. Bahat O et al: Preservation of ridges utilizing hydroxylapatite, *Int J Periodontol Res Dent* 6:35, 1987.

14. Lekovic V et al: A bone regenerative approach to alveolar ridge maintenance following tooth extraction. Report of 10 cases, *J Periodontol* 68:563, 1997.

15. Spear FM: Maintenance of the interdental papilla following anterior tooth removal, *Pract Periodont Aesthet Dent* 11:21, 1999.

16. Perel ML: A modified sanitary pontic, *J Prosthet Dent* 28:589, 1972.

17. Hood JA, Farah JW, Craig RG: Stress and deflection of three different pontic designs, *J Prosthet Dent* 33:54, 1975.

18. Shillingburg HT et al: *Fundamentals of fixed prosthodontics,* ed 2, Chicago, 1981, Quintessence Publishing, p 387.

19. Eissmann HF et al: Physiologic design criteria for fixed dental restorations, *Dent Clin North Am* 15:543, 1971.

20. Tripodakis AR, Constandinides A: Tissue response under hyperpressure from convex pontics, *Int J Perio Rest Dent* 10:409, 1990.

21. Cavazos E: Tissue response to fixed partial denture pontics, *J Prosthet Dent* 20:143, 1968.

22. Henry PJ et al: Tissue changes beneath fixed partial dentures, *J Prosthet Dent* 16:937, 1966.

23. Jacques LB et al: Tissue sculpturing: an alternative method for improving esthetics of anterior fixed prosthodontics, *J Prosthet Dent* 81:630, 1999.

24. Hirshberg SM: The relationship of oral hygiene to embrasure and pontic design: a preliminary study, *J Prosthet Dent* 27:26, 1972.

25. McLean JW: *The science and art of dental ceramics,* vol 2, Chicago, 1980, Quintessence Publishing, p 339.

26. Harmon CB: Pontic design, *J Prosthet Dent* 8:496, 1958.

27. Henry PJ: Pontic form in fixed partial dentures, *Aust Dent J* 16:1, 1971.

28. Allison JR, Bhatia HL: Tissue changes under acrylic and porcelain pontics, *J Dent Res* 37:66 (abstract no. 168), 1958.

29. Silness J et al: The relationship between pontic hygiene and mucosal inflammation in fixed bridge recipients, *J Periodont Res* 17:434, 1982.

30. Gildenhuys RR, Stallard RE: Comparison of plaque accumulation on metal restorative surfaces, *Dent Surv* 51(1):56, 1975.

31. Keenan MP et al: Effects of cast gold surface finishing on plaque retention, *J Prosthet Dent* 43:168, 1980.

32. Ørstavik D et al: Bacterial growth on dental restorative materials in mucosal contact, *Acta Odontol Scand* 39:267, 1981.

33. Clayton JA, Green E: Roughness of pontic materials and dental plaque, *J Prosthet Dent* 23:407, 1970.

34. Tolboe H et al: Influence of pontic material on alveolar mucosal conditions, *Scand J Dent Res* 96:442, 1988.

35. Smith DE: The pontic in fixed bridgework, *Pacific Dent Gaz* 36:741, 1928.

36. Ante IH: Construction of pontics, *J Can Dent Assoc* 2:482, 1936.

37. Beke AL: The biomechanics of pontic width reduction for fixed partial dentures, *J Acad Gen Dent* 22(6):28, 1974.

38. Ferracane JL, Condon JR: Post-cure heat treatments for composites: properties and fractography, *Dent Mater* 8:290, 1992.

39. Rothfuss LG et al: Resin to metal bond strengths using two commercial systems, *J Prosthet Dent* 79:270, 1998.

40. Wise MD, Dykema RW: The plaque-retaining capacity of four dental materials, *J Prosthet Dent* 33:178, 1975.

CHAPTER TWENTY-ONE

RETAINERS FOR REMOVABLE PARTIAL DENTURES

KEY TERMS

base

clip

guide plane

intracoronal rest

minor connector

occlusal rest

parallel attachment

passive

precision attachment

reciprocal arm

reciprocation

removable partial denture

survey line

surveyor

undercut

wrought retention clasp

Different philosophies exist regarding the need for restoration of abutment teeth in fabricating a **removable partial denture** (RPD). Some authors advocate making removable prostheses with a minimum of mouth preparation. They do not suggest the routine use of cast restorations for abutment teeth but prefer to modify the remaining natural dentition through enamoplasty and/or composite resin. This has the advantages of reducing the time and expense of treatment. Other authors point to the advantages of using cast restorations on abutment teeth, suggesting the masticatory and retentive forces can be directed more favorably through precisely shaped **occlusal rests** and **guide planes**. In addition the use of cast retainers permits **intracoronal rests** or **precision attachments**, which may afford significant esthetic advantages and the possibility of splinting to reduce the mobility of abutment teeth.[1]

The correct choice of treatment for any patient depends on a thorough history and examination and an accurate diagnosis and prognosis. Decisions concerning the restoration of abutment teeth involve many factors—caries, existing restorations, tooth vitality, shape and angulation, oral hygiene, and cost and experience—and these must all be assessed and evaluated. Only then is the selected treatment likely to achieve the planned outcome based on the functional requirements of the patient.

◼ TREATMENT PLANNING

The fabrication of a precisely fitting removable partial denture is one of the more challenging tasks in restorative dentistry. Without a careful all-inclusive diagnosis and well-designed treatment plan, the chances of success are minimal. Patients who require a removable prosthesis (Fig. 21-1) usually have sustained extensive damage as a consequence of caries, periodontal disease, or trauma. They also may exhibit acquired or congenital intraoral defects. As a result of prolonged loss of arch integrity, there may be drifting or tipping, and the occlusion is often less than ideal.

Treatment plans that include a removable prosthesis may require additional diagnostic procedures besides those described in Chapters 1 and 2. The importance of accurate diagnostic casts mounted in centric relation can hardly be overemphasized. If all posterior teeth are absent, it will be much more difficult to relate opposing diagnostic casts, and stable record bases must be made under these circumstances (Fig. 21-2).

The use of a dental **surveyor** (Fig. 21-3) is essential during treatment planning for the following reasons:

1. To help assess the relative alignment of the long axes of teeth that support an RPD.
2. To help determine the optimum path of placement and removal.
3. To help evaluate tissue **undercuts** and their influence on RPD design.

The most appropriate anteroposterior and mediolateral tilt of the cast needs to be selected. Careful analysis is essential because a compromise often must be made between the requirements of an ideal tooth preparation (see Chapter 7) and the requirements for a particular tooth to be used as an abutment to support and retain an RPD. The path of insertion is the single most important factor in determining how much tooth reduction is needed to meet mechanical and esthetic requirements simultaneously (Fig. 21-4).

When surveying the diagnostic cast, the anteroposterior tilt should be established first. The lateral inclination is then determined. The operator should focus on the relative alignment of selected abutment teeth, any tissue undercuts, and the available

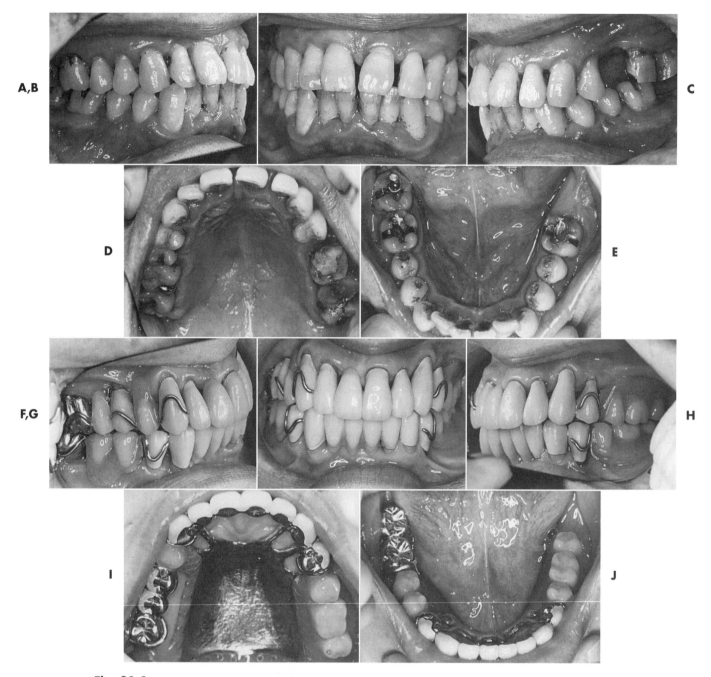

Fig. 21-1. **A** to **E,** This patient presented with extensive periodontal disease; several posterior teeth were removed. **F** to **J,** Restoration completed. A combination of fixed and removable prostheses was used.

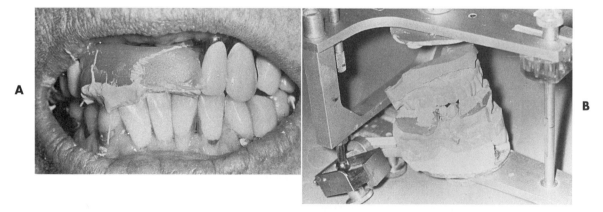

Fig. 21-2. Where multiple teeth are missing, a clasp-retained record base with wax rims (used here with ZOE paste) should be used to ensure accurate articulation. This minimizes the risk of tipping of the casts relative to one another.

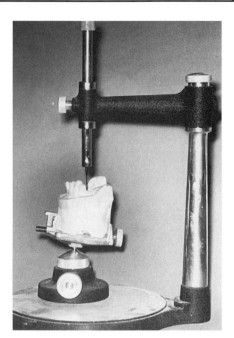

Fig. 21-3. A dental surveyor is essential during treatment planning and in designing retainers for RPDs.

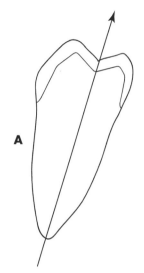

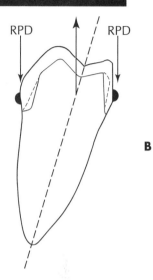

> The tooth preparation must allow for guide planes and occlusal rests.

A

B

Fig. 21-4. **A,** Normal tooth preparation for a complete cast crown. The path of withdrawal is in the long axis of the tooth. **B,** Modified tooth preparation for an RPD retainer with lingual guide planes. This preparation has a more buccal path of withdrawal.

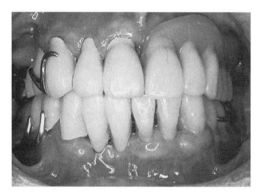

Fig. 21-5. The appearance of an anterior RPD is improved by careful selection of the path of insertion.

occlusocervical dimension for anticipated proximal and reciprocal guide planes. The feasibility of recontouring axial walls and the possible consequences of such recontouring must also be considered. For instance, it may be necessary to treat a malposed tooth orthodontically or endodontically if recontouring is not feasible. Similarly, removal of a tooth that unnecessarily complicates RPD design should be considered and carefully weighed against its effect on the stability of the prosthesis. If future loss of an already compromised tooth would render the RPD useless, it may be better to remove that tooth before initiating any prosthetic treatment.

When a patient has missing anterior teeth, the path of insertion of an RPD should be parallel to the proximal surfaces of the abutment teeth adjacent to the space (Fig. 21-5). This results in superior esthetics because it minimizes the space between the artificial and natural teeth. Sometimes esthetics can be improved by using a rotational insertion path.[2]

Apparently complex decisions as to the best tooth preparation–path of withdrawal combination can be greatly simplified by using diagnostic tooth preparation, waxing, and denture tooth setting (Figs. 21-6 and 21-7). These trial procedures on diagnostic casts help determine how to arrive at the best mechanical and esthetic result without deviating from the principles of occlusion or making excessively bulky restorations that inevitably causes periodontal complications. The concept is to determine before treatment the precise end point in re-

gard to occlusion and appearance with interchangeably articulator-mounted casts of the pre- and posttreatment condition. These cross-mounted casts also enable the treatment sequence to be simplified by allowing one arch to be treated at a time. The restorations on the first arch to be restored are fabricated against the diagnostically waxed opposing cast (Fig. 21-8 and Fig. 3-34).

PREREQUISITES FOR SUCCESS

The clinician and laboratory technician must have a good understanding of RPD design (Fig. 21-9). To

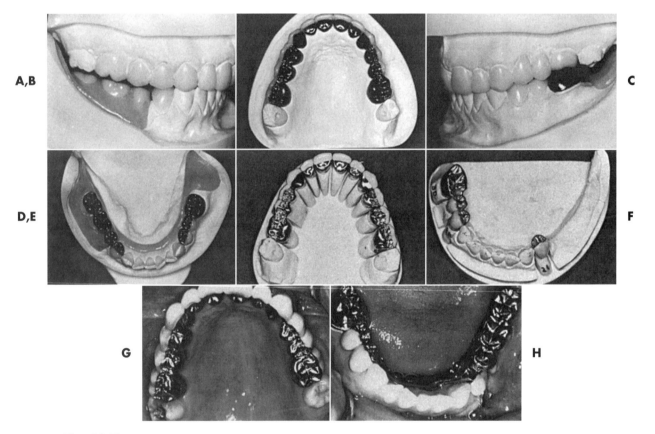

Fig. 21-6. Diagnostic mounted casts and waxing are essential prerequisites for extensive prosthodontic care. **A,** Diagnostically mounted casts. **B,** Diagnostic tooth arrangement.
(Courtesy Dr. N.L. Clelland.)

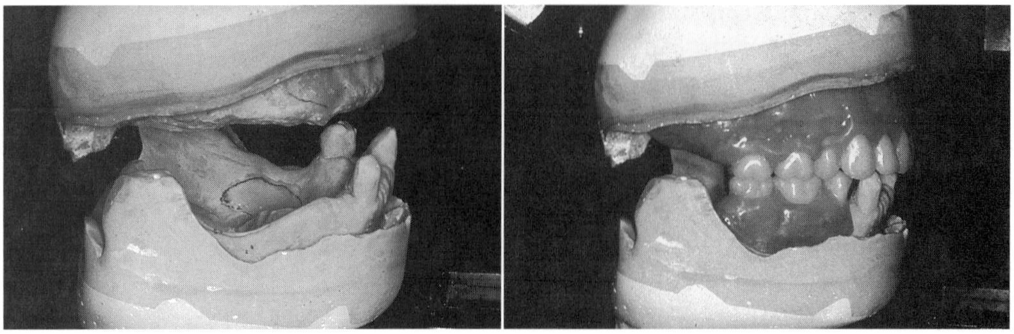

Fig. 21-7. Diagnostic tooth preparation is especially valuable in treating patients requiring a combination of fixed and removable prosthodontics. **A to D,** Diagnostic waxing. **E and F,** Fixed prostheses. **G and H,** Completed restorations. Mandibular RPD has cast metal occlusal surfaces.
(Courtesy Dr. J.H. Bailey.)

embark on an in-depth discussion of the approaches to framework design is beyond the scope of this text. We therefore will primarily consider the modifications that must be incorporated in the cast restoration to accommodate an RPD.

Design. Many concepts of removable partial denture design have been advocated. Regardless of the concept selected, the operator needs a keen understanding of the requirements placed on fixed retainers. The design should allow the forces developed

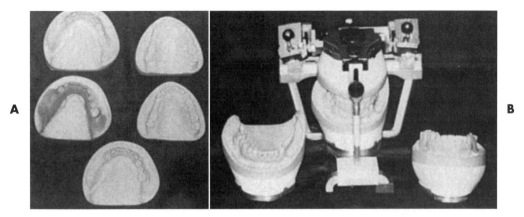

Fig. 21-8. Cross-mounted casts are used to simplify complex prosthodontic treatments. One set of casts is waxed to the end point of treatment, whereas the other set is left unaltered to enable the working casts to be mounted. An additional cast is needed for surveying a removable prosthesis. **A,** Casts needed for treating a patient requiring a maxillary fixed prosthesis opposed by mandibular fixed and removable prostheses (see Fig. 21-7). **B,** The duplicated casts are mounted in the identical relationship on an articulator. Treatment can now be undertaken in phases. First the mandibular teeth are prepared, and a working cast is obtained. This is mounted against the maxillary unaltered cast, which is then replaced by the identically oriented, diagnostically waxed cast for the laboratory fabrication of the mandibular fixed prosthesis. (See also Fig. 3-34.)
(Courtesy Dr. J.H. Bailey.)

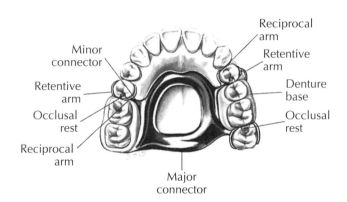

Fig. 21-9. Design of a removable partial denture. The component parts are labeled.

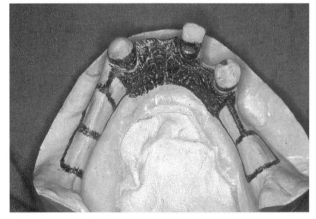

Fig. 21-10. Initial RPD design sketched on the diagnostic cast.
(Courtesy Dr. N.L. Clelland.)

during placement, removal, and function to be so directed as to cause the least harm to the remaining dentition. The proposed design (Fig. 21-10) should be carefully sketched at the initial treatment planning stage. Generally this reveals any existing problems. Each fixed restoration should be designed to be fully compatible with the removable prosthesis while fulfilling the functional requirements of mastication and facilitating the performance of oral hygiene.

Denture Bases. The denture **base** areas are shaped to avoid interference with the abutment retainer during placement and removal. Therefore the

fixed prosthesis determines the denture base configuration, rather than vice versa.

Occlusal Rests (Fig. 21-11). The rests of an RPD should fit precisely into the corresponding rest seats on the abutment retainers. To reduce laterally directed forces, the rest seats should be spoon shaped. The junction between the internal aspect of the rest seat and the proximal guide plane should be rounded to minimize stress on the framework and thereby reduce the chance of fracture.

The size of the rest seat has been a matter of controversy. Ordinarily a no. 8 round bur produces an

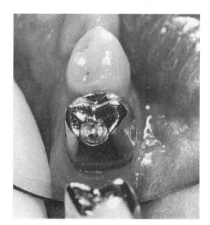

Fig. 21-11.   Cross section through an occlusal rest seat.

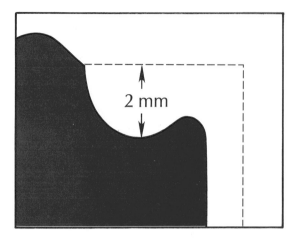

Fig. 21-12.   Distal rest seat on a mandibular second premolar.

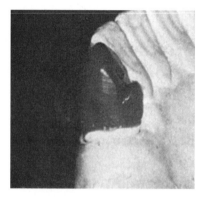

Fig. 21-13.   V-shaped cingulum rest seat.

adequate rest in the wax pattern. On small teeth under normal loading, a no. 6 round bur can provide adequate space (Fig. 21-12). On anterior teeth a cingulum rest seat should be created to support the partial denture. It should be convex mesiodistally and resemble a V-shaped groove labiolingually (Fig. 21-13). This configuration prevents displacement of

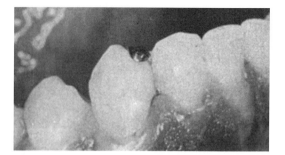

Fig. 21-14.   Incisal rest on a mandibular canine. *(Courtesy Dr. M.T. Padilla.)*

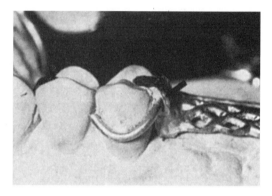

Fig. 21-15.   Minor connector of a cast RPD *(arrow)* closely adapted to the proximal guide plane.

the abutment while simultaneously transmitting forces parallel to its long axis. Unfortunately a distinct cingulum rest can rarely be placed in the cingulum of an unrestored tooth without penetrating the enamel.[3] Sometimes a pin-retained or resin-bonded restoration[4] is used to provide a cingulum rest.* An incisal rest may be used on unrestored mandibular canines (Fig. 21-14). This provides good support for the RPD but may be unacceptable esthetically. When a rest is placed on a metal-ceramic restoration, adequate thickness of metal must remain between the occlusal rest seat and the porcelain-metal junction. About 1 mm is sufficient. To minimize the risk of fracture, an occlusal rest seat should not be placed directly on porcelain.

Minor   Connectors (Fig. 21-15). The **minor connectors** of an RPD join the rests and the clasps to the major connector and should fit intimately against the proximal guide plane. The guide plane should be as long as possible occlusocervically and should follow the normal configuration of the tooth buccolingually. All proximal guide planes should be parallel to each other.

---

*NOTE: Porcelain labial veneers (see Chapter 25) or composite resin have also been used for providing undercuts for RPD retention.[5, 6]

Retention. The amount of retention is related to, among other things, the configuration of the retentive arm of the clasp of an RPD, the material from which the clasp is made, and the extent of the undercut into which it is placed and from which it is dislodged when the RPD is taken out of the mouth.

Partial denture frameworks are usually fabricated of base metal alloys, although some operators prefer an ADA Type IV gold alloy. In addition to conventional cast clasps, **wrought retention clasp** arms can be made of a platinum-gold-palladium or nickel-chromium alloy.

The modulus of elasticity of the base metals is considerably higher than that of a Type IV gold alloy. Hence shallower retentive undercuts, on the order of 0.12 to 0.25 mm (0.005 to 0.010 in), can be used with the former. Undercuts of 0.25 to 0.50 mm (0.010 to 0.020 in) can routinely be used with clasps made of either Type IV gold or wire.

When a clasp is in its normal position with the removable partial denture fully seated, it should fit in a **passive** manner against the retainer; simultaneously it should be at least 2 mm occlusal to the crest of the free gingiva so as not to interfere with maintenance of periodontal health. This means the **survey line** must not be placed too far cervically.

Likewise, the height of contour must not be placed too far occlusal, or binding of the retentive arm may occur during placement. Ideally it should be within the middle third of the retentive surface of the retainer. A properly contoured surface permits the retentive arm to flex gradually along the path of placement. Only the terminal third of the retentive arm should be placed gingival to the survey line (Fig. 21-16). If more than the terminal third of the retentive arm is placed cervical to the height of contour, this may impede placement and removal of the RPD.

A typical survey line has an undulating configuration similar to the letter *S*, with its most gingival portion adjacent to the minor connector for occlusally approaching clasps. If a gingivally approaching clasp is used, the undercut may be located immediately adjacent to the proximal guide plane, although with the popular RPI design it is placed at or mesial to the midline of the tooth.[7] Several factors—rest seat location, origin of the clasp, tissue undercuts, and degree of clasp encirclement—influence the actual configuration of the survey line for individual retainers.

Reciprocation (Fig 21-17). The **reciprocal arms**, or reciprocal clasps, of an RPD have two functions: they guide the prosthesis to place upon insertion, and they support the abutments against horizontal forces exerted by the flexing retentive arms. The re-

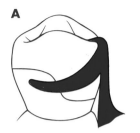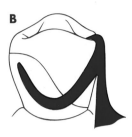

Fig. 21-16. The shape of the survey line is influenced by the material selected for the clasp. **A,** Cast clasp. Only the terminal third engages the undercut. **B,** Wrought clasp. The terminal half is retentive.

> To minimize lateral loading, the reciprocal arm should engage before the retentive arm starts to flex.

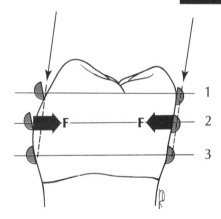

Fig. 21-17. Reciprocal arms prevent harmful lateral forces from being generated by the retentive arms during placement of an RPD. *1,* Initial contact of the retentive arm; the reciprocal arm is in passive contact. *2,* Maximum flexure of the retentive arm; the forces exerted *(F)* are resisted by the reciprocal clasp. *3,* The RPD fully seated; both the retentive and the reciprocal clasps should be in passive contact.

tentive arms should flex rather than displace the abutments laterally. Guide planes are needed on the crowns to allow for successful **reciprocation**. These should extend from the proximal guide plane to an area directly opposite the terminal position of the retentive arm. Reciprocal arms must contact the guide plane before the retentive arms start to flex so the periodontium is protected against excessive lateral loading.

◼ TOOTH PREPARATION

After the proposed path of insertion for the RPD has been determined and any necessary enamel modifications made, the teeth requiring abutment crowns can be prepared (Fig. 21-18). Often making complete crowns is necessary, but when facial contour does not require modification, partial coverage may sometimes be used.

PATH OF WITHDRAWAL

Careful planning is required when selecting the path of withdrawal of tooth preparations for RPD retainers. Although conventional crowns generally have a path in the long axis of the tooth, RPD retainers may not. Surfaces where both guide planes and reciprocal planes are planned, as well as areas that require survey lines in the gingival third, typically need to be "overprepared" relative to the ideal conservative technique used on individual teeth. Because of the lingual inclination of mandibular molars, reducing them slightly more in the occlusal two thirds of the lingual axial surface is often necessary.

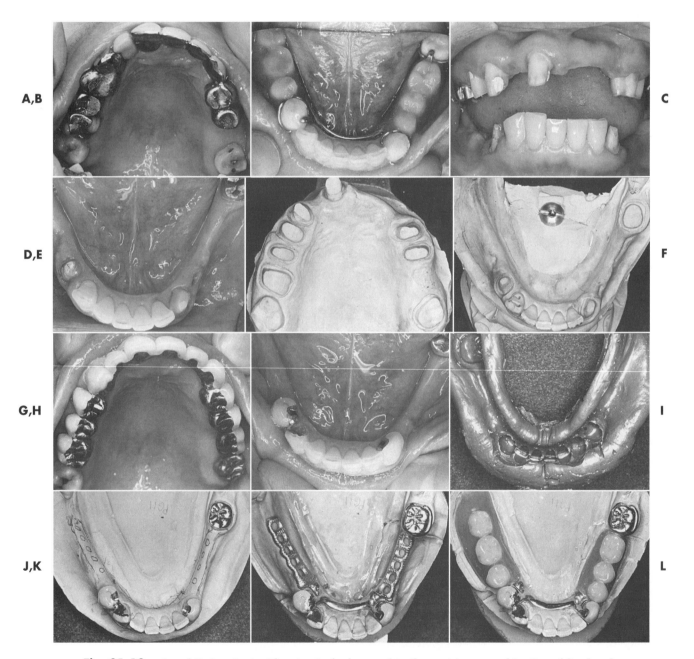

Fig. 21-18. **A** and **B,** A patient with extensively damaged teeth requiring a combination of fixed and removable prostheses. **C** and **D,** The teeth prepared for fixed retainers. **E** and **F,** Working casts. **G** and **H,** Fixed labainers at try-in. **I,** The impression for an RPD. **J** to **L,** Castings, framework, and the completed denture on altered master cast. The tissue surfaces have been modified with a wash impression.

Continued

Similarly, the axial reduction of surfaces adjacent to an edentulous ridge often involves removal of additional tooth structure. Care must be taken that these modifications do not lessen the retention form excessively, because during denture removal the retainers are usually subjected to forces parallel to their path of withdrawal, and retention becomes even more important. Frequently the use of additional features (e.g., grooves, boxes, pinholes) is needed. It is certainly not mandatory that all retainers for an RPD have identical paths of withdrawal.

REST SEATS

An adequate amount of tooth structure must be removed to allow for a minimum metal thickness of 1 mm in the area of an occlusal rest seat. To achieve adequate reduction, some operators prepare a rest seat in the tooth before starting the retainer preparation. They then use 1-mm reduction grooves to ensure adequate thickness. Although this approach can work well, problems may occur if it becomes necessary to alter the position of the rest seat during the laboratory phase. Preference therefore should be given to the slightly less conservative approach seen in Figure 21-19 because it can be extremely helpful to be able to move the rest seat. Often esthetic needs, such as the interproximal extent of a cutback for a metal-ceramic restoration, can be assessed only on the laboratory bench during waxing procedures.

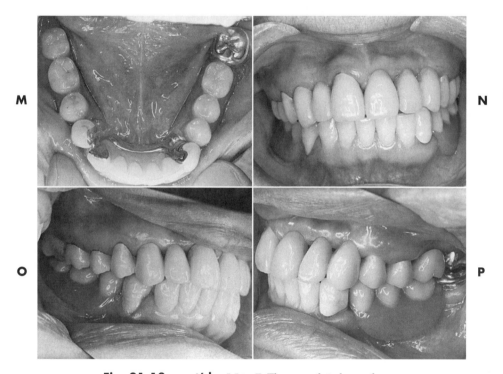

Fig. 21-18, cont'd. M to P, The completed prostheses.

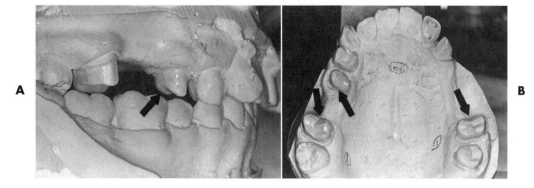

Fig. 21-19. Teeth prepared for RPD retainers. The rest seat preparation (*arrows*) allows some adjustment of rest seat location during the waxing phase.

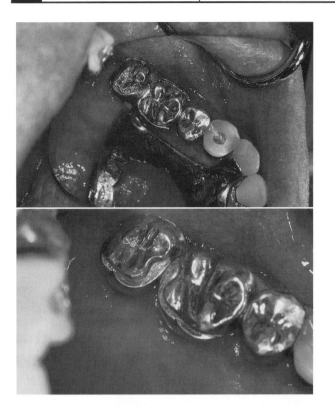

Fig 21-20. Abutment crowns contoured to precisely receive the RPD clasp.
(Courtesy Drs. K. Seckler and J. Jankowski.)

AXIAL CONTOURS

When a crown is to serve as an RPD abutment, modifications may be necessary in the normal axial reduction. The planned RPD design should be evaluated (see Fig. 21-9).

Additional tooth reduction is necessary if a retainer must be undercontoured with respect to the original tooth form to accommodate proximal or reciprocal guide planes and allow the nonretentive part of an occlusally approaching clasp to be positioned as far gingivally as possible. (A diagnostic waxing procedure can prove helpful in assessing the need for additional axial reduction.)

An advantage of providing an abutment crown is the opportunity to contour the axial contours to accommodate the RPD clasps within the normal crown contours (Fig. 21-20). Although this approach requires additional axial reduction, it allows for a less bulky removable prosthesis contour. The use of a precision machine-tool milling device (see Fig. 21-27) is essential for these restorations.

IMPRESSION MAKING

Because of the relative interdependence of RPD abutment preparations, a diagnostic irreversible hydrocolloid impression should be made after the preparations have been completed. This is poured

in accelerated-setting stone or plaster. The cast is then surveyed and the need for any further modifications is determined. These modifications can then be incorporated with minimum loss of chair time. The casts can also be used for fabricating the provisional restorations (see Chapter 15). A definitive impression is obtained with either an elastomeric or a reversible hydrocolloid technique, as described for conventional restorations (see Chapter 14).

OCCLUSAL RECORDS

A record base with wax rims is needed to articulate the casts unless an adequate number of posterior teeth are present to relate the opposing casts with a conventional centric relation record.

Because a record base is stable only on the cast from which it was made, it should not be fabricated in advance. Therefore an additional patient visit must be planned to obtain an interocclusal record. The maxillary cast orientation is transferred by means of a facebow to the articulator, and the mandibular cast is articulated in the usual manner.

WAX PATTERN FABRICATION

Waxing partial denture abutments can be difficult, even for experienced operators. Often the needs of good occlusion, anatomic form, and proper contours for plaque control appear to conflict with the need for guide planes and retentive undercuts. Careful analysis is essential at the treatment planning stages, when a diagnostic waxing procedure can prove helpful. An organized approach to waxing abutment retainers must be maintained. The wax patterns are made in the usual way (see Chapter 18), creating normal axial form and embrasures and allowing for optimum distribution of the forces of occlusion. This is followed by adjustments for the survey line, guide planes, and rest seats.

SURVEY LINE (FIG. 21-21)

When normal coronal contour has been established in wax, the cast is removed from the articulator and placed on the surveyor. The preliminary path of insertion that was established during the treatment-planning and tooth-preparation phases may require slight modification. However, a minor alteration is all that should be necessary, and it often compensates for small, previously unrecognized errors in the tooth-preparation stage.

A survey line can be relocated by tilting the cast (e.g., a mesial undercut enlarged by increasing the mesial tilt, a buccal survey line moved further occlusally by increasing the tilt toward the buccal surface). When the cast tilt for the final path of placement has been selected, the cast is marked at three

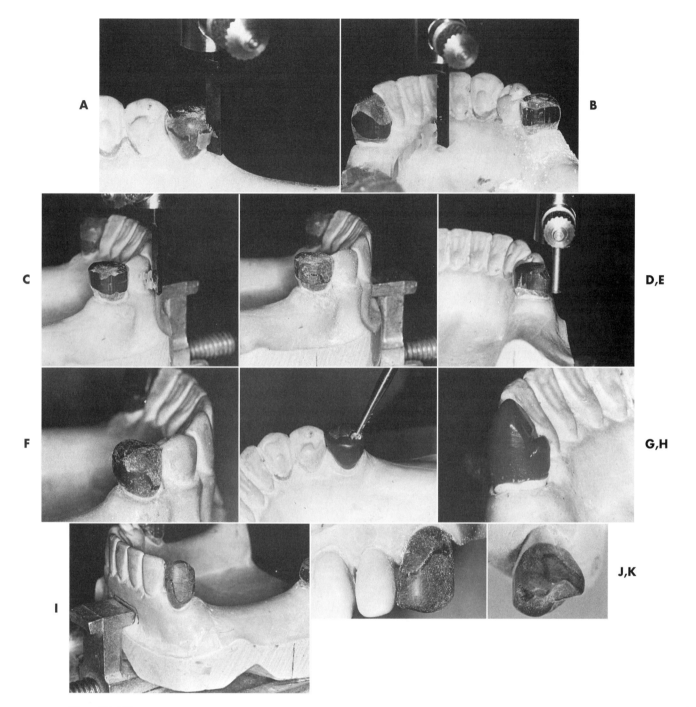

Fig. 21-21. Waxing RPD retainers. **A,** After the path of insertion has been established, the carving attachment of the surveyor is used to make a 2- to 4-mm-wide band on the pattern. **B,** Note that the band includes the proximal and lingual walls of the pattern where the proximal and reciprocal guide planes, respectively, will be established. **C,** The band is carried onto the facial surface, where the retentive clasp is to be placed. Viewed from the occlusal when complete, the band remains within the normal anatomic contour. **D,** The pattern is dusted with zinc stearate or powdered wax, and the desired survey line is scribed. **E,** After excess wax has been carved away occlusally and gingivally to create the desired contour, the undercut gauge is used to verify that the proper amount of wax has been removed. **F,** After smoothing of the various surfaces, the pattern is again dusted with powder, and the configuration of the final survey line is verified. **G,** Then a round bur is used to place the occlusal rest seat. On premolars a no. 6 bur is adequate; on molars a no. 8 may be used. **H,** A cingulum rest seat on a canine pattern can be carved with conventional waxing instruments. The lingual aspect of the rest seat must withstand lingual displacement. Mesiodistally the rest seat is slightly curved, with the highest point in the middle of the pattern. **I,** Typical survey line for a wrought clasp. Note that the distal half of the clasp can easily be placed above the height of contour. The terminal half engages the undercut. A sufficiently long trajectory must remain above the height of contour to permit gradual flexing of the clasp. **J** and **K,** The completed patterns for the maxillary canine and molar. Note the deviations from normal contour to accommodate the requirements of the RPD.

points. This "tripodizing" allows the selected path to be reestablished with minimum inconvenience. Additional wax is added until the pattern is slightly overcontoured in the area of the desired survey line and proximal and reciprocating guide planes.

The surveyor carving attachment is used. Some dental surveyors have a movable arm, which makes wax carving easier. Identical results can usually be obtained with the rigid-arm type, but more care is required to prevent fracture of the wax pattern or tilting of the surveyor table. With the carving attachment, a parallel band is scraped on the surface of the pattern, and this is inspected for the possible need of additional wax. The desired survey line is then marked, after which excess wax occlusal and cervical to the line is removed with a wax carver to obtain the correct contour.

The final evaluation of the survey contour consists of dusting the pattern with zinc stearate or waxing powder, marking the height of contour with the analyzing rod, and measuring with the undercut gauge.

GUIDE PLANES (FIG. 21-22)

The proximal and reciprocal guide planes are formed by trimming all excess wax from the patterns. Cervicoocclusally the typical guide plane should remain within normal contours. Cervically it should follow the configuration of the remaining tooth structure at the margin.

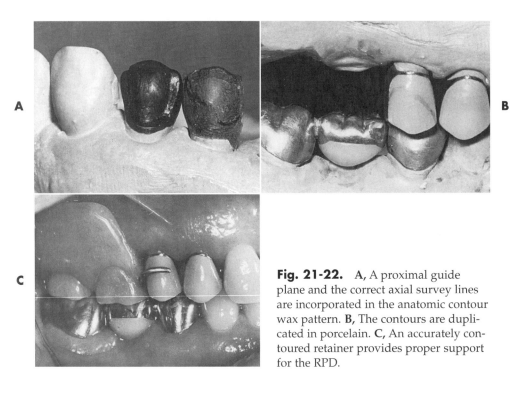

Fig. 21-22. **A,** A proximal guide plane and the correct axial survey lines are incorporated in the anatomic contour wax pattern. **B,** The contours are duplicated in porcelain. **C,** An accurately contoured retainer provides proper support for the RPD.

Lingual view

Buccal view

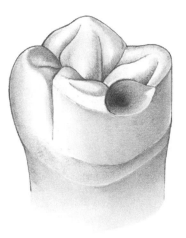
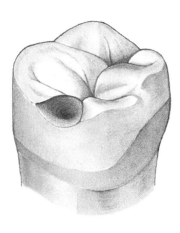

Fig. 21-23. Completed wax pattern for an RPD retainer with occlusal rest seat, distobuccal retention, and proximal and lingual guide planes.

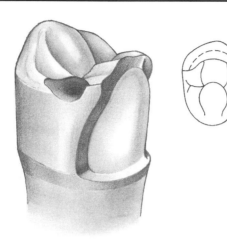

Fig. 21-24. Maxillary premolar wax pattern after cutting back for the porcelain application. The rest seat should be at least 1 mm from the metal-ceramic junction. The guide plane continues in the porcelain.

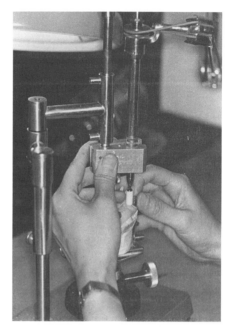

Fig. 21-26. Handpiece holder for milling guide planes. The holder attaches a conventional straight handpiece to a dental surveyor.

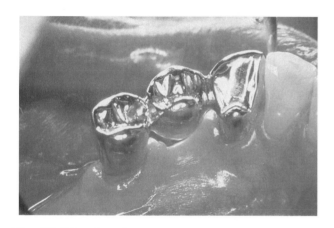

Fig. 21-25. Cingulum rest seat on a mandibular canine. *(Courtesy Dr. X. Lepe.)*

The minimum cervicoocclusal length for guide planes is that which allows the reciprocal arms of the clasps to make initial contact and remain in contact during seating of the partial denture (see Fig. 21-17).

OCCLUSAL REST SEATS (FIG. 21-23)

Occlusal rest seats are most commonly located in the interproximal marginal ridge area and can easily be cut into the wax patterns with a handheld round bur (see Fig. 21-21, G). When metal-ceramic restorations are the retainers, the rest seat should be located in metal at least 1 mm from the metal-ceramic junction (Fig. 21-24). When a rest is placed in a wax pattern for a metal-ceramic restoration, this is best done after the pattern has been cut back for the metal-ceramic veneer.

Cingulum rest seats (Figs. 21-13 and 21-25) are placed with a carver. Buccolingually they have a V

configuration in cross section; mesiodistally they are slightly curved, with the highest point in the center of the tooth.

■ SPECIAL FINISHING PROCEDURES

After the wax patterns have been invested and eliminated and the retainers have been cast, the restoration is carefully seated on the die. When the individual fit is satisfactory, it is transferred to the surveyor for milling.

MILLING

Many precision parallel milling devices are available commercially. The simplest consists of a clamp that holds a conventional straight handpiece parallel to the shaft of the surveyor (Fig. 21-26). This works satisfactorily when used carefully. Expensive machine-tool milling devices are also available that can be controlled with great precision and are particularly useful for extensive attachment prostheses (Fig. 21-27).

Cylindrical carbide burs without crosscuts are recommended for refining the proximal and reciprocal guide planes. Light pressure should be used throughout the milling procedure. Once an acceptable contour has been obtained, only minimum finishing with paper disks or rubber wheels is necessary. A complete- or partial-coverage crown is finished through the normal sequence of abrasives

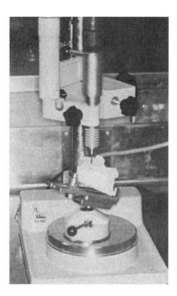

Fig. 21-27. Machine tool-milling device allows precise control of the milling process.

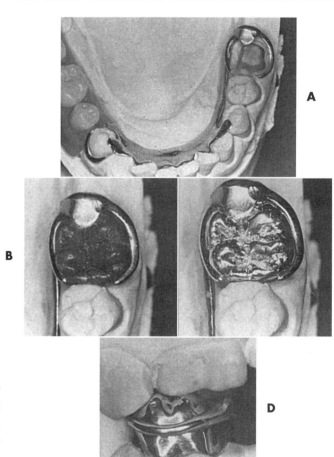

Fig. 21-28. Crown fabricated to fit an existing RPD using the indirect procedure. **A,** After a pick-up impression the RPD is fitted to the working cast. **B,** Wax pattern. **C** and **D,** Completed crown.
(Courtesy Dr. M.T. Padilla.)

until a high polish has been attained. If the retainer is a metal-ceramic crown, the veneering surface is prepared after completion of the milling procedure. Then the desired survey line and retentive undercuts are established in porcelain.

The operator should use caution when scribing survey lines on a bisque bake of porcelain. Red or green pigments must be used because they do not contaminate. Graphite from a soft lead pencil produces discoloration in the fired porcelain and must be avoided (see Fig. 21-22, *B*).

TRY-IN AND CEMENTATION

The prosthesis is tried in and evaluated as is done for any restoration. It should have good marginal integrity and proper axial contour, and it should be stable with accurate occlusal and proximal contact.

When these criteria have been met, a precementation irreversible hydrocolloid impression is poured in fast-setting stone, and the cast is analyzed on the surveyor. Any change in contour that may have occurred during finishing is easily detected at this time, when corrective action is still possible. For a metal-ceramic restoration, recontouring and reglazing may be necessary.

Cementation procedures for survey crowns are identical to those for conventional restorations (see Chapter 31). When multiple restorations involving prefabricated attachments are to be cemented, postponing cementation of the retainers until after the completion of the RPD is sometimes advantageous.

FABRICATION OF A CROWN FOR AN EXISTING RPD

Occasionally a patient has a defective abutment crown of an otherwise satisfactory removable partial denture. Although on many occasions a new RPD might be the more appropriate choice, at least 14 different methods have been described for making a crown fit an existing RPD.[8,9] These can be classified as direct, direct-indirect, or indirect procedures. When a direct-indirect procedure is used, a pattern is fabricated from autopolymerizing acrylic resin duplicating the axial contours of the original abutment crown. Margins are refined in wax on a die. The indirect procedure consists of a "pick-up" impression of the prepared tooth and seated RPD. This is poured in the conventional way after any undercuts in the denture have been waxed out. The crown is fabricated in the conventional way, removing and replacing the RPD on the cast to establish appropriate contours. Additional wax (or porcelain for a metal-ceramic crown) is added where the retentive undercut is needed (Fig. 21-28). A disadvan-

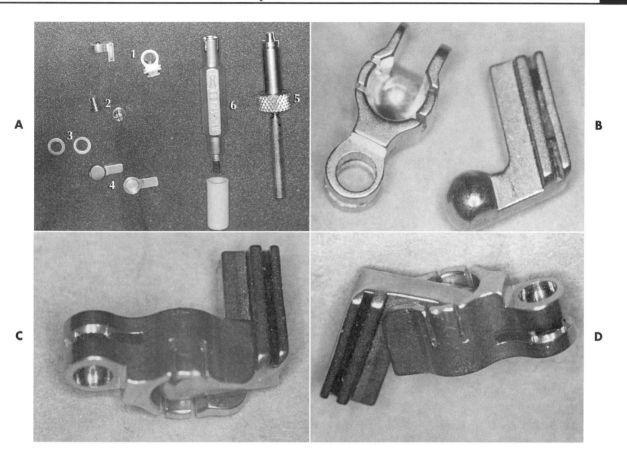

Fig. 21-29. Prefabricated extracoronal attachments. **A,** The Ceka. *1,* Female; *2,* male; *3,* spacer; *4,* male RPD connector; *5,* positioning mandrel; *6,* adjustment tool. **B** to **D,** The Stern nonrigid. This attachment provides some movement between male and female components.

tage of this technique compared to the direct approach is that the RPD is required in the laboratory. This may not be acceptable to the patient.

ATTACHMENTS

A wide range of prefabricated attachments are available for use with removable partial dentures.[10,11] Most of these consist of two components: one is incorporated in the abutment, and the other becomes part of the RPD. Both extracoronal and intracoronal designs are available.

Generally a limited use of attachments, whether extracoronal or intracoronal, is recommended. Attachments add to the complexity and cost of the restorative service and often necessitate remaking the fixed retainers when the attachments wear out. In a recent study, only 22 of 57 prostheses were complication-free during the first 2 years.[12] When used with distal extensions, attachments lead to higher stresses in the abutment teeth.[13] Nevertheless, their use can be justified, in particular to enhance appearance.

EXTRACORONAL ATTACHMENTS (FIG. 21-29)

Careful judgment is needed in deciding when to use extracoronal attachments (e.g., Ceka* or Stern†) because they place unfavorable stresses on the abutment teeth, similar to those stresses exerted by a cantilever. In addition, they make oral hygiene more difficult. In some instances, however, extracoronal attachments offer esthetic advantages that may outweigh their biologic and mechanical disadvantages (Fig. 21-30). Resin bonding has been used for the retention of extracoronal attachments using the same principles as resin-retained FPDs.[14] That the retention obtained is adequate to prevent eventual dislodgment of the attachment is doubtful.

INTRACORONAL ATTACHMENTS

Intracoronal attachments can be prefabricated as well as made in a laboratory.

*APM/Sterngold: Attleboro, Mass.
†Ney Dental International: Bloomfield, Conn.

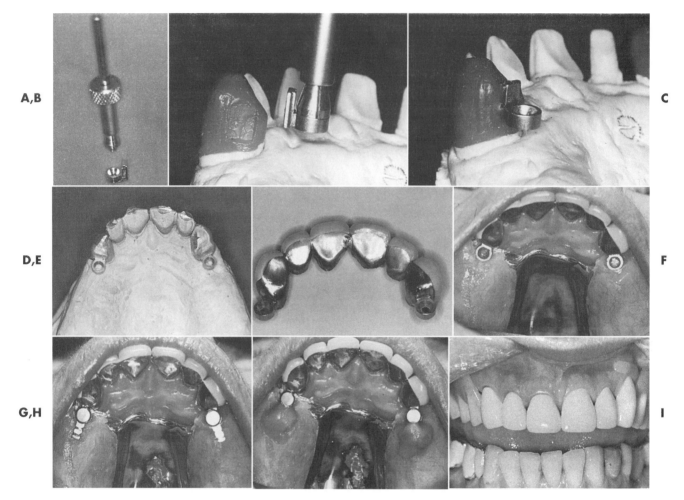

Fig. 21-30. Use of Ceka extracoronal attachments to retain a distal extension RPD. **A** to **C,** The female attachment is positioned in relation to the wax pattern by means of a mandrel in the dental surveyor. **D,** Substructures are cast directly onto the attachments. **E,** Anterior prosthesis assembled. Porcelain has been applied. **F,** Fixed splint and RPD at try-in. **G,** Male attachments in place. **H,** Attachments bonded to the RPD base. **I,** The completed prosthesis.

Prefabricated Types (Fig. 21-31). The more commonly used prefabricated intracoronal attachments (e.g., Stern* or Ney-Cheyes no. 9†) typically consist of a precision-milled male-female assembly similar to the dovetail configuration described for nonrigid connectors (see Chapter 28).

The tolerance between accurately fitting components of an intracoronal precision attachment is so fine that retention results from the frictional fit. An intracoronal attachment RPD is not readily dislodged, because it can be removed only in one direction, which may become a liability in patients with limited dexterity. However, retention can be significantly reduced after wear of the retentive sur-

faces. Most precision attachments are made of platinum-palladium alloys, which withstand the high temperature associated with casting of metal-ceramic alloys.

The female attachment is incorporated in a wax pattern, and the assembly is invested. After wax elimination the restoration is cast directly onto the attachment. Although multiple **parallel attachments** can be fabricated in this manner, most technicians prefer to solder a second or third attachment to the respective retainer(s). This allows for verification of alignment with the attachment in the first retainer.

A tray may be incorporated in the secondary retainer for added flexibility during positioning of the second attachment parallel to the first attachment. The secondary retainer is luted into place, invested, and soldered. Male components can then be in-

*APM/Sterngold: Attleboro, Mass.
†Ney Dental International: Bloomfield, Conn.

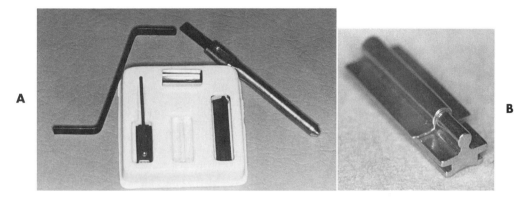

Fig. 21-31. Prefabricated intracoronal attachments. **A,** The Ney-Cheyes no. 9. **B,** The Stern.

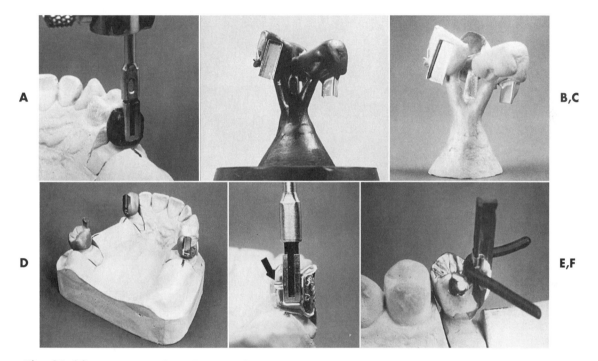

Fig. 21-32. Intracoronal attachment technique. **A,** The female attachment is tried in the proximal tray, which has been luted to the anatomic contour wax pattern. **B,** Sprued wax patterns. The extruding portion of the tray provides retention for the investment. **C,** The retainers have been cast directly on the tray. Casting directly onto the female attachment is also possible. **D,** Retainers seated on the master cast. **E,** After preliminary finishing, the female attachment is positioned and luted in the tray. Note the lingual channel *(arrow)* through which solder will be fed. **F,** A carbon insert is placed in the female attachment, and sprue wax is added to create airways in the soldering assembly.

Continued

serted. After the RPD framework has been made, the male attachments are either soldered to the frame or attached to the acrylic resin denture base with autopolymerizing resin (see Fig. 21-30 and Fig. 21-32).

The preceding paragraph condenses an intricate sequence of technically demanding steps. The less experienced operator is strongly cautioned not to underestimate the high level of skill and meticulous attention to detail that are required.

The biggest advantage of intracoronal attachments is they eliminate the need for an often unesthetic facial clasp. Simultaneously the size of most precision intracoronal attachments limits their application, especially on vital teeth. To facilitate maintaining the health of supporting tissues, the proximal surface of the restoration should not be overcontoured. Therefore the optimum placement of attachments is within the normal contours of the restoration. However, this is usually possible only

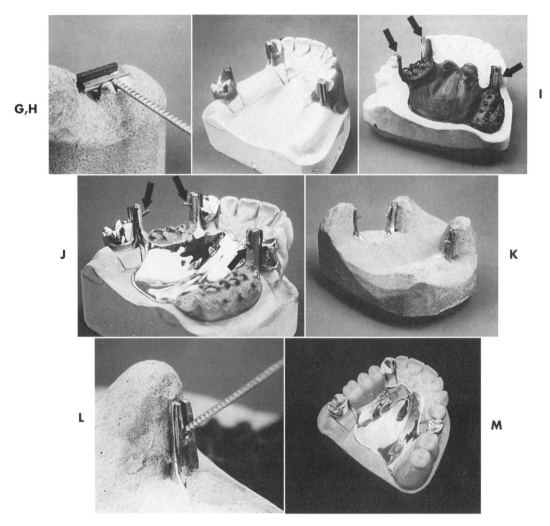

Fig. 21-32, cont'd. **G,** After investing and burnout, the female is soldered to the tray. Note that the carbon rod provides positional stability of the female attachment. **H,** Master cast with completed retainers ready for duplicating the refractory cast. **I,** Removable partial denture waxed. Note the plastic patterns incorporated adjacent to the attachments *(arrows)*. **J,** The partial denture cast and seated. The females have been positioned and their locator wires bent to extrude through the proximal plate *(arrows)*. **K,** RPD invested. It is now ready for burnout. However, before soldering, the locator wires (connected to the female attachments with low-fusing solder) should be removed. **L,** Solder is fed in through the slot in the proximal plate. **M,** The completed RPD ready for try-in.
(Courtesy Ney Dental International.)

on large teeth. On small teeth, few intracoronal precision attachments can be kept within the confines of normal tooth contour without endodontic treatment. Additionally, sufficient clinical crown must exist for adequate cervicoocclusal length to allow a positive friction fit (4 mm or more is recommended).

Laboratory-made Types. Many laboratory-made (semiprecision) attachments are in use today. Often they are referred to as *dovetails* because of the shape of their interlocking components. They can be made by incorporating a prefabricated plastic insert in the wax pattern, which is then invested and eliminated, and the pattern is cast (Fig. 21-33). The fe-

male dovetail also can be milled, after which the male component is waxed and cast.

An alternative method of fabrication is to use a tapered metal mandrel (e.g., Ticon*) that is heated and inserted in the wax pattern. When the wax is eliminated after investing, the exposed portion of the mandrel in the mold oxidizes. The crown is then cast directly onto the mandrel, which is later removed. A male attachment can be waxed and cast separately. After seating, the attachment is soldered to the RPD (Fig. 21-34).

---

*Ticonium Co.: Albany, N.Y.

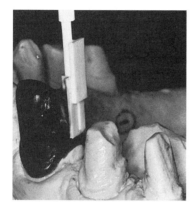

Fig. 21-33. Plastic prefabricated pattern for an intracoronal rest. *(Courtesy Dr. F. Hsu.)*

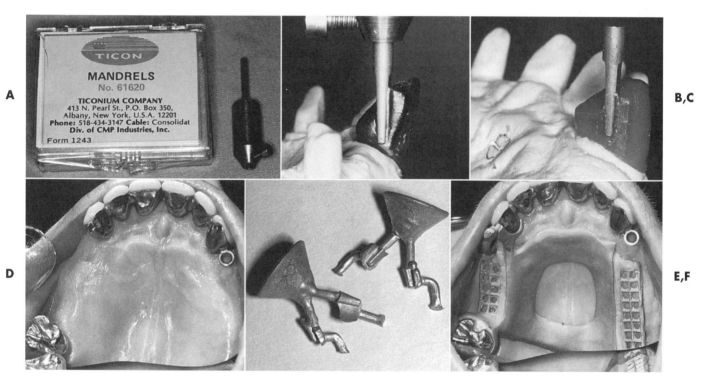

Fig. 21-34. **A,** Ticon mandrels for intracoronal rests. **B,** The mandrel is positioned with a dental surveyor. **C,** Mandrel luted to the wax pattern. The assembly (pattern and mandrel) is invested, and the metal is cast directly against the mandrel. The mandrel is then removed, creating the intracoronal rest, after which porcelain is applied in the conventional manner. **D,** Fixed prosthesis at try-in. **E,** The male attachment is waxed and cast independently. **F,** Framework and male attachment at try-in. After this, the components are soldered together. *(B to D and F courtesy Dr. F. Hsu.)*

Because of the inaccuracies inherent in their fabrication, most laboratory-made attachments have a limited amount of frictional retention compared to the commercially available precision attachments. The majority are tapered for ease of fabrication and therefore require the use of lingual clasps for positive retention.

When attachments are used with a metal-ceramic restoration, adequate metal must remain between the female component and the facial veneer of dental porcelain. A minimum material thickness of 1 mm is recommended between any intracoronal attachment and the metal-ceramic interface (Fig. 21-35).

BARS, STUDS, AND MAGNETS (FIG. 21-36)

Stud attachments[15] and magnets[16] are sometimes used to retain overdentures. They are incorporated in post-retained castings or implant abutments and offer the advantage of allowing increased occlusal force[17] (Fig. 21-37). A bar-retained RPD or overdenture can be very stable while it braces individual abutment teeth. The bar should attach to the retainer without interfering with oral hygiene.

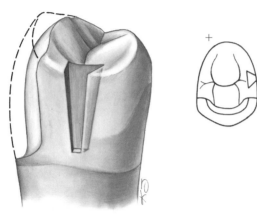

Fig. 21-35. Female intracoronal rest incorporated in a metal-ceramic restoration. The attachment should be at least 1 mm from the metal-ceramic junction. Retention is provided by a lingual undercut into which a clasp engages. Reciprocation is provided internally by the rest seat.

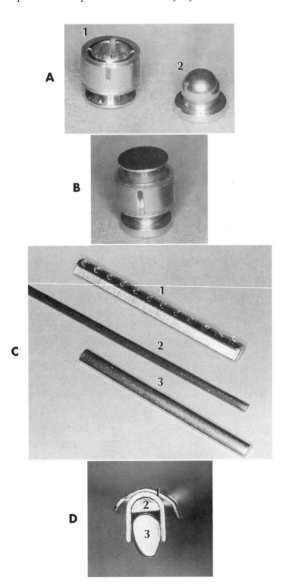

Fig. 21-36. **A,** The Stern stud attachment. *1,* Female component; *2,* male component. **B,** Stud attachment assembled. **C** and **D,** The Stern bar attachment. *1,* Sleeve; *2,* spacer; *3,* bar.

Considerable vertical space is needed for stud attachments and bar-supported RPDs.

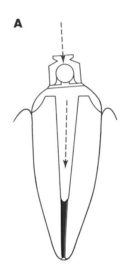

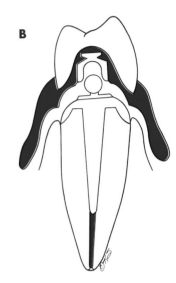

Fig. 21-37. **A,** Post-retained casting incorporating a male component of a stud attachment. The design allows for slightly different paths of insertion *(arrows)* of the post and overdenture. **B,** The female component is attached to the overdenture with acrylic resin.

Generally this means considerable coronal length is necessary for the bar to produce an acceptable result. The bar should not be placed in contact with an edentulous ridge (Fig. 21-38).

◼SUMMARY

Along with conventional diagnostic procedures, an in-depth survey analysis of the diagnostic cast must be performed for any patient requiring a removable partial denture. The coronal surfaces of the abutment teeth should be shaped to allow for optimum retention and stability of the RPD during function. Simultaneously, proximal and reciprocal guide planes should be established to guide and stabilize the prosthesis during placement and to minimize horizontal forces on the abutment teeth.

To achieve harmony with the necessary RPD design, making cast restorations on otherwise intact and caries-free teeth is sometimes necessary. Unaltered crowns of natural teeth may not have suitable contours or axial configuration for the best clasp design.

The amount of tooth reduction needed to fabricate restorations with the desired survey contours is often slightly greater than that needed if the respective abutment teeth are prepared for conventional

Considerable vertical space is needed for stud attachments and bar-supported RPDs.

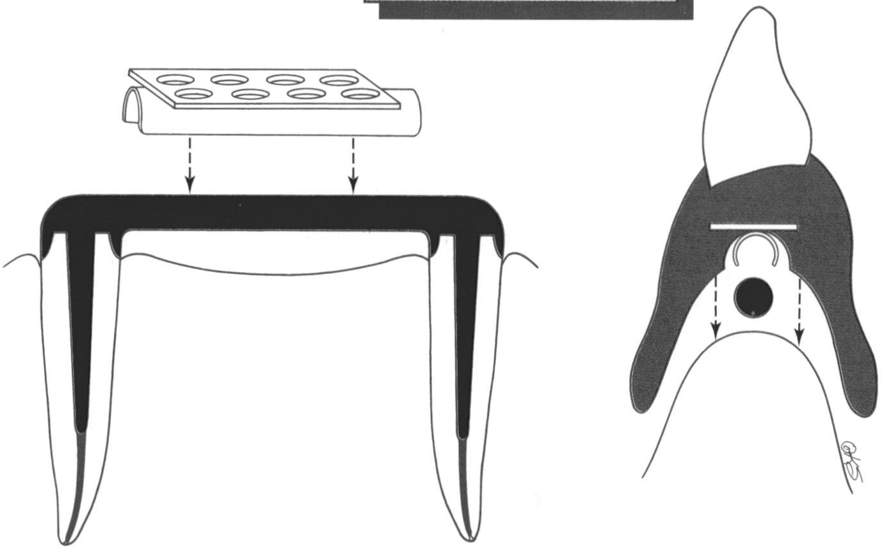

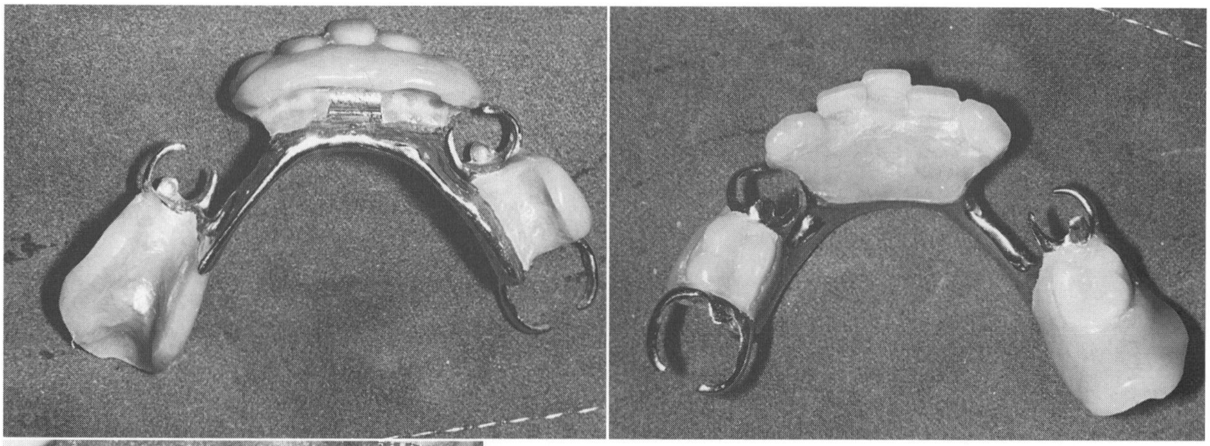

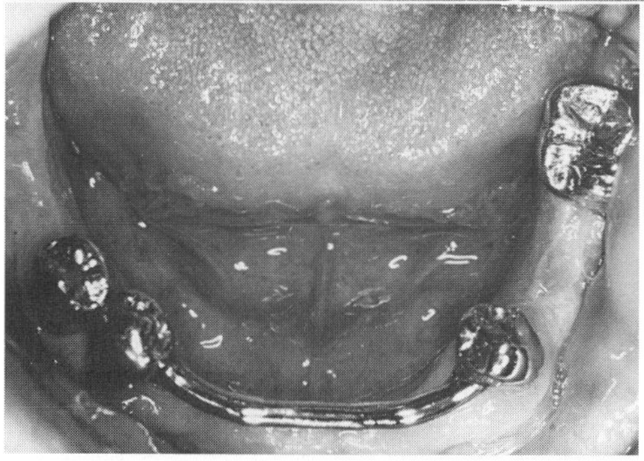

Fig. 21-38. Bar attachment. **A,** The bar is retained by posts or conventional fixed restorations. The clip provides support and retention for the RPD. **B,** Sufficient incisogingival height is needed to accommodate a bar prosthesis. **C,** Internal view of the bar-retained RPD. **D,** Occlusal view. **E,** Cemented fixed prosthesis with a bar to accommodate an RPD.

restorations. Allowances must be made for occlusal rest seats and guide planes.

Intracoronal attachments are often more esthetic than conventional clasps. They work well if kept within the normal contours of the teeth (Fig. 21-39).

Extracoronal attachments should be used minimally because of their unfavorable loading of abutment teeth and the associated oral hygiene problems.

Attachments and occlusal rest seats in metal-ceramic restorations should be placed at least 1 mm from the metal-ceramic interface.

Survey crowns require finishing procedures for which special milling equipment is needed.

A precementation impression should be obtained for verifying the best coronal contours have been created in harmony with the removable partial denture.

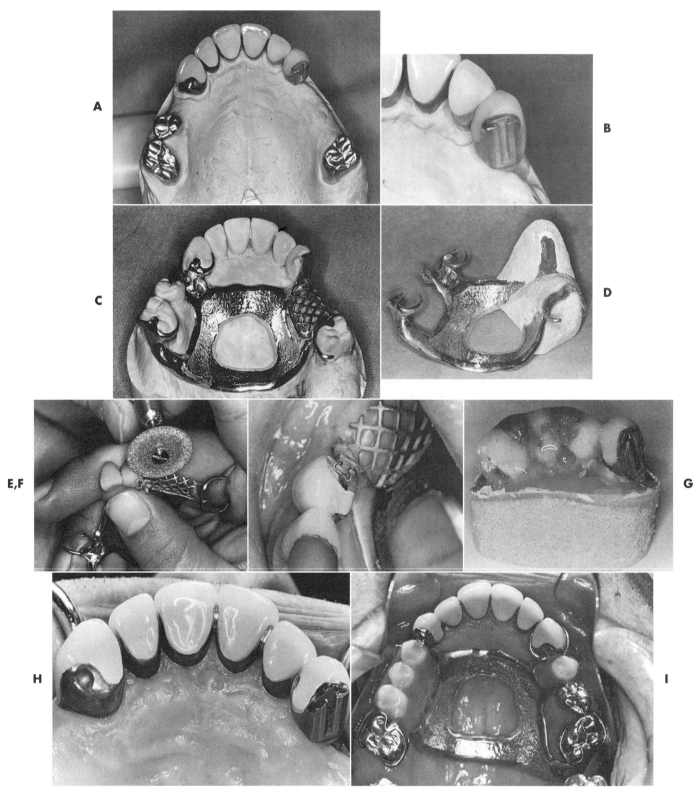

Fig. 21-39. Integration of fixed and removable prosthodontics. **A,** The retainers for an RPD have been fabricated. **B,** An intracoronal precision attachment has been incorporated into a cantilevered pontic. Note that it is still in the bisque stage. **C,** The RPD framework has been fabricated. **D,** After indexing intraorally, the male attachment is invested for soldering onto the RPD. **E,** After assembly, the excess length is removed following try-in. At this time the anterior guidance is refined on the fixed prosthesis. **F,** After glazing of the lateral incisor and canine, an autopolymerizing resin soldering index is made. **G,** The anterior splint is post-ceramic soldered. **H,** The anterior FPD in place. **I,** The completed restoration of the maxillary arch.
(Courtesy Dr. X. Lepe.)

Study Questions

1. Explain the principles underlying reciprocation and their impact on the coronal contour of individual retainers.
2. Discuss the principles that govern the determination of the location of height of contour and the survey line on the retentive surface of a retainer that is to support a removable partial denture.
3. How does tooth preparation for a retainer for a removable partial denture differ from a conventional tooth preparation for the same tooth? What are the various factors that must be considered, and how do they influence the result?
4. What is the recommended fabrication sequence of a wax pattern for a retainer for a removable partial denture?
5. Discuss the classification of attachments and the respective indications, contraindications, advantages, and disadvantages.

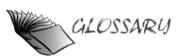

GLOSSARY

cingulum rest: a portion of a partial denture that contacts the prepared or natural cingulum of the tooth, termed the *cingulum rest seat.*

Dolder bar: [Eugene J. Dolder, Zurich, Switzerland prosthodontist] eponym for one of many bar attachments that splint teeth or roots together while acting as removable partial denture abutments. The bar is straight with parallel sides and a round top. The sleeve or clip that fits over the bar gains retention by friction only. The bar is of variable sizes and is pear shaped in cross section, as is its accompanying sleeve. This clip allows for some measure of rotational movement about the bar (Dolder EJ. The bar joint mandibular denture. *J Prosthet Dent* 1961; 11:689-707).

fulcrum line *1:* a theoretical line passing through the point around which a lever functions and at right angles to its path of movement *2:* an imaginary line, connecting occlusal rests, around which a removable partial tends to rotate under masticatory forces. The determinants for the fulcrum line are usually the cross-arch occlusal rests located adjacent to the tissue borne components.

indirect retention: the effect achieved by one or more indirect retainers of a removable partial denture that reduces the tendency for a denture base to move in an occlusal direction or rotate about the fulcrum line.

infrabulge clasp: a removable partial denture retentive clasp that approaches the retentive undercut from a cervical or infrabulge direction.

internal attachment: see *precision attachment*

keyway: *n* an interlock using a matrix and patrix between the units of a fixed partial denture. It may serve two functions: 1) to hold the pontic in the proper relationship to the edentulous ridge and the opposing teeth during occlusal adjustment on the working cast (during application of any veneering material) and 2) to reinforce the connector after soldering.

mill in: *v 1:* the procedure of refining occluding surfaces through the use of abrasive materials *2:* the machining of boxes or other forms in cast restorations to be used as retainers for fixed or removable prostheses.

minor connector: the connecting link between the major connector or base of a removable partial denture and the other units of the prosthesis, such as the clasp assembly, indirect retainers, occlusal rests, or cingulum rests.

occlusal rest: a rigid extension of a removable partial denture that contacts the occlusal surface of a tooth or restoration, the occlusal surface of which may have been prepared to receive it.

partial denture retention: the ability of a partial denture to resist movement away from its foundation area and/or abutments.

precision attachment: *1:* a retainer consisting of a metal receptacle (matrix) and a closely fitting part (patrix); the matrix is usually contained within the normal or expanded contours of the crown on the abutment tooth and the patrix is attached to a pontic or the removable partial denture framework *2:* an interlocking device, one component of which is fixed to an abutment or abutments, and the other is integrated into a removable prosthesis to stabilize and/or retain it.

reciprocation: *n* (1561) *1:* the mechanism by which lateral forces generated by a retentive clasp passing over a height of contour are counterbalanced by a reciprocal clasp passing along a reciprocal guiding plane *2:* a mutual exchange *3:* an alternating motion—reciprocative *adj.*

survey line: a line produced on a cast by a surveyor marking the greatest prominence of contour in relation to the planned path of placement of a restoration.

surveyor: *n* (15c): a paralleling instrument used in construction of a prosthesis to locate and delineate the contours and relative positions of abutment teeth and associated structures.

[1]undercut: *n* (1859) *1:* the portion of the surface of an object that is below the height of contour in relationship to the path of placement *2:* the contour of a cross-sectional portion of a residual ridge or dental arch that prevents the insertion of a prosthesis *3:* any irregularity in the wall of a prepared tooth that prevents the withdrawal or seating of a wax pattern or casting.

[2]undercut: *v* (ca. 1598): to create areas that provide mechanical retention for materials placement.

wrought: *adj* (13c) *1:* worked into shape; formed *2:* worked into shape by tools; hammered.

REFERENCES

1. Altay OT et al: Abutment teeth with extracoronal attachments: the effects of splinting on tooth movement, *Int J Prosthodont* 3:441, 1990.

2. Krol AJ, Finzen FC: Rotational path removable partial dentures. II. Replacement of anterior teeth, *Int J Prosthodont* 1:135, 1988.

3. Jones RM et al: Dentin exposure and decay incidence when removable partial denture rest seats are prepared in tooth structure, *Int J Prosthodont* 5:227, 1992.

4. Seto BG et al: Resin bonded etched cast cingulum rest retainers for removable partial dentures, *Quintessence Int* 16:757, 1985.

5. Dixon DL et al: Use of a partial coverage porcelain laminate to enhance clasp retention, *J Prosthet Dent* 63:55, 1990.

6. Davenport JC et al: Clasp retention and composites: an abrasion study, *J Dent* 18:198, 1990.

7. Berg T: I-bar: myth and countermyth, *Dent Clin North Am* 28:371, 1984.

8. Tran CD et al: A review of techniques of crown fabrication for existing removable partial dentures, *J Prosthet Dent* 55:671, 1986.

9. Elledge DA, Schorr BL: A provisional and new crown to fit into a clasp of an existing removable partial denture, *J Prosthet Dent* 63:541, 1990.

10. Becerra G, MacEntee M: A classification of precision attachments, *J Prosthet Dent* 58:322, 1987.

11. Burns DR, Ward JE: Review of attachments for removable partial denture design. I. Classification and selection, *Int J Prosthodont* 3:98, 1990.

12. Owall B, Jonsson L: Precision attachment-retained removable partial dentures. III. General practitioner results up to 2 years, *Int J Prosthodont* 11:574, 1998.

13. Chou TM et al: Photoelastic analysis and comparison of force-transmission characteristics of intracoronal attachments with clasp distal-extension removable partial dentures, *J Prosthet Dent* 62:313, 1989.

14. Doherty NM: In vitro evaluation of resin-retained extracoronal precision attachments, *Int J Prosthodont* 4:63, 1991.

15. Mensor MC: Removable partial overdentures with mechanical (precision) attachments, *Dent Clin North Am* 34:669, 1990.

16. Gillings BR, Samant A: Overdentures with magnetic attachments, *Dent Clin North Am* 34:683, 1990.

17. Sposetti VJ et al: Bite force and muscle activity in overdenture wearers before and after attachment placement, *J Prosthet Dent* 55:265, 1986.

INVESTING AND CASTING

The lost-wax **casting** technique has been used since ancient times to convert **wax patterns** to cast metal. It was first described[1,2] at the end of the nineteenth century as a means of making dental castings.

The process consists of surrounding the wax pattern with a mold made of heat-resistant **investment** material, eliminating the wax by heating, and then introducing molten metal into the mold through a channel called the **sprue**. In dentistry the resulting casting must be an accurate reproduction of the wax pattern in both surface details and overall dimension. Small variations in **investing** or casting can significantly affect the quality of the final restoration. Successful castings depend on attention to detail and consistency of technique.

An understanding of the exact influence of each variable in the technique is important so rational decisions can be made to modify the technique as needed for a given procedure.

PREREQUISITES

When the wax pattern has been completed and its margin has been reflowed (see p. 478), it is carefully evaluated for smoothness, finish, and contour (see Chapter 18). The pattern is inspected under magnification, and any residual flash is removed. A sprue is attached to the pattern, then removed from the die and fitted to a **crucible former** (Fig. 22-1). The wax pattern should be invested immediately because any delay leads to distortion of the pattern due to stress relief of the wax.[3]

SPRUE (FIG. 22-2)

Sprue design varies depending on the type of restoration being cast, the **alloy** used, and the **casting machine.** There are three basic requirements, as follows:

1. The sprue must allow the molten wax to escape from the mold.

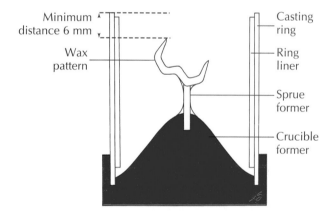

Fig. 22-1. Wax pattern attached to the crucible former with a sprue ready for investing. A ring liner is in place.

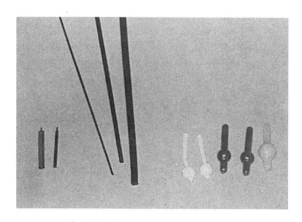

Fig. 22-2. Prefabricated sprues.

2. The sprue must enable the molten metal to flow into the mold with as little turbulence as possible.

3. The metal within it must remain molten slightly longer than the alloy that has filled the mold. This provides a reservoir to compensate for the shrinkage that occurs during solidification of the casting.

The shape of the channel in the **refractory mold** is determined by the sprue connecting the wax pattern to the crucible former. The sprue can be wax, plastic, or metal. Wax sprues are preferred for most castings because they melt at the same rate as the pattern and thus allow easy escape of the molten wax. Solid plastic sprues soften at a higher temperature than the wax pattern and may block the escape of wax, resulting in increased casting roughness. However, plastic sprues can be useful when casting fixed partial dentures (FPDs) in one piece because their added rigidity minimizes distortion. Also, hollow plastic sprues are available that permit the escape of wax.

If a metal sprue is used, it should be made of non-rusting metal to avoid possible contamination of the wax. Metal sprues are often hollow to increase contact surface area and strengthen the attachment between the sprue and pattern. They are usually removed from the investment at the same time as the crucible former. Special care must be taken to examine the orifice for small particles of investment that may break off when such a sprue is removed because these can cause an incomplete casting if undetected (see p. 585).

Diameter. In general, a relatively large-diameter sprue is recommended because this improves the flow of molten metal into the mold and ensures a reservoir during solidification.[4,5]

A 2.5-mm (10-gauge) sprue is recommended for molar and metal-ceramic patterns. A smaller 2.0-mm (12-gauge) is adequate for premolars and partial-coverage restorations.

In some casting techniques other than the commonly used centrifugal technique, a narrow sprue is essential. For instance, with air-pressure machines the melt is made directly in the depression created by the crucible former and then forced into the mold by the sudden change in air pressure. With this technique a narrow sprue prevents the molten metal from flowing into the mold prematurely.

Location. The sprue should be attached to the bulkiest part of the pattern, away from margins and occlusal contacts. Normally the largest noncentric cusp is used. The point of attachment should permit

a stream of metal to be directed to all parts of the mold without having to flow opposite the direction of the casting force (Fig. 22-3). The sprue must also allow for proper positioning of the pattern in the ring. This can be critical because expansion within the mold is not uniform.[6,7] For example, spruing on the cusp tip can give good results, but spruing on the proximal contact may produce a casting that is too wide mesiodistally and too short occlusocervically (Fig. 22-4).

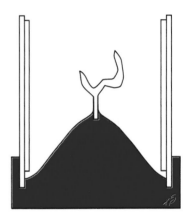

Fig. 22-3.   Correct sprue placement on the bulkiest noncentric cusp allows molten alloy to flow to all parts of the mold.

Incorrect sprue placement. The gold needs to change direction at an angle of almost 90 degrees after entering the mold. Better placement is at a 45-degree angle on the thickest portion of the pattern.

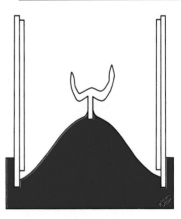

Fig. 22-4.   Incorrect sprue placement in the central fossa obliterates occlusal anatomy and may result in poor mold filling because the molten metal is not pushed into the cusp tips by centrifugal force.

Attachment.   The sprue's point of attachment to the pattern should be carefully smoothed to minimize turbulence. The attachment area should not be restricted because necking increases casting **porosity** and reduces mold filling.[8]

Venting.   Small auxiliary sprues or vents have been recommended to improve casting of thin patterns. Their action may help gases escape during casting[9] or ensure that solidification begins in critical areas by acting as a heat sink[10] (Fig. 22-5).

CRUCIBLE FORMER (FIG. 22-6)

The sprue is attached to a crucible former,* usually made of rubber, which constitutes the base of the **casting ring** during investing. The exact shape of the crucible former depends on the type of casting machine used. With most modern machines, the crucible former is tall to allow use of a short sprue and allow the pattern to be positioned near the end of the casting ring.

---

*Sometimes also referred to as a *sprue former*.

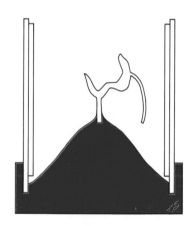

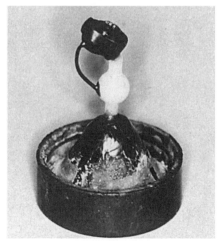

Fig. 22-5.   The thin auxiliary sprue may help gases escape and ensure the casting solidifies in a critical area.

CASTING RING AND LINER

The casting ring holds the investment in place during setting and restricts the expansion of the mold. Normally a liner is placed inside the ring to allow for more expansion. At one time asbestos was used as the liner, but this has been replaced by other materials to avoid the health risks associated with asbestos fibers. Wetting the liner increases the **hygroscopic expansion** of the mold, but because an absorbent dry liner removes water from the investment and makes a thicker mix, the total expansion increases.[11,12] Care must be taken not to squeeze the liner against the ring to prevent expansion restriction. Increased expansion can be obtained by placing the mold in a water bath. This is because of hygroscopic expansion (Fig. 22-7).

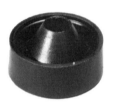
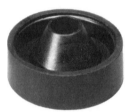

Fig. 22-6.   Rubber crucible formers. *(Courtesy Whip Mix Corporation.)*

Various methods to influence the amount of *setting expansion* of the investment.

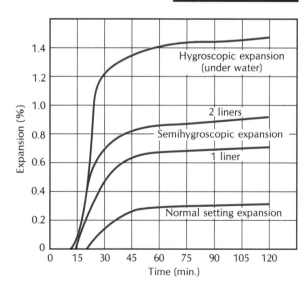

Fig. 22-7.   Setting expansions of dental casting investments. Note that expansion can be increased by a hygroscopic technique as well as by the particular type of ring liner used.
(Courtesy Whip Mix Corporation.)

The position of the pattern in the casting ring affects expansion, so for consistent results a single **crown** should be positioned within the ring equidistant from its walls. When fixed prostheses are cast as one piece, greater accuracy is achieved if the pattern is placed near the center of a large or special oval ring, rather than near the edge of a smaller ring.[6]

RINGLESS INVESTMENT TECHNIQUE (FIG. 22-8)

With the use of higher-strength, phosphate-bonded investments, the ringless technique has become quite popular.[13] The method uses a paper or plastic casting ring and is designed to allow unrestricted expansion.[14]

SPRUING TECHNIQUE

Armamentarium (Fig. 22-9)

- Sprue
- Sticky wax
- Rubber crucible former
- Casting ring
- Ring liner
- Bunsen burner
- Pattern cleaner
- Scalpel blade
- Forceps

Step-by-step Procedure for a Single Casting. A 2.5-mm-diameter (10-gauge) sprue form is recommended for molar crowns or metal-ceramic castings, although a 2-mm (12-gauge) sprue is adequate for premolar and partial-coverage restorations. The procedure is as follows:

1. Attach a 12-mm wax sprue to the bulkiest non-centric cusp of the wax pattern, and angle it so it is obtuse to the adjacent axial walls and occlusal surface (Fig. 22-10, *A*). This angle is usually about 135 degrees to the axial walls, and it facilitates filling of the mold.
2. Add wax to the point of attachment and smooth it to prevent turbulence during casting.

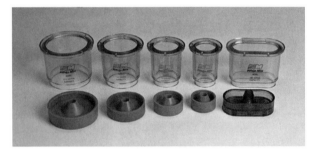

Fig. 22-8. Ringless investment technique. Crucible formers and cone-shaped plastic rings for a ringless casting system. The crucible former and plastic ring are removed before wax elimination, leaving the invested wax pattern. The systems are designed to achieve expansion that is unrestricted by a metal ring.
(Courtesy Whip Mix Corporation.)

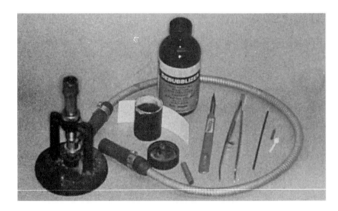

Fig. 22-9. Armamentarium for spruing the wax pattern.

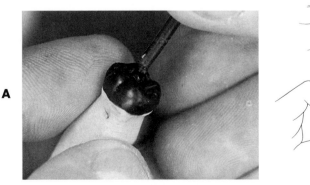

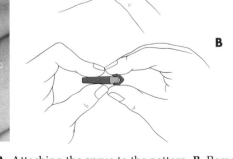

Fig. 22-10. Spruing technique for a single casting. **A,** Attaching the sprue to the pattern. **B,** Removing the pattern from the die.

Continued

3. Remove the pattern from the die, using extreme caution not to distort it (Fig. 22-10, *B*).

4. Insert the sprue into the hole in the crucible former, holding it with forceps (Fig. 22-10, *C*). It should now be luted into place with wax and the junction between sprue and **crucible** should be smoothed. Use of a surfactant greatly enhances wetting of the pattern during investing (Fig. 22-10, *D*).

5. Line the casting ring, keeping it flush with the open end, and moisten the liner (Fig. 22-10, *E*).

6. Place the ring over the pattern to ensure it is sufficiently long to cover the pattern with about 6 mm of investment (Fig. 22-10, *F*). If necessary, the sprue may be shortened, or a longer ring may be chosen as an alternative.

Procedure for Multiple Castings (Fig. 22-11). When more than two units are being cast together, each is joined to a runner bar. A single sprue is used to feed the runner bar. Two units may be cast with a runner bar, or each unit may be fed from a separate sprue.

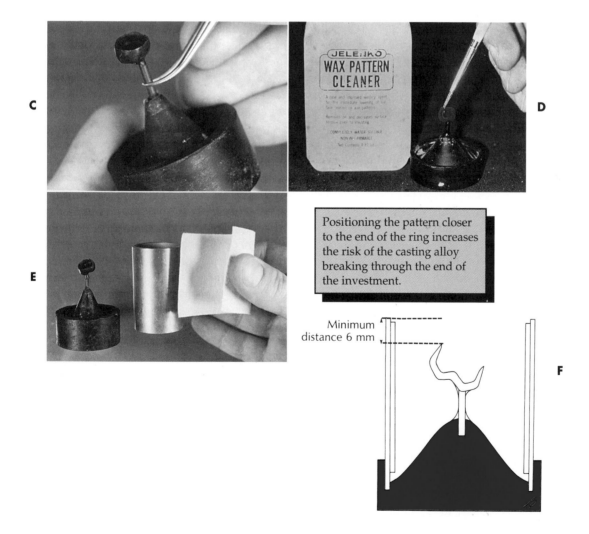

Fig. 22-10, cont'd. **C,** Positioning the pattern on the crucible former. **D,** Application of surfactant. **E,** A ring liner increases the setting expansion. **F,** The pattern must be positioned sufficiently away from the end of the ring.

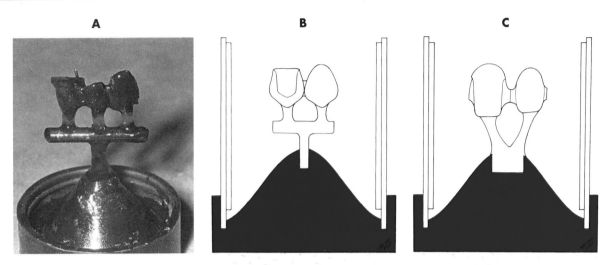

Fig. 22-11. Spruing multiple units. **A,** For more than two castings a runner bar is used. **B** and **C,** For two castings a runner bar may be used, or each casting may be fed through a separate sprue.

MATERIALS SCIENCE

M. H. Reisbick

Several investment materials are available for fabricating a dental casting mold. Typically these consist of a **refractory** material (usually silica) and a binder material, which provides strength. Additives are used by the manufacturer to improve handling characteristics.

When classifying investments by binder, three groups are recognized: gypsum-bonded, phosphate-bonded, and silica-bonded investments. Each has specific applications. The gypsum-bonded investments are used for castings made from ADA Type II, Type III, and Type IV gold alloys. The phosphate-bonded materials are recommended for metal-ceramic frameworks. The silica-bonded investments are for high-melting **base metal** alloys used in removable partial denture castings. However, because of their limited application in fixed prosthodontics, silica-bonded investments are not included in the following discussion.

Gypsum-bonded Investments

Gypsum is used as a binder, along with **cristobalite** or **quartz** as the refractory material, to form the mold. The cristobalite and quartz are responsible for the **thermal expansion** of the mold during **wax elimination.** Because gypsum is not chemically stable at temperatures exceeding 650° C (1200° F), these investments are typically restricted to castings of conventional Type II, III, and IV gold alloys.

Expansion. Three types of expansion can be influenced to obtain the desired size of casting: setting, hygroscopic, and thermal.

Setting Expansion. As the gypsum investment sets after mixing, it expands and slightly enlarges the mold. The pattern, metal casting ring, and compressibility of the ring liner all influence this expansion.

The water–powder ratio can be altered to reduce or increase the amount of **setting expansion.** The use of less water increases the setting expansion and results in a slightly larger casting. Use of an additional ring liner increases the setting expansion, as will a slight increase in mixing time. If a smaller casting is desired, more water can be used or the liner can be eliminated, both of which curtail the amount of expansion. When attempting to alter setting expansion, do not deviate more than minimally from the manufacturer's recommendations to ensure there will be no changes in the essential properties of the investment.

Hygroscopic Expansion. Hygroscopic expansion occurs when water is added to the setting gypsum investment immediately after the ring has been filled. Usually this is accomplished by submerging the ring in a water bath at 37° C (100° F) for up to 1 hour immediately after investing. A significant amount of additional setting expansion results, permitting the use of a slightly lower burnout temperature. A wet ring liner also contributes hygroscopic expansion to that portion of the mold with which it is in contact (see Fig. 22-7).

Thermal Expansion (Fig. 22-12). As the mold is heated to eliminate the wax, thermal expansion occurs. The **silica** refractory material is principally responsible for this because of solid-state phase transformations. Cristobalite changes from the α to the β (high-temperature) form between 200° C (392° F) and

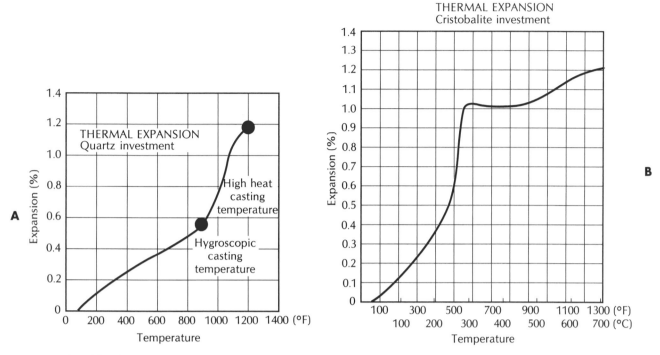

Fig. 22-12. Thermal expansions of quartz-based **(A)** and cristobalite-based **(B)** investments. *(Courtesy Whip Mix Corporation.)*

270° C (518° F); quartz transforms at 575° C (1067° F). These transitions involve a change in crystal form, an accompanying change in bond angles and axis dimension, and a decreased density, producing a volume increase in the refractory components.

PHOSPHATE-BONDED INVESTMENTS

Because most metal-ceramic alloys fuse at around 1200° C (2300° F) (as opposed to conventional gold alloys at 925° C [1700° F]), additional shrinkage occurs when the casting cools to room temperature. To compensate for this, a larger mold is necessary. The added expansion can be obtained with phosphate-bonded investments.

The principal difference between gypsum-bonded and phosphate-bonded investments is the composition of the binder and the relatively high concentration of silica refractory material in the latter. The binder consists of magnesium oxide and an ammonium phosphate compound. Contrary to gypsum-bonded products, this material is stable at burnout temperatures above 650° C (1200° F) (Fig. 22-13), which allows for additional thermal expansion. Most phosphate-bonded investments are mixed with a specially prepared suspension of colloidal silica in water. (Some, however, can be mixed with water alone.)

Some phosphate-bonded investments contain carbon and therefore are gray in color. Carbon-

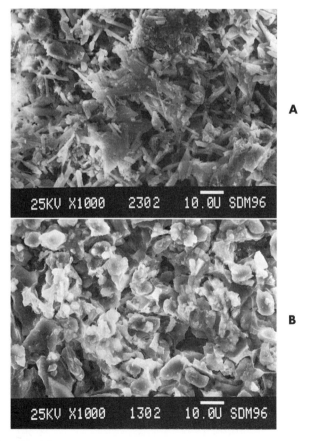

Fig. 22-13. Scanning electron micrographs of a gypsum-bonded **(A)** and a phosphate-bonded investment **(B)**, each heated to 700° C (1292° F).

containing materials should not be used for casting base metals because the carbon residue affects the final alloy composition. They may be used for casting high-gold or palladium content alloys.

Expansion. Compared to gypsum-bonded investments, phosphate-bonded investments offer greater flexibility in controlling the amount of expansion. The liquid–powder ratio needs only slight modification to effect a significant change in setting expansion. Increasing the proportion of special liquid (colloidal silica) also increases expansion.

Working Time. Phosphate-bonded investments have a relatively short working time compared to gypsum materials. Their exothermic setting reaction accelerates as the temperature of the mix rises during manipulation. The filled ring feels warm to the touch even shortly after it has been filled. A longer mixing time significantly accelerates the setting reaction and temperature and thus reduces the working time even further. The addition of water to the colloidal silica suspension increases the working time, with some loss of setting expansion. Many technicians therefore vary the quantity of special liquid and water between batches and make trial mixes for each new shipment. This has been a reliable means of adjusting expansion.[15] Gas is formed during the reaction and must be removed for a sufficiently long period to minimize nodules on the casting.[16] Maintaining a vacuum for about 60 seconds appears to be adequate for this.

• • •

SELECTION OF MATERIALS

SELECTING A CASTING ALLOY

The choice of casting alloy largely determines the selection of investment and casting techniques and therefore is discussed first.

The number and variety of alloys suitable for casting have expanded dramatically, largely because of changes in the price of gold. Many alloys are available, especially for metal-ceramic restorations (see Chapter 19). The dentist must be able to make a rational choice based on current information.

Factors to Be Considered

Intended Use. Traditionally alloys for casting were classified on the basis of their intended use, as follows:
Type I: Simple inlays
Type II: Complex inlays
Type III: Crowns and FPDs
Type IV: RPDs and pinledges
Porcelain: Metal-ceramic alloys

Physical Properties. In 1965 the ADA adopted the specifications of the Fédération Dentaire Internationale (FDI), which classified casting alloys according to their physical properties (specifically their hardness), as follows:
Type I: Soft
Type II: Medium
Type III: Hard
Type IV: Extra hard
Porcelain-type alloys with a high **noble metal** content were found to have similar hardness to Type III alloys, and base metal alloys were found to be harder than Type IV alloys (see Chapter 19).

Color. Manufacturers place considerable emphasis on the color of their alloys, and color preference is often given to gold over silver. The patient's views on the subject should be sought if the metal will be visible in the mouth; otherwise, the color of the alloy is irrelevant.

Color is not a good guide to gold content: 9-**carat** jewelry alloy with only 37.5% gold looks considerably more yellow than a metal-ceramic alloy with 85% gold but no copper.

Composition. To be accepted by the ADA as an alloy suitable for dental restorations,[17] the manufacturer must list the percentage composition by weight of the three main ingredients and any noble metal percentage(s). Traditionally the functional characteristics of corrosion resistance and tarnish resistance were predicted on the basis of gold content. In general, if at least half the atoms in the alloy are gold (which would be 75% by weight), good resistance to corrosion and tarnish can be predicted. Nevertheless clinical evaluations have failed to show statistically significant differences in the tarnish resistance of high-gold (77%) and low-gold (59.5% to 27.6%) alloys.[18] However, a poorly formulated alloy, even of high gold content, can rapidly tarnish intraorally.

Cost. Treatment plans are often modified to suit the financial capabilities of the patient or a third party. Base metal alloys have found favor principally because of their low cost. Similarly, alloys containing approximately 50% gold have been found to offer some economic advantage (although the savings are not proportional to the reduced gold content of the

---

*At the time of writing, palladium is considerably more expensive at $560 per ounce than gold ($280 per ounce). However, it is less dense (12.0 g/ml compared to 19.3 g/ml so an ounce of metal will yield more restorations).

alloy). Alloys containing primarily palladium* and only a small percentage of gold offer an alternative for use in the metal-ceramic technique, although soldering procedures may be less predictable.

When calculating the intrinsic metal cost of a restoration, determine the volume of the casting rather than its weight. Dental casting alloys can vary considerably in density from 8 g/ml to almost 19 g/ml (see Table 19-1). An "average" restoration has a volume of 0.08 ml; an all-metal pontic may have a volume reaching 0.25 ml.[19] Therefore, it is conceivable that the cost of a large pontic cast in a low-density alloy would be equal to or less than the cost of a complete cast crown fabricated from a high-density alloy. When noble metal prices are high, more sophisticated techniques of scrap recovery become economically attractive. These can range from installing conventional metal catchers in all areas where castings are finished to equipping all work stations with filtered suction machines.

Clinical Performance. In most respects, clinical performance (biologic and mechanical) is more important than cost. Biologic properties that can be evaluated include gingival irritation, recurrent caries, plaque retention, and allergies. Mechanical properties include wear resistance and strength, marginal fit, ceramic bond failure, connector failure, and tarnish and corrosion.

A risk in choosing a new alloy is that defective clinical performance may fail to appear in laboratory testing or short-term animal and clinical trials. For example, manufacturers introduced copper-based casting alloys with very poor corrosion resistance[20] when the price of gold was rapidly rising.* Although the clinically established alloys all have disadvantages, their performance is likely to have been well documented, and the prognosis of restorative treatment can be more accurately predicted.

Laboratory Performance. Sound laboratory data are essential in the selection of a casting alloy. Important areas of consideration are casting accuracy, surface roughness, strength, sag resistance, and metal-ceramic bond strength. Presently available data suggest that nickel-chromium alloys have lower casting accuracy[21] and greater surface roughness[22] than gold alloys (Fig. 22-14) but higher strength and sag resistance because of their higher melting ranges.[23]

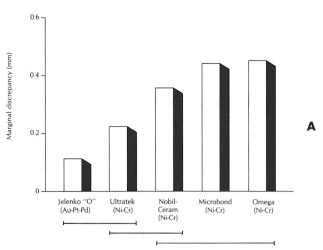

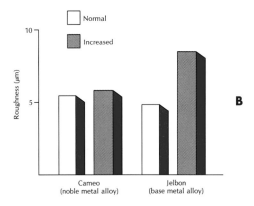

Fig. 22-14. **A,** Comparison of casting accuracies with different alloys. **B,** Influence of metal casting temperature and alloy selection on casting roughness. *(A from Duncan JD: J Prosthet Dent 47:63, 1982; **B** from Ogura H et al: J Prosthet Dent 45:529, 1981.)*

Handling Properties. The ease with which an alloy can be manipulated may influence its selection. An alloy that produces satisfactory clinical results, but only under extremely critical conditions or with expensive equipment, may be rejected in favor of one that produces acceptable results with less critical manipulation.

The ability to burnish an alloy to reduce marginal gap width and thus reduce the exposed thickness of the luting agent is important,[24] although the areas where marginal adaptation is clinically most important (interproximally and subgingivally) are usually not very accessible for such manipulation.

Biocompatibility. All materials for intraoral use should be biocompatible. In addition, it should be possible to handle them safely in the office or laboratory. Many hazardous materials are commonly used in dentistry, such as mercury, chloroform, silver

---

*In fact, these formulations were very similar to aluminum-bronze alloys sold as dental gold in the 1920s.

cyanide, and hydrofluoric acid. Consequently, restrictions have been imposed on their shipping and use. For instance, asbestos in casting ring liners and uranium salts in dental porcelain are no longer used. There is also concern[25] for the possible health hazards (see Chapter 19) associated with alloys containing nickel and beryllium. Although no definite conclusions can be drawn, appropriate safety precautions are advisable when grinding these alloys. Filtered suction units and appropriate barriers (masks) should be used. The ADA[26] requires nickel-containing alloys to carry a precautionary label stating that their use should be avoided in patients with a known nickel allergy (Fig. 22-15).

SELECTING AN INVESTMENT MATERIAL
After the choice of casting alloy has been made, the investment material can be selected.

Ideal Properties. An ideal investment should incorporate the following features:
- Controllable expansion to compensate precisely for shrinkage of the cast alloy during cooling
- The ability to produce smooth castings with accurate surface reproduction without nodules
- Chemical stability at high casting temperatures
- Adequate strength to resist casting forces
- Sufficient porosity to allow for gas escape
- Easy recovery of the casting

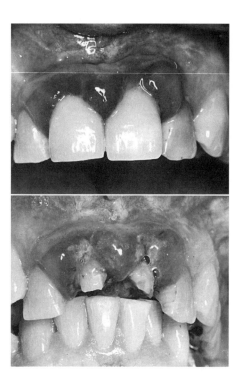

Fig. 22-15. Dramatic gingival reaction to nickel-containing metal-ceramic restorations. *(Courtesy Dr. W.V. Campagni.)*

Gypsum-bonded Investments. Gypsum-bonded investments satisfy most of the requirements for an ideal material, although they are not suitable for casting metal-ceramic alloys because the gypsum is unstable at the high temperatures required. Additionally, with some materials, obtaining adequate expansion may be difficult. This can be critical when casting complete crowns. A casting that is slightly oversized (in a controlled manner) is advantageous for accurate seating (see Chapter 7). Factors that increase expansion[27] of gypsum-bonded investments include the following:

1. Use of a full-width ring liner
2. Prolonged spatulation
3. Storage at 100% humidity
4. Lower water–powder ratio
5. Use of a dry liner
6. Use of two ring liners
7. Hygroscopic technique with the pattern in the upper part of the ring[28]

Phosphate-bonded Investments. Phosphate-bonded investment materials offer certain advantages over gypsum-bonded investments. They are more stable at high temperatures and thus are the material of choice for casting metal-ceramic alloys. They expand rapidly at the temperatures used for casting alloys, and their size can be conveniently controlled. The increased expansion that they exhibit results from a combination of the following factors:

1. Heat from the setting reaction softens the wax and allows freer setting expansion.
2. The increased strength of the material at high temperatures restricts shrinkage of the alloy as it cools.
3. The powder mixed with colloidal silica reduces the surface roughness of the castings and also increases expansion. Thus expansion can be conveniently controlled by slightly diluting the colloidal silica with distilled water.

However, castings made with phosphate-bonded investments are rougher than those made with gypsum-bonded investments[29] and are more difficult to remove from the investment.[30] Because phosphate-bonded investments have lower porosity,[31] complete mold filling becomes more difficult. Castings also are more likely to have surface nodules, which must be removed. (**Vacuum mixing** and a careful investing technique help reduce but do not eliminate the occurrence of nodules.)

■ INVESTING

Vacuum mixing of investment materials (Fig. 22-16) is highly recommended for consistent results in casting with minimal surface defects, especially when phosphate-bonded investments are used. Good results are possible with brush application of vacuum-mixed investment or when the investment is poured into the ring under vacuum. Vacuum mixing with brush application of the investment is the suggested mode. To expedite the procedure and minimize distortion, all necessary items and materials should be prepared before the wax pattern is reflowed and removed from the die.

Armamentarium (Fig. 22-17)
- Vacuum mixer and bowl
- Vibrator
- Investment powder (gypsum or phosphate bonded)
- Water or colloidal silica
- Spatula
- Brush

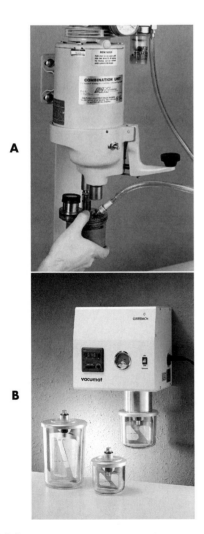

Fig. 22-16. Vacuum investing machines. **A,** The Whip Mix combination unit. **B,** Girrbach Vacumat. *(A courtesy Whip Mix Corporation; B courtesy Girrbach Dental GmbH.)*

- Surfactant
- Casting ring and liner

Step-by-Step Procedure

Brush Technique. In this technique, the pattern is first painted with surface tension reducer; the surface must be wet completely. The procedure is as follows:

1. Add investment powder to the liquid in the mixing bowl and quickly incorporate it by hand (Fig. 22-18, *A*). Residual material from the spatula is wiped onto the mechanical mixing blade. The powder–liquid ratio is critical for accurate control of expansion. The mixing bowl can either be wiped completely dry or shaken dry. If shaken dry, remember the residual water will add about 1 ml to the mix.

2. Attach the vacuum hose to the bowl, evacuate the bowl, and mechanically spatulate (Fig. 22-18, *B*). The mixing should be carefully timed in accordance with the manufacturer's instructions and the type of mixing bowl used (high speed versus low speed). If phosphate-bonded investments are used, additional vibration under vacuum helps minimize nodules.

3. Coat the entire pattern with investment, pushing the material ahead of the brush from a single point (Fig. 22-18, *C*). Gently vibrate throughout the application of investment, being especially careful to coat the internal surface and the margin of the pattern (Fig. 22-18, *D*).

NOTE: A finger positioned under the crucible former on the table of the vibrator minimizes the risk of excessive vibration and possible breaking of the pattern from the sprue. After the pattern has been completely coated, the ring is immediately filled by vibrating the remaining investment out of the bowl.

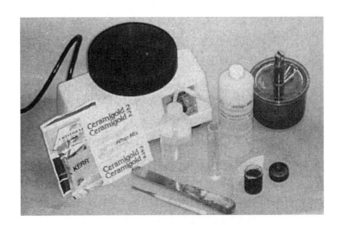

Fig. 22-17. Investing armamentarium.

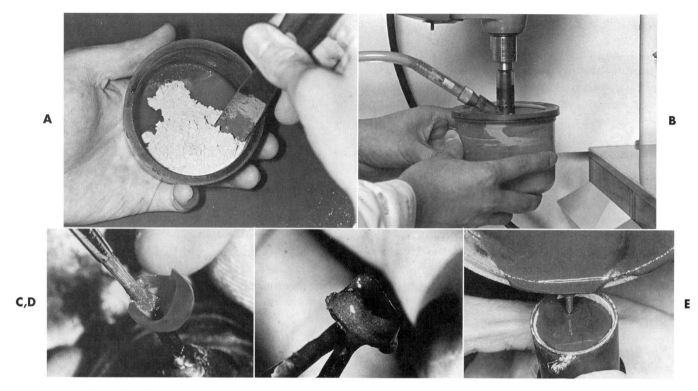

A

B

C,D

E

Fig. 22-18. Investing procedure: brush technique. **A,** Hand spatulate the mix to incorporate powder quickly. **B,** Vacuum mix the investment according to manufacturer's recommendations. **C,** Carefully coat the wax pattern, teasing the investment ahead of the brush. **D,** Be sure the margins are covered as well as the axial and occlusal surfaces. **E,** Slowly fill the ring, holding it on the vibrator. Tilt the ring from side to side to avoid trapping air under the pattern.

4. Place the lined casting ring over the pattern and with the aid of vibration, pour the investment down the side of the ring. Fill the ring slowly, starting from the bottom and moving up (Fig. 22-18, *E*).

5. When the investment reaches the level of the pattern, tilt the ring several times to cover and uncover the pattern, thereby minimizing the possible entrapment of air. Investing must be performed quickly within the working time of the investment. If the investment begins to set too soon, rinse it off quickly with cold water. The wax pattern can then be replaced on the die, and its margins can be reflowed again.

6. After the ring is filled to the rim, allow the investment to set.

7. If the hygroscopic technique is used, the ring is placed in a 37° C (100° F) water bath for 1 hour.

VACUUM TECHNIQUE
1. First, hand spatulate the mix (Fig. 22-19, *A*).
2. With the crucible former and pattern in place, attach the ring to the mixing bowl (Fig. 22-19, *B*).
3. Attach the vacuum hose and mix according to the manufacturer's recommendations (Fig. 22-19, *C* and *D*).

4. Invert the bowl and fill the ring under vibration (Fig. 22-19, *E*).
5. Remove the vacuum hose before shutting off the mixer (Fig. 22-19, *F*).
6. Remove the filled ring and crucible former from the bowl (Fig. 22-19, *G*).
7. Immediately clean the bowl and mixing blade under running water (Fig. 22-19, *H*).

WAX EXAMINATION
Wax elimination or burnout consists of heating the investment in a thermostatically controlled furnace (Fig. 22-20) until all traces of the wax are vaporized. The temperature reached by the investment determines the thermal expansion.

All water in the investment must be driven off during wax elimination. The temperature to which the ring is heated during wax elimination must be sufficiently high. It should be maintained long enough ("heat soak") to minimize a sudden drop in temperature upon removal from the oven. Such a drop could result in an incomplete casting because of excessively rapid solidification of the alloy as it enters the mold. Once the investment is heated during the wax-elimination procedure, heating must be continued, and casting must be completed. Cooling

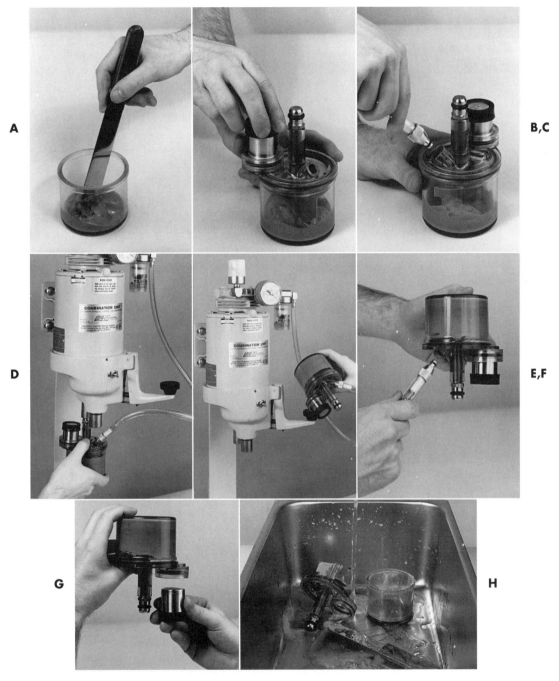

Fig. 22-19. Investing procedure: vacuum technique. **A,** Hand spatulate the mix. **B,** With the crucible former in place, attach the ring to the mixing bowl. **C,** Attach the vacuum hose. **D,** Mix according to manufacturer's recommendations. **E,** Invert the bowl and fill the ring under vibration. **F,** Remove the vacuum hose before shutting off the mixer. **G,** Remove the filled ring and crucible former from the bowl. **H,** Immediately clean the bowl and mixing blade under running water.
(Courtesy Whip Mix Corporation.)

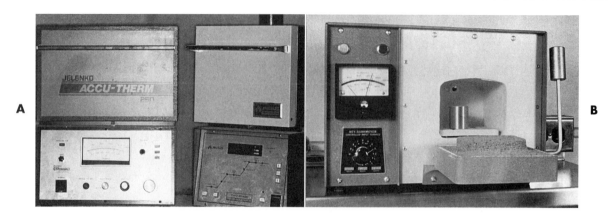

Fig. 22-20. **A,** Burnout ovens are available with manual, semiautomatic, or fully programmable controls. **B,** Ring positioned for burnout.

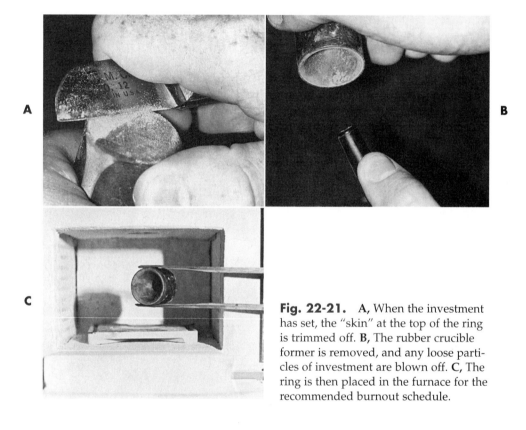

Fig. 22-21. **A,** When the investment has set, the "skin" at the top of the ring is trimmed off. **B,** The rubber crucible former is removed, and any loose particles of investment are blown off. **C,** The ring is then placed in the furnace for the recommended burnout schedule.

and reheating of the investment can cause casting inaccuracy because the refractory and binder will not revert to their original forms (hysteresis). Inadequate expansion and cracking of the investment are typical results.

STEP-BY-STEP PROCEDURE (FIG. 22-21)

1. Allow the investment to set for the recommended time (usually 1 hour) and then remove the rubber crucible former. If a metal sprue is used, remove it as well. The ring should be placed in a humidor if stored overnight. The smooth skin that forms on the ring with phosphate-bonded investments should be removed, and any loose particles of investment should be blown off with compressed air.

2. Reexamine the ring for any residual particles and then place it with the sprue facing down in the furnace on a ribbed tray. The tray allows the molten wax to flow out freely.

3. Bring the furnace to 200° C (400° F) and hold this temperature for 30 minutes. Most of the wax is eliminated by this time.

4. Increase the heat to the final burnout temperature (generally 650° C [1200° F] or 480° C [900° F] if a hygroscopic technique is used; follow the manufacturer's instructions) and hold for 45 minutes. Because the heating rate affects the

expansion,[32] it also should be standardized as part of the investing and casting protocol for accurately fitting castings. The mold is now ready for casting, although a large casting ring usually requires increased heating time. If preferred, two burnout furnaces can be set at 200° C and 650° C or 480° C, or a programmable two-stage furnace can serve equally well. However, the investment should not be overheated or kept at temperature too long. Gypsum-bonded investments are not stable above 650° C (1200° F). Also, some carbon in carbon-containing investments burns off, causing increased surface roughness of the casting[22] (see Table 22-1).

When transferring the casting ring to the casting machine, a quick visual check of the sprue in shaded light is helpful to see whether it is properly heated. It should be a cherry-red color.

ACCELERATED CASTING METHOD

Conventional casting techniques require considerable time, typically 1 hour bench set for the investment and 1 to 2 hours for the wax elimination. Accelerated casting procedures have been proposed that reduce this time to 30 to 40 minutes.[33-35] Initially suggested as a way to make cast post-and-core restorations in a one-visit procedure,* the procedure has been found to produce castings with accuracy and surface roughness similar to traditional methods.[36,37] The technique uses a phosphate-bonded investment that is given approximately 15 minutes bench set (generally judged as the time taken for the

---

*Also for castings made for dental licensure examinations.

investment to reach its maximum exothermic setting reaction temperature) and a 15-minute wax elimination by placing the ring in a furnace preheated to 815° C (1500° F).

CASTING

CASTING MACHINES (FIG. 22-22)
A casting machine requires a heat source to melt the alloy and a casting force. For a complete casting, the casting force must be high enough to overcome the high surface tension of the molten alloy[38] as well as the resistance of the gas within the mold.

The heat source can be either the reducing flame of a torch or electricity. Conventional alloys can be melted with a gas-air torch (Fig. 22-23, A and B), but the metal-ceramic alloys in a higher melting range need a gas-oxygen torch (Fig. 22-23, C). Base metal alloys need a multiorifice gas-oxygen (Fig. 22-23, D) or oxyacetylene torch. Electric heating can occur by convection from a heating muffle or by generation of an induction current in the alloy. Advocates of the latter[39] maintain that heating can be more evenly controlled, preventing undesirable changes in alloy composition caused by volatilization of the lower-melting point elements. In general, the electric machines are expensive and more appropriate for larger dental laboratories, whereas a torch may be the method of choice for smaller laboratories and dental offices.

Present-day casting machines still use either air pressure or centrifugal force to fill the mold, which were first proposed in the early days of lost-wax castings.[2,40] Some machines evacuate the mold before it is filled with metal, and vacuum has been shown to improve mold filling,[41] although it is not clear if the difference is clinically significant.[42]

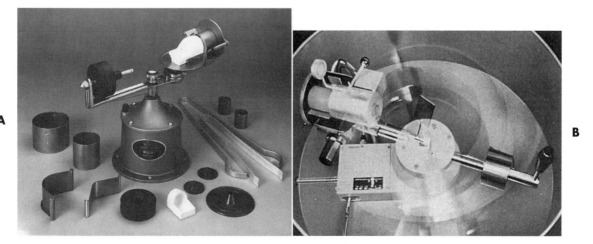

Fig. 22-22. Casting machines. A, Kerr Broken-Arm. B, Degussa Model TS-1.
(*A courtesy Kerr Manufacturing Co; B courtesy Degussa Corporation.*)

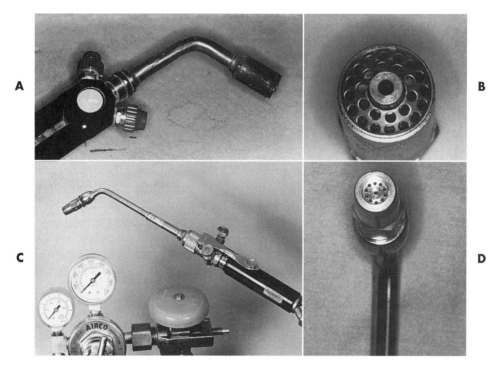

Fig. 22-23.   **A,** Gas-air π **B,** Gas-air tip. **C,** Gas-oxygen casting torch. **D,** Multiorifice tip.

CASTING TECHNIQUE

The mold is not removed from the burnout furnace until the alloy has been melted and is ready to cast.

Cleaning a previously cast alloy is necessary to remove investment debris and oxides before its reuse. Noble metal alloys can be melted on a charcoal block with a gas-air torch, which provides a reducing atmosphere, and remaining impurities are removed through pickling and ultrasonic or steam cleaning. Alloys from different manufacturers should not be mixed, even if they are similar. Overheated or otherwise abused alloys, as well as grindings and old restorations, should be returned to the manufacturer as scrap materials, rather than being reused.

Armamentarium (Fig. 22-24)
- Broken-arm (Kerr) centrifugal casting machine
- Crucible
- Blowtorch
- Protective colored goggles
- Tongs
- Casting alloy
- Flux

Procedure.   The casting machine is given three clockwise turns (four if using metal-ceramic alloys) and locked in position with the pin. The cradle and counterbalance weights are checked for the appro-

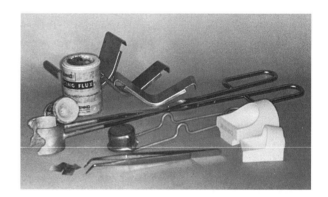

Fig. 22-24.   Casting armamentarium.

priate size of the casting ring. A crucible for the alloy being cast is placed in the machine. The torch is lit and adjusted (gas-air for regular alloys, gas-oxygen for metal-ceramic). For metal-ceramic alloys, a pair of colored goggles should be worn to protect the eyes and also to permit direct viewing of the melt.

The crucible is preheated (Fig. 22-25, *A*), particularly in the area that will be in contact with the alloy, and the alloy is added. Preheating avoids excessive slag formation during casting. Also, when metal-ceramic alloys are cast, a crucible that is too cool can "freeze" the alloy, resulting in an incomplete casting. Sufficient mass of alloy must be present to sustain adequate casting pressure. With a high-density

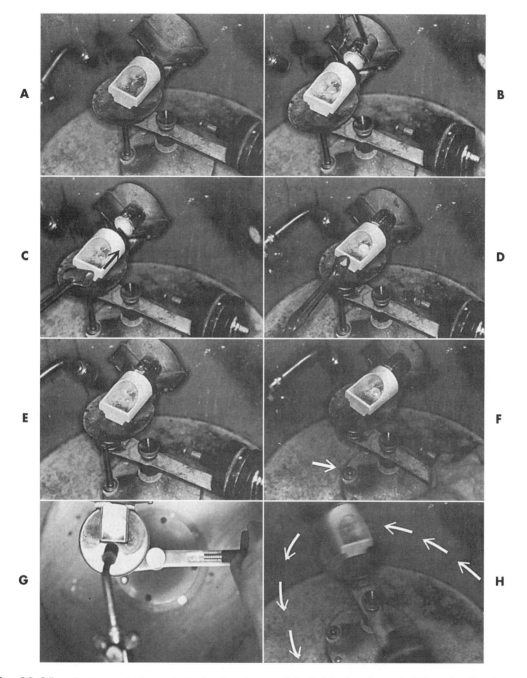

Fig. 22-25. Casting technique. **A,** Preheating the crucible. **B,** Making the melt. When the alloy is molten, the casting ring is removed from the furnace and placed in the cradle. **C,** Tongs are used to slide the crucible platform into contact with the casting ring *(arrow)*. **D,** The orifice of the crucible aligns with the sprue. **E,** Heating continues for a few seconds so the melting is complete and casting can proceed. **F,** The casting arm is pulled forward until the pin drops *(arrow)*. **G,** Casting machine immediately before release. **H,** Centrifugal force carries the melt into the mold cavity *(arrows show the direction of spin)*.

noble metal alloy, 6 g (4 dwt*) is typically adequate for premolar and anterior castings, 9 g (6 dwt) is adequate for molar castings, and 12 g (8 dwt) is adequate for pontics.

---

*Pennyweight (*d* is an abbreviation for *denarius*, a Roman copper coin).

The alloy is heated in the reducing part of the flame until it is ready to cast. A little **flux** can be added to conventional gold alloys (not metal-ceramic alloys). Gold alloys ball up and have a mirrorlike shiny surface that appears to be spinning. Nickel-chromium and cobalt alloys are ready to cast when the sharp edges of the ingot

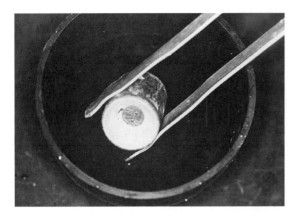

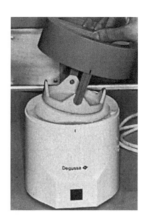

Fig. 22-26. The ring is quenched in cold water in a plaster bowl. Gypsum-bonded investments readily disintegrate; phosphate-bonded investments are much stronger and need careful devestment.

Fig. 22-27. Nonfuming pickling acid can be used in conjunction with this covered pickling unit.

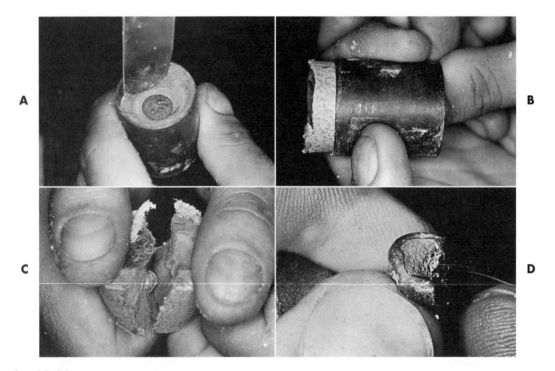

Fig. 22-28. Recovery of a casting from phosphate-bonded investment. **A,** Trimming is done from the button end of the ring. **B,** Investment is being pushed out of the casting ring. **C,** The mold is broken open. **D,** Investment is removed from the casting. Care must be taken to avoid damaging the margin.

round over. The mold is placed in the cradle of the casting machine (Fig. 22-25, *B*) and kept on the alloy with the reducing flame until the crucible is moved into position (Fig. 22-25, *C* to *G*). The casting machine arm is then released to make the casting (Fig. 22-25, *H*). The machine is allowed to spin until it has slowed enough that it can be stopped by hand, and the ring is removed with casting tongs.

Recovery of the Casting. After the red glow has disappeared from the button, the casting ring is plunged under running cold water into a large rubber mixing bowl (Fig. 22-26).

Gypsum-bonded investments quickly disintegrate, and elimination of residue is easily accomplished with a toothbrush. Final traces can be removed ultrasonically. Oxides are removed by pickling in 50% hydrochloric acid (or preferably a nonfuming substitute) (Fig. 22-27). Phosphate-bonded investments do not disintegrate and must be forcibly removed from the casting ring (Fig. 22-28). They can be handled as soon as they are sufficiently cooled under running water.

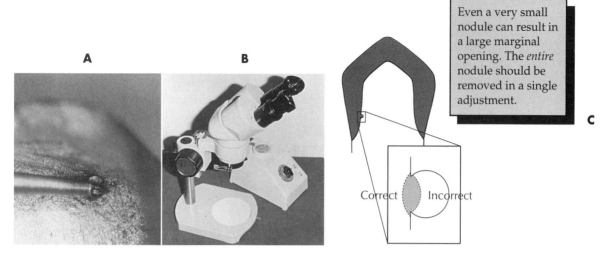

Fig. 22-29. Removing casting nodules. Small nodules are frequently present, particularly with phosphate-bonded investments. They interfere with seating and must be identified before the casting is placed on the die. **A,** Once they are identified, a small, round bur can be used to remove them. **B,** Magnification is helpful for this. **C,** Remove slightly more, rather than less, metal than the size of the nodule to ensure the casting does not bind during seating.

A knife is used to trim the investment at the button end of the ring (Fig. 22-28, *B*). The other end is not trimmed for fear of damaging the margin. When the ring liner is exposed, the investment can be pushed out of the ring (Fig. 22-28, *C*). It is then broken apart under running water (because it is still hot). The remaining investment is carefully removed with a small blunt instrument (Fig. 22-28, *D*), and any traces are dissolved in hydrofluoric acid or a less caustic substitute. Care must be taken to prevent scratching of the internal surface of the casting or damage to the margins.

Evaluation. The casting is never fitted on the die until the inner surface has been carefully evaluated under magnification; even tiny imperfections can cause damage to the stone die. *A die may be rendered useless in a matter of seconds if a casting is fitted prematurely.*

Defects in the Casting. Investing and casting requires meticulous attention to detail to obtain a successful, properly fitting casting. Table 22-1 summarizes and provides examples of the more common causes of various problems.

Roughness. The surface of a casting should be smooth, although finishing and **polishing** are still required (see Chapter 29). Lines or grooves in the casting were usually present but overlooked in the wax pattern. They may necessitate a remake, particularly if they were positioned near the margin or on

the fitting surface. Generalized casting roughness may indicate a breakdown of the investment from excessive burnout temperature.

Nodules. Bubbles of gas trapped between the wax pattern and the investment produce nodules on the casting surface. Even minute nodules can limit the seating of the casting to a considerable degree. When they are large or situated on a margin, they usually necessitate remaking of the restoration. When small, they can often be removed with a no. $\frac{1}{4}$ or $\frac{1}{2}$ round bur (Fig. 22-29). A binocular microscope is extremely helpful to detect and remove nodules. Remove a slight excess of metal to ensure the nodule does not interfere with complete seating.

The key to avoiding nodules is a careful investing technique, a surfactant, vacuum spatulation, and careful coating of the wax pattern with investment. Castings made with phosphate-bonded investment are especially prone to such imperfections, and experience and care are required to produce castings that are routinely free of nodules.

Fins. Fins are caused by cracks in the investment that have been filled with molten metal. These cracks can result from a weak mix of investment (high water-powder ratio), excessive casting force, steam generated from too-rapid heating, reheating an invested pattern, an improperly situated pattern (too close to the periphery of the casting ring), or even premature or rough handling of the ring after investing.

Incompleteness.   If an area of wax is too thin (less than 0.3 mm), which occurs occasionally on the veneering surface of a metal-ceramic restoration, an incomplete casting may result. Thickening of the wax in these areas is recommended. Incomplete casting of normal-thickness wax patterns may result from inadequate heating of the metal, incomplete wax elimination, excessive cooling ("freezing") of the mold, insufficient casting force, not enough metal, or metal spillage.

Voids or Porosity.   Voids in the casting (in particular in the margin area) may be caused by debris trapped in the mold (usually a particle of the invest-

Common Causes of Casting Failure		TABLE 22-1
Problem	Possible Causes	Appearance
Rough casting	Improper finishing of wax pattern Excess surfactant Improper W/P ratio Excessive burnout temperature	
Large nodule	Air trapped during investing procedure	
Multiple nodules	Inadequate vacuum during investing Improper brush technique Lack of surfactant	
Nodules on occlusal surface	Excessive vibration	
Fins	Increased W/P ratio Pattern too near edge of investment Premature heating (mold still wet) Too-rapid heating Dropped mold	

ment undetected before wax elimination). A well-waxed smooth sprue helps prevent this. Porosity resulting from solidification shrinkage ("suck back") occurs if the metal in the sprue solidifies before the metal in the mold, as may happen when a sprue is too narrow, too long, or incorrectly located or when a large casting is made in the absence of a chill vent.

Gases may dissolve in the molten alloy during melting and leave porosity defects. **Back pressure porosity**[43] may be caused by air pressure in the mold as the molten metal enters. Its occurrence is reduced by using a more porous investment, locating the pattern near the end of the ring (6 to 8 mm), and casting with a vacuum technique.

Common Causes of Casting Failure, cont'd

TABLE 22-1

Problem	Possible Causes	Appearance
Incomplete casting	Wax pattern too thin Cool mold or melt Inadequate metal	
Incomplete casting with shiny, rounded defect	Incomplete wax elimination	
"Suck-back" porosity	Improper pattern position Narrow, long sprue	
Inclusion porosity	Particle of investment dislodged during casting	
Marginal discrepancy	Wax pattern distortion Uneven expansion	
Inadequate or excessive expansion	Improper W/P ratio Improper mixing time Improper burnout temperature	

Marginal Discrepancies. Inaccuracies of fit at the margin can be caused by distortion during removal of the wax pattern from the die. They may also result from increased setting expansion (hygroscopic technique) following uneven expansion of the mold.

Dimensional Inaccuracies. The casting can be either too small or too large. Attention to detail is essential for an accurately expanded mold. A standardized procedure is needed in regards to liquid–powder ratio, spatulation, the ring liner, the amount of liquid added, and mold heating.

REVIEW OF TECHNIQUE

The following list summarizes the steps involved in investing and casting (Fig. 22-30) and should prove helpful in reviewing the material covered in this chapter:

1. A sprue 2 or 2.5 mm in diameter (10- or 12-gauge) is attached to the bulkiest noncentric cusp (the larger size for molar and metal-ceramic patterns, the smaller size for premolar and partial coverage). Multiple units can be sprued with a runner bar (Fig. 22-30, *A*).

2. The pattern is carefully removed from the die and attached to a crucible former (sprue length should be 6 mm or less) (Fig. 22-30, *B*).
3. The pattern is painted with surface tension reducer (Fig. 22-30, *C*) and then carefully coated with vacuum mixed investment (Fig. 22-30, *D*).
4. The ring is filled, and the investment is allowed to bench set for a minimum of 1 hour.
5. After wax elimination, the casting machine is prepared, and the crucible is preheated. The alloy is melted, the ring is transferred, and the casting is made promptly (Fig. 22-30, *E*).
6. The casting is recovered from the investment (Fig. 22-30, *F*).
7. Defects are identified and corrected if possible (Fig. 22-30, *G*).

SUMMARY

Investing and casting, a series of highly technique-sensitive steps, converts the wax pattern into a metal casting. Accurate and smooth restorations can be obtained if the operator pays special attention to each step in the technique. When initial attempts at casting produce errors or defects, appropriate corrective measures must be taken so they do not recur.

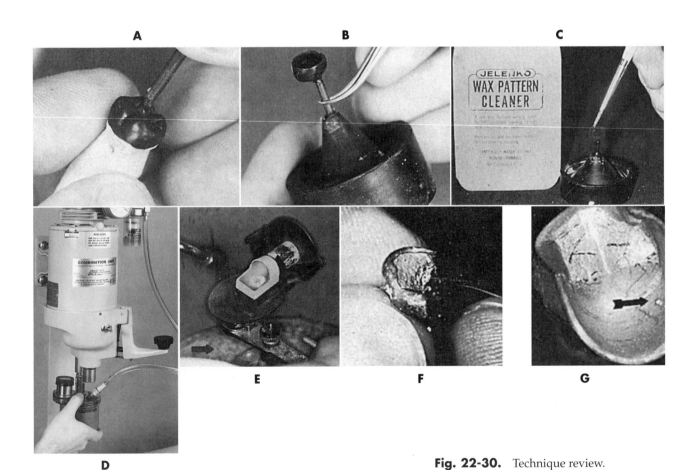

Fig. 22-30. Technique review.

Study Questions

1. Discuss in detail the requirements of a sprue and the factors and special considerations involved in selecting the sprue position.
2. Discuss gypsum-bonded and phosphate-bonded investments and explain the various ways that investment expansion can be influenced, including pertinent materials science considerations.
3. What is the difference between gypsum- and phosphate-bonded investments?
4. What determines investment selection? What are the ideal properties of an investment material?
5. What factors can result in rough castings, nodules on castings, finning of a casting, or incomplete castings?
6. Identify the various types of casting porosity. What are the causes for each?

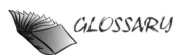

GLOSSARY

alloy: *n* (14c): a mixture of two or more metals or metalloids that are mutually soluble in the molten state; distinguished as binary, ternary, quaternary, etc., depending on the number of metals within the mixture. Alloying elements are added to alter the hardness, strength, and toughness of a metallic element, thus obtaining properties not found in the pure metal. Alloys may also be classified on the basis of their behavior when solidified.

back pressure porosity: porosity produced in dental castings thought to be due to the inability of gases in the mold to escape during the casting procedure.

base metal: any metallic element that does not resist tarnish and corrosion.

casting: *n* (14c): something that has been cast in a mold; an object formed by the solidification of a fluid which has been poured or injected into a mold.

casting ring: the inferior portion of a refractory flask that provides a negative likeness or dimple into which a metal is cast in the refractory investment.

compressive stress: the internal induced force that opposes the shortening of a material in a direction parallel to the direction of the stresses; any induced force per unit area that resists deformation caused by a load that tends to compress or shorten a body.

cristobalite: *n:* a allotropic form of crystalline silica used in dental casting investments.

crucible: *n* (15c): a vessel or container made of any refractory material (as porcelain) used for melting or calcining any substance that requires a high degree of heat.

crucible former: the base to which a sprue former is attached while the wax pattern is being invested in refractory investment; a convex rubber, plastic, or metal base that forms a concave depression or crucible in the refractory investment.

dental casting investment: a material consisting principally of an allotrope of silica and a bonding agent. The bonding substance may be gypsum (for use in lower casting temperatures) or phosphate and silicas (for use in higher casting temperatures).

devest: *vb:* the retrieval of a casting or prosthesis from an investing medium.

flux: *n* (14c) *1:* in physics, the rate of flow of a liquid, particles or energy *2:* in ceramics, an agent that lowers the fusion temperature of porcelain *3:* in metallurgy, a substance used to increase fluidity and to prevent or reduce oxidation of a molten metal *4:* any substance applied to surfaces to be joined by brazing, soldering or welding to clean and free them from oxides and promote union.

hygroscopic expansion: expansion due to the absorption of moisture

investing: *v* the process of covering or enveloping, wholly or in part, an object such as a denture, tooth, wax form, crown, etc., with a suitable investment material before processing, soldering, or casting.

investment: *n:* see Dental Casting I., Refractory I.

occluded gas porosity: a porosity produced in castings due to the inability of gasses in the mold to escape.

¹pickle: *n* (15c): a solution or bath for preserving or cleaning; any of various baths used in cleaning or processing.

²pickle: *vt* **pickled; pickling:** (1552): to treat, preserve, or clean in or with an agent.

¹polish: *vb* (14c): to make smooth and glossy, usually by friction; giving luster; the act or process of making a denture or casting smooth and glossy.

²polish: *n* (1704): a smooth, glossy surface; having luster.

polishing: *v, obs 1:* to make smooth and glossy, usually by friction; to give luster to (GPT-1) *2: obs:* the act or process of making a denture or casting smooth and glossy (GPT-1).

porosity: *n, pl* **ties:** (14c) *1:* the presence of voids or pores within a structure *2:* the state or quality of having minute pores, openings or interstices.

proportional limit: that unit of stress beyond which deformation is no longer proportional to the applied load.

quartz: *n* (ca. 1631): an allotropic form of silica; the mineral SiO_2 consisting of hexagonal crystals of colorless, transparent silicon dioxide.

refractory: *adj* (1606): difficult to fuse or corrode; capable of enduring high temperatures

refractory investment: an investment material that can withstand the high temperatures used in soldering or casting.

refractory mold: a refractory cavity into which a substance is shaped or cast.

setting expansion: the dimensional increase that occurs concurrent with the hardening of various materials, such as plaster of paris, dental stone, die stone, and dental casting investment.

shrink-spot porosity: an area of porosity in cast metal that is caused by shrinkage of a portion of the metal as it solidifies from the molten state without flow of additional molten metal from surrounding areas.

silica: *n* (ca 1301): silicon dioxide occurring in crystalline, amorphous, and usually impure forms (as quartz, opal, and sand, respectively).

solidification porosity: a porosity that may be produced by improper spruing or improper heating of either the metal or the investment.

sprue: *n* (1880) *1:* the channel or hole through which plastic or metal is poured or cast into a gate or reservoir and then into a mold *2:* the cast metal or plastic that connects a casting to the residual sprue button.

sprue button: the material remaining in the reservoir of the mold after a dental casting.

thermal expansion: expansion of a material caused by heat.

vacuum casting: the casting of a metal or plastic in the presence of a partial vacuum.

vacuum investing: the process of investing a pattern within a partial vacuum.

vacuum mixing: a method of mixing a material such as plaster of paris or casting investment under subatmospheric pressure.

wax elimination: the removal of wax from a mold, usually by heat.

wax expansion: a method of expanding a wax pattern to compensate for the shrinkage of gold during the casting process.

References

1. Philbrook D: Cast fillings, *Iowa State Dent Soc Trans* 277, 1897.
2. Taggart WH: A new and accurate method of making gold inlays, *Dent Cosmos* 49:1117, 1907.
3. Anusavice KJ: *Phillips' science of dental materials,* ed 10, Philadelphia, 1996, WB Saunders.
4. Ryge G et al: Porosities in dental gold castings, *J Am Dent Assoc* 54:746, 1957.
5. Johnson A, Winstanley RB: The evaluation of factors affecting the castability of metal ceramic alloy–investment combinations, *Int J Prosthodont* 9:74, 1996.
6. Mahler DB, Ady AB: The influence of various factors on the effective setting expansion of casting investments, *J Prosthet Dent* 13:365, 1963.
7. Takahashi J et al: Nonuniform vertical and horizontal setting expansion of a phosphate-bonded investment, *J Prosthet Dent* 81:386, 1999.
8. Verrett RG, Duke ES: The effect of sprue attachment design on castability and porosity, *J Prosthet Dent* 61:418, 1989.
9. Strickland WD, Sturdevant CM: Porosity in the full cast crown, *J Am Dent Assoc* 58:69, 1959.
10. Rawson RD et al: Photographic study of gold flow, *J Dent Res* 51:1331, 1972.
11. Earnshaw R: The effect of casting ring liners on the potential expansion of a gypsum-bonded investment, *J Dent Res* 67:1366, 1988.
12. Davis DR: Effect of wet and dry cellulose ring liners on setting expansion and compressive strength of a gypsum-bonded investment, *J Prosthet Dent* 76:519, 1996.
13. Engelman MA et al: Oval ringless casting: simplicity, productivity, and accuracy without the health hazards of ring liners, *Trends Tech Contemp Dent* 6:38, 1989.
14. Shell JS: Setting and thermal expansion of investments. III. Effects of no asbestos liner, coating asbestos with petroleum jelly, and double asbestos liner, *J Alabama Dent Assoc* 53:31, 1969.
15. Ho EK, Darvell BW: A new method for casting discrepancy: some results for a phosphate-bonded investment, *J Dent* 26:59, 1998.
16. Lacy AM et al: Incidence of bubbles on samples cast in a phosphate-bonded investment, *J Prosthet Dent* 54:367, 1985.
17. American Dental Association: *Dentist's desk reference: materials, instruments and equipment,* ed 1, Chicago, 1981, The Association.
18. Sturdevant JR et al: The 8-year clinical performance of 15 low-gold casting alloys, *Dent Mater* 3:347, 1987.
19. Goldfogel MH, Nielsen JP: Dental casting alloys: an update on terminology, *J Prosthet Dent* 48:340, 1982.
20. Johansson BI et al: Corrosion of copper, nickel, and gold dental casting alloys: an in vitro and in vivo study, *J Biomed Mater Res* 23:349, 1989.
21. Duncan JD: The casting accuracy of nickel-chromium alloys for fixed prostheses, *J Prosthet Dent* 47:63, 1982.
22. Ogura H et al: Inner surface roughness of complete cast crowns made by centrifugal casting machines, *J Prosthet Dent* 45:529, 1981.
23. Moffa JP et al: An evaluation of nonprecious alloys for use with porcelain veneers. I. Physical properties, *J Prosthet Dent* 30:424, 1973.
24. Moon PC, Modjeski PJ: The burnishability of dental casting alloys, *J Prosthet Dent* 36:404, 1976.

25. Moffa JP et al: An evaluation of nonprecious alloys for use with porcelain veneers. II. Industrial safety and biocompatibility, *J Prosthet Dent* 30:432, 1973.

26. American Dental Association Council on Dental Materials, Instruments, and Equipment: biological effects of nickel-containing dental alloys, *J Am Dent Assoc* 104:501, 1982.

27. Lacy AM et al: Three factors affecting investment setting expansion and casting size, *J Prosthet Dent* 49:52, 1983.

28. Vieira DF, Carvalho JA: Hygroscopic expansion in the upper and lower parts of the casting ring, *J Prosthet Dent* 36:181, 1976.

29. Cooney JP, Caputo AA: Type III gold alloy complete crowns cast in a phosphate-bonded investment, *J Prosthet Dent* 46:414, 1981.

30. Chew CL et al: Investment strength as a function of time and temperature, *J Dent* 27:297, 1999.

31. Abu Hassan MI et al: Porosity determination of cast investment by a wax-infiltration technique, *J Dent* 17:195, 1989.

32. Papadopoulos T, Axelsson M: Influence of heating rate in thermal expansion of dental phosphate-bonded investment material, *Scand J Dent Res* 98:60, 1990.

33. Campagni WV, Majchrowicz M: An accelerated technique for casting post-and-core restorations, *J Prosthet Dent* 66:155, 1991.

34. Campagni WV et al: A comparison of an accelerated technique for casting post-and-core restorations with conventional techniques, *J Prosthodont* 2:159, 1993.

35. Bailey JH, Sherrard DJ: Post-and-core assemblies made with an accelerated pattern elimination technique, *J Prosthodont* 3:47, 1994.

36. Konstantoulakis E et al: Marginal fit and surface roughness of crowns made with an accelerated casting technique, *J Prosthet Dent* 80:337, 1998.

37. Schilling ER et al: Marginal gap of crowns made with a phosphate-bonded investment and accelerated casting method, *J Prosthet Dent* 81:129, 1999.

38. Henning G: The casting of precious metal alloys in dentistry: a rational approach, *Br Dent J* 133:428, 1972.

39. Preston JD, Berger R: Some laboratory variables affecting ceramo-metal alloys, *Dent Clin North Am* 21:717, 1977.

40. Jameson A: British patent no. 19801, 1907.

41. Hero H, Waarli M: Effect of vacuum and supertemperature on mold filling during casting, *Scand J Dent Res* 99:55, 1991.

42. Eames WB, MacNamara JF: Evaluation of casting machines for ability to cast sharp margins, *Operative Dent* 3:137, 1978.

43. Anusavice KJ: op.cit., p 521.

CHAPTER TWENTY-THREE

COLOR SCIENCE, ESTHETICS, AND SHADE SELECTION

KEY TERMS

achromatic	metamerism
chroma	Munsell color order system
CIELAB color system	opalescence
color blindness	photopic vision
color rendering index	reflectance
color temperature	rod
complementary colors	saturation
cones	scotopic vision
electromagnetic spectrum	shade
esthetics	value
fluorescence	visible spectrum
hue	wavelength

An understanding of the nature of light and how the eye perceives and the brain interprets light as color is important for successful esthetic restorations, particularly when metal-ceramic or all-ceramic restorations are being made. Errors in **shade** matching can be a problem in these procedures and are a source of frustration for the dentist and technician and a source of dissatisfaction for the patient. This chapter outlines some of the principles of light and color and how they relate to shade selection and esthetics.

◼ LIGHT AND COLOR

Without light, color does not exist. An object that we perceive as a certain color absorbs all light waves corresponding with other colors and reflects only those waves that we interpret as that object's color. For example, an object that absorbs blue and green light and reflects red appears red. The apparent color of an object is influenced by its physical properties, the nature of the incident light to which the object is exposed, the relationship to other colored objects, and the subjective assessment of the observer. These factors can cause a single tooth to look very different among different observers. Saleski[1] has pointed out that although lighting standards are available in industries as diverse as automobile and

textile manufacturing, there is no standard for lighting in dentistry.

DESCRIPTION OF LIGHT

Scientifically, light is described as visible electromagnetic energy whose **wavelength** is measured in nanometers (nm) or billionths of a meter. The eye is sensitive only to the visible part of the **electromagnetic spectrum**, a narrow band with wavelengths of 380 to 750 nm. At the shorter wavelengths lie ultraviolet, x, and gamma rays; at the longer wavelengths are infrared radiation, microwaves, and television and radio transmissions (Fig. 23-1).

Pure white light consists of relatively equal quantities of electromagnetic energy over the visible range. When it is passed through a prism (Fig. 23-2), it is split into its component colors because the longer wavelengths are bent (refracted) less than the shorter ones.

Quality of Light. The most common light sources in dental offices are incandescent and fluorescent, neither of which are pure white light. An ordinary incandescent light bulb emits relatively higher concentrations of yellow light waves than of blue and blue-green, whereas fluorescent ceiling fix-

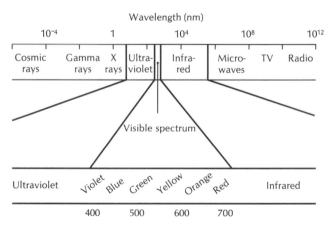

Fig. 23-1. Electromagnetic energy spectrum. A nanometer (nm) is 10^{-9} meter.

tures give off relatively high concentrations of blue waves.

Artists have traditionally chosen studios illuminated by northern daylight, which can be close to full-spectrum white light and often is used as the "normal" standard for judging light from other sources (Fig. 23-3). It has a **color rendering index** (CRI) close to 100. The color rendering index, on a scale of 1 to 100, indicates how well a particular light source renders color as compared to a specific standard source.

Although daylight is often used as the standard against which other light sources are compared, tooth shades should never be selected in direct sunlight. The distribution of light waves from the sun depends on the time of day and on humidity and pollution. During morning and evening hours, the shorter light waves (blues and greens) are scattered, and only the longer ones (at the red end of the spectrum) penetrate the atmosphere. Consequently, incident daylight at dawn and dusk is rich in yellow and orange but lacking in blue and green. Northern daylight around the noon hour on a bright day is considered ideal because there is a harmonious balance of the full **visible spectrum**. Nevertheless, circumstances may dictate the use of artificial light for shade selection. In these cases, color-corrected fluorescent lighting is recommended because it approaches the necessary type of balance. Bergen and McCasland[2] have reported that two commercially available, color-corrected fluorescent tubes are acceptable full-spectrum sources with a CRI of greater than 90.* Another light source reference standard is **color temperature**, which is related to the color of a standard black body when heated. Color tempera-

ture is reported in degrees Kelvin (K), or absolute (0° K = −273° C). Accordingly, 1000° K is red; 2000° K is yellow; 5555° K is white; 8000° K is pale blue. Northern daylight has an average color temperature of around 6500° K, but this varies with the time of day, cloud cover, humidity, and pollution.

DESCRIPTION OF COLOR

Just as a solid body can be described by three dimensions of physical form (length, width, and depth), color has three primary attributes that allow it to be described with the same precision. Describing these attributes, however, depends on the color system used.

Munsell Color Order System.[3]   The most popular method for describing color is the Munsell system. Despite certain disadvantages, the Munsell system has been widely used in the dental literature.[4,5] The three attributes of color in this system are called *Hue*, *Value*, and *Chroma*.*

Hue.   *Hue* is defined as the particular variety of a color, shade, or tint. The Hue of an object can be red, green, yellow, and so on, and is determined by the wavelength of the reflected and/or transmitted light observed. The place of that wavelength (or wavelengths) in the visible range of the spectrum determines the Hue of the color. The shorter the wavelength, the closer the Hue will be to the violet portion of the spectrum; the longer the wavelength, the closer it will be to the red portion.

In the Munsell color system, Hues are divided into 10 gradations: yellow, yellow-red, red, red-purple, purple, purple-blue, blue, blue-green, green,

---

*The common cool white fluorescent tubes have a CRI of between 50 and 80 and are therefore not suitable for shade selection.

*When used in reference to the Munsell coordinates, these terms are capitalized.

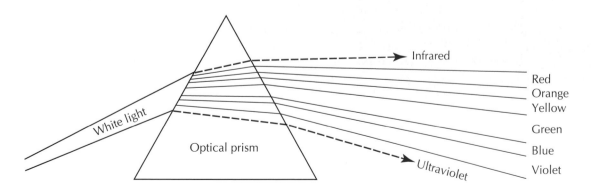

Fig. 23-2.   A prism bends or refracts short wavelengths of light more than longer wavelengths, thereby separating the colors.

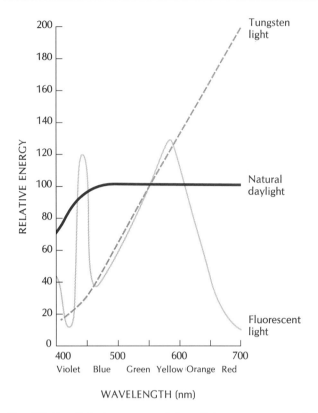

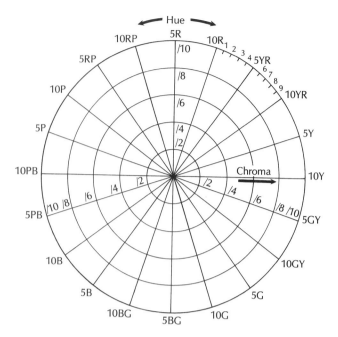

Fig. 23-4. Arrangement of Hue and Chroma in the Munsell system: *R*, Red; *YR*, yellow-red; *Y*, yellow; *GY*, green-yellow; *G*, green; *BG*, blue-green; *B*, blue; *PB*, purple-blue; *P*, purple; *RP*, red-purple.

Fig. 23-3. Relative energy of three light sources: natural daylight has an even spectral distribution; tungsten filament light is high in orange and red wavelengths; fluorescent tube light has peaks of blue and yellow.

and green-yellow. These are arranged in a wheel (Fig. 23-4). Each gradation is subdivided; for example, red can be written *1R, 2R, 3R . . . 9R, 10R*, followed by *1YR, 2YR, 3YR . . . 9YR, 10YR*, followed by *1Y, 2Y, 3Y*, and so on. These can be further subdivided (e.g., a particular Hue might be *4.3Y* or *8.1YR*). Most natural teeth fall into a range between yellow and yellow-red. In a study of 95 extracted anterior teeth, O'Brien et al[6] found that the average Hue was 1.2 Y for the gingival third, 1.3 Y for the middle third, and 1.4 Y for the incisal third (Fig 23-5).

Chroma. Chroma is defined as the intensity of a Hue. The terms ***saturation*** and *Chroma* are used interchangeably in the dental literature; both mean the strength of a given Hue or the concentration of pigment.

A simple way to visualize differences in Chroma is to imagine a bucket of water. When one drop of ink is added, a solution of low Chroma results. Adding a second drop of ink increases the Chroma, and so on, until a solution is obtained that is almost all ink and consequently of high Chroma. In the Munsell color system, maximum Chroma depends on the particular Hue but can range from 10 to 14. **Achromatic** shades have a Chroma near 0 (Fig.

23-6). Natural teeth are found with Chroma ranges from 0.5 to 4 (see Fig 23-5).

Value. Value is defined as the relative lightness or darkness of a color or the brightness of an object. The brightness of any object is a direct consequence of the amount of light energy the object reflects or transmits.

Light energy is measured in photons, and it is possible for objects of different Hues to reflect the same number of photons and thus have the same brightness or Value. A common example is the difficulty experienced in trying to tell a green from a blue object in a black and white photograph. The two objects will reflect the same amount of light energy and therefore will appear identical in the picture. This fact created a popular misconception that the Value of a color quantified the amount of grayness.

In the Munsell method of describing color, Value is divided into 10 gradations, with 0 being black and 10 being white. Natural teeth range in Value from 5.5 to 8.5 (see Fig 23-5). A restoration that has too high a Value (is too bright) may be easily detected by an observer and is a common esthetic fault in metal-ceramic prosthodontics.

CIELAB Color System. Determined by the Commission Intérnationale de l'Éclairage in 1978, this method of evaluating color continues to gain

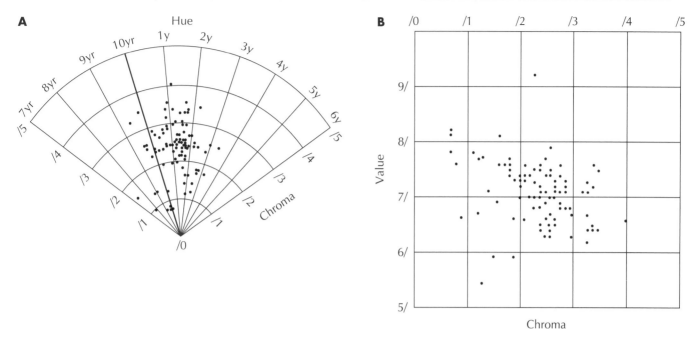

Fig. 23-5. The Munsell plots of the middle third of 95 incisor teeth. **A,** Munsell Hue and Chroma.
B, Munsell Value and Chroma.
(From O'Brien WJ et al: Dent Mater 13:179, 1997.)

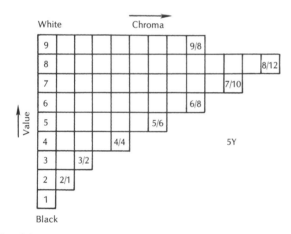

Fig. 23-6. Arrangement of Value and Chroma in the
Munsell system.

acceptance in dental research.[7-10] In both the Munsell and the CIELAB color order systems, the location in the color space of a particular shade is defined by three coordinates: Value, Hue, and Chroma
for Munsell; L*, a*, and b* for CIELAB. Value and L*
are proportional to each other and represent the
lightness, brightness, or black/white character of
the color. Colors with high Value or L* (such as
tooth colors) are located near the top of the color
space as depicted in Figure 23-7. The chromatic, or
non–black/white characteristics of a color are represented in the Munsell system by Hue and Chroma
and in CIELAB by a* and b.* In each system, these
two coordinates define the location of color on a

plane of given lightness, such as the one depicting
color B in Fig. 23-7. In Munsell, the color is identified by one polar coordinate (Hue) and one linear,
or Cartesian, coordinate (Chroma); in CIELAB, both
coordinates (a* and b*) are Cartesian. For an anal-
ogy, consider how the location of a house in a city
might be described. One could say that one lived
a distance of 11.85 miles (linear coordinate) in the
north-northwest direction (polar coordinate) from
downtown. This is analogous to describing a color
in the Munsell system. The identical location could
also be defined as being 10.6 miles north and 5.3
miles west of downtown (two Cartesian coordinates) (Fig. 23-8). This is analogous to describing a
color in CIELAB. They represent the same location
in space. However, unlike Munsell, the CIELAB coordinates define the color space in approximately
uniform steps of human color perception. This means
that equal distances across the CIELAB color space
(color differences or ΔE) represent approximately
equally perceived shade gradations, an arrangement that makes interpretation of color measurements more meaningful.

L.* L* is a lightness variable proportional to Value
in the Munsell system. It describes the achromatic
character of the color.

a and b*.* The a* and b* coordinates describe the
chromatic characteristics of the color. Although they
do not correlate directly with Munsell's Hue and
Chroma, they can be converted by numerical parameters[11] (see Fig. 23-7). The a* coordinate corresponds

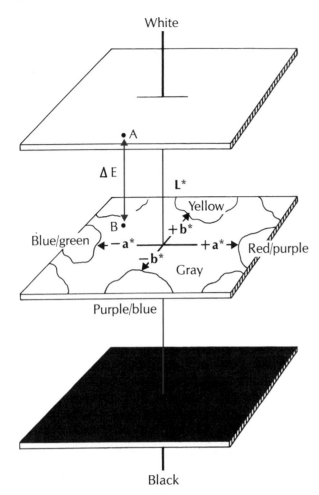

Fig. 23-7. *L*a*b** color space. Any color can be defined in terms of these coordinates. L* (the vertical axis) defines the lightness or darkness of the color and corresponds to Value in the Munsell system; a* and b* define the chromatic characteristic. The color difference (ΔE) between two colors (*A* and *B*) can be calculated from the sum of the squares of the differences among the three coordinates. The system is arranged so that a color difference of 1 is perceivable by 50% of observers with normal color vision.[42]
(From Rosenstiel SF, Johnston WM: J Prosthet Dent 60:297, 1988.)

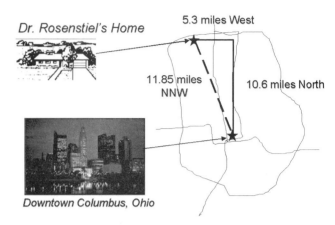

Fig. 23-8. Locations in space can be defined in polar or Cartesian coordinates.

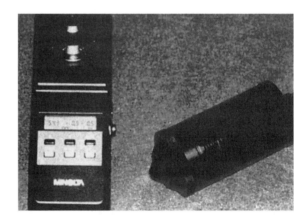

Fig. 23-9. Colorimeters are used for color matching in industry and are useful in dental research.

to the red-purple/blue-green axis in the Munsell color space. A positive a* relates to a predominantly red-purple color, whereas a negative a* denotes a color that is more blue-green. Similarly, the b* coordinate corresponds to the yellow-purple/blue axis.

COLOR-MEASURING INSTRUMENTS (FIG. 23-9)
Color selection for dental restorative materials is generally done visually by matching a shade sample. In industry, electronic color measuring equipment is used. This equipment consists of spectrophotometers that measure light reflectance at wavelength intervals over the visible spectrum and colorimeters that provide direct color coordinate

specifications without mathematical manipulation. This is accomplished by sampling light reflected from an object through three color filters that simulate the response of the color receptors in the eye. These instruments have been used extensively in dental research.[12-15] Recently, a color measuring system* has been introduced to guide the practicing dentist (Fig. 23-10). This instrument appears to have comparable accuracy to subjective assessment.[16]

PERCEPTION OF COLOR
Light from an object enters the eye and acts on receptors in the retina (**rods** and **cones**). Impulses from these are passed to the optical center of the brain, where an interpretation is made. Shade selection is very subjective—different individuals will have different interpretations of the same stimulus.

The Eye. Under low lighting conditions, only the rods are used (**scotopic vision**). These receptors

---

*ShadeEye-EX, Shofu, Inc.: Menlo Park, Calif.

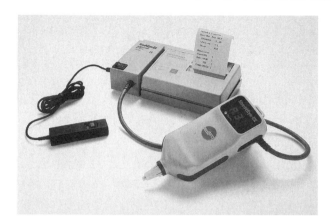

Fig. 23-10. ShadeEye-EX Chroma Meter. This device uses a colorimeter to measure tooth color and processes the information into formulae for fabricating a metal-ceramic restoration.
(Courtesy Shofu, Inc.)

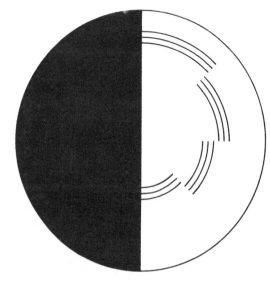

Fig. 23-11. The Benham disk. When it rotates, red, green, and blue rings are seen. The order of the colors is reversed if the disk rotates in the opposite direction. This is a purely sensory phenomenon caused by afterimages.

allow an interpretation of the brightness (but not the color) of objects to be made. They are most sensitive to blue-green objects. Color vision is dependent on the cones, which are active under higher lighting conditions (**photopic vision**). The change from photopic to scotopic vision is called *dark adaptation* and takes about 40 minutes.[17]

The area with the most cones is in the center of the retina, which is free of rods. The rods begin to predominate toward the periphery. This means that the central field of vision is more color perceptive. Although the exact mechanism of color vision is not known, there are three types of cones—sensitive to red, green, and blue light[18]—which form an image in much the same way as the additive effect of the pixels in a television picture.

Color Adaptation. Color vision decreases rapidly as an object is observed. The original color appears to become less and less saturated until it appears almost gray. Simultaneously, the chroma (intensity) of **complementary colors** appears greater. This phenomenon explains the suggestion that shade selection can be enhanced if operatory walls are painted pale blue (complementary to yellow) or that a pale gray-blue surface should be glanced at periodically while viewing color choices.

Deceptive Color Perception. The brain can be tricked in how it perceives color. The classic example is the Benham disk (Fig. 23-11). When this black and white disk is illuminated and rotated at an appropriate speed, it appears to be highly colored.

Color is also influenced by surrounding colors, particularly complementary ones (those diametrically opposed in Fig. 23-4). For example, when blue and yellow are placed side by side, their chroma may appear to be increased. The color of teeth can also look different if the patient is wearing brightly colored clothing or lipstick.

Metamerism. Two colors that appear to be a match under a given lighting condition but have different spectral reflectance (Fig. 23-12) are called *metamers,* and the phenomenon is known as **metamerism.** For example, two objects that appear to be an identical shade of yellow may absorb and reflect light differently. Normally a yellow object reflects yellow light, but some may actually absorb yellow light and reflect orange and green. To an observer, the orange and green combination looks yellow, although when the lighting is changed, the metamers no longer match. This means that a sample that appears to match under the operatory light, for example, may no longer be satisfactory in daylight. The problem of metamerism can be avoided by selecting a shade and confirming it under different lighting conditions (e.g., natural daylight and fluorescent light).

Fluorescence. Fluorescent materials, such as tooth enamel, re-emit radiant energy at a lower frequency than it is absorbed.[19] For example, ultraviolet radiation is re-emitted as visible light. In theory, a mismatch can occur if the dental restoration has different **fluorescence** than the natural tooth. In practice, fluorescence does not play a significant role in color matching dental restorations.[20]

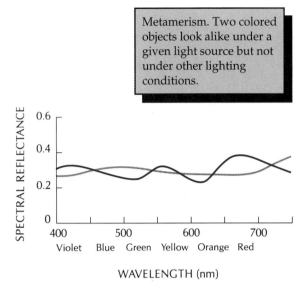

Metamerism. Two colored objects look alike under a given light source but not under other lighting conditions.

Fig. 23-12. Spectral reflectance curves of a metameric pair. The two objects represented will appear to match under some lighting conditions but not under others.

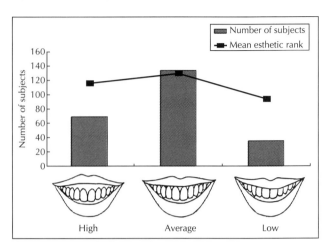

Fig. 23-13. Number of subjects and mean esthetic rank for three upper lip positions.
(From Dong JK et al: Int J Prosthodont 12:9, 1999.)

Opalescence. Natural teeth, particularly at their incisal edges, exhibit a light-scattering effect* that creates the appearance of bluish-white colors as the teeth are seen at different angles. This is similar to the bluish-white background seen in opal gemstones (this explains the term *opalescence*). Manufacturers try to match this effect when formulating dental porcelains.[21,22]

Color Blindness. Defects in color vision affect about 8% of the male population and less of the female population.[23] Different types exist, such as achromatism (complete lack of hue sensitivity), dichromatism (sensitivity to only two primary hues—usually either red or green are not perceived), and anomalous trichromatism (sensitivity to all three hues with deficiency or abnormality of one of the three primary pigments in the retinal cones). Dentists should therefore have their color perception tested. If any deficiency is detected, the dentist should seek assistance when selecting tooth shades.[24]

ESTHETICS

Esthetics is the study of beauty. A knowledge of esthetics helps the dentist achieve a pleasing appearance or effect. A successful prosthodontic restoration will provide the patient with excellent long-term function. It should also produce an at-

tractive smile—esthetics is often the primary motivating factor for patients to seek dental care.[25] In fact, correction of esthetic problems has a positive effect on self-esteem.[26]

ANATOMY OF A SMILE

Most people feel they can recognize an attractive smile, but individual opinion will vary, particularly when cultural factors are considered. Research is conducted by showing test subjects photographs or computer-manipulated images of various smiles and having them graded for attractiveness[27,28] (Fig. 23-13).* Such research is quantified in the standard dental esthetic index (DAI), an orthodontic treatment need index based on perceptions of dental esthetics in the United States.[29] In general, an extensive smile that showed the complete outline of the maxillary anterior teeth and teeth posterior to the first molar was considered the most attractive and youthful. (A smile in an aging individual shows less of the maxillary incisors and more of the mandibular incisors.) In smiles that were considered the most attractive, the incisal edges of the maxillary teeth were parallel to the lower lip (Fig. 23-14), a factor that should be considered when shaping restorations.

PROPORTION

Esthetics depends largely on proportion. An object is considered beautiful if it is properly proportioned, and unattractive if it is top-heavy, squat, or out of proportion. Concepts of proportion are probably based on what is found in nature. Leaves,

---

*Called *Mie scattering* after the German physicist, Gustav Mie, 1868-1957.

*See also www.dent.ohio-state.edu/restsurvey/

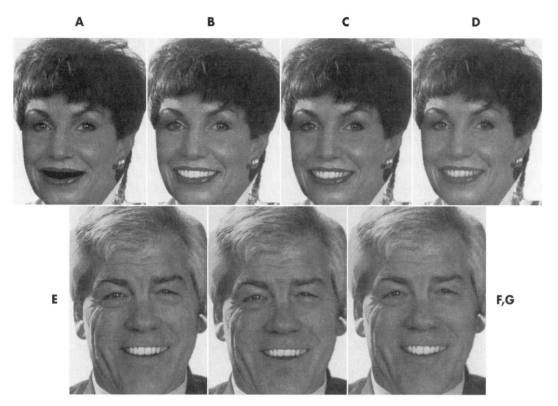

A   **B**   **C**   **D**

E   **F,G**

Fig. 23-14.   Computer image manipulation was used to determine the attractiveness of various smiles. Light colors and oval-shaped teeth in women and rectangular teeth in men were considered the most attractive.
(From Carlsson GE et al: Int J Prosthodont 11:248, 1998.)

flowers, shells, and pinecones normally develop in proportion. Their growth is closely related to a mathematical progression (called the *Fibonacci* series*) in which each number is the sum of the two immediately preceding it (i.e., 1, 1, 2, 3, 5, 8, 13, 21, 34, 55, 89, 144, and so on). The ratio between succeeding terms converges on approximately 1.618 to 1, known as *the golden proportion*. When a line is bisected in the golden proportion, the ratio of the smaller section to the larger section is the same as the ratio of the larger section to the whole line (Fig. 23-15). The golden proportion was used extensively in ancient Greek architecture and is exemplified in the Parthenon.

Claims have been made[30] that the golden proportion exists in natural dentitions in the ratio of the widths of incisors and canines as seen from the front. Special calipers† can be used that always extend to the golden proportion, which may be helpful in designing a well-proportioned prosthesis (Fig. 23-16). Others have attempted to apply mathematical concepts to dental esthetics.[31]

*After the Italian mathematician, Leonardo Fibonacci, who devised it in the thirteenth century.
†Available from Dr. Edwin I. Levin: 42 Harley St., London W1N 1AB, U.K.

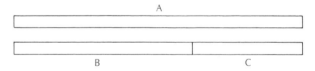

A

B   C

Fig. 23-15.   The golden proportion. The ratio of *A* to *B* (1.618 to 1) is the same as that of *B* to *C*.

BALANCE

Balance, including the location of the midline (Fig. 23-17), is an important prosthodontic concept.[32] The observer expects the left and right sides of the mouth to balance out, if not to match precisely. An obvious restoration on one side may be balanced if there is a diastema or a large tooth on the other side. If something is out of balance, the brain infers that there is an unreciprocated force and the arrangement is unstable; a balanced arrangement implies stability and permanence.

MIDLINE

Coincidence of facial and incisal midlines is stressed when assessing orthodontic treatment planning and should be carefully evaluated when treatment-planning prosthodontics. Studies have shown that

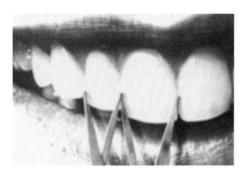

Fig. 23-16. The calipers always extend to the golden proportion.
(From Levin EI: J Prosthet Dent 40:244, 1978.)

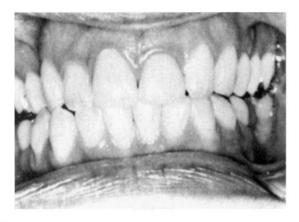

Fig. 23-17. Poor esthetics resulting from a lack of balance. The differences in central incisor height, unilateral cross-bite, and misaligned midline contribute to lack of symmetry.

the mean threshold for acceptable dental midline deviation is 2.2 /-1.5 mm.[33]

SHADE SELECTION

Because shade matching is subjective, consistency is difficult to achieve. Considerable variation exists among dentists.[34,35] Some dentists are unable to duplicate even their own shade selection from one patient to the next. Fortunately, a lifelike restoration does not have to be an exact color duplicate of the adjacent or contralateral teeth. It should, however, blend with the teeth as a result of the distribution of ceramic materials in the restoration. Shade selection can be improved by applying the principles of light and color and dental ceramic techniques.

GENERAL PRINCIPLES

Regardless of which system of shade selection is used, there should be general adherence to the following principles:

1. The patient should be viewed at eye level so that the most color-sensitive part of the retina will be used.

2. Shade comparison should be made under different lighting conditions. Normally the patient is taken to a window, and the color is confirmed in natural daylight after initial selection under incandescent and fluorescent lighting.

3. The teeth to be matched should be clean. If necessary, stains should be removed by prophylaxis.

4. Shade comparisons should be made at the beginning of a patient's visit. Teeth increase in value when they are dry, particularly if rubber dam has been used.

5. Brightly colored clothing should be draped and lipstick removed. The operatory walls should not be brightly painted.

6. Shade comparisons should be made quickly, with the color samples placed under the lip directly next to the tooth being matched. This will ensure that the background of the tooth and the shade sample are the same, which is essential for accurate matching. The dentist should be aware of eye fatigue, particularly if very bright fiber-optic illumination has been used. The eyes should be rested by focusing on a gray-blue surface immediately before a comparison, because this balances all the color sensors of the retina and resensitizes the eye to the yellow color of the tooth.

COMMERCIAL SHADE GUIDES (FIG. 23-18)

The most convenient method for selecting a shade is a commercially available porcelain shade guide. Each shade-tab (Fig. 23-19) has an opaque backing color, neck color, body color, and incisal color. Shade selection consists of picking the shade tab that looks the most natural and reproducing this in a laboratory with materials and techniques recommended by the manufacturer. The procedure is easier if specimens of the same hue are grouped together in the shade guide. In the past, shade guides were produced in response to the demand for denture teeth rather than on the range of natural tooth color.[36] More recently, shade guides have covered the color space occupied by natural teeth,* such as the Vitapan 3D-Master shade guide (Fig. 23-18, C).

Hue Selection. In the popular Vita Lumin vacuum shade guide (Fig. 23-18, A), A1, A2, A3, A3.5, and A4 are similar in hue, as are the B, C, and D shades. Choosing the nearest hue first and then selecting the appropriate match of chroma and value from the tabs available is the recommended technique.

---

*Shades that match artificially bleached teeth are also available.

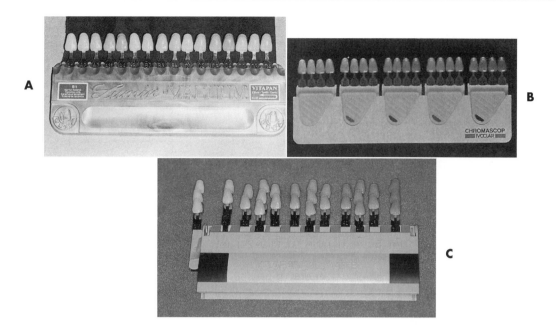

Fig. 23-18. Commercial shade guides. **A,** The Vita Lumin vacuum shade guide. **B,** Ivoclar Chromo-scop shade guide. **C,** Vitapan 3D-Master shade guide.

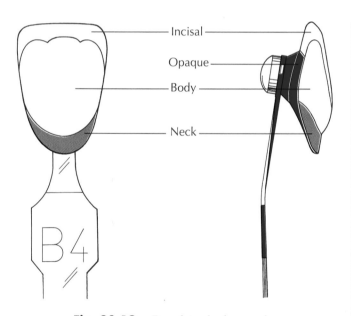

Fig. 23-19. Porcelain shade sample.

Average Color Measurements for Vita Lumin Vacuum Shade Guides			TABLE 23-1
Shade	Lightness (Value)	Chroma	Hue (degrees)
A1	53.3	5.3	87.9
A2	53.1	7.2	92.1
A3	51.5	8.9	87.4
A3.5	50.0	11.9	85.8
A4	49.1	13.0	85.4
B1	53.4	3.9	98.3
B2	52.8	6.2	89.7
B3	49.4	11.2	86.1
B4	49.8	12.8	90.9
C1	49.7	7.0	94.9
C2	49.7	8.9	91.5
C3	48.1	9.0	89.6
C4	46.0	11.5	86.0
D2	50.7	3.3	96.3
D3	47.2	7.0	85.4
D4	47.4	6.6	88.6

Data from Dr. A.M. Peregrina.

If its chroma or intensity is low, accurately determining a given hue may be difficult. Therefore, the region with the highest chroma (i.e., the cervical region of canines) should be used for initial hue selection (Fig. 23-20, *A*).

Chroma Selection. Once the hue is selected, the best chroma match is chosen. For example, if a B hue is determined to be the best match for color variety, there are four available gradations (tabs) of that hue: B1, B2, B3, and B4 (Fig. 23-20, *B*). Several comparisons are usually necessary when determining which sample best represents the hue and its corresponding chroma (saturation) level. Between comparisons, glancing at a blue object will rest the operator's eye and help avoid retinal cone fatigue.

Table 23-1 presents color measurement values made from a Vita Lumin vacuum shade guide with

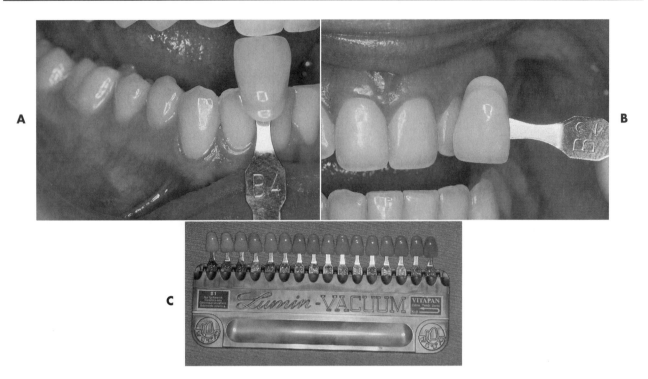

Fig. 23-20.   Shade selection using the Lumin Vacuum shade guide. **A,** Selecting hue by matching samples with high chroma (e.g., A4, B4, C4, D3) to a tooth with high chroma (i.e., canine). **B,** Selecting chroma from within the hue group (e.g., B1, B2, B3 or B4). **C,** Value-ordered shade guide is used to check lightness.

a small-area colorimeter. Manufacturer claims about hue consistency within a letter group have not been confirmed by these measurements, which is one of the main difficulties with commercial shade guides.

Value Selection.   Finally, value is determined with a second commercial guide whose samples are arranged in order of increasing lightness (Fig. 23-20, C). (The lightness readings in Table 23-1 can be used as a guide to the sample sequencing.) By holding the second shade guide close to the patient, the operator should be able to determine whether the value of the tooth is within the shade guide's range. Attention is then focused on the range of shade that best represents the value of the tooth and how that range relates to the tab matching for hue and saturation. An individual will be able to assess the value most effectively by observing from a distance, standing slightly away from the chair, and squinting the eyes. By squinting, the observer can reduce the amount of light that reaches the retina. Stimulation of the cones is reduced, and a greater sensitivity to achromatic conditions may result.[37] While squinting, the observer concentrates on which disappears from sight first—the tooth or the shade tab. The one that fades first has the lower value.

When the proper value selection has been made, it will be the exception rather than the rule for this to co-incide with the determinations for hue and chroma. The operator must decide whether to change the previously selected shade sample. If the independent value determination is lower than the value of the sample selected for hue and chroma, a change is usually necessary, because increasing the value of an object by adding surface stain (which always reduces brightness) is not possible. If the value determination is higher than the hue determination, the operator should decide whether this difference can be bridged through internal or surface staining of the restoration. The final decisions about hue, chroma, and value are then communicated to the laboratory.

VITAPAN 3D-MASTER SHADE GUIDE* (FIG 23-21, A)

The manufacturer of this recently introduced shade system claims that it covers the entire tooth color space. The shade samples are grouped in six lightness levels,† each of which has chroma and hue variations in evenly spaced steps (Fig. 23-21, B). The shade guide is spaced in steps (ΔE) of 4 CIELAB units in the lightness dimension and 2 CIELAB units in the hue and chroma dimensions. The differ-

---

*Vident: Brea, Calif.
†The "0" brightness level is used to match bleached teeth.

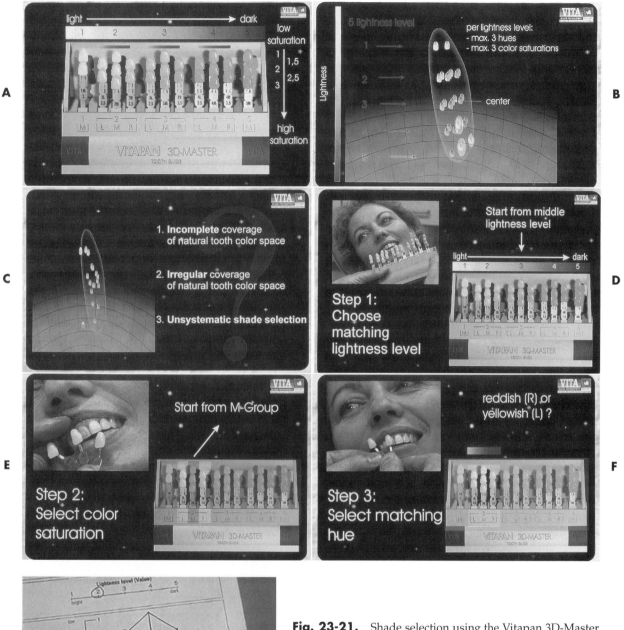

Fig. 23-21. Shade selection using the Vitapan 3D-Master shade guide. **A,** The shade guide is arranged in five lightness levels (plus an additional level for bleached teeth). Each lightness level has sufficient variations in chroma and hue to cover the natural tooth color space (**B**). **C,** This contrasts with traditional shade guides, which are not uniformly spaced. **D,** Lightness is selected first, then chroma or saturation (**E**) and finally hue (**F**). **G,** The color communication form allows convenient laboratory shade prescription and intermediate shades if necessary. *(Courtesy Vident).*

ence between lightness and color steps seems a logical approach to reducing the number of shade samples needed in the guide because of the way the CIELAB units are visually perceived. It seems to match the color difference formula of the Colour Measurement Committee (CMC) of the Society of Dyers and Colourists.[38] Because the guide is evenly spaced, intermediate shades can be predictably formulated by combining porcelain powders.

The manufacturer recommends selecting the lightness level first with this system (Fig. 23-21, *D*) and then selecting the chroma or saturation (Fig.

23-21, *E*) and finally the hue (Fig. 23-21, *F*). A form is available to facilitate the laboratory shade prescription, which can include intermediate steps (Fig. 23-21, *G*).

EXTENDED RANGE SHADE GUIDES

Most commercial shade systems cover a more limited range than the colors found in natural teeth, and the steps in the guide are greater than can be perceived visually.[39] Some porcelain systems are available with extended range shade guides, and other manufacturers have extended their range over the years. The use of two shade guides is a practical way to extend the range of commercial guides.

DENTIN SHADE GUIDES

When using a translucent all-ceramic system for a crown or veneer (see Chapter 25), communicating the shade of the prepared dentin to the dental labo-

ratory is helpful. One system* provides specially colored die materials that match the dentin shade guide and enable the technician to judge restoration esthetics (Fig. 23-22).

CUSTOM SHADE GUIDE

Unfortunately, certain teeth may be impossible to match to commercial shade samples. In addition, difficulties may be encountered in reproducing the shade guides in the final restorations. The extensive use of surface staining has severe drawbacks, because the stains increase surface reflection and prevent light from being transmitted through the porcelain.[40]

One approach to this problem is to extend the concept of a commercial shade guide by making a custom shade guide (Fig. 23-23). An almost infinite

*IPS Empress, Ivoclar North America: Amherst, N.Y.

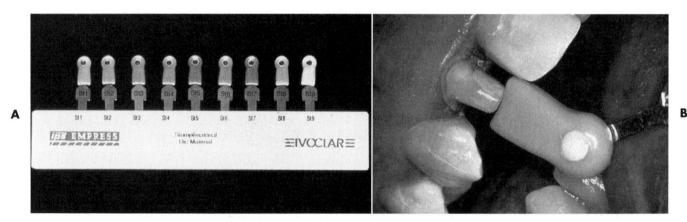

Fig. 23-22. Dentin shade guide is used to communicate the color of the prepared tooth to the technician when translucent ceramic systems are used.
(Courtesy Ivoclar North America.)

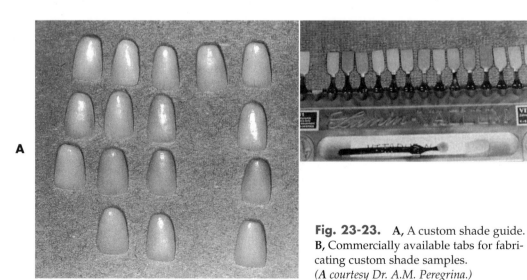

Fig. 23-23. **A,** A custom shade guide. **B,** Commercially available tabs for fabricating custom shade samples.
(A courtesy Dr. A.M. Peregrina.)

number of samples can be made by using different combinations of porcelain powders in varying distributions. However, the procedure is time consuming and is generally confined to specialty practice.

Shade Distribution Chart (Fig. 23-24). Shade distribution charting is a practical approach to accurate shade selection and is recommended even when a fairly good match is available from the commercial shade sample.

The tooth is divided into three regions: cervical, middle, and incisal. Each region is matched independently, either to the corresponding area of a commercial shade sample or to a single color porcelain chip. Because only a single color is matched, intermediate shades can usually be estimated rather easily and duplicated by mixing porcelain powders. The junctions between these areas are normally distinct and can be communicated to the laboratory in the form of a diagram. The shade distribution and thickness of the enamel porcelain are particularly important.[41] Individual characteristics are marked on such a sketch and will allow the ceramist to mimic details like hairline fractures, hypocalcification, and proximal discolorations.

SUMMARY

An understanding of the science of color and color perception is crucial to success in the ever-expanding field of esthetic restorative dentistry. Although limitations in materials and techniques may make a perfect color match impossible, a harmonious restoration can almost always be achieved. Shade selection should be approached in a methodical and organized manner. This will enable the practitioner to make the best choice and communicate it accurately to the laboratory. Newly developed shade systems and instruments may help the practitioner achieve a reliable restoration match.

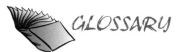

GLOSSARY

achromatic: *adj* (1766) *1:* lacking in hue and saturation, therefore falling into a series of colors that varies only in lightness or brightness *2:* possessing no hue; being or involving black, gray or white.

additive color mixture: the perceived color that results when the same area of the retina of the eye is illuminated by lights of different spectral distribution such as by two colored lights.

chroma: *n* (1889) *1:* the purity of a color, or its departure from white or gray *2:* the intensity of a distinctive hue; saturation of a hue *3:* chroma describes the strength or saturation of the hue (color).

CIE LAB system: CIE LAB relates the tristimulus values to a color space. This scale accounts for the illuminant and the observer. By establishing a uniform color scale, color measurements can be compared and movements in color space defined.

color: *n 1:* a phenomenon of light or visual perception that enables one to differentiate otherwise identical objects *2:* the quality of an object or substance with

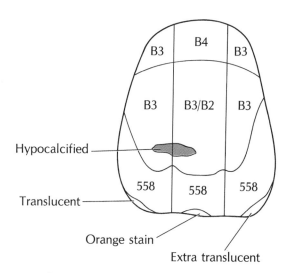

Fig. 23-24. Shade distribution chart.

respect to light reflected or transmitted by it. Color is usually determined visually by measurement of hue, saturation, and luminous reflectance of the reflected light 3: a visual response to light consisting of the three dimensions of hue, value, and saturation.

color blindness: abnormal color vision or the inability to discriminate certain colors, most commonly along the red-green axis.

color deficiency: a general term for all forms of color vision that yield chromaticity discrimination below normal limits, such as monochromatism, dichromatism, and anomalous trichromatism.

color temperature: the temperature in degrees Kelvin (Celsius plus 273°) of a totally absorbing or black body (object) that produces colors as the temperature changes. The range is from a dull red to yellow to white to blue. This term is sometimes used incorrectly to describe the color of "white" light sources. The correct term to describe the color of light sources is correlated color temperature

complementary colors: two colors that, when mixed together in proper proportions, result in a neutral color. Colored lights that are complementary when mixed in an additive manner form white light and follow the laws of additive color mixture. Colorants that are complementary when mixed together form black or gray and follow the laws of subtractive colorant mixture 2: colors located in directly opposite positions on the color wheel. Colorants that are complementary when mixed together form black or gray and follow the laws of subtractive color.

continuous spectrum: a spectrum or section of the spectrum in which radiations of all wavelengths are present; opposed to line spectra or band spectra.

delta E: total color difference computed by use of a color difference equation. It is generally calculated as the square root of the sums of the squares of the chromaticity difference and the lightness difference. It signifies the difference between sample and standard.

dichromatic vision: defective color vision characterized by the interpretation of wavelengths from the red portion of the spectrum matching a given green. There are two known subclassifications. One requires red light to be approximately 10 times brighter than the red selected by the other to achieve a similar color mismatch.

dimensions of color: terms used to describe the three dimensional nature of color. In the Munsell Color Order System, the dimensions are named hue, value, and chroma. These are used to describe the color family (hue), the lightness/darkness (value), and the purity or strength (chroma).

electromagnetic spectrum: the range of energy waves that extend from gamma rays to radio waves. The eye is sensitive to a very narrow band of wavelengths between about 380 and 760 nm.

fluorescence: *n* (1852): a process by which a material absorbs radiant energy and emits it in the form of radiant energy of a different wavelength band, all or most of whose wavelengths exceed that of the absorbed energy. Fluorescence, as distinguished from phosphorescence, does not persist for an appreciable time after the termination of the excitation process.

hue: *n* (bef. 12 c): often referred to as the basic color, hue is the quality of sensation according to which an observer is aware of the varying wavelengths of radiant energy. The dimension of color dictated by the wavelength of the stimulus that is used to distinguish one family of color from another—as red, green, blue, etc. The attribute of color by means of which a color is perceived to be red, yellow, green, blue, purple, etc. White, black, and grays possess no hue. (Munsell AH. A color notation. Baltimore: Munsell Color Co. Inc., 1975:14-6.)

Kelvin temperature: [Thomson W. (Lord Kelvin), Scottish mathematician and physicist (1824-1907)]: absolute temperature indicated by the symbol K. Zero Kelvin = −273° C.

light: *n* (bef. 12 c): the aspect of electromagnetic radiation of which the human observer is aware through the visual sensations that arise from the stimulation of the retina of the eye.

metameric pair: a pair of objects whose colors match when viewed in a described way, but which do not match if the viewing conditions are changed. Thus a metameric pair of samples exhibit the same tristimulus values for a described set of viewing conditions (observer, light source, geometry of the illumination and viewing arrangement) but have different spectral distributions. Hence, they exhibit a match that is conditional.

metamerism: *n* (1877): pairs of objects that have different spectral curves but appear to match when viewed in a given illuminant exhibit metamerism. Metamerism should not be confused with the terms *flair* or *color constancy*, which apply to apparent color change exhibited by a single color when the spectral distribution of the light source is changed or when the angle of illumination or viewing is changed.

monochromatic vision: vision in which there is no color discrimination.

Munsell color order system: [Alfred H. Munsell, Massachusetts, U.S. artist and teacher, 1858-1918]: eponym for a color order system; developed in 1905, it places colors in an orderly arrangement encompassing the three attributes of hue, value, and chroma (Munsell AH. A color notation. Baltimore: Munsell Color Co., 1975:14-6).

natural color system: a color order system derived by Anders Hard that defines six color perceptions using the concept of percentage for localizing nuances within the three-part system. The six perceptions are white, black, red, green, yellow, and blue. The dimensions of hue, blackness or whiteness, and chroma are used to relate colors within this system.

partitive color mixing: color mixing in which both additive and subtractive principles are involved. The eye interprets tiny dots of subtractive color too small to be individually resolved at the viewing distance. The resultant color will be the average of the colors used.

perceived color: attribute of visual perception that can be described by color names: white, gray, black, yellow, orange, brown, red, green, blue, purple, etc., or by a combination of names.

phosphorescence: *n* (1796): a form of photoluminescence based on the properties of certain molecules to absorb energy (either near ultra violet or visible), and emit it in the form of visible radiation at a higher wave length. Distinguished from fluorescence in that light continues to be emitted for some time after the exciting energy has ceased.

photopic vision: vision as it occurs under illumination sufficient to permit the full discrimination of colors. It is the function of the retinal cones and is not dependent on the retinal rods—called also daylight vision as contrasted with twilight or scotopic vision.

photoreceptor process: that specific process that is set in motion in a visual sensory end organ or other photic receptor by the incidence of its adequate stimulus, i.e., light.

primary colors: three basic colors used to make most other colors by mixture, either additive mixture of lights or subtractive mixture of colorants.

reflectance: *n* (1926): the ratio of the intensity of reflected radiant flux to that of the incident flux. In popular usage, it is considered as the ratio of the intensity of reflected radiant flux to that reflected from a defined reference standard. Specular reflection is the angle of reflection equal to the angle of incidence. Surface reflection is associated with objects having optically smooth surfaces. These objects are usually termed *glossy.*

refraction: *n* (1603): the deflection of light or energy waves from a straight path that occurs when passing obliquely from one medium into another in which its velocity is different.

rod: *n* (bef. 12th cent.): the photoreceptor in the retina that contains a light-sensitive pigment capable of initiating the process of scotopic vision, i.e., low intensity for achromatic sensations only.

saturation: *n* (1554): the attribute of color perception that expresses the degree of departure from gray of the same lightness. All grays have zero saturation.

scotopic vision: vision that occurs in faint light or dark adaptation and is attributable to the retinal rods.

The maximum of the relative spectral visual sensitivity is shifted to 510 nm and the spectrum is seen uncolored.

shade: *n 1:* a term used to describe a particular hue, or variation of a primary hue, such as a greenish shade of yellow *2:* a term used to describe a mixture with black (or gray) as opposed to a tint that is a mixture with white.

spectrum: *n 1:* band of colors produced when sunlight is passed through a prism *2:* spatial arrangements of components of radiant energy in order of their wavelengths, wave numbers, or frequency— **spectral** *adj.*

standard light source: a reference light source whose spectral power distribution is known.

subtractive color system: the system whereby light is removed by filtration or absorption from a white source. The primary colors of the subtractive system are magenta, cyan, and yellow—called also *pigment mixture color system.*

subtractive primary colors: the primary colorant substances for pigment and filtering mixtures typically evoking responses of cyan (blue-green), magenta (red-blue), and yellow (red-green). The complementary colors of the subtractive primary colors are red, green, and blue. Magenta is a mixture of red and blue and is the complement of green. Cyan is a mixture of blue and green and is the complement of red. Yellow is a mixture of red and green and is the complement of blue.

tooth color selection: the determination of the color and other attributes of appearance of an artificial tooth or set of teeth for a given individual.

trichromatic system: a system for specifying color stimuli in terms of the tri-stimulus value based on matching colors by additive mixtures of three primary colored lights.

uniform color space: color space in which equal distances are intended to represent threshold or above threshold perceived color differences of equal size.

value: *n:* the quality by which a light color is distinguished from a dark color, the dimension of a color that denotes relative blackness or whiteness (grayness, brightness). Value is the only dimension of color that may exist alone (Munsell, AH. A color notation. Baltimore: Munsell Color Co., 1975:14-7.)

visible spectrum: the section of the electromagnetic spectrum that is visible to the human eye. It ranges from 380 nm to 760 nm.

wave length: the distance at any instant between two adjacent crests (or identical phases) of two series of waves that are advancing through a uniform medium. The wave length varies inversely with the vibration rate or number of waves passing any given point per unit period of time.

REFERENCES

1. Saleski CG: Color, light, and shade matching, *J Prosthet Dent* 27:263, 1972.

2. Bergen SF, McCasland J: Dental operatory lighting and tooth color discrimination, *J Am Dent Assoc* 94:130, 1977.

3. Munsell AH: *A color notation,* ed 11, Baltimore, 1961, Munsell Color Co.

4. Sproull RC: Color matching in dentistry. II. Practical applications of the organization of color, *J Prosthet Dent* 29:556, 1973.

5. Hammad IA, Stein RS: A qualitative study for the bond and color of ceramometals. II. *J Prosthet Dent* 65:169, 1991.

6. O'Brien WJ et al: Color distribution of three regions of extracted human teeth, *Dent Mater* 13: 179, 1997.

7. Seghi RR et al: Spectrophotometric analysis of color differences between porcelain systems, *J Prosthet Dent* 56:35, 1986.

8. Rosenstiel SF, Johnston WM: The effects of manipulative variables on the color of ceramic metal restorations, *J Prosthet Dent* 60:297, 1988.

9. Okubo SR et al: Evaluation of visual and instrument shade matching, *J Prosthet Dent* 80:642, 1998.

10. Rinke S et al: Colorimetric analysis as a means of quality control for dental ceramic materials, *Eur J Prosthodont* 4:105, 1996.

11. Wyszecki G, Stiles WS: *Color science: concepts and methods, quantitative data and formulae,* ed 2, p. 840, New York, 1982, Wiley & Sons.

12. Seghi RR: Effects of instrument-measuring geometry on colorimetric assessments of dental porcelains, *J Dent Res* 69:1180, 1990.

13. Rosenstiel SF et al: Randomized clinical trial of the efficacy and safety of a home bleaching procedure, *Quintessence Int* 27:413, 1996.

14. Yannikakis SA et al: Color stability of provisional resin restorative materials, *J Prosthet Dent* 80: 533, 1998.

15. Douglas RD: Precision of in vivo colorimetric assessments of teeth, *J Prosthet Dent* 77: 464, 1997.

16. Wee AG et al: Colorimetric analysis of porcelain disks by different shade matching systems, *J Dent Res* 79:540, 2000 (abstract no. 3175).

17. Wyszecki G, Stiles WS: op. cit., p 519.

18. Land EH: The retinex theory of color vision, *Sci Am* 237:108, 1977.

19. Wyszecki G, Stiles WS: op cit., p 236.

20. Seghi RR, Johnston WM: Estimate of colorimetric measurement errors associated with natural tooth fluorescence, *J Dent Res* 71:303, 1992 (abstract no. 1578).

21. Yamamoto M: Newly developed opal ceramic and its clinical use with respect to relative breaking indices. I. Significance of opalescence and development of opal ceramic, *Quintessenz Zahntech* 15:523, 1989.

22. Hegenbarth EA: Opalescence effects in low melting ceramic, *Quintessenz Zahntech* 17:1415, 1991.

23. Rushton WAH: Visual pigments and color blindness, *Sci Am* 232:64, 1975.

24. Davison SP, Myslinski NR: Shade selection by color vision defective dental personnel, *J Prosthet Dent* 63:97, 1990.

25. Elias AC, Sheiham A: The relationship between satisfaction with mouth and number and position of teeth, *J Oral Rehabil* 25:649, 1998.

26. Davis LG et al: Psychological effects of aesthetic dental treatment, *J Dent* 26:547, 1998.

27. Dong JK et al: The esthetics of the smile: a review of some recent studies, *Int J Prosthodont* 12:9, 1999.

28. Carlsson GE et al: An international comparative multicenter study of assessment of dental appearance using computer-aided image manipulation, *Int J Prosthodont* 11:246, 1998.

29. Proffit EG: *Contemporary orthodontics,* ed 2, St. Louis, 1995, Mosby.

30. Levin EI: Dental esthetics and the golden proportion, *J Prosthet Dent* 40:244, 1978.

31. Ahmad I: Geometric considerations in anterior dental aesthetics: restorative principles, *Pract Periodont Aesthet Dent* 10:813, 1998.

32. Lombardi RE: The principles of visual perception and their clinical application to denture esthetics, *J Prosthet Dent* 29:358, 1973.

33. Beyer JW, Lindauer SJ: Evaluation of dental midline position, *Semin Orthodont* 4:146, 1998.

34. Culpepper WD: A comparative study of shade-matching procedures, *J Prosthet Dent* 24:166, 1970.

35. Geary JL, Kinirons MJ: Colour perception of laboratory-fired samples of body-coloured ceramic, *J Dent* 27:145, 1999.

36. Hall NR: Tooth colour selection: the application of colour science to dental colour matching, *Aust Prosthodont J* 5:41, 1991.

37. McPhee ER: Light and color in dentistry. I. Nature and perception, *J Mich Dent Assoc* 60:565, 1978.

38. Ragain JC: *Matching the optical properties of direct esthetic dental restorative materials to those of human enamel and dentin,* PhD dissertation, The Ohio State University, 1998.

39. O'Brien WJ et al: Coverage errors of two shade guides, *Int J Prosthodont* 4:45, 1991.

40. McLean JW: *The science and art of dental ceramics,* vol 2, p 308, Chicago, 1980, Quintessence Publishing.

41. Blackman RB: Ceramic shade prescriptions for work authorizations, *J Prosthet Dent* 47:28, 1982.

42. Kuehni FG, Marcus RT: An experiment in visual scaling of small color differences, *Color Res Appl* 4:83, 1979.

CHAPTER • TWENTY-FOUR

METAL-CERAMIC RESTORATIONS

KEY TERMS

bisque bake	opaque
ceramic	pigment
devitrification	porcelain
feldspar	quartz
firing	silica
frit	substructure
glaze	thermal expansion
opacity	translucency

HISTORICAL PERSPECTIVE

Ceramic objects have been constructed for thousands of years. The earliest techniques usually consisted of shaping the item in clay or soil and then baking it to fuse the particles together. The initial attempts resulted primarily in coarse and somewhat porous products, such as goblets and other forms of pottery. Later developments led to very detailed stoneware items. The Egyptian faiences are the first known effort to enamel a **substructure** with a ceramic veneer (Fig. 24-1). Their typical blue-green hues result from metal oxides created during the **firing** process.

Fig. 24-1. Glazed Egyptian faience tile from the Western Doorway or Gate of the Mortuary Temple of Ramses III, with a "Rekhyet" bird worshipping the cartouche of Ramses III, "Lord of the Two Lands" (circa 1182-1151 BCE), Dynasty XX, excavated at Medinet Habu by the Oriental Institute. *(Courtesy the Oriental Institute, The University of Chicago.)*

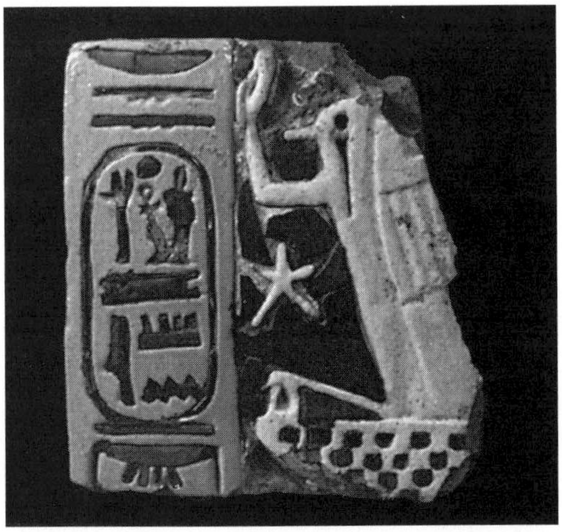

More recently, although still in antiquity, Chinese ceramists developed **porcelain**, which was characterized by vitrification, **translucency**, hardness, and impermeability. European attempts at developing porcelain of similar quality were conducted in the seventeenth century. These efforts spread the knowledge of porcelain's basic components: kaolin and **feldspar**.

As early as the second half of the eighteenth century, Pierre Fauchard and others attempted to use porcelain in dentistry. Their efforts were largely unsuccessful. However, porcelain was successfully used for dental prostheses by the end of the 1800s, when the technique to fire all-porcelain jacket crowns on a platinum matrix was first developed.[1] It was not until the mid-1950s that a dental porcelain was developed with a coefficient of **thermal expansion** similar to that of dental casting alloys. The metal-ceramic restoration first became available commercially during the later 1950s.[2] Today this technique is considered a routine procedure with high predictability.

OVERVIEW

The metal-ceramic restoration (Fig. 24-2) consists of a metal substructure (see Chapter 19) supporting a ceramic veneer that is mechanically and chemically bonded to it. The chemical component of the bond is achieved through firing (baking).

Porcelain powders of varying composition and color are applied and fired to produce the desired appearance. The first ceramic layer, the **opaque**, masks the dark metal oxide and is the primary source of color for the completed restoration. The opaque is covered with slightly translucent body porcelain, which is then veneered with a more translucent enamel overlay that contains only a few **pigments**. Achieving an accurate appearance match may warrant incorporating either translucent or highly pigmented powders into selected areas of the buildup. The shiny, lifelike appearance of the completed metal-ceramic restoration results from a surface **glaze** formed during an additional firing after the restoration has been shaped.

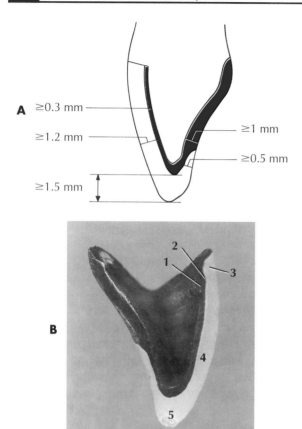

Fig. 24-2. **A,** Longitudinal section through a metal-ceramic crown. Note the minimum dimensions. **B,** Sectioned metal-ceramic restoration. *1,* Metal substructure; *2,* opaque porcelain; *3,* gingival porcelain; *4,* body porcelain; *5,* incisal porcelain.

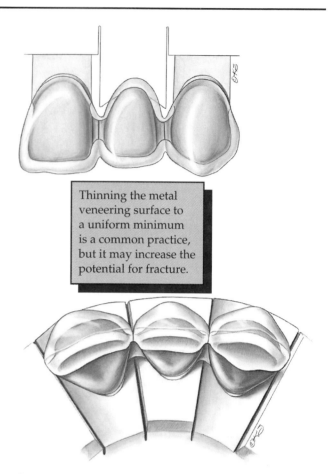

Thinning the metal veneering surface to a uniform minimum is a common practice, but it may increase the potential for fracture.

Fig. 24-3. Substructure design for an anterior FPD. The metal should be shaped to support an even thickness of porcelain.

Historically, the metal-ceramic restoration was fabricated with metal margins, and the veneer was limited to visible areas. More recently, however, the use of porcelain on occlusal and lingual surfaces has become common.[3] Several techniques[4,5] have been developed to obtain porcelain margins on the facial aspect of the restoration. The latter technique is common for anterior teeth, whereas the metal collar is commonly used in areas with a lesser esthetic demand.

METAL PREPARATION

SHAPE

Sharp angles or pits on the veneering surface of a metal-ceramic restoration should be avoided because they can contribute to internal stress in the final porcelain.[6] Convex surfaces and rounded contours should be created so that the porcelain will be supported without development of stress concentrations (Fig. 24-3). In addition, a smooth surface will facilitate wetting the framework by the porcelain slurry.

The intended metal-ceramic junction should be as definite (90-degree angle) and as smooth as possible to make finishing easier during all fabrication stages (Fig. 24-4). The metal framework must be sufficiently thick to prevent distortion during firing. A minimum of 0.3 mm is advocated for the noble metal alloys; 0.2 mm is sufficient for base metal alloys, which can be finished thinner and still withstand distortion because of their higher melting ranges, moduli of elasticity, and yield strengths (see Chapter 19).

The mechanical properties of a metal-ceramic restoration depend largely on the design of the substructure that supports the ceramic veneer. The metal-ceramic interface must be at least 1.5 mm from all centric occlusal contacts and must be distinct to facilitate the removal of excess porcelain. The veneering surface must be finished to a smooth texture with rounded internal angles to allow proper wetting by the opaque porcelain.

INVESTMENT REMOVAL

After the framework has been cast, all investment should be removed ultrasonically with airborne

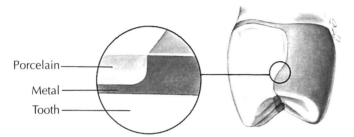

Porcelain
Metal
Tooth

Fig. 24-4. The metal substructure should have a distinct margin for finishing the veneer.

particle abrasion or with steam (follow the alloy manufacturer's directions). The phosphate-bonded investments, which must be used with the high-fusing metal-ceramic alloys, are more difficult to remove from the metal surface than conventional gypsum-bonded investments. Hydrofluoric acid will dissolve the refractory **silica** material of the investment. However, this material is extremely dangerous and must be handled very cautiously.[7] A small spill on the skin will result in painful acid burns, and slight exposure to the fumes may produce severe corneal damage. Less dangerous substitute solutions (e.g., No-San*) are available.

Careful examination of the internal aspect of the framework may reveal small investment particles. Several cycles of ultrasonic cleaning may be required to eliminate all residual investment. If air-abrasion is used for investment removal, the margins of the framework must be protected to prevent the removal of metal and investment.[8]

OXIDE REMOVAL

The oxide layer that has been formed on the metal surface during casting must be removed with either acid or air-abrasion. For maximal metal-porcelain bonding, the alloy manufacturer's directions should be followed, because the bonding depends on a controlled thickness of the metal-oxide layer.

METAL FINISHING

Care is needed when grinding the veneering surface to avoid dragging the metal over itself, which could entrap air and grinding debris (which later results in bubbling or contamination of the porcelain). Finishing the surface in one direction and using light pressure will help avoid trapping debris between folds of the metal, which is a problem when using high-gold content alloys with high elongation values (Fig. 24-5).

Surface finishing should be performed with ceramic-bound stones, because the organic binders used in conventional rotary instruments are a po-

Careful metal preparation is essential before porcelain application.

A

CORRECT

B

INCORRECT

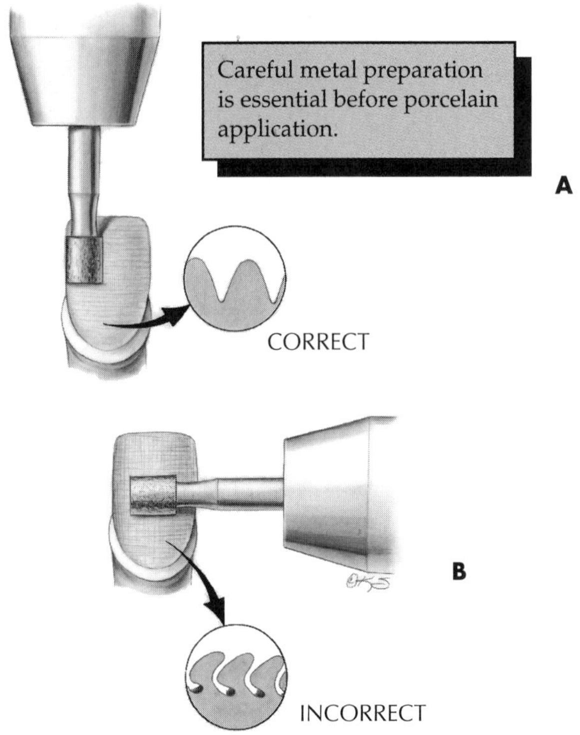

Fig. 24-5. **A,** Correct way to prepare the veneer area. The metal should be ground in the same direction. **B,** Incorrect multidirectional grinding can trap debris in the high-noble alloys.

tential source of contamination. Carbide burs also may be used safely. After the surface has been smoothed, it should be air-abraded with aluminum oxide according to manufacturer instructions. This will create a satin finish on the veneering surface that is easily wettable by the porcelain slurry (Fig. 24-6).

Thickness. A dial (or metric) caliper is invaluable for verifying that the metal substructure con-forms to all specified minimum dimensions (Fig. 24-7). Metal thickness less than 0.3 mm may lead to distortion during firing. Sometimes the margin is thinned to a knife edge so that a metal line is not visible. There is no evidence that thinning the margin adversely affects the fit of restorations cast in contemporary alloys.[9,10] The all-porcelain labial margin design can provide a

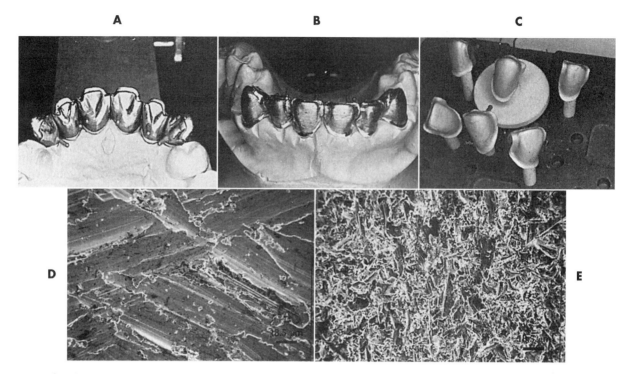

Fig. 24-6. Metal preparation. **A** and **B,** Castings prepared by grinding. **C,** Satin finish obtained by air-abrasion. **D** and **E,** Scanning electron micrographs of metal after grinding with a stone **(E)** and with air-abrasion **(F).**
*(**D** and **E** courtesy Dr. J. L. Sandrik.)*

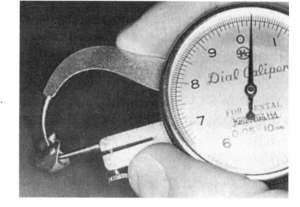

Fig. 24-7. Dimensions should be verified with calipers.

better appearance, particularly where a high smile line and thin gingival margins make good esthetics at the labial margin essential.

Finishing. Finishing of the metal-ceramic interface is a difficult laboratory procedure and requires attention to detail. The axial surfaces and visible portion of the metal collar should be contoured and finished to a rubber wheel stage before preparation of the veneering surface is attempted

(Fig. 24-8, *A* and *B*). At this time, the margin itself is left untouched. Round stones and carbides can be used to finish the veneering surface at the metal-ceramic interface (Fig. 24-8, *C*), and the desired right-angle configuration is then easily obtained. Any remaining irregularities can be blended easily with barrel-shaped stones (Fig. 24-8, *D*).

When the grinding phase is completed, a satin finish is obtained by air-abrading the veneering surface with a fine grit alumina (Fig. 24-8, *E* and *F*).

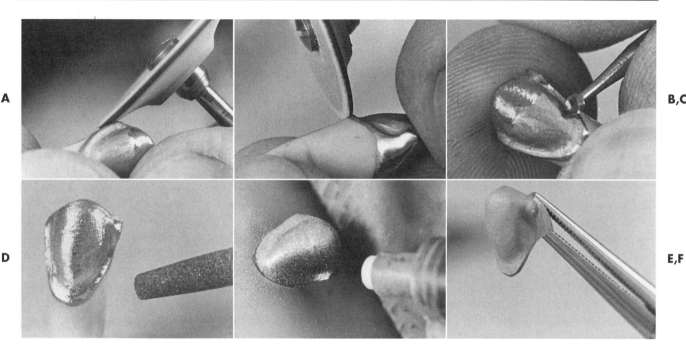

Fig. 24-8. Preparing the substructure. **A** and **B,** Nonveneering surface finished to the rubber wheel stage. **C,** Metal-ceramic junction delineated with a stone or tungsten carbide bur. **D,** Veneering surface dressed with a ceramic-bound stone. (NOTE: To avoid perforation, check the metal thickness regularly with calipers.) **E,** Air-abrasion of the veneering area. The margins have been protected by soft wax. **F,** The completed substructure ready for oxidizing.

Cleaning. Although a properly prepared framework will appear smooth to the naked eye, its appearance is still quite rough when viewed with a microscope. Small particles, grinding debris, oil, and finger grease must be removed because they will interfere with the wetting process, which is critical to a good metal-to-ceramic bond.

The substructure can be cleaned by immersion in a general-purpose cleaning solution in an ultrasonic unit. The duration of the cleaning cycle will depend on the unit, but 5 minutes is adequate in most cases. Residual soap can be removed by rinsing the substructure in distilled water. Some manufacturers recommend following this with a rinse in 92% alcohol (conventional 70% isopropyl alcohol should not be used because it contains aromatic and mineral oils, which could cause contamination). Steam cleaning is an excellent and timesaving alternative to ultrasonic cleaning. To prevent further contamination, the veneering surface should not be touched once the cleaning procedures have been completed.

Oxidizing (Fig. 24-9). To establish the chemical bond between metal and porcelain, a controlled oxide layer must be created on the metal surface. In noble-metal alloys, iron, tin, indium, and galium are the base elements used for oxide formation (see p. 617).

The oxide layer is typically obtained by placing the substructure on a firing tray, inserting it into the

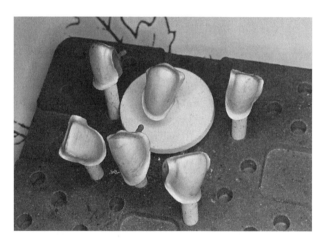

Fig. 24-9. Metal-ceramic substructure after cleaning and before oxidizing in the porcelain furnace.

muffle of a porcelain furnace, and raising the temperature to a specified level that sufficiently exceeds the firing temperature of the porcelain. A vacuum is created in the firing chamber which, although insufficient to remove adherent gases, reduces the thickness of the oxide layer. The incorrect term *degassing* often is used interchangeably with *oxidizing* (see p. 618).

The specific procedure may vary slightly depending on the alloy used. High-gold content ceramic alloys usually are held at the oxidizing temperature for several minutes. The first porcelain application can be performed as soon as the casting has cooled to room temperature after it is removed from the furnace.

Many of the lower-gold content alloys contain more base elements, which can result in a thicker oxide layer. Some of these systems therefore do not require the work to be held at the oxidizing temperature for any length of time. To reduce excessive surface oxides, some manufacturers recommend briefly air-abrading the casting with alumina or placing it in hydrofluoric acid after firing.

Because of lower costs, the use of non-noble or base metal alloys for metal-ceramic restorations is now widespread. These alloy systems undergo continuous oxide formation. Although the techniques for different systems vary, most manufacturers prefer not to oxidize substructures made of base metal alloys. Instead, they recommend performing the first porcelain application immediately after cleaning. Because the extent of oxide formation cannot be easily controlled, there is a potential for failure through the thick and brittle oxide layer with these alloy systems. However, it may be of no significance with other alloy systems.

◼ MATERIALS SCIENCE

Isabelle L. Denry

Leon W. Laub

Dental ceramics are generally classified into three groups, according to their maturation or fusion range: high-fusing (1290° to 1370° C; 2350° to 2500° F), medium-fusing (1090° to 1260° C; 2000° to 2300° F), and low-fusing (870° to 1070° C, 1600° to 1950° F). In contrast to denture teeth and the original porcelain jacket crowns, which are fired in the medium- and high-fusing ranges, metal-ceramic veneer restorations are fired in the range of 950° to 1020° C (1750° to 1860° F). This discussion is limited to these low-fusing porcelains.

PORCELAIN MANUFACTURE

Dental porcelain is produced from a blend of **quartz** (SiO_2), feldspar (potassium aluminum silicate orthoclase, sodium aluminum silicate albite), and other oxides. During manufacture, the materials are heated to high temperature to form a glassy mass and then rapidly cooled by quenching them in water, which causes the glassy mass to fracture. The resulting product is called a *frit*. This process may be repeated several times, after which the frit is ball-milled until the desired particle size distribution is obtained. Because fritting takes place at temperatures much higher than those used in the fabrication of a dental restoration, most of the chemical reactions between raw materials occur before they are used in the dental laboratory. Typical compositions are provided in Table 24-1, although the actual compositions will vary depending on the proposed use of the end product. Most formulations designed for metal-ceramic use are similar to that described by Weinstein et al.[11,12] They consist of a mixture of two frits: a low-fusing glass frit and a high-expansion frit consisting of crystalline leucite ($KAlSi_2O_6$) (Fig. 24-10) with tetragonal symmetry (Fig. 24-11). This combination overcomes the two principal difficulties in veneering metal with ceramic: having a porcelain firing temperature well below the melting range of the metal and having a sufficiently high thermal expansion compatible with the metal. After firing in the laboratory, dental ceramics consist of about 20 volume percent tetragonal leucite crystals dispersed in a glassy matrix.[13] The structure of this glassy matrix is a random Si-O network. The silicon atom combines with four oxygen atoms in a tetrahedral configuration (Fig. 24-12). These tetrahedra may be linked into a chain with both covalent and ionic bonds, leading to a stable structure. However, such a Si-O network would have a very high melting point. Usually, potassium and sodium are added to the glass composition to help break down

Composition of High-, Medium-, and Low-Fusing Body Porcelains (Weight Percent)

TABLE **24-1**

	High-fusing	Medium-fusing	Low-fusing (Vacuum Fired)	Metal-ceramic
SiO_2	72.9	63.1	66.5	59.2
Al_2O_3	15.9	19.8	13.5	18.5
Na_2O	1.68	2.0	4.2	4.8
K_2O	9.8	7.9	7.1	11.8
B_2O_3	—	6.8	6.6	4.6
ZnO	—	0.25	—	0.58
ZrO_2	—	—	—	0.39

Modified from Yamada HN, Grenoble PB: *Dental porcelain: the state of the art—1977*, Los Angeles, 1977, University of Southern California School of Dentistry.

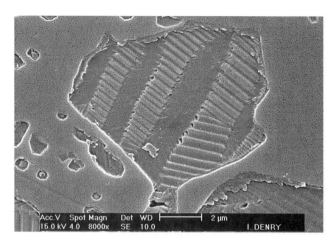

Fig. 24-10. Scanning electron micrograph of polished and etched leucite-containing dental ceramic showing a tetragonal leucite crystal.

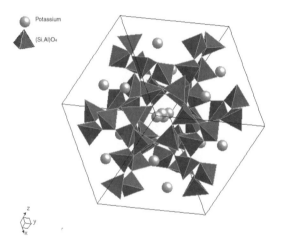

Fig. 24-11. Crystalline structure of low-temperature (tetragonal) leucite.

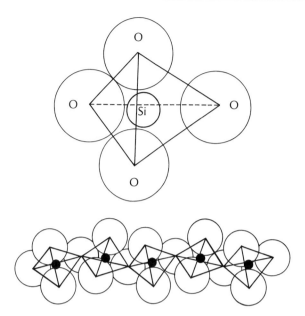

Fig. 24-12. The Si-O tetrahedral configuration. *(Redrawn from Gilman JJ: Sci Am 217:113, 1967.)*

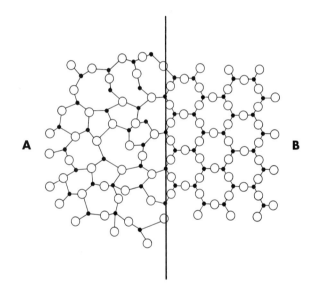

Fig. 24-13. Change in the Si-O network structure from a glassy (A) to a crystalline (B) form.
(Modified from Kingery WD et al: Introduction to ceramics, ed 2, New York, 1976, Wiley & Sons.)

the Si-O network and are therefore known as *glass modifiers*. In dental ceramics, potassium and sodium are initially provided by the feldspars. Two desirable consequences result: (1) the softening temperature of the glass is reduced, and (2) the coefficient of thermal expansion is increased. The manufacturer adjusts the oxide content so that the dental ceramic's coefficient of thermal expansion will be close to the corresponding value for the alloys used to make the substructure. If the composition of the glass is not properly adjusted, extensive breakdown and reorganization of the Si-O network may occur, leading to a crystallization of the glass (also called *devitrification*). The change in lattice structure from a vitreous to a crystalline form (devitrification) is shown schematically in Figure 24-13. This phenomenon may occur partially in dental ceramics if a ceramic restoration is fired too often, and it is typically associated with an increase in the coefficient of thermal expansion and **opacity**.

Feldspar also contains alumina (Al_2O_3), which acts as an intermediate oxide to increase the viscosity and hardness of the glass. As a result, dental porcelain has a good resistance to slump or pyroplastic flow, which is necessary to obtain the desired configuration of the restoration.

PORCELAIN TECHNIQUE
Dental porcelain is usually received from the manufacturer in powder form, which is mixed with either water or a water-based glycerin-containing liquid to form a paste of workable consistency. This mixture

is then used to make a restoration with the required configuration. Several condensation techniques (e.g., vibration and blotting) are used to remove as much excess water as possible. The porcelain particles are drawn together during condensation by capillary action. Proper condensation minimizes steam generation during the drying phase of firing. When the mass is heated, individual porcelain particles conglomerate by sintering. The viscous flow of unfused particles results in wetting and bridging between such particles (Fig. 24-14). Consequently, a loss of interstitial space occurs, accompanied by as much as a 27% to 45% volumetric shrinkage after firing.[14]

TYPES OF PORCELAIN

The following porcelain blends are produced for the different roles they play in the fabrication of metal-ceramic restorations: opaque, body, and incisal porcelains.

Opaque Porcelain. This is applied as a first ceramic coat and performs two major functions: it masks the color of the alloy, and it is responsible for the metal-ceramic bond.

The density of the oxides is greater than that of the glass matrix. Consequently, the oxides of tin, titanium, and zirconium have a higher refractive index than the components of the glass matrix (feldspar and quartz): 2.01 to 2.61 and 1.52 to 1.54, respectively. When a specific range of oxide particle sizes is used, most of the incident light is scattered and reflected rather than transmitted through the porcelain, effectively masking the color of the alloy substrate.

A scanning electron microscope (SEM) view of the alloy-porcelain interface[15] for a high noble metal alloy is shown in Fig. 24-15. When the region around the interface is examined for specific elements (a technique known as *elemental mapping*), the concentrations of aluminum and titanium can be identified. These appear as dense regions in the figure, indicating that discrete oxide particles of Al and Ti are in the opaque porcelain, probably just be-

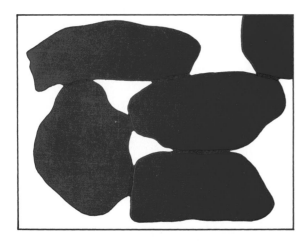

Fig. 24-14. Vitreous sintering. Glass flow (dark regions) leads to bonding of unfused particles.
(Modified from Van Vlack LH: Elements of materials science, ed 2, Reading, Mass, 1964, Addison-Wesley.)

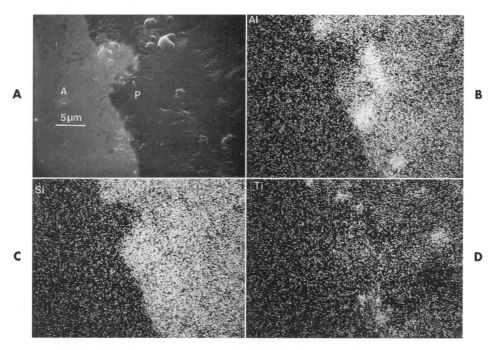

Fig. 24-15. Alloy-porcelain interface for a high noble metal alloy system, Degudent U (Degussa), and Vita normal (Vident). **A,** SEM of the interface. **B** to **D,** Elemental maps of aluminum, silicon, and titanium.
(From Laub LW et al: J Dent Res 57:A293, 1978 [abstract no. 874]).

neath the surface. By comparing the elemental map with the photomicrograph of the interface, identifying the distribution and size of the subsurface opacifying oxide particles is possible. Silicon examined in this way also demonstrates a uniform porcelain distribution, which is to be expected.

The oxides of titanium, zirconium, tin, or cerium are added to the original porcelain blend to help mask the color of the alloy. Because these oxides have an optical index of refraction different from the other components, they cause incident light to scatter and thereby mask the alloy substrate.

Body Porcelain. Body porcelain is fired onto the opaque layer, usually in conjunction with the incisal porcelain. It provides some translucency and contains oxides that aid in shade matching. Body porcelains are available in a wide selection of shades to match adjacent natural teeth. Most porcelain manufacturers provide an opaque shade for each body shade. Although porcelains of different manufacturers are given the same nominal shade (e.g., the popular Vita Lumin Vacuum shade guide), there is significant color variation among manufacturers,[16,17] and a dentist should know which brands the technician uses.

Incisal Porcelain. Incisal porcelain is usually translucent. As a result, the perceived color of the restoration is significantly influenced by the color of the underlying body porcelain.

• • •

PORCELAIN-ALLOY BONDING

William A. Brantley

Leon W. Laub

The formation of a strong bond between the opaque porcelain layer and the cast alloy is essential for the longevity of the metal-ceramic restoration. Extensive research over the past three decades has provided insight into the important factors for achieving metal-ceramic bonding. Early work[18] established the importance of wetting the alloy surface by the porcelain at the firing temperature. Although similar measurements of contact angles have not been reported for current dental porcelains and casting alloys, good wetting is essential to minimize porosity at the metal-ceramic interface. A detailed relationship between the elevated-temperature contact angle and metal-ceramic bonding has not been established, but the research by O'Brien and Ryge[18] indicates that perfect wetting (a contact angle of 0°) does not occur.

The model by Borom and Pask[19] considers idealized continuous lattice structure across the metal-ceramic interface for chemical bonding. This is achieved by incorporating certain oxidizable ele-

ments that become dissolved in the porcelain into the casting alloy composition. Recent research[20,21] has shown that the structure of the oxidized regions for high-palladium alloys is highly complex, and similar results would be anticipated for detailed studies of other types of oxidized casting alloys. The existence of multiple phases in the oxidized region of the alloy indicates that the proposed continuity[19] of atomic bonds cannot generally be achieved across the metal-ceramic interface, except possibly at sites where the glass matrix of the porcelain is in contact with the solid solution matrix of the alloy.

Manufacturers incorporate in the casting alloy composition small amounts of certain base metals that form oxides[22,23] and contribute chemical bonding to the metal-ceramic adherence. Studies using the electron microprobe and scanning electron microscope (SEM)[15,24-29] have shown that these elements accumulate at the metal-ceramic interface and form an interfacial oxide layer. For noble metal alloys, elements having a major role for porcelain adherence are iron (high-gold alloys), tin and indium (lower gold content, palladium-silver, silver-palladium, and high-palladium alloys), and gallium (high-palladium alloys). For base metal alloys where the principal elements are nickel and cobalt, chromium oxidation provides chemical bonding for porcelain adherence, whereas titanium oxidation fulfills this role for the titanium casting alloys.

Figure 24-16, *A*, is an SEM photomicrograph of the interface for a high-palladium alloy bonded to dental porcelain. This alloy undergoes complex external and internal oxidation during the porcelain firing cycles. The internal oxide particles in the palladium solid solution grains are too small (less than 1 to 2 μm diameter) for accurate compositional determinations with x-ray energy-dispersive spectroscopic analysis with the SEM. X-ray diffraction[20] has shown that $CuGa_2O_3$, SnO_2, and Cu_2O are present in the oxidation region when the alloy surface receives standard airborne particle abrasion with 50 μm aluminum oxide before oxidation. Figure 24-16, *B* shows line scans obtained with the SEM for major elements in the metal and ceramic near the interface. Variations in the x-ray counts occurred when the line scan crossed a region of internal oxidation.

FACTORS AFFECTING THE BOND

Most metal-ceramic systems require that the cast alloy be subjected to an initial oxidation step before the several layers of dental porcelain are fired. (A notable exception is the Pd-Cu-Ga high-palladium alloy *Freedom Plus*,* in which the oxidation step

---

*Jelenko: Armonk, N.Y.

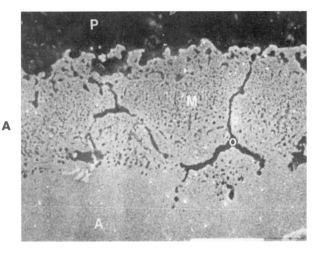

A

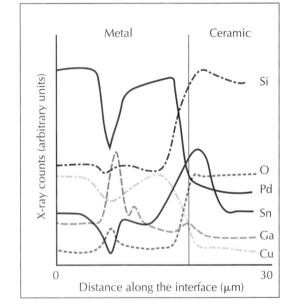

B

Fig. 24-16. **A,** Secondary electron image (SEM) photomicrograph of the metal-ceramic interface for Liberty (Jelenko) Pd-Cu-Ga high-palladium alloy bonded to Vita VMK 68 (Vident) dental porcelain. The grain boundaries of the alloy (M) have been widened by the formation of oxide (O) deposits, and there are numerous very small oxide particles within the grains. Scale bar = 10 μm. **B,** Elemental line scans perpendicular to the metal-ceramic interface obtained by x-ray energy-dispersive spectroscopic analyses for the Liberty alloy. Because the raw SEM data have not received matrix corrections, the relative elemental concentrations (x-ray counts) are qualitative, but the indicated trends are appropriate.
(From Papazoglou E et al: Int J Prosthodont 9:315, 1996.)

does not need to be performed before firing the opaque porcelain layer.) This step has also been called a *conditioning bake* or *degassing.* The latter term, which is frequently used in the dental laboratory industry, is inaccurate, because this procedure's purpose is to oxidize the metal surface for subsequent adherence to the fired porcelain. Historically, some individuals thought that the heating cy-

cle might result in loss of gases incorporated in the alloy during melting. However, this occurs during solidification because of the much greater solubility of atmospheric gases in the molten alloy compared to the solidified alloy; it results in the formation of microscopic porosity[30] in the casting.

The oxide layer between the metal and ceramic should have an optimum thickness for a strong metal-ceramic interfacial bond. This was demonstrated in the 1970s for selected noble and base metal alloys.[31] Research has shown that particular care is required with the base metal casting alloys to avoid excessively thick oxide layers.[32] Beryllium is added to some Ni-Cr alloy compositions to lower the melting range; beryllium also has an effect on the thickness of the oxide layer.[32] Some systems require the application of a bonding agent before firing of the opaque porcelain. Certain formulations consist of colloidal gold suspensions that are fired on silver-colored, gold-based ceramic alloys for esthetic purposes. SEM examination of the interfaces has shown that in Ni-Cr alloys, the bonding agents may increase or decrease the width of the interaction zone between the metal and ceramic.[28] An analysis of bonding agents for several Ni-Cr alloys indicates that they contain elements found in porcelain (e.g., aluminum, tin, and silicon).[33] For certain specific brands of Ni-Cr alloys, the bonding agent appears to increase the adherence between the alloy and the opaque porcelain. The manufacturer will indicate whether a bonding agent is necessary or beneficial.

Airborne particle abrasion with aluminum oxide (alumina) is routinely performed on the alloy castings to create surface irregularities and to provide mechanical interlocking with the opaque dental porcelain, which has sufficiently low viscosity in the firing temperature range to flow into these microscopic openings. Early studies found no effect of such surface roughening in the interfacial resistance of Au-Pt-Pd,[34] Au-Pd-Ag, and Ni-Cr[35] systems to shear loading. More recent research with a Pd-Cu-Ga high-palladium alloy showed that controlled amounts of mechanical surface roughening that yielded greater notch depth for the irregularities increased the metal-ceramic bond strength, with greater improvements from coarse roughening.[36]

The linear coefficients of thermal expansion for the metal (α_M) and ceramic (α_C) must closely match to achieve a strong interfacial bond. Typically, α_M values range from 13.5 to 14.5 x 10^{-6}/° C; α_C values range from 13.0 to 14.0 x 10^{-6}/° C.[37] The slightly higher coefficient for the metal causes the ceramic to be in a beneficial state of residual compressive stress at room temperature (Fig. 24-17). (The thermal con-

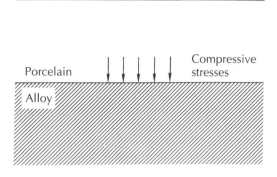

Fig. 24-17. Porcelain in a state of compression at the alloy interface.

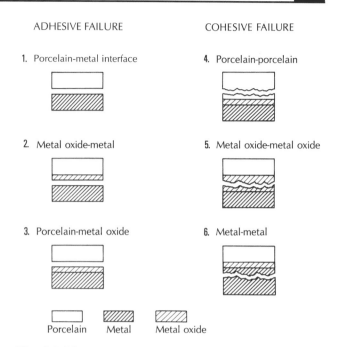

Fig. 24-18. Possible modes of failure of alloy-porcelain restorations.
(Modified from O'Brien WJ: In Valega TM Sr: Alternatives to gold alloys in dentistry, DHEW publ. no. (NIH) 77-1227, Washington, D.C., 1977, U.S. Government Printing Office.)

traction and expansion coefficients are assumed to be equal, and residual stress is only developed in the ceramic below its glass transition temperature where viscous flow is no longer possible.) Porcelain is much stronger in compression than tension, and residual tensile stress in the porcelain must be avoided to prevent fracture of the restoration.

Adherence between the alloy casting and porcelain is very important in fixed prosthodontics, and investigators have used a variety of test configurations with shear, tensile, flexural, and torsional loading to determine the metal-ceramic bond strength. Ideally, the interfacial bond is strong enough so that fracture of the test specimen occurs entirely within the porcelain (cohesive failure). In one early study,[38] no significant difference was found in the diametral tensile strength of commercial dental porcelains for air-firing and vacuum-firing. Lower-strength values of 28 MPa (4100 psi) for opaque porcelain compared to 42 MPa (6100 psi) for gingival porcelain were attributed to greater porosity and the inclusion of opacifying oxides in the latter. In addition, vacuum-firing appeared to have little effect on the porosity of the opaque porcelain. Based on this research, the tensile strength of the metal-ceramic bond should exceed 28 MPa to have cohesive failure through the porcelain rather than failure at the interface. Measurement of the shear strength of dental porcelain[39] allows a similar prediction for the minimum interfacial shear strength required for cohesive shear failure through the ceramic. Results from several studies[33,40,41] that measured the tensile bond strength of metal-ceramic systems were consistent with these concepts. Cohesive failure within the porcelain occurred at 15 to 39 MPa (2200 to 5700 psi), whereas bond strengths measured in shear ranged from 55 to 103 MPa (8000 to 15,000 psi). For many of the shear bond strength determinations, a mixed mode of failure was observed, where adhesive failure at the metal-ceramic interface extended into the porcelain, which fractured cohesively.

In more recent years, the focus has been directed toward measurement of porcelain adherence rather than determination of metal-ceramic bond strength. A finite element analysis of the tests used to measure metal-ceramic bond strength (e.g., pull-shear, three-point bending, and four-point bending) by Anusavice et al[42] revealed two major problems with all the tests: the stress varied with position along the metal-ceramic interface (particularly near porcelain termination sites), and there was a lack of the pure shear stress conditions that were considered to simulate the loading expected to cause clinical failure most effectively. Furthermore, the small mismatch between the thermal coefficients of the metal (α_M) and ceramic (α_C) results in an unknown amount of residual stress at the interface, and an idealized value of metal-ceramic bond strength assumes the presence of a residual stress-free interface.

To avoid these problems, O'Brien[43,44] proposed a completely different approach, focusing on the mode of failure of metal-ceramic specimens or restorations. The adhesive and/or cohesive failure can occur at six possible sites or combinations of those sites (Fig. 24-18). Adhesive failure can occur at the porcelain-metal interface (1) if no oxide layer is present, and at the metal oxide-metal interface (2) and the porcelain-metal oxide interface (3). Cohesive failure can occur through the porcelain (4), which is the desirable mode, and through the metal oxide layer (5) and metal (6).* This philosophy has been adopted in the American National Standards Institute/American Dental Association (ANSI/ADA) specification no. 38 for metal-ceramic systems,[45] although the method of microscopic measurement has not been specified.

A quantitative x-ray spectrometric method was developed by Ringle et al[46] to measure porcelain adherence. The fracture surfaces of metal-ceramic specimens loaded to failure in biaxial flexure are examined with the SEM, using x-ray energy-dispersive analysis. The x-ray spectrometric method is based on the principle that silicon is a major element in dental porcelain but is largely absent in dental alloys (except as contaminants from investments or polishing abrasives used to prepare specimens). The amount of dental porcelain remaining on the metal surface of the fractured specimen is readily determined by measuring the Si Kα signal, with necessary calibration measurements on the oxidized alloy surface before porcelain application and on the porcelain surface before testing the specimen. This technique has been used to measure the oxide adherence to a variety of ceramic alloys[47] and was recently used to measure the porcelain adherence to high-palladium alloys.[48,49]

Another philosophical change in the recommended method for evaluating the metal-ceramic bond appears to be underway with the introduction of ISO (International Organization for Standardization) standard no. 9693 for dental porcelain fused to metal restorations,[50] which contains a three-point bending test. Lenz et al[51] have performed a finite element analysis for this test, considering the stress concentrations that arise at the porcelain termination sites, although the effect of unknown residual stresses arising from the mismatch between α_M and α_C could not be included.[52] A recent study using several Pd-Ga high-palladium alloys with identical values of elastic modulus found no correlation between the porcelain adherence measured by the x-ray spectrometric method[46,48] and the force to failure using the three-point bending test in ISO standard no. 9693[50] and the Lenz et al analysis.[51] These experimental results cast doubt on the x-ray spectrometric technique's[46,48] effectiveness in measuring porcelain adherence. Future experimental research in this area may use a fracture-mechanics approach to evaluate the metal-ceramic interfacial bond.

Other important factors that affect the metal-ceramic bond are the surface treatment of the alloy before firing the porcelain and the atmosphere of the

porcelain furnace during firing. As previously mentioned, air-abrasion of the cast alloy is typically performed before the oxidation step to help remove surface contaminants that remain from devesting and to help clean the casting and provide microscopic surface irregularities for mechanical retention of the ceramic. The oxidation step for the alloy can be performed in air or by using the reduced atmospheric pressure (approximately 0.1 atm) available in dental porcelain furnaces. A much thinner oxide layer will be formed if the alloy is oxidized at this reduced atmospheric pressure compared to the thickness for oxidation in air. One manufacturer (Jelenko) recommends performing the oxidation step in air and then carefully reducing the thickness of the oxide layer before firing the opaque porcelain. Manufacturer recommendations for the oxidation of the alloy and the porcelain firing cycles must be followed. An early study[53] showed that the shear bond strength of porcelain-gold alloy specimens was 60% greater when air firing was employed; another study at that time[54] reported that the tensile bond strength varied according to the furnace atmosphere used. The shear bond strength of porcelain-nickel-based alloy specimens was greater when firing was performed in oxidizing atmospheres, compared to nonoxidizing or reducing atmospheres.[55] More recently, Wagner et al[36] found that the use of a reducing atmosphere severely reduced the bond strength of a Pd-Cu-Ga high-palladium alloy, which confirmed the role of alloy oxidation during the standard porcelain firing cycles.

• • •

SELECTION CRITERIA

Most manufacturers of modern dental porcelains specify the alloy systems with which a material is compatible. Usually that compatibility refers to the relative coefficients of thermal expansion. The shade selected clinically determines which powders to combine. Depending on the characteristics of the color to be matched, several powders can be combined for the desired esthetic result. Commercially available porcelains can be divided into fine grain and coarse grain types. The typical particle size of a fine-grain porcelain ranges from 5 to 110 μm; the particle size for a coarse-grain porcelain can be as large as 200 μm.

OPAQUE PORCELAIN

For a proper mechanical bond and chemical interaction at the interface, opaque porcelain must wet the surface easily. It becomes the primary source of color of the restoration and must mask the color of the metal, even in thin layers. Opaque thickness generally should not exceed 0.1 mm; otherwise, achieving

---

*Metal fracture is highly unlikely but is included in this model for completeness.

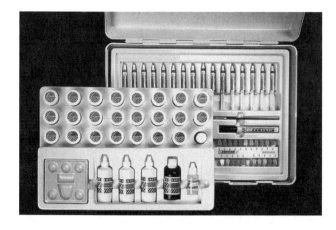

Fig. 24-19. Metal-ceramic porcelain. Opaque porcelains are available as powders or pastes. *(Courtesy Ivoclar North America.)*

an esthetic result without overcontouring the restoration becomes impossible, although a greater thickness may be needed to mask the darker oxide of some alloys.[56] Small amounts of zirconium oxide and titanium oxide, in conjunction with alumina, act as the opacifying agents to block the darker color of the oxidized metal. Some of these oxides are also present in the body porcelain. Manufacturers supply opaque porcelains in paste and powder form (Fig. 24-19).

BODY AND INCISAL PORCELAINS
As with opaque porcelain, the selection of body and incisal porcelains is based largely on their esthetic properties. However, the amount of shrinkage that occurs when these powders are fired must also be considered. Body and incisal porcelains usually shrink as much as 27% to 45% of their volume during a first firing[14]; opaque porcelain, on the other hand, may exhibit some cracking during an initial bake, but it will remain relatively stable dimensionally. Recently, lower-fusing metal-ceramic porcelains* have become popular.[57] These materials should be considered when opposing enamel wear is likely to be a problem, because in vitro they tend to exhibit lower abrasiveness than conventional formulations.[58]

⊡ FABRICATION

For optimum esthetics, custom-mixing body and enamel powders to achieve desired color variations is recommended.

PORCELAIN APPLICATION
Armamentarium (Fig. 24-20)
- Porcelain modeling liquid

- Paper napkin
- Glass slab or palette
- Tissues or gauze squares
- Two cups of distilled water
- Glass spatula
- Serrated instrument
- Porcelain tweezers or hemostat
- Ceramist's sable brushes (no. 2, 4, and 6) and whipping brush
- Razor blade or modeling knife
- Cyanoacrylate resin
- Colored pencil or felt marker
- Articulating tape
- Ceramic-bound stones
- Flexible thin diamond disk (about 20 mm in diameter)

Step-by-step Procedure. After the metal substructure has been oxidized, it must be inspected carefully. An uninterrupted oxide layer should cover the entire surface to be veneered.

Opaque Porcelain (Fig. 24-21)
1. When selecting the opaque bottle, shake it to mix the powder thoroughly. Then place it on the bench to allow the smaller pigment particles to settle. Over time, all porcelain powders will segregate into layers of different particle size if left undisturbed.
2. Dispense a small amount of powder on a glass slab or palette. Add some modeling liquid and mix it with the spatula. Metal instruments should not be used in mixing, because metal particles could rub off and act as contaminants. The proper opaque consistency should "hold an edge" for a few seconds.
3. Moisten the substructure with some of the liquid and pick up a small bead of opaque with the tip of the brush or spatula. Apply it to the coping, which should be held with the porcelain tweezers.
4. Use light vibration to spread the material thinly and evenly. Moving the serrated instrument back and forth over the handle of the tweezers will create the necessary disturbance. Excess moisture that comes to the surface can be blotted off with a clean tissue. Vibration may not be as necessary with the so-called paint opaques.
5. Apply a second bead on top of the first and spread it in a similar manner. To minimize the entrapment of air when the two masses meet, do not apply opaque porcelain adjacent to the initial mass. If the moisture content is properly controlled, condensing will pose little difficulty. A mix that is too wet will slump and

*Finesse: Ceramco; Omega 900: Vident.

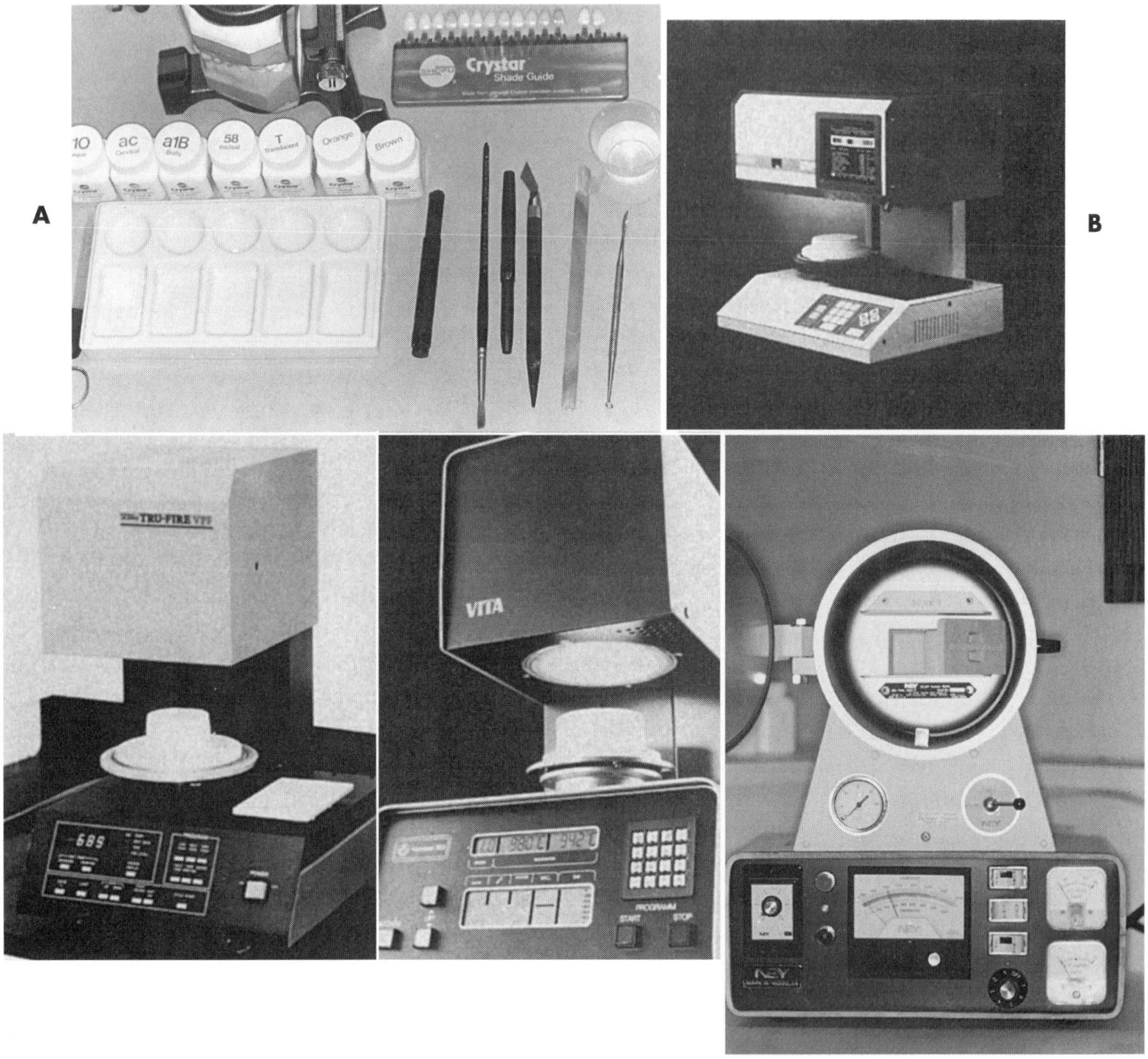

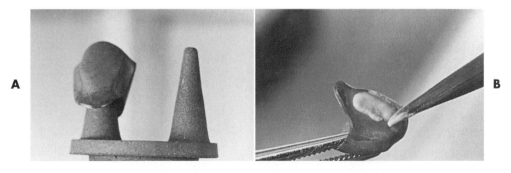

Fig. 24-20. **A,** Armamentarium for porcelain application. **B,** CMP KC 2000. Vacuum porcelain furnaces **C,** Jelenko Tru-Fire VPF; **D,** Vita Vacumat; **E,** Ney Mark III.
*(**B** courtesy CMP Industries, Inc. **D** courtesy Vident.)*

Fig. 24-21. Opaque porcelain application. **A,** Substructure is oxidized. **B,** Porcelain is applied.

Continued

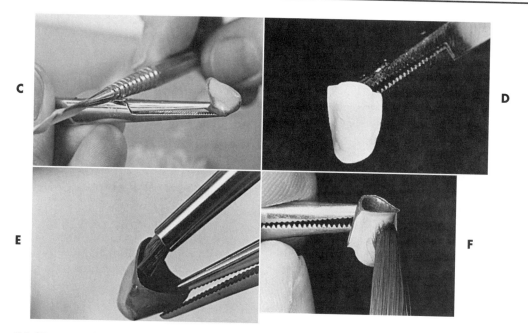

Fig. 24-21, cont'd.   **C,** Vibration can be used to help spread the opaque into an even, thin film. **D,** After drying in front of the furnace, the opaque powder should have a uniform matte-white appearance. **E,** Excess must be removed before firing. Use a stiff brush. **F,** If a second application is necessary, the surface should be wetted and additional opaque added.

produce too thick a layer on the substructure, especially in the concave areas near the porcelain-metal junction.

6. Once the veneering surface is covered, add more material to a dry base. Wetting the initial application before adding more porcelain may be necessary. If not, the moisture will be absorbed immediately by the dry base layer before a new material can be properly condensed and distributed, which will result in a porous and weakened application (similar to constructing a sand castle with wet sand on a dry beach). The addition of more liquid and further vibration will resolve the problem.

7. When the entire veneering surface has been covered, remove any excess material from other surfaces with the side of a slightly moistened brush. If the metal immediately adjacent to the veneer has been properly prepared and smoothed, the excess porcelain will not be difficult to remove. However, this critical task is often overlooked and can make metal polishing much more difficult.

8. After removing any excess porcelain, carefully inspect the inside of the restoration for porcelain particles. A stiff, dry, short-bristle brush can be used to remove the particles.

9. Before firing, inspect the opaque application to see that it satisfies the following criteria:

- The entire veneering surface is evenly covered with a smooth layer that masks the color of the metal.
- There is no excess anywhere on the veneering surface.
- There is no opaque on any external surface adjacent to the veneer.
- There is no opaque on the internal aspect of the substructure.

If these criteria have been met, the coping is transferred to a sagger tray and placed near the open muffle of the porcelain furnace for several minutes. This allows moisture to evaporate. When drying is completed, (this varies according to specific manufacturer's recommendations), reinspect the work for any residual excess opaque powder. Material that was previously overlooked will be clearly visible, because the chalky white porcelain contrasts with the darker oxidized metal. A stiff, short-bristle brush can again be used to remove any remaining porcelain. The opaque is then fired according to manufacturer recommendations.

10. After the first firing, remove the work from the muffle and set it aside to cool to room temperature.

11. At this time, inspect the opaque veneer for cracks, thin spots, and general adequacy of coverage. When the veneer is removed from the furnace, it will appear yellow; however, when it has cooled, the more representative

matte-white color is apparent. Fired opaque should have an eggshell appearance. If necessary, a second application of opaque can be made. Small cracks and fissures are common after the first firing. This problem can be resolved by applying moisture, followed by a thin mix of opaque carefully condensed into the fissures. When correcting a thin area where the color of the metal has not been masked completely, the surface should be moistened before a second coat is applied (to facilitate wetting).

12. After firing, check that the opaque application (Fig. 24-22) meets the following criteria:
- Relatively smooth even layer masking the color of the framework
- Eggshell appearance
- No excess on any external or internal surface of the restoration (which would prevent it from seating fully on the die)

Body and Incisal Porcelains (Fig. 24-23). When a satisfactory opaque layer has been fired, the body and incisal porcelains can be applied. The use of several porcelains in one restoration is common. Body porcelains with increased opacity* may be used where less translucency is required (e.g., gingival area of the pontic, incisal mamelons) to mimic existing anatomic features of adjacent natural teeth. Special neck powders can be applied on the cervical third, and incisal powders on the incisal edge, to simulate natural enamel. Generally, the restoration is built to anatomic contour; when it is acceptable, a cut-back similar to that made during the waxing stage will allow for a veneer of the more translucent incisal porcelain.

1. Dispense the neck, body, incisal, and other powders on a glass slab or palette. If the same

---

*Often called *opacious dentins.*

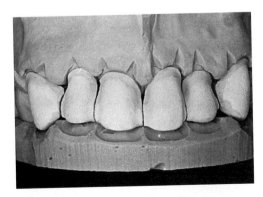

Fig. 24-22.   Evaluation of the opaque porcelain.

---

slab was used for the opaque porcelain, any opaque residue must be removed.

2. Mix the powders with the recommended liquid or distilled water. The moisture content for these powders should be the same as for opaque porcelain. Specially formulated liquids are available that allow longer manipulation than is possible with conventional glycerin-containing liquids.

3. Wet the previously fired opaque layer with a small amount of the liquid and place a bead of neck powder on the cervical portion of the veneering surface. Gentle patting with a brush and light tapping on the cast will produce adequate vibration during the preliminary stage of condensation. A tissue is held close for removal of excess surface moisture. During the entire buildup procedure, the facial surface should not be blotted with tissue, because the smaller pigment particles might be removed. Blotting consistently from the lingual aspect is recommend and will result in superior esthetics.

4. After placing the neck powder and sculpting it, build the veneer to anatomic contour with body porcelain. Use the adjacent and opposing teeth as a guide. Where contact is anticipated between the wet buildup and stone cast, the cast can be coated with a small amount of cyanoacrylate resin, immediately blown into a thin layer. This will seal the surface and prevent the absorption of moisture from the buildup.

5. To compensate for the firing shrinkage that results when the particles fuse, slightly overbuild the porcelain. A typical metal-ceramic anterior crown will shrink 0.6 mm at the incisal edge and 0.5 mm midfacially[59] (Fig. 24-24).

6. When the body buildup is completed, assess it for proper mesiodistal, faciolingual, and incisogingival contour.

7. Depending on the desired appearance, make a cut-back for the more translucent incisal powder. Some manufacturers recommend carrying the incisal veneer all the way to the cervical portion of the restoration, while others suggest limiting it to the incisal third. An almost infinite variety of possibilities exist, and only with experience can the dentist predict the finished product's appearance. Whether the cut-back is made with a razor blade, scalpel, or modeling instrument, condensing the body buildup well before cutting back is necessary. This will minimize the risk of fracture during the process. Furthermore, to minimize the chance of damaging the unsupported

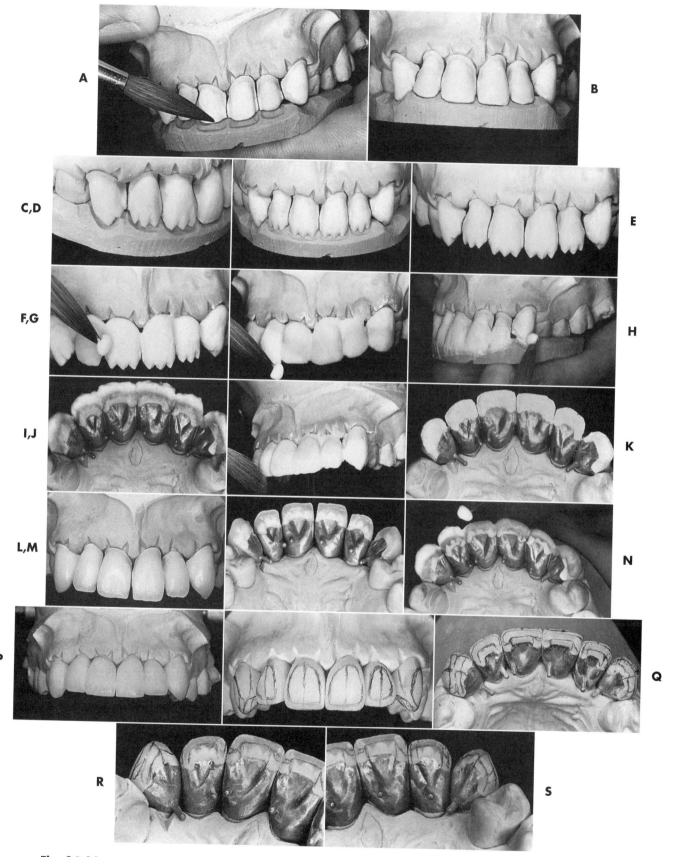

Fig. 24-23. Body and incisal porcelain application. **A** to **E,** Development of incisal mamelons with opacious dentin. The incisal plaster index is made from the anatomic contour wax patterns (see Chapter 18) and serves as a guide to developing proper incisal edge position. **F** and **G,** Cervical and body powders are added to the contour. **H,** Alternatively, the incisal index can be used to establish incisal edge position. This is especially helpful for extensive restorations. **I,** Restorations are slightly overbuilt. **J,** The buildup is smoothed with a whipping brush. **K,** Restorations are separated with a razor blade before firing. Additional porcelain is added to the proximal contacts. **L** and **M,** Restorations after firing of the first body bake. **N,** Porcelain is added in areas of deficient contour. **O,** After firing, the proximal contacts are carefully adjusted, and the restorations are seated on the cast. **P** to **S,** Restorations are contoured by grinding. Careful attention is paid to the shape and position of line angles and incisal edges. When completed, the restorations are ready for try-in and final contouring intraorally (see Chapter 30).

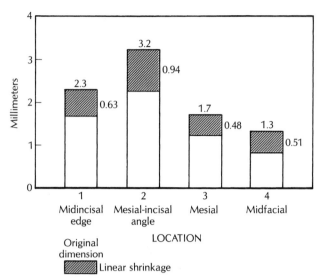

Fig. 24-24. Mean shrinkage values from firing of a typical maxillary central incisor metal-ceramic crown. *(From Rosenstiel SF: Br Dent J 162:390, 1987.)*

incisal portion of the buildup, the cut-back should be made from incisal to cervical. Adequate space must exist for the incisal veneer in the interproximal area.

8. Apply the incisal powder in the same manner and overbuild the restoration as described for body porcelain. The remaining body powder must be wet before application of the incisal powder, and, again, intermittent light vibration will help achieve an acceptable level of condensation. Prolonged condensation should be avoided. It will not reduce porosity[60] or increase fracture toughness[61] and may lead to unwanted redistribution of the pigmented particles.

9. Mark the opposing teeth on the stone cast with a red or green felt tip marker. These markings will not be absorbed if the cast first has been coated with cyanoacrylate resin. The articulator can then be closed to allow the antagonists to contact the wet porcelain. If this is done carefully, the markings will be transferred onto the buildup without fracturing, and it can be modified to the necessary occlusal scheme. Only red or green dyes, which burn off without leaving a residue, should be used for these markings. Blue or black pigments usually contain metal oxides or carbon, which after firing can discolor the porcelain.

10. Moisten the proximal contact areas immediately before removing the completed buildup from the cast. This reduces the risk of fracturing that portion of the buildup.

11. After the coping has been removed from the cast, fill in the proximal contact areas. At this

time, the work should be reinspected for any excess material beyond the veneering area (which, as before, must be removed before firing). The internal aspect of the coping should be reinspected even more carefully, because enamel powders are quite transparent in thin layers and are not easily detected after firing.

12. Place the restoration on a sagger tray close to the open muffle at the drying temperature recommended by the manufacturer. A drying time of 6 to 10 minutes is usually sufficient. If a restoration is fired prematurely, the residual moisture in the buildup may generate steam, and the accompanying vapor pressure will cause the buildup to explode. After the drying process, once it has been determined that no undesired excess material remains, proceed with firing. When the bake is completed, the work should cool to room temperature before further handling. Follow the manufacturer's recommendations concerning the cooling rate after firing. Incorrect cooling rates may lead to residual stresses that will eventually result in porcelain fracture during function. Thermal expansion will increase after slow cooling, because additional (high-expansion) leucite will crystallize.[62] In general, alloys with high thermal expansion coefficients require more rapid cooling than alloys with low coefficients.[63]

13. Be especially critical when evaluating the first (or low bisque) bake. If the surface is fissured, grind the porcelain before adding any more (Fig. 24-25). The shape of the restoration should conform to the standards set by dental anatomy and the predetermined occlusal scheme for the patient.

14. Remove all excess material with ceramic-bound stones. A flexible diamond disk is imperative for proper shaping of the embrasure spaces. To extend its life, the disk should be kept moist.

15. When the restoration has been contoured and all the necessary areas reduced, certain portions will probably require a second application of porcelain.

16. Before a second corrective bake (also referred to as a *patch bake*), clean the restoration ultrasonically to remove any grinding debris.

17. Place the second body and incisal layers directly on the slightly moistened low **bisque bake**. Evaluate the color at this time, keeping the restoration moist. Sometimes another bake will be needed, particularly for an extensive prosthesis. However, multiple firing

A   **B**   **C**   **D**

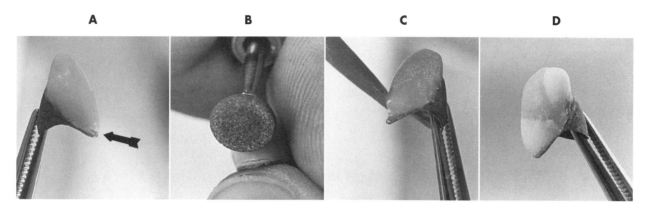

Fig. 24-25. **A,** This restoration had a defect *(arrow)* at the gingival margin after the first firing. **B,** Access for the repair has been made with a stone. **C,** The area is moistened where porcelain is to be added. **D,** The porcelain has been added, and the restoration is ready for the second firing.

will lead to devitrification of the porcelain, with a loss of translucency and a decrease in the restoration's fracture resistance.[64]

INTERNAL CHARACTERIZATION

Internal or intrinsic characterization or staining may be accomplished by incorporating colored pigments in the opaque, body, or incisal powder. These pigments are ceramic in nature and have physical properties similar to the porcelain powders.

Most commercially available porcelains have colored opaque modifiers that can be selectively mixed with the opaque to increase the saturation of the desired pigment. A variation of this approach is to use opacified dentin powders that produce a finished restoration with a slightly higher chroma than one prepared with the more translucent dentin powders. Similarly, a translucent powder can be used to enhance incisal translucency (Fig. 24-26). Highly colored glazes, commonly used as surface **stains**, may be layered within the buildup powders to create special effects (Fig. 24-27).

The use of internal stains presents little technical difficulty for operators familiar with metal-ceramic procedures. However, because the pigment is built into the material, if the desired effect is not obtained through internal staining, the porcelain must be stripped from the substructure.

Another technique for internal characterization is to fire the body powders initially, carve them into the desired mamelon shape, and then apply the subsequent enamel powders (Fig. 24-28). A disadvantage of this approach is that an additional firing is needed.

CONTOURING

The appearance of the finished restoration depends on its color, shape, and surface texture, which can be altered by shaping and characterizing dental porce-

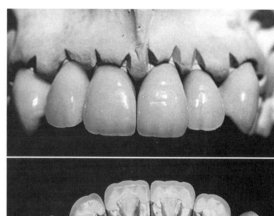

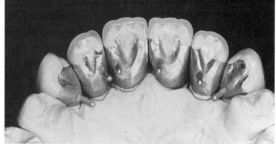

Fig. 24-26. Incisal translucency has been achieved through subtle layering of porcelains of different shades.

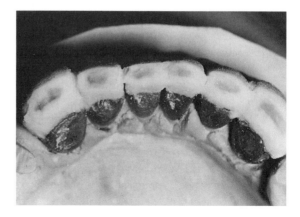

Fig. 24-27. Porcelain stain was applied intrinsically to create the effect of discolored dentin in these mandibular incisors seen before firing.

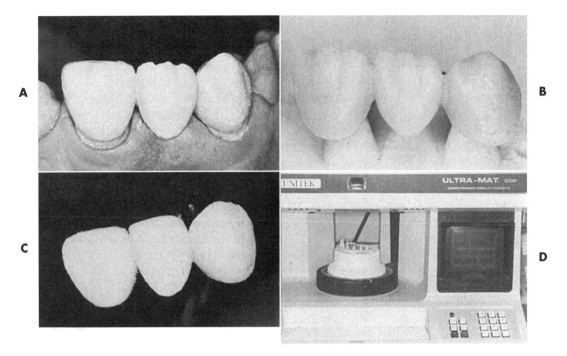

Fig. 24-28. **A,** Body powder is sculpted in the desired shape. **B,** Mamelon configuration is carved in the fired body bake. **C,** Additional enamel powder is added, and the buildup is slightly overcontoured. **D,** Second firing of the anatomical contour buildup. *(Courtesy Dr. M. Chen.)*

lain to mimic the appearance of natural teeth (see Fig. 24-23, *P* to *S*).

The appearance of restorations can be influenced considerably through the selected use of optical illusion (see Chapter 20). The human eye is capable of discerning differences in height and width, but its depth perception is far less developed. Even trained observers experience difficulty when attempting to recognize subtle differences in the third dimension.

Through selective contouring, the apparent shape of a restoration can be made to look quite different from its actual configuration. The perceived size of a tooth depends on the reflection of its line angles and the relative position and spacing of these reflections. Even though an edentulous area on one side may be slightly larger than a space occupied by the corresponding tooth on the contralateral side, a restoration can be made to appear similar (or even identical) through careful mimicking of the line angle distribution and contours immediately adjacent to the line angles. An illusion is created that the restoration is narrower than it really is (Fig. 24-29). In addition, by simulating the normal distance between line angles superimposed on a pontic in an edentulous area that is otherwise too narrow, it is possible to create the illusion that teeth are of normal size but merely crowded. Careful application of these principles may trick the casual observer into concluding that the teeth overlap and that a portion

of the tooth (or restoration) is behind an adjacent tooth when, in reality, it does not exist.

The surface texture of a metal-ceramic restoration should resemble that of the adjacent teeth, including selected characterizing irregularities that exist on those teeth. Several rules of light reflection must be remembered when attempting to accomplish this:

1. A flat surface will reflect primarily parallel light bundles.
2. A convex surface will result in divergence of reflected light, whereas a concave surface will create a convergent light bundle.
3. Sharp transitions (e.g., geometric line angles) will result in line reflections, but smooth, gently flowing curved surfaces will create a reflection pattern with greater surface area.

Thus a smooth restoration can appear larger than one of identical size that has been characterized or textured. Careful study of adjacent teeth and an understanding of how their reflective patterns should be simulated before characterization are essential. Care must also be taken not to "overcharacterize," which would draw attention to the restoration and reveal that it is artificial.

GLAZING AND SURFACE CHARACTERIZATION

Metal-ceramic restorations are glazed to create a shiny surface similar to that of natural teeth (Fig. 24-30).* The glazing cycle can be performed concur-

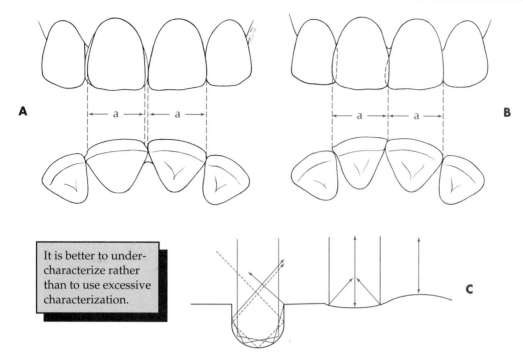

It is better to under-characterize rather than to use excessive characterization.

Fig. 24-29. **A** and **B,** The esthetics of an abnormally sized restoration can be improved by matching the location of the line angles and adjusting the interproximal areas. **C,** The pattern of light reflection depends on the surface texture of the restoration.
(A and B redrawn from Blancheri RL: Rev Asoc Dent Mex 8:103, 1959.)

rently with any necessary surface characterization (see Chapter 30).

In *autoglazing* the contoured bisque bake is raised to its fusion temperature and maintained for a time before cooling. A pyroplastic surface flow occurs, and a vitreous layer or surface glaze is formed. Sharp angles and edges are rounded slightly during this process. Consequently, occlusal contact in porcelain will be altered slightly during glazing.

By contrast, in *overglazing,* a separate mix of powder and liquid is applied to the surface of a shaped restoration, and the restoration is subsequently fired. The firing procedure is similar to that for autoglazing, although there are variations among brands. Because most metal-ceramic restorations use low-fusing porcelain, overglazing is not currently in widespread use.

EXTERNAL CHARACTERIZATION

Surface stains are highly pigmented glazes, which can be mixed with glycerin and water (supplied with most commercially available staining kits).

By moistening the bisque firing, mimicking the appearance of the glazed restoration is made possi-

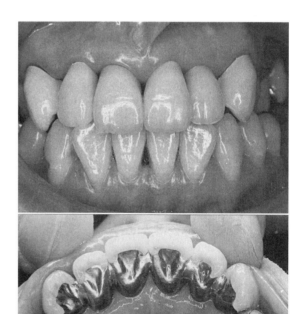

Fig. 24-30. Glazed and polished restorations.

ble. After the desired effect has been obtained by placing selected stains on the surface, the restoration is held outside the open muffle of the glazing furnace, and the stain is allowed to dry.

---

*An acceptable alternative is to polish the ceramic (see Chapter 30).

When it turns white and chalky, any excess that may have been accidentally applied to the metal surface is removed, and the restoration is fired. During this staining and glazing bake, a pyroplastic surface flow occurs, and a glassy layer (or autoglaze) forms on the surface in which the stains are incorporated.

PORCELAIN LABIAL MARGINS

Many patients object to the grayness at the margin associated with metal-ceramic restorations. However, hiding the margin subgingivally may not be possible. If esthetics is of prime importance, a collarless metal-ceramic crown (Fig. 24-31) should be considered. Collarless crowns have a facial margin of porcelain and lingual and proximal margins of metal* (Fig. 24-32).

ADVANTAGES AND DISADVANTAGES

The collarless crown's most obvious advantage is the esthetic improvement it offers compared to the conventional metal-ceramic restoration. Plaque removal also is easier when gingival tissues are in contact with vacuum-fired glazed porcelain than when they are contacting highly polished gold. Therefore, porcelain would appear to be the material of choice for restorations that will be in contact with gingival tissues.

---

*Some technicians fabricate a 360° porcelain margin to optimize light transmission in the gingival area and provide optimal esthetics. The technique is quite demanding. Preparation for these restorations is similar to an all-ceramic crown (see Chapter 11) with a circumferential shoulder with rounded internal line angles.

The difficulties encountered during fabrication, however, limit its application. Although a technically comparable result is feasible,[65,66] the marginal adaptation of these restorations (as presently produced by most commercial laboratories) is slightly inferior to that of cast metal. Due to careless handling, fracture of the unsupported margin is sometimes a problem during try-in or cementation. Fracture during function is rarely a problem, because the labial margin is not subjected to high tensile stresses.[67] In addition, the collarless metal-ceramic restoration is more time consuming and therefore more costly to make.

INDICATIONS AND CONTRAINDICATIONS

A porcelain labial margin is indicated when a conventional metal-ceramic restoration will not create the desired esthetic result. It is contraindicated when an extremely smooth, 1-mm-wide shoulder cannot be prepared in the area of the ceramic veneer. (In this respect, the conventional metal-ceramic restoration is somewhat more "forgiving.") Although multiple porcelain margins may be used in one fixed prosthesis without sacrificing marginal adaptation, the limitations of the operator and the technical auxiliaries should be carefully and objectively assessed before the dentist and patient commit themselves to a fixed prosthesis consisting of multiple collarless retainers.

FRAMEWORK DESIGN FOR LABIAL MARGIN

Various framework designs have been proposed with different facial framework reductions[68] (Fig. 24-33). In general, the more metal reduction, the better the esthetic result. However, the technical proce-

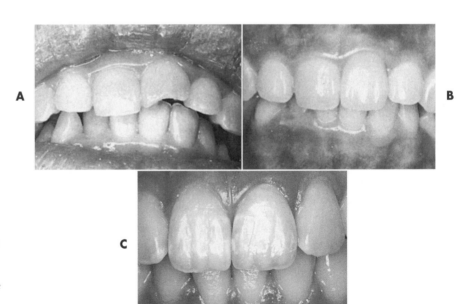

Fig. 24-31. **A** and **B,** A porcelain labial margin was used on this metal-ceramic restoration of a maxillary left central incisor. **C,** Multiple restorations with porcelain labial margins.

dures become more demanding. Removal of up to 2 mm of the labial framework has been shown not to decrease the fracture resistance of the restoration.[69,70]

METHODS OF FABRICATION

Several techniques have been proposed to fabricate porcelain labial margins in metal-ceramic restorations: platinum foil matrix, direct lift or cyanoacrylate resin, and porcelain wax.

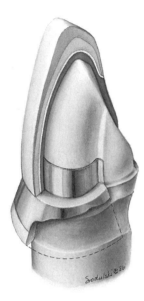

Fig. 24-32. Schematic of a collarless restoration fabricated with the platinum foil technique. To support the foil during burnishing, a "skirt" of a suitable blockout material has been added to the facial aspect of the die adjacent to the proposed porcelain labial margin. This will prevent distortion of the foil upon removal from the die. Alternatively, a blocked-out die can be duplicated in epoxy resin or electroplated.

Platinum Foil Matrix Technique. The platinum foil technique[4] uses a platinum matrix that is spot-welded to the metal substructure. Its primary purpose is to support the porcelain during firing.

Step-by-step Procedure (Fig. 24-34)

1. Wax the metal substructure and cast it in the conventional manner. Some technicians prefer to cast a conventional restoration and trim the collar off the casting; others wax the substructure exactly as desired and cast it.

2. To prevent the foil from becoming distorted on removal, block out undercuts apical to the margin. Modeling compound is suitable for this step. Any excess that may have covered the shoulder of the tooth preparation must be carefully cleaned off. Some prefer to use epoxy or electroplated dies so that more pressure can be applied during burnishing without the risk of chipping.

3. Burnish a small piece of platinum foil onto the facial portion of the die where the porcelain margin is to be placed, and extend it a few millimeters onto the axial wall of the preparation.

4. After burnishing, trim it so there is a 2- to 3-mm "skirt" lying cervical to the margin.

5. Carefully place the coping over the foil and, if necessary, scrape the die in the cervical area (on the facial aspect only) to allow the casting to seat. To help stabilize the foil, a drop of sticky wax may be applied.

6. Remove the casting from the die, together with the foil, and position the assembly between the electrodes of an orthodontic spot

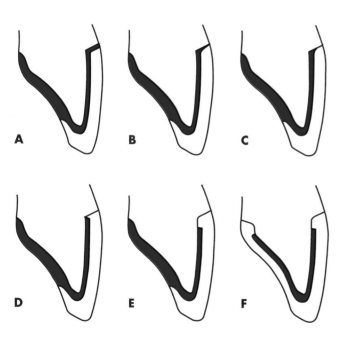

Fig. 24-33. Labial margin designs for metal-ceramic restorations. **A,** A thin metal band provides excellent adaptation but is very unesthetic unless it can be hidden subgingivally. For esthetic reasons, this design is rarely used for anterior teeth. **B,** "Disappearing" margin, sometimes called a *conventional margin,* is commonly used and is esthetically acceptable in some patients. However, the metal often causes unacceptable greyness of the gingival tooth surface. **C** to **E,** Various cut-back designs for labial porcelain margin restorations. Reducing the metal will provide better esthetics but makes the laboratory phase more demanding and may result in margin chipping. **F,** A 360-degree porcelain margin provides excellent light transmission in the gingival area and optimal esthetics; however, the laboratory fabrication is very demanding. This design requires a preparation design that is similar to an all-ceramic crown (see Chapter 11) with a circumferential rounded shoulder. Close cooperation between dentist and technician is essential in determining the best labial margin design.

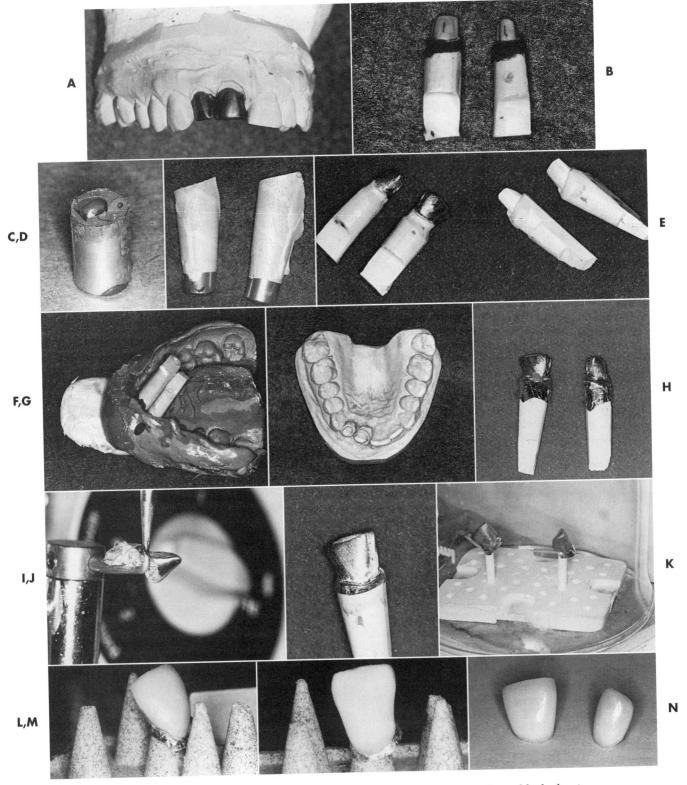

Fig. 24-34. The platinum foil matrix technique. **A,** Wax patterns. **B,** Cervical area blocked out. **C** to **E,** Dies duplicated. **F,** Dies located in the master impression. **G,** The master cast with modified removable dies. **H,** Castings seated over the platinum foil. **I,** Spot welding the foil to the metal substructure. **J,** The trimmed matrix. **K,** Oxidation. **L,** The first body firing has a cervical ditch. **M,** The ditch is filled on the second firing. **N,** The completed restorations.

welder. The foil can now be welded to the framework, which should be done as close as possible to the edge of the metal. Four or five welds are usually adequate to attach the foil to the substructure. The restoration is then fabricated in a conventional manner, although the facial margin is similar to that for the porcelain jacket crown. After oxidizing,* the metal is opaqued. The foil itself is not covered with opaque at this time, however. The restoration is built to contour, and the marginal portion is ditched as for the porcelain jacket crown. Some technicians prefer to paint a thin coat of separating liquid on the foil instead of ditching.

7. When the coronal portion has been shaped to a satisfactory contour, burnish the foil and fill in the ditched portion with cervical porcelain.

8. When the desired contour has been obtained after firing, trim the platinum skirt.

9. Leave the platinum that covers the shoulder portion of the preparation and seat the crown on the original die for final cervical contouring. During subsequent staining and glazing, the platinum foil will remain in place to support the porcelain and minimize rounding of the margin during firing.

---

*Before the oxidation step, applying a framework-repair metal paste (e.g., Vita Metall-Corrector) to the junction between the foil and framework may be helpful. This material fuses during the oxidation firing and helps support the foil during subsequent procedures.

10. When satisfied with characterization, staining, and glazing, remove the foil and cement the restoration after verifying the fit one more time.

Direct Lift (Cyanoacrylate) Technique. Because this technique is less time consuming[5] and easier to perform than the platinum foil technique, it is more widely used. The substructure is fabricated in the same manner, but the die is coated with a layer of cyanoacrylate resin, and the porcelain is condensed directly onto it (because the die no longer absorbs moisture from the wet ceramic buildup). Separation is achieved with a porcelain release agent. As with most techniques, a second bake is usually necessary for satisfactory marginal adaptation.

The principal difficulty associated with the cyanoacrylate technique occurs during the staining and glazing firing. Because the porcelain is not supported as in the platinum foil technique, the margin tends to round off slightly; therefore, special shoulder powders are needed.

Step-by-step Procedure (Fig. 24-35)

1. Apply cyanoacrylate resin to the labial margin area of the die. This acts as a sealant of the porous stone. Compressed air should be used to minimize the thickness of the film.

2. Apply porcelain release agent to the shoulder of the prepared die.

3. Seat the opaqued casting on the die.

4. Mix shoulder porcelain and apply it directly to the die and the opaque porcelain. Light tapping will assist in condensation and

A   B   C

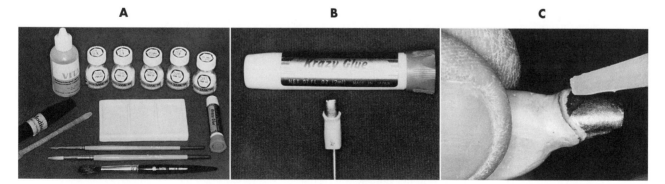

Fig. 24-35. The direct lift technique for a porcelain labial margin. **A,** Armamentarium. **B,** Cyanoacrylate resin serves as a sealant of the porous stone die. **C,** The resin is applied to the die where the porcelain will be in direct contact with the die. Compressed air is used to minimize film thickness. *Continued*

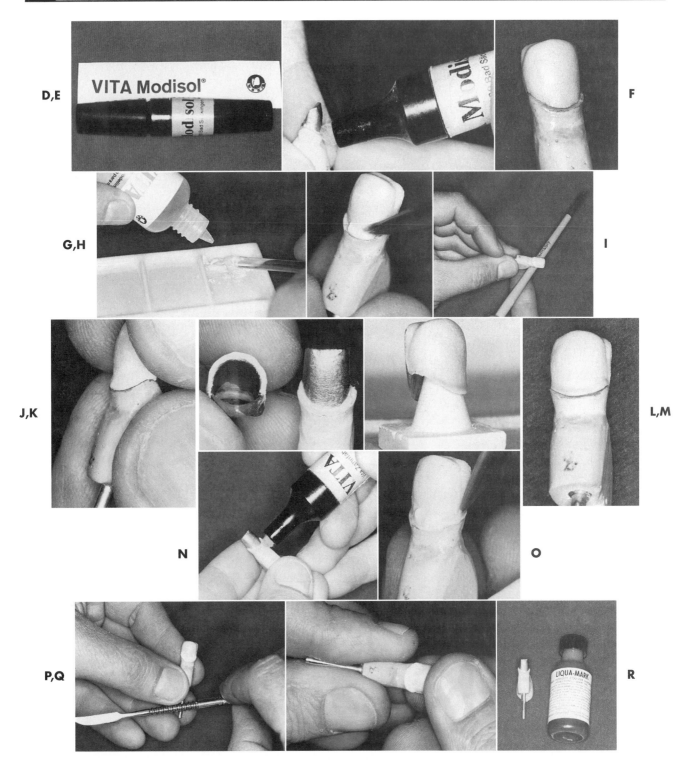

Fig. 24-35, cont'd.   **D,** Recommended separating medium. **E,** The separating liquid is applied to the shoulder of the prepared die. **F,** The opaqued casting seated on the prepared die. **G,** Mixing the shoulder porcelain. **H,** Shoulder porcelain is applied in direct contact with the die and opaque porcelain. **I,** Light tapping is used to assist in condensation. **J,** Separating the dry buildup from the die. **K,** The buildup before firing. **L,** First firing of the shoulder porcelain completed. **M,** The fixed restoration is reseated on the die. Note the minor marginal discrepancy. **N,** Before additional porcelain application, the die is relubricated. **O,** Second application of shoulder porcelain. **P,** Vibration. **Q,** Separating after the second shoulder application. **R,** Water-soluble marking agent for detecting premature contact.

Continued

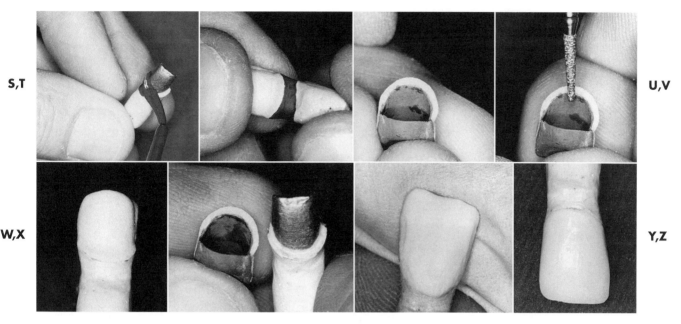

Fig. 24-35, cont'd. **S,** The marking agent is applied to the shoulder. **T,** The fired restoration is gently tried on the die. **U,** Markings are visible on the porcelain and on the internal aspect of the casting. **V,** Excess porcelain is removed. **W,** The seated restoration. **X,** Internal view of the completed shoulder. **Y,** Conventional buildup with body and incisal powders. **Z,** The glazed restoration.

should be done before separating the dry buildup from the die.

5. After the first firing of the shoulder porcelain, reseat the crown on the die. At this time, the restoration should be examined for margin discrepancies. A second shoulder firing is usually necessary.

6. Relubricate the die, reseat the crown, and apply a thinner mix of shoulder powder to the margin. Vibration will help the porcelain fill the defect completely. After blotting, the restoration can be separated from the die.

7. When the firing is completed, use a water-soluble marking agent to detect premature contacts. The marking agent is applied to the shoulder, and the restoration is then gently tried on the die. The markings will be visible on the porcelain and the inner aspect of the casting.

8. Adjust any areas of contact of the restoration and proceed with the conventional buildup of body and incisal porcelains, followed by glazing of the final restoration.

Porcelain Wax Technique. A mixture of body porcelain and wax (6:1 by weight)[71] is applied to the die for final adaptation of the porcelain labial margin of the metal-ceramic restoration.

Step-by-step Procedure (Fig. 24-36)

1. After coating the substructure with opaque porcelain, lubricate the die with a porcelain release agent.

2. Apply the porcelain-wax mixture to the cervical shoulder. Use an electric waxing instrument to flow it into the proper areas.

3. With a conventional wax-carving instrument, shape the material and blend it into the opaque. It will separate easily from the die and can be fired in the conventional manner.

4. A second application will be needed. Using the electric waxing instrument, keep the mixture liquid long enough so that capillary action can draw it into the marginal discrepancies. The restoration is completed in the conventional manner. If rounding of the margins is experienced during glazing, using a shoulder porcelain rather than a body porcelain in the wax mixture is recommended. Advantages and disadvantages of each technique are summarized in Table 24-2.

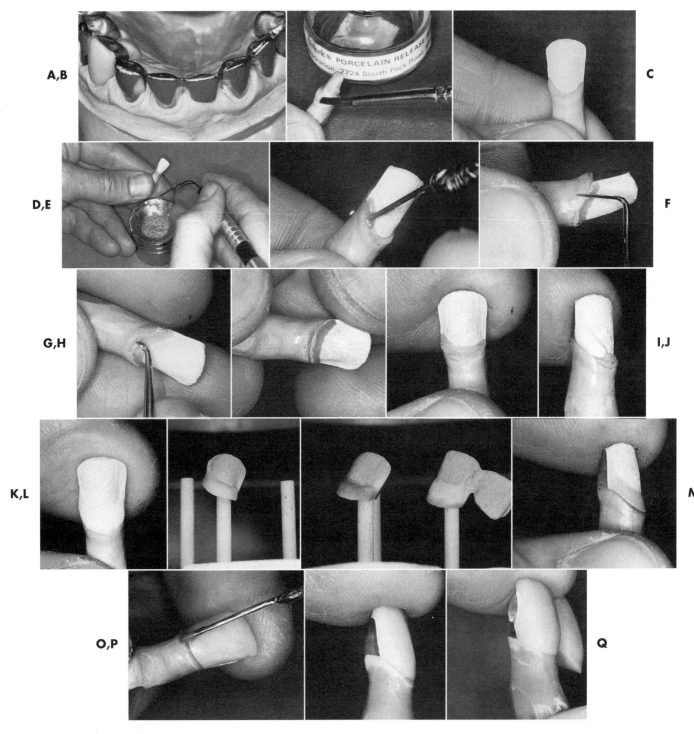

Fig. 24-36. The porcelain wax technique. **A,** Castings are prepared for porcelain labial margins. **B,** Release agent is applied to the die. **C,** Opaqued casting. **D,** The porcelain-wax mixture is carried to the restoration with an electric instrument. **E,** The mixture is flowed to place. **F,** A conventional carving instrument shapes the material. **G,** The material is carved into a rounded cervical configuration. **H,** Removal of the casting from the die. **I,** Reseated on the die. **J,** Shoulder porcelain is applied. **K,** Application is completed. **L** and **M,** The restorations before firing. **N,** The restorations are tried on the die after firing. Note the minor marginal discrepancy. **O,** Second application of the porcelain-wax mixture. **P** and **Q,** Restorations after firing.

Continued

R
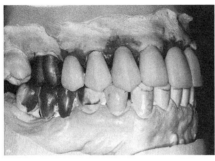
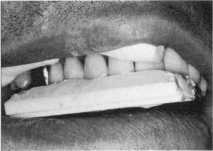
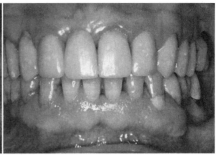
S,T

Fig. 24-36, cont'd.   **R,** The completed restorations before try-in. **S,** Soldering index. **T,** The finished prosthesis in place.
(Courtesy Dr. A. G. Gegauff.)

Advantages and Disadvantages of Fabrication Techniques — TABLE 24-2

Method	Advantages	Disadvantages
Platinum foil	No shoulder porcelain (best esthetics)[72] Good marginal adaptation Smooth surface[72] Low plaque accumulation[72]	Time consuming Technically difficult
Wax suspension	Separates easily	Shoulder porcelain needed Less accurate fit[73]
Direct lift	Least time consuming	Shoulder porcelain needed Rougher margins[72]

Common Reasons for Failure of Metal-Ceramic Restorations — TABLE 24-3

Failure	Reason
Fracture during bisque bake	Improper condensation Improper moisture control Poor framework design Incompatible metal-porcelain combination
Bubbles	Too many firings Air entrapment during building of restoration Improper moisture control Poor metal preparation Poor casting technique
Unsatisfactory appearance	Poor communication with technician Inadequate tooth reduction Opaque too thick Excessive firing
Clinical fracture	Poor framework design Centric stops too close to metal-ceramic interface Improper metal preparation

TROUBLESHOOTING

Technical failures can occur in the complex metal-ceramic system and are difficult to diagnose. Different errors may lead to problems that appear similar. Table 24-3 summarizes some of these.

CRACKS

Surface cracks and fractures in the opaque porcelain are usually of little concern. They can be patched be-fore the body firing begins. Fractures during the bisque bake, however, often are the result of improper condensation, overly rapid drying, or haphazard moisture control. Poor substructure design, resulting in areas of unsupported porcelain, also can lead to porcelain failure (see Chapter 19). After cementation, pinpointing the cause of failure may be difficult. If the substructure is properly designed and the porcelain-metal interface is kept away from

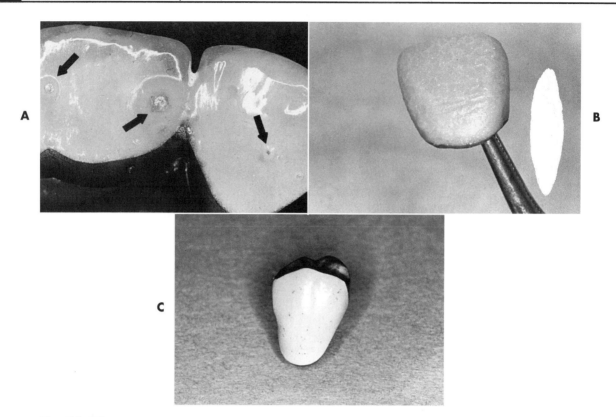

Fig. 24-37. **A,** Bubbles *(arrows)* have made this metal-ceramic restoration unacceptable. **B,** Devitrified porcelain on a metal-ceramic restoration, the result of an excessive number of firings. **C,** Contamination of the porcelain surface has made this prosthesis unacceptable.

direct occlusal contact, cracks and fractures should not develop during normal function.

BUBBLES

Even the most experienced ceramist will sometimes trap air between the metal and the opaque. Usually this is of little concern. However, if a restoration is fired too many times, the trapped air may appear as blisters that rise to the surface. If this occurs, the porcelain must be stripped, and the procedure is started over.

If bubbles appear after only a few firings, improper casting technique, insufficient metal preparation, and haphazard moisture control can usually be isolated as the cause (Fig. 24-37).

UNSATISFACTORY APPEARANCE

Poor esthetic results are often due to poor communication between the operator and the dental technician (see Chapter 16). An opaque application that is too thick can result in opacity of the veneer. Inadequate tooth reduction, especially in the cervical third and the interproximal areas, is one of the more common causes of a poor esthetic result. Careful communication, based on a thorough understand-

ing and knowledge of relevant laboratory procedures and color science, is essential.

◼ REVIEW OF TECHNIQUE

Fabricating a metal-ceramic restoration involves the following steps:
1. Patterns are waxed to anatomical contour.
2. The cut-back is completed and verified with an index made from the anatomical waxing.
3. The patterns are cast (see Chapter 22) and seated on the die.
4. After finishing (and clinical evaluation if desired [see Chapter 30]), the substructures are opaqued to mask the metal color.
5. Body powders are added to build to contour and cut back to standardize the amount of enamel powder that is added.
6. Enamel powder is added, and the buildup is slightly overcontoured to compensate for firing shrinkage.
7. After preliminary contouring, the bisque bake can be evaluated clinically. The incisal edge position is adjusted for function, esthetics, and phonetics.

8. After contouring, the restorations are glazed, and the metal is polished before cementation.

SUMMARY

Substructure design for metal-ceramic restorations must be based on an understanding of fundamental material properties. Restorations should be waxed to anatomic contour and then cut back in the area that is to be veneered. This will allow an even porcelain thickness, which is not only a means of obtaining superior mechanical properties in the completed restoration, but also simultaneously helps standardize shade matching.

Metal-ceramic restorations with excellent appearance and good mechanical properties are obtainable if the techniques of metal preparation, framework design, porcelain manipulation, drying, and firing are carefully followed. Lifelike effects can be achieved by layering cervical, body, and incisal porcelains and by the judicious use of internal characterization and special dentin powders with relatively higher concentrations of opacifiers. Although it may create esthetic problems in many patients, the simplest way to obtain good marginal fit is to use a narrow, 0.2- to 0.3-mm facial collar.

Whenever optimum appearance is desired, the procedures described in this chapter for fabricating a labial porcelain margin should be considered. However, the level of expertise needed to produce excellent marginal adaptation with these techniques is higher than those that use a cast margin; this should be considered in treatment planning. When failure occurs, all technical steps and materials should be reevaluated.

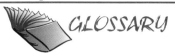

GLOSSARY

bisque bake: a series of stages of maturation in the firing of ceramic materials relating to the degree of pyrochemical reaction and sintering shrinkage occurring before vitrification (glazing)—called also *biscuit bake.*

ceramic: *adj* (1850): of or relating to the manufacture of any product made essentially from a nonmetallic mineral (as clay) by firing at a higher temperature.

collarless metal ceramic restoration: a metal ceramic restoration whose cervical metal collar has been eliminated. Porcelain is placed directly in contact with the prepared finish line.

¹coping: *n 1:* a long, enveloping ecclesiastical vestment *2a:* something resembling a cope (as by concealing or covering) *2b:* coping.

²coping: *n* (ca. 1909): a thin covering or crown.

¹craze: *vb* **crazed; crazing:** *vt:* to produce minute cracks on the surface or glaze of; to develop a mesh of fine cracks.

²craze: *n* (1534): a crack in a surface or coating (as of glaze or enamel).

degas: *vt;* **degassed:** *pt; pp;* **degassing:** *ppr* (1920) *1:* to remove gas from an object or substance *2:* the process commonly used to denote the first heat cycle in fabrication of a metal ceramic restoration used to remove surface impurities from the metallic component before the application of opaque porcelain.

devitrification: *n* (1832): to eliminate vitreous characteristics partly or wholly; to recrystallize.

feldspar: *n* (1757) *1:* any one of a group of minerals, principally aluminosilicates of sodium, potassium, calcium, or barium, that are essential constituents of nearly all crystalline rocks *2:* a crystalline mineral of aluminum silicate with sodium, potassium, barium,

Study Questions

1. Discuss the types of dental porcelains used in the fabrication of a metal-ceramic restoration. What are the composition differences among the various powders? How does the handling differ?
2. What are the prerequisites for casting preparation before the initial firing?
3. What is the role of a vacuum in firing a metal-ceramic restoration? Which procedures require a vacuum and which are performed without it?
4. How do firing schedules vary as a function of the alloy used?
5. What is vitrification? What is devitrification?
6. Discuss the porcelain-metal bond. Which components of the alloy are involved? Which components of the dental porcelain are involved?
7. Discuss two different techniques for fabricating a porcelain labial margin.
8. Describe the causes for fractures and air bubbles during the bisque bake.

and/or calcium; a major constituent of some dental porcelains.

firing: the process of porcelain fusion, in dentistry, specifically to produce porcelain restorations.

glaze: *vb* **glazed; glazing:** *vt* **1:** to cover with a glossy, smooth surface or coating **2:** the attainment of a smooth and reflective surface **3:** the final firing of porcelain in which the surface is vitrified and a high gloss is imparted to the material **4:** a ceramic veneer on a metal porcelain restoration after it has been fired, producing a nonporous, glossy or semiglossy surface.

intrinsic coloring: coloring from within; the incorporation of a colorant within the material of a prosthesis or restoration.

metal ceramic restoration: a fixed restoration that uses a metal substructure on which a ceramic veneer is fused.

microcrack: *n:* in porcelain, one of the numerous surface flaws that contributes to stress concentrations and results in strengths below those theoretically possible.

modifier: *n:* a substance that alters or changes the color or properties of a substance.

natural glaze: the production of a glazed surface by the vitrification of the material itself and without addition of other fluxes or glasses.

opacity: *n* (1611): the quality or state of a body that makes it impervious to light.

opaque: *adj* (1641): the property of a material that absorbs and/or reflects all light and prevents any transmission of light.

overglaze: *adj* (1879): the production of a glazed surface by the addition of a fluxed glass that usually vitrifies at a lower temperature.

pigment: *n:* finely ground, natural or synthetic, inorganic or organic, insoluble dispersed particles (powder), which, when dispersed in a liquid vehicle, may provide, in addition to color, many other essential properties such as opacity, hardness, durability, and corrosion resistance. The term is used to include extenders and white or color pigments. The distinction between powders that are pigments and those that are dyes is generally considered on the basis of solubility—pigments being insoluble and dispersed in the material, dyes being soluble or in solution as used.

platinum foil: a precious-metal foil with a high fusing point that makes it suitable as a matrix for various soldering procedures as well as to provide an internal form for porcelain restorations during their fabrication.

porcelain: *n* (known in Europe, ca. 1540): a ceramic material formed of infusible elements joined by lower fusing materials. Most dental porcelains are glasses and are used in the fabrication of teeth for dentures, pontics and facings, metal ceramic restorations, crowns, inlays, onlays, and other restorations.

porcelain labial margin: the extension of ceramic material to the finish line of the preparation without visible metal substructure in the marginal area.

quartz: *n* (ca. 1631): an allotropic form of silica; the mineral SiO_2 consisting of hexagonal crystals of colorless, transparent silicon dioxide.

silica: *n* (ca 1301): silicon dioxide occurring in crystalline, amorphous, and usually impure forms (as quartz, opal, and sand, respectively).

stain: *vb* **1:** to suffuse with color **2:** to color by processes affecting chemically or otherwise the material itself **3:** in dentistry, to intentionally alter ceramic or resin restorations through the application of intrinsic or extrinsic colorants to achieve a desired effect.

thermal expansion: expansion of a material caused by heat.

translucency: *n* (1611): having the appearance between complete opacity and complete transparency; partially opaque.

REFERENCES

1. Ernsmere JB: Porcelain dental work, *Br J Dent Sci* 43:547, 1900.

2. Johnston JF et al: Porcelain veneers bonded to gold castings: a progress report, *J Prosthet Dent* 8:120, 1958.

3. MacEntee MI, Belser UC: Fixed restorations produced by commercial dental laboratories in Vancouver and Geneva, *J Oral Rehabil* 15:301, 1988.

4. Goodacre CJ et al: The collarless metal-ceramic crown, *J Prosthet Dent* 38:615, 1977.

5. Toogood GD, Archibald JF: Technique for establishing porcelain margins, *J Prosthet Dent* 40:464, 1978.

6. Warpeha WS, Goodkind RJ: Design and technique variables affecting fracture resistance of metal-ceramic restorations, *J Prosthet Dent* 35:291, 1976.

7. Moore PA, Manor RC: Hydrofluoric acid burns, *J Prosthet Dent* 47:338, 1982.

8. Felton DA et al: Effect of air abrasives on marginal configurations of porcelain-fused-to-metal alloys: an SEM analysis, *J Prosthet Dent* 65:38, 1991.

9. Hamaguchi H et al: Marginal distortion of the porcelain-bonded-to-metal complete crown: an SEM study, *J Prosthet Dent* 47:146, 1982.

10. Richter-Snapp K et al: Change in marginal fit as related to margin design, alloy type, and porcelain proximity in porcelain-fused-to-metal restorations, *J Prosthet Dent* 60:435, 1988.

11. Weinstein M et al: *Fused porcelain-to-metal teeth.* U.S. Patent No. 3,052,982, September 11, 1962.

12. Weinstein M, Weinstein AB: *Porcelain-covered metal-reinforced teeth.* U.S. Patent No. 3,052,983, September 11, 1962.

13. Barreiro MM et al: Phase identification in dental porcelains for ceramo-metallic restorations, *Dent Mater* 5:51, 1989.

14. Rasmussen ST et al: Optimum particle size distribution for reduced sintering shrinkage of a dental porcelain, *Dent Mater* 13:43, 1997.

15. Laub LW et al: The metal-porcelain interface of gold crowns, *J Dent Res* 57:A293, 1978 (abstract no. 874).

16. Seghi RR et al: Spectrophotometric analysis of color differences between porcelain systems, *J Prosthet Dent* 56:35, 1986.

17. Rosenstiel SF, Johnston WM: The effects of manipulative variables on the color of ceramic metal restorations, *J Prosthet Dent* 60:297, 1988.

18. O'Brien WJ, Ryge G: Contact angles of drops of enamels on metals, *J Prosthet Dent* 15:1094, 1965.

19. Borom MP, Pask JA: Role of "adherence oxides" in the development of chemical bonding at glass-metal interfaces, *J Am Ceram Soc* 49:1, 1966.

20. Brantley WA et al: X-ray diffraction studies of oxidized high-palladium alloys, *Dent Mater* 12:333, 1996.

21. Kerber SJ et al: The complementary nature of x-ray photoelectron spectroscopy and angle-resolved x-ray diffraction. II. Analysis of oxides on dental alloys, *J Mater Eng Perform* 7:334, 1998.

22. Cascone PJ: The theory of bonding for porcelain-metal systems. In Yamada HN, Grenoble PB, editors: *Dental porcelain: the state of the art—1977,* Los Angeles, 1977, University of Southern California School of Dentistry, p. 109.

23. Cascone PJ: Oxide formation on palladium alloys and its effects on porcelain adherence, *J Dent Res* 62:255, 1983 (abstract no. 772).

24. Lautenschlager EP et al: Microprobe analyses of gold-porcelain bonding, *J Dent Res* 8:1206, 1969.

25. Payan J et al: Changes in physical and chemical properties of a dental palladium-silver alloy during metal-porcelain bonding, *J Oral Rehabil* 13:329, 1986.

26. Hong JM et al: The effect of recasting on the oxidation layer of a palladium-silver porcelain alloy, *J Prosthet Dent* 59:420, 1988.

27. Anusavice KJ et al: Adherence controlling elements in ceramic-metal systems. I. Precious alloys, *J Dent Res* 56:1045, 1977.

28. Anusavice KJ et al: Adherence controlling elements in ceramic-metal systems. II. Nonprecious alloys, *J Dent Res* 56:1053, 1977.

29. Papazoglou E et al: New high-palladium casting alloys. Studies of the interface with porcelain, *Int J Prosthodont* 9:315, 1996.

30. Anusavice KJ: *Phillips' science of dental materials,* ed 10, Philadelphia, 1996, WB Saunders, p. 517.

31. Caputo AA: Effect of surface preparation on bond strength of nonprecious and semi-precious alloys, *J Calif Dent Assoc* 6:42, 1978.

32. Baran GR: The metallurgy of Ni-Cr alloys for fixed prosthodontics, *J Prosthet Dent* 50:639, 1983.

33. Laub LW et al: The tensile and shear strength of some base metal/ceramic interfaces, *J Dent Res* 56:B178, 1977 (abstract no. 504).

34. Shell JS, Nielsen JP: Study of the bond between gold alloys and porcelain, *J Dent Res* 41:1424, 1962.

35. Carpenter MA, Goodkind RJ: Effect of varying surface texture on bond strength of one semi-precious and one nonprecious ceramo-alloy, *J Prosthet Dent* 42:86, 1979.

36. Wagner WC et al: Effect of interfacial variables on metal-porcelain bonding, *J Biomed Mater Res* 27:531, 1993.

37. Craig RG, editor: *Restorative dental materials,* ed 10, St. Louis, 1997, Mosby, p. 485.

38. Meyer JM et al: Sintering of dental porcelain enamels, *J Dent Res* 55:696, 1976.

39. Johnston WM, O'Brien WJ: The shear strength of dental porcelain, *J Dent Res* 59:1409, 1980.

40. Nally JN: Chemico-physical analysis and mechanical tests of the ceramo-metallic complex, *Int Dent J* 18:309, 1968.

41. Kelly M et al: Tensile strength determination of the interface between porcelain fused to gold, *J Biomed Mater Res* 3:403, 1969.

42. Anusavice KJ et al: Comparative evaluation of ceramic-metal bond tests using finite element stress analysis, *J Dent Res* 59:608, 1980.

43. O'Brien WJ: Cohesive plateau theory of porcelain-alloy bonding. In Yamada HN, Grenoble PB, editors: *Dental porcelain: the state of the art—1977,* Los Angeles, 1977, University of Southern California School of Dentistry, p. 137.

44. O'Brien WJ: The cohesive plateau stress of ceramic-metal systems, *J Dent Res* 56:B177, 1977 (abstract no. 501).

45. ANSI/ADA specification no. 38 for metal-ceramic systems, Chicago, 1991, American Dental Association.

46. Ringle RD et al: An x-ray spectrometric technique for measuring porcelain-metal adherence, *J Dent Res* 62:933, 1983.

47. Mackert JR et al: Measurement of oxide adherence to PFM alloys, *J Dent Res* 63:1335, 1984.

48. Papazoglou E et al: Porcelain adherence to high-palladium alloys, *J Prosthet Dent* 70:386, 1993.

49. Papazoglou E et al: Effects of dental laboratory processing variables and in vitro testing medium on the porcelain adherence of

high-palladium casting alloys, *J Prosthet Dent* 79:514, 1998.

50. International Organization for Standardization: ISO standard no. 9693: *Dental porcelain fused to metal restorations,* Geneva, Switzerland, 1991.

51. Lenz J et al: Bond strength of metal-ceramic systems in three-point flexure bond test, *J Appl Biomater* 6:55, 1995.

52. Papazoglou E, Brantley WA: Porcelain adherence vs. force to failure for palladium-gallium alloys: critique of metal-ceramic bond testing, *Dent Mater* 14:112, 1998.

53. Leone EF, Fairhurst CW: Bond strength and mechanical properties of dental porcelain enamels, *J Prosthet Dent* 18:155, 1967.

54. Knap FJ, Ryge G: Study of bond strength of dental porcelain fused to metal, *J Dent Res* 45:1047, 1966.

55. Sced IR, McLean JW: The strength of metal/ceramic bonds with base metals containing chromium, *Br Dent J* 13:232, 1972.

56. Terada Y et al: The masking ability of an opaque porcelain: a spectrophotometric study, *Int J Prosthodont* 2:259, 1989.

57. McLaren EA: Utilization of advanced metal-ceramic technology: clinical and laboratory procedures for a lower-fusing porcelain, *Pract Periodont Aesthet Dent* 10:835, 1998.

58. Metzler KT et al: In vitro investigation of the wear of human enamel by dental porcelain, *J Prosthet Dent* 81:356, 1999.

59. Rosenstiel SF: Linear firing shrinkage of metal-ceramic restorations, *Br Dent J* 162:390, 1987.

60. Evans DB et al: The influence of condensation method on porosity and shade of body porcelain, *J Prosthet Dent* 63:380, 1990.

61. Rosenstiel SF, Porter SS: Apparent fracture toughness of metal ceramic restorations with different manipulative variables, *J Prosthet Dent* 61:185, 1989.

62. Mackert JR Jr, Evans AL: Effect of cooling rate on leucite volume fraction in dental porcelains, *J Dent Res* 70:137, 1991.

63. Asaoka K, Tesk JA: Transient and residual stress in a porcelain-metal strip, *J Dent Res* 69:463, 1990.

64. Barghi N et al: Comparison of fracture strength of porcelain-veneered-to-high noble and base metal alloys, *J Prosthet Dent* 57:23, 1987.

65. Abbate MF et al: Comparison of the marginal fit of various ceramic crown systems, *J Prosthet Dent* 61:527, 1989.

66. Belser UC et al: Fit of three porcelain-fused-to-metal marginal designs in vivo: a scanning electron microscope study, *J Prosthet Dent* 53:24, 1985.

67. Anusavice KJ, Hojjatie B: Stress distribution in metal-ceramic crowns with a facial porcelain margin, *J Dent Res* 66:1493, 1987.

68. Touati B, Miara P: Light transmission in bonded ceramic restorations, *J Esthet Dent* 5:11, 1993.

69. O'Boyle K et al: An investigation of new metal framework design for metal ceramic restorations, *J Prosthet Dent* 78:295, 1997.

70. Lehner CR et al: Variable reduced metal support for collarless metal ceramic crowns: a new model for strength evaluation, *Int J Prosthodont* 8:337, 1995.

71. Prince J et al: The all-porcelain labial margin for ceramometal restorations: a new concept, *J Prosthet Dent* 50:793, 1983.

72. Koidis PT et al: Color consistency, plaque accumulation, and external marginal surface characteristics of the collarless metal ceramic restoration, *J Prosthet Dent* 65:391, 1991.

73. Belles DM et al: Effect of metal design and technique on the marginal characteristics of the collarless metal ceramic restoration, *J Prosthet Dent* 65:611, 1991.

CHAPTER TWENTY-FIVE

ALL-CERAMIC RESTORATIONS

Isabelle L. Denry, contributing author

All-ceramic inlays, onlays, veneers, and crowns can provide some of the most esthetically pleasing restorations currently available. They can be made to match natural tooth structure accurately in terms of color, surface texture, and **translucency.** Well-made all-ceramic restorations can be virtually indistinguishable from unrestored natural teeth (Fig. 25-1).

Traditionally, ceramic crowns have been made on a platinum matrix and were referred to as porcelain jacket crowns. More recently, improved materials and techniques have been introduced in an attempt to overcome disadvantages inherent in that traditional method. These improvements, particularly the use of higher-strength ceramics and adhesives for bonding the ceramic restoration to tooth structure, have led to a resurgence of interest in all-ceramic restorations, including the more conservative inlays and veneers. With increasing demand for esthetics, all-ceramic restorations are an important part of contemporary dental practice.

This chapter reviews the historical background of ceramic restorations and more recent developments. It outlines the laboratory procedures necessary for the fabrication of all-ceramic inlays, veneers, and crowns and compares the alternatives.

The importance of the design of the tooth preparation to the success of ceramic restorations cannot be overemphasized (see Chapter 11).

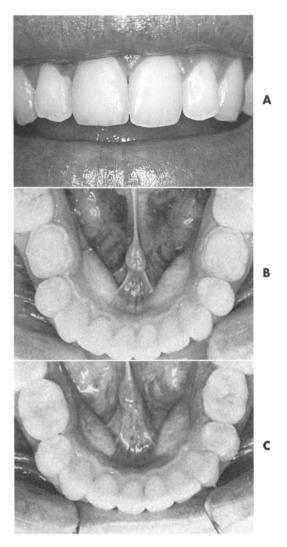

Fig. 25-1. **A,** All-ceramic crown restoring the maxillary central incisors. **B** and **C,** Retained deciduous mandibular second molars restored with ceramic inlays. (**B** *and* **C** *courtesy Dr. R.B. Miller.*)

◼ HISTORICAL BACKGROUND

The first attempt to use ceramics for making denture teeth was by Alexis Duchateau in 1774. More than a hundred years later, C.H. Land made the first ceramic crowns and inlays with a **platinum foil** matrix technique and was granted a patent in 1887.[1] The popularity of ceramic restorations declined with the introduction of acrylic resin in the 1940s and continued to be low until the disadvantages of resin veneering materials (increased wear, high permeability leading to discoloration and leakage) were realized.[2-4] In 1962 Weinstein and Weinstein patented a leucite-containing porcelain frit for use in metal-ceramic restorations.[5] The presence of leucite, an aluminosilicate with high thermal expansion, allowed a match between the thermal expansion of the ceramic and that of the metal (see Chapter 24). The appearance of ceramic restorations was improved by the introduction of **vacuum firing,** which considerably reduced the amount of **porosity** and therefore resulted in denser and more translucent restorations than could be achieved with **air firing**.[6]

HIGH-STRENGTH CERAMICS

The chief disadvantage of the early restorations was their low strength, which limited their use to low-stress situations, such as anterior teeth. Even so, fracture was a fairly common occurrence, which prompted the development of higher-strength materials.[7] These developments have followed two paths. One approach uses two ceramic materials to fabricate the restoration. A high-strength but nonesthetic **ceramic core** material is veneered with a lower-strength, esthetic porcelain. The approach is similar to the metal-ceramic technique (see Chapter 24), although the color of the ceramic core is more easily masked than a metal substructure. The other approach is the development of a ceramic that combines good esthetics with high strength. This has the obvious attraction of not needing the additional thickness of material to mask a high-strength core. However, at present, the strongest dental ceramics are nonesthetic core materials.[8]

STRENGTHENING MECHANISMS OF DENTAL CERAMICS

In spite of their excellent esthetic qualities and outstanding biocompatibility, dental ceramics, like all ceramic materials, are brittle. They are susceptible to fracture at the time of placement or during function. Methods used to improve the strength and clinical performance of dental ceramics include crystalline reinforcement, chemical strengthening, and thermal tempering. Brittle materials such as ceramics contain at least two flaws: fabrication defects and surface cracks.

FABRICATION DEFECTS
Fabrication defects are created during processing and consist of voids or inclusions generated during sintering. Condensation of a ceramic slurry by hand before sintering may introduce porosity. Sintering under vacuum reduces the porosity in dental ceramics from 5.6 to 0.56 vol%.[9] Porosity on the internal side of clinically failed **glass-ceramic** restorations has been shown to constitute a fracture-initiation site.[10] Also, **microcracks** develop within the ceramic upon cooling in leucite-containing ceramics and are due to thermal contraction mismatch between the crystals and the glassy matrix.[11]

SURFACE CRACKS
Surface cracks are induced by machining or grinding. The average natural flaw size varies from 20 to 50 μm.[12] Usually, fracture of the ceramic takes place from the most severe flaw, which effectively determines the fracture resistance of the restoration. Ceramic engineers analyze failure with a statistical approach, looking at flaw size and spatial distribution.[13]

CRYSTALLINE REINFORCEMENT
Strengthening by crystalline reinforcement involves the introduction of a high proportion of crystalline phase into the ceramic to improve the resistance to crack propagation. The crystals can deflect the advancing crack front to increase the fracture resistance of two-phase materials. Microstructural features that typically lead to crack deflection include (1) weakened interfaces between grains in single phase materials that may be due to incomplete sintering and (2) residual strains in two-phase materials.[14] The latter constitutes a major issue in dental ceramics.

A crystalline phase with *greater* thermal expansion coefficient than the matrix produces tangential *compressive* stress (and radial tension) near the crystal-matrix interface. Such tangential stresses tend to divert the crack around the particle. Leucite particles have a greater thermal expansion coefficient than the surrounding glassy matrix. Upon cooling, compressive stresses will develop at the leucite crystal-matrix interface.

CHEMICAL STRENGTHENING
Chemical strengthening is another method used to increase the strength of glasses and ceramics. The principle of chemical strengthening relies on the exchange of small alkali ions for larger ions below the strain point of the ceramic. Because stress relaxation is not possible in this temperature range, the exchange leads to the creation of a compressive layer at the surface of the ceramic.[15] Finally, any applied load must first overcome this built-in compression

layer before the surface can be placed into tension, resulting in an increase in fracture resistance. This technique involves the use of alkali salts with a melting point lower than the glass transition temperature of the ceramic material. Ion-exchange strengthening has been reported to increase the flexural strength of feldspathic dental porcelain up to 80%, depending on the ionic species involved and the composition of the porcelain.[16,17] The depth of the ion-exchanged layer can be as high as 50 μm.[18] However, this technique is diffusion driven, and its kinetics are limited by time, temperature, and ionic radius of the exchanged ions.

THERMAL TEMPERING

Thermal tempering occurs when a glass is rapidly cooled from near the softening temperature. The cooling leads to compressive stress being generated in the glass surface, which must be overcome before cracks can propagate and fracture can occur. Thermal tempering is used to strengthen automobile windshields, and under experimental conditions it has been an effective strengthener for dental ceramics.[19]

GLAZING

The addition of a surface **glaze** can also be used to strengthen ceramics. The principle is the formation of a low-expansion surface layer formed at high temperature. Upon cooling, the low-expansion glaze places the surface of the ceramic in compression and reduces the depth and width of surface flaws. With contemporary dental ceramics, self-glazing is the standard technique. This consists of an additional firing in air following the original firing, without application of a low-expansion glaze. However, self-glazing does not significantly improve the flexure strength of feldspathic dental porcelain.[20,21]

PREVENTION OF STRESS CORROSION

The strength of ceramics is reduced in moist environments. This weakening is due to a chemical reaction between water and the ceramic at the tip of the strength-controlling crack, resulting in an increase in the crack size—a phenomenon called **stress-corrosion** or *static fatigue*.[22] According to Michalske and Freiman,[23] the reaction steps involve the following:

- The adsorption of water to a strained Si-O-Si bond
- A concerted reaction involving simultaneous proton and electron transfer
- The formation of surface hydroxyls

Sherrill and O'Brien[24] reported a reduction in fracture strength of about 30% when dental porcelains were fractured in water, and others have concluded that stress-corrosion is important in the performance of dental ceramic restorations.[25,26] Ceramic systems such as Captek* that place a metal foil on the internal surface may reduce fracture incidence by reducing moisture exposure to the internal surface of the ceramic, from where the fracture is thought to initiate.[11] In industry, coatings are used to reduce stress-corrosion of glass and ceramics, such as optical fibers. Similar coatings have been tried experimentally for their effect on dental ceramics.[27]

ALL-CERAMIC SYSTEMS

The microstructure of some ceramic systems discussed in this chapter is illustrated in Figure 25-2, and their properties are summarized in Table 25-1.

---

*Captek Division, Precious Chemicals USA: Longwood, Fla.

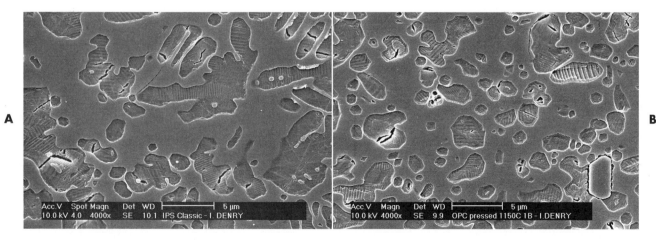

Fig. 25-2.   Representative dental ceramics etched to reveal microstructure. **A,** A feldspathic porcelain (IPS Classic). **B,** A pressable high leucite (OPC). *Continued*

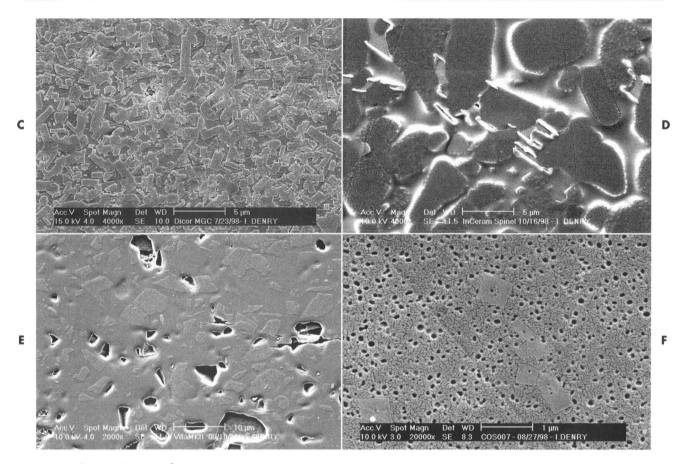

Fig. 25-2, cont'd.   **C,** A fluormica machinable (Dicor MGC). **D,** A slip-cast spinel (In-Ceram Spinell). **E,** A feldspathic machinable (Vita Mark II). **F,** A lithium phosphate pressable (Empress Cosmo).

Comparison of Available All-ceramic Systems

Brand	Captek	Ceramco	Cerinate	Dicor MGC	Empress	Empress 2	Empress Cosmo	Finesse
Manufacturer	Precious Chemicals	Dentsply	Den-Mat	Dentsply	Ivoclar	Ivoclar	Ivoclar	Dentsply
Crystalline phase	Leucite	Leucite	Leucite	Tetrasilicic fluormica	Leucite	Lithium disilicate	Lithium phosphate	Leucite
Recommended usage	Crowns	Inlays Onlays Veneers	Inlays Onlays Crowns Veneers	Inlays Onlays	Inlays Onlays Crowns Veneers	3-unit FPDs Crowns	Endodontic foundation	Inlays Onlays Crowns Veneers
Fabrication	Metal core or sintered	Sintered	Sintered	CAD/CAM	Heat-pressed	Heat-pressed	Heat-pressed	Heat-pressed
Strength	Low	Low	Medium	High	Medium	High	Medium	Medium
Fracture toughness	Medium	Medium	Medium	Medium-high	Medium	High	Medium	Medium
Translucency	Opaque	Medium	Medium	Medium	Medium	Medium	Opaque	Medium
Enamel abrasiveness	Medium	Medium	High	Low	Medium	Low	*	Medium
Marginal fit	Good	Fair	Fair	Fair	Fair	Fair	*	*

*Not tested.

ALUMINOUS CORE CERAMICS

The high-strength ceramic core was first introduced to dentistry by McLean and Hughes[28] in 1965. They advocated using aluminous porcelain, which is composed of **aluminum oxide** (alumina) crystals dispersed in a glassy matrix. Their recommendation was based on the use of alumina-reinforced porcelain in the electrical industry[29] and the fact that alumina has a high fracture toughness and hardness.[30]

The technique devised by McLean[31] used an **opaque** inner core containing 50% by weight alumina for high strength. This core was veneered by a combination of esthetic body and enamel porcelains with 15% and 5% crystalline alumina, respectively[32] (Fig. 25-3) and matched thermal expansion. The resulting restorations were approximately 40% stronger than those using traditional feldspathic porcelain.[23]

Fabrication Procedure. Although declining in popularity with the introduction of innovative all-ceramic products, a technician skilled in the fabrication of the aluminous core porcelain jacket crown produces an exceptionally esthetic restoration. The procedure is outlined in Figs. 25-4 to 25-6.

SLIP-CAST CERAMICS

High-strength core frameworks for all-ceramic restorations can be produced with a slip-casting procedure[33] such as the In-Ceram.* Slip-casting is a traditional technique in the ceramic industry and is used to make sanitary ware. The starting media in slip-casting is a slip that is an aqueous suspension of fine alumina particles in water with

*Vident: Brea, Calif.

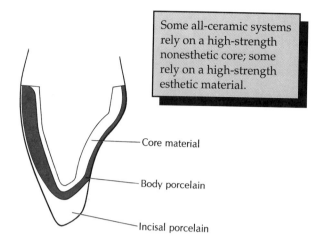

Some all-ceramic systems rely on a high-strength nonesthetic core; some rely on a high-strength esthetic material.

Fig. 25-3. The strength of an aluminous jacket crown comes from its high-alumina content core, onto which esthetic body and incisal porcelains are fired. This is analogous to the metal-ceramic crown, whose strength comes from a metal substructure.

Core material
Body porcelain
Incisal porcelain

TABLE **25-1**

Helioform	In-Ceram	In-Ceram Spinell	In-Ceram Zirconia	Mark II	Optimal	ProCad	Procera	Metal Ceramic
Vident	Vident	Vident	Vident	Vident	Jeneric/ Pentron	Ivoclar	Nobel Biocare	Various
Leucite	Alumina	Alumina Spinel	Zirconia/ alumina	Feldspar	Leucite	Leucite	Alumina	Leucite
Crowns	Crowns Veneers	Crowns Veneers	3-unit FPDs	Inlays Onlays Crowns	Inlays Onlays Crowns Veneers	Inlays Onlays Crowns	Crowns	Crowns FPDs
Electro-formed gold core or sintered	Slip-cast core or sintered	Slip-cast core or sintered	Slip-cast core or sintered	CAD/CAM	Heat pressed	CAD/CAM	CAD/CAM	Cast framework or sintered
Low	High	High	Very high	Medium	Medium	Medium	Very high	Very high
Medium	High	High	Very high	Medium	Medium	Medium	Very high	Medium
Opaque	Opaque	Medium	Opaque	Medium	Medium		Opaque	Opaque
Medium	High	High	High	Medium	Low	*	Medium	Medium
Good	Fair	Fair	Fair	Fair	Fair	Fair	Fair	Good

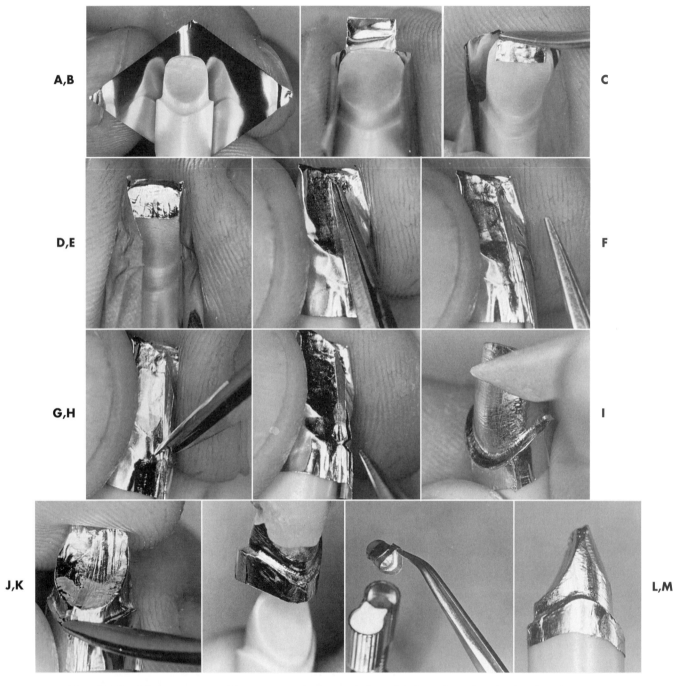

Fig. 25-4. Platinum matrix fabrication. **A,** A diamond-shaped foil is adapted to the facial surface (a cutting guide is provided with the foil). **B,** Two cuts are made, one to each incisal corner, and a triangle of foil is removed by cutting at 45 degrees toward the corners. **C,** The foil is folded onto the lingual surface and burnished. **D** and **E,** It is then gathered on the lingual surface with tweezers and adapted with finger pressure. **F,** The foil is trimmed to follow the lingual contour evenly. The two ends are separated, and one is trimmed to exactly half the width of the other. **G** and **H,** The long end is folded over the short, and relieving cuts are made (see Fig. 25-5). Then the three-thickness joint is folded toward the short end. **I,** The foil is adapted with a wooden point, always starting from the incisal edge and working toward the margin. **J,** A beaver-tail burnisher is used to adapt the margin, working the foil toward the internal angle to prevent a perforation. Better adaptation can be achieved by swaging at this stage. The matrix is removed with sticky wax **(K)** and annealed in a Bunsen flame **(L)** to relieve work hardening. **M,** The completed platinum foil matrix.

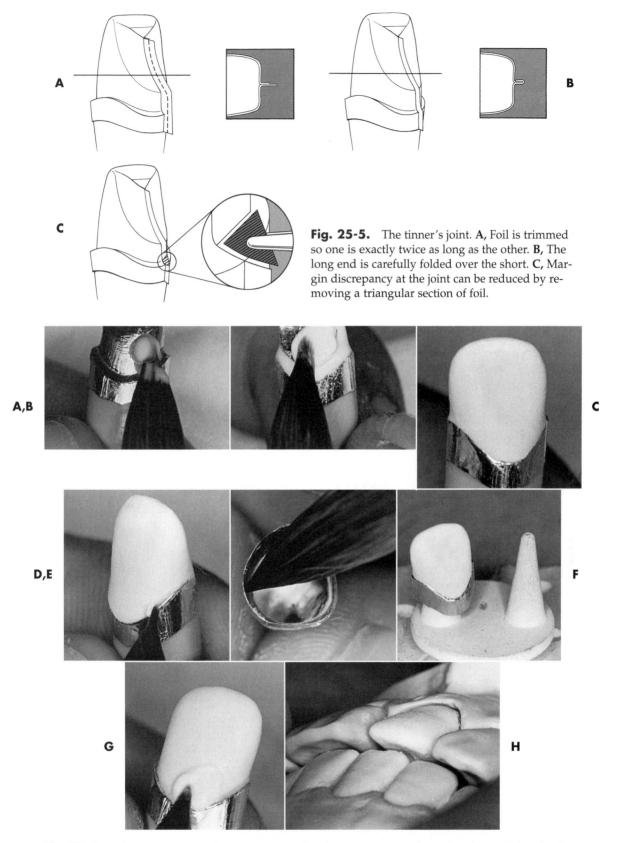

Fig. 25-5. The tinner's joint. **A,** Foil is trimmed so one is exactly twice as long as the other. **B,** The long end is carefully folded over the short. **C,** Margin discrepancy at the joint can be reduced by removing a triangular section of foil.

Fig. 25-6. Aluminous core technique. **A** to **C,** The platinum matrix is heated to drive off dissolved gases, and the core porcelain is built up. **D,** A thin blade is used to form a cervical ditch, which will prevent the matrix from becoming distorted during the first firing. **E,** There must be no porcelain particles on the inner aspect. **F,** The fired core should be checked with a thickness gauge. Often additional core material will be needed to obtain the recommended dimensions. **G,** The foil is readapted to the margin, and the ditch is filled with additional porcelain. This lingual view shows where the core should be thickest. For esthetic reasons the core is much thinner on the facial surface. **H,** The core is seated on the working cast before the application of body and incisal porcelains.

dispersing agents. The slip is applied onto a porous refractory die, which absorbs the water from the slip and leads to the condensation of the slip on the die. The piece is then fired at high temperature (1150° C). The refractory die shrinks more than the condensed slip, which allows easy separation after firing. The fired porous core is later glass-infiltrated, a unique process in which molten glass is drawn into the pores by capillary action at high temperature.[34] Materials processed by slip-casting tend to exhibit lower porosity and less processing defects than traditionally sintered ceramic materials. The strength of In-Ceram is about three to four times greater than earlier alumina core materials,[35,36] a finding that has prompted its use in high-stress situations such as FPDs (Fig. 25-7). Two modified porcelain compositions for the In-Ceram technique have been introduced: In-Ceram Spinell* contains a magnesium spinel ($MgAl_2O_4$) as the major crystalline phase, which improves the translucency of the final restoration (Fig. 25-8). In-Ceram Zirconia contains zirconium oxide (ZrO_2) and is said to provide the highest strength.[37,38] Marginal fit of In-Ceram has been reported as very good[39] or good[40] but also poor,[41] emphasizing the technique sensitivity of the process and the need to select a skilled dental laboratory.

Fabrication Procedure

1. Duplicate the working die with an elastomeric impression material (Fig. 25-9, *B*) and pour it with the special refractory die material. Any undercuts must be blocked out first, and two coats of die-spacer must be applied. When the die material has fully set (2 hours), remove the die, mark the **margins,** and apply the wetting agent (Fig. 25-9, *C*).

2. Mix the appropriate shade of alumina slip with ultrasonic agitation (Fig. 25-9, *D*), place the mixture under a vacuum, brush apply it to the plaster die (Fig. 25-9, *E*), and shape it with a blade, trimming back to the margins carefully.

3. The slip is fired in a special furnace (Fig. 25-9, *F*), initially through a prolonged drying cycle to 120° C (248° F) that dries the die material, which shrinks away from the core. Then the alumina is fired at 1120° C (2048° F). The resulting core is porous and weak at this stage but can be carefully transferred to the master die after the die spacer is removed. The relatively low sintering shrinkage (about 0.3%) is compensated for by an expansion of the refractory material.

4. Paint a thick coat of the appropriate shade of glass mixture onto the surface of the core (Fig. 25-9, *G*) and fire at 1100° C (2012° F). As the glass melts, it is drawn into the interstices of the alumina by capillary action, producing a dense composite structure with excellent strength properties.

5. Remove excess glass from the core by grinding (Fig. 25-9, *H*) and airborne particle abrasion. Body and incisal porcelain is applied to the core in a manner similar to that for metal-ceramic crowns, as shown in Figure 25-10. Powder distribution is governed by a detailed prescription of the patient's shade (see Chapter 23). With experience the practitioner will be able to mix different powders to match almost any shade. If necessary, test firings can be used to help select the correct blend in difficult situations.

6. After moistening the core, mix the powder with modeling liquid and apply in increments with a brush (Fig. 25-10, *A* to *C*).

7. Remove moisture with a paper tissue held against the lingual surface. The capillary action will condense the porcelain particles. Slight vibration brings further moisture to the surface before the next increment is added. To prevent voids from forming between increments, always add to a moist surface.

8. When the crown has the correct shape, cut it back to allow room for incisal porcelain (Fig. 25-10, *D*).

9. Apply incisal porcelain, overbuilding the incisal edge by 1 or 1.5 mm to allow for firing shrinkage (Fig. 25-10, *E*).

10. Lightly condense the buildup with a large whipping brush. Absorb excess moisture with a tissue.

11. Remove the crown from the working cast and add material interproximally to allow for shrinkage (Fig. 25-10, *F*).

12. Dry the crown and fire it (Fig. 25-10, *G,H*).

HOT-PRESSED CERAMICS

Leucite based. Hot-pressed ceramics are becoming increasingly popular in dentistry. The restorations are waxed, invested, and pressed in a manner somewhat similar to gold casting. Marginal adaptation seems to be better with hot-pressing

---

*NOTE: The product *In-Ceram Spinell* is spelled differently than the mineral spinel.

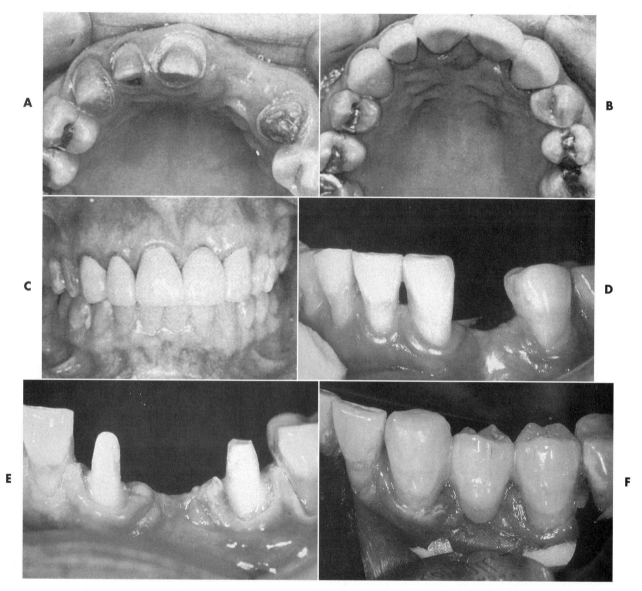

Fig. 25-7.   **A** to **C**, All-ceramic FPD replacing the maxillary left central incisor using the In-Ceram system. **D** to **F**, All-ceramic FPD replacing the mandibular left first premolar using the Empress 2 system. (*D to F courtesy Ivoclar North America.*)

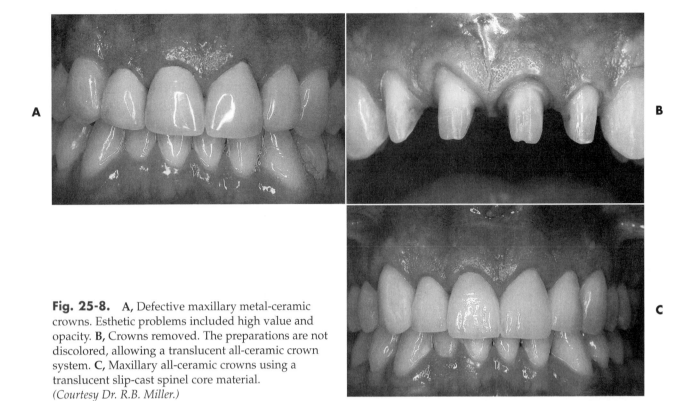

Fig. 25-8. **A,** Defective maxillary metal-ceramic crowns. Esthetic problems included high value and opacity. **B,** Crowns removed. The preparations are not discolored, allowing a translucent all-ceramic crown system. **C,** Maxillary all-ceramic crowns using a translucent slip-cast spinel core material. *(Courtesy Dr. R.B. Miller.)*

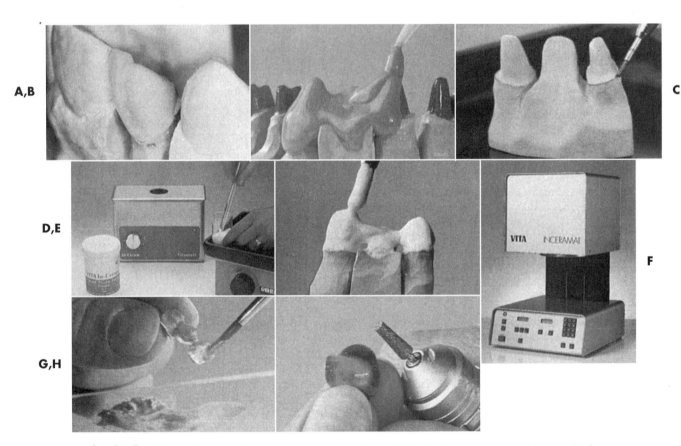

Fig. 25-9. Fabrication of a slip-cast alumina restoration. **A,** The In-Ceram system relies on a high-strength core veneered with an esthetic feldspathic porcelain. **B,** The master cast is duplicated with a special elastomer. **C,** The special plaster die. **D,** The alumina slip is ultrasonically mixed and applied to the plaster die **(E). F,** The Vita Inceramat special porcelain furnace. **G,** A special colored infiltration glass is painted on the porous sintered alumina and fired. **H,** Excess glass is carefully removed by grinding and air abrasion.

(A courtesy Morehead Dental Laboratories; B to H courtesy Vident.)

than with the high-strength alumina core materials,[39] although the results from individual dental laboratories may not support the research. Most hot-pressed materials contain leucite as a major crystalline phase, dispersed in a glassy matrix. The crystal size varies from 3 to 10 μm, and the leucite content varies from about 35% to about 50% by volume depending on the material. Leucite is used as a reinforcing phase due to the tangential stresses it creates within the porcelain.

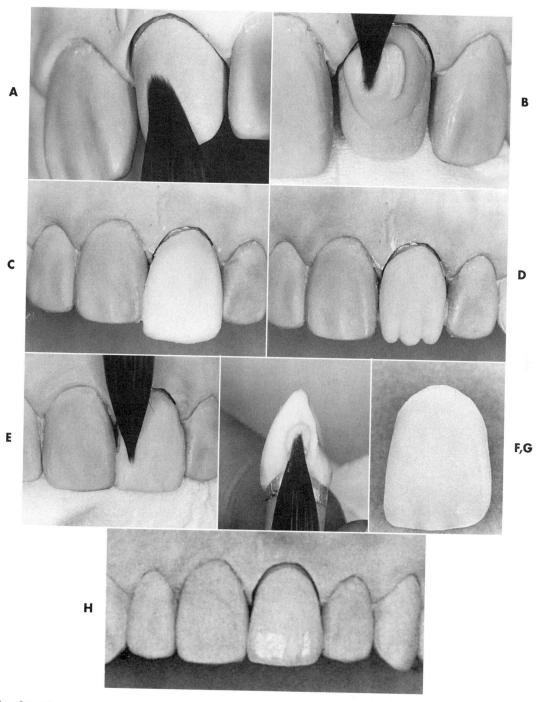

Fig. 25-10. Body and incisal porcelain application. **A,** Moistening the high-strength core. **B** and **C,** Applying gingival and body porcelains. **D,** Cutback for the incisal porcelain. **E,** The incisal porcelain. **F,** Adding to the interproximal areas. **G,** The completed buildup. **H,** The fired crown is seated on the master cast.

Ceramic ingots are pressed at high temperature (from 900° C to 1165° C [1650° F to 2130° F] depending on the material) into a refractory mold made by the lost-wax technique. The ceramic ingots are available in different shades. Two finishing techniques can be used: a characterization technique (surface **stain** only) and a layering technique, involving the application of a veneering porcelain (see Fig. 25-11, *G* and *H*). The two techniques lead to comparable mean flexure strength values for the resulting porcelain composite.[42] The thermal expansion coefficient of the core material for the veneering technique is usually lower than that of the material for the staining technique to be compatible with the thermal expansion coefficient of the veneering porcelain. Among the currently available leucite-containing materials for hot-pressing are IPS Empress,* Optimal Pressable Ceramic,† and two lower fusing materials, Cerpress‡ and Finesse.§

Lithium Silicate based.   IPS Empress 2* is a recently introduced hot-pressed ceramic. The major crystalline phase of the core material is a lithium disilicate. The material is pressed at 920° C (1690° F)

---

*Ivoclar North America Inc: Amherst, N.Y.
†Jeneric/Pentron, Inc: Wallingford, Conn.
‡Leach & Dillon Dental Products: San Diego, Calif.
§Dentsply/Ceramco Division: Burlington, N.J.

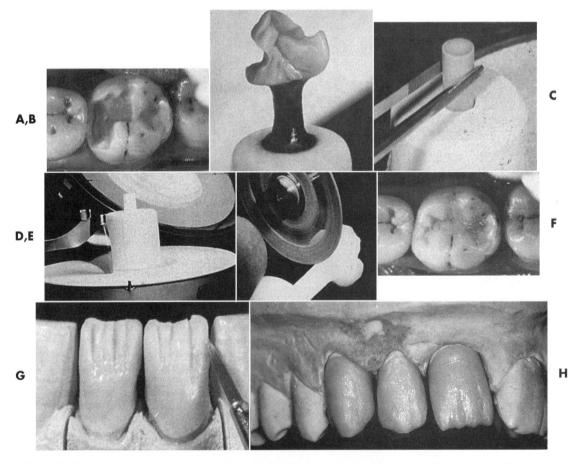

Fig. 25-11.   Heat-pressed ceramic technique. **A,** Inlay preparation for a mandibular molar. **B,** A wax pattern is made in a similar manner to conventional gold castings. **C,** After investing the pattern, it is burned out, and a ceramic ingot and alumina plunger are placed in the heated mold. **D,** The pressing is done under vacuum at 1150° C. **E,** Sprue removal. **F,** The cemented restoration. **G** and **H,** For esthetic anterior restorations, only the dentin-colored ceramic is pressed. The incisal porcelain is brush applied in the conventional manner.
(Courtesy Ivoclar North America, Inc.)

Continued

and layered with a glass containing some dispersed apatite crystals.[43] The initial results from clinical trials seem quite promising[44] and may have application for anterior three-unit fixed partial dentures (FPDs).

Fabrication Procedure

1. Wax the restoration to final contour, sprue, and invest as with conventional gold castings (Fig. 25-11, *A*). If the veneering technique is used, only the body porcelain shape is waxed.

2. Heat the investment to 800° C (or recommended temperature) to burn out the wax pattern.
3. Insert a ceramic ingot of the appropriate shade and alumina plunger in the sprue (Fig. 25-11, *B*) and place the refractory in the special pressing furnace.
4. After heating to 1150° C, the softened ceramic is slowly pressed into the mold under vacuum (Fig. 25-11, *C*).
5. After pressing, recover the restoration from the investment by airborne particle abrasion, remove

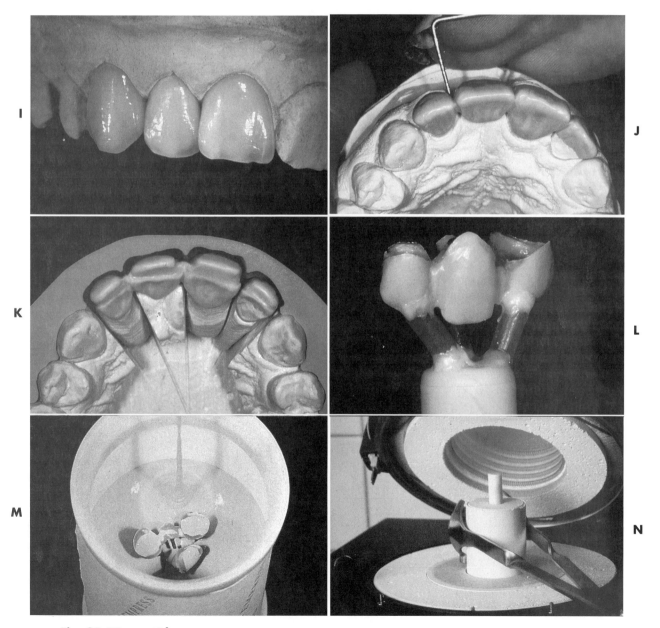

Fig. 25-11, cont'd.   **I,** Three-unit FPD and veneer waxed to anatomic contour. **J,** Ensure the connector size is adequate (4 × 4 mm). **K,** Use a silicone matrix to aid in cut-back of the wax pattern.
L, Framework sprued and invested (**M**). **N,** The lithium-silicate ceramic is pressed into the mold.

Continued

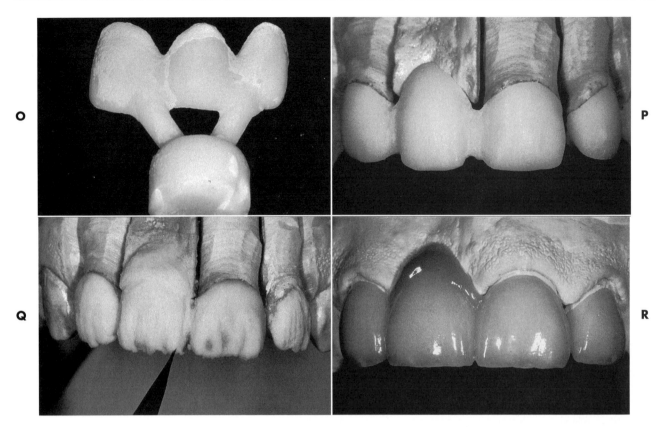

Fig. 25-11, cont'd.   **O,** The pressed restoration. **P,** Framework on master cast. **Q,** Applying veneering porcelain. **R,** Completed restorations.
(Courtesy Ivoclar North America, Inc.)

the sprue (Fig. 25-11, *D*), and refit it to the die. Esthetics can be enhanced by applying an enamel layer of matching porcelain (Fig. 25-11, *E* to *H*) or by adding surface characterization. The procedure for an FPD is similar (Fig. 25-11, *I* to *R*).

MACHINED CERAMICS

The evolution of **CAD/CAM** systems for the production of machined inlays, onlays, veneers, and crowns led to the development of a new generation of ceramics that are machinable.

Cerec System. The Cerec system* has been marketed for several years with the improved Cerec 2 system introduced in the mid-1990s. The equipment consists of a computer integrated imaging and milling system, with the restorations designed on the computer screen (Fig. 25-12, *A*). At least three materials can be used with this system: Vita Mark II,† Dicor MGC,‡ and ProCad.§ Vita

*Sirona Dental Systems:Bensheim, Germany.
†Vident: Brea, Calif.
‡Dentsply International, Inc: York, Pa.
§Ivoclar North America, Inc: Amhurst, N.Y.

Mark II contains sanidine ($KAlSi_3O_8$) as a major crystalline phase within a glassy matrix. Dicor MGC is a mica-based machinable glass-ceramic that contains 70 volume percent of crystalline phase.[45,46] The unique "house of cards" microstructure found in Dicor MGC is due to the interlocking of the small platelet-shaped mica crystals with an average size of 1 to 2 μm. This particular microstructure leads to multiple crack deflections and ensures a greater strength than leucite-containing ceramics.[47] ProCad is a leucite-containing ceramic designed for making machined restorations. Weaknesses of the earlier Cerec system include the poor marginal fit of the restorations[48] and the lack of sophistication in the machining of the occlusal surface. The marginal adaptation of Cerec 2 is improved,[49] and the occlusal anatomy can be shaped.

Fabrication Procedure

1. Tooth preparation follows typical all-ceramic guidelines.
2. Coat the preparation with opaque powder.
3. Image the preparation with the optical scanner, aligning the camera with the path of insertion of the restoration (Fig. 25-12, *B*).

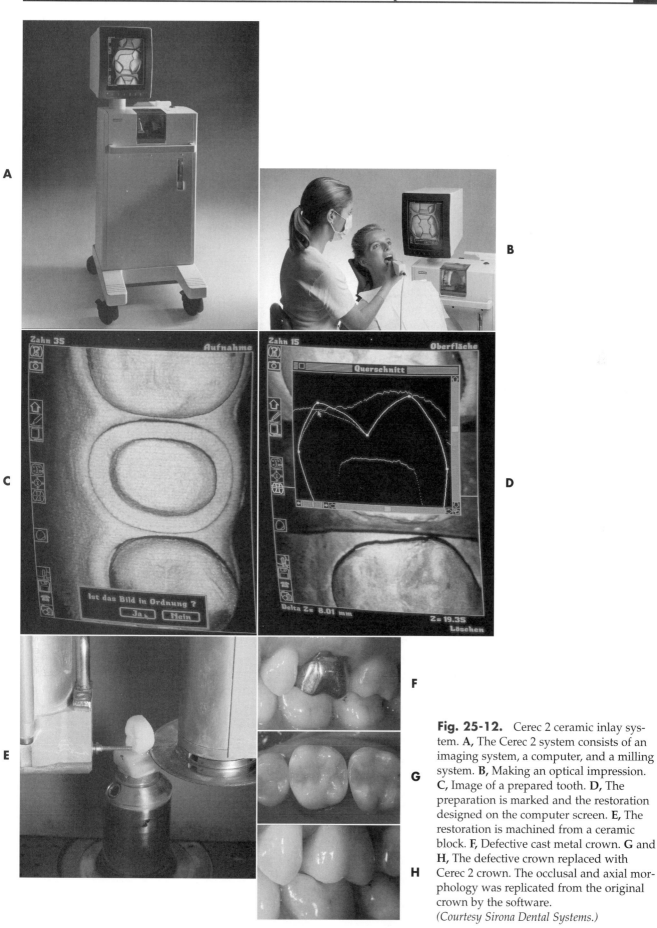

Fig. 25-12. Cerec 2 ceramic inlay system. **A,** The Cerec 2 system consists of an imaging system, a computer, and a milling system. **B,** Making an optical impression. **C,** Image of a prepared tooth. **D,** The preparation is marked and the restoration designed on the computer screen. **E,** The restoration is machined from a ceramic block. **F,** Defective cast metal crown. **G** and **H,** The defective crown replaced with Cerec 2 crown. The occlusal and axial morphology was replicated from the original crown by the software. *(Courtesy Sirona Dental Systems.)*

When the best view is obtained, it is stored in the computer (Fig. 25-12, *C*).

4. Identify and mark the margins and contours on the computer screen. The computer software assists with this step (Fig. 25-12, *D*).
5. Insert the appropriate shade of ceramic block in the milling machine. The fabrication time for a crown is about 20 minutes (Fig. 25-12, *E*). Additional characterization is achieved with stains.
6. Try the restoration back in the mouth, etch, and silanate and lute it to place as described in Chapter 31.

Celay System (Fig. 25-13). The Celay system* uses a copy milling technique to manufacture ceramic inlays or onlays.[50] A resin pattern is fabricated directly on the prepared tooth or on a master die, then the pattern is used to mill a porcelain restoration.[51] As with the Cerec system, the starting material is a ceramic blank available in different shades† (extracted human teeth have also been used experimentally[52]). This material is similar to Vita Mark II ceramic, used with the Cerec 2 system. Alternatively, blanks of the InCeram Alumina or InCeram Spinell materials can be used.[53] Marginal accuracy seems to be good, a little better than the Cerec 2 system.[54]

Procera AllCeram System (Fig. 25-14). The Procera AllCeram system involves an industrial CAD/CAM process.[55,56] The die is mechanically scanned by the technician, and the data are sent to a work station where an enlarged die is milled using a computer-controlled milling machine. This enlargement is necessary to compensate for the sintering shrinkage. Aluminum oxide powder is then compacted onto the die, and the coping is milled before sintering at very high temperature (>1550° C). The coping is further veneered with an aluminous ceramic‡ with matched thermal expansion. The restorations seem to have good clinical performance[57] and marginal adaptation,[58] provided the scanning is done skillfully. They may be suitable for posterior crowns and FPDs, although long-term data are needed.[59]

Step-by-step Procedure

1. Tooth preparation (Fig. 25-14, *A*) follows all-ceramic guidelines.

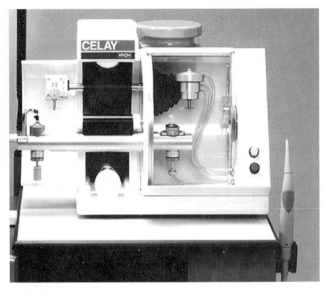

Fig 25-13. The Celay system. The pattern on the left is copied milling the restoration from the ceramic block *(right)*.
(Courtesy Vident.)

2. The cast is made in the conventional way, but the die is ditched to make the margin easier to identify during scanning (Fig. 25-14, *B*).
3. The die is mapped using a contact scanner (Fig. 25-14, *C* and *D*).
4. The shape of the prepared tooth is transferred to the computer screen (Fig. 25-14, *E*).
5. The design of the restoration is transferred to the manufacturer via computer line.
6. The production process starts with milling an enlarged die to compensate for the sintering shrinkage (Fig. 25-14, *F* and *G*).
7. An enlarged high-alumina coping is milled that shrinks to the desired shape after sintering (Fig. 25-14, *H*).
8. The coping is returned to the laboratory, and body and incisal porcelains are applied in the conventional manner (Fig. 25-14, *I* and *J*).

METAL REINFORCED SYSTEMS

High-gold substructure systems are designed to overcome some of the disadvantages inherent in the porcelain jacket crown technique. The systems rely on different ways of creating a thin coping onto which the ceramic is fired. In strictest terms, therefore, they are metal-ceramic as opposed to **all-ceramic crowns.**

---

*Mikrona Technologie: Spreitenbach, Switzerland.
†Vita-Celay, Vident: Brea, Calif.
‡Procera Porcelain All Ceramic, Nobel Biocare, Inc: Yorba Linda, Calif.

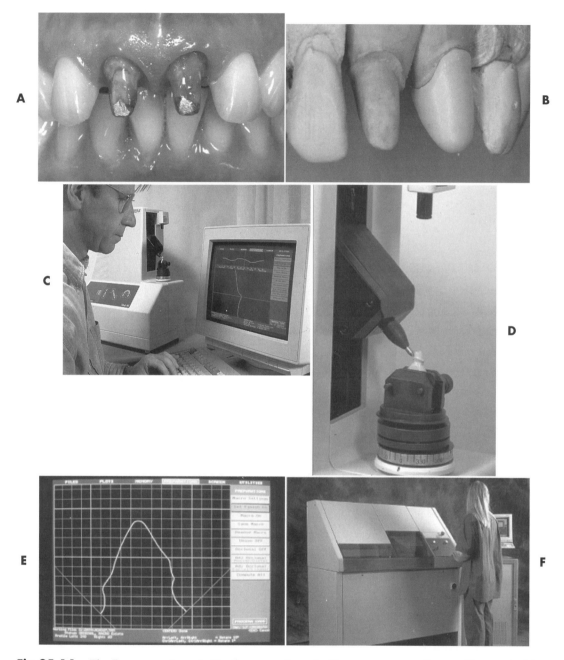

Fig 25-14. The Procera system. **A,** Tooth preparations for Procera crown on the maxillary central incisors. **B,** The die is ditched to make the margin easier to identify during scanning. **C** and **D,** The die is mapped using a contact scanner. **E,** The shape of the prepared tooth is transferred to the computer screen. **F,** Milling machine.   *Continued*
(Courtesy Nobel Biocare USA, Inc.)

The Captek System.   In the Captek* system the coping is produced from two metal-impregnated

*Captek Division, Precious Chemicals USA: Longwood, Fla.

wax sheets that are adapted to a die and fired. The first sheet forms a porous gold-platinum-palladium layer that is impregnated with 97% gold when the second sheet is fired.[60] Advantages of the system include excellent esthetics and marginal adaptation.[61]

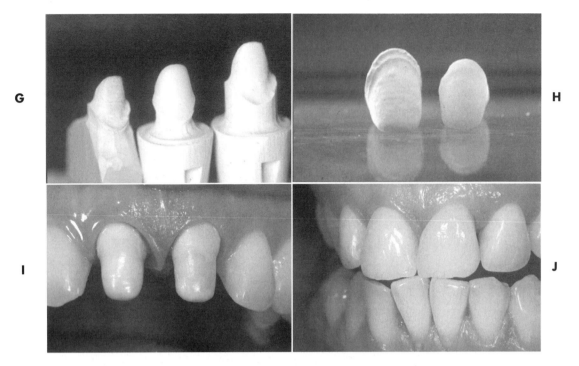

Fig 25-14, cont'd. **G,** Enlarged die compensates for the sintering shrinkage. **H,** High-alumina coping before and after sintering. **I,** Body and incisal porcelains application. **J,** Cemented restorations.

Fabrication Procedure

1. Duplicate the working die in the special refractory material (Fig. 25-15, *A*).
2. Cut a piece of the gold-platinum-palladium impregnated wax sheet (Fig. 25-15, *B*).
3. Adapt the foil to the die (Fig. 25-15, *C*). Then it is fired to 1075° C (1965° F), forming a porous metal coping (Fig. 25-15, *D*).
4. Adapt the second gold-impregnated wax (Fig. 25-15, *E*) and refire (Fig. 25-15, *F*). Capillary action draws the gold into the porous gold-platinum-palladium structure to form the finished coping.
5. Build up the opaque body and incisal porcelains in a manner similar to that for a conventional metal-ceramic crown.
6. Glaze the completed restoration and polish the metal foil at the margin (Fig. 25-15, *I*). The procedure has been adapted for FPDs (Fig. 25-15, *J*).

Electroformed. The Helioform HF 600 system* (Fig. 25-16) uses an electroforming technique to produce a thin pure gold coping. The gold is deposited on polyurethane dies that are coated with a silver spacer using computer-controlled plating equipment to control thickness. The coping is coated with a noble metal paste primer before porcelain application. Electroforming enables very good marginal adaptation (better than conventional casting[62]). The system has been adapted for FPDs.

Step-by-step Procedure

1. Duplicate the working die with the polyurethane material.
2. Drill the polyurethane and glue the electrode into the die.
3. Apply an even coat of the silver spacer to the preparation and allow it to dry.
4. Insert the dies into the plating equipment (Fig. 25-16, *B*). A magnetic stirrer ensures circulation of the cyanide-free gold sulfite solution.
5. Turn on the electric current, and gold will be deposited on the die at an approximate rate of 0.02 mm per hour.

*Vident: Brea, Calif.

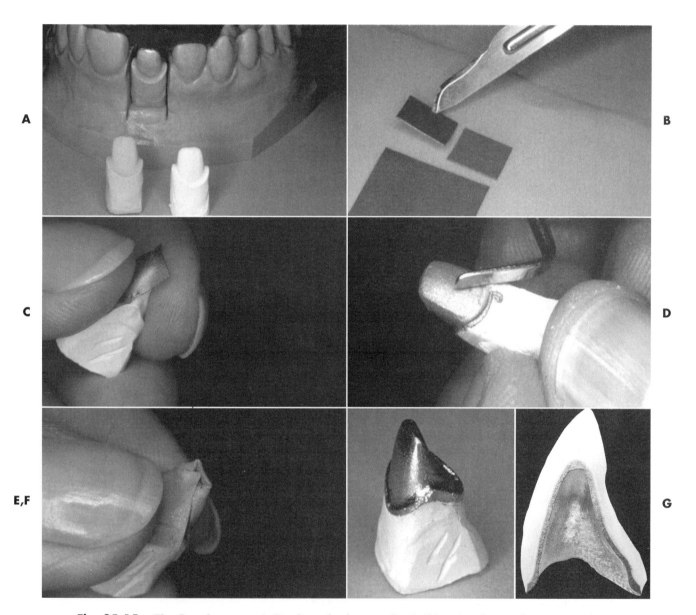

Fig. 25-15. The Captek system. **A,** Duplicated refractory die. **B,** Trimming the metal-impregnated wax sheet. **C,** Adapting first sheet to the die. **D,** First layer is fired to form a porous coping. **E,** Adapting second metal-impregnated wax sheet. **F,** Fired framework. **G,** Sectioned Captek crown showing coping design. *Continued*

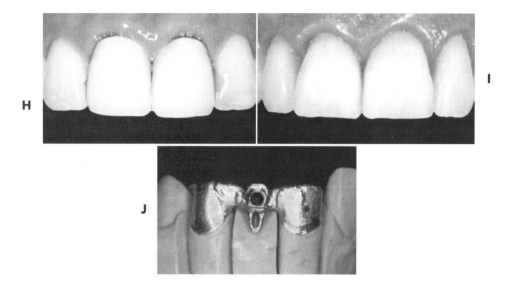

Fig. 25-15, cont'd.   **H,** Defective metal ceramic crown on the maxillary incisors replaced with Captek crowns **(I). J,** Fixed partial denture frameworks can be fabricated with special pontic components, incorporating unique framework design.
(Courtesy Captek Division, Precious Chemicals, Inc.)

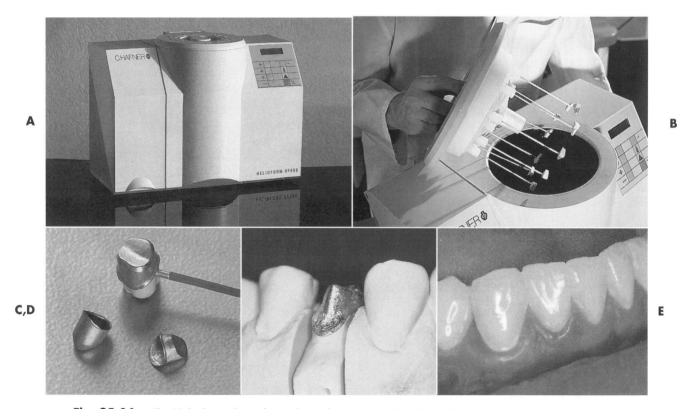

Fig. 25-16.   The Helioform electroformed metal system. **A,** The electroforming equipment. **B,** Inserting the polyurethane dies. **C,** The electroformed copings. **D,** Coping on the die. **E,** Restoration of mandibular canine and lateral with Helioform crowns.
(Courtesy Vident.)

6. Remove the plated copings (Fig. 25-16, *C*) by heating the dies and remove the silver spacer with nitric acid or air abrasion.
7. Trim flash from the margin with an abrasive silicone wheel and seat the coping on the die (Fig. 25-16, *D*).
8. Air-abrade the surface and apply the special bonding paste before porcelain application (Fig. 25-16, *E*).

SELECTION OF ALL-CERAMIC SYSTEMS

The primary purpose in recommending an all-ceramic restoration is to achieve the best possible esthetic result. Typically this will be at the risk of reduced restoration longevity due to the potential for fracture of the ceramic, and the restoration may have a slightly inferior marginal adaptation than a metal-ceramic crown.

FRACTURE RESISTANCE
Most hazards of restoration failure will be removed if these restorations are confined to lower-stress anterior teeth, and patients are carefully evaluated for evidence of parafunctional activity. Although laboratory testing of strength and fracture toughness has identified promising materials,[34,63] clinical studies have consistently shown good performance on anterior teeth yet poor performance on molars and for FPDs.[64-66] Although the newer materials, such as Empress 2 and In-Ceram Zirconia, promise higher strength (see Table 25-1), the long-term data are lacking to determine whether they are satisfactory, particularly for FPDs.[43,67,68]

ESTHETICS
A knowledge of the available ceramic systems is needed to select a material that will provide the best esthetics for a particular patient. This is especially important when matching a single maxillary incisor to an adjacent tooth. Careful consideration should also be given to the availability of laboratory support, because no dental laboratory invests in the expensive equipment needed for all the various systems. The marginal adaptation of the system is very important, even when resin bonding is used. When selecting a system, the dentist should carefully evaluate the internal and marginal adaptation using an elastomeric detection paste.* Although research studies have identified differences among the vari-

ous systems[69] (see Table 25-1), these results may not represent an individual laboratory's results. The translucency of the adjacent teeth and discoloration of the tooth being restored also must be considered when selecting the most appropriate system.[70] Highly translucent teeth would not be best restored with a more opaque, high-strength core, ceramic system (e.g., In-Ceram or Procera). However, these might be the best choice if the tooth exhibits discoloration that would not be well masked by a more translucent material. Conversely, when concern exists about fracture, the higher-strength materials should normally be the first choice (see Table 25-1).

ABRASIVENESS
One concern with ceramic restorations is the potential for abrasion of the opposing enamel, particularly in patients with parafunctional habits. Whenever possible, a low-abrasion material should be considered. Abrasiveness has been studied in vitro,[71-76] and the results are summarized in Table 25-1.

PORCELAIN LABIAL VENEER

Porcelain labial veneers (see Chapter 11) can be fabricated using a refractory die technique (Fig. 25-17) as well as on a platinum matrix.* The platinum matrix technique is tedious and somewhat tricky to learn, but once acquired it enables veneers to be made with better marginal adaptation than the refractory technique.[77] Therefore the platinum matrix technique will be described here. Many of the steps are similar to the porcelain jacket crown technique (see Fig. 25-4).

Step-by-step Procedure
1. Modify the working die by blocking out tooth undercuts with modeling plastic.
2. Adapt the platinum foil (0.025 mm) in the same manner as described for the porcelain jacket crown, covering the entire tooth. Some technicians prefer to adapt the foil to the facial surface only, but distortion of the foil during firing of the porcelain seems to lead to inferior marginal adaptation if this is done.[73] Careful adaptation is essential for good fit, especially at the proximal incisal margin, where the tinner's joint is made.
3. Remove, clean, and degas the foil. Airborne particle abrasion can be used for this step.

---

*This must be thoroughly removed before bonding the restoration.

*Porcelain labial veneers can also be made with hot-pressed ceramics and the machinable systems.

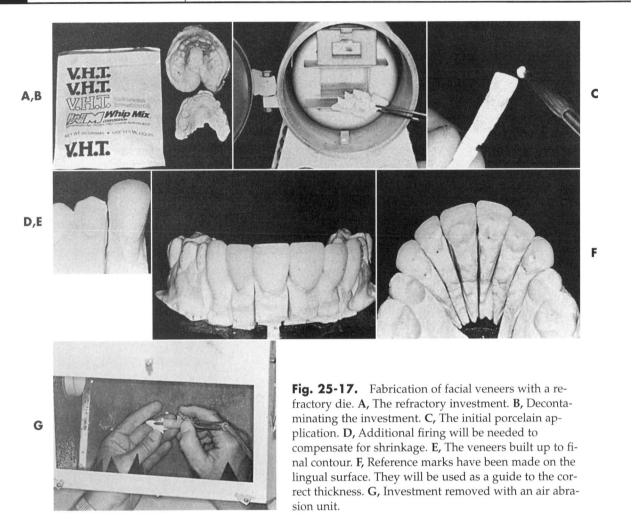

Fig. 25-17. Fabrication of facial veneers with a refractory die. **A,** The refractory investment. **B,** Decontaminating the investment. **C,** The initial porcelain application. **D,** Additional firing will be needed to compensate for shrinkage. **E,** The veneers built up to final contour. **F,** Reference marks have been made on the lingual surface. They will be used as a guide to the correct thickness. **G,** Investment removed with an air abrasion unit.

4. Build up and fire the veneers. This is generally done in two or three layers, particularly if the veneer is required to mask tetracycline staining and a more opaque initial layer is applied. Sometimes tetracycline staining can be more effectively masked by incorporating the complementary hue in the ceramic buildup, rather than fabricating a veneer that is unesthetically opaque looking. With experience, a technician can achieve excellent results with porcelain labial veneers. Special formulations of porcelain are available for veneers. Some are based on traditional jacket or metal-ceramic porcelain systems; higher-strength, high-leucite content formulations are also available. Fracture of porcelain labial veneers is sometimes encountered in practice, even though the restorations are generally placed in low-stress situations. At present, there are little data about the incidence of veneer fracture or whether a high-strength ceramic has better performance than a traditional formulation. When a fracture

does occur, the broken pieces are often still firmly bonded to the tooth. At that point, it is probably not necessary to replace the restoration unless the fracture line is stained or the ceramic is chipped.

5. Contour and glaze the facings. The veneers should be shaped to final contour at this stage.

6. Remove the foil before try-in. The steps for **etching**, silanating, and luting the veneers are presented in Chapter 31.

◼ INLAYS AND ONLAYS

REFRACTORY DIES

Ceramic restorations are normally made using a refractory die rather than with a platinum foil matrix. This is specified by the manufacturer of some ceramic systems (e.g., Cerinate), and other materials can be used according to the technician's preference. Marginal adaptation can be excellent, depending more on the technician than the ceramic material used.[78]

STEP-BY-STEP PROCEDURE

1. Pour an elastomeric impression of the prepared teeth in Type IV or V stone; then repour it or duplicate it in ceramic refractory, using an appropriate removable die system (Fig. 25-18, A). The Di-Lok (see Chapter 17) or a similar system is convenient for this technique. The dies need to be separated very carefully because the refractory is friable and will break if mishandled.
2. Trim the **refractory cast** as far as possible to minimize the quantity of ammonia released during decontamination.
3. Mark the margins lightly with a special pencil (V.H.T.*)
4. Decontaminate the cast by firing according to the manufacturer's instructions. Normally this will be done in two stages: the first in a burnout furnace, the second under vacuum in a porcelain furnace.

*Whip Mix Corp: Louisville, Ky.

5. Allow the cast to cool and then soak it in soaking liquid or distilled water for 5 minutes. This will seal the die and prevent moisture from being drawn out of the porcelain buildup.
6. Apply an initial layer of porcelain to the refractory cast (Fig. 25-18, B) and fire according to the manufacturer's directions. With some systems, a higher-strength core material is used as the initial coat.
7. Build up the restorations onto moist dies; for inlays, leave short of the margins.
8. Make a relieving cut through the central fossa (Fig. 25-18, C) and fire the porcelain (Fig. 25-18, D).
9. Fill in the central fossa area and build up to the margins (Fig. 25-18, E and F).
10. Contour and refine occlusion and proximal contacts. Glaze according to the manufacturer's instructions.
11. Remove the investment with a bur (Fig. 25-18, G) and 50-μm alumina in an airborne particle abrasion unit. Transfer the restorations to the master dies on the mounted cast (Fig. 25-18, H).

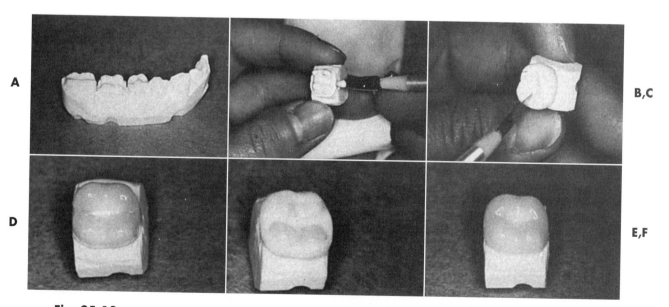

Fig. 25-18. Fabrication of a ceramic onlay using the refractory die technique. **A,** A refractory die is produced as a duplicate of the stone die. **B,** After decontamination and soaking, an initial layer of porcelain is added to the die. **C,** A relieving cut through the central fossa is made to prevent the porcelain pulling away from the margin during sintering. **D,** The onlay after the first porcelain firing. **E,** Additional porcelain is added to the central fossa and margins. **F,** Restoration after second porcelain firing. *(Courtesy Den-Mat Corporation.)*

Continued

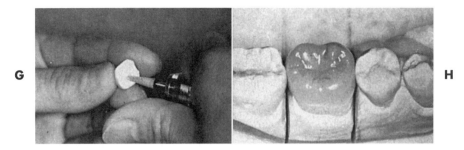

Fig. 25-18, cont'd. **G,** After contouring and adjustment of occlusion the refractory is removed with a stone and air abrasion. **H,** Completed restoration ready for try-in.
(Courtesy Den-Mat Corporation.)

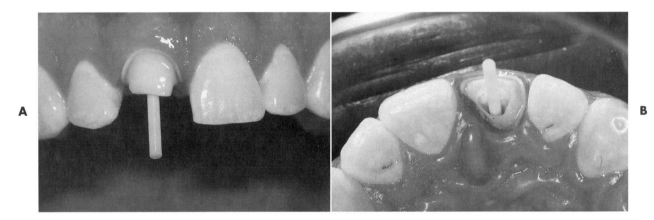

Fig. 25-19. Fabrication of an all-ceramic post-and-core. **A** and **B,** Zirconia post seated in prepared tooth.   *Continued*
(Courtesy Dr. J.A. Holloway.)

12. If necessary, adjust the restoration margins and occlusion with fine-grit diamond stones. Polish with diamond **polishing** paste.

ALL-CERAMIC FIXED PARTIAL DENTURES

All-ceramic FPDs have a checkered history. They were attempted with aluminous porcelain by connecting alumina cores with pure alumina rods. these restorations were usually unsuccessful; either they fractured, or the restorations encroached excessively into the embrasures, resulting in hygiene deficiencies. Leucite-containing heat-pressed ceramics do not appear to possess adequate strength for FPDs, except in very low-stress situations. Clinical trials of posterior ceramic FPDs have reported disastrous results.[28,79] The recently introduced InCeram Zirconia has much higher laboratory strength than these materials and might be suitable for FPD frameworks. In-Ceram alumina was somewhat successful for anterior FPDs (see Fig. 25-7). The more recent lithium disilicate, heat-pressed ceramic, Empress 2, and the CAD/CAM Procera systems have also been recommended as suitable for anterior

FPDs. Although the newer materials might be successful for FPDs, their manufacturers recommend a design with substantial connectors (typically 4 × 4 mm, as opposed to 2 × 3 mm recommended for metal connectors). These dimensions can lead to problems with adequate access for cleaning and poor esthetics.

ALL-CERAMIC FOUNDATION RESTORATIONS

All-ceramic materials have been used as foundation restorations for endodontically treated teeth[80,81] to overcome esthetic problems associated with metal post-and-core systems (see Chapter 12). The post is made of zirconia,* chosen for its excellent strength,[82] and depending on the system, the core material can be composite resin or a pressable ceramic† (Fig. 25-19).

---

*CosmoPost, Ivoclar North America; Biopost Incermed SA: Lausanne, Switzerland; TZP-post, Maillefer: Ballaigues, Switzerland.
†Empress, Cosmo: Ivoclar North America, Inc.: Amherst, N.Y.

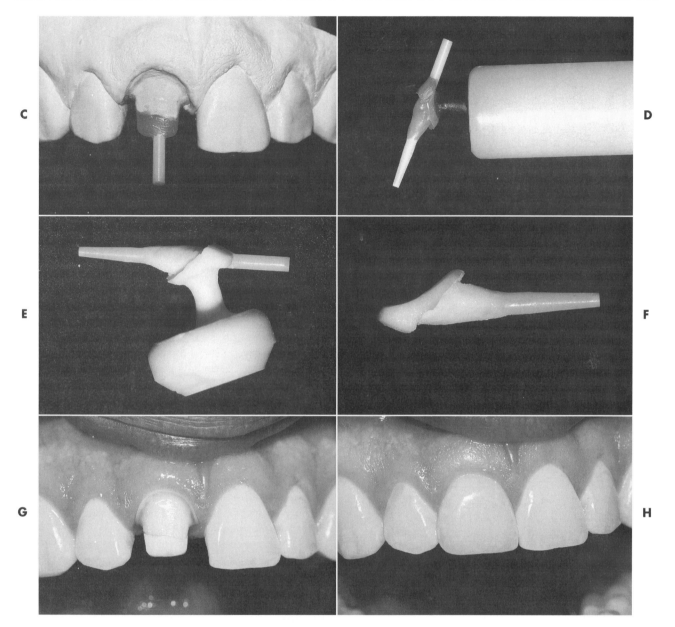

Fig. 25-19, cont'd. C, Zirconia post fitted to the working cast and the core waxed to shape. D, Sprued pattern before investing. E, Core ceramic is hot-pressed and trimmed to shape. F and G, Seated all-ceramic post-and-core. H, Completed all-ceramic crown.

RESIN-BONDED CERAMICS

The performance of all-ceramic restorations has been enhanced by the use of resin bonding. This technique was first devised for the porcelain laminate veneer technique[83,84] and has been applied to other ceramic restorations. The technique uses hydrofluoric acid or a less toxic substitute to etch the ceramic and a **silane** coupling agent to bond a resin luting agent to the ceramic. The luting agent is bonded to enamel after etching with phosphoric acid as with resin-retained FPDs (see Chapter 26) and bonded to dentin with a dentin-bonding agent.

Significant reduction in the fracture incidence of some types of ceramic crowns has been reported when an adhesive cement has been used,[85] although a recent retrospective study failed to find an improvement compared to traditional cements.[86] Resin bonding does not appear to improve the fracture resistance of the high-strength alumina core materials such as In-Ceram and Procera. Nevertheless, for feldspathic and leucite-reinforced ceramics, resin-bonding is now the recommended procedure and is also used extensively for luting ceramic inlays and onlays.[87]

ETCHING AND SILANATING THE RESTORATION

1. Support the restoration in soft wax with the fitting surface uppermost.
2. Apply a 1-mm coat of the etching gel* to the fitting surface only.
3. The etching time will depend on the ceramic material. Feldspathic porcelain is typically etched for 5 minutes.
4. Very carefully rinse away the gel under running water. The gel is very caustic; it should not be allowed to contact skin or eyes.
5. Continue to rinse until all the gel color has been removed.
6. Dry the ceramic with oil-free air. A hair dryer is recommended to ensure that the ceramic is not contaminated.
7. Apply the silane according to the manufacturer's recommendations. Some manufacturers recommend a heat-cured silane coupling agent for increased bond strength, rather than a chemically-activated silane. Heat curing is normally done by the laboratory, and care must be taken to clean the fitting surface thoroughly with alcohol before cementation.

The cementation procedures are presented in Chapter 31.

▪SUMMARY

For many years porcelain jacket crowns have been the most esthetic of fixed restorations. Unfortunately, they incorporate a number of disadvantages compared to the more popular metal-ceramic crowns, including inferior mechanical properties and increased technical difficulties associated with obtaining adequate margin fit.

---

*Ceram-Etch Gel (9.5% hydrofluoric acid), Gresco Products, Inc: Stafford, Tex. (or the ceramic manufacturer's recommended product).

Improved materials and the bonded ceramic technique have renewed interest in all-ceramic restorations. Porcelain laminate veneers have proved to be conservative and esthetic alternatives to complete coverage. Porcelain inlays and onlays may provide a durable alternative to posterior composite resins without the extensive tooth preparation needed for crowns. The highest-strength materials may be suitable for high-stress applications, including FPDs. However, they are relatively new and still lack the support of long-term clinical experience and research.

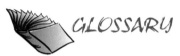

GLOSSARY

aluminum oxide *1:* a metallic oxide constituent of dental porcelain that increases hardness and viscosity *2:* a high-strength ceramic crystal dispersed throughout a glassy phase to increase its strength as in aluminous dental porcelain used to fabricate aluminous porcelain jacket crowns *3:* a finely ground ceramic particle (frequently 50 μm) often used in conjunction with airborne particle abrasion of metal castings before the application of porcelain as with metal ceramic restorations.

bisque bake: a series of stages of maturation in the firing of ceramic materials relating to the degree of pyrochemical reaction and sintering shrinkage occurring before vitrification (glazing)—called also *biscuit bake.*

CAD-CAM: acronym for *Computer Aided Design-Computer Aided Manufacturer (or Computer Assisted Machining).*

castable ceramic: for dental applications, a glass-ceramic material that combines the properties of a restorative material for function with the capability to be cast using the lost wax process.

ceram: *n:* a heat treatment process that converts a specially formulated glass into a fine grained glass-ceramic material.

Study Questions

1. Discuss the advantages and disadvantages, indications, and contraindications of all-ceramic crowns.
2. Which all-ceramic system might be considered for a fixed partial denture? What are the limitations with all-ceramics in this application?
3. Compare the fabrication steps for a slip cast versus a heat-pressed ceramic system. What are the advantages of each?
4. What are the advantages and disadvantages of using a ceramic system as a post-and-core restoration?
5. Describe the fabrication steps for laminate veneers.
6. What are the currently available CAD/CAM systems? What are the advantages and limitations of these restorations?

ceramic: *adj* (1850): of or relating to the manufacture of any product made essentially from a non-metallic mineral (as clay) by firing at a higher temperature.

¹coping: *n* **1:** a long, enveloping ecclesiastical vestment **2a:** something resembling a cope (as by concealing or covering) **2b:** coping.

²coping: *n* (ca. 1909): a thin covering or crown.

etching: *vt* (1632) **1:** the act or process of selective dissolution **2:** in dentistry, the selective dissolution of the surface of tooth enamel, metal, or porcelain through the use of acids or other agents (etchants) to create a retentive surface.

feldspar: *n* (1757) **1:** any one of a group of minerals, principally aluminosilicates of sodium, potassium, calcium, or barium, that are essential constituents of nearly all crystalline rocks **2:** a crystalline mineral of aluminum silicate with sodium, barium, and/or calcium; a major constituent of some dental porcelains.

firing: the process of porcelain fusion, in dentistry, specifically to produce porcelain restorations.

fluorescence: *n* (1852): a process by which a material absorbs radiant energy and reemits it in the form of radiant energy of a different wavelength band, all or most of whose wavelengths exceed that of the absorbed energy. Fluorescence, as distinguished from phosphorescence, does not persist for an appreciable time after the termination of the excitation process.

glass-ceramic: a solid material, partly crystalline and partly glassy, formed by controlled crystallization of a glass.

glaze *vb* **glazed; glazing:** *vt* **1:** to cover with a glossy, smooth surface or coating **2:** the attainment of a smooth and reflective surface **3:** the final firing of porcelain in which the surface is vitrified and a high gloss is imparted to the material **4:** a ceramic veneer on a metal porcelain restoration after it has been fired, producing a nonporous, glossy or semiglossy surface.

hydroxyapatite ceramic: a composition of calcium and phosphate in physiologic ratios to provide a dense, nonresorbable, biocompatible ceramic used for dental implants and residual ridge augmentation.

inlay: *n* (1667): a fixed intracoronal restoration; a dental restoration made outside of a tooth to correspond to the form of the prepared cavity, which is then luted into the tooth.

intrinsic coloring: coloring from within; the incorporation of a colorant within the material of a prosthesis or restoration.

ion exchange strengthening: the chemical process whereby the surface of a glass is placed in compression by the replacement of a small ion by a larger one while maintaining chemical neutrality.

microcrack: *n:* in porcelain, one of the numerous surface flaws that contributes to stress concentrations and results in strengths below those theoretically possible.

natural glaze: the production of a glazed surface by the vitrification of the material itself and without addition of other fluxes or glasses.

opacity: *n* (1611): the quality or state of a body that makes it impervious to light.

opaque: *adj* (1641): the property of a material that absorbs and/or reflects all light and prevents any transmission of light.

overglaze *adj* (1879): the production of a glazed surface by the addition of a fluxed glass that usually vitrifies at a lower temperature.

pigment: *n* (14 cent.): finely ground, natural or synthetic, inorganic or organic, insoluble dispersed particles (powder), which, when dispersed in a liquid vehicle, may provide, in addition to color, many other essential properties such as opacity, hardness, durability, and corrosion resistance. The term is used to include extenders and white or color pigments. The distinction between powders that are pigments and those that are dyes is generally considered on the basis of solubility—pigments being insoluble and dispersed in the material, dyes being soluble or in solution as used.

platinum foil: a precious-metal foil with a high fusing point that makes it suitable as a matrix for various soldering procedures as well as to provide an internal form for porcelain restorations during their fabrication.

porcelain: *n* (known in Europe, ca. 1540): a ceramic material formed of infusible elements joined by lower fusing materials. Most dental porcelains are glasses and are used in the fabrication of teeth for dentures, pontics and facings, metal ceramic restorations, crowns, inlays, onlays, and other restorations.

porosity *n, pl* **-ties:** (14 cent.) **1:** the presence of voids or pores within a structure **2:** the state or quality of having minute pores, openings or interstices.

refractory cast: a cast made of a material that will withstand high termperatures without disintegrating-called also investment cast.

silica: *n* (ca 1301): silicon dioxide occurring in crystalline, amorphous, and usually impure forms (as quartz, opal, and sand, respectively).

stain: *vb* **1:** to suffuse with color **2:** to color by processes affecting chemically or otherwise the material itself **3:** in dentistry, to intentionally alter ceramic or resin restorations through the application of intrinsic or extrinsic colorants to achieve a desired effect.

translucency: *n* (1611): having the appearance between complete opacity and complete transparency; partially opaque.

References

1. Ernsmere JB:Porcelain dental work, *Br J Dent Sci* 43:547, 1900.

2. Ehrlich A: Erosion of acrylic resin restorations (letter), *J Am Dent Assoc* 59:543, 1959.

3. Söremark R, Bergman B: Studies on the permeability of acrylic facing material in gold crowns, a laboratory investigation using Na, *Acta Odontol Scand* 19:297, 1961.

4. Lamstein A, Blechman H: Marginal seepage around acrylic resin veneers in gold crowns, *J Prosthet Dent* 6:706, 1956.

5. Weinstein M, Weinstein AB: Fused porcelain-to-metal teeth, U.S. Patent No. 3,052,982, Sept 11, 1962.

6. Vines RF, Semmelman JO: Densification of dental porcelain, *J Dent Res* 36:950, 1957.

7. Hondrum SO: A review of the strength properties of dental ceramics, *J Prosthet Dent* 67:859, 1992.

8. Denry IL: Recent advances in ceramics for dentistry, *Crit Rev Oral Biol Med* 7:134, 1996.

9. Jones DW, Wilson HJ: Some properties of dental ceramics, *J Oral Rehab* 2:379, 1975.

10. Kelly JR et al: Fracture surface analysis of dental ceramics: clinically failed restorations, *Int J Prosthodont* 3:430, 1990.

11. Mackert JR Jr: Isothermal anneal effect on microcrack density around leucite particles in dental porcelain, *J Dent Res* 73:1221, 1994.

12. Anusavice KJ et al: Influence of initial flaw size on crack growth in air-tempered porcelain, *J Dent Res* 70:131, 1991.

13. Weibull W: A statistical theory of the strength of material, *Ing Vetensk Akad Proc* 151:1, 1939.

14. Davidge RW, Green TJ: The strength of two-phase ceramic/glass materials, *J Mater Sci* 3:629, 1968.

15. Dunn B et al: Improving the fracture resistance of dental ceramic, *J Dent Res* 56:1209, 1977.

16. Seghi RR et al: The effect of ion-exchange on the flexural strength of feldspathic porcelains, *Int J Prosthodont* 3:130, 1990.

17. Denry IL et al: Enhanced chemical strengthening of feldspathic dental porcelain, *J Dent Res* 72:1429, 1993.

18. Anusavice KJ et al: Strengthening of porcelain by ion exchange subsequent to thermal tempering, *Dent Mater* 8:149, 1992.

19. Anusavice KJ, Hojjatie B: Effect of thermal tempering on strength and crack propagation behavior of feldspathic porcelains, *J Dent Res* 70:1009, 1991.

20. Fairhurst CW et al: The effect of glaze on porcelain strength, *Dent Mater* 8:203, 1992.

21. Griggs JA et al: Effect of flaw size and auto-glaze treatment on porcelain strength, *J Dent Res* 74:219, 1995 (abstr. no. 1658).

22. McLean JW, Kedge MI: High-strength ceramics, *Quintessence Int* 18:97, 1987.

23. Michalske TA, Freiman SW: A molecular interpretation of stress corrosion in silica, *Nature* 295:511, 1982.

24. Sherrill CA, O'Brien WJ: Transverse strength of aluminous and feldspathic porcelain, *J Dent Res* 53:683, 1974.

25. Morena R et al: Fatigue of dental ceramics in a simulated oral environment, *J Dent Res* 65:993, 1986.

26. Rosenstiel SF et al: Stress-corrosion and environmental aging of dental ceramics, *J Dent Res* 71:208, 1992 (abstr. no. 823).

27. Rosenstiel SF et al: Fluoroalkylethyl silane coating as a moisture barrier for dental ceramics, *J Biomed Mater Res* 27:415, 1993.

28. McLean JW, Hughes TH: The reinforcement of dental porcelain with ceramic oxides, *Br Dent J* 119:251, 1965.

29. Batchelor RW, Dinsdale A: Some physical properties of porcelain bodies containing corundum. In *Transactions, Seventh International Ceramics Congress,* p. 31, London, 1960.

30. Dinsdale A et al: The mechanical strength of ceramic tableware, *Trans Br Ceram Soc* 66:367, 1967.

31. McLean JW: A higher strength porcelain for crown and bridge work, *Br Dent J* 119:268, 1965.

32. Jones DW: Ceramics in dentistry. II. *Dent Techn* 24:64, 1971.

33. Claus H: Vita In-Ceram, a new procedure for preparation of oxide-ceramic crown and bridge framework, *Quintessenz Zahntech* 16:35, 1990.

34. Pröbster L, Diehl J: Slip-casting alumina ceramics for crown and bridge restorations, *Quintessence Int* 23:25, 1992.

35. Seghi RR et al: Flexural strength of new ceramic materials, *J Dent Res* 69:299, 1990.

36. Wolf WD et al: Mechanical properties and failure analysis of alumina-glass dental composites, *J Amer Ceram Soc* 79:1769, 1996.

37. McLaren EA: All-ceramic alternatives to conventional metal-ceramic restorations, *Compend Contin Educ Dent* 19:307, 1998.

38. Sorensen JA et al: Core ceramic flexural strength from water storage and reduced thickness, *J Dent Res* 78:219, 1999 (abstr. no. 906).

39. Shearer B et al: Influence of marginal configuration and porcelain addition on the fit of In-Ceram crowns, *Biomaterials* 17:1891, 1996.

40. Pera P et al: In vitro marginal adaptation of alumina porcelain ceramic crowns, *J Prosthet Dent* 72:585, 1994.

41. Sulaiman F et al: A comparison of the marginal fit of In-Ceram, IPS Empress, and Procera crowns, *Int J Prosthodont* 10:478, 1997.

42. Lüthy H et al: Effects of veneering and glazing on the strength of heat-pressed ceramics, *Schweiz Monatssch Zahnmed* 103:1257, 1993.

43. Culp L: Empress 2. First year clinical results, *J Dent Technol* 16:12, 1999.

44. Sorensen JA et al: A clinical investigation on three-unit fixed partial dentures fabricated with a lithium disilicate glass-ceramic, *Pract Periodontics Aesthet* 11:95, 1999.

45. Mörmann WH et al: CAD/CAM ceramic inlays and onlays: a case report after 3 years in place, *J Amer Dent Assoc* 120:517, 1990.

46. Grossman DG: Structure and physical properties of DICOR-MGC glass-ceramic. In Mörmann WH, ed: International symposium on computer restorations: state of the art of the CEREC-method, Chicago, 1991, Quintessence.

47. Grossman DG: Biaxial flexure strength of CAD/CAM materials, *J Dent Res* 70:433, 1991 (abstr. no. 1341).

48. Anusavice KJ: Recent developments in restorative dental ceramics, *J Am Dent Assoc* 124:72, 1993.

49. Mörmann WH, Schug J: Grinding precision and accuracy of fit of CEREC 2 CAD-CIM inlays, *J Am Dent Assoc* 128:47, 1997.

50. Trushkowsky RD: Ceramic inlay fabrication with three-dimensional copy milling technology—Celay, *Compend Contin Educ Dent* 19:1077, 1998.

51. Eidenbenz S et al: Copy milling ceramic inlays from resin analogs: a practicable approach with the Celay system, *Int J Prosthodont* 7:134, 1994.

52. Moscovich H, Creugers NH: The novel use of extracted teeth as a dental restorative material—the "Natural Inlay," *J Dent* 26:21, 1998.

53. Jacot-Descombes Y et al: Copy-milled and resin-bonded full-ceramic structures. A further development of the Celay/In-Ceram System, *Schweiz Monatsschr Zahnmed* 108:1184, 1998.

54. Congdon RW et al: Marginal adaptation of ceramic copings manufactured by CAD/CAM techniques, *J Dent Res* 78:473, 1999 (abstr. no. 2941).

55. Hegenbarth EA: Procera aluminum oxide ceramics: a new way to achieve stability, precision, and esthetics in all-ceramic restorations, *Quintessence Dent Technol* 19:21, 1996.

56. Andersson M et al: Procera: a new way to achieve an all-ceramic crown, *Quintessence Int* 29:285, 1998.

57. Oden A et al: Five-year clinical evaluation of Procera AllCeram crowns, *J Prosthet Dent* 80:450, 1998.

58. May KB et al: Precision of fit: the Procera AllCeram crown, *J Prosthet Dent* 80:394, 1998.

59. Smedberg JI et al: Two-year follow-up study of Procera-ceramic fixed partial dentures, *Int J Prosthodont* 11:145, 1998.

60. Shoher I: Vital tooth esthetics in Captek restorations, *Dent Clin North Am* 42:713, 1998.

61. Zappala C et al: Microstructural aspects of the Captek alloy for porcelain-fused-to-metal restorations, *J Esthet Dent* 8:151, 1996.

62. Holmes JR et al: Marginal fit of electroformed ceramometal crowns, *J Prosthodont* 5:111, 1996.

63. Seghi RR et al: Relative fracture toughness and hardness of new dental ceramics, *J Prosthet Dent* 74:145, 1995.

64. Kelsey WP et al: 4-year clinical study of castable ceramic crowns, *Am J Dent* 8:259, 1995.

65. Hankinson JA, Cappetta EG: Five years' clinical experience with a leucite-reinforced porcelain crown system, *Int J Periodont Restor Dent* 14:138, 1994.

66. Sorensen JA et al: In-Ceram fixed partial dentures: three-year clinical trial results, *J California Dent Assoc* 26:207, 1998.

67. Pospiech P et al: Clinical evaluation of Empress-2 bridges: first results after two years, *J Dent Res* 79:334, 2000 (abstr. no 1527).

68. Sorensen JA et al: A clinical investigation on three-unit fixed partial dentures fabricated with a lithium disilicate glass-ceramic, *Pract Periodontics Aesthet Dent* 11:95, 1999.

69. Sulaiman F et al: A comparison of the marginal fit of In-Ceram, IPS Empress, and Procera crowns, *Int J Prosthodont* 10:478, 1997.

70. Holloway JA, Miller RB: The effect of core translucency on the aesthetics of all-ceramic restorations, *Pract Periodontics Aesthet Dent* 9:567, 1997.

71. Seghi RR et al: Abrasion of human enamel by different dental ceramics in vitro, *J Dent Res* 70:221, 1991.

72. Hacker CH et al: An in vitro investigation of the wear of enamel on porcelain and gold in saliva, *J Prosthet Dent* 75:14, 1996.

73. Metzler KT et al: In vitro investigation of the wear of human enamel by dental porcelain, *J Prosthet Dent* 81:356, 1999.

74. al-Hiyasat AS et al: Investigation of human enamel wear against four dental ceramics and gold, *J Dent* 26:487, 1998.

75. Ramp MH et al: Evaluation of wear: enamel opposing three ceramic materials and a gold alloy, *J Prosthet Dent* 77:523, 1997.

76. Sorensen JA et al: Three-body in vitro wear of enamel against dental ceramics, *J Dent Res* 78:219, 1999 (abstr. no. 909).

77. Wall JG et al: Cement luting thickness beneath porcelain veneers made on platinum foil, *J Prosthet Dent* 68:448, 1992.

78. Dietschi D et al: In vitro evaluation of marginal fit and morphology of fired ceramic inlays, *Quintessence Int* 23:271, 1992.

79. Christensen R, Christensen G: Service potential of all-ceramic fixed prostheses in areas of varying risk, *J Dent Res* 71:320, 1992 (abstr. no. 1716).

80. Kakehashi Y et al: A new all-ceramic post-and-core system: clinical, technical, and in vitro results, *Int J Periodont Restor Dent* 18:586, 1998.

81. Zalkind M, Hochman N: Esthetic considerations in restoring endodontically treated teeth with posts and cores, *J Prosthet Dent* 79:702, 1998.

82. Asmussen E et al: Stiffness, elastic limit, and strength of newer types of endodontic posts, *J Dent* 27:275, 1999.

83. McLaughlin G: Porcelain fused to tooth-a new esthetic and reconstructive modality, *Compend Contin Educ Gen Dent* 5:430, 1984.

84. Calamia JR: Etched porcelain veneers: the current state of the art, *Quintessence Int* 16:5, 1985.

85. Malament KA, Grossman DG: Bonded vs. non-bonded DICOR crowns: four-year report, *J Dent Res* 71:321, 1992 (abstr. no. 1720).

86. Sjögren G et al: Clinical evaluation of all-ceramic crowns (Dicor) in general practice, *J Prosthet Dent* 81:277, 1999.

87. Schaffer H, Zobler C: Complete restoration with resin-bonded porcelain inlays, *Quintessence Int* 22:87, 1991.

CHAPTER TWENTY-SIX

RESIN-RETAINED FIXED PARTIAL DENTURES

Van Thompson

Resin-retained fixed partial dentures have had a variable popularity since the technique for splinting mandibular anterior teeth with a perforated metal casting was described by Rochette in 1973.[1] His work suggested an alternative to conventional metal-ceramic fixed partial dentures (FPDs) and its substantial removal of tooth structure needed to create strong, anatomically contoured, and esthetic restorations (see Chapter 7). A prosthesis that requires minimal removal of tooth structure is appealing, particularly for abutment teeth that are intact and caries free. The primary goal of the resin-retained fixed partial denture is the replacement of missing teeth and maximum conservation of tooth structure.

The advent of **electrolytic etching** of the metal surface to provide micromechanical **retention** for metal adhesion to enamel led to the technique's broad application.[2] The restoration is simple in concept and consists of one or more pontics supported by thin metal **retainers** bonded lingually and proximally to the enamel of the abutment teeth (Fig. 26-1). These conservative prostheses depend on bonding between etched enamel and the metal casting and require precise and defined metal engagement of the abutment. The early use of these bonded retainers tested the limits of its application. There was a limited understanding of the treatment planning required and the degree of resistance and **retention form** necessary. In general use, poor de-

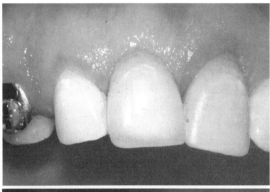

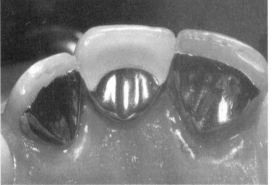

Fig. 26-1. **A,** Facial view of resin-bonded retainer replacing the right central incisor, which was lost as a result of trauma. **B,** Lingual view of above. Note the extension of the retainer over the marginal ridges of both abutment teeth, which is an aspect of all designs for anterior retainers.

sign of the early retainers (with some only bonded to lingual enamel), was compounded by the difficulty of properly etching the metal. As a result, several failures occurred, and the technique was used more conservatively from 1986 to 1996. During and since that period, design parameters have been enumerated and tested clinically.[3-6] These designs, combined with new technologies for adhesive bonding of resin to the metal, have led to a more reliable prosthetic procedure that complements the dentist's prosthodontic armamentarium.

DEVELOPMENT OF RESIN-RETAINED FPDs

BONDED PONTICS

The earliest resin-retained prostheses were extracted natural teeth or acrylic teeth used as pontics bonded to the proximal and lingual surfaces of abutment teeth with composite resin.[7-9] The composite resin connectors were brittle and required supporting wire or a stainless steel mesh framework. These bonded pontics were limited to short anterior spans and had a limited lifetime with degradation of the composite resin bond to the wire or mesh and subsequent fracture. Such restorations should only be presented to patients as short-term replacements.[10-12]

CAST PERFORATED RESIN-RETAINED FPDs (MECHANICAL RETENTION)

In 1973, Rochette[1] introduced the concept of bonding metal to teeth using flared perforations of the metal casting to provide mechanical retention. He used the technique principally for periodontal splinting but also included pontics in his design. Howe and Denehy[6] recognized the metal framework's improved retention (as compared to bonded pontics) and began using FPDs with cast-perforated metal retainers bonded to abutment teeth and metal-ceramic pontics to replace missing anterior teeth. Their design recommendation, extending the framework to cover a maximum area of the lingual surface, suggested little or no tooth preparation. Patient selection limited these FPDs to mandibular teeth or situations with an open occlusal relationship. The restorations were bonded with a heavily filled composite resin as a luting medium.

This concept was expanded to replacement of posterior teeth by Livaditis. Perforated retainers were used to increase resistance and retention.[13] The castings were extended interproximally into the edentulous areas and onto occlusal surfaces. The design included a defined occlusogingival path of insertion by tooth modification, which involved lowering the proximal and lingual height of contour of the enamel on the abutment teeth. These restorations were placed in normal occlusion; many have survived and have been seen on recall for up to 13 years (Fig. 26-2). Despite this success, the perforation technique presents the following limitations:

- Weakening of the metal retainer by the perforations
- Exposure to wear of the resin at the perforations
- Limited adhesion of the metal provided by the perforations[14]

Clinical results with the perforated technique were followed for 15 years in a study at the University of Iowa.[15] The results from this well-controlled

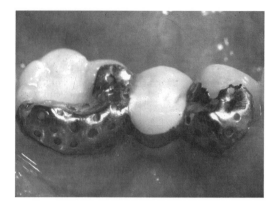

Fig. 26-2. Lingual view of an early perforated resin-bonded FPD replacing a premolar at the 13-year recall. Note the loss of resin from the perforations, the poor gingival embrasures, and the generalized wear of the occlusal composite resin restoration on the molar abutment.

study suggest that for anterior fixed partial dentures, 63% of the perforated retainer prostheses fail in about 130 months.[16] Later data[15] indicate that 50% fail in about 110 months (Table 26-1).

ETCHED CAST RESIN-RETAINED FPDs (MICROMECHANICAL RETENTION—"MARYLAND BRIDGE")

Based on the work of Tanaka et al[17] on pitting corrosion for retaining acrylic resin facings and the metal etching studies of Dunn and Reisbick,[18] Thompson and Livaditis at the University of Maryland developed a technique for the electrolytic etching of Ni-Cr and Cr-Co alloys.[19,20] Etched cast retainers have definite advantages over the cast-perforated restorations:

- Retention is improved because the resin-to-etched metal bond can be substantially stronger than the resin-to-etched enamel. The retainers can be thinner and still resist flexing.
- The oral surface of the cast retainers is highly polished and resists plaque accumulation.

During the course of this work, the need for a composite resin with a low film thickness for luting the casting became apparent. This led to the first generation of resin **cements**, which permitted **micromechanical bonding** into the **undercuts** in the metal casting created by etching while providing adequate strength and allowing complete seating of the cast retainers. Comspan,* the first of these cements, was moderately filled (60% by weight) with

---

*Caulk, Dentsply: Milford, Del.

Estimate Time to 50% Failure (Debonds) in Studies with at Least 10-year Mean	TABLE 26-1
Study	Months to 50% Failure
University of Iowa	
Perforated design	110
Etched metal*	250
University of Maryland	
Etched metal†	190

*Boyer et al, 1993: 143 anterior and 30 posterior FPDs.[16]
†de Rijk et al, 1996: 61 anterior and 84 posterior FPDs.[76]

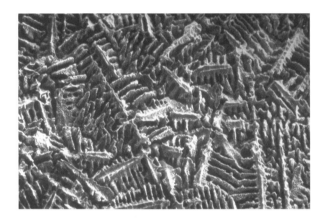

Fig. 26-3. Scanning electron micrograph (SEM) at 1000× magnification of a Ni-Cr-Mo-Al-Be alloy electrolytically etched. The microstructure is selectively removed to create a highly undercut surface that can be wet by hydrophobic composite resins.

a film thickness of approximately 20 μm.[21] Such cements are not chemically adhesive to the metal.

Electrolytic etching of **base metal** alloys proved to be critically dependent on the base metal alloy and attention to detail in the laboratory. Initial etching methods were developed for a Ni-Cr alloy* and a Ni-Cr-Mo-Al-Be alloy.†[2] These methods were followed by simplified techniques,[22] chemical etching,[23] or attempts at gel etching.[24] They all yield similar results, provided the technique is optimized for a specific alloy.[25] Proper etching requires evaluation of the alloy surface with a scanning electron microscope. The degree of undercut created by this etching process can be seen in Figure 26-3. Lack of attention to detail can result in electropolishing or surface contamination.[26] With time, both severely degrade bond strengths in a moist environment.

Highly variable results were reported for dental laboratories when etching the same alloy.[27] Etching

and bonding techniques were adopted based on bond strength testing of specimens only subjected to 24 hours or 7 days of water exposure. When resin-to-metal test specimens were aged for 6 months in water and then thermally stressed by 10,000 or more thermal cycles, large reductions in bond strengths were recorded.[28-30] Therefore, data from specimens that have not been aged and thermally stressed should be viewed skeptically. Even particle abrasion will provide initially high resin-to-metal bonds, which can degrade to almost zero with time.[31]

Well-researched and tested resin systems for direct adhesion to metal surfaces have now completely supplanted metal etching as retention mechanisms.[32] This is discussed subsequently.

MACROSCOPIC MECHANICAL RETENTION RESIN-RETAINED FPDS ("VIRGINIA BRIDGE")

As a result of concerns about etching base metal and the desire to use alternative alloys, several methods have been developed to provide visible macroscopic mechanical undercuts on the inner surface of FPD retainers. The first was developed at the Virginia Commonwealth University School of Dentistry and is known as the "Virginia Bridge."[33] It involves a "lost salt crystal" technique. On the working cast, the abutments are coated with a model spray, and a lubricant is then applied. Within the outlines of the retainers, specially sized salt crystals* (150 to 250 μm) are sprinkled over the surface in a uniform monolayer, leaving a 0.5-mm border without crystals at the periphery of the pattern. This is followed by application of a resin pattern. After pattern investment, the salt crystals are dissolved from the surface of the pattern. Adequate bond strengths are possible with this method,[34] but the thickness of the casting must be increased to allow for the undercut thickness. Although no long-term results have been reported with this technique, it does permit the use of almost any metal-ceramic alloy.

*Biobond C & B, Dentsply International: York, Pa.
†Rexillium III, Jeneric/Pentron: Wallingford, Conn.

*Virginia technique kit: Richmond, Va.

An alternative technique for macroscopic retention is the use of a cast mesh pattern on the internal surface of the retainers.[35,36] The mesh, usually made of nylon,* should be adapted to the lingual and proximal surfaces of the abutments. The mesh is then covered by wax or resin; this must be done carefully to prevent occluding the mesh with the pattern material. Investing and casting then follow (Fig. 26-4). This method is technique sensitive but can provide adequate retention with a resulting thick lingual casting. The cast mesh and the lost salt crystal method have been supplanted by direct adhesion with resin, which is possible for most casting alloys if the correct surface treatment is provided.

CHEMICAL BONDING RESIN-RETAINED FPDS (ADHESION BRIDGES)

While etched castings were the method of choice for retention of resin-retained FPDs during the 1980s and early 1990s, extensive research was underway

---

*Klett-O-Bond, Denerica Dental Corporation: Batavia, Ill.

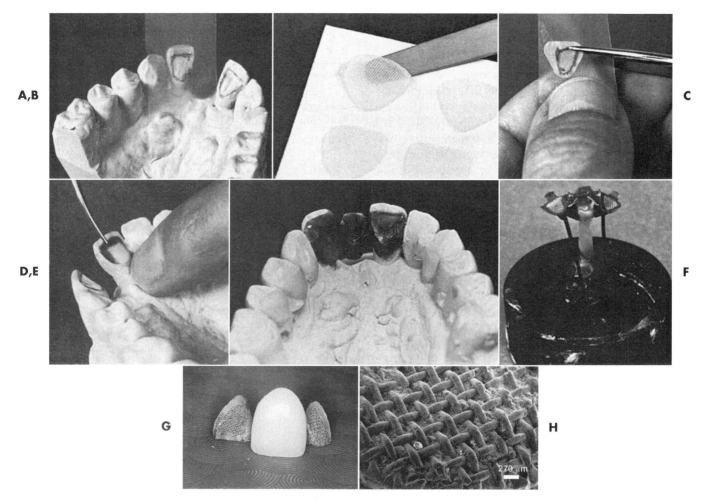

Fig. 26-4. Fabrication of a resin-retained FPD that uses macroscopic retention. **A,** The retainers are outlined in pencil, and the wax backing sheet is marked. **B,** Prefabricated plastic mesh patterns. **C,** A pattern is trimmed on the backing sheet and is luted to the cast **(D). E,** The framework is waxed and cut back. **F,** The pattern is sprued, ready for investing. **G,** The completed fixed partial denture. H, Scanning electron micrograph of the retentive surface.
(A to F courtesy 3M-Unitek Corporation; G courtesy Dr. P. Hasiakos; H courtesy Dr. J.L. Sandrik.)

in Japan to develop adhesive systems for direct bonding of metal for this application. The first of these resin systems* is based on a formulation of a methyl methacrylate polymer powder and MMA liquid modified with the adhesion promoter 4-META (4-methacryloxyethyl-trimellitic anhydride).[37] It was developed with a unique tri-n-butylborane catalyst system that is added to the liquid before combining with the powder. On base metal alloys, Super-Bond has the highest initial bond strengths of any adhesive resin system. Unfortunately, there is some concern about the hydrolytic stability of these bonds over time,[38] which depends on the alloy's Cr-Ni ratio.[39] Its advantages include its lower elastic modulus and higher fracture toughness when compared to BISGMA-based resin cements,[40, 41] which could result in less brittleness and better clinical results with less well-adapted castings.[42] This resin system has been under development in Japan since 1982, when a book detailing its clinical usefulness was published.[37] This system has shown poor clinical results with bonding high gold alloy retainers to abutment teeth.[43] However, alloy primers are being developed to provide a more stable bond to noble alloy surfaces.[44, 45]

Super-Bond's introduction was followed by a BISGMA-based composite resin luting cement† that is modified with the adhesion promoter MDP.‡ MDP's chemical structure and use are described in the literature.[46]

Panavia has shown excellent bonds to air-abraded Ni-Cr and Cr-Co alloys[46-49] as well as tin-plated gold and gold palladium-based alloys.[25,50,51]

Panavia has a tensile bond to etched enamel (10 to 15 MPa) comparable to the traditional BISGMA low-film thickness composites (e.g., Comspan and Conclude). The combination of metal electrolytic etching, followed by application of an adhesive such as Panavia, does not improve the tensile bond to the alloy and is actually slightly lower than the bond of Panavia to airborne-particle—abraded (sandblasted) base metal alloys.[51] The most recent version of Panavia, Panavia F, is a dual cure system (chemical and visible light) that releases fluoride. It also incorporates a self-etching primer system (ED Primer) for bonding to enamel and dentin.

Tin-plating of noble alloys allows resin-to-metal bond tensile bond strengths only slightly lower than

those for either the electrolytically etched or air-abraded Ni-Cr-Be alloys (18 to 30 MPa). However, tensile bond strengths are certainly greater than the bond to etched enamel.[25,50,52,53] Tin-plating of the metal surface also requires particle abrasion of the alloy surface for adequate tin nucleation sites (Fig. 26-5). Tin-plating can be completed in the dental laboratory, chairside, or intraorally to achieve metal bonding. Particle abrasion of the alloy surface just before the plating procedure is critically important.[54, 55] One common tin-plating system* (Fig. 26-6, A) uses a tin amide solution, which is applied to the metal surface with a saturated cotton pledget held on the end of a battery-powered probe (4 volts). The probe is grounded elsewhere on the metal (Fig. 26-6, B). Tin-plating times are usually 5 to 10 seconds and produce a light gray surface. Plating is followed by copious rinsing with water and drying; the adhesive resin is then applied.

Particle abrasion of the alloy surface with 50 μm alumina before bonding or tin- plating not only creates a roughened, higher surface area substrate for bonding, but it also creates a molecular coating of alumina.[56] The alumina on the surface aids in oxide bonding of the phosphate-based adhesive systems (e.g., Panavia to alloy surfaces). Studies of this bonding mechanism are also reinforced by laboratory data on bonding to alumina and zirconia surfaces.[57-59]

These adhesive systems have now shown nearly the same degree of long-term clinical bonding (since 1983 in Japan) as the conventional composites on etched metal (since 1981 in the United States).[19] Laboratory data support their efficacy. The favorable findings for direct adhesion to metal make alloy etching and macroscopic retention mechanisms obsolete.[3,60] This simplifies the laboratory and clinical procedures for placement of resin-retained FPDs.

Laboratory systems for adhesive bonding resin to metal have been developed. One method first involves the flame application of a silica-carbon layer to the metal surface. This treated metal is then silane-coated, which provides a surface to which composite resin will bond. The system (burner-aspirator-timer and associated chemistry) was initially marketed to the dental laboratory industry as the *Silicoater*.† It has since evolved to an oven method to bake the silica-carbon layer to the alloy surface and is now called the *Silicoater MD system*. Subsequently, the critical aspects of sandblasting before treatment in the oven have been investigated.[61]

---

*Super-Bond C&B, Sun Medical: Osaka, Japan (also known as C&B. Metabond, Parkell: Farmingdale, N.Y.)
†Panavia, Kuraray Company: Osaka, Japan.
‡10-methacryloxydecyl dihydrogen phosphate.

---

*Tin Plater, Danville Engineering: San Ramon, Calif.
†3M-Dental Products Division: St. Paul, Minn.

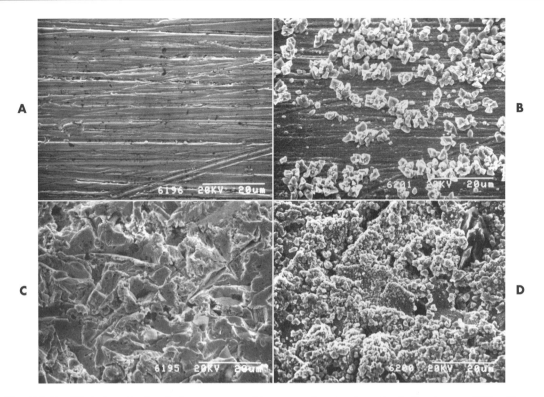

Fig. 26-5. Variations in tin-plating patterns with two surface treatments. **A,** Sandpaper (600 grit) prepared gold alloy* surface. **B,** Tin-plating exhibiting local clumping and random distribution of tin particles. **C,** Gold alloy surface after 50 μm alumina particle abrasion. **D,** Particle-abraded gold alloy surface after tin-plating with an even distribution of fine tin particles.

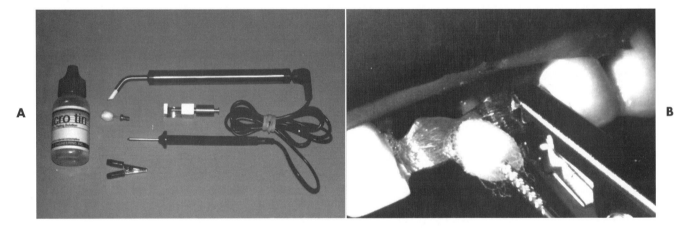

Fig. 26-6. Intraoral tin-plating. **A,** Tin-plating system where direct current is used to deposit tin from an amide solution†. **B,** Tin plater in use intraorally. Note the gray color change. The tin is being deposited from the solution and carried to the metal in the cotton pledget affixed to one electrode of the plater; the circuit is completed with the alligator clip, which is in electrical contact with the prosthesis.

Another laboratory method for resin bonding is the Rocatec System.‡ In this method, the metal surface is initially particle-abraded with 120 μm alumina. This is followed by abrasion with a special silicate particle-containing alumina (Fig. 26-7). This second particle abrasion step deposits a molecular coating of silica and alumina on the alloy surface. Silane is then applied to the surface, making it adhesive to composite resin. The various silane application techniques have been compared by Norling et al.[62] The Silicoater and the Rocatec systems have been compared to Panavia for bonding to a range of surfaces and are adequate in this regard.[28-30,56,63]

---

*Firmilay, Jelenko: Armonk, N.Y.
†Tin Plater, Danville Engineering: San Ramon, Calif.
‡ESPE: Norristown, Pa.

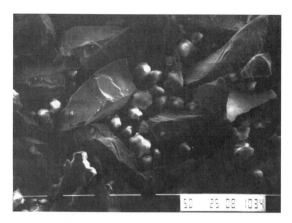

Fig. 26-7. SEM of air abrasion particles* composed of a mixture of 50 μm alumina *(dark irregular particles)* and smaller silicate particles *(light color)* used for final abrasion of metals during which a molecular coating of silicate is tribochemically deposited on the metal. This silicate layer on the metal allows reaction with a silane-priming solution for subsequent bonding of resin to the metal.

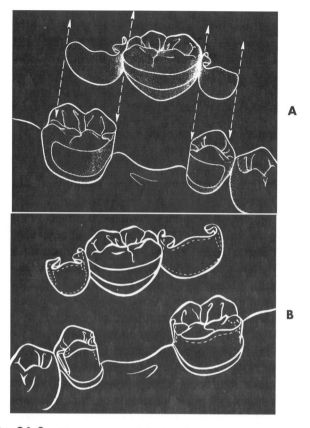

Fig. 26-8. Comparison of initial and contemporary posterior resin-bonded FPD designs. **A,** Original design. Minimal modification of lingual and proximal enamel allowed sufficient buccal extension of the metal. Once seated, the retainer could not be displaced from buccal to lingual. **B,** More extensive enamel preparation is now used with proximal grooves at the buccal-proximal line angles of the edentulous space. Note that with this design, the abutment teeth cannot be displaced from the retainer.

However, they require careful laboratory technique and are generally confined to bonding composite resin veneers to alloy castings because of the concern that the silane-treated surface may become contaminated before or during the clinical bonding procedures.

Changing the method of attachment of the resin to the metal framework does not change the design of the framework itself, because the limiting factor in the system is still the bond of resin to enamel. The evolution of Japanese designs for resin-retained FPDs[64] have paralleled those in North America and Europe. There is an almost universal agreement concerning the need for mechanical retention of the framework to limit the stress on the bond interfaces (resin-to-metal and resin-to-enamel) and in the composite resin, which can become fatigued with time.[65-67]

DESIGN CONCEPTS

The guidelines for optimum design of resin-retained FPDs have been empirically derived. The underlying principle for these restorations has always been that it is necessary to cover as much enamel surface as possible, as long as occlusion, esthetics, or periodontal health are not compromised. To emphasize the significance of maximum enamel coverage, Crispin et al[68] reported 3-year failure rates

of up to 50% when using small bonded areas and minimal retention designs.

The initial designs of etched cast retainers included an "interproximal wraparound" concept developed to resist occlusal forces and provide a broader area for bonding. Enamel preparations consisted of creating occlusal clearance, placement of occlusal/cingulum rests, and lowering the lingual and proximal height of contour, thus creating proximal extensions.

Frameworks should seat in an occlusogingival direction and should have no facial-lingual displacement (Fig. 26-8, *A*). The contemporary design has improved retention with well-placed and precise **grooves** on abutment teeth (Fig. 26-8, *B*). They will be detailed in the following paragraphs. Contemporary mouth preparations, in an effort to minimize failures, do not preserve as much tooth structure as their predecessors; nevertheless, they are still limited to enamel and adhere to conservative

*Rocatec Special - ESPE America: Norristown, Pa.

ADVANTAGES AND DISADVANTAGES OF RESIN-RETAINED FIXED PARTIAL DENTURES			BOX 26-1
Advantages	**Disadvantages**	**Indications**	**Contraindications**
Minimal removal of tooth structure	Reduced restoration longevity	Replacement of missing anterior teeth in children and adolescents	Parafunctional habits
Minimal potential for pulpal trauma	Enamel modifications are required	Short span	Long edentulous spans
Anesthesia not usually required	Space correction is difficult	Unrestored abutments	Restored or damaged abutments
Supragingival preparation	Good alignment of abutment teeth is required	Single posterior teeth	Compromised enamel
Easy impression making	Esthetics is compromised on posterior teeth	Significant crown length	Significant pontic width discrepancy
Provisional not usually required		Excellent moisture control	Deep vertical overlap
Reduced chair time			Nickel allergy
Reduced patient expense			
Rebond possible			

design principles. The new designs have been tested in laboratory studies.[69, 70]

Three principles are fundamental to achieve predictable results with resin-retained FPDs: proper patient selection, correct enamel modification, and framework design. The treatment is not a panacea, and if any of the contraindications are present, the patient should be treated with a conventional FPD or an implant-supported prosthesis.

ADVANTAGES

When used appropriately, resin-bonded FPDs offer several advantages over conventional fixed prosthodontics (Box 26-1). Due to the unique preparation design, minimal tooth structure needs to be removed. In general, the preparation is confined to enamel only. Because of the conservative nature of the preparation, the potential for pulpal trauma is minimized. Anesthesia is not routinely used during tooth preparation (without anesthesia, it is possible to monitor the proximity of the preparation to the DEJ by the patient's comfort level). The prosthesis can often be kept entirely supragingival; as a result, periodontal irritation is kept to a minimum. In a periodontal evaluation of restorations that averaged 10 years in service, the periodontal response was not significantly different from unrestored contralateral teeth.[71] Only when the retainer gingival margins were less than 0.5 mm from the gingival crest was there a correlation with a gingival response. Concurrently, impression making is simplified due to the supragingival margins. Because the abutment teeth are maintained with normal proximal contacts, in addition to being nonsensitive, fabrication of traditional provisional

restorations (Chapter 15) is usually not required other than in selected patients. However, judicious placement of composite resin is important to maintain occlusal clearances after the final impression and until the final restoration is bonded.[72] (See Fig. 26-15.) Chair time is significantly reduced as compared to conventional fixed prosthodontics, and the cost incurred by the patient is less. Both may be reduced by as much as 50 percent.[73]

The restoration can be rebonded, which is a dental operatory procedure that uses particle abrasion and adhesive resin systems (as long as the debonding occurred with no sequela to the abutment teeth). If one retainer remains bonded, it can be gently loosened with a monobevel, single-ended instrument and a soft mallet. Any deformation of the metal framework relative to the tooth structure can cause a crack to propagate through the luting composite resin. The monobevel chisel is located at an incisal or occlusal edge at an oblique angle to the long axis of the tooth along a mesial or distal line angle. The mallet should be used lightly (limited by patient response); repeated tapping will cause a debond. However, with mechanically retentive designs, which employ grooves and slots, the framework may require sectioning and removal of the sections with the procedure just discussed (Fig. 26-9). As an alternative, ultrasonic scalers have been proposed to help remove partially debonded prostheses.[74] Special ultrasonic scalers with special tips are available. They are applied at the incisal and gingival margins, but the procedure requires a high-power setting and can take considerable time. The debond rate with rebonded restorations is high,[75] and design modifications and a new or alternative restoration should be considered.

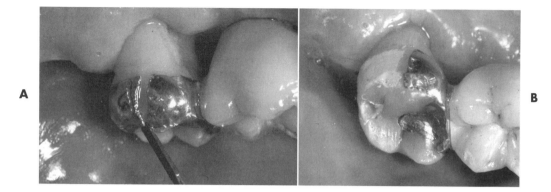

Fig. 26-9.   Removal of a retainer with a contemporary design. **A,** The retainer has been sectioned with a carbide bur to allow separation of the mesial and distal retentive features. The monobevel chisel is oriented to provide a wedging action between the metal and the enamel, which will allow a crack to propagate though the brittle resin. **B,** The cracking of the resin has propagated a debond between the metal and the resin. The mesial retainer half can now be removed in a similar manner. This retainer was removed because of fatigue fracture of the metal at the junction of the pontic metal with the premolar retainer arm (not shown), where the retainer was thinner than 1 mm. The poor periodontal support of the molar abutment allowed large lateral movements of the pontic and molar during function.

DISADVANTAGES

The primary disadvantage associated with resin-bonded FPDs relates to the fact that the longevity of the prosthesis is less than for conventional prostheses. This has been the subject of considerable investigation. Studies of first-generation etched metal FPDs at the University of Iowa (more anterior prostheses than posterior) and the University of Maryland (more posterior prostheses than anterior), with an average service time of more than 10 years, have been relatively successful. The results estimate that 50% will fail after 250 months and 190 months, respectively (see Table 26-1).[16,76,77] These studies also indicate that the rate of debonds does not increase with time.

In a study conducted in a private-practice setting, contemporary designs with a mean service time of 6 years achieved a 93% success rate.[3] This differs with the findings in a multicenter study in Europe, where debonding rates increased with the time after placement (almost 50% at 5 years) and were related to preparation design, luting agent selection, and the area of placement within the dental arch.[78] Another European study found retention rates of 60% at 10 years for early designs. In one study, posterior and mandibular resin-retained FPDs demonstrated higher dislodgment rates,[79] which may have resulted from occlusal forces (see Chapter 4) and increased isolation difficulty during the bonding procedure.[75,80] In light of these studies, the likelihood of eventual debonding should be discussed with the patient before treatment. By comparison, a meta-analysis of conventional FPD clinical studies indicated a doubling of the failure rate for every 5 years

of service from 0 to 15 years.[81] When these results are projected from 15 years to 20 years, a 50% failure rate for conventional fixed partial dentures would take about 20 years.[77]

Extensive enamel modifications are required with retentive design to the proximal and lingual surfaces of the abutment teeth (see Fig. 26-8, *B*). If the restoration is removed, composite resin bonding could restore the enamel contours, but transition to a more traditional prosthesis is likely. Enamel is limited in thickness, which requires precision in design and preparation with attention to detail.[82] Enamel lingual surfaces of anterior teeth are almost always thinner than 0.9 mm.[83]

Space correction is difficult with resin-retained FPDs. When the pontic space is greater or less than the dimensions of a normal tooth, achieving an esthetic result with this restoration is difficult. As with conventional fixed prostheses, treatment of diastemas is demanding, although a cantilever option may be appropriate.

Good alignment of abutment teeth is required because the prosthesis' path of insertion is limited by potential penetration of the enamel thickness. However, some posterior teeth, which are mesially or mesiolingually tilted, can be onlayed with a bonded retainer (see Figs. 26-19 and 26-21).

Esthetics is compromised on posterior teeth. Posterior resin-retained FPD design requires the extension or the metal framework onto the occlusal surface of posterior teeth. These occlusal rests and occasional onlaying of cusps are visible, which might be objectionable to some patients (see Fig. 26-19).

Clinical indications and contraindications are quite specific. In the presence of any contraindications, a conventional FPD or an implant-supported crown should be considered.

INDICATIONS

In the treatment plan for any fixed prosthesis, the patient's individual needs must be properly identified. The presence of any existing disease, its etiology, and how it relates to the treatment prognosis must be assessed. Periodontal and general dental health must be reestablished, and the proposed abutment teeth should not exhibit mobility; however, periodontal splinting of teeth with a resin-retained FPD has been successful with strict provision of mechanical retention of each tooth within the alloy framework.

Resin-retained restorations have been used for many years to replace missing anterior teeth in children (Fig. 26-10).[75,80] Conventional fixed prosthodontic techniques are generally contraindicated in young patients because of management problems, inadequate plaque control, the large size of the pulps, and the fact that children routinely participate in sports. Anteriorly, one or two teeth with mesial and distal abutments can generally be replaced with a resin-bonded FPD. Depending on the circumstances, a greater number of teeth can be involved.

Sound teeth or those with minimal restorations are suitable as an abutment with a resin-bonded retainer. When bonding to anterior teeth, the presence of Class III restorations is not a contraindication to a bonded retainer. However, large multiple restorations or a Class IV restoration would limit the bonding and the abutment's mechanical integrity. In the posterior region, existing Class II lesions proximal to the edentulous space can be incorporated into the retainer design. Minimal or moderate alloy restorations in the abutment teeth should be replaced with dentin bonding and composite resin, or they can sometimes be incorporated into the preparation design. The incorporation of an MO amalgam into the retainer design is shown in Fig. 26-11 and was placed before the advent of high-strength dentin bonding systems. The 9-year recall of the restoration is also presented.

As demonstrated in clinical studies, single posterior teeth can be replaced with resin-bonded FPDs.[3,76]

Significant clinical crown length should be present to maximize retention and **resistance form**. In addition to replacing missing teeth, the resin-bonded prosthesis can be used for periodontal splinting and postorthodontic fixation.

The restorations may be used both anteriorly and posteriorly. However, excellent moisture control must be practiced during **cementation**.

Proper patient selection also requires an aggressive and ongoing follow-up program to detect debonding and the presence of caries resulting from

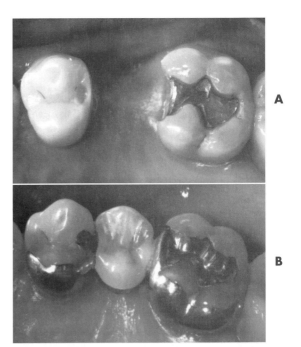

Fig. 26-11. **A,** Preparation for resin-retained FPD incorporating an existing amalgam restoration by use of a shallow inlay preparation where the amalgam reduction is short of the depth of the DEJ (with current dentin bonding technology, a composite resin base would be substituted for the amalgam). Note the shallow distal rest on the premolar and the lack of mesiolingual slot/groove preparation on the premolar abutment. **B,** Nine-year recall of the restoration where luting resin is still present as a sealant in the molar lingual groove.

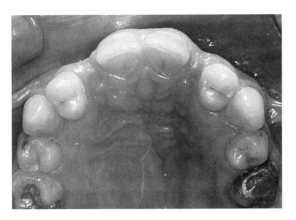

Fig. 26-10. Resin-retained FPDs are particularly useful in the treatment of young patients with congenitally missing teeth. Note the unusual tooth pattern with the first premolar in the canine space and the missing laterals.

a debond. However, caries rates on bonded retainers are low.[84,85]

CONTRAINDICATIONS

Because of the apparent advantages of resin-retained restorations, they have often been used in inappropriate circumstances, leading to failures that reduced patient (and dentist) confidence in the technique. Fortunately, these failures were usually correctable by more conventional methods. If any of the following contraindications exist in a particular clinical situation, an alternative approach to treatment should be selected.

Patients with parafunctional habits should be approached cautiously when the use of resin-retained FPDs is considered, because the resistance to displacement of these retainers is lower than in conventional FPDs. They should be used judiciously where above-average lateral forces are likely to be applied (e.g., in a patient with parafunctional habits or in a patient who requires an anterior tooth replacement in the presence of an unstable or nonexistent posterior occlusion). In these instances, all means of mechanical retention of the framework (grooves, occlusal rests, interproximal extension of metal) (see Fig. 26-8, B) should be used. The patient should be informed about the possibility of debonding. Periodontal splints can also be fabricated, but they require strict attention to mechanical retention.[4,5,86]

Long edentulous spans should be avoided because they place excessive force on the metal retention mechanism; with repeated loading, fatigue of the bonding interfaces or even the metal is possible.

Retention is dependent on an adequate surface area of enamel and sufficient clinical crown for proximal contouring and placement of grooves. This can be difficult if the abutment teeth have short

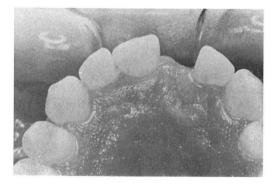

Fig. 26-12. Minimal crown length is available for preparations of adequate retention due to hyperplastic gingival tissues. Surgical crown lengthening is indicated.

clinical crowns (Fig. 26-12). Surgical crown lengthening may therefore be necessary as a way to increase the bondable surface area and because subgingival margins must be avoided.

Extensively restored or damaged teeth are unsuitable as abutments. One sound abutment and one extensively restored abutment can be incorporated into a combination FPD. In one retrospective clinical study with restorations in function for an average of more than 10 years, combination FPDs with one conventional retainer and one bonded retainer were very successful.[77]

Compromised enamel on abutment teeth as a result of hypoplasias, demineralizations, or congenital problems (e.g., amelogenesis imperfecta or dentinogenisis imperfecta) will adversely affect resin bond strength.

As previously mentioned, edentulous spaces that are larger or smaller than normal tooth size or diastemas are not easily accommodated. The labiolingual thickness of anterior abutment teeth and translucency of the enamel should be assessed to determine whether the shade of the abutment teeth will be changed (a consequence of reduction of tooth translucency by the metal retainer.[72,87]) Graying of the abutments can be eliminated with opaque resins and by limiting the incisal extent of the metal on the lingual surface. Translucent resins cause optical coupling of the metal to the tooth; appreciable graying of the enamel will result. A trial insertion of the metal with water between the metal and the tooth provides a preview of the possible graying. Similarly, when custom-staining the pontic of a resin-retained FPD, a trial resin (which will not polymerize) should be used to visualize the final shade of the abutment teeth with the metal backing (Fig. 26-13).

The presence of a deep vertical overlap prevents adequate enamel reduction and can place excessive forces on resin-retained FPDs; this situation should be approached cautiously.

Nickel-based alloys have been the primary metal for resin-retained FPDs. Patients who are allergic to nickel should be identified and offered an alternative.[88] Tin-plating and laboratory-applied bonding systems allow the use of noble alloys. However, with the reduced elastic modulus of most noble alloys, the metal thickness should be increased approximately 30% to 50% to make the stiffness of the **noble metal** framework equal to that of base metal.[89] This is an important factor in treatment planning and can influence the amount of occlusal clearance required for the metal (which is critical in patients with a deep vertical overlap).

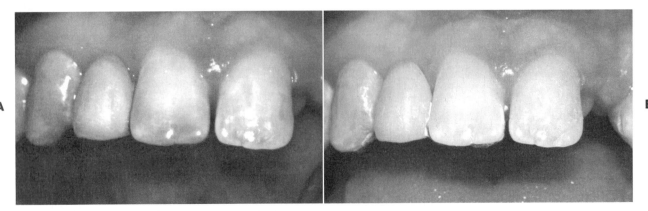

Fig. 26-13. **A,** Try-in of resin-retained FPD for staining of the pontic showing extensive graying of the central incisor abutment when translucent resin optically couples the dark metal to the tooth. **B,** Use of opaque resin prevents the darkening of the abutment and raises the value slightly. Opaque and translucent resins can be combined to provide the correct shade for the abutment; the pontic can then be characterized accordingly.

FABRICATION

In the fabrication of resin-retained FPDs, attention to detail in the following three phases is necessary for predictable success:

1. Preparation of the abutment teeth
2. Design of the restoration
3. Bonding

PREPARATION OF THE ABUTMENT TEETH

Whether anterior or posterior teeth are prepared, common principles dictate tooth-preparation design. A distinct path of insertion must exist, proximal undercuts must be removed to provide "planes of metal" on the lingual and proximal surfaces, occlusal rest seats and proximal groove/slots must provide resistance form, and a definite and distinct margin gingival margin should be established wherever possible (Fig. 26-14).

On anterior teeth, the procedure is similar in many ways to the lingual reduction needed for a pinledge preparation (see Chapter 10), but the amount of reduction is less because the enamel must not be penetrated. If necessary, the opposing teeth can be recontoured to increase interocclusal clearance. There must be sufficient enamel area for successful bonding, and the metal retainers must encompass enough tooth structure and have sufficient resistance form to prevent the individual abutment tooth from being displaced in any direction out of the framework.

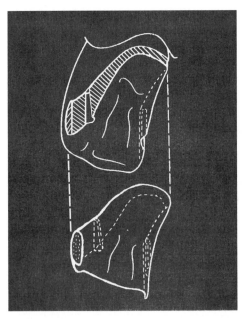

Fig. 26-14. Preparation design for anterior resin retainer FPD. Note the lowering of the height of contour in the interproximal, the slight extension of the metal toward the facial (but not so much that it will compromise esthetics), and the use of small but distinct proximal grooves.

Bur selection depends on operator preference. Gingival margins and circumferential preparation are easily accomplished with a chamfer or round-tipped diamond. Occlusal rest seats and cingulum notches can be prepared with a diamond or carbide inverted cone bur. The other critical retentive features (e.g., slots, grooves) can be made with a tapered fissure bur.

The dentist should determine the restoration design before beginning tooth preparation. This may include surveying the abutment teeth and making trial modifications on a cast.

Step-by-step Procedure

1. Leave the margins about 1 mm from the incisal or occlusal edge, and, if possible, 1 mm from the gingival margin. Definite rests and grooves will provide resistance form for the retainers and will assist in positive seating during cementation. Small, defined gingival margins (where possible) will guide the laboratory as to the gingival extent of the retainer. To enhance resistance, more than half the circumference of the tooth should be prepared (i.e., the concept of greater than 180-degree wraparound, which is particularly important for posterior teeth).

2. Make an accurate impression. Marginal fit is as critical for a resin-retained restoration as for a conventional FPD. Bond strengths are reduced with thick resin layers.[42]

3. Provide temporary occlusal stops. Significant supraocclusion of the abutment teeth can occur rapidly, particularly in younger patients or patients with reduced periodontal support. This can be avoided on anterior teeth by placing a small amount of composite resin on the opposing lower teeth. This is rarely needed for posterior teeth unless significant onlaying of the abutment is planned (in which case small composite resin stops can be bonded to the enamel) (Fig. 26-15). The resin is removed just before placement of the resin-retained FPD.

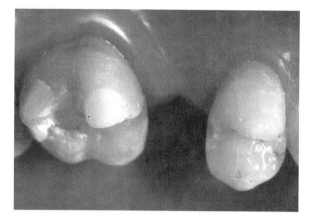

Fig. 26-15. Temporary replacement of occlusal stops is critical whenever they have been removed as a result of enamel recontouring. The composite resin stops shown here will be removed when this posterior inlay/**onlay** resin-retained FPD is bonded.

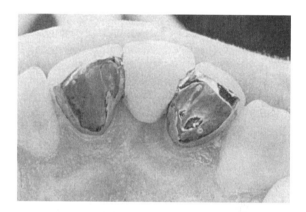

Fig. 26-16. Clinical view of an anterior prosthesis demonstrating the extent of coverage of the metal retainer, which forms planes on the mesial and distal lingual surfaces.

ANTERIOR TOOTH PREPARATION AND FRAMEWORK DESIGN

When designing the anterior prosthesis, use the largest possible surface area of enamel that will not compromise the esthetics of the abutment teeth. The retentive retainers (wings) should extend one tooth mesial and distal if a single tooth is replaced (Fig. 26-16). If two teeth are replaced, double abutments on either side can be considered, but only if the periodontal support of the abutments is compromised. With proper mechanically retentive designs, two maxillary incisors pontics can be retained by two lateral incisors, unless the laterals have short clinical crowns or a deep vertical overlap is present. If a combination of tooth replacement and splinting is used, the framework may cover more teeth.

Cantilevering pontics with resin-retained FPDs is also possible. This has been successful in selected situations in the anterior region[90] and is particularly useful for replacement of lateral incisors where **cantilevers** from either the central incisor or canine are possible. The retainer design is critical and requires adequate mechanical engagement of the abutment tooth.

The gingival margin should be designed so that a slight supragingival chamfer exists that delineates the gingival extension of the preparation. Any undercut enamel is removed at this time. The chamfer finish line should extend incisally through the distal marginal ridge area so that mesial, lingual, and distal "planes" are created (see Fig. 26-16). Abutments should have parallel proximal surfaces whenever possible.

The finish line on the proximal surface, adjacent to the edentulous space, should be placed as far facially as practical. A 0.5-mm-deep slot, prepared with a tapered carbide bur, should be placed slightly lingual to the labial termination of the proximal reduction (Fig. 26-17). Great care in paralleling the proximal grooves is required. A paralleling instrument is very helpful during this procedure* and has demonstrated its importance in highly successful clinical studies.[4,6] This device is also helpful when many teeth are to be incorporated in the framework (e.g., an extensive periodontal splint).

The occlusion is assessed to ensure at least 0.5 mm of interocclusal clearance for the metal retainers in the intercuspal position and throughout the lateral and protrusive excursive pathways. If inadequate clearance exists, selective enameloplasty is performed. Occasionally, additional clearance can be obtained by reducing the opposing teeth. However, this is contraindicated if there is wear or attrition on the incisal edges.

---

*Parallelometer, Coltène/Whaledent: Brooklyn, N.Y.

The restoration must extend labially past the proximal contact point. To optimize esthetics, the proximal wrap in the anterior region may be achieved in part with the porcelain pontic[82,91] (see Fig. 26-16).

Preparation of mandibular anterior teeth is similar to that for the maxillary incisors. Lingual enamel thickness is 11% to 50% less than for maxillary teeth, and tooth preparation must therefore be more conservative.[82] Combinations of periodontal splinting and tooth replacement are commonly used in the mandibular anterior region (Fig. 26-18). This presents a challenge for providing mechanical retention for the abutment and splinted teeth.

POSTERIOR TOOTH PREPARATION AND FRAMEWORK DESIGN

The basic framework for the posterior resin-retained FPD consists of three major components: the occlusal rest (for resistance to gingival displacement), the retentive surface (for resistance to occlusal displacement), and the proximal wrap and proximal slots (for resistance to torquing forces) (see Fig. 26-8, *B*).

A spoon-shaped occlusal rest seat, similar to that described for a removable partial denture (RPD) (see Chapter 21), is placed in the proximal marginal

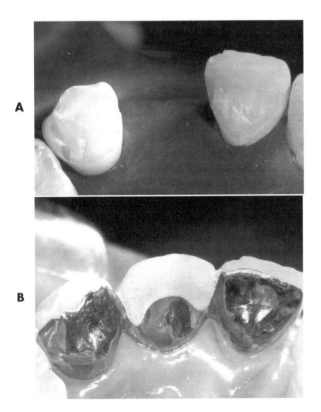

Fig. 26-17. **A,** Preparation design for an anterior prosthesis. Proximal grooves have been prepared on the mesial and distal surfaces of the abutment teeth. This mechanical retention is particularly important on the canine, where a distinct wear facet is seen. **B,** The gold alloy retainer is thicker than if a base metal alloy had been used. Note the extent of the metal into the canine distal proximal embrasure while the central mesial extension has been limited because of the incisor diastema.

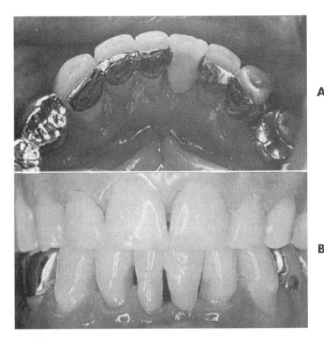

Fig. 26-18. **A** and **B,** Lingual and labial view of a resin-retained FPD that combines periodontal splinting and replacement of the left lateral incisor. Note the lack of distal metal extension on the left canine and the lack of metal extension into the proximal embrasures. This lingual bonding with lack of mechanical retention on teeth with limited periodontal support can lead to debonds.

ridge area of the abutments adjacent to the edentulous space. An additional rest seat may be placed on the opposite side of the tooth (Fig. 26-19). The rest is an important retention feature for resistance to both occlusal and lateral forces and should be designed to function as a shallow "pin."

To resist occlusal displacement, the restoration is designed to maximize the bonding area without unnecessarily compromising periodontal health or esthetics. Proximal and lingual axial surfaces are reduced to lower their height of contour to approximately 1 mm from the crest of the free gingiva. The proximal surfaces are prepared so that parallelism results without undercuts. In the interproximal area, no gingival chamfer is necessary to prevent penetration of the enamel, resulting in a knife-edge margin. Occlusally, the framework should be extended high on the cuspal slope, well beyond the actual area of enamel recontouring (provided it does not interfere with the occlusion) (Fig. 26-20).

Resistance to lingual displacement is more easily managed in the posterior region of the mouth. A single path of insertion should exist. The alloy framework should be designed to engage at least 180 degrees of tooth structure when viewed from the occlusal. This proximal wrap enables the restoration to resist lateral loading by engaging the underlying tooth structure and is assisted in this regard by grooves in the proximal just lingual to the buccal line angle. Distal to the edentulous space, the retainer resistance is augmented by a groove at the lingual proximal line angle. Moving a properly designed resin-bonded FPD in any direction except parallel to its path of insertion should not be possible, nor should it be possible to displace any tooth to the buccal from the framework (see Figs. 26-8, B, 26-19, and 26-20).

In general, preparation differs between maxillary and mandibular molar teeth only on the lingual surfaces. The lingual wall of the mandibular tooth may be prepared in a single plane. The lingual surface of the maxillary molars requires a two-plane reduction due to occlusal function and the taper of these functional cusps in the occlusal two thirds. However, the mandibular lingual retainer may be carried over the lingual cusps to augment resistance and retention form on short clinical crowns of mesially and

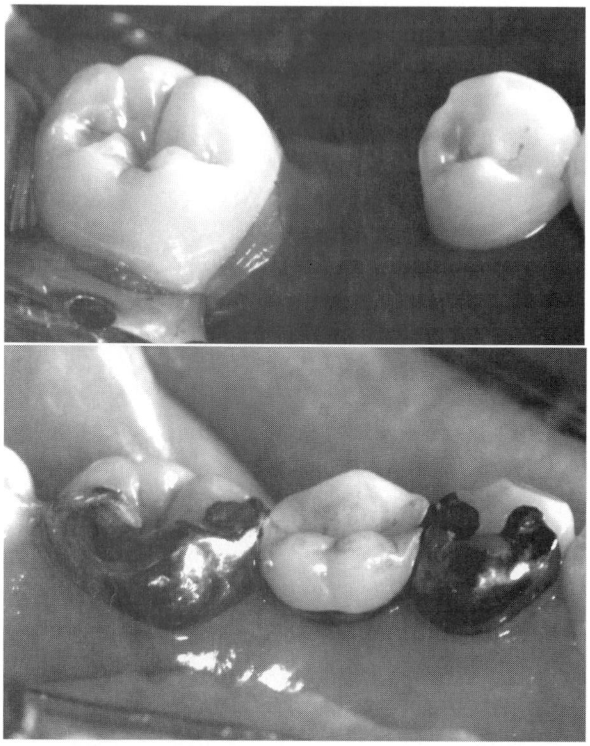

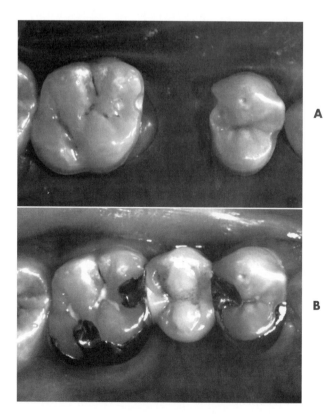

Fig. 26-19. **A,** Preparation for large premolar pontic. The first premolar has been prepared with mesial and distal rests and a distobuccal groove. **B,** The final restoration, which displays extensive metal on the occlusal surface of the premolar. This may be esthetically unacceptable for some patients.

Fig. 26-20. **A,** Preparation for a maxillary premolar prosthesis. A groove has been placed at the mesial extension of the premolar retainer arm to eliminate the use of a mesial occlusal rest. This could compromise esthetics. Note that the lingual groove preparation on the molar extends gingivally as the preparation is carried down the buccal slope of the groove, which adds mechanical retention. **B,** The completed prosthesis.

lingually inclined molars (this may require a two-plane modification [82,92]) (Fig. 26-21).

A wide range of extensions of the casting onto the occlusal surfaces of posterior teeth is possible. They include shoeing of cusps, encircling of cusps, and extensions of metal through the central fossa from mesial to distal with the lingual cusps exposed. The clinician is limited only by imagination, available enamel, occlusion, and the display of metal tolerated by the patient. Several examples of preparations and restorations are presented in Figs. 26-22 and 26-23.

Occasionally, a combination restoration can be used. This type of FPD includes a resin-bonded retainer on one of the abutment teeth and a conventional cast restoration on the other. As previously noted, this type of FPD has been very successful in clinical studies.[77,93] Periodontal splinting is the most demanding of the restoration designs; splints and splint-FPD combinations require care in designing adequate mechanical retention. An example of multiple rest design with interproximal extension of the metal is shown in Fig. 26-24. The posterior FPD/splint uses multiple rests and distinct mechanical retention of the abutment in the retainer, which can be important when the abutment is the most distal tooth in the arch (Fig. 26-25). The anterior splint must engage as much enamel as possible to aid in retention (Fig. 26-26) and is more demanding in tooth alignment and preparation design.

LABORATORY PROCEDURES

1. Wax the framework and cast it in a nickel-chromium or noble metal-ceramic alloy (see Fig. 26-4).

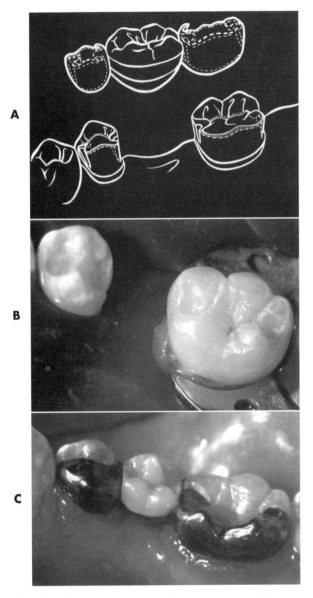

Fig. 26-21. **A,** Schematic of a resin-retained FPD onlay design. A thin veneer of metal is extended onto the occlusal surface of the teeth with approximately 0.5 mm reduction of the enamel where necessary. **B,** Preparation of molar and premolar. The lingual cusp of the premolar is covered to add additional mechanical retention on this short clinical crown. **C,** Completed restoration. The lingual cusps of the molar could also have been onlayed. However, the mesial and distal rests were deemed sufficient in this situation.

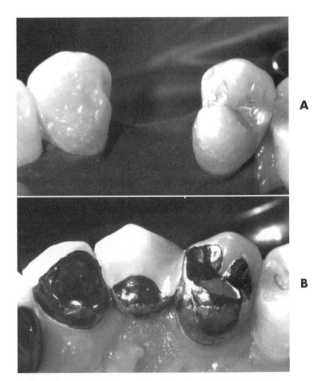

Fig. 26-22. **A,** Preparations for a premolar resin-retained FPD. The distal of the canine had a small Class III composite resin restoration. This has been replaced and modified to create a distal slot for the retainer. The premolar has both mesial and distal occlusal rest preparations. **B,** Bonded prosthesis. The gingival margin of the restoration is very close to the free gingival crest (the ideal is 1 mm above the gingival crest). Careful plaque control will be essential.

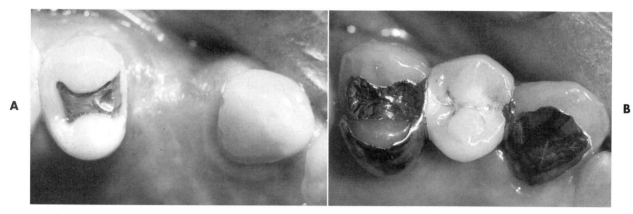

Fig. 26-23. **A,** Incorporation of an amalgam restoration into a resin-retained FPD. Note the margin placement at the gingival level, the use of two distal grooves, and a distinct gingival finish line on the canine abutment. **B,** Another completed resin-retained FPD with an inlay component.

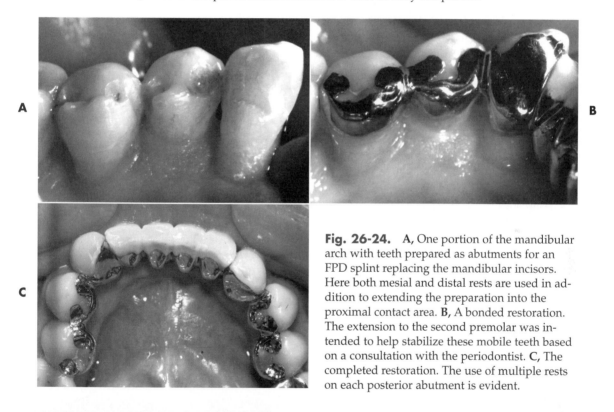

Fig. 26-24. **A,** One portion of the mandibular arch with teeth prepared as abutments for an FPD splint replacing the mandibular incisors. Here both mesial and distal rests are used in addition to extending the preparation into the proximal contact area. **B,** A bonded restoration. The extension to the second premolar was intended to help stabilize these mobile teeth based on a consultation with the periodontist. **C,** The completed restoration. The use of multiple rests on each posterior abutment is evident.

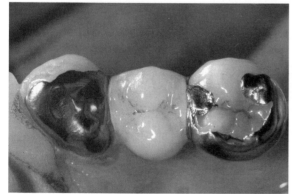

Fig. 26-25. Long-term recall of a resin-retained FPD. Particular care has been exercised in providing mechanical engagement of the second premolar—the most distal abutment in the arch.

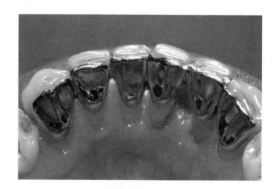

Fig. 26-26. Anterior splint seen at 12-year recall. Note the extension of the metal to engage as much lingual enamel as possible, extending over marginal ridges and into the interproximal areas wherever possible.

Different alloys require different surface preparation or tin-plating; the dentist should use an alloy that has been well tested with the adhesive composite resin of choice (see below).

2. Build up the pontic in porcelain, fire it, and contour it.
3. Evaluate the restoration clinically; when the fit is satisfactory, characterize and glaze it. As previously noted, opaque resins are necessary to prevent metal from graying the abutment teeth. Depending on the opacity of the resin and the teeth, the value of the abutment may be increased. Try-in for anterior teeth should involve a try-in paste for proper characterization of the pontic. Any remaining try-in paste will be burned out during the glaze firing. After this is completed, the restoration can be polished. Regular finishing compound is suitable.
4. Clean the fitting surface with a particle abrasion unit, using aluminum oxide (50 μm at a minimum of 40 psi [0.3 MPa] pressure); rinse thoroughly with water and dry. If the restoration is tried-in again, particle abrasion should be repeated just before bonding.

BONDING THE RESTORATION

Cements (Bonding Agents). Composite resins play an important role in bonding the metal framework to etched enamel. A variety of resin adhesives have been introduced specifically for this purpose. Conventional BIS-GMA type resins (e.g., Comspan*) originally used for luting resin-retained FPDs have been replaced by these more recently developed resin-metal adhesives, which continue to improve.

As mentioned earlier in this chapter, Panavia† is an adhesive monomer (MDP), glass-filled BIS-GMA composite with a long history of successful application (see Fig. 26-27, *B*). Panavia exhibits excellent bond strengths to base metal alloys and tin-plated noble metals. It has an anaerobic setting reaction and will not set in the presence of oxygen. To ensure a complete cure, the manufacturer provides a polyethylene glycol gel‡ that can be placed over the restoration margins. The gel creates an oxygen barrier and can be washed away after the material has completely set. The latest version of this cement§ is both chemically and light cured; as an alternative to the Oxyguard II, a curing light can be used to poly-

merize the margins. Panavia is supplied in opaque and tooth-colored (TC) forms. Because of the anaerobic setting reaction, both types can be mixed and will not set until air is excluded (as in seating of the restoration). This allows the application of opaque to the lingual of an anterior retainer and the translucent tooth color to the interproximal so that an opaque line is not visible from the facial. Both types can be mixed ahead of time and applied to the bonding surfaces of the retainer at a convenient time (see Fig. 26-27, *C*). This method makes it possible to mask the unesthetic metallic gray retainer, thus preventing it from showing through translucent enamel.[94]

STEP-BY-STEP BONDING PROCEDURES
Step-by-step Procedure with Panavia Resin Adhesive Cement (Fig. 26-27).

As for any adhesive cement system, the manufacturer's instructions must be closely followed to maximize the cemented restoration's physical properties.

1. Clean the teeth with pumice and water. Isolate them with the rubber dam and acid etch with 37% phosphoric acid for 30 seconds. Rinse, dry, and maintain air drying until the primer is applied (see Fig. 26-27, *A*). The assistant should dispense and mix the Panavia cement during the etching process and set it aside until step 3. The assistant should then mix the Panavia ED Primer and give it to the operator, who is keeping the etched teeth dry.
2. Apply the ED Primer to the etched surface. NOTE: although ED Primer is a "self-etching" primer, it should not be used without enamel etching, because bonded retainer surfaces are not "freshly prepared enamel." Since preparation, they have acquired a salivary pellicle, which limits the self-etching capabilities of this type of product.[95]
3. Apply the premixed Panavia cement (both opaque and tooth-colored if it is an anterior retainer) to the inner surface of the casting (Fig. 26-27, *C*).
4. Dry the ED Primer to ensure evaporation of the solvent (this should remain on the enamel surface for 30 seconds before drying).
5. Seat the casting firmly and maintain pressure while removing the excess resin cement with a brush or pledget. The cement will set within 60 to 90 seconds under the casting but not at the margins, which are exposed to air (Fig. 26-27, *D*).
6. Light-cure the margins or apply Oxyguard II to exclude air (Fig. 26-27, *E*).

---

*Dentsply Caulk: Milford, Del.
†J. Morita USA, Inc: Irvine, Calif.
‡Oxyguard II.
§Panavia F.

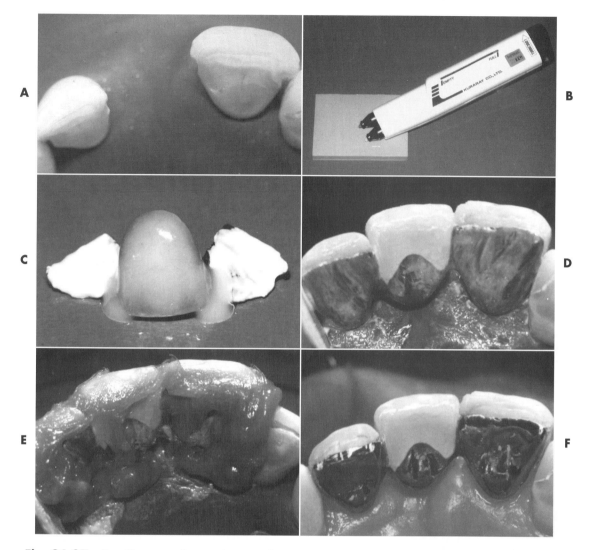

Fig. 26-27. Bonding procedures using an adhesive resin. **A,** Anterior resin-retained FPD preparation with mesial and distal groove retention based on the presence of incisal wear facets. Note the use of rubber dam for moisture control. **B,** Anaerobic-setting adhesive composite resin paste-dispensing system. **C,** Use of both opaque and translucent composite resin with the opaque on the lingual and the translucent in the interproximal for esthetics. **D,** The restoration has been seated, and the excess resin has been removed while the resin between the retainers and the enamel sets anaerobically. The margin resin and excess remain nonsetting. **E,** Oxygen-barrier gel is applied for margin resin setting. **F,** The final restoration, which was cast from a high-gold alloy and tin-plated. To provide good mechanical retention, the casting is increased in thickness by 50% as compared to a higher stiffness (elastic modulus) base metal alloy.

7. Rinse away Oxyguard II after 2 minutes and remove residual cement with a sharp hand instrument (Fig. 26-27, *F*). Major finishing, polishing, and occlusal adjustments should be performed before bonding the restoration. The tensile strength of the bonded prosthesis can be adversely affected by the heat or vibrations produced with rotary instruments.[82]

However, minor adjustments and removal of excess resin can be accomplished with judicious use of these instruments.

POSTOPERATIVE CARE

All resin-bonded restorations should be scrutinized at the regular recall examinations (see Chapter 32).

Since debonding or partial debonding can occur without complete loss of the prosthesis, visual examination and gentle pressure with an explorer should be performed to confirm such a complication. Because debonding is most commonly associated with biting or chewing hard food,[96] patients should be warned about this danger. If the patient perceives any changes in the restoration, he or she should seek early attention. Early diagnosis and treatment of a partially debonded prosthesis can prevent significant caries (Fig. 26-28).[97]

The restoration can usually be rebonded successfully. NOTE: The bonding surface should be cleaned with air abrasion and the enamel surface refreshed by carefully removing the remaining resin with rotary instruments, followed by etching. If a prosthesis debonds more than twice, reevaluating the preparation and remaking the prosthesis is probably necessary.

Attention to periodontal health is critical, because this retainer design has the potential to accumulate excess plaque as a result of lingual overcontouring and the gingival extent of the margins.[71] The patient should be taught appropriate plaque-control measures (see Chapter 32). Calculus removal with hand instruments is recommended over ultrasonic scalers to reduce the chance of debonding.

REVIEW OF TECHNIQUE

The following list summarizes the steps involved in preparation and placement of a resin-bonded FPD:
1. Patient selection is generally limited to sound abutments with minimal or no restorations. Occlusion must be stable.
2. Tooth preparations consist of creating a large lingual bonding area with proximal wrap; a definite, single path of insertion; occlusal, incisal, or cingulum rest seats; and proximal grooves/slots.
3. An accurate elastomeric impression material should be used.
4. Careful laboratory technique is necessary to ensure a well-fitting and esthetic casting.
5. Specially formulated resin-luting agents that are capable of adhering to metal should be used to bond the prosthesis.

SUMMARY

One of the basic principles of tooth preparation for fixed prosthodontics is conservation of tooth structure. This is the primary advantage of resin-retained fixed partial dentures. Precision and attention to detail are just as important in resin-retained fixed partial dentures as they are in conventional prostheses. To provide a long-lasting prosthesis, the practitioner must plan and fabricate a resin-retained restoration with the same diligence used for conventional restorations. The techniques can be very rewarding but must be approached carefully. Careful patient selection is an important factor in predetermining clinical success.

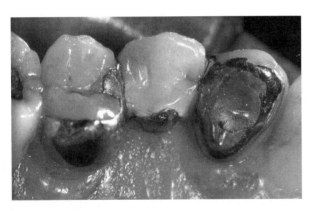

Fig. 26-28. Maxillary three-unit, resin-retained FPD. The distal retainer became debonded but was not detected promptly, resulting in a carious lesion.

Study Questions

1. Discuss the indications and contraindications of resin-retained fixed partial dentures.
2. When the replacement of a congenitally missing lateral incisor with a resin-retained fixed prosthesis is planned, a cantilevered design is considered. Is a single abutment better or worse than a two-abutment design? Why?
3. List the various bonding techniques used for resin-retained fixed partial dentures. Which one is currently recommended? Why?
4. Discuss the tooth preparations needed for anterior resin-retained fixed partial dentures. How does the preparation differ for posterior abutments?

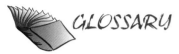

GLOSSARY

airborne particle abrasion: the process of altering the surface of a material through the use of abrasive particles propelled by compressed air or other gases.

anterior open occlusal relationship: the lack of anterior tooth contact in any occluding position of the posterior teeth.

autopolymerizing resin: a resin whose polymerization is initiated by a chemical activator.

base metal: any metallic element that does not resist tarnish and corrosion.

cantilever fixed partial denture: a fixed partial denture in which the pontic is cantilevered, i.e., is retained and supported only on one end by one or more abutments.

catalyst: *n* (1902): a substance that accelerates a chemical reaction without affecting the properties of the materials involved.

cementation: *obs 1:* the process of attaching parts by means of a cement *2:* attaching a restoration to natural teeth by means of a cement (GPT-4).

etching: *vt* (1632) *1:* the act or process of selective dissolution *2:* in dentistry, the selective dissolution of the surface of tooth enamel, metal, or porcelain through the use of acids or other agents (etchants) to create a retentive surface.

groove: *n:* a long narrow channel or depression, such as the indentation between tooth cusps or the retentive features placed on tooth surfaces to augment the retentive characteristics of crown preparations.

guiding planes: vertically parallel surfaces on abutment teeth oriented so as to contribute to the direction of the path of placement and removal of a removable partial denture.

¹lute: *n:* a substance, such as cement or clay, used for placing a joint or coating a porous surface to make it impervious to liquid or gas.

²lute: *vt:* luted; luting: to fasten, attach, or seal.

noble metal: those metal elements that resist oxidation, tarnish, and corrosion during heating, casting, or soldering and when used intraorally; examples include gold and platinum.

nonprecious metal: see Base Metal.

parallelometer: *n 1:* an instrument used for determining the exact parallel relationships of lines, structures, and surfaces in dental casts and prostheses *2:* an apparatus used for making one object parallel with another object, as in paralleling attachments and abutments for fixed partial dentures or precision attachments for removable partial dentures.

precious metal alloy: an alloy predominantly composed of elements considered precious, i.e., gold, the six metals of the platinum group (platinum, os-mium, iridium, palladium, ruthenium, and rhodium), and silver.

resin-bonded prosthesis: a prosthesis that is luted to tooth structure, primarily enamel, which has been etched to provide micromechanical retention for the resin cement.

resistance form: the features of a tooth preparation that enhance the stability of a restoration and resist dislodgment along an axis other than the path of placement.

retainer: *n* (1540): any type of device used for the stabilization or retention of a prosthesis.

retention: *n* (15 cent.): that quality inherent in the prosthesis acting to resist the forces of dislodgment along the path of placement.

retention form: the feature of a tooth preparation that resists dislodgment of a crown in a vertical direction or along the path of placement.

semiprecious metal alloy: an alloy composed of precious and base metals. There is no distinct ratio of components separating semiprecious alloys from another group.

span length: the length of a beam between two supports.

¹undercut: *n* (1859) *1:* the portion of the surface of an object that is below the height of contour in relationship to the path of placement *2:* the contour of a cross-sectional portion of a residual ridge or dental arch that prevents the insertion of a prosthesis *3:* any irregularity in the wall of a prepared tooth that prevents the withdrawal or seating of a wax pattern or casting.

²undercut: *v* (ca. 1598): to create areas that provide mechanical retention for materials placement.

REFERENCES

1. Rochette A: Attachment of a splint to enamel of lower anterior teeth, *J Prosthet Dent* 30:418, 1973.

2. Livaditis G, Thompson V: Etched castings: an improved retentive mechanism for resin-bonded retainers, *J Prosthet Dent* 47:52, 1982.

3. Barrack G, Bretz WA: A long-term prospective study of the etched-cast restoration, *Int J Prosthodont* 6:428, 1993.

4. Marinello CP, Meyenberg KH: In Degrange M, Roulet J-F, editors: *Minimally invasive restorations with bonding,* Chicago, 1997, Quintessence.

5. Marinello C, Schärer P: Tooth preparation in adhesive dentistry, *Dent Today* 2:46, 1991.

6. Brabant A: In Degrange M, Roulet J-F, editors: *Minimally invasive restorations with bonding,* Chicago, 1997, Quintessence.

7. Portnoy J: Constructing a composite pontic in a single visit, *Dent Surv* 39:30, 1973.

8. Ibsen R: Fixed prosthetics with a natural crown pontic using an adhesive composite, *J South Calif Dent Assoc* 41:100, 1973.

9. Ibsen R: One-appointment technique using an adhesive composite, *Dent Surv* 37:30, 1973.

10. Jordan R et al: Temporary fixed partial dentures fabricated by means of the acid-etch resin technique: a report of 86 cases followed for up to three years, *J Am Dent Assoc* 96:994, 1978.

11. Heymann H: Resin-retained bridges: the natural-tooth pontic, *Gen Dent* 31:479, 1983.

12. Heymann H: Resin-retained bridges: the acrylic denture-tooth pontic, *Gen Dent* 32:113, 1984.

13. Livaditis G: Cast metal resin-bonded retainers for posterior teeth, *J Am Dent Assoc* 101:926, 1980.

14. Williams VD et al: The effect of retainer design on the retention of filled resin in acid-etched fixed partial dentures, *J Prothet Dent* 48:417, 1982.

15. Wang J et al: Survival of resin-bonded prostheses with different retention mechanisms, *J Dent Res* 74:109, 1995 (abstract no. 784).

16. Boyer DB et al: Analysis of debond rates of resin-bonded prostheses, *J Dent Res* 72:1244, 1993.

17. Tanaka T et al: Pitting corrosion for retaining acrylic resin facings, *J Prosthet Dent* 42:282, 1979.

18. Dunn B, Reisbick M: Adherence of ceramic coatings on chromium-cobalt structures, *J Dent Res* 55:328, 1976.

19. Thompson VP et al: Resin bond to electrolytically etched non-precious alloys for resin bonded prostheses, *J Dent Res* 60:377, 1981.

20. Livaditis GJ et al: Etched casting resin bonded retainers I. Resin bond to electrolytically etched non-precious alloys, *J Prosthet Dent* 50:771, 1983.

21. Levine W: An evaluation of the film thickness of resin luting agents, *J Prosthet Dent* 62:175, 1989.

22. McLaughlin G, Masek J: Comparison of bond strengths using one-step and two-step alloy etching techniques, *J Prosthet Dent* 53:516, 1985.

23. Livaditis G: A chemical etching system for creating micromechanical retention in resin-bonded retainers, *J Prosthet Dent* 56:181, 1986.

24. Doukoudakis A et al: A new chemical method for etching metal frameworks of the acid-etched prosthesis, *J Prosthet Dent* 58:421, 1987.

25. Re G et al: Shear bond strengths and scanning electron microscope evaluation of three different retentive methods for resin-bonded retainers, *J Prosthet Dent* 59:568, 1988.

26. Wiltshire WA: Tensile bond strengths of various alloy surface treatments for resin bonded bridges, *Quintessence Dent Technol* 10:227, 1986.

27. Sloan KM et al: Evaluation of laboratory etching of cast metal resin-bonded retainers, *J Dent Res* 63:305, 1983 (abstract no. 1220).

28. Kern M, Thompson VP: Tensile bond strength of new adhesive systems to pure titanium, *J Dent Res* 72:368, 1993.

29. Kern M, Thompson VP: Influence of prolonged thermal cycling and water storage on the tensile bond strength of composite to NiCr alloy, *Dent Mater* 10:19, 1994.

30. Kern M, Thompson VP: Durability of resin bonds to a cobalt-chromium alloy, *J Dent* 23:47, 1995.

31. Thompson VP, Pfeiffer P: Bonded bridge techniques: electrolytic etching of NiCr alloy, *Dtsch Zahnarztl Z* 41:829, 1986.

32. Ozcan M et al: A brief history and current status of metal-and ceramic surface-conditioning concepts for resin bonding in dentistry, *Quintessence Int* 29:713, 1998.

33. Moon P: Resin bonded bridge tensile bond strength utilizing porous patterns, *J Dent Res* 63:320, 1984.

34. Moon P: Bond strengths of the lost salt procedure: a new retention method for resin-bonded fixed prostheses, *J Prosthet Dent* 57:435, 1987.

35. Taleghani M et al: An alternative to cast etched retainers, *J Prosthet Dent* 58:424, 1987.

36. Taleghani M, Gerbo LR: Using a mesh framework for resin-bonded retainers, *Compend Contin Educ Dent* 8:166, 1987.

37. Masuhara E: *A dental adhesive and its clinical application*, vol 1, Tokyo, 1982, Quintessence.

38. Ohno H et al: The adhesion mechanism of dental adhesive resin to alloy relationship between Co-Cr alloy surface structure analyzed by ESCA and bonding strength of adhesive resin, *Dent Mater J* 5:46, 1986.

39. Salonga JP et al: Bond strength of adhesive resin to three nickel-chromium alloys with varying chromium content, *J Prosthet Dent* 72:582, 1994.

40. Asmussen E et al: Adherence of resin-based luting agents assessed by the energy of fracture, *Acta Odontol Scand* 51:235, 1993.

41. Northeast SE et al: Tensile peel failure of resin-bonded Ni/Cr beams: an experimental and finite element study, *J Dent* 22:252, 1994.

42. Degrange M et al: Bonding of luting materials for resin-bonded bridges: clinical relevance of in vitro tests, *J Dent* 22:S28, 1994.

43. Hannsson O: Clinical results with resin-bonded prostheses and an adhesive cement, *Quintessence Int* 25:125, 1994.

44. Matsumura H et al: Adhesive bonding of noble metal alloys with a triazine dithiol derivative primer and an adhesive resin, *J Oral Rehabil* 26:877, 1999.

45. Matsumura H et al: Bonding of silver-palladium-copper-gold alloy with thiol derivative

primers and tri-n-butylborane initiated luting agents, *J Oral Rehabil* 24:291, 1997.

46. Yamashita A: *A dental adhesive and its clinical application.* In Masuhura E, editor: Vol 2, Tokyo, 1983, Quintessence.

47. Omura I et al: Adhesive and mechanical properties of a new dental adhesive, *J Dent Res* 63:233, 1984.

48. Omura I, Yamauchi J: Correlation between molecular structure of adhesive monomer and adhesive property, *Internat Congr Dent Mater,* Hawaii, 1989, Internat Conference Center, Univ Hawaii, Honolulu, Hawaii, November, Department of Medical and Dental Development, Kuraray Company Ltd., Kurashiki, Japan, 710, 1989.

49. Tjan A et al: Bond strength of composite to metal mediated by metal adhesive promoters, *J Prosthet Dent* 57:550, 1987.

50. Imbery TA et al: Tensile strength of three resin cements following two alloy surface treatments, *Int J Prosthodont* 5:59, 1992.

51. Thompson V: Total patient care. In Wei SHY, editor: *Textbook of pediatric dentistry,* Philadelphia, 1988, Lea & Febiger.

52. Breeding LC, Dixon DL: The effect of metal surface treatment on the shear bond strengths of base and noble metals bonded to enamel, *J Prosthet Dent* 76:390, 1996.

53. Dixon DL, Breeding LC: Shear bond strengths of a two-paste system resin luting agent used to bond alloys to enamel, *J Prosthet Dent* 78:132, 1997.

54. Wood M et al: Repair of porcelain/metal restoration with resin bonded overcasting, *J Esthet Dent* 4:110, 1992.

55. Bertolotti RL et al: Intraoral metal adhesion utilized for occlusal rehabilitation, *Quintessence Int* 25:525, 1994.

56. Kern M, Thompson VP: Sandblasting and silica-coating of dental alloys: volume loss, morphology and changes in the surface composition, *Dent Mater* 9:151, 1993.

57. Kern M, Thompson VP: Bonding to glass infiltrated alumina ceramic: adhesive methods and their durability, *J Prosthet Dent* 73:240, 1995.

58. Kern M, Strub JR: Bonding to alumina ceramic in restorative dentistry: clinical results over up to 5 years, *J Dent* 26:245, 1998.

59. Kern M, Wegner SM: Bonding to zirconia ceramic: adhesion methods and their durability, *Dent Mater* 14:64, 1998.

60. Barrack G: A look back at the adhesive resin-bonded cast restoration, *J Esthet Dent* 7:263, 1995.

61. Mukai M et al: Relationship between sandblasting and composite resin-alloy bond strength by a silica coating, *J Prosthet Dent* 74:151, 1995.

62. Norling B et al: Resin-metal bonding via three silica deposition processes, *J Dent Res* 70:390, 1991.

63. Kern M, Thompson VP: Effects of sandblasting and silica-coating procedures on pure titanium, *J Dent* 22:300, 1994.

64. Yamashita A, Yamami T: Adhesive cements and techniques. In Gettleman L et al, editors: *Adhesive prosthodontics,* Nijmegen (The Netherlands), 1988, Eurosound.

65. Saunders W: The effect of fatigue impact forces upon the retention of various designs of resin-retained bridgework, *Dent Mater* 3:85, 1987.

66. Zardiakas L et al: Tensile fatigue of resin cements to etched metal and enamel, *Dent Mater* 4:163, 1988.

67. Aquilino S et al: Tensile fatigue limits of prosthodontic adhesives, *J Dent Res* 70:208, 1991.

68. Crispin B et al: Etched metal bonded restoration: three years of clinical follow-up, *J Dent Res* 65:311, 1986.

69. Pegoraro LF, Barrack G: A comparison of bond strengths of adhesive cast restorations using different designs, bonding agents, and luting resins, *J Prosthet Dent* 57:133, 1987.

70. el Salam Shakal MA et al: Effect of tooth preparation design on bond strengths of resin-bonded prostheses: a pilot study, *J Prosthet Dent* 77:243, 1997.

71. Romberg E et al: 10-year periodontal response to resin-bonded bridges, *J Periodontol* 66:973, 1995.

72. Simonsen R et al: *Etched cast restorations: clinical and laboratory techniques,* Chicago, 1983, Quintessence.

73. Creugers NH, Kayser AF: A method to compare cost-effectiveness of dental treatments: adhesive bridges compared to conventional bridges, *Community Dent Oral Epidemiol* 20:280, 1992.

74. Krell KV, Jordon RD: Ultrasonic debonding of anterior etched-metal resin bonded retainers, *Gen Dent* 34:378, 1986.

75. Creugers NH et al: Risk factors and multiple failures in posterior resin-bonded bridges in a 5-year multi-practice clinical trial, *J Dent* 26:397, 1998.

76. de Rijk WG et al: Maximum likelihood estimates for the lifetime of bonded dental prostheses, *J Dent Res* 75:1700, 1996.

77. Thompson VP et al: In Degrange M, Roulet J-F, editors: *Minimally invasive restorations with bonding,* Chicago, 1997, Quintessence.

78. Creugers NH et al: Long-term survival data from a clinical trial on resin-bonded bridges, *J Dent* 25:239, 1997.

79. De Kanter RJ et al: A five-year multi-practice clinical study on posterior resin-bonded bridges, *J Dent Res* 77:609, 1998.

80. Olin PS et al: Clinical evaluation of resin-bonded bridges: a retrospective study, *Quintessence Int* 22:873, 1991.

81. Creugers NHJ et al: A meta-analysis of durability on conventional fixed bridges, *Community Dent Oral Epidemiol* 22:448, 1994.

82. Eshleman J et al: Tooth preparation designs for resin-bonded fixed partial dentures related to enamel thickness, *J Prosthet Dent* 60:18, 1988.

83. Shillingburg HT, Grace GS: Thickness of enamel and dentin, *J South Calif Dental Assoc* 41:33, 1973.

84. Wood M et al: Resin-bonded fixed partial dentures. II. Clinical findings related to prosthodontic characteristics after approximately 10 years, *J Prosthet Dent* 76:368, 1996.

85. Djemal S et al: Long-term survival characteristics of 832 resin-retained bridges and splints provided in a post-graduate teaching hospital between 1978 and 1993, *J Oral Rehabil* 26:302, 1999.

86. Marinello CP et al: First experiences with resin-bonded bridges and splints—a cross-sectional retrospective study. II. *J Oral Rehabil* 15:223, 1988.

87. Wood M, Thompson VP: In Aschheim KW, Dale BG, editors: *Esthetic dentistry: a clinical approach to techniques and materials,* St. Louis, 2000, Mosby.

88. Blanco-Dalmau L: The nickel problem, *J Prosthet Dent* 48:99, 1982.

89. Nakabayashi N et al: Relationship between the shape of adherend and the bond strength, *Dent Mater J* 6:422, 1987.

90. Briggs P et al: The single unit, single retainer, cantilever resin-bonded bridge, *Br Dent J* 181:373, 1996.

91. Simonsen R et al: General considerations in the framework design and tooth modification, *Quintessence Dent Technol* 7:21, 1983.

92. Simonsen R et al: Posterior design principles in etched cast restorations, *Quintessence Int* 3:311, 1983.

93. Wood M et al: Ten-year clinical and microscopic evaluation of resin-bonded restorations, *Quintessence Int* 27:803, 1996.

94. Caughman WF et al: A double-mix cementation for improved esthetics of resin-bonded prostheses, *J Prosthet Dent* 58:48, 1987.

95. Kanemara N et al: Tensile bond strength to and SEM evaluation of ground and intact enamel surfaces, *J Dent* 27:523, 1999.

96. Creugers NHJ et al: Clinical performance of resin-bonded bridges: a 5-year prospective study. III. Failure characteristics and survival after rebonding, *J Oral Rehabil* 17:179, 1990.

97. Gilmour ASM: Resin-bonded bridges: a note of caution, *Br Dent J* 167:140, 1988.

CHAPTER • TWENTY-SEVEN

FIBER-REINFORCED COMPOSITE FIXED PROSTHESES

Martin A. Freilich

A. Jon Goldberg

KEY TERMS

all-polymer prosthesis
braided
fiber architecture
fiber-reinforced composite (FRC)
flexure strength

glass fiber
polyethylene
unidirectional
woven

Fiber-reinforced fixed prostheses are an innovative alternative to traditional metal-ceramic restorations. They should be considered for certain patients be-cause they provide a conservative approach to re-placing missing teeth and overcome some of the drawbacks of conventional prostheses. The restoration consists of a **fiber-reinforced composite (FRC)** substructure veneered with a particulate composite material. The substructure provides strength, and the veneer, because it is laboratory processed, exhibits better physical properties and esthetics than direct placement composite restoratives (Fig. 27-1). The following topics are included in this chapter:

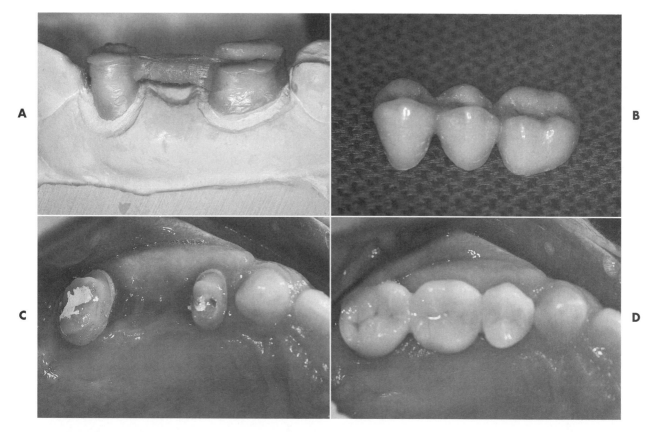

Fig. 27-1. **A,** FRC substructure. **B,** Completed polymer fixed prosthesis consisting of the substructure and particulate composite veneer material. **C,** Teeth prepared for three-unit fiber-reinforced FPD. **D,** Completed prosthesis.

697

1. The advantages of the clinical use of an FRC prosthesis
2. A description of the composition, mechanical properties, and handling characteristics of FRC materials
3. A review of the clinical applications and limitations of these materials in fixed prosthodontics

ADVANTAGES AND DISADVANTAGES

As discussed in Chapter 24, the most common fixed prostheses are composed of a metal substructure veneered with a ceramic material. The substructure provides mechanical integrity, whereas the ceramic imparts the necessary esthetics. This metal-ceramic prosthesis has an excellent clinical service record but continues to exhibit several drawbacks. Although the metal substructure is strong and durable, there are biological concerns, especially when base metal alloys (commonly used in clinical practice) are selected. They may exhibit corrosion[1-3] and/or may elicit an allergic reaction from some patients.[4-8] Certain constituents of some base metal alloys may even cause acute and chronic health hazards to laboratory personnel.[9,10] In addition, the metal framework is opaque with a dark oxide layer, which is not esthetically pleasing. This must be covered with a porcelain veneer to produce a lifelike appearance.

Porcelain is a brittle material and can fracture, which is a leading cause of restoration failure.[11-14] When this occurs, porcelain can sometimes be repaired with silane coupling agents or 4-META to promote bonding with acrylic or composite resin[15-18] (see Chapter 32). Porcelain is also abrasive to opposing enamel and can severely damage unrestored opposing teeth.[19-23] Porcelain has been implicated in severe occlusal wear, particularly when it is not glazed or highly polished (see Chapter 19). In one survey, less wear on opposing teeth was cited as the single major need for change in posterior tooth-colored crowns.[24]

Because of these problems and concerns, alternatives to metal-ceramic materials continue to be explored. All-ceramic and all-particulate composite prostheses have been described in dental literature.[25,26] Recorded problems include low resilience and toughness, resulting in clinical failure.

As with the porcelain surface of metal-ceramic prostheses, the surfaces of the all-ceramic prostheses are abrasive to tooth enamel and can potentially damage unrestored opposing teeth. Conversely, the composite materials have historically exhibited less than adequate occlusal wear resistance and color stability over time, but newer composites continue to improve with regard to these characteristics. Light-, heat-, and vacuum-polymerized laboratory processed particulate composite materials are now commercially available and use new polymer formulations with improved filler particle distribution.[27] These improved materials demonstrate better physical properties, such as hardness and wear resistance. However, particulate composites are brittle and need the support of a substructure with good flexure properties.

Fiber-reinforced composites (FRCs) have good **flexure strength** and other physical characteristics that make them suitable fixed prosthesis substructure materials.[28-30] In addition, the FRC substructure is translucent and requires no opaque masking. This permits a relatively thin layer of particulate covering composite and excellent esthetics. FRCs have been used to make two-phase **all-polymer prostheses** composed of an internal **glass fiber**-reinforced composite substructure covered by a particulate composite (Fig. 27-2).

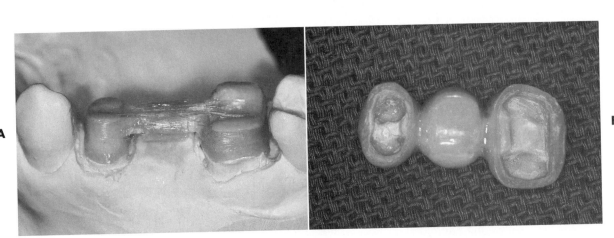

Fig. 27-2. **A,** FRC substructure for a three-unit polymer FPD. **B,** Internal surface of FRC-reinforced polymer FPD.

AVAILABLE MATERIALS

FRC materials are categorized according to the following characteristics:

1. Type of fiber
2. Fiber orientation
3. Whether the fiber impregnation is performed by the dentist or laboratory technician or preimpregnated by the manufacturer
4. Whether the material is formed by hand or with a machine

The most commonly used fibers in dental applications are glass, **polyethylene,** and carbon. **Fiber architectures** in dentistry include **"unidirectional"** patterns, in which all fibers are parallel, as well as **braided** and **woven** patterns. Commercially available nonimpregnated materials include polyethylene weaves (e.g., Ribbond* and Connect†) and glass weaves (e.g., GlasSpan‡). These products are hand formed. Preimpregnated materials include Vectris§, which is machine formed and available in both a unidirectional and woven-glass form; FiberKor,‖ which is hand formed and available as a unidirectional glass material; Splint-It,‖ which is also hand-formed and available in both a unidirectional and woven glass form (Fig. 27-3).

---

*Ribbond, Inc: Seattle, Wash.
†Kerr: Orange, Calif.
‡GlasSpan, Inc: Exton, Pa.
§Ivoclar North America: Amherst, N.Y.
‖Jeneric/Pentron, Inc: Wallingford, Conn.

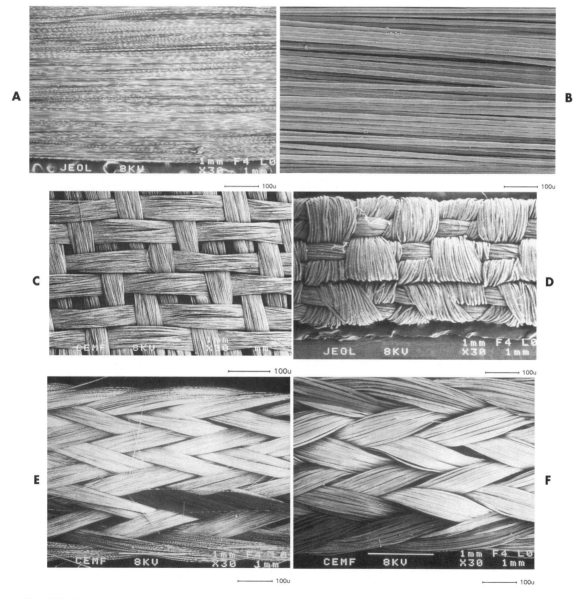

Fig. 27-3. Scanning electron micrographs. **A,** Unidirectional long glass fiber FRC (Fibrekor: Jeneric/Pentron). **B,** Unidirectional long glass fiber FRC (Vectris pontic: Ivoclar). **C,** Woven glass fiber FRC (Vectris frame: Ivoclar). **D,** Woven polyethylene FRC (Ribbond: Ribbond). **E,** Braided glass fiber FRC (GlasSpan: GlasSpan). **F,** Braided polyethylene FRC (Connect: Kerr).

Flexure Properties of Commercial Fiber-Reinforced Composites

TABLE 27-1

Material	Fiber Type	Fiber Architecture	Flexural Strength MPa	Flexural Modulus GPa
FibreKor	Glass	Unidirectional	539 (68)	28.3 (2.7)
GlasSpan	Glass	Braid	321 (28)	13.9 (1.1)
Connect	Polyethylene	Braid	222 (23)	8.3 (0.5)
Ribbond	Polyethylene	Leno weave	206 (15)	3.9 (0.7)

Different FRC materials exhibit different handling and mechanical properties. Fiber type, fiber orientation, and the quality of fiber impregnation with the resin matrix have a substantial impact on handling characteristics and physical properties. As seen in Table 27-1, glass materials with a unidirectional architecture exhibit flexural properties that are superior to the polyethylene materials with a woven or braided architecture. These glass materials have a flexural strength that is more than twice the strength of polyethylene materials and a flexural modulus almost eight times as great.[16] Because of their good handling characteristics, the braided and woven polyethylene products may be useful for other dental applications (e.g., operatory fabrication of periodontal splints).

◼ INDICATIONS

Indications for selecting a fiber-reinforced polymer prosthesis include the following factors:
1. The need for a restoration with excellent appearance
2. The need to decrease wear of the opposing dentition
3. The use of conservative intracoronal abutment tooth preparations
4. The potential for bonding the prosthesis retainer to the abutment teeth
5. The desire for a metal-free, nonporcelain prosthesis (this is especially important for individuals with metal allergies)

These materials can be used anywhere in the mouth where esthetics is important. The lack of metal or opaque materials provides good translucency and a very natural appearance. This natural appearance at the cervical aspect of the prosthesis retainer eliminates the need to hide margins subgingivally, where they may create periodontal problems for the patient. Supragingival margins of this polymer prosthesis blend in easily with the nonprepared tooth structure apical to the tooth preparation finish line, just as the overall prosthesis blends in with the adjacent natural teeth. Resin composite luting materials that bond to the internal aspect of the polymer prosthesis retainers and to the dentin and enamel of the abutment teeth improve retention of the prosthesis. This feature may provide critical retention of a polymer prosthesis on abutment teeth that cannot be made to exhibit optimum geometric retention form; however, the bonding process requires careful control of moisture and soft tissues.

◼ CONTRAINDICATIONS

Contraindications for selecting an FRC fixed prosthesis include the following factors:
1. Inability to maintain good fluid control (e.g., patients with chronic or acute gingival inflammation or when margins would be placed deeply into the sulcus)
2. Long span (i.e., two or more pontics)
3. Patients with parafunctional habits
4. Patients with unglazed porcelain or removable partial denture frameworks that would oppose the restoration
5. Patients who abuse alcoholic substances

Patient-selection criteria are summarized in Table 27-2. Composite resin luting materials and an adhesive cementation technique can only be used in situations where the operator can maintain a contamination-free field. Rubber dam isolation is ideal and should be used whenever possible. At this time, FPDs that replace more than two teeth are not recommended because the material's ability to support greater edentulous spans has not been documented. An increased susceptibility to wear or fracture may occur in patients who brux or clench, and surface degradation of the particulate composite is likely to be a problem in alcoholics. Because there are no clinical data to substantiate how the FRC fixed prosthesis would perform when subjected to these conditions, it should not be considered until more information is available.

NOTE: There are no long-term clinical data regarding the overall success of the FRC prosthesis. Primary concerns are the wear and potential fracture of the composite veneer materials. Short-term data indicate that the adequacy of tooth preparation (Fig. 27-4) and the shape and volume of the FRC framework are instrumental factors in the performance of an FRC fixed prosthesis.

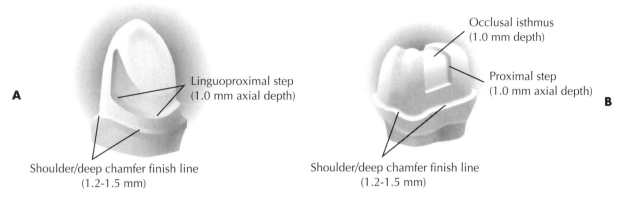

A

Linguoproximal step
(1.0 mm axial depth)

Shoulder/deep chamfer finish line
(1.2-1.5 mm)

Occlusal isthmus
(1.0 mm depth)

Proximal step
(1.0 mm axial depth)

B

Shoulder/deep chamfer finish line
(1.2-1.5 mm)

Fig. 27-4. Abutment tooth preparations made for hand-fabricated FRC prostheses. **A,** Anterior. **B,** Posterior.

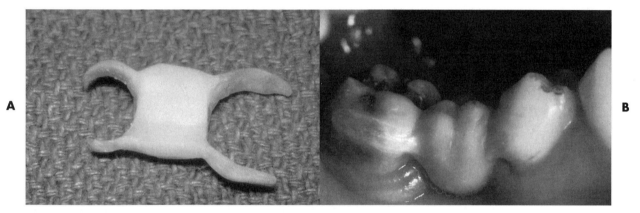

A   **B**

Fig. 27-5. Early prosthodontic application of an experimental thermoplastic unidirectional FRC. **A,** A bonded FPD made with polycarbonate FRC. **B,** A polycarbonate FRC prosthesis after delivery.

Patient Selection for Fiber-Reinforced FPDs	TABLE **27-2**
Indications	**Contraindications**
• Optimal esthetic result	• Inability to maintain fluid control
• Metal free	• Long span needed
• Conservative abutment preparation	• Patients with parafunctional habits
• Decreased wear to opposing teeth	• Unglazed opposing porcelain
• Use of an adhesive luting technique	• Patients who abuse alcohol

An early prosthodontic application of an experimental thermoplastic unidirectional FRC[31-33] was the fabrication of a single tooth replacement bonded FPD.[34] These prostheses were formed in the laboratory and then bonded to the teeth (Fig. 27-5).

EXTRACORONAL COMPLETE-COVERAGE FIXED PROSTHESES

Newer, lighter, heat/vacuum laboratory polymerized FRC formulations have been developed and tested. They demonstrate excellent esthetics, good handling characteristics, and good flexure properties.[29,35-38] Commercial products have been based on these formulations. The fabrication of a complete-

coverage prosthesis with a commercially available, preimpregnated unidirectional FRC (FibreKor: Jeneric/Pentron) and a hand-fabricated technique is shown in Fig. 27-6. The fabrication of a prosthesis with commercially available, preimpregnated woven and unidirectional FRCs (Vectris: Ivoclar) and the use of an equipment-fabricated technique are shown in Fig. 27-7.

INTRACORONAL PARTIAL-COVERAGE FIXED PROSTHESES

The FRC partial-coverage FPD allows a conservative design when the abutment teeth are unrestored or have modest intracoronal restorations. When an

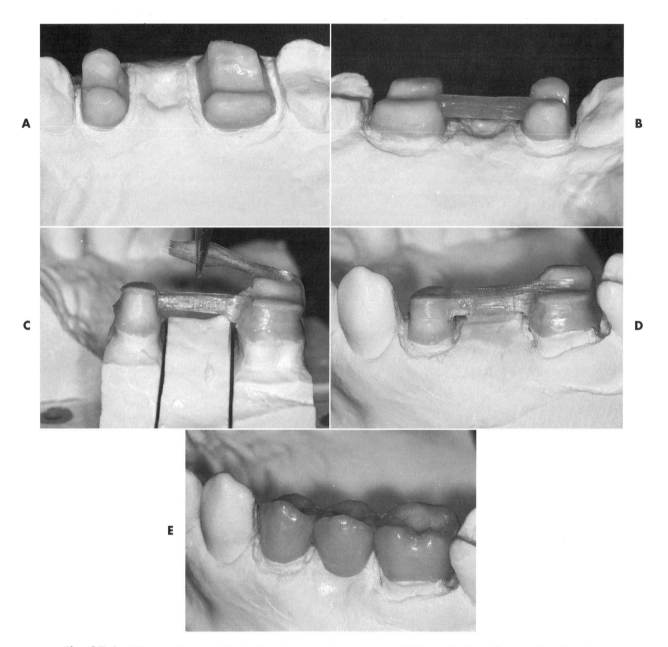

Fig. 27-6. The step-by-step fabrication of a complete-coverage FRC prosthesis with a unidirectional glass material (FibreKor: Jeneric/Pentron) using a hand-fabricated technique. **A,** Thin coping of opacious body particulate composite adapted to the die. **B,** Bar of multiple layers of FRC spanning the pontic region, bonding the copings together. **C,** Continuous strip of FRC bonded to one end of the pontic bar and then wrapped around the axial surfaces of the copings while being polymerized. **D,** Buccal view of the completed FRC substructure. **E,** Completed prosthesis.

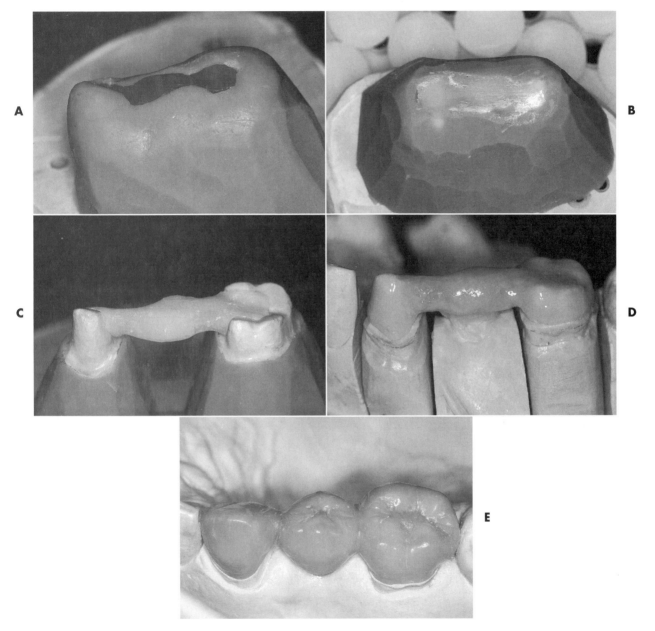

Fig. 27-7. The step-by-step fabrication of a complete-coverage FRC prosthesis with both unidirectional and woven glass components (Vectris: Ivoclar) and the use of an equipment-fabricated technique. **A,** Wax pattern of bar covered by a silicone index. **B,** Unidirectional FRC in silicone index after polymerization. **C,** Already polymerized unidirectional "pontic" bar after contouring with acrylic burs. **D,** Completed FRC substructure with woven FRC covering unidirectional pontic bar. **E,** Completed prosthesis.

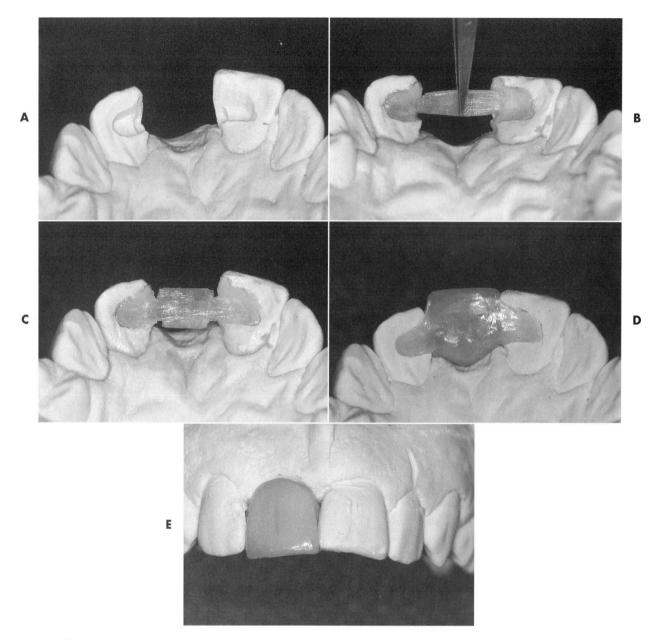

Fig. 27-8. The tooth preparation and step-by-step fabrication of a partial-coverage, intracoronal FRC prosthesis with a unidirectional glass material (FibreKor: [Jeneric/Pentron]) and a hand-fabricated technique. **A,** Intracoronal tooth preparation. **B,** Placement of the unidirectional FRC bar into unpolymerized opacious body particulate composite. **C,** Completed FRC substructure. **D,** Completed prosthesis as viewed from the lingual surface. **E,** Facial surface.

implant is not possible, an etched metal resin-retained FPD (see Chapter 26) is the only other conservative fixed treatment alternative. However, these prostheses have problems with retention, graying of abutment teeth (due to metal showing through), and overcontoured retainers. The advantages discussed for the complete-coverage FPD (esthetics, metal-free framework, ease of laboratory fabrication, and use of an adhesive cementation technique) also apply to the partial-coverage FPD.

The fabrication of a partial-coverage, intracoronal prosthesis with a commercially available, preimpregnated unidirectional FRC (FibreKor: Jeneric/Pentron) and a hand-fabricated technique are shown in Fig. 27-8.

TRY-IN AND CEMENTATION

As with any restoration, the dentist must check proximal contacts, occlusion, anatomical form, and shade. Any necessary adjustments should be made (see Chapter 31). Proximal contacts can be added by using a hybrid restorative composite after roughening the surface and placing an unfilled resin on the FRC's overlay particulate composite. As with porcelain veneers, (see Chapter 31) the shade of the prosthesis should be assessed with a try-in, water-soluble paste that corresponds to the selected luting composite. Minor adjustments can be obtained by selecting darker or lighter luting resins. The translucency of the FRC/prosthesis allows the luting composite to play a role in the final shade.

Luting an FRC/prosthesis involves those procedures that accompany any bonded restorative procedure: isolation of the abutment teeth, treatment of the inner surface of the FRC retainers, and treatment of the abutment teeth.

SUMMARY

The natural, esthetic appearance of this metal-free prosthesis and its inherent adhesive nature make the fiber-reinforced prosthesis a successful fixed tooth replacement. Its adhesive qualities may permit the use of abutment teeth that do not exhibit classic geometric retention and resistance form without the need for elective endodontics, surgical crown-lengthening procedures, and the apical placement of finish margins. Furthermore, its favorable strength, esthetics, and adhesive properties make the intracoronal fiber-reinforced prosthesis uniquely qualified for the minimally invasive replacement of a single missing tooth adjacent to unrestored or minimally restored abutment teeth. Multiyear clinical studies are currently in progress to determine the value and efficacy of the fiber-reinforced composite prosthesis as a long-term tooth replacement.

REFERENCES

1. Johansson BI et al: Corrosion of copper, nickel, and gold dental casting alloys: an in vitro and in vivo study, *J Biomed Mater Res* 23:349, 1989 (supplement).

2. Hani H: Corrosive changes of dental alloys in oral environment--scanning electron microscopic observation and electron probe microanalysis on crown surfaces (in Japanese), *Kokubyo Gakkai Zasshi* 60:372, 1993.

3. Ludwig K: Homogeneity and corrosion resistance of cast dental precious metal alloys compared with uncast alloys (in German), *Dtsch Zahnarztl Z* 44:905,1989.

4. American Dental Association, Council on Dental Materials, Instruments and Equipment: Biological effects of nickel-containing dental alloys, *J Am Dent Assoc* 104:501, 1982.

5. Association Report: Classification system for cast alloys, *J Am Dent Assoc* 109:838, 1984.

6. American Dental Association, Council on Dental Materials, Instruments, and Equipment: Report on base metal alloys for crown and bridge applications: benefits and risks, *J Am Dent Assoc* 111:479, 1985.

7. Covington JS et al: Quantization of nickel and beryllium leakage from base metal casting alloys, *J Prosthet Dent* 54:127, 1985.

8. Marcusson JA: Contact allergies to nickel sulfate, gold sodium thiosulfate and palladium chloride in patients claiming side-effects from dental alloy components, *Contact Derm* 34:320, 1996.

9. Moffa JP et al: Allergic response to nickel containing dental alloys, *J Dent Res* 56:1378, 1977 (abstract no. 107).

10. Morris HF: Veterans Administration Cooperative Studies Project No. 147. IV. Biocompatibility of base metal alloys, *J Dent* 58:1, 1987.

11. Walton JN et al: A survey of crown and fixed partial denture failures: length of service and reasons for replacement, *J Prosthet Dent* 56:416, 1986.

12. Libby G et al: Longevity of fixed partial dentures, *J Prosthet Dent* 78:127, 1997.

13. Sundh B, Odman P: A study of fixed prosthodontics performed at a university clinic 18 years after insertion, *Int J Prosthod* 10:513, 1997.

14. Priest GF: Failure rates of restorations for single-tooth replacement, *Int J Prosthod* 9:38, 1996.

15. Robbins JW: Intraoral repair of the fractured porcelain restoration, *Oper Dent* 23:203,1998.

Study Questions

1. Compare a fiber-reinforced composite fixed prosthesis with a metal-ceramic FPD. Discuss the advantages and disadvantages of each.
2. Discuss tooth preparation designs for fiber-reinforced composite fixed prostheses and specify how they differ from conventional preparations.
3. Current fiber-reinforced prostheses use either glass or polyethylene. Compare the performance and architecture of each.

16. Chung KH, Hwang YC: Bonding strengths of porcelain repair systems with various surface treatments, *J Prosthet Dent* 78:267, 1997.

17. Kupiec KA et al: Evaluation of porcelain surface treatments and agents for composite-to-porcelain repair, *J Prosthet Dent* 76:119, 1996.

18. Pameijer CH et al: Repairing fractured porcelain: how surface preparation affects shear force resistance, *J Am Dent Assoc* 127:203, 1996.

19. Monasky GE, Taylor DF: Studies on the wear of porcelain, enamel, and gold, *J Prosthet Dent* 25:299, 1971.

20. Ekfeldt A, Øilo G: Occlusal contact wear of prosthodontic materials, *Acta Odontol Scand* 46:159, 1988.

21. Kelly JR et al: Ceramics in dentistry: historical roots and current perspectives, *J Prosthet Dent* 75:18, 1996.

22. Hacker CH et al: An in vitro investigation of the wear of enamel on porcelain and gold in saliva, *J Prosthet Dent* 75:14, 1996.

23. Ramp MH et al: Evaluation of wear: enamel opposing three ceramic materials and a gold alloy, *J Prosthet Dent* 77:523, 1997.

24. Christensen GJ: The use of porcelain-fused-to-metal restorations in current dental practice: a survey, *J Prosthet Dent* 56:1, 1986.

25. Kern M, Knode H, Strubb JR: The all-porcelain resin bonded bridge, *Quintessence Int* 22:257, 1991.

26. Dickerson WG: The Concept bridge, *Dent Econ* 84:67, 1994.

27. Yang Z, Jia W, Prasad A: *Non-diluent dental composite,* Las Vegas, 1997, ACS National Meeting.

28. Karmaker AC, DiBenedetto AT, Goldberg AJ: *Fiber reinforced composite materials for dental appliances,* Indianapolis, 1996, Society of Plastic Engineers ANTEC.

29. Freilich MA et al: Flexure strength of fiber-reinforced composites designed for prosthodontic application, *J Dent Res* 76:138, 1997 (abstract no. 999).

30. Freilich MA et al: Flexure strength and handling characteristics of fiber-reinforced composites used in prosthodontics, *J Dent Res* 76:184, 1997 (abstract no. 1561).

31. Goldberg AJ et al:Flexure properties and fiber architecture of commercial fiber reinforced composites, *J Dent Res* 77:226, 1998 (abstract no. 967).

32. Goldberg AJ et al: Screening of matrices and fibers for reinforced thermoplastics intended for dental applications, *J Biomed Mat Res* 28:167, 1994.

33. Jancar J, DiBenedetto AT: Thermoplastic fiber reinforced composites for dentistry. II. Effect of moisture on flexural properties of unidirectional composites, *J Mater Sci* 4:562, 1993.

34. Altieri JV et al: Longitudinal clinical evaluation of fiber-reinforced composite fixed partial dentures: a pilot study, *J Prosthet Dent* 71:16, 1994.

35. Goldberg AJ, Burstone CJ: The use of continuous fiber reinforcement in dentistry, *Dent Mater* 8:197,1992.

36. Karmaker AC, DiBenedetto AT, Goldberg AJ: Extent of conversion and its effect on the mechanical performance of Bis-GMA/PEGDMA-based resins and their composites with continuous glass fibers, *J Mater Sci* 8:369, 1997.

37. Freilich MA et al: Preimpregnated, fiber-reinforced prostheses. I. Basic rationale and complete-coverage and intracoronal fixed partial denture designs, *Quintessence Int* 29:689, 1998.

38. Freilich MA et al: Development and clinical applications of a light-polymerized fiber-reinforced composite, *J Prosthet Dent* 80:311, 1998.

CONNECTORS FOR FIXED PARTIAL DENTURES

KEY TERMS

antiflux
cast connector
fineness
index
infrared radiation
mortise
nonrigid connectors

soldered connector
soldering flux
stabilization
tenon
welding
wetting

Connectors are those parts of a fixed partial denture (FPD) or splint that join the individual retainers and pontics together. Usually this is accomplished with rigid connectors (Fig. 28-1), although **nonrigid connectors** are used occasionally. The latter are usually indicated when it is impossible to prepare a common path of insertion for the abutment preparations for an FPD (Fig. 28-2, *A* and *B*).

RIGID CONNECTORS

Rigid connections in metal can be made by casting, soldering, or welding. **Cast connectors** are shaped in wax as part of a multiunit wax pattern. Cast connectors are convenient and minimize the number of steps involved in the laboratory fabrication. However, the fit of the individual retainers may be adversely affected because distortion more easily results when a multiunit wax pattern is removed from the die system. **Soldered connectors** involve the use of an intermediate metal alloy whose melting temperature is lower than that of the parent metal (Fig. 28-3). The parts being joined are not melted during soldering but must be thoroughly wettable by liquefied solder.[1] Dirt or surface oxides on the connector surfaces can reduce **wetting** and impede successful soldering; for example, the solder may melt

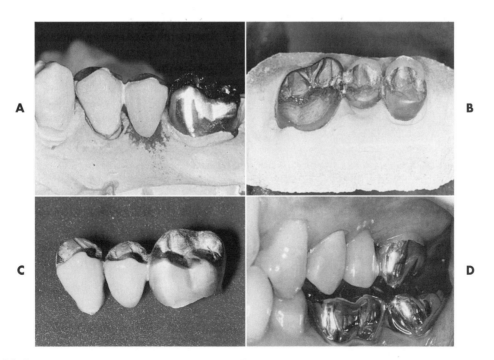

Fig. 28-1. Rigid connectors: A three-unit FPD replacing the maxillary second premolar. **A,** The anterior abutment and the pontic are connected with a rigid cast connector. These two FPD components are fabricated separately from the posterior abutment, which is cast in gold. **B,** The components are related to one another by a soldering assembly. **C,** The connected components. **D,** The fixed prosthesis in place.

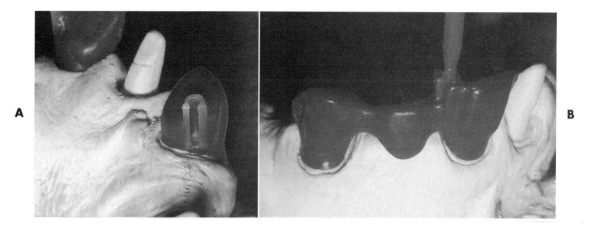

Fig. 28-2.   FPD with nonrigid connector. **A,** Mortise pattern (female) positioned on distal of the canine retainer. **B,** FPD assembled with prefabricated resin tenon (male) on mesial of pontic. *(Courtesy Dr. M. Chen.)*

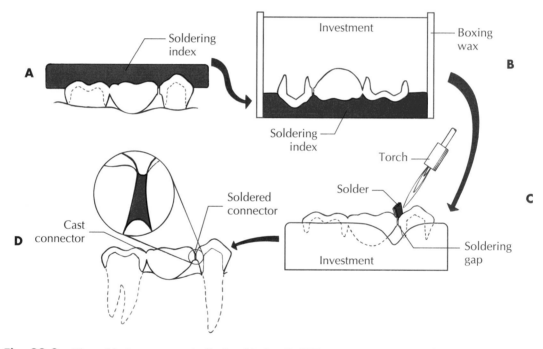

Fig. 28-3.   The soldering process. **A,** Occlusal index. **B,** FPD components invested. **C,** Torch soldering. **D,** Clinical evaluation.

but will not flow into the soldering gap. *Welding* is another method of rigidly joining metal parts. Here the connection is created by melting adjacent surfaces with heat or pressure. A filler metal whose melting temperature is about the same as that of the parent metal can be used during welding.

In industrial metalworking, a distinction is made between *soldering,* in which the filler metal has a melting point below 450° C (842° F), and *brazing,* in which the filler has a melting point above 450° C.[2] Rigid connections in dentistry are generally fabricated above 450° C, but the process has almost always been referred to in the dental literature as *soldering.* However, a proposed international standard uses the term *brazing.* With time the latter term may

become more generally accepted. In this text, however, the term *soldering* will be used.

NONRIGID CONNECTORS

Nonrigid connectors are indicated when it is not possible to prepare two abutments for an FPD with a common path of placement. Segmenting the design of large, complex FPDs into shorter components that are easier to replace or repair individually is advisable. This can be helpful if there is uncertainty about an abutment's prognosis. If the abutment fails, only a portion of the FPD may need to be remade. In the mandibular arch, nonrigid connectors are indicated when a complex FPD consists

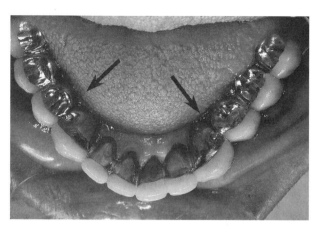

Fig. 28-4. To accommodate the stresses that potentially result from mandibular flexure, this complex FPD has been segmented through the use of nonrigid connectors on the distal of the two canines *(arrows)*. *(Courtesy Dr. F. Hsu.)*

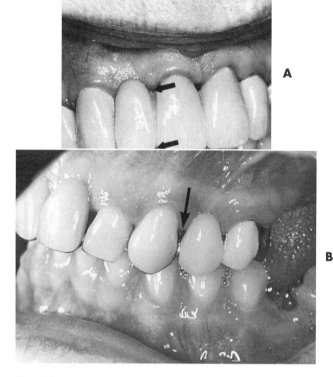

Fig. 28-5. Restorative failure. **A,** Incisocervically an excessively large connector *(arrows)* impedes proper plaque control and has led to periodontal breakdown. **B,** Although it may be acceptable from a biologic and mechanical perspective, a connector *(arrow)* that displays metal can prove to be esthetically unacceptable.

of anterior and posterior segments. During the mandibular opening and closing stroke, th mandible flexes mediolaterally.[3] Rigid fixed partial dentures have been shown to inhibit mandibular flexure, and extensive splints have been shown to flex during forced opening.[4] The associated stresses can cause dislodgment of complex FPDs. Segmenting complex mandibular FPDs can minimize this risk (Fig. 28-4).

Nonrigid connectors are generated through incorporation of prefabricated inserts in the wax pattern or through custom milling procedures after the first casting has been obtained. The second part is then custom-fitted to the milled retainer and cast. They are often made with prefabricated plastic patterns. The retainers are then cast separately and fitted to each other in metal.

CONNECTOR DESIGN

The size, shape, and position of connectors all influence the success of the prosthesis. Connectors must be sufficiently large to prevent distortion or fracture during function but not too large; otherwise, they will interfere with effective plaque control and contribute to periodontal breakdown over time. Adequate access (i.e., embrasure space) must be available for oral hygiene aids cervical to the connector. If a connector is too large incisocervically, hygiene is impeded, and over time periodontal failure will occur (Fig. 28-5, *A*). For esthetic FPDs, a large connector or inappropriate shaping of the individual retainers may result in display of the metal connector, which may compromise the appearance of the restoration and lead to patient dissatisfaction (Fig. 28-5, *B*).

In addition to being highly polished, the tissue surface of connectors is curved faciolingually to facilitate cleansing. Mesiodistally, it is shaped to create a smooth transition from one FPD component to the next. A properly shaped connector has a configuration similar to a meniscus formed between the two parts of the prosthesis.

In a buccolingual cross section, most connectors have a somewhat elliptical shape. Such an elliptical connector is strongest if the major axis of the ellipse parallels the direction of the applied force. Unfortunately, because of anatomic considerations, this can not always be achieved. In fact, due to space constraints, most connectors have their greatest dimension perpendicular to the direction of applied force, which tends to result in a weaker connector. For ease of plaque control, the connectors should occupy the normal anatomic interproximal contact areas because encroaching on the buccal, gingival, or lingual embrasure restricts access. However, to improve appearance without significantly affecting plaque control, anterior connectors are normally placed toward the lingual. Figure 28-6 depicts typical locations for connectors on selected teeth.

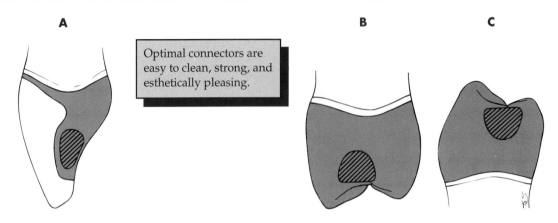

A

Optimal connectors are easy to clean, strong, and esthetically pleasing.

B   **C**

Fig. 28-6. Cross sections through FPD connectors. **A,** Maxillary anterior. **B,** Maxillary posterior. **C,** Mandibular posterior. Note the convexity of the gingival aspect of the connectors. To prevent excessive display of metal, anterior connectors should be placed toward the lingual.

Pulp size and clinical crown height can be limiting factors in the design of nonrigid connectors. Most prefabricated patterns require the preparation of a fairly sizable box. This allows incorporation of the **mortise** in the cast restoration without overcontouring of the interproximal emergence profile. Short clinical crowns do not provide adequate occlusocervical space to ensure adequate strength. Most manufacturers recommend 3 to 4 mm of vertical height.

■ TYPES OF CONNECTORS

RIGID CONNECTORS

Rigid connectors must be shaped and incorporated into the wax pattern after the individual retainers and pontics have been completed to final contour but before reflowing of the margins for investing (see Chapter 18).

Cast Connectors. Connectors to be cast are also waxed on the master cast before reflowing and investing of the pattern. The presence of a cast connector makes the latter somewhat more awkward. Access to the proximal margin is impeded, and the pattern cannot be held proximally during removal from the die. Restricting cast connectors to complete coverage restorations is therefore advisable, which can be gripped buccolingually. Partial-coverage wax patterns are easily distorted when they are part of a single-cast FPD. One-piece castings often appear to simplify fabrication but tend to create more problems than do soldered connectors, especially as pattern complexity increases.

Soldered Connectors. As with cast connectors, connectors to be soldered are waxed to final shape but are then sectioned with a thin ribbon saw (Fig. 28-7, *A* and *B*); therefore, when the components are cast, the surfaces to be joined will be flat, parallel, and a controlled distance apart. This allows accurate soldering with a minimum of distortion.[5] Molten solder will flow toward the location where the temperature is highest. In metal, the two flat surfaces previously created in wax retain heat, ensuring that the highest temperature is in the connector area.

Soldering Gap Width. As gap width increases, soldering accuracy decreases.[6] Extremely small gap widths can prevent proper solder flow and lead to an incomplete or weak joint.[7] An even soldering gap of about 0.25 mm is recommended. If a connector area has an uneven soldering gap width, obtaining a connector of adequate cross-sectional dimension without resulting distortion is more difficult.

Loop Connectors (Fig. 28-8). Although they are rarely used, loop connectors are sometimes required when an existing diastema is to be maintained in a planned fixed prosthesis. The connector consists of a loop on the lingual aspect of the prosthesis that connects adjacent retainers and/or pontics. The loop may be cast from sprue wax that is circular in cross section or shaped from a platinum-gold-palladium (Pt-Au-Pd) alloy wire. Meticulous design is important so that plaque control will not be impeded.

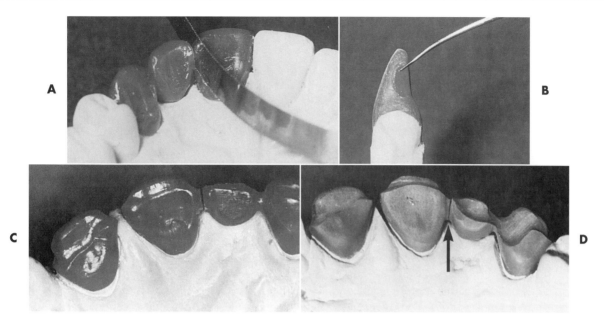

Fig. 28-7.   Connector design. **A,** A ribbon saw is used to section the wax pattern. **B,** The sectioned surface should be flat and located sufficiently far incisally and lingually to permit adequate hygiene and esthetics of the completed FPD. **C,** A three-unit FPD after sectioning. **D,** Ready for porcelain application. Note the uniform gap width *(arrow)*.

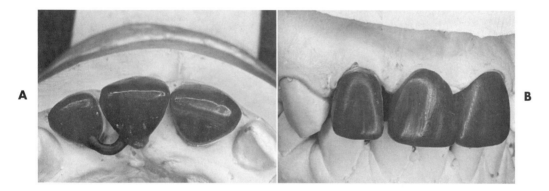

Fig. 28-8.   In the presence of a diastema that is to be maintained, a loop connector is indicated. **A,** Incisal view of the anatomic contour wax pattern of a three-unit FPD with a loop connector. **B,** Labial view. Note that the diastema between the lateral and central incisors is maintained.

NONRIGID CONNECTORS

The design of nonrigid connectors that are incorporated in the wax pattern stage consists of a mortise (also referred to as the *female component*) prepared within the contours of the retainer and a **tenon** (male) attached to the pontic (Fig. 28-9). The mortise is usually placed on the distal aspect of the anterior retainer. Accurate alignment of the dovetail or cylindrically shaped mortise is critical; it must parallel the path of withdrawal of the distal retainer (see Fig. 28-2). Paralleling is normally accomplished with a dental surveyor. When aligning the cast, the path of placement of the retainer that will be contiguous with the tenon is identified. The mortise in the other retainer is then shaped so its path of insertion permits concurrent seating of the tenon and its corresponding retainer.

The mortise can be prepared freehand in the wax pattern or with a precision milling machine. Another approach is to use prefabricated plastic components for the mortise and tenon of a nonrigid connector (Fig. 28-10). As an alternative, a special mandrel can be embedded in the wax pattern (Fig. 28-11) and the abutment retainer can be cast, with refinement of the female component as necessary; the male key is then fabricated of autopolymerizing acrylic resin and attached to the pontic.

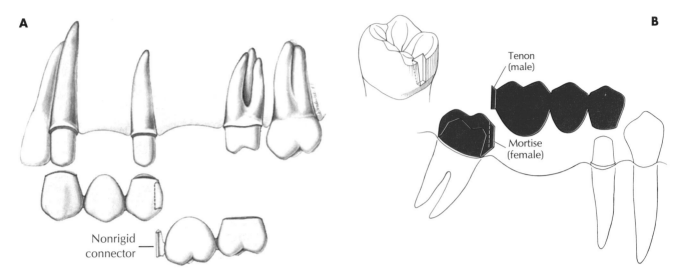

Fig. 28-9. Fixed partial dentures with nonrigid connectors. This type of connector may be indicated to overcome problems with intermediate or pier abutments **(A)** and abutment alignment **(B).**

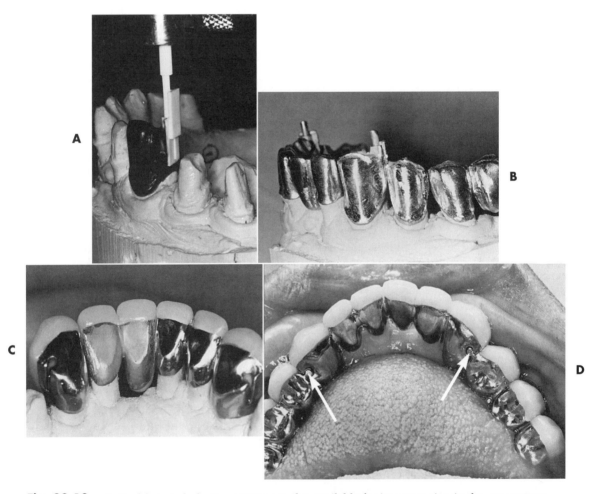

Fig. 28-10. **A,** Prefabricated plastic patterns are also available for incorporation in the wax pattern. **B,** The metal substructure. **C,** The anterior component of the prosthesis. **D,** The cemented prosthesis incorporates bilateral nonrigid connectors *(arrows).*
(Courtesy Dr. F. Hsu.)

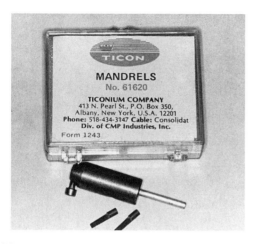

Fig. 28-11. Ticon mandrels are prefabricated inserts embedded in the wax pattern. The retainer is cast directly onto the mandrel to form the female component of the connector.
(Courtesy Dr. F. Hsu.)

▄ MATERIALS SCIENCE

M.H. Reisbick
Solder

Dental gold solders are given a **fineness** designation to indicate the proportion of pure gold contained in 1000 parts of alloy. For example, a 650-fine solder contains 65% gold. An earlier designation[8] assigned the solder a carat number, which indicated the gold content of the castings that were to be joined with the solder; an 18-carat solder could be used to solder castings fabricated of an alloy containing 75% gold. Because numerous alloys other than Type IV gold are available today, many of which contain platinum-group metals, the carat designation is of little value.

Modern casting alloys have become so metallurgically complex that most manufacturers now recommend specifically formulated solders. One manufacturer (Jelenko) classifies traditional gold-containing solders as group I and others (termed *special solders*) as group II. Most of these have the brand name with a *pre* or *post* designation to indicate whether the solder is to be used for joining the components before or after porcelain application. The preceramic solders are obviously high-fusing alloys, sometimes fusing only slightly beneath the softening point of the parent alloy to be joined. Ideally they should flow well above the fusion range of the subsequently applied porcelain. Postceramic solders must flow well below the pyroplastic range of the porcelain. For example, one popular silver-palladium (Ag-Pd) casting alloy has a specified melting range

between 1232° C and 1304° C (2280° F to 2384° F). The recommended special presolder melts at 1110° C to 1127° C (2030° F to 2061° F), whereas the postsolder melts at 710° C to 743° C (1310° F to 1369° F). The porcelain fuses at about 982° C (1800° F), depending on time and temperature.

The composition of the solder determines its melting range, among other things. Some typical compositions and melting ranges are given in Table 28-1. Solder's main requirement is to fuse safely below the sag or creep temperature of the casting to be soldered. Newer palladium casting alloys, by virtue of their higher melting ranges, have somewhat increased the reliability of the preceramic application soldering technique.[9]

However, preceramic soldering is relatively difficult and can be structurally hazardous (Fig. 28-12). This may be due to the volatilization of base metal solder constituents that occurs with overheating.[10] Volatilization then results in microporosity or pitting. The melting range of presolders is quite narrow, because silver and copper (the usual modifiers of temperature range) cannot be used in the alloy. These elements discolor porcelain on contact. Another consideration is the oxide necessary for the chemical adherence of porcelain. Porcelain does not chemically bond equally well to all solders.

Other requirements of solders are their ability to resist tarnish and corrosion, to be free flowing, to match the color of the units that will be joined, and to be strong. These factors also depend on the chemical composition of the solder.

Resistance to tarnish and corrosion is determined by a solder's noble or precious metal content and its Ag/Cu ratio.[11] In addition, if the compositions of the solder and workpiece differ, galvanic corrosion may occur.

During the soldering procedure, the solder must flow freely over clean and smooth surfaces. These surfaces should be smoothed with abrasive disks, not with rubber wheels or polishing compounds. The phenomenon of free flow is termed *wetting*, during which remelting or realloying of the surface of the units to be joined must not occur.[12] Solder flow is increased by the addition of silver and decreased by the presence of copper. Fig. 28-13 demonstrates a properly made solder joint. Note that the filler metal has joined the surfaces of the two castings without penetrating either one.

Lower-fineness gold solders are often more fluid and are generally chosen for joining castings. If necessary, proximal contacts with a higher-fineness solder can also be added, because this tends to flow less freely. However, the exact minimally acceptable

| Composition (%) and Flow Temperatures of Dental Solders | | | | | | TABLE 28-1 |
Fineness	Gold (Au)	Silver (Ag)	Copper (Cu)	Tin (Sn)	Zinc (Zn)	Flow temperature (°C)
490	49.0	17.5	23.0	4.5	6.0	780
585	58.5	14.0	19.0	3.5	4.5	780
615	61.5	13.0	17.5	3.5	4.5	790
650	65.0	12.0	16.0	3.0	4.0	790
730	73.0	9.0	12.5	2.5	3.0	830

Courtesy Williams Dental Co.

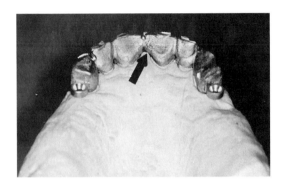

Fig. 28-12. Metal substructure for an anterior prosthesis. The preceramic soldering procedure has led to partial melting of the framework (*arrow*), which can result in distortion and/or premature failure.

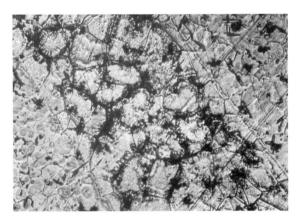

Fig. 28-13. Photomicrograph of a properly made solder joint connecting two castings.

fineness necessary for resisting tarnish and corrosion has not been conclusively established; 615 or 580 fineness is probably the lower limit of clinical acceptability.

The last requirement, strength, is easily satisfied by most solders and is usually greater than that of the soldered parent metal, provided the procedure is followed carefully.[7] In addition, most solders harden during cooling because of the "order-disorder" transformation and the formation of other intermetallic phases, which occur at grain boundaries. Brittleness is frequently encountered with gold-based copper-containing solders. As with Type III and Type IV gold casting alloys, the gold-copper–order-disorder (or discontinuous phase-hardening) mechanism will cause similar changes in the solder's microstructure.[13] Simply stated, with these solders, cooling to room temperature results in a brittle joint. The joints are strong but have no ductility. Some solder joints are weakened by notches.[14] This means soldered connectors should be well-polished to prevent fracture.

Fixed partial dentures fabricated of Type III gold alloys and joined interproximally with traditional gold-based solders are usually water quenched 4 to 5 minutes after soldering is complete. Quenching immediately after soldering causes the FPD to warp; failure to quench will create a joint with little or no ductility. A brittle joint may easily fracture. Thus, a disadvantage of postceramic soldering is the loss of joint ductility. Because the components are partially porcelain, quenching is not possible because porcelain fracture will occur.

SOLDERING FLUX AND ANTIFLUX

Soldering Flux. This substance is applied to a metal surface to remove oxides or prevent their formation. When the oxides are removed, the solder is free to wet and spread over the clean metal surface.

Borax glass ($Na_2B_4O_7$) is frequently used with gold alloys because of its affinity for copper oxides. An often-cited soldering flux formula[15] is borax glass (55 parts), boric acid (35 parts), and silica (10 parts). These ingredients are fused together and then ground into a powder.

Fluxes are available in powder, liquid, or paste form. The paste is popular because it can be easily placed and confined. Pastes are made by mixing the flux powder with petrolatum. The petrolatum excludes oxygen during heating and eventually carbonizes and then vaporizes.

New fluxes are available for use with nongold-based alloys. Their formulas are not generally published. At present, none of the new fluxes are totally capable of preventing oxide formation during heating of the base metal or nonnoble alloys. An exam-

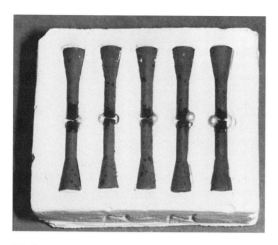

Fig. 28-14. Simulated base metal-to-base metal postceramic soldering procedure. Excessive oxide formation has prevented wetting by the solder.
(From Sloan RH et al: J Prosthet Dent 48:688, 1982.)

ple of a rapidly forming oxide on a base metal occurring during a simulated postceramic application soldering can be seen in Fig. 28-14. Soldering of base metal alloys is still unpredictable.[16]

All fluxes should be kept from contacting porcelain-veneered surfaces. The contact will cause pitting and porcelain discoloration.

Soldering Antiflux. Antiflux is used to limit the spreading of solder. It is placed on a casting before the flux application to limit the flow of molten solder. When the metal surfaces are clean, any excess solder introduced into the work gap will tend to flow into unwanted areas. The antiflux helps prevent this.

Graphite (from a pencil) is often used as an antiflux. However, the carbon easily evaporates at higher temperature, leaving the workpiece unprotected. A more reliable antiflux is iron oxide (rouge) in a suitable solvent such as turpentine, which can be painted on the casting with a small bristle brush.

SOLDERING INVESTMENT

Soldering investments are similar in composition to casting investments (see Chapter 22). Casting investments, both gypsum and phosphate bonded, mixed with water only, have been used for soldering. However, note that the refractory component in casting investments usually creates unwanted thermal expansion and therefore excessively separates the units to be joined. Soldering investments should ideally contain fused quartz (the lowest thermally expanding form of silica) as their refractory component.

Invested units expand during heating, and they should do so at the same rate as the castings. The

units must be correctly gapped so that they do not touch. When the work units are allowed to touch, distortion and porous inadequate joints result.[8] Alternatively, excessive gap spaces cause undersized mesiodistal fixed partial denture widths because of solder solidification shrinkage. However, Ryge[8] has shown that the gap space closes somewhat during heating, so it is doubtful that the alloy and investment truly expand equally or at the same rates. Several commercial soldering investments are available; these should be used whenever possible. A list of reliable investments appears in Appendix A.

• • •

◼ SELECTION OF SOLDERING TECHNIQUE

When FPDs are assembled by soldering, the relative position of the components is recorded with a soldering **index** on the working cast or intraorally. If pontics are made individually, they can be difficult to position properly relative to the abutment teeth. Although a positioning index made previously upon completion of the wax pattern can be helpful (Fig. 28-15), they should be connected to one of the retainers with a cast connector because this stabilizes them and makes accurate positioning relative to the other retainer much easier. To understand the selection of soldering technique, a thorough knowledge of the fusing ranges of all materials involved in the FPD is essential (Fig. 28-16).

Soldering of all metal FPDs consisting of Type III or IV gold units requires the use of a low-fusing solder. The procedure is referred to as *conventional soldering*. By using the same low-fusing solder, regular gold retainers can also be connected with metal ceramic components. A gas-air torch is used for either of these procedures.

For FPDs consisting of metal-ceramic units, the soldered connectors may be made either before the ceramic application with high-fusing solder (approximately 1100° C, or 2012° F) or after the ceramic application with lower-fusing solder (750° C, or 1382° F). Soldering before ceramic application is called *preceramic application soldering* or *presoldering*. Soldering of metal-ceramic crowns after their completion is referred to as *postsoldering*. Many alloys can be combined using either preceramic or postceramic soldering. However, presoldering has been found to be less reliable,[7] with a number of apparently sound connectors exhibiting negligible tensile strength. Considerable variation in solder joint strength has also been recorded after laboratory

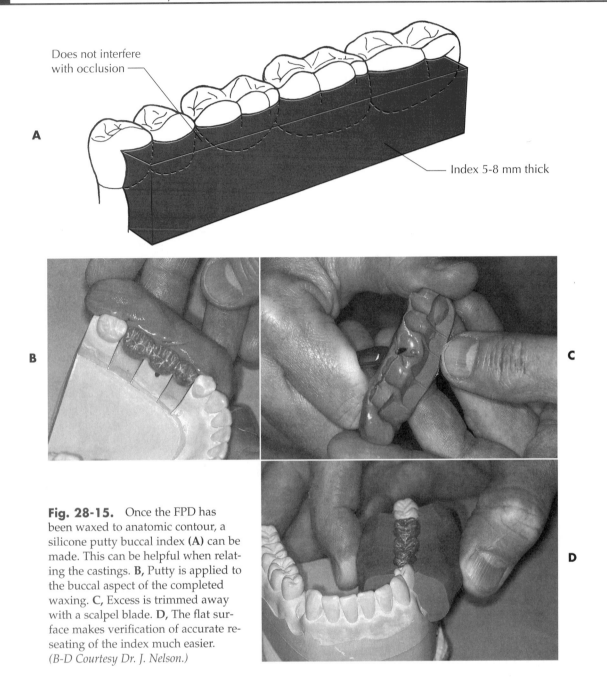

Does not interfere
with occlusion

A

Index 5-8 mm thick

B

C

D

Fig. 28-15. Once the FPD has been waxed to anatomic contour, a silicone putty buccal index **(A)** can be made. This can be helpful when relating the castings. **B,** Putty is applied to the buccal aspect of the completed waxing. **C,** Excess is trimmed away with a scalpel blade. **D,** The flat surface makes verification of accurate reseating of the index much easier. *(B-D Courtesy Dr. J. Nelson.)*

testing,[17] which emphasizes the special care needed to avoid defective connections.

Base metal alloys can be difficult to solder because they oxidize; this must be controlled with special fluxes, although excessive fluxing can lead to undesirable inclusions and weak connectors. One study[18] found that 20% of postceramic soldered joints involving base metal alloys had to be resoldered because they were so weak that they broke with finger pressure. Another study[19] showed great variability in solder joint quality with these alloys, with no consistent relationship of strength to gap width. These authors found that most failures oc-

curred through the solder and were attributable to voids caused by gas entrapment or localized shrinkage. With experience and careful adherence to the manufacturer's recommended techniques and materials, reliable base metal alloy soldered connectors are possible.[20] However, because of the problems of soldering base metal alloys, various alternative procedures have been advocated. These include making the soldered joint through the center of the pontic to increase the area soldered[21] and connecting the parts by a second casting procedure, with the molten metal flowing into undercuts in the sectioned pontic.[22]

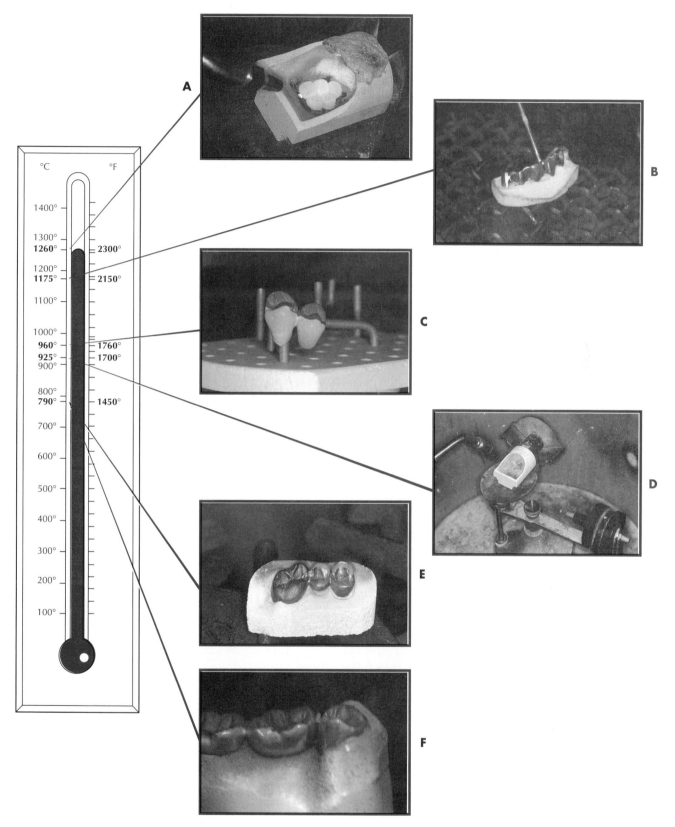

Fig. 28-16. **A,** Casting metal-ceramic alloys. **B,** Presoldering. **C,** Porcelain firing. **D,** Casting Type III and Type IV gold alloy. **E,** Post-ceramic soldering. **F,** Conventional soldering.

SOLDERING ALL-METAL FPDs

Type III and IV gold retainers of fixed partial dentures are soldered with gold solder ranging from 615 to 650 fineness. An occlusal plaster index or autopolymerizing resin index is fabricated intraorally or in the dental laboratory; after investing, a gas-air torch can be used to solder the components. A disadvantage of the soldering procedure is that it requires an additional step, compared to a one-piece casting. However, soldering simplifies the manipulation of wax patterns. For instance, when a three-abutment FPD with two splinted abutments (e.g., two premolars) is fabricated, access to the interproximal margins of the two splinted abutments is often very difficult during the reflowing and finishing steps. Soldering such retainers permits the retainers to be shaped and adjusted individually with improved access for finishing procedures. Conventional soldering requires a gas-air torch; soldering can also be performed in a furnace.

SOLDERING METAL-CERAMIC FPDs

Preceramic Soldering. Once a metal-ceramic framework has been assembled by preceramic application soldering, the subsequent procedures are the same as if it had been cast in one piece. This has the advantage of allowing the connected prosthesis to be tried in the mouth in the unglazed state. Any necessary adjustments can be made to the porcelain, which fuses at a lower temperature than the preceramic soldered connector. However, with preceramic soldering, contouring the proximal embrasures so the units resemble natural teeth may be more difficult. A very thin diamond disk is helpful for this.

A disadvantage results from having to apply the porcelain to a longer structure, which needs support during firing to prevent high-temperature deformation or sag. Sag can be a particular problem with the high-gold content ceramic alloys because they have a lower melting range. High palladium-content or base metal alloys exhibit little sag during firing. Presoldering requires a gas-oxygen torch.

Postceramic Soldering. Postceramic soldering is necessary when regular gold and metal-ceramic units are being combined in an FPD. The regular gold will melt if it is subjected to the high temperatures needed for porcelain application; therefore all porcelain adjustment and firing, including that for the final staining and glazing, must be completed before the soldering. If further corrective adjustment is needed after soldering, the porcelain will have to be polished, or the joint will have to be separated, after which additional porcelain can be

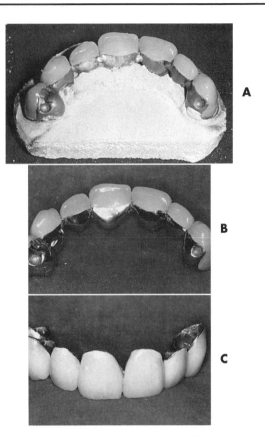

Fig. 28-17. **A,** This anterior fixed prosthesis was fabricated in individual units and assembled by postceramic soldering. **B,** Note the connectors placed sufficiently lingual for good facial embrasure form. **C,** The assembled splint.

added as needed, the restorations can be reglazed, a new index can be made, and the FPD can be resoldered.

Because the proximal areas are shaped before soldering, a postsoldered connector can often be made to look more natural than a presoldered or cast connector (Fig. 28-17). In addition, customized firing supports are not needed because sag is not a problem (the lengths of the individual components are shorter). Postsoldering is performed either in a porcelain furnace or with a gas-air torch.

█ HEAT SOURCES

TORCH SOLDERING

When a gas-air torch is used as the heat source to melt the solder, metal-ceramic restorations are preheated in an oven to avoid cracking of the porcelain veneer. Oxidization of the joint surfaces is prevented by using the reducing portion of the flame (Fig. 28-18) and by applying an appropriate flux (some soldering fluxes are unsuitable because they discolor the porcelain). To prevent uneven heat distribution, which could result in fracture, the flame is

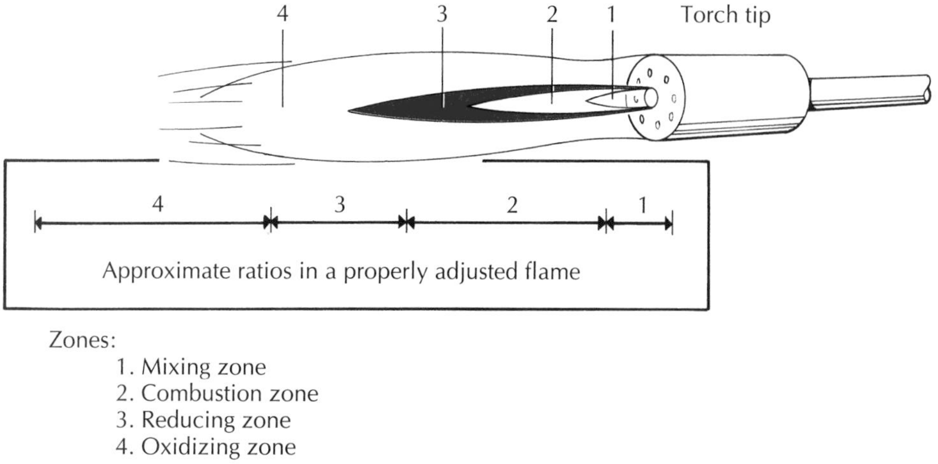
4
3
2
1
Torch tip
4
3
2
1
Approximate ratios in a properly adjusted flame
Zones:
1. Mixing zone
2. Combustion zone
3. Reducing zone
4. Oxidizing zone

Fig. 28-18. Gas-air torch adjusted for soldering.

never concentrated in one area but is kept in constant motion.

Some dentists believe the flow of solder is more controllable during torch soldering because a slight temperature differential can be created and the solder always flows toward the hotter point. This makes torch soldering useful when the connector has not been well designed in wax and a minor temperature difference can deliberately be created in the assembly to help direct the flow of the molten solder to ensure an adequate connection.

Oven Soldering

Furnace or oven soldering is performed under vacuum or in air. A piece of solder is placed at the joint space, and the casting and solder are heated simultaneously.

Criticism of the technique has been based on earlier observations[23] that less porosity resulted when castings were brought to soldering temperature before the solder was applied. The method does not allow the moment of solder fusion to be observed.* This may be important, because the longer the solder remains molten, the more it will dissolve the parent metal and consequently weaken the joint.[8] Nevertheless, joints of similar or superior strength to the parent metal have been demonstrated[7] when oven soldering was used.

A different technique may be appropriate if the porcelain furnace has a horizontal muffle with a fixed floor. The soldering assembly is heated above the fusion point of the solder, the muffle door is opened, and the solder is fed into the joint space (Fig. 28-19).

*Some porcelain furnaces have an observation window for postsoldering.

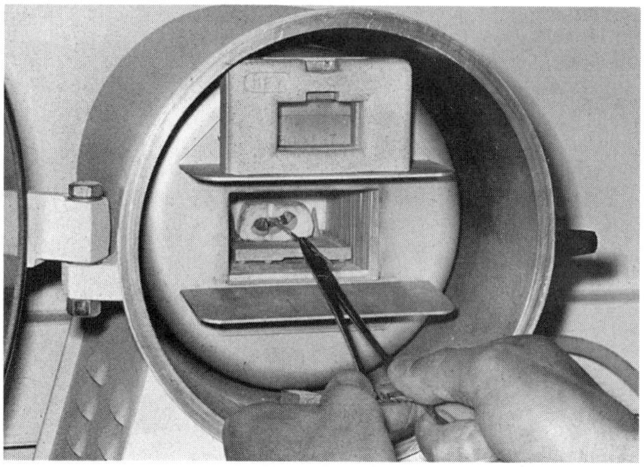

Fig. 28-19. Oven soldering a three-unit FPD. *(Courtesy Dr. A.G. Gegauff.)*

Infrared Soldering (Fig. 28-20)

Infrared soldering can be used for low-fusing connectors as well as preceramic soldered joints. A specially designed unit that uses an infrared light as its heat source is used. The connector area of the soldering assembly must be positioned precisely relative to the focal point of the reflector that concentrates the heat. The operator observes the soldering procedure through a dark screen and cuts off the electrical supply when solder flow is observed. Good accuracy is possible with the system.[24] The joints have similar strength to conventional soldering,[24] although weaker joints have been reported with infrared presoldering of gold-platinum-palladium alloys.[25]

Laser Welding (Fig. 28-21)

Laser energy is extensively used for welding in many industries and has been described in dentistry

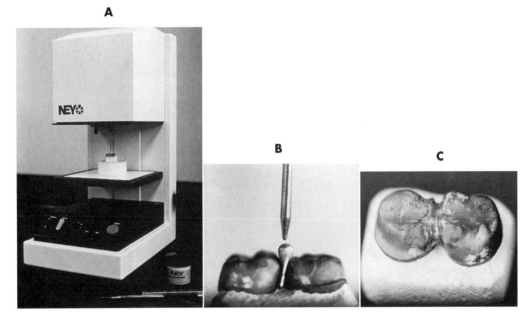

Fig. 28-20. Infrared soldering.
(Courtesy Ney Dental International.)

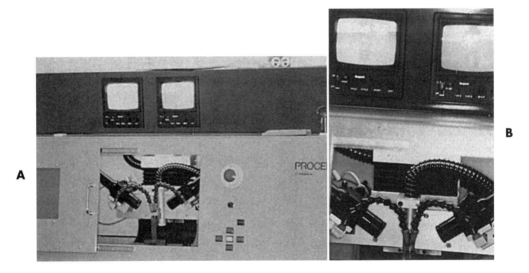

Fig. 28-21. Laser welding. Individual titanium components are carefully aligned in the laser welding unit. The joining procedure is monitored by high-magnification video.
(Courtesy Dr. M. Chen.)

since the 1970s.[26,27] Interest has continued in laser assembly of fixed prostheses with reported higher strength[28] and reduced corrosion[29] in comparison to conventional soldering, although laser welding does seem as susceptible as conventional soldering to fatigue failure.[30] Laser welding may be a practical way to join cast titanium components (e.g., if these are to be used for implant superstructures[31,32]).

SOLDERING ACCURACY

Controversy exists as to the relative accuracy of fixed partial dentures that are cast in one piece, preceramic soldered, or postceramic soldered. An individual laboratory technician will often obtain consistently better results with one particular technique, but scientific evidence is conflicting.[33,34] When evaluating clinical work to determine whether cast or soldered connectors provide better results, the determining factor should be the fit of the individual abutment castings. This should be optimized through the investing and casting processes (see Chapter 22) to minimize the risks of incomplete seating or excessive luting agent space. In some situations it may be impossible to cast a long-span FPD with ideal retainer dimensions and ideal inter-abutment dimensions; the challenge lies in obtaining enough interabutment expansion without making the retainers too loose. In such circumstances, a soldered connector may provide better accuracy. The situation is reversed when fabricating frameworks for implant-supported prostheses (see Chapter 13). Here the fit of the individual units is determined by the implant manufacturer. Only the overall abutment-to-abutment fit is under the control of the technician. However, an accurate, passively fitting implant superstructure is critical to avoid damaging forces. It is not yet clear if accurate implant superstructures are most effectively made with one-piece castings or sectioned and soldered units.[35]

◼ SOLDERING TECHNIQUE

Armamentarium
- Autopolymerizing acrylic resin
- Zinc oxide–eugenol paste
- Impression plaster
- Mixing bowl
- Spatula
- Small brush
- Waxing instrument
- Sticky wax
- Baseplate wax
- Sprue wax
- Soldering investment
- Glass slab
- Soldering tripod
- Flux
- Solder
- Tongs
- Pickling solution

Step-by-step Procedure
Occlusal Soldering Index (Fig. 28-22; see Fig. 28-3).   An intraoral plaster or ZOE impression is made of the occlusal surfaces of the FPD to capture the relative relationship of the individual FPD components and transfer this to the laboratory. This procedure can also be performed in the laboratory if the technician is satisfied that the individual components are seated completely on an accurate master cast. An advantage of an occlusal index is that after the soldering procedure has been completed, the FPD can be reseated in the index and soldering ac-

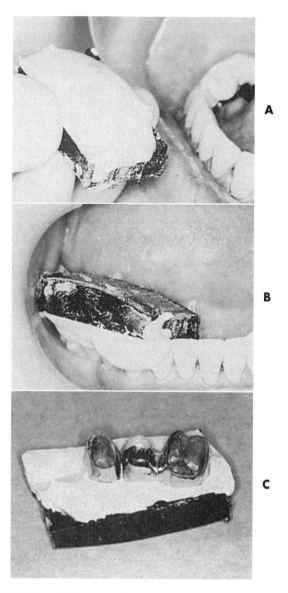

Fig. 28-22.   Soldering index (plaster) for posterior FPDs. **A,** A suitable carrier (e.g., baseplate wax) is trimmed to proper shape before making a registration with impression plaster **(B). C,** The plaster occlusal registration.

curacy can be verified (sometimes a small amount of plaster must be removed in the area where the solder has been added to ensure seating).

1. Grind the connector surfaces of the finished castings with a stone to remove surface oxides. Then fully seat the castings on the working cast or in the mouth. Postceramic application joints are best indexed intraorally after the contour and appearance have been perfected. If necessary, the soldering gap can be adjusted at this time (gap distance 0.25 mm).

2. Make an impression plaster registration in a small tray or on a sheet of baseplate wax for the occlusal index. As an alternative, an index can

be made with ZOE paste, a technique that has shown[36] consistent and accurate recordings. The index should not cover the margins of regular gold retainers because these are to be embedded in the investment to prevent their accidental melting during soldering.

3. Trim the index to fully expose the margins before investing (Fig. 28-23).

Investing

4. Seat each casting into the index and lute it to place with sticky wax.
5. Flow wax into the connector area to prevent the investment from entering.
6. To create a space that will help the solder spread, adapt sprue wax gingival to the solder joint. Burying the units completely in the investment makes soldering difficult because the unnecessary bulk of the investment prevents rapid heating of the castings.

7. Protect any glazed porcelain from contacting the investment by coating it with wax before investing. To protect regular gold margins from the soldering flame, they should be embedded in the investment; otherwise, they may become overheated and melt. For the same reason, all margins should be embedded in the investment before preceramic application soldering.
8. Box the assembly with a suitable sheet wax.
9. Mix the investment carefully and flow it into the castings without trapping any air. Only slight vibration is used so the castings will not be displaced from the index.
10. Allow the invested block to bench set before removing the wax and preheating.

Autopolymerizing Resin Soldering Index (Fig. 28-24). A plaster or ZOE occlusal index is less suitable for the registration of anterior restorations. The thinness of the incisal edges of these units makes

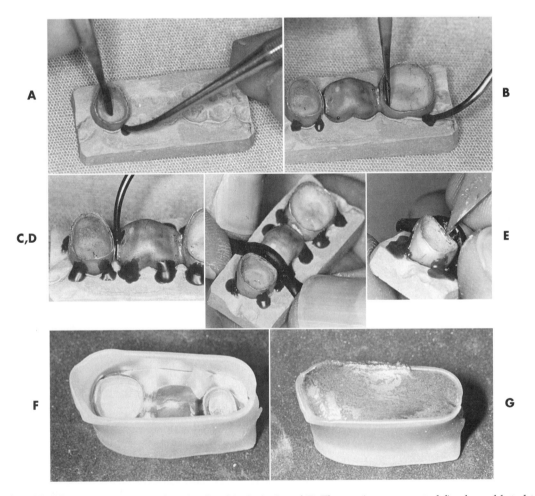

Fig. 28-23. Investing procedure (occlusal index). **A** and **B,** The castings are seated firmly and luted to place with sticky wax. **C,** The wax is flowed into the connector areas and is adapted gingivally to each connector to create an airway **(D). E,** There must be no wax on the internal surface of the casting. **F,** The soldering assembly is boxed and filled with soldering investment **(G).** There must be no air bubbles in the investment.

them less stable, and accurate repositioning is more difficult. For this reason, autopolymerizing resin is recommended, although the resin burns off during the procedure. Therefore, the accuracy of the soldering procedure can only be verified intraorally.

1. Join the completed units together with autopolymerizing resin. The resin will later burn out, leaving no residue that could interfere with the casting.

2. Apply the resin with a bead technique. This will minimize the distortion from polymerization shrinkage. Excessive bulk of resin reduces the accuracy of the technique,[37] but sufficient material must be present to ensure that the components do not break (because they cannot then be accurately reseated in the index). NOTE: The resin should extend onto the incisal edges of the retainers.

3. When the resin has fully hardened, carefully loosen the prosthesis from the abutments. Then replace it and check whether distortion has occurred. This is done in the same way as the try-

in of a finished FPD. It must be stable with no marginal discrepancies (see Fig. 28-24, C).

Investing (Fig. 28-25).

4. Warm a sheet of wax and push the cervical aspect of the restorations through it. Then seal it along the axial wall with a warmed instrument. This will protect the porcelain from contact with the soldering investment.

5. Fill the castings with soldering investment and blot excess water from the remaining investment, forming it into a patty on a slab or tile.

6. Seat the restorations on the patty. When a joint is to be oven-soldered, the restoration should be angled forward so that the solder can be placed above the joint before the block is set inside the furnace.

Wax Removal and Preheating (Fig. 28-26)

1. If a plaster or ZOE index was used, remove it after the investment has fully set. This is most effectively accomplished after removing the wax

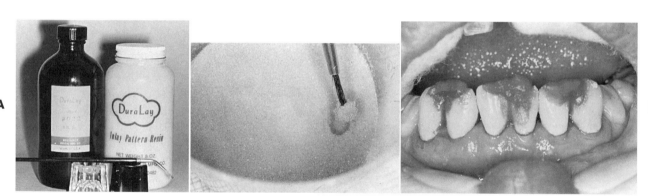

Fig. 28-24. Soldering index (autopolymerizing resin). **A,** Armamentarium. **B,** A small brush dipped in resin monomer is touched to the polymer powder. This forms a bead. **C,** The restorations are thus connected, with resin extending onto the incisal edges of all the retainers.

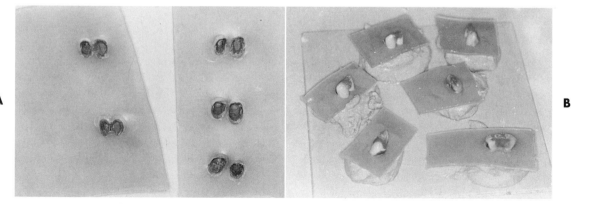

Fig. 28-25. Investing procedure (autopolymerizing resin). **A,** The castings pressed firmly into a softened sheet of wax. Note that the internal walls of the castings are exposed; the wax seals them. **B,** Castings filled with soldering investment and then inverted onto a patty of investment.

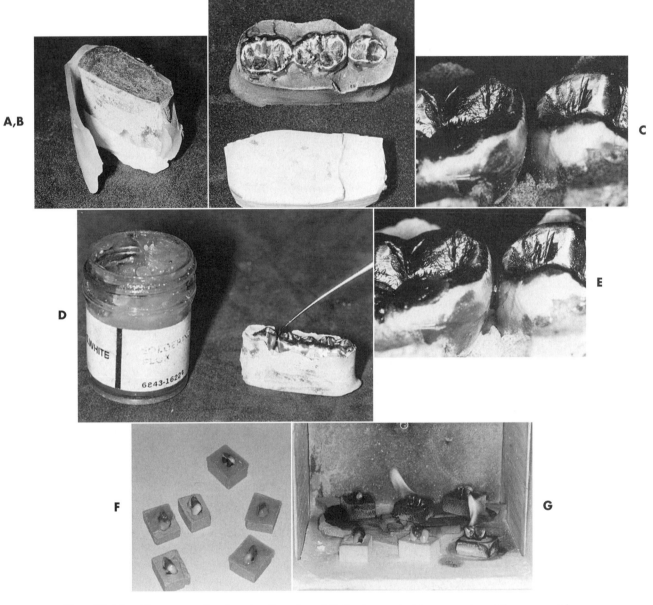

Fig. 28-26. Wax removal and preheating. **A** and **B,** Boxing material removed and the wax residue flushed out with boiling water. **C,** The connector area must be free of contaminants. **D,** A small amount of soldering flux is applied while the assembly is still warm. **E,** The flux is carried into the connector areas by capillary action. Then the assembly is placed in the burnout furnace. **F** and **G,** Autopolymerizing resin indexes. These are burned off directly in the furnace after wax elimination.

with boiling water. The joint space must be free of investment. Flowing a little flux into the joint space while the soldering block is still warm from wax removal is recommended. This will prevent small particles from inadvertently falling into the gap. Be aware that many special soldering investments have low strength, and the assembly is easily broken at this stage.

2. Preheat the investment in a burnout furnace to 650° C (for low-heat soldering) or 850° C (for preceramic soldering) (1202° F or 1562° F).

Acrylic resin indexes are removed by heating slowly to 300° C (572° F), at which time most of the resin will have burned away.

3. Heat the block to 650° C (1202° F) until all traces of wax and resin have vaporized and then transfer it to the soldering stand or porcelain furnace.

Torch Soldering (Low Heat) (Fig. 28-27)

1. Transfer the assembly to a soldering stand with a Bunsen flame underneath and place a piece of solder above the gap. Adjust the gas-air torch to

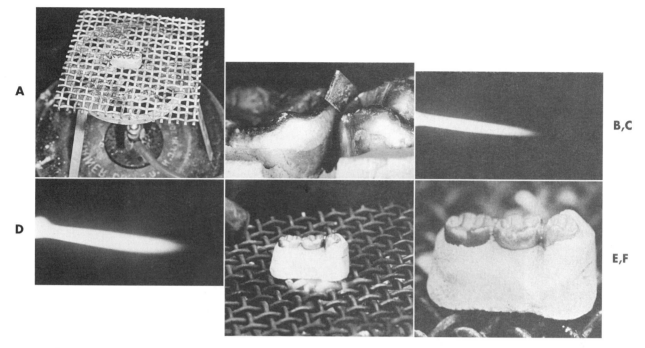

Fig. 28-27. Low-heat torch soldering. **A,** The assembly positioned on a wire mesh over a Bunsen burner. **B,** A flexed piece of solder placed into the connector area. **C,** A sharply defined flame is preferable for casting procedures. **D,** A brush flame is more suitable for soldering. This can be obtained by slightly reducing the amount of air. **E,** The assembly is heated evenly until the solder melts. The solder must "spin" in the connector area to form a complete connection **(F).**

give a sharp blue cone (as for casting) and then reduce the air for a softer "brush" flame. The reducing zone of the flame is used to heat the investment block. The flame is directed at the lingual aspect of the block rather than at the casting.

2. Heat evenly and slowly, moving the tip of the flame constantly. This is particularly important in postceramic application soldering because the porcelain may easily crack. When the metal glows brightly, the solder will melt and flow into the joint space.

3. Quickly move the flame to the facial. When the solder "spins" in the joint, remove the flame.

4. Extinguish the flame and let the soldered prosthesis cool for 4 or 5 minutes before quenching (unless there is porcelain on the restoration, in which case it should cool to room temperature). Earlier quenching may lead to distortion, whereas prolonged bench cooling increases the brittleness of the joint.

Torch Soldering (High Heat) (Fig. 28-28).

1. Wear dark glasses for eye protection (Fig. 28-29). Gas-oxygen torches for high-heat preceramic soldering use a miniature needle tip so that the flame can be pinpointed on the joint space.

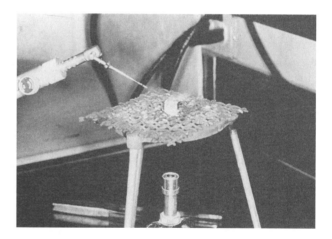

Fig. 28-28. High-heat (preceramic application) torch soldering with gas-oxygen and a miniature needle tip.

2. Place the solder above the gap and concentrate the reducing zone of the flame on the joint space.

3. When the solder melts, draw it into the joint and quickly "chase" it around with the flame (Fig. 28-30). The preceramic solder may have a melting point close to that of the parent metal, and there is danger of melting a thin framework unless the flame is concentrated on the joint space (see Fig. 28-12).

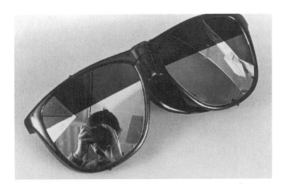

Fig. 28-29. Eye protection is essential for high-heat soldering and the casting of high-fusing alloys.

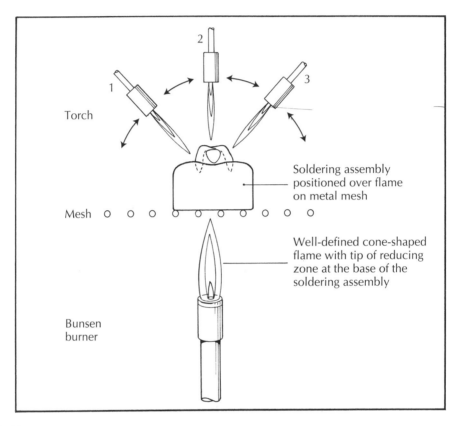

Fig. 28-30. The flame is directed at the connector immediately when the solder melts and is moved around from position 1 to positions 2 and 3. This ensures that a complete meniscus is formed.

Oven Soldering

1. Prepare a piece of solder by dipping it in liquid flux and melting it in a Bunsen flame to form a ball. The size of the ball will be determined by the connector size and the joint gap.
2. Leave a short tail attached to the ball to help position it above the joint space. As an alternative, the solder can be fed into the joint area as shown in Fig. 28-19.
3. Put the assembly in the furnace and increase the temperature to fuse the solder. A vacuum is not needed for oven soldering of noble metal alloys. Air firing is preferred by some technicians be-

cause in a vacuum there is always the chance of drawing entrapped gases to the surface of glazed porcelain, causing localized swelling or bloating.

Infrared Soldering (see Fig. 28-20)

1. Invest the assembly in the customary manner, using the appropriate material.
2. After wax elimination, position the assembly in the heat focus of the soldering machine. A pointer is used to ensure proper positioning of the connector area relative to the heat source. The connector area is fluxed, and the solder is positioned as described for oven soldering.

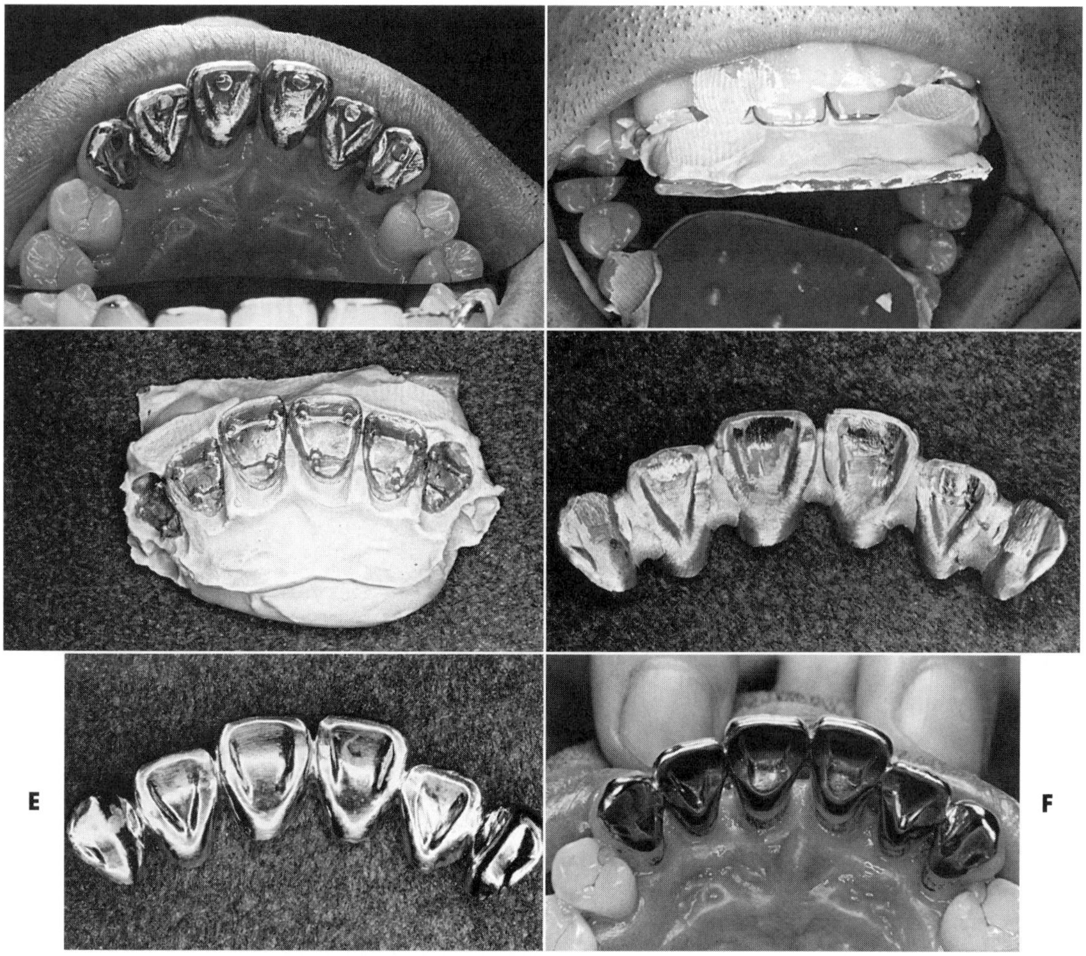

Fig. 28-31. **A,** A fixed splint was indicated in this patient to prevent drifting of teeth with compromised periodontal support. **B** and **C,** Plaster soldering index. **C,** The assembled prosthesis after soldering. **E,** Note that the connectors have been considerably reduced in size during the finishing procedure. Splinted teeth do not require as large connectors as do FPDs. **F,** The completed prosthesis.

3. Lower the protective shield to prevent eye injury, and activate the heat source. When a complete connector has formed after the fusing point of the solder is reached, the heat source is shut off, and the assembly is removed from the soldering platform.

EVALUATION

If the solder fails to flow during torch soldering but forms a ball above the joint area, heating should be discontinued. The solder has oxidized, and further heating will melt the castings. If the solder has flowed properly, the completed joint can be evaluated for size before removal of the investment and, if necessary, reheated while still hot, with additional solder added. Excessive solder must be ground away during the finishing procedure (Fig. 28-31).

If the connector has been designed properly and the solder has been properly positioned, no solder should run onto the occlusal surface or cover the margins. To prevent stray flow, a small amount of antiflux (rouge dissolved in turpentine) can be painted on critical areas before the assembly is heated. After bench cooling for about 5 minutes, the assembly is quenched (not porcelain) and the investment broken away (Fig. 28-32). The connector is then carefully inspected. If signs of an incomplete joint are evident (e.g., visible porosity in the solder), they are removed by grinding with a fine disk; the units are then reinvested and resoldered.

The joints must be tested for strength (Fig. 28-33). Any connector that can be broken by force of hand will not serve adequately in the mouth. Because broken connectors cannot be easily repaired intraorally once the prosthesis has been cemented, the entire restoration usually must be remade.

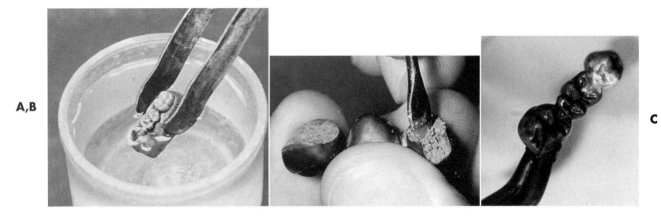

A,B

C

Fig. 28-32. **A,** The assembly is quenched after bench cooling for approximately 5 minutes. **B,** Investment removed from the castings. **C,** Surface oxides dissolved in a pickling solution.

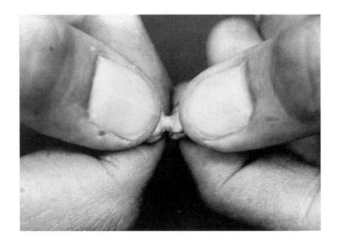

Fig. 28-33. Solder joints should always be tested for strength.

⬛REVIEW OF TECHNIQUE

Figure 28-34 summarizes the steps involved in FPD connector fabrication and should be referred to when the material is reviewed.

1. The design of connectors is determined in the wax pattern (Fig. 28-34, *A*).
2. All soldered connections require clean parallel surfaces. Gap width should be 0.25 mm (Fig. 28-34, *B*).
3. The units are indexed either from the master cast or in the mouth (Fig. 28-34, *C*).
4. Wax is added to the indexed restorations to shape the soldering assembly. For metal-

ceramic restorations, it is added to protect the porcelain (Fig. 28-34, *D*).

5. The units are invested, and the investment is allowed to bench set (Fig. 28-34, *E*).
6. If a plaster or ZOE index is used, wax is eliminated with boiling water or chloroform, the joint is fluxed, and the assembly is preheated in a burnout furnace (Fig. 28-34, *F*).
7. If a resin index has been used, it is placed directly in the burnout furnace (Fig. 28-34, *G*).
8. The connectors are soldered with a torch or in a porcelain furnace (Fig. 28-34, *H*).

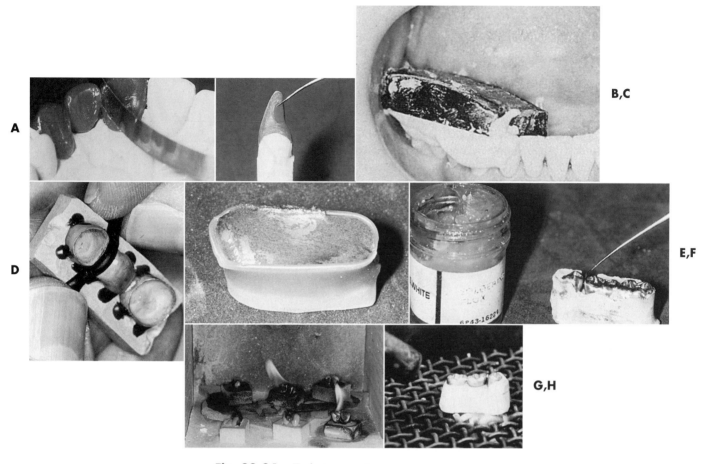

Fig. 28-34. Technique review.

Study Questions

1. Contrast soldering, brazing, and welding.
2. Discuss how biologic, mechanical, and esthetic considerations affect connector size and position for each of the following classes of teeth: incisors, premolars, and molars.
3. When and why would a nonrigid connector be used? A loop connector?
4. Discuss fineness and carat. What is their importance to dental soldering?
5. How do soldering investments differ from conventional casting investments? Why?
6. What is flux? Antiflux? How do they work? Give several examples of each.
7. What are the fundamental differences among conventional soldering, postceramic soldering, and preceramic soldering? When contrasting the last two techniques, what are the advantages and limitations associated with their use?
8. Describe the step-by-step procedures for two techniques to make a soldering index for a fixed partial denture. What are the respective advantages and limitations?

SUMMARY

Connectors join individual retainers and pontics. Rigid or nonrigid connectors can be used. Connector size, shape, and position influence the success of an FPD. The use of soldered connectors can simplify the fabrication of larger fixed prostheses, which may be cast separately in groups of one or two units and assembled after their individual fit has been verified. The technical procedures involved in soldering are not difficult. If the joint surfaces have been correctly designed and soldering gap width has been carefully controlled, the procedures are routine. All debris must be removed from the connector area because it interferes with surface wetting.

Conventional soldering involves the assembly of Type II and Type IV gold castings. Presoldering is the assembly of metal ceramic substructures before porcelain application. Postsoldering is the assembly of metal ceramic units after porcelain application. Heat sources used for soldering procedures include gas-air torches, gas-oxygen torches, furnaces, infrared, and laser units.

If the basic principles are understood and the technique has been mastered, these procedures are entirely reliable.

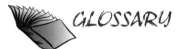 GLOSSARY

abrasive: *n* (1853): a substance used for abraiding, smoothing, or polishing.

antiflux: *n:* a material that prevents or confines solder attachment or flow.

connector *n:* in fixed prosthodontics, the portion of a fixed partial denture that unites the retainer(s) and pontics—*usage:* see nonrigid c., rigid c.

fineness: *n:* the proportion of pure gold in a gold alloy; the parts per 1000 of gold.

flux: *n* (14 cent.) **1:** in physics, the rate of flow of a liquid, particles or energy **2:** in ceramics, an agent that lowers the fusion temperature of porcelain **3:** in metallurgy, a substance used to increase fluidity and to prevent or reduce oxidation of a molten metal **4:** any substance applied to surfaces to be joined by brazing, soldering or welding to clean and free them from oxides and promote union.

index: *n* (1571): a core or mold used to record or maintain the relative position of a tooth or teeth to one another, to a cast, or to some other structure.

infrared radiation: electromagnetic radiation of wavelengths between 760 nm and 1000 nm.

nonrigid connector: any connector that permits limited movement between otherwise independent members of a fixed partial denture.

rigid connector: a cast, soldered, or fused union between the retainer(s) and pontic(s).

solder *n* **solder** *v,* **soldered; soldering, solderability:** *n*—**solderer** *n:* to unite, bring into, or restore to a firm union; the act of uniting two pieces of metal by the proper alloy of metals.

stabilization: *n, obs:* the seating of a fixed or removable denture so that it will not tilt or be displaced under pressure (GPT-1).

weld: *vb:* to unite or fuse two pieces by hammering, compression, or by rendering soft by heat with the addition of a fusible material.

REFERENCES

1. Anusavice KJ: *Phillips' science of dental materials,* ed 10, Philadelphia, 1996, WB Saunders.
2. British Standard Institute: *British standard glossary of dental terms,* London, 1983, British Standard Institute.
3. Goodkind RJ, Heringlake CB: Mandibular flexure in opening and closing movements, *J Prosthet Dent* 30:134, 1973.
4. Fischman BM: The influence of fixed splints on mandibular flexure, *J Prosthet Dent* 35:643, 1976.
5. Steinman RR: Warpage produced by soldering with dental solders and gold alloys, *J Prosthet Dent* 4:384, 1954.
6. Willis LM, Nicholls JI: Distortion in dental soldering as affected by gap distance, *J Prosthet Dent* 43:272, 1980.
7. Stade EH et al: Preceramic and postceramic solder joints, *J Prosthet Dent* 34:527, 1975.
8. Ryge G: Dental soldering procedures, *Dent Clin North Am* 747, 1958.
9. Rasmussen EJ et al: An investigation of tensile strength of dental solder joints, *J Prosthet Dent* 41:418, 1979.
10. Craig RG: *Restorative dental materials,* ed 10, St Louis, 1997, Mosby.
11. Tucillo JJ: Compositional and functional characteristics of precious metal alloys for dental restorations. In Valega TM, ed: *Alternatives to gold alloys in dentistry,* U.S. DHEW publ. no. (NIH) 77-1227, p. 40, Washington, DC, 1977.
12. El-Ebrashi MK et al: Electron microscopy of gold soldered joints, *J Dent Res* 47:5, 1968.
13. Leinfelder KF et al: Hardening of dental gold-copper alloys, *Dent Res* 51:900, 1972.
14. Chaves M et al: Effects of three soldering techniques on the strength of high-palladium alloy solder, *J Prosthet Dent* 79:677, 1998.
15. Phillips RW: *Skinner's science of dental materials,* ed 8, Philadelphia, 1982, WB Saunders.
16. Sloan RM et al: Postceramic soldering of various alloys, *J Prosthet Dent* 48:686, 1982.
17. Beck DA et al: A quantitative study of preporcelain soldered connector strength with palladium-based porcelain bonding alloys, *J Prosthet Dent* 56:301, 1986.
18. Staffanou RS et al: Strength properties of soldered joints from various ceramic-metal combinations, *J Prosthet Dent* 43:31, 1980.
19. Anusavice KJ et al: Flexure test evaluation of presoldered base metal alloys, *J Prosthet Dent* 54:507, 1985.
20. Sobieralski JA et al: Torch versus oven preceramic soldering of a nickel-chromium alloy, *Quintessence Int* 21:753, 1990.

21. Ferencz JL: Tensile strength analysis of midpontic soldering, *J Prosthet Dent* 57:696, 1987.

22. Fehling AW et al: Cast connectors: an alternative to soldering base metal alloys, *J Prosthet Dent* 55:195, 1986.

23. Saxton PL: Post-soldering of nonprecious alloys, *J Prosthet Dent* 43:592, 1980.

24. Byrne G et al: The fit of fixed partial dentures joined by infrared soldering, *J Prosthet Dent* 68:591, 1992.

25. Louly AC et al: Tensile strength of preceramic solder joints formed using an infrared heat source, *Int J Prosthodont* 4:428, 1991.

26. Gordon TE, Smith DL: Laser welding of prostheses- an initial report, *J Prosthet Dent* 24:472, 1970.

27. Preston JD, Reisbick MH: Laser fusion of selected dental casting alloys, *J Dent Res* 54:232, 1975.

28. Kasenbacher A, Dielert E: Tests on laser-welded or laser-soldered gold and Co/Cr/Mo dental alloys, *Dtsch Zahnarztl Z* 43:400, 1988.

29. Van Benthem H, Vahl J: Corrosion behavior of laser-welded dental alloys, *Dtsch Zahnarztl Z* 43:569, 1988.

30. Wiskott HW et al: Mechanical and elemental characterization of solder joints and welds using a gold-palladium alloy, *J Prosthet Dent* 77:607, 1997.

31. Sjögren G et al: Laser welding of titanium in dentistry, *Acta Odontol Scand* 46:247, 1988.

32. Ortorp A et al: Clinical experiences with laser-welded titanium frameworks supported by implants in the edentulous mandible: a 5-year follow-up study, *Int J Prosthodont* 12:65, 1999.

33. Gegauff AG, Rosenstiel SF: The seating of one-piece and soldered fixed partial dentures, *J Prosthet Dent* 62:292, 1989.

34. Sarfati E, Harter J-C: Comparative accuracy of fixed partial dentures made as one-piece castings or joined by solder, *Int J Prosthodont* 5:377, 1992.

35. Wee AG et al: Strategies to achieve fit in implant prosthodontics: a review of the literature, *Int J Prosthodont* 12:167, 1999.

36. Harper RJ, Nicholls JI: Distortions in indexing methods and investing media for soldering and remount procedures, *J Prosthet Dent* 42:172, 1979.

37. Moon PC et al: Comparison of accuracy of soldering indices for fixed prostheses, *J Prosthet Dent* 40:35, 1978.

CHAPTER TWENTY-NINE

FINISHING THE CAST RESTORATION

KEY TERMS

airborne particle abrasion	intaglio
aluminum oxide	polishing
Beilby layer	rouge
finishing	

A cast metal restoration is not ready for try-in and cementation merely because it has been stripped of its investment. The unpolished surface is relatively rough, and a series of **finishing** procedures are needed to produce highly polished axial surfaces. This will limit the accumulation[1,2] and retention[3] of plaque and facilitate maintenance of health of the supporting periodontal tissues. The sprue needs to be removed, and the area of its attachment needs to be recontoured. Any nodules or other minor irregularities remaining on the cast surface must be eliminated.

Metal finishing for metal-ceramic restorations is similar to cast metal. The discussion in this chapter is applicable to both restoration types. In practice, the final polishing of metal-ceramic restorations is not done until after characterization and glazing (see Chapter 30).

◼ OBJECTIVES AND PROCEDURES

The objectives and procedures for finishing are different for each part of the cast restoration. The following discussion is sequentially divided into corresponding phases; each are identified as zones (Fig. 29-1).

ZONE 1: INTERNAL MARGIN

Objective. To minimize any dissolution of the luting agent, a 1-mm-wide band of metal must be obtained that is closely adapted to the tooth surface.[4] A defect within this zone can significantly reduce a restoration's longevity. Good adaptation is obtained by carefully reflowing the wax pattern (Fig. 29-2). With careful standardization of technique, the dentist can achieve predictable and consistent results.

Procedure. If a defect occurs in the marginal area, the restoration will have to be remade. This may require an additional patient visit to make the new impression. Defects can be prevented or minimized by paying particular attention to reflowing the margins of the wax pattern and through careful investing (see Chapter 22).

Even small nodules can prevent a casting from seating completely. Careful examination under ample magnification will help identify interferences. Small nodules, if far enough away from the margin itself, can be removed under a binocular microscope with exceptionally cautious use of very small rotary instruments (e.g., a no. $\frac{1}{4}$ round bur). However, great care is needed to avoid damage to the margin and annoying remakes.

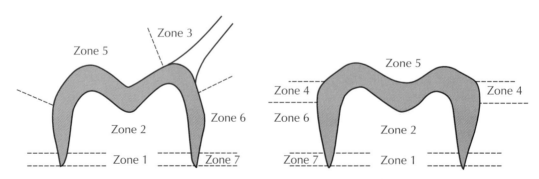

Fig. 29-1. Recommended sequence for finishing of a cast restoration. All procedures for a zone should be completed before the next zone is started. *Zone 1* is the internal margin; *Zone 2*, the internal surface; *Zone 3*, the sprue; *Zone 4*, the proximal contacts; *Zone 5*, the occlusal surface; *Zone 6*, the axial walls; and *Zone 7*, the external margins.

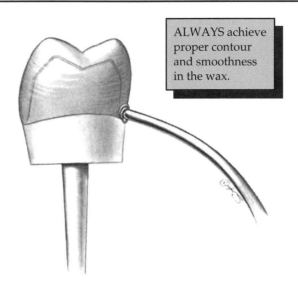

ALWAYS achieve proper contour and smoothness in the wax.

Fig. 29-2. Reflowing the wax pattern. The objective is to create a well-adapted 1-mm zone to prevent cement dissolution. Proper reflowing before investing is a prerequisite to accomplish this.

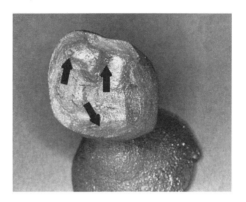

Fig. 29-3. Multiple nodules on a casting (*arrows*) have resulted from improper investing. To permit complete seating of the casting, even small ones such as these must be removed entirely.

NEVER force the casting onto the die; use great caution when fitting the casting.

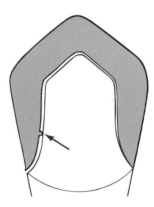

Fig. 29-4. A relatively small nodule (*arrow*) will result in a substantial open margin.

ZONE 2: INTERNAL SURFACE (INTAGLIO)

Objective. No contact should exist between the die and the internal surface of the casting. A uniform space of 25 to 35 μm is necessary for the luting agent to spread evenly. Any contact(s) must be identified and relieved by careful selective grinding of the internal surface.

Procedure. Under normal circumstances, a casting's internal surface does not require finishing. It should, however, be examined for nodules (Fig. 29-3) before the restoration is seated on the die. Nodules can be removed with a small round carbide bur, which can be time consuming because it may need to be repeated several times. If the internal surface needs to be adjusted more than occasionally, the investing procedure should be reexamined for flaws.

Even a very small nodule can result in significant increase of the marginal gap width (Fig. 29-4). A binocular microscope is especially helpful in identifying nodules. High-quality loupes are an acceptable alternative. Great care should be exercised when seating a casting on its die. Any significant force will abrade or chip the die so that the casting will seat on the die but will not seat fully on the prepared tooth. Overlooking this at the cementation appointment will result in a restoration with open margins and a poor prognosis. If a casting does not seat, a nodule may have been overlooked and may have scratched the die. A little stone may have been

picked up in the process. Close examination of the internal surface of the casting or the axial walls of the die (Fig. 29-5) will reveal this. Corrective action is often relatively simple, and the casting may be acceptable. Care must be taken not to seat a faulty casting repeatedly, thereby abrading the die. After a die has been abraded by a casting, it should not be used for rewaxing a restoration. If this is necessary, a new impression will be required.

When a nodule is removed from the internal aspect of a casting, deliberately removing a slightly greater amount of alloy in the area is recommended. Once the casting has been adjusted, determining the exact location of the nodule will no longer be

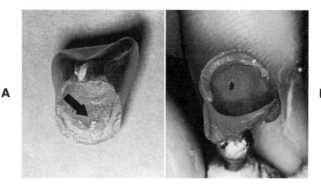

Fig. 29-5. **A,** Internal surface of a casting. Note the stone *(arrow)* adhering where the die has been abraded by the casting. **B,** A suitable marking agent (e.g., rouge and chloroform) can be used to detect areas that must be relieved to allow complete seating.

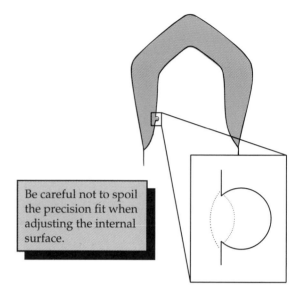

Be careful not to spoil the precision fit when adjusting the internal surface.

Fig. 29-6. When removing a nodule, remove slightly more than the defect to ensure complete seating of the restoration.

possible. Therefore, the nodule should be removed entirely in one step, rather than through sequential relief of the internal surface (Fig. 29-6).

Indiscriminately removing material from the internal aspect of any casting is not an acceptable alternative. This will result in excessive loss of retention and resistance form, and the restoration will need to be remade.

Marking Agents. Several agents are commercially available to facilitate identification of the seating interference between the casting and the die. These include water-soluble dies (e.g., Liqua-Mark*), solvent-based dies (e.g., Accufilm IV†), and powdered sprays (e.g., Occlude‡). A suspension of rouge in chloroform or an elastomeric detection paste (e.g., Fit Checker)§ can also be used as an alternative.[5,6] These agents should be applied as a thin film to the internal surface of the casting. High magnification of the casting after seating will reveal initial contact for grinding. Regardless of the method used, the internal surface of the casting should always be thoroughly cleaned before the luting procedure (see Chapter 31).

ZONE 3: THE SPRUE
Objective. To reestablish proper coronal morphology and function, the sprue must be sectioned, and the casting must be recontoured in the area of its attachment.

---

*The Wilkinson Company: Post Falls, Idaho.
†Parkell Products: Farmingdale, N.Y.
‡Pascal Co, Inc: Bellevue, Wash.
§GC America, Inc: Chicago, Ill.

Procedure. Once the fit of the casting has been verified on the die and it has been found to be acceptable, the sprue is sectioned, and the area of its attachment to the casting (Fig. 29-7) is reshaped.

A carborundum separating disk is used to cut through the sprue. Cutting should be performed circumferentially, maintaining a small area in the center of the sprue. This last connection is broken by twisting and separating it from the casting. Wire cutters are not recommended, because they may lead to distortion of the casting. Any excess in the area of the sprue attachment is removed with the disk, and the area is refined with stones and sandpaper disks.

ZONE 4: PROXIMAL CONTACTS
Objective. The proximal contact areas are adjusted in the laboratory so that they will be correct (or slightly too tight) when the casting is evaluated in the mouth.

Procedure. Special care is needed to prevent the finishing procedures from producing an overreduced and consequently inadequate proximal contact. Although this can be corrected with solder (see p. 747), it is a time-consuming and unnecessary procedure.

A slightly excessive contact, however, may be corrected easily during clinical evaluation. The proximal contacts on the stone cast can be minimally relieved by careful scraping with a scalpel (Fig. 29-8). The casting is then adjusted until it just seats. When adjacent castings are made, they should not be ad-

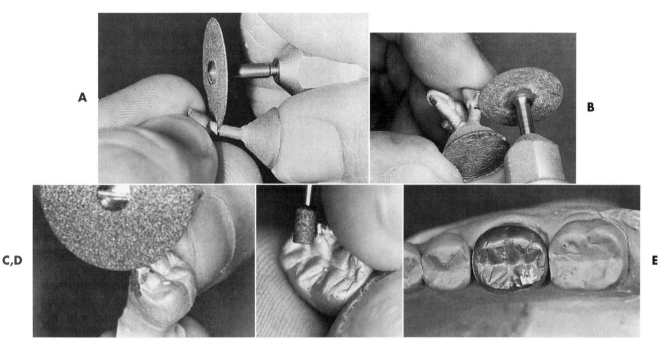

Fig. 29-7. **A,** The button is most effectively removed by cutting around the sprue and then twisting it off. **B,** With multiple castings made simultaneously, access is more difficult. When it is necessary to sever a sprue completely, care must be taken not to damage the margin inadvertently. **C** and **D,** Disks and stones are used for gross recontouring. **E,** The recontoured casting before finishing.

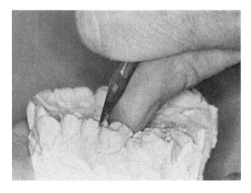

Fig. 29-8. Rather than risk a deficient proximal contact at evaluation, the technician may reduce the cast slightly by scraping the adjacent teeth with a blade.

justed to seat on the working cast simultaneously. Under these circumstances, the proximal contacts should be left slightly too tight in the dental laboratory. For such multiple castings, clinical evaluation is done sequentially and on an individual basis. Adjustments are made for each casting independently.

When adjusting proximal contacts, placing a thin Mylar articulating film between adjacent castings or between the casting and the adjacent tooth is helpful (Fig. 29-9). Doing this allows the areas where binding contact occurs to be adjusted through selective adjustment where markings result.

Connectors. When an FPD is being finished, the connectors require special attention. Unless they are properly contoured and highly polished, periodontal health will invariably be affected, even in the presence of the most meticulous oral hygiene. Ideally, a properly finished connector has a parabolic configuration (Fig. 29-10). Rotary instruments such as rubber wheels, which allow access to the cervical aspect of the connector for finishing while not jeopardizing the margin, are essential in these situations. In cases of root proximity between adjacent teeth, this can be quite problematic. After preliminary finishing with rubber wheels, a piece of twine can be used to impart the final polish to the cervical aspect of the connector (Fig. 29-11).

ZONE 5: OCCLUSAL SURFACE

Objective. Occlusal contacts are reestablished in static and dynamic relationships to the opposing arch. Obtaining accurate and stable contacts does not require highly polished metal occlusal surfaces. A satin finish is acceptable. Occlusal morphology must ensure positional stability and satisfy all functional requirements (see Chapter 4).

Procedure. The occlusal contacts are checked with thin Mylar articulating film (Fig. 29-12) to ensure that they match the design in the waxing stage. If they do not, the occlusion must be adjusted. Wax

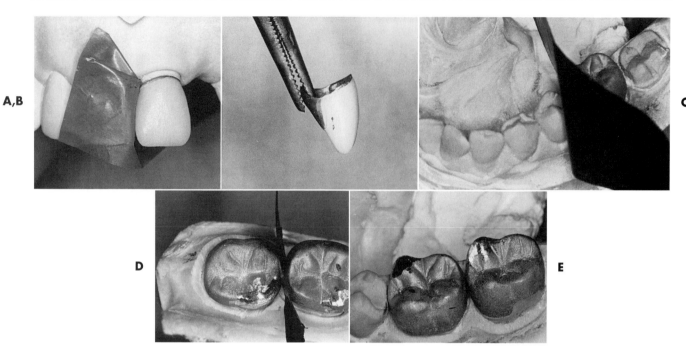

Fig. 29-9. **A,** Thin articulating film interposed between a metal-ceramic restoration and the adjacent tooth. **B,** The area of contact that prevents complete seating is readily apparent. **C** to **E,** Articulating film is used to detect the location of an excessive proximal contact on cast metal.

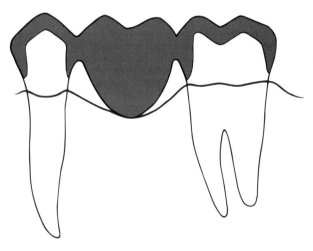

Fig. 29-10. Cross sections showing properly finished connectors.

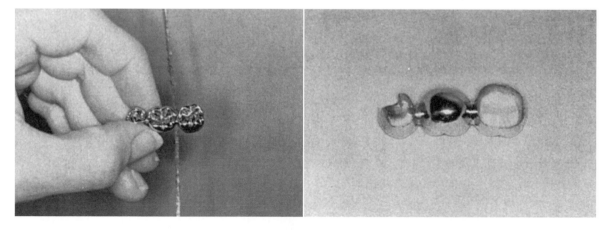

Fig. 29-11. Polishing connector areas. Twine impregnated with polishing compound is an efficient way to polish this hard-to-reach area.

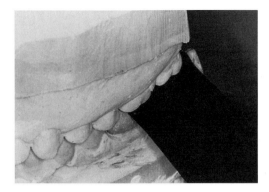

Fig. 29-12. After complete seating is verified, the initial point of contact is marked.

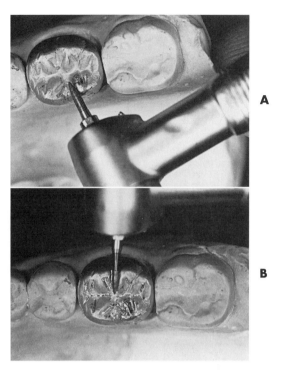

Fig. 29-14. **A,** Occlusal adjustment is readily accomplished with a pointed diamond or carbide. **B,** The grooves and fissures are concurrently refined.

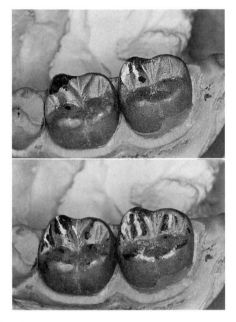

Fig. 29-13. Occlusal prematurities are generally the result of excessively heavy contact on the wax pattern.

is subject to elastic recovery. If an occlusal contact is heavy in wax, it will spring back slightly when the articulator is opened and will produce an occlusal prematurity in the casting (Fig. 29-13). If "pinpoint" contacts are established carefully during the waxing phase, significant occlusal adjustment should not be necessary.

Occlusal adjustments can be performed with flame-shaped finishing burs or diamonds (Fig. 29-14). A large stone will create unwanted concavities in the occlusal surface. The correct technique for occlusal adjustment is to redevelop the anatomy of the entire ridge or cusp rather than grinding only the point of interference. Simultaneously, any nodules can be removed, and grooves can be defined with a finishing bur or small round bur.

Before starting any adjustment, the practitioner should use a thickness gauge on the metal. If only minimum clearance was established at the tooth-preparation stage, indiscriminate adjustment will lead to inadequate thickness of the casting (Fig. 29-15) and possible perforation. Although soldering such a hole in a casting is possible, the occurrence of this complication usually indicates an earlier error that requires correction (e.g., inadequate clearance necessitates additional reduction of the tooth preparation).

After the occlusal contacts have been refined, they must not be altered by extensive polishing. A high polish may be essential for plaque control on axial surfaces (Zones 6 and 7), but its benefit is questionable on the occlusal surface of metal castings. In fact, an accurate occlusion so painstakingly established in wax can be rapidly destroyed by overzealousness to make a casting "look pretty."

If the wax pattern has been carefully finished, a smooth casting will have resulted, and removing surface oxides with a soft wire brush wheel will be sufficient. The surface can then be polished with **rouge** on a soft brush wheel (which removes only 5 μm from the surface of the casting[7]) (see Fig. 29-18).

Some authorities[8] recommend producing a matte finish on the occlusal surfaces to aid in the initial identification of wear facets during function, which will show up as shiny marks on an otherwise dull

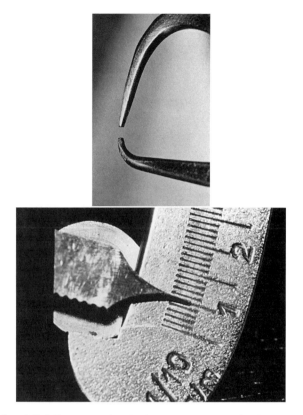

Fig. 29-15. As occlusal adjustments are made, the residual thickness is continually monitored with an appropriately designed thickness gauge. For structural durability, 0.5 mm is inadequate metal thickness and is the result of insufficient occlusal reduction.

surface. This type of finish is usually achieved with an airborne particle abrasion unit and 25- to 50-μm Al$_2$O$_3$ (alumina) particles. However, a 5-second blast with 50-μm alumina at 500 kPa* (73 psi) pressure will remove about 20 μm of metal from the air-abraded surfaces[9]; therefore, the margins should be protected.[10] An exposure of about 1 second will usually produce a smooth satin finish. If this cannot be accomplished, it is likely that the preparation before this step was deficient. Further refinement will be necessary.

Zone 6: Axial Walls

Objective. When axial wall finishing is completed, the walls should be smoothly contoured and highly polished, enabling the patient to carry out optimum plaque control.

Procedure. Surface defects are removed by grinding with abrasive particles bound into a grinding stone or rubber wheel, on a paper disk, or ap-

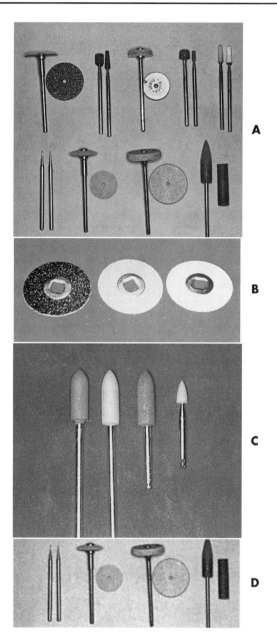

Fig. 29-16. Abrasives for finishing. A sequence of progressively finer grades is used to attain the desired surface. Carborundum disks and stones of varying degrees of coarseness **(A)** are typically used first; these are followed by garnet paper and sandpaper disks **(B)**, rubber points and white Arkansas stones **(C)**, and rubber wheels and points along with small carbide burs for removing nodules **(D)**.

plied as an abrasive paste (Fig. 29-16). Each particle acts as a cutting tool on the metal surface.

The most efficient method of polishing[11] is a sequence of progressively finer abrasives (Fig. 29-17), each removing the scratches made by the previous grade. Time is wasted if the progression to a finer-grade abrasive is too rapid, because the coarser grits will remove material much more efficiently.

---

*Kilopascals are equal to 1000 newtons/m².

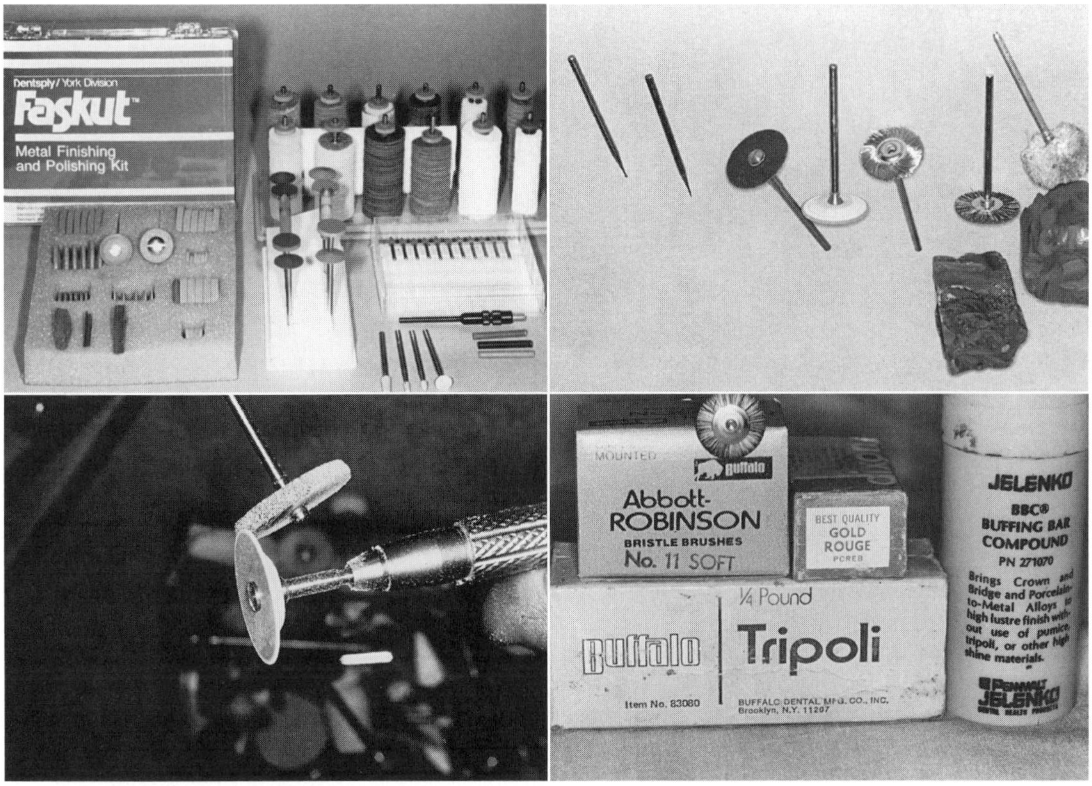

Fig. 29-17. Finishing armamentarium. **A,** Assorted abrasives, sandpaper disks, rubber points, and polishing wheels. **B,** Instruments used range from small carbides (for removing nodules) and a steel wire brush (for occlusal surface smoothing) to buffing wheels and compounds. **C,** A coarse wheel is used to true and thin the edge of a rubber wheel. **D,** Buffing compounds applied on a felt wheel or bristle brush.

Light pressure is applied when using abrasives, and the instrument must be kept rotating; otherwise, the surface of the casting will be ground into a series of facets that ultimately will impede plaque control. When all surface irregularities have been removed and the progression through the series of abrasives has left a finish with only minute scratches, the axial surfaces of the restoration are polished. Jeweler's rouge will rapidly produce a high polish on a well-prepared surface of a dense casting (Fig. 29-18, *K*). This is carried on a wheel or brush, with heavier pressures and higher rotational speeds than were used in finishing (Fig. 29-18).

ZONE 7: EXTERNAL MARGINS

Objective. Margin finishing is critical to a restoration's longevity and therefore deserves special attention. The objective of all cast restoration finishing is a highly polished metal surface without ledges or steps as the transition is made from restoration to unprepared tooth. Failure to accomplish this will compromise plaque control.

Procedure. Where access permits, cavosurface margins should be finished directly on the tooth

(see Fig. 30-10). Unfortunately, the areas where access for finishing is restricted (e.g., proximally or subgingivally) are precisely where plaque control will present the most problems. Therefore, only the least critical areas can be finished intraorally. An advantage of partial-coverage restorations over complete crowns is that they allow better access for finishing margins and for subsequent plaque control.

Those parts of the margin that cannot be finished on the tooth are finished on the die (Fig. 29-19). Care must be taken not to remove more metal than is strictly necessary. Excessive finishing creates problems similar to those caused by incomplete polishing. This raises the issue of how much material can be removed from the surface of a casting without compromising the ultimate fit and emergence profile of the finished restoration.

A stone die from a polysulfide impression is approximately 25 μm wider than the tooth because of polymerization and thermal shrinkage of the impression material and expansion of the gypsum.[12] In theory, therefore, if 12.5 μm is removed during finishing, the casting will be flush with the tooth surface. Although these values cannot be measured on a day-to-day basis in a dental office, they illustrate

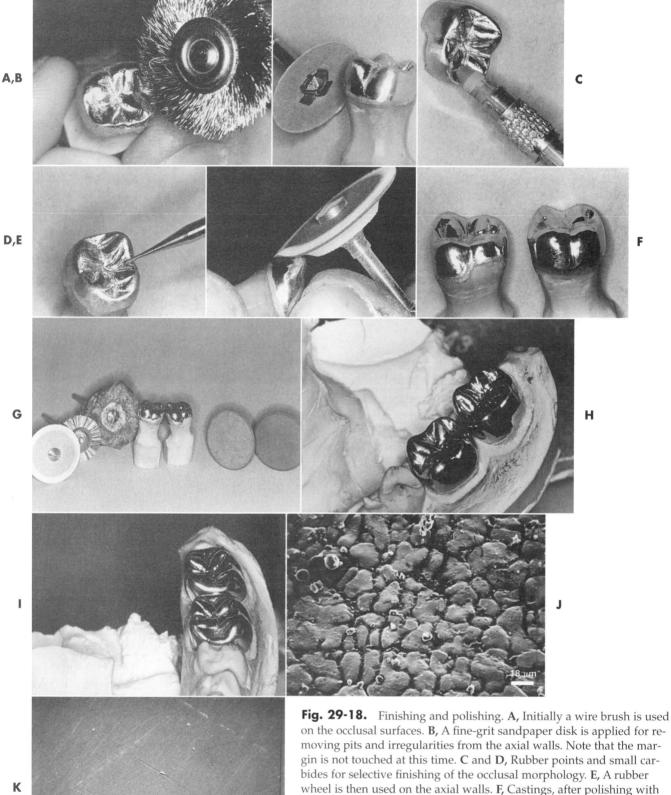

A,B

C

D,E

F

G

H

I

J

K

Fig. 29-18.   Finishing and polishing. **A,** Initially a wire brush is used on the occlusal surfaces. **B,** A fine-grit sandpaper disk is applied for removing pits and irregularities from the axial walls. Note that the margin is not touched at this time. **C** and **D,** Rubber points and small carbides for selective finishing of the occlusal morphology. **E,** A rubber wheel is then used on the axial walls. **F,** Castings, after polishing with buffing compound, immediately before clinical evaluation. **G,** When the fit has been verified clinically, the margins are polished. **H** and **I,** The completed castings immediately before cementation. **J,** Scanning electron micrograph of a gold alloy in the "as-cast" state. **K,** The same casting after finishing and polishing with a series of abrasives culminating in rouge.

(*J* and *K* courtesy Dr. J.L. Sandrik.)

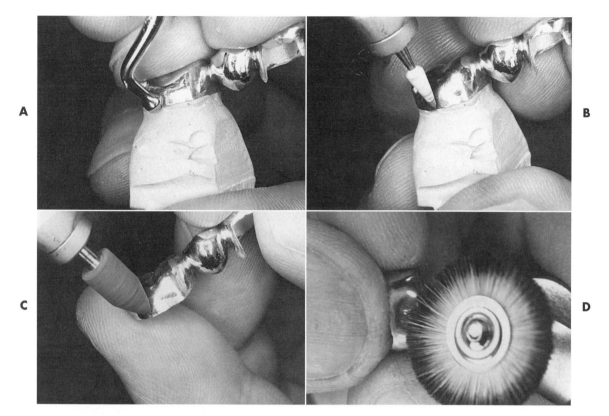

Fig. 29-19. When subgingival margins do not allow access, final finishing is performed on the die. During final polishing, the margin is carefully supported with a finger.

the tolerances of, and restrictions imposed by, the materials that are presently in use.

The edge of the margin must not be distorted during finishing, although carefully rubbing a smooth instrument along the length of the margin (burnishing) (Fig. 29-19, *A*) may improve the margin,[13,14]* but only when softer alloys are used.[15]

Finishing should be performed by gently brushing a fine-grit stone over the surface to remove casting roughness (Fig. 29-19, *B*). This is followed by a soft rubber wheel or point (Fig. 29-19, *C*) and finally by rouge on a brush. The margin should be supported with a finger during final polishing (Fig. 29-19, *D*).

When the casting is smooth on all critical surfaces, any remaining polishing compound can be removed with a soft toothbrush, by ultrasonic cleaning in an appropriate solution, or by steam cleaning (see Chapter 31).

---

*Unfortunately, burnishing will not make a poorly fitting margin acceptable.

REVIEW OF TECHNIQUE

Fig. 29-20 presents the steps involved in finishing a restoration and should be consulted when techniques are reviewed.

1. The internal margin is inspected to confirm that the casting accurately reproduces the prepared tooth and is intimately adapted to the prepared surfaces adjacent to the margin (Fig. 29-20, *A*).
2. The internal surface is inspected under magnification and adjusted as necessary with small stones and carbide burs. Adjustments are restricted to areas where binding contacts occur (Fig. 29-20, *B*).
3. The casting should seat completely without force and without noticeable rocking or instability (Fig. 29-20, *C*).
4. The sprue is removed (Fig. 29-20, *D*).
5. The area of its attachment is reshaped (Fig. 29-20, *E*).
6. The proximal contact areas are adjusted (Fig. 29-20, *F*).

7. On the cast, proximal contacts can be left slightly tight before the clinical evaluation appointment (Fig. 29-20, *G*).
8. The occlusal surfaces are evaluated and adjusted. No centric or excursive interferences should remain (Fig. 29-20, *H*).

9. The axial surfaces are finished and polished. Finishing the cervical aspect of axial walls on metal-ceramic restorations is postponed until after final glazing and characterization. In addition, if a soldering procedure is anticipated, the marginal area is left unfinished until the

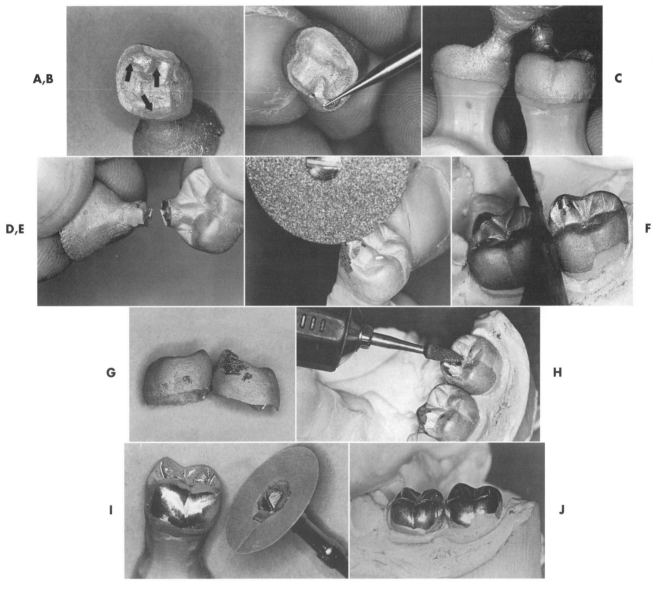

Fig. 29-20. Technique review.

Study Questions

1. What is the purpose of finishing and polishing the margin of a cast restoration? The occlusal surface? The proximal contact area?
2. What is the recommended procedure for severing a sprue?
3. What is the recommended procedure for removing a nodule?
4. What is the recommended procedure for shaping and finishing a connector for a fixed partial denture?
5. Discuss the uses and limitations of air particle abrasion in finishing cast restorations (gold and metal-ceramic).

soldering has been completed and the fit of the assembled prosthesis is acceptable (Fig. 29-20, *I*).

10. The polished restoration is cleaned. A steam cleaner or ultrasonic cleaner (with the appropriate solutions) can be used (Fig. 29-20, *J*). The cleaned castings are seated on the master cast (Fig. 29-20, *J*).

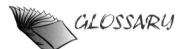

GLOSSARY

airborne particle abrasion: the process of altering the surface of a material through the use of abrasive particles propelled by compressed air or other gases.

aluminum oxide: *1:* a metallic oxide constituent of dental porcelain that increases hardness and viscosity *2:* a high-strength ceramic crystal dispersed throughout a glassy phase to increase its strength as in aluminous dental porcelain used to fabricate aluminous porcelain jacket crowns *3:* a finely ground ceramic particle (frequently 50 μm) often used in conjunction with airborne particle abrasion of metal castings before the application of porcelain as with metal ceramic restorations.

Beilby layer [Sir George Thomas Beilby, British chemist, 1850-1924]: eponym for the molecular disorganized surface layer of a highly polished metal. A relatively scratch-free microcrystalline surface produced by a series of abrasives of decreasing coarseness.
Beilby GT. Aggregation and flow of solids, 1921.

devest: *vb:* the retrieval of a casting or prosthesis from an investing medium.

intaglio: *n, pl* **-ios** (1644) *1:* an incised or engraved figure in stone or any hard material depressed below the surface of the material such that an impression from the design would yield an image in relief *2:* something carved in intaglio.

intaglio surface: the portion of the denture or other restoration surface that has its contour determined by the impression; the interior or reversal surface of an object.

polishing: *v, obs 1:* to make smooth and glossy, usually by friction; to give luster to (GPT-1) *2: obs:* the act or process of making a denture or casting smooth and glossy (GPT-1).

rouge: *n* (1753): a compound composed of ferric oxide and binders used for imparting a high luster to a polished surface, glass, metal, or gems.

REFERENCES

1. Gildenhuys RR, Stallard RE:Comparison of plaque accumulation on metal restorative surfaces, *Dent Surv* 51:56, 1975.
2. Shafagh I: Plaque accumulation on cast gold complete crowns polished by a conventional and an experimental method, *J Prosthet Dent* 55:339, 1986.
3. Keenan MP et al: Effects of cast gold surface finishing on plaque retention, *J Prosthet Dent* 43:168, 1980.
4. Mesu FP: Degradation of luting cements measured in vitro, *J Dent Res* 61:665, 1982.
5. White SN et al: Improved marginal seating of cast restorations using a silicone-disclosing medium, *Int J Prosthodont* 4:323, 1991.
6. Troendle GR, Troendle KB: Polyvinyl siloxane as a disclosing medium, *J Prosthet Dent* 68:983, 1992.
7. Phillips RW: *Skinner's science of dental materials,* ed 8, Philadelphia, 1982, WB Saunders.
8. Shillingburg HT et al: *Fundamentals of fixed prosthodontics,* ed 2, Chicago, 1981, Quintessence Publishing.
9. Adams HF: Effect of abrasive blasting on castings of gold alloys, *Op Dent* 6:11, 1981.
10. Felton DA et al: Effect of air abrasives on marginal configurations of porcelain-fused-to-metal alloys: an SEM analysis, *J Prosthet Dent* 65:38, 1991.
11. Troxell RR: The polishing of gold castings, *J Prosthet Dent* 9:668, 1959.
12. Rosenstiel SF: *The marginal reproduction of two elastomeric impression materials,* master's thesis, 1977, Indiana University.
13. Eames WB, Little RM: Movement of gold at cavosurface margins with finishing instruments, *J Am Dent Assoc* 75:147, 1967.
14. Goretti A et al: A microscopic evaluation of the marginal adaptation of onlays in gold, *Schweiz Monatsschr Zahnmed* 102:679, 1992.
15. Sarrett DC et al: Scanning electron microscopy evaluation of four finishing techniques on margins of gold castings, *J Prosthet Dent* 50:784, 1983.

CLINICAL PROCEDURES PART TWO

CHAPTER THIRTY

EVALUATION, CHARACTERIZATION, AND GLAZING

KEY TERMS

castings

characterize

emergence profile

glaze

intrinsic coloring

natural glaze

overglaze

pigment

remount procedure

stains

◼ EVALUATION

When the laboratory procedures have been completed, the restoration is ready to be evaluated in the patient's mouth before final finishing and cementation. The completed prosthesis is cleaned either ultrasonically or with a steam cleaner to remove any residual polishing compound and then disinfected. Metal **castings** need to be evaluated in terms of proximal contacts, margin integrity, stability, internal fit, external contours, occlusion, and surface finish.

Metal-ceramic restorations often require a separate metal evaluation stage, when the margin integrity, stability, occlusion and substructure design are evaluated. Especially important at this appointment is the assessment of the cut-back area. Minor adjustments can be made, for instance by extending the veneering surface slightly interproximally to enhance the appearance of the completed prosthesis. During the subsequent bisque evaluation, the marginal integrity and stability are reassessed to determine whether any distortion has occurred during firing. Proximal contacts also are evaluated during this stage, as are porcelain contours, stability, and the shade, texture, and **glaze**. For fixed partial dentures (FPDs), tissue contact of the pontics and the location and shape of connectors need careful assessment. Otherwise, tissue irritation may occur. Primarily because of the inevitable inaccuracies that result during the indirect technique and the high degree of precision needed for a successful fixed prosthesis, only rarely will the restoration not require some chairside adjustment.

PROVISIONAL RESTORATION AND LUTING AGENT

The provisional restoration is removed with gentle application of hemostats or a Backhaus towel clamp. Special band removers (Fig. 30-1) may also be used. Most of the luting agent or temporary cement will adhere to the provisional when it is taken out of the mouth. Any remaining cement should be loosened from the prepared tooth surface with an explorer followed by careful application of a water-pumice mixture* in a prophylaxis cup. Slow speed and relatively light pressure are essential. Polishing the preparation is undesirable because it may lessen retention. The preparations are rinsed with water and air spray, and after drying the area is inspected. All residual luting agent must have been removed because even a very small particle of temporary cement can prevent a casting from seating completely.

EVALUATION SEQUENCE

Following a logical sequence during the evaluation procedures is important if mistakes are to be avoided. The recommended sequence is as follows:

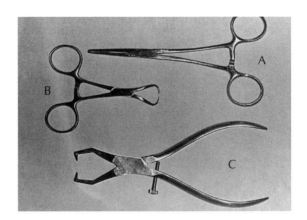

Fig. 30-1. Hemostats *(A)*, Backhaus towel clamp forceps *(B)*, and Baade-type band removers *(C)*.

---

*As an alternative, the pumice can be mixed with an antimicrobial such as Consepsis (Ultradent Products, Inc.), which may reduce postcementation sensitivity.

1. Proximal contacts
2. Marginal Integrity
3. Stability
4. Occlusion
5. Characterization and glazing

The proximal contacts are evaluated first because excessive contact here will prevent the restoration from seating, leading to a marginal discrepancy. Similarly, if a restoration is not seating completely, assessing stability and sectioning, or adjusting the occlusion, is contraindicated.

PROXIMAL CONTACTS

The location, size, and tightness of a restoration's proximal contacts should resemble those of the natural teeth. Typically, textbooks refer to contacts that allow unwaxed floss to "snap" through "relatively easily." Although this is not a very scientific definition, the use of floss is a convenient method to compare the contacts with others in the dentition. If the floss will not pass, the contact is excessively tight; if it goes through too easily, food impaction may result (Fig. 30-2). The use of shim stock (thin Mylar film) is probably a more reliable indicator of proximal contact. The ideal contact should allow for positional stability of the abutments and adjacent teeth as well as easy maintenance of the supporting structures. Most patients will give reliable information as to a tight proximal contact when asked if they "feel as though they have a seed between their teeth," provided a local anesthetic has not been administered. A deficient contact is easily overlooked but will invariably result in patient complaints as food becomes impacted.

Excessive Tightness

All-metal Restorations. If a tight contact prevents the seating of an all-metal restoration, adjustments are readily made with a rubber wheel. The satin finish produced helps identify where binding

occurs, because a shiny spot (Fig. 30-3) will appear where adjustment is necessary.

When a contact is too tight, the restoration is removed from the mouth, adjusted, and then reevaluated intraorally. Remember to allow a small degree of excessive tightness for polishing.

Porcelain Restorations. A tight proximal contact in unglazed porcelain is easily adjusted with a cylindrical mounted stone. The area of contact (Fig. 30-4) can be identified with red pencil or thin marking tape.

After glazing, a slight change in the contact may be observed because of the pyroplastic surface flow that occurs during firing. If adjustment of a glazed restoration is needed, it can be repolished with diamond-impregnated silicone points, pumice, or diamond-polishing paste.

Deficiency

All-metal Restorations. A gold casting with a deficient proximal contact can usually be corrected by soldering (Fig. 30-5). The procedure is simple and can be performed in the dental office in a matter of minutes. However, soldering a proximal

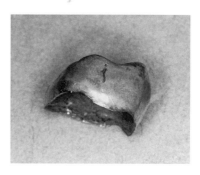

Fig. 30-3. Identifying the location of a tight proximal contact. The metal is given a matte finish by grinding with a rubber wheel. A shiny mark will be formed where the contact is excessive.

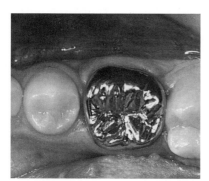

Fig. 30-2. Deficient mesial contact, which could allow food to become impacted.

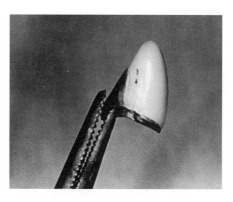

Fig. 30-4. The location of tight porcelain contacts can be identified with thin marking tape.

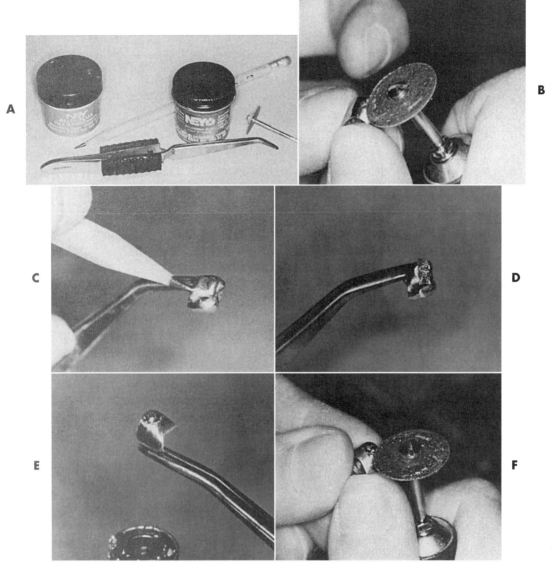

Fig. 30-5. Adding a proximal contact with gold solder. **A,** Armamentarium. **B,** Roughening the deficient proximal surface. **C,** Adding antiflux (graphite or rouge/chloroform) to the margin. **D,** Segment of solder positioned with paste flux. **E,** Heated over a Bunsen burner flame until the solder just melts. **F,** Proximal contact readjusted.

contact should not be routinely necessary. After soldering, the restoration will require repolishing.

Armamentarium (Fig. 30-5, *A*)
- Soldering tweezers
- Gold solder
- Paste flux
- Bunsen burner
- Antiflux
- Polishing armamentarium

Step-by-step Procedure
1. Roughen the deficient area with a disk (Fig. 30-5, *B*).
2. Protect the margin of the casting with a graphite pencil (or another suitable antiflux) (Fig. 30-5, *C*).

3. Coat a small piece of solder with flux and position it on the previously roughened surface (Fig. 30-5, *D*).
4. Hold the casting with the soldering tweezers in a properly adjusted flame of the Bunsen burner to position the solder at the height of the reducing portion of the flame (Fig. 30-5, *E*).
5. Observe the solder carefully as it heats up. As the solder starts to fuse, it will rapidly spread. With a little practice the casting can be tipped to help the solder flow in the desired direction. The casting is then immediately removed from the flame.
6. Pickle the casting and adjust the addition with disks (Fig. 30-5, *F*) before repolishing and cleaning.

A   **B**   **C**

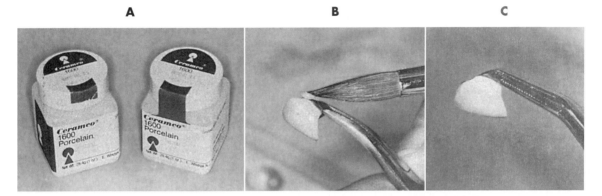

Fig. 30-6. Correction of a defective proximal contour with low fusing, add-on porcelain **(A). B,** Applying the porcelain. **C,** Corrected proximal contours.

Porcelain Restorations. A deficient proximal contact in porcelain requires additional firing. At the bisque stage, this is time consuming, but additional porcelain is not a problem. However, if a restoration has been completely finished, glazed, and stained at the time the deficient contact is discovered, a lower-fusing "add-on" or correction porcelain can be used to solve the problem (Fig. 30-6).

This is a mixture of body porcelain and **overglaze** with additional modifiers to produce a maturation temperature as low as 850° C (1562° F). Minor corrections can thus be made with little risk of dimensional change to any other part of the restoration. Major corrections should be made by performing an additional firing with the conventional body and incisal powders, although there are limits to the number of times a restoration can be fired if devitrification is to be avoided (see p. 638).

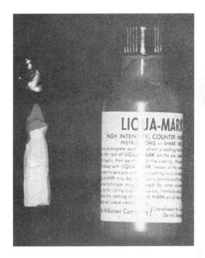

Fig. 30-7. Water-soluble marking agent.

MARGIN INTEGRITY

The completed restoration should go into place without binding of its internal aspect against the occlusal surface or the axial walls of the tooth preparation; in other words, the best adaptation should be at the margins. If the indirect procedure is handled properly, there should be no noticeable difference between the fit of a restoration on the die and that in the mouth.

Several techniques have been used to detect where a casting binds against an occlusal or axial wall—including disclosing waxes, a suspension of rouge in turpentine or acetic acid, air abrasion to form a matte finish surface, powdered sprays, water-soluble marking agents (Fig. 30-7), and special elastomeric detection pastes. However, none has proved entirely satisfactory. Most techniques are rather messy and time consuming and should not be needed on a routine basis.

Nevertheless, elastomeric paste (Fig. 30-8) has some advantages. The material is similar to a sili-

cone impression material and is obtained as a two-paste system. It has a similar viscosity to the final luting agents, so it can be used not only to identify unwanted internal contacts but also to assess adequate marginal fit. The degree of clinically acceptable marginal opening (i.e., the discrepancy unlikely to have an adverse effect on the prognosis) is hard to define. Margin integrity has been the subject of many laboratory and clinical evaluations. Obviously, to limit dissolution of the luting agent, the thickness of the cement film at the margins should be kept minimal. Through careful technique, a marginal adaptation below 30 μm can be obtained consistently.[1,2]

Assessment. Fig. 30-9 illustrates some of the possibilities that may be encountered when verifying margin integrity. The presence of a small ledge does not necessarily mean the restoration must be remade. It may merely require additional finishing where accessibility permits.

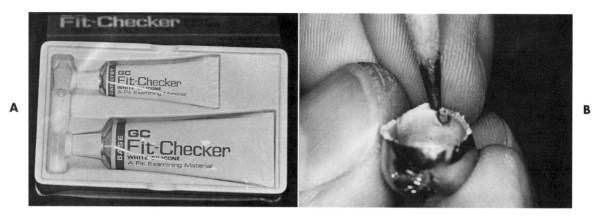

Fig. 30-8. **A,** Elastomeric detection paste, recommended for evaluating the internal surface of a restoration. **B,** The interference is seen as a perforation in the film of silicone material, which can be marked with a colored pencil. NOTE: The residual film of silicone should be thoroughly removed before cementing the restoration.
(Courtesy Dr. J.H. Bailey.)

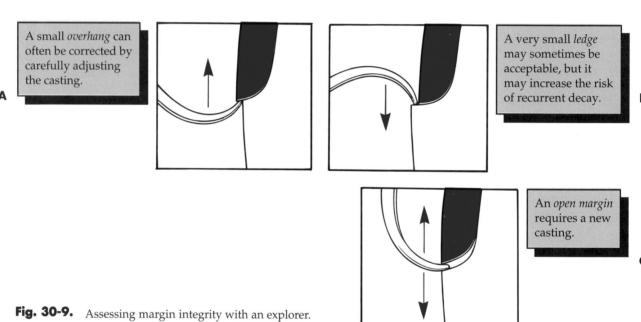

A small *overhang* can often be corrected by carefully adjusting the casting.

A very small *ledge* may sometimes be acceptable, but it may increase the risk of recurrent decay.

An *open margin* requires a new casting.

Fig. 30-9. Assessing margin integrity with an explorer. **A,** An overhang. **B,** A ledge. **C,** An open margin.

A sharp explorer moved from restoration to tooth and from tooth to restoration can be used in evaluating the marginal adaptation. If resistance is encountered in both directions, a gap or open margin exists whose cause must be determined. If the gap is the result of an excessive proximal contact or of residual provisional luting agent that prevents the casting from being seated, corrective action can be easily taken and the situation remedied. However, an obviously inaccurate restoration should be quickly rejected. Avoid trying to "make it fit," because a new impression is a better use of time.

Finishing. Subgingival margins are not accessible for finishing in the mouth. They must be fin-

ished on the die. Because clinical examination of subgingival margins is not always easy, a precementation radiograph may be justified.

Supragingival margins are generally finished with the casting seated on the tooth. White stones and cuttle disks rotating from restoration to tooth structure should result in a suitably finished margin (Fig. 30-10), which, provided the casting is properly adapted, will be virtually undetectable with the tip of a sharp explorer.[3]

Accessible margins can also be burnished during the cementation procedure before initial setting of the cement.[4] However, the less accessible proximal margins are the critical ones in terms of prognosis. They are the most common site of recurring caries

A   **B**   **C**

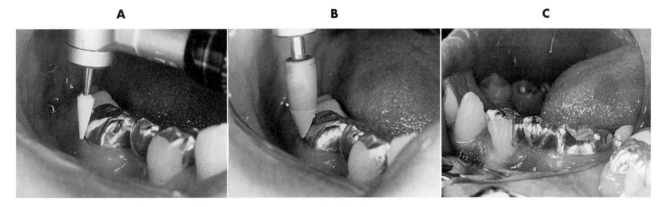

Fig. 30-10. Supragingival margins allow access for finishing the restoration directly on the tooth. **A,** Fine-grit white stone. **B,** Rubber point. **C,** Completed restoration.

and periodontal disease, and they can neither be evaluated readily nor finished easily. It has also been demonstrated[5,6] that correcting a poorly fitting cast restoration with finishing procedures is not possible.

STABILITY

The restoration should then be assessed for stability on the prepared tooth. It should not rock or rotate when force is applied. Any degree of instability is likely to cause failure during function. If instability is due to a small positive nodule, this can usually be corrected; however, if it is due to distortion, a new casting will be necessary.

OCCLUSION

After the restoration has been seated and the margin integrity and stability are acceptable, the occlusal contact with the opposing teeth is carefully checked. The criteria for these relationships, both static and dynamic, have been discussed in Chapters 4 and 18. Any undesirable eccentric contacts as well as centric interferences must be identified. NOTE: minor adjustment of eccentric contacts may be needed if a semiadjustable (as opposed to a fully adjustable) articulator is used.

Evaluation and Adjustment
Armamentarium

- Hemostats
- Miller forceps
- Marking ribbon or tape
- Thin Mylar shim stock
- Diamond rotary instruments
- White stones

Only restorations in supraocclusion can be adjusted. For those that are out of occlusion, no satisfactory solution exists other than remaking (if in metal) or refiring (if in porcelain).

Step-by-step Procedure (Fig. 30-11)

1. Before seating the casting, assess the contact relationship between maxillary and mandibular teeth. The most convenient way to do this is to cut a narrow strip of Mylar shim stock, hold it in hemostats or forceps, and have the patient open and close with the strip between opposing teeth. A "tug" can be felt on the Mylar, indicating occlusal contact (Fig. 30-12). Ideally, contact should be as evenly distributed as possible, but it is not uncommon to find one or more areas of relatively light contact between opposing teeth.

2. Seat the restoration, have the patient close, and reassess the contacts. The new restoration should hold the shim stock and yet not alter the existing tooth relationships. If a discrepancy is detected, a decision must be made whether this can be adjusted intraorally or whether a **remount procedure** will be necessary.

3. Mark any interferences that are detected. Have the patient close on articulating ribbon or tape.

4. Adjust these with the diamond rotary instrument or white stone, always checking the thickness of the casting with calipers before an adjustment is made. On occasion, adjusting an opposing cusp rather than cementing a restoration that is too thin may be the preferred method, although performing such adjustment at the tooth preparation stage is recommended. Explaining the procedure and its rationale to the patient before grinding an opposing tooth is essential. Options, such as increasing occlusal clearance by repreparing the tooth, should be presented to the patient before proceeding.

5. Be careful not to misinterpret occlusal markings. Note that a true interocclusal contact leaves a mark with a clean center (like a bull's-eye), but a false contact leaves a smudge.

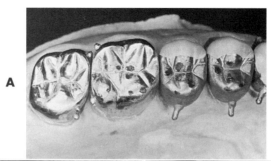

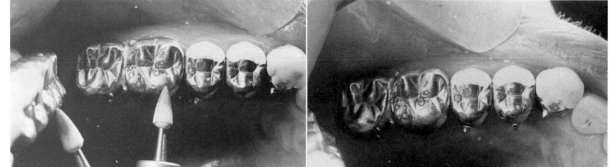

Fig. 30-11. Evaluating and adjusting the occlusion. **A,** Refinement on the articulator before evaluation. **B,** Testing the occlusal relationship with shim stock and marking with tape. Typically some adjustment will be needed, especially in more complex treatments, but this should not be extensive unless an error has been made. **C,** After adjustment, the occlusal contacts should always be verified with shim stock because ribbon markings can be misinterpreted.

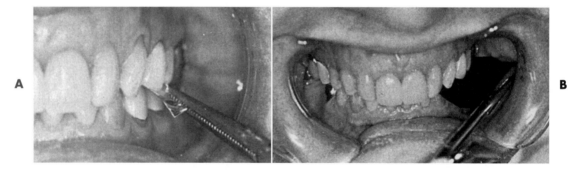

Fig. 30-12. **A,** Use Mylar shim stock to identify presence or absence of occlusal contacts. **B,** Use articulating tape to identify the location of occlusal contact.

Shim stock is a more reliable indicator than ribbon or tape of the presence or absence of an occlusal contact and should be used to evaluate when the end point has been reached. Marking ribbon or tape is better to help determine the location of an interference.

6. Use two colors of ribbon for the different types of movement. Excursive movements and interferences are first marked in one color (e.g., green). Then a different color (e.g., red) is inserted for centric contacts. Any interferences are adjusted with the diamond or white stone.

An alternative technique requires the use of an airborne particle abrasion unit with aluminum oxide (Fig. 30-13). A matte finish is obtained on the oc-clusal surfaces of the casting in question, and the patient is asked to close. Where shiny marks appear, an adjustment is made. This technique, however, presents the following disadvantages:

- Differentiating between centric and excursive contacts is not possible.
- The technique is more time consuming.
- It is applicable only to cast-metal occlusal surfaces.

Gross occlusal adjustment involving dental porcelain is better done in the bisque stage, because interferences are more easily marked on a bisque surface than on glazed porcelain. Minor adjustments will be needed after glazing because of the pyroplastic flow of the porcelain.[7] After adjustment,

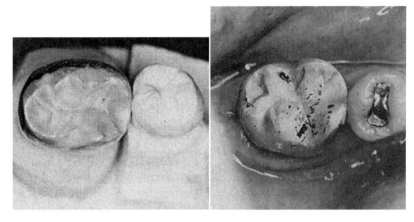

Fig. 30-13. Occlusal prematurities can be identified by giving the casting a matte finish with an air-abrasion unit. The prematurities will appear as shiny areas. *(Courtesy Dr. M.T. Padilla.)*

the porcelain can be polished with silicone wheels or diamond-polishing paste.

Remount. If there is a need for significant occlusal adjustment, a remount procedure[8] may be recommended. It is typically used when extensive restorative dentistry has been performed, and it serves to convey the relationships of the restorations and teeth to the dental laboratory (Fig. 30-14). Detailed adjustments can then be made in an organized manner. Any inaccuracy (e.g., slight tooth movement, previous mounting discrepancies, or small dimensional change inherent with the indirect process) can be compensated for relatively easily, thus reducing the amount of chair time needed for precementation adjustment.

Intraoral occlusal refinement is limited because of visibility and access difficulties. Laboratory adjustments offer optimum access and visibility and the opportunity to evaluate lingual contact relationships.

The remount procedure consists of making an impression of the castings in the patient's mouth, with an occlusal index in place. The index is made with reinforced resin or impression plaster and provides the opportunity to accurately reposition the castings back into the impression after it has been removed from the patient's mouth. A new master cast can then be fabricated. To enable easy removal of the castings from the newly fabricated master cast, resin is usually poured into the castings, after which the rest of the impression is poured in conventional Type IV stone (Fig. 30-15). The cast can then be articulated with a conventional facebow transfer and occlusal registration techniques (see Chapter 2).

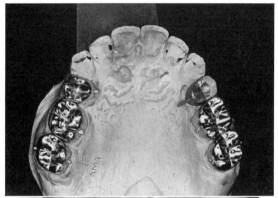

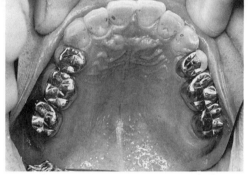

Fig. 30-14. Accurate transmission of occlusal relationships to the laboratory should be the rule when a careful technique has been followed. If discrepancies occur, they are often better corrected by a remount procedure in the laboratory.

Armamentarium (Fig. 30-16)
- Impression trays *(A)*
- Irreversible hydrocolloid *(B)*
- Rubber bowl and spatula *(C)*
- Provisional luting agent *(D)*
- Petrolatum *(E)*
- Autopolymerizing resin *(F)*

Although it is complex, a remount procedure will save considerable chair time when an error in articulation requires any significant occlusal adjustment.

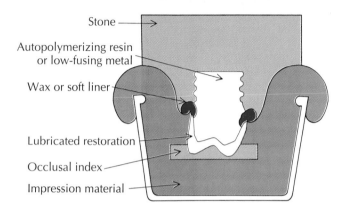

Stone
Autopolymerizing resin or low-fusing metal
Wax or soft liner
Lubricated restoration
Occlusal index
Impression material

Fig. 30-15.   Cross-sectional schematic of the remount procedure.

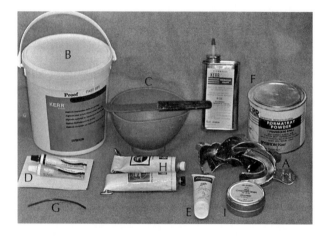

Fig. 30-16.   Armamentarium for a remount procedure.

- Stiff wire (e.g., coat hanger wire) *(G)*
- ZOE occlusal registration paste *(H)*
- Inlay wax or light-bodied reversible hydrocolloid *(I)*
- Facebow transfer equipment
- Centric relation recording

Step-by-step Procedure *(Fig. 30-17)*

1. Use autopolymerizing resin (e.g., custom tray resin) to make an occlusal index of the restorations on the working cast. Reinforce the index with stiff wire. The index should not extend beyond the occlusal table of the restored teeth, and its thickness must not be greater than 5 mm. It should fit the cast passively.

2. Grind the occlusal aspect of the index until only shallow indentations of the cusp tips remain.

3. Seat the restorations on the prepared teeth (Fig. 30-17, *B*). To prevent dislodgment, use a small amount of provisional luting agent mixed with petrolatum. FPDs that have yet to be assembled can be stabilized with autopolymerizing resin applied by the brush-bead technique (see Chapter 28).

4. After the fit of the index has been verified, cover the surfaces of the restorations with a thin coating of petrolatum and apply ZOE registration paste to the occlusal aspect of the index. Then seat it in the patient's mouth. As an alternative, impression plaster can be used (Fig. 30-17, *C*).

5. Make an orientation impression over the index and the restorations with an elastomeric impression material in a stock tray, making sure the index is not displaced (Fig. 30-17, *D*).

6. Make a conventional opposing impression if no restorations were made for that arch. If restorations have been made for both arches, repeat the procedure described previously.

7. Remove the restorations from the mouth, replace the provisionals, and reschedule the patient.

8. Clean the internal aspects of the restoration of any residual cement or debris, reseat the restoration in the index, and apply a thin coating of petrolatum.

9. Cover the margins of the restoration with wax or soft lining resin. As an alternative, reversible hydrocolloid impression material can be applied around them with a syringe. NOTE: Crowns with long retentive axial walls can be partially filled with reversible hydrocolloid to aid in their subsequent removal.

10. Pour the internal surface of the casting with autopolymerizing resin or low-fusing metal, adding retention (Fig. 30-17, *E*). ADA Type IV stone can be used, but the casting must be lubricated carefully; special care must be taken to prevent fracture when the casting is removed.

11. Complete the maxillary cast (Fig. 30-17, *F*) and articulate it with a facebow transfer technique (see Fig. 30-17, *G*).

12. Make a new centric relation record at the vertical dimension of occlusion.

13. Save the index to confirm accuracy after the remount is poured.

This completes the remount procedure. The restoration can now be reassessed and adjusted in the dental laboratory. Although a remount procedure is

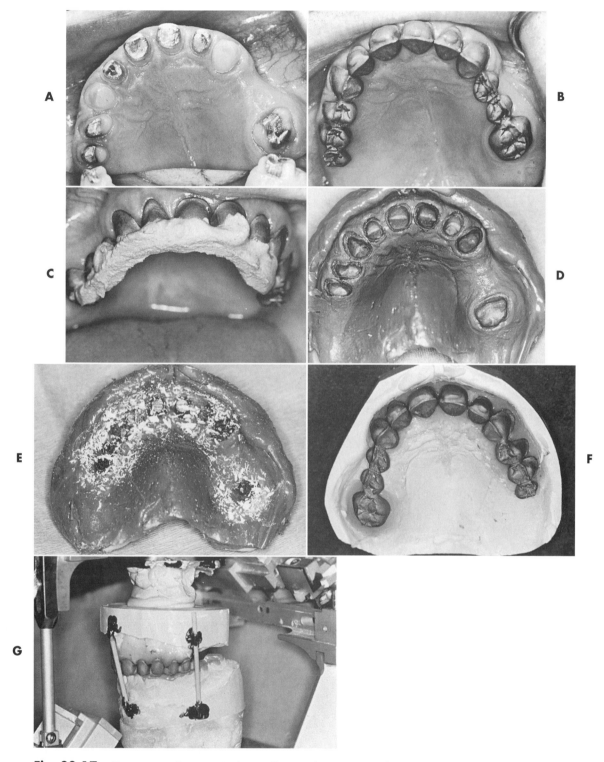

Fig. 30-17.   Remount technique. **A,** A maxillary arch is prepared for metal-ceramic crowns and fixed partial dentures. **B,** The metal substructure is evaluated clinically; a remount procedure is needed. **C,** Impression plaster is used to register the location of each unit. **D,** The registration is picked up with an elastomeric material. **E,** Restorations are lubricated, and soft lining resin is painted around them. Their internal surfaces are filled with hard resin. Acrylic chips provide retention for the soft resin. Small wood screws are inserted into the hard acrylic, which are also for retention. **F** and **G,** The remainder of the cast is poured and articulated in the usual way.
(Courtesy Dr. J.H. Bailey.)

not routinely needed, it may be advantageous with an extensive restoration to reduce the amount of chair time required for occlusal adjustment.

CERAMIC RESTORATIONS

Ceramic restorations need certain additional steps during evaluation to satisfy esthetic, biologic, and mechanical requirements. Achieving an esthetic result depends on the contour of the restoration, surface characterization, and color match.

Contouring
Armamentarium (Fig. 30-18)
- Flexible diamond disk
- Porcelain grinding wheel
- Ceramic-bound stones
- Diamonds

When contouring a restoration that is to be evaluated during the bisque stage, it should be moistened first with water or saliva. The moist surface reflects light in the same manner as the glazed restoration.

Step-by-step Procedure
1. Check the proximal contact relationship (adjust as necessary) and verify the marginal fit of the restoration.
2. Verify the contour of the gingival third and make any necessary adjustments. Excessive bulk in this area is a common fault and is often associated with periodontal disease (Fig. 30-19). When adjustment of porcelain is needed, the porcelain and metal should not be ground simultaneously because small metal particles may be transferred to the porcelain, causing discoloration and a black spotty appearance after the restoration has been glazed. If grinding both porcelain and metal simultaneously is absolutely necessary, the direction of grinding should be parallel to the metal-ceramic junction

(Fig. 30-20). A thin, flexible disk may be used to reduce any overcontoured interproximal area (Fig. 30-21).
3. Identify and adjust any occlusal interferences on the posterior teeth. As mentioned, porcelain occlusal contacts will need readjustment after glazing because of the pyroplastic flow of porcelain.
4. On anterior teeth, establish the proper position and shape of the incisal edge. This is a key step in achieving good esthetics and function. Unfortunately, it is hard to obtain in the laboratory because the soft tissues of the patient's lips and cheeks are not present on the articulator. A stone cast of a well-adjusted provisional restoration (made from the diagnostic cast or waxing procedure) helps the technician because it can be duplicated when the porcelain is applied. However, as a general rule, the restoration should be tried in the patient's mouth with the incisal edges slightly longer than intended; their shape should be refined in the mouth.

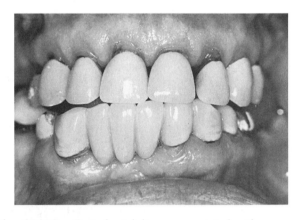

Fig. 30-19. Periodontal disease associated with excessively contoured restorations.

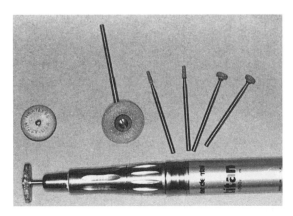

Fig. 30-18. Armamentarium for porcelain adjustment.

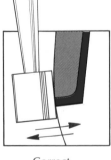
Correct

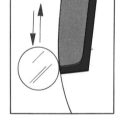
Incorrect

Fig. 30-20. If it is necessary to grind at the metal-porcelain junction, the stone should be held perpendicular to the junction. Otherwise, metal particles may contaminate the porcelain.

NOTE: If too much adjustment is made, the incisal porcelain layer will be ground away, and the esthetic effect will be spoiled. Incisal edge position is important in obtaining good esthetics and function. Specific criteria for what constitutes "normal" are hard to define, but an average of 1 to 2 mm of the clinical crown should be visible on maxillary central and lateral incisors when the upper lip is relaxed. Additional help in contouring the incisal edges can be obtained by looking at the patient's smile and listening to speech characteristics. Ideally, the incisal edges of the maxillary anterior teeth will follow the curvature of the lower lip when the patient smiles.[9] Ordinarily the incisal edges of the lateral incisors (Fig. 30-22) are 1 to 2 mm shorter than the central incisors, which may touch the internal aspect of the lower lip when it is relaxed.

5. Evaluate the *negative space*, the name given to the shape of the incisal embrasures[10] (see Chapter 1). Proper embrasures (Fig. 30-23) significantly enhance the apparent separation between restorations, whereas their absence draws attention to the prosthesis and reveals its artificial nature (Fig. 30-23, *C*). Similarly, when viewed from the incisal, interproximal embrasures should be as narrow and deep as possible to enhance the shadows between components of the fixed prosthesis. If these are absent, even the casual observer will recognize the teeth as artificial.

6. Have the patient enunciate the consonants. *F* sounds are particularly helpful because they are made with the incisal edge of the maxillary central incisors touching at the junction of the moist and dry surfaces of the vermilion border of the lower lip ("wet-dry line").[11]

7. Mark the line angles directly on the porcelain restoration in the bisque stage with a colored pencil and compare these to the line angles of adjacent and contralateral teeth. NOTE: Red pencil is preferred because blue or black pencil may discolor the porcelain. The position of the line angles is probably one of the more critical procedures for achieving good esthetics because the line angles delineate the shape of the tooth to an observer. (Line angles on wax patterns are discussed in Chapter 18.) By superimposing normal line angle distribution over teeth that are otherwise too large or too narrow,[12] creating the impression that the left and right sides are identical is possible (see Chapter 23).

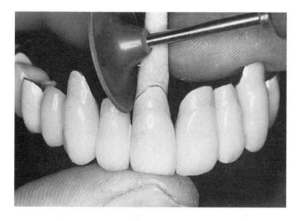

Fig. 30-21. Adjusting the axial contour.

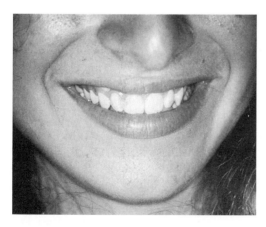

Fig. 30-22. Typical incisal edge position.
(From Monteith BD: J Prosthet Dent 54:81, 1985.)

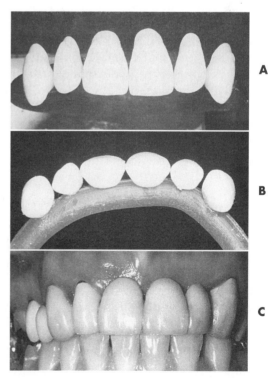

Fig. 30-23. *A* and *B,* Properly shaped incisal embrasures. *C,* Inadequate embrasures. Note the unnatural look.

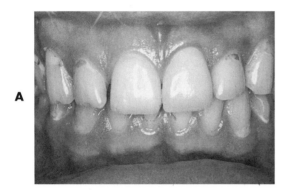

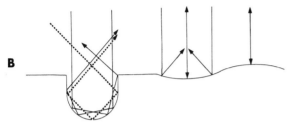

Fig. 30-24. **A,** Restoration texture should closely match natural enamel. **B,** Sharp grooves should not be cut into the ceramic surface because these "trap" light. A curved surface looks more natural and results in either converging or diverging reflections.

8. Evaluate the overall contour to see that it matches the shape of the adjacent teeth. With experience, most operators quickly develop an appreciation for evaluating "normal" contours and detecting areas that need correction. Moistening the teeth and observing light reflections may help. It also helps to have the patient stand up to be checked at normal conversational distance as opposed to the extreme close-up of a dental examination.

Surface Texture Characterization. When the contour of the restoration has been finalized, the next goal is to duplicate the surface detail of the patient's natural teeth.

Armamentarium
* Diamond disk
* Carborundum stones
* Diamond stones

Step-by-step Procedure
1. Dry the teeth and examine their surfaces carefully. Perikymata and defects can be simulated by grinding the porcelain with a diamond stone of appropriate texture. (Be careful not to overemphasize such details.) Flat or concave areas will reflect light in a characteristic manner, producing highlights (Fig. 30-24).

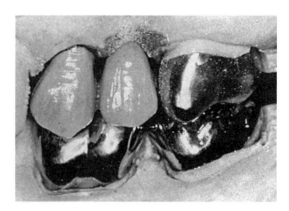

Fig. 30-25. The texture of these metal-ceramic units has been overemphasized, leading to an artificial appearance.

2. Copy the details and carefully blend them with the adjacent area.
3. Similarly, mimic any vertical defects with careful grinding.
4. Be careful to avoid "overcharacterizing" restorations, which is a common error (Fig. 30-25).

On occasion, altering the apparent size of a restoration by these techniques may be possible. A smooth tooth appears larger than one that is identical in size but has intensive surface texture characterization.

CHARACTERIZATION AND GLAZING

The surface luster or degree of gloss of a porcelain restoration depends on the autoglazing procedure (see Chapter 24). Both time and temperature must be carefully controlled. During a glazing heat treatment, the surface layers of porcelain melt slightly, coalescing the particles and filling in surface defects.

The restoration should not be glazed in a vacuum because included air may be drawn to the surface and result in bubbling. Because air-fired glazing furnaces are relatively compact and inexpensive, some dentists prefer to glaze porcelain restorations in the operatory. This is particularly convenient if surface **stains** are to be used. The glazing step is straightforward; the degree of glaze depends on furnace temperature and the time the restoration is held at that temperature. Excessively glazed anterior teeth will look unnatural. The patient should moisten the restoration because saliva affects its appearance. A dry crown will look misleadingly underglazed. Underglazing and refiring a restoration is better than overglazing it. If a restoration is not sufficiently glazed, it will retain more plaque and may be more liable to fracture. After glazing, the metal surfaces of the restoration are polished.

An alternative to glazing is to polish the porcelain surfaces of the restoration.[13] This provides greater control of the surface luster and distribution than glazing.[14] For example, having a higher gloss on the cervical area and a lower one on the incisal is possible. This is not possible with glazing because the entire crown is subjected to the same time-temperature combination.

Polishing dental ceramics has long been advocated as an expedient way of restoring luster after adjusting by grinding. A number of commercially available polishing kits are available for this purpose. If used correctly (i.e., without omitting the successively finer grits), most are capable of producing smooth porcelain surfaces.[15,16] As an alternative, finishing wheels followed by pumice is satisfactory.[17] More recently, ceramists have advocated polishing as a way to improve luster control. To achieve the precise degree and distribution of luster required, the porcelain is polished rather than glazed.

Despite the esthetic advantages of polishing, there is concern as to whether the strength of a polished restoration might be reduced or its abrasiveness increased. Glazing has been cited as strengthening a dental restoration,[18] presumably because it causes a reduction of the flaws that initiate fracture. However, polishing also reduces flaws, and in laboratory studies, polishing has not been found to result in reduced physical properties as compared to glazing.[19-23] Laboratory studies have shown that polished porcelain is no more abrasive than glazed porcelain.[24] However, unpolished porcelain is much more abrasive on opposing enamel and is more plaque retentive than polished or glazed porcelain.

EXTERNAL COLOR MODIFICATION AND CHARACTERIZATION

Stuart H. Jacobs

The accomplishment of a perfect color match using the basic shades supplied in the porcelain kits, without the need for chairside modification, is the goal of all dental ceramists. However, there are difficulties and inaccuracies inherent in the metal-ceramic technique. There are also difficulties in duplicating the appearance of a patient's tooth without the patient actually being present in the dental laboratory. These problems make perfect shade matching impossible to achieve routinely. In many situations, a restoration that does not blend well with the adjacent teeth can be improved by simple chairside color modification or characterization procedures.[25] These are done with final glazing, and it is therefore recommended that restorations be tried in the pa-

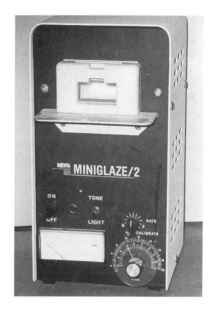

Fig. 30-26. Ney Miniglaze/2 glazing furnace.

tient's mouth contoured but unglazed (bisque stage).

Armamentarium

- Porcelain furnace (a small air-fired furnace is suitable for the operatory) (Fig. 30-26).
- Clean glass slab
- Sable hair brush
- Distilled water
- Tissue
- Stain kit

A number of stain kits are available from porcelain manufacturers, and most contain a fairly wide range of colors. The stains themselves are highly pigmented surface colorants that contain a small amount of glass, allowing the color to fuse into the porcelain surface.

The popular Vitachrom L kit* is illustrated in Fig. 30-27. It comes with sample-color laminae of the stains in the appropriate range. Additional colors can be made by mixing the stains with each other; the color intensity can also be toned down with a colorless porcelain.

Step-by-step Procedure The application of stain has advantages and disadvantages. One advantage is that the dentist or technician can modify the color after a restoration is completed with the patient present. The greatest disadvantage is that the color can be applied only to the surface, so it is ineffective in producing characterizations that look

*Vident: Brea, Calif.

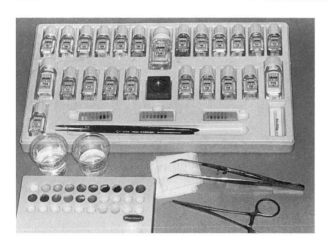

Fig. 30-27. The Vitachrom L stain kit.

realistic (i.e., deep within the tooth). Also, if surface characterization is applied excessively,[26] it can cause a loss of fluorescence in the finished restoration as well as an increase in the metameric effect (shade mismatch is more apparent under some lighting conditions). Furthermore, a characterized crown is slightly rougher than an autoglazed one[27] and the stain will eventually wear away under normal toothbrushing[28,29] (10 to 12 years).

Three aspects of characterization may be used singly or in combination to achieve a natural appearance: shade modification (increasing the chroma, changing the hue, or reducing the value); specific characterization (e.g., hypocalcified areas or cracks); and special illusions of form or position (Fig. 30-28).

1. Mix the stain with the liquid provided in the kit (normally a glycerin-water mixture) to a creamy, stiff consistency (Fig. 30-28, *A*). If the mixture is too thin, it will run over the restorations and pool in certain areas. An even coat is essential for producing the best results.
2. Apply stain to the restorations with the clean moist sable brush (Fig. 30-28, *B*). When moist, the brush becomes easier to draw to a point, and application of the stain is greatly facilitated.
3. When the effect has been created, make a note of which stain was used and where. This procedure usually must be duplicated because absolute cleanliness is essential; in addition, placing a unit in the mouth without some contamination is difficult. Removing the restorations without smudging is also difficult.
4. Take the restorations out of the mouth, wash them, and recreate the characterization (Fig. 30-28, *C*).

5. After the characterization is complete, transfer the restorations to a firing tray and place it in front of the muffle of the furnace until the stain is dry and the surface appears chalky white (Fig. 30-28, *D*).
6. Remove the prosthesis and examine it to ensure no stain has run inside (Fig. 30-28, *E*).
7. Remove any excess with a dry brush and place the crown in the furnace.
8. Increase the heat to the maturation temperature of the porcelain and hold it there according to the degree of glaze required (Fig. 30-28, *F*).
9. Remove the restorations, allow them to cool, and retry them in the patient's mouth.

Shade Modification (see Chapter 23). When a porcelain shade is being altered with external stain, certain limitations must be considered, particularly because surface characterization causes a loss of fluorescence and increases the effect of metamerism. It cannot be used to make major corrections or compensate for gross errors.

When assessing the correctness of shade, simulating the appearance of glazed porcelain is necessary. This can be done by painting on some of the liquid provided in the stain kit. It may also help to paint the adjacent natural tooth to prevent dehydration during the characterization procedure, which would increase the value of the tooth.

Chroma and Hue Adjustment. Increasing the chroma (saturation) is one of the simplest shade alterations to achieve.[30] The addition of yellow stain increases the chroma of a basically yellow shade, whereas adding orange has the same effect on a yellow-red shade. When an alteration in hue is necessary, pink-purple moves yellow toward yellow-red, whereas yellow decreases the red content of a yellow-red shade. These are the only two modifications that should be necessary because the hue of a natural tooth always lies in the yellow-red to yellow range.

A metal-ceramic restoration that has too high a chroma is difficult to modify. Choosing a shade with a lower chroma is always better, which allows it to be altered easily. Using the complementary color of a restoration reduces its chroma: yellow requires violet, and orange requires blue or green. However, the addition of these stains lowers the value of the restoration and increases the metameric effect; it is rarely successful in practice.

Value Adjustment. Value can be reduced by adding a complementary color (see Chapter 23). Violet is used on yellow restorations and has the

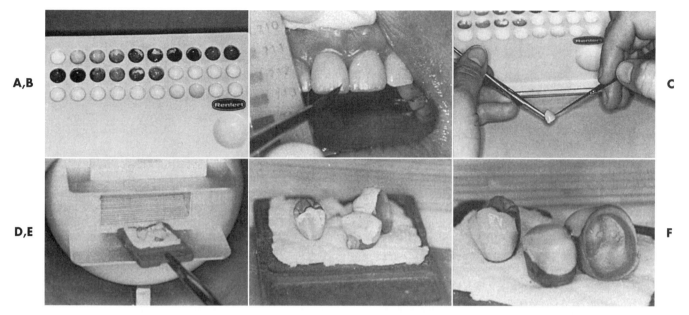

Fig. 30-28. Characterization and glazing technique. **A,** The colored stains are mixed to a stiff consistency on a suitable palette. **B,** A thin brown check line is made by painting a line of stain on the porcelain. This is reduced to the desired width by wiping a clean brush on each side of it. **C,** Often the procedure is repeated, or modifications are made after removal from the mouth. **D** and **E,** Stain is dried to a chalky consistency in front of the furnace muffle. **F,** Characterized and glazed restorations after firing.

added effect of increasing the translucency. Gray is not encouraged because it tends to reduce translucency and makes the surface cloudy.

Attempting to increase the value is generally less successful, although value can be increased if the dominant color added has a higher lightness ranking. For example, a crown can be stained with white, but opacity will be greatly increased.

Characterization. Characterization is the art of reproducing natural defects, and it can be particularly successful in making a crown blend with the adjacent natural teeth. In general, defects should be reproduced to a slightly lesser extent on the restoration than as they appear on the natural teeth. The temptation to overcharacterize is strong but must be resisted.

Characterization looks slightly more natural and is more permanent if applied intrinsically during the buildup of the restoration (see Chapter 24) rather than by subsequent extrinsic application.[31] However, communicating to the laboratory the exact characterization needed may be difficult; therefore, copying natural defects at chairside may be more practical.

Hypocalcified Areas. These are produced with white stain and may be some of the easiest and most commonly made modifications.

Proximal Coloration. Many natural teeth exhibit proximal characterization. By reproducing this in the restoration, the dentist is able to create the illusion of depth and separation and is also able to tone down excessive opacity at the cervical area. The stains used are brown and orange. They are applied lightly to the proximal area and extended slightly onto the buccal surface apical to the contact. Proximal coloring is particularly useful in creating the illusion of separate units of an FPD.

Enamel Cracks. This characterization is better if done intrinsically, although it can be added extrinsically. A linear vertical crack interrupts the light transmission across the tooth surface, causing a shadow. Thus both the highlight and the shadow of the crack must be simulated for an authentic result.

The highlight is developed with white and yellow mixed in the ratio of 4:1, and gray stain is used for the shadow. A thin line is drawn with a brush in the desired area with the white and yellow stains. Then a thin line of gray is placed distal to the first line to create the illusion of a shadow.

Stained Crack Line (Fig. 30-29). Cracked enamel stains quickly on natural teeth. An orange-brown mixture applied in as thin a line as possible will effectively simulate a crack.

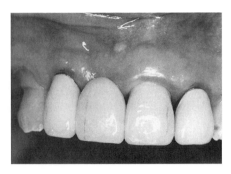

Fig. 30-29. Thin brown check lines have been added to enhance the appearance of this prosthesis.

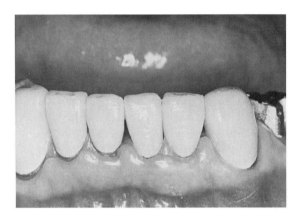

Fig. 30-30. Exposed incisal dentin has been mimicked with brown and orange characterization on these mandibular incisor crowns.

Exposed Incisal Dentin (Fig. 30-30). This is usually seen on the mandibular incisors of older patients and is due to enamel wear. The incisal edge should be "cupped out," with orange and brown colorants used to reproduce the dentinoenamel junction.

Incisal Halo. Translucent incisal edges are more common on the incisors of younger patients. Often, although the incisal area is translucent, the edge will be totally opaque. This may be difficult to reproduce internally. A mixture of white and yellow stains in the ratio of 4:1 is placed in the linguoincisal area, with an extension just onto the labial, to give the halo effect.

Translucency. Translucency can be mimicked with violet stain, although the results are usually disappointing compared to those achieved with correct application of the incisal porcelain. For optimum results both labial and lingual surfaces should be coated. Decreasing the translucency is accomplished by adding the dominant hue over the labiolingual surface.

Staining Procedures		TABLE **30-1**
	Basic Colors	Vitachrom L Stain No.
Chroma increase	Yellow and yellow-red	709, 710
Chroma decrease	Violet and blue-green	721, 720
Hue adjustment	Pink-purple or yellow	704/721, 709
Value adjustment	Violet and (white)*	721 (701)*
Hypocalcification	White	701
Proximal coloration	Brown and orange	715, 712
Enamel cracks	White-yellow and gray	701/702, 708
Stained crack line	Orange-brown	712, 713
Exposed incisal dentin	Orange and brown	712, 715
Incisal halo	White-yellow	701/702
Translucency	(Violet)*	(721)*
Cervical staining		
A shades	Orange-browns	716, 717
B shades	Greenish-browns	718, 716
C shades	Greenish-browns	719, 718
D shades	Greenish-browns	718

*Modification may not be successful.

Special Illusions. Form and position are undoubtedly the most important factors in achieving an attractive result. However, restoring the original form may not always be possible. Loss of supporting tissue, the size of a pontic space, or a poor occlusal position may impede the attempt.

An FPD pontic may be very long because of loss of supporting bone. Simulating a root surface can partially improve the appearance. The root extension is contoured for length and width, and then an orange-brown mixture is placed over the extension. Pink stain can be used to simulate gingival tissue, but results are better with pink body porcelain.

Recommended characterization procedures are summarized in Table 30-1.

▣ SUMMARY

When a restoration is tried in the mouth, the proximal contacts, margin integrity, and occlusion must be verified. Minor occlusal discrepancies can usually be adjusted intraorally. For extensive restorative procedures, a remount may be needed and will reduce the chair time needed for an optimum occlusal scheme in the restoration.

With a metal-ceramic restoration, proper contouring of the porcelain in the cervical third is critical to facilitating maintenance of health of the supporting structures. Proper shaping of the gingival and incisal embrasures, along with contouring and characterization, will significantly improve the esthetic result. Small corrections and subtle changes can be made with surface stains.

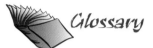

Glossary

characterize: to distinguish, individualize, mark, qualify, singularize, or differentiate something.

emergence profile: the contour of a tooth or restoration, such as a crown on a natural tooth or dental implant abutment, as it relates to the adjacent tissues.

glaze: *vb* **glazed; glazing** *vt* (14 cent.) *1:* to cover with a glossy, smooth surface or coating. *2:* the attainment of a smooth and reflective surface. *3:* the final firing of porcelain in which the surface is vitrified, creating a high gloss to the material. *4:* a ceramic veneer on a metal porcelain restoration after it has been fired, producing a nonporous, glossy, or semiglossy surface.

intrinsic coloring: coloring from within; the incorporation of a colorant within the material of a prosthesis or restoration.

natural glaze: the production of a glazed surface by the vitrification of the material itself without addition of other fluxes or glasses.

overglaze: *adj* (1879) the production of a glazed surface by the addition of a fluxed glass that usually vitrifies at a lower temperature.

pigment: *n* (14 cent.) finely ground, natural or synthetic, inorganic or organic, insoluble dispersed particles (powder), which, when dispersed in a liquid vehicle, may provide, in addition to color, many other essential properties such as opacity, hardness, durability, and corrosion resistance. The term is used to include extenders and white or color pigments. The distinction between powders that are pigments and those that are dyes is generally considered on the basis of solubility (pigments are insoluble and dispersed in the material; dyes are soluble or in solution).

remount procedure: any method used to relate restorations to an articulator or analysis and/or to assist in development of a plan for occlusal equilibration or reshaping.

stain: *vb* (14 cent.) *1:* to suffuse with color. *2:* to color by processes affecting chemically or otherwise the material itself. *3:* in dentistry, to intentionally alter ceramic or resin restorations through the application of intrinsic or extrinsic colorants to achieve a desired effect.

References

1. Byrne G et al: Casting accuracy of high-palladium alloys, *J Prosthet Dent* 55:297, 1986.
2. Schilling ER et al: Marginal gap of crowns made with a phosphate-bonded investment and accelerated casting method, *J Prosthet Dent* 81:129, 1999.
3. Christensen GJ: Marginal fit of gold inlay castings, *J Prosthet Dent* 16:297, 1966.
4. Goretti A et al: A microscopic evaluation of the marginal adaptation of onlays in gold, *Schweiz Monatsschr Zahnmed* 102:679, 1992.
5. Lofstrom LH, Asgar K: Scanning electron microscopic evaluation of techniques to extend deficient cast gold margins, *J Prosthet Dent* 55:416, 1986.
6. Eames WB: Movement of gold at cavosurface margins with finishing instruments (letter), *J Prosthet Dent* 56:516, 1986.
7. Hobo S: Distortion of occlusal porcelain during glazing, *J Prosthet Dent* 47:154, 1982.
8. Huffman RW, Regenos JW: *Principles of occlusion,* ed 4, London, Ohio, 1973, H & R Press.
9. Monteith BD: A cephalometric method to determine the angulation of the occlusal plane in edentulous patients, *J Prosthet Dent* 54:81, 1985.
10. Matthews TG: The anatomy of a smile, *J Prosthet Dent* 39:128, 1978.
11. Rahn AO, Heartwell CM: *Textbook of complete dentures,* ed 5, Philadelphia, 1993.

Study Questions

1. What is the recommended sequence in which to evaluate a gold crown at the time of clinical try-in? Why? Which additional steps are necessary for a metal-ceramic restoration?
2. How is a tight proximal contact most effectively identified and corrected?
3. Discuss the addition of a proximal contact for a gold crown and a metal-ceramic crown.
4. What is a remount procedure? Discuss the steps involved.
5. What is the "negative space"?
6. When shade modification is desired, how is chroma increased? What hue adjustments are feasible? How is value adjusted?

12. Blancheri RL: Optical illusion and restorative dentistry, *Rev Asoc Dent Mex* 8:103, 1950.

13. al-Wahadni A, Martin DM: Glazing and finishing dental porcelain: a literature review, *J Can Dent Assoc* 64:580, 1998.

14. Hubbard JR: Natural texture and lustre in ceramics. In Preston JD, editor: *Perspectives in dental ceramics,* Chicago, 1988, Quintessence.

15. Goldstein GR et al: Profilometer, SEM, and visual assessment of porcelain polishing methods, *J Prosthet Dent* 65:627, 1991.

16. Fuzzi M et al: Scanning electron microscopy and profilometer evaluation of glazed and polished dental porcelain, *Int J Prosthodont* 9:452, 1996.

17. Newitter DA et al: An evaluation of adjustment and postadjustment finishing techniques on the surface of porcelain-bonded-to-metal crowns, *J Prosthet Dent* 48:388, 1982.

18. Binns DB: The physical and chemical properties of dental porcelain. In Yamada HN, editor: *Dental porcelain: the state of the art 1977. A compendium of the colloquium held at the University of Southern California School of Dentistry on Feb. 24-26, 1977, Los Angeles, 1977,* The University.

19. Levy H: Effect of laboratory finishing technics and the mechanical properties of dental ceramic, *Inf Dent* 69:1039, 1987.

20. Rosenstiel SF et al: Comparison of glazed and polished dental porcelain, *Int J Prosthodont* 2:524, 1989.

21. Brackett SE et al: An evaluation of porcelain strength and the effect of surface treatment, *J Prosthet Dent* 61:446, 1989.

22. Fairhurst CW et al: The effect of glaze on porcelain strength, *Dent Mater* 8:203, 1992.

23. Giordano R et al: Effect of surface finish on the flexural strength of feldspathic and aluminous dental ceramics, *Int J Prosthodont* 8:311, 1995.

24. al-Hiyasat AS et al: The abrasive effect of glazed, unglazed, and polished porcelain on the wear of human enamel, and the influence of carbonated soft drinks on the rate of wear, *Int J Prosthodont* 10:269, 1997.

25. Abadie FR: Porcelain surface characterization and staining in the office, *J Prosthet Dent* 51:181, 1984.

26. Weiner S: Staining porcelain veneer restorations, *J Prosthet Dent* 44:670, 1980.

27. Cook PA et al: The effect of superficial colorant and glaze on the surface texture of vacuum-fired porcelain, *J Prosthet Dent* 51:476, 1984.

28. Aker DA et al: Toothbrush abrasion of color-corrective porcelain stains applied to porcelain-fused-to-metal restorations, *J Prosthet Dent* 44:161, 1980.

29. Bativala F et al: The microscopic appearance and effect of toothbrushing on extrinsically stained metal-ceramic restorations, *J Prosthet Dent* 57:47, 1987.

30. Lund TW et al: Spectrophotometric study of the relationship between body porcelain color and applied metallic oxide pigments, *J Prosthet Dent* 53:790, 1985.

31. Winings JR: A method of making decalcifications in the porcelain build up, *J Dent Technol* 15:13, 1998.

LUTING AGENTS AND CEMENTATION PROCEDURES

PROVISIONAL CEMENTATION

On many occasions, cementing a restoration provisionally is advised so that the patient and dentist can assess its appearance and function over a longer time than a single visit. However, these trial cementations should be managed cautiously. On one hand, removing the restoration for definitive cementation may be difficult, even when temporary zinc oxide eugenol (ZOE) **cement** is used. To avoid this problem, the provisional cement can be mixed with a little petrolatum or silicone grease and applied only to the margins of the restoration to seal them while allowing subsequent removal without difficulty. On the other hand, a provisionally cemented restoration may come loose during function. If a single unit is displaced, it can be embarrassing or uncomfortable for the patient. If one abutment of a fixed partial denture becomes loose, the consequences can be more severe. If the patient does not promptly return for recementation, caries may develop very rapidly. Provisional cementation should not be undertaken unless the patient is given clear instructions about the objectives of the procedure, the intended duration of the trial cementation, and the importance of returning if an abutment loosens. If removing a provisionally cemented fixed prosthesis is difficult, the use of a crown-removal device such as the Coronaflex* (see Chapter 32) is recommended.

DEFINITIVE CEMENTATION

CONVENTIONAL CAST RESTORATIONS

Definitive cementation often does not receive the same attention to detail as other aspects of restorative dentistry. Careless cement selection can result in margin discrepancies and improper occlusion and may even require cutting the restoration from the patient's mouth and making a new one. The choice of cement depends first on whether a conventional casting or an adhesively bonded restoration, such as a ceramic inlay or resin-retained FPD, is to be cemented. Traditional dental cements can be used for cast crowns and FPDs, but not where adhesion is needed. Adhesive resins are necessary for some restorations, but they can be difficult to use; in addition, there are no long-term data to justify more general use with conventional castings.

DENTAL CEMENTS

Most **luting agents** traditionally used for cast restorations are dental cements (Fig. 31-1). These consist of an acid combined with a metal oxide base to form a salt and water. The setting mechanism results from the binding of unreacted powder particles by a matrix of salt to harden the mass. However, because they are ionic, these agents are susceptible to acid attack and are therefore somewhat soluble in oral fluids.[1-4] Traditionally, the success of restorations cemented with these luting agents has been attributed to excellent adaptation between the casting and the prepared tooth. In vitro, however, cement dissolution is independent of the marginal width up to a certain critical value. After that, it increases only slightly, which is explained by Fick's first law of diffusion.*[5] This study and others identify dissolution (rather than physical disintegration) as the mechanism for cement erosion.[6] They explain the success of cast restorations, despite the prevalence of relatively large subgingival marginal discrepancies, which are difficult to detect even at 0.1 mm.[7]

---

*KaVo America: Lake Zurich, Ill.

*Fick's first law states that the flux of a component of concentration across a membrane of unit area, in a predefined plane, is proportional to the concentration differential across that plane.

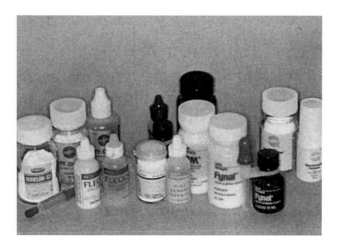

Fig. 31-1. Luting agents.

Zinc Phosphate Cement. This traditional luting agent continues to be popular for cast restorations. It has adequate strength, a **film thickness** of about 25 μm[8] (Fig. 31-2) (which is within the tolerance limits required for making cast restorations), and a reasonable working time. Excess material can be easily removed.

The toxic effects of zinc phosphate, or more specifically phosphoric acid, are well documented.[9] However, the successful use of the material over many years suggests that its effect on the dental pulp is clinically acceptable as long as normal precautions are taken and the preparation is not too close to the pulp.

Zinc Polycarboxylate Cement. One advantage of this luting agent is its relative biocompatibility,[10] which may stem from the fact that the polyacrylic acid molecule is large and therefore does not penetrate into the dentinal tubule.

Zinc polycarboxylate cement also exhibits specific adhesion to tooth structure because it chelates the calcium (although it has no adhesion to gold castings). Because of its high viscosity, zinc polycarboxylate cement can be difficult to mix, but this problem is mainly encountered by inexperienced operators.

In clinical trials, polycarboxylate performs as well or slightly better than zinc phosphate.[11,12] However, dentists have reported varying success rates, and claims of inferior long-term retention have been made. These problems may be related to the powder/liquid ratio. At manufacturers' recommended powder/liquid ratios, mixed polycarboxylate cement is very viscous. Some dentists may prefer a more fluid working consistency for reliable seating during cementation. However, polycar-

boxylate cements have different rheological or flow properties than zinc phosphate, exhibiting thinning with increased shear rate.[13] This means that they are capable of forming low film thicknesses despite their viscous appearance. When the dentist unnecessarily reduces the powder/liquid ratio, the **solubility** of the cement increases dramatically (as much as threefold).[14] This may be the cause of increased clinical failures. By fabricating luting agents, including polycarboxylate in encapsulated form, manufacturers have reduced problems due to manipulative variables.*

The working time of polycarboxylate is much shorter than that of zinc phosphate (about 2.5 minutes compared to 5 minutes). This may be a problem when cementing multiple units. Residual zinc polycarboxylate is more difficult to remove than zinc phosphate, and there is some evidence[15,16] that it provides less retention than zinc phosphate (Fig. 31-3). Its application therefore should probably be limited to restorations with good retention and resistance form where minimum pulp irritation is wanted. Its use as a base material and to block out minor undercuts in preparations on vital teeth may also be worth considering.

Glass Ionomer Cement. This cement adheres to enamel and dentin and exhibits good biocompatibility. In addition, because it releases fluoride,[17,18] it may have an anticariogenic effect, although this has not been documented clinically.[19] The set cement is somewhat translucent, which is an advantage when it is used with the porcelain labial margin technique (see Chapter 24).

The mechanical properties of glass ionomer cement are generally higher than those of zinc phosphate and polycarboxylate cements (Fig. 31-4). A disadvantage is that during setting, glass ionomer appears particularly susceptible to moisture contamination[20] and should be protected with a foil or resin coat or by leaving a band of cement undisturbed for 10 minutes.[21] The water changes the setting reaction of the glass ionomer as cement-forming cations are washed out and water is absorbed, leading to erosion.[22] Nevertheless, zinc phosphate has also demonstrated significant early erosion when exposed to moisture.[18] Glass ionomers should not be allowed to desiccate during this critical initial setting period. The newer resin-modified glass ionomers are less susceptible to early moisture.[23]

---

*Durelon Maxicap: ESPE North America: Norristown, Pa.

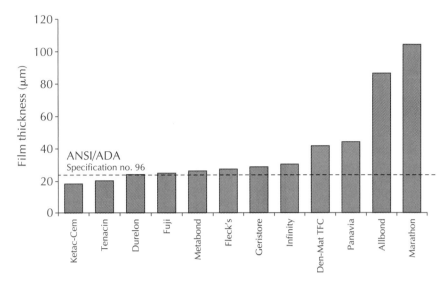

Fig. 31-2. The film thickness of a range of luting agents was tested according to ADA specification No. 8 for zinc phosphate cement (Now ANSI/ADA specification No. 96) by White and Yu.[56] Some of the adhesive materials possessed unacceptably high film thicknesses, which may translate into clinical problems for complete restoration seating.
(From Rosenstiel SF et al: J Prosthet Dent *80:280, 1998.)*

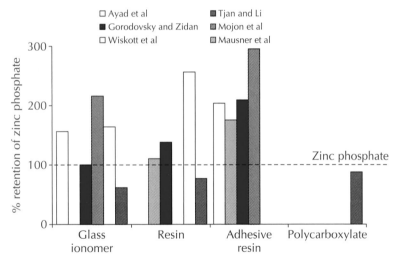

Fig. 31-3. **Crown-retention** studies. Effect of luting agent. These six in vitro studies evaluated the effect of luting agent on crown retention. The data were normalized as a percentage of the retention value with zinc phosphate cement. Adhesive resins had consistently greater retention than zinc phosphate. Conventional resins and glass ionomers yielded less consistent results.
(From Rosenstiel SF et al: J Prosthet Dent *80:280, 1998.)*

Although glass ionomers have been reported to cause sensitivity,[24] there appears to be little pulpal response at the histological level,[25] particularly if the remaining dentin thickness exceeds 1 mm.[26] Side-effects such as post-treatment sensitivity thought to result from a lack of biocompatibility may actually be a result of desiccation or bacterial contamination[27] of the dentin rather than irritation by the cement. The anecdotal reports that glass ionomer causes more post-treatment sensitivity have not been supported by clinical trials. Authors have reported little association between the choice of zinc phosphate or glass ionomer cement and increased pulpal sensitivity, provided manufacturers' recommendations were followed[28-30] (Fig. 31-5). If postcementation sensitivity becomes a problem, dentists should carefully evaluate their technique, particularly avoiding desiccation of the prepared dentin surface. Resin-modified glass-ionomer materials have been reported to exhibit less post-treatment sensitivity. Again, this information is anecdotal. A desensitizing agent may prevent sensitivity, although it may also

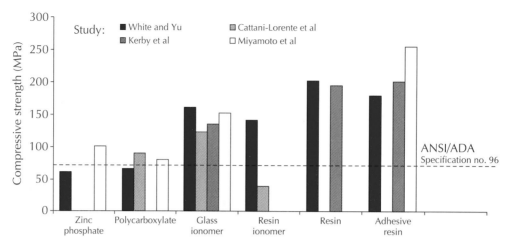

Fig. 31-4. Compressive strength of luting agents. Higher strength values were reported in these studies with the resin cements and glass ionomers than with zinc phosphate or polycarboxylate. Resin-modified glass ionomer exhibited greater variation than other cements.
(From Rosenstiel SF et al: J Prosthet Dent *80:280, 1998.)*

Fig. 31-5. Clinical trials that evaluated postcementation sensitivity of crowns cemented with zinc phosphate or glass ionomer cement. Contrary to anecdotal evidence, glass ionomer cemented crowns did not exhibit increased postcementation sensitivity.
(From Rosenstiel SF et al: J Prosthet Dent *80:280, 1998.)*

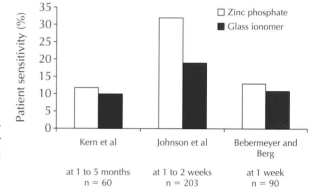

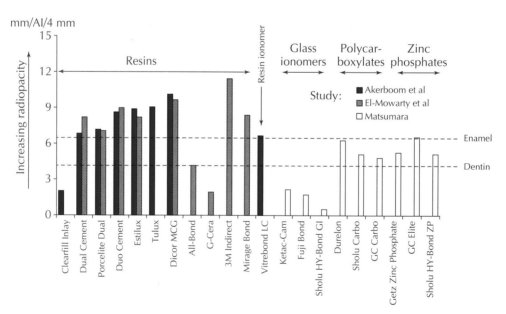

Fig. 31-6. Radiopacity of luting agents. These three in vitro studies compared the radiographic appearance of various luting agents to aluminum. The data were normalized to account for different specimen thicknesses used by the investigators. Excess luting agent will be more difficult to detect if materials with lower values are chosen. In addition, margin gaps and recurrent caries will be more difficult to diagnose.
(From Rosenstiel SF et al: J Prosthet Dent *80:280, 1998.)*

reduce retention, at least with some luting cements.[16,31] Some formulations of glass ionomer and resin cements are radiolucent (Fig. 31-6), which may prevent the practitioner from distinguishing between a cement line and recurrent caries, as well as detecting cement overhangs.[32] The use of a glass ionomer luting agent in general practice has been favorable, with low recurrent caries, excellent casting retention, and acceptable pulpal response.[33]

Zinc Oxide-eugenol with and without EBA. Reinforced ZOE cement is extremely biocompatible and provides an excellent seal. However, its physical properties are generally inferior to those of other cements, which limits its use.[34] In terms of **compressive strength,** solubility, and film thickness, another luting agent (e.g., zinc phosphate) should be used. The 2-ethoxybenzoic acid (EBA) modifier replaces a portion of the eugenol in conventional ZOE cement, although the change improves compressive strength without affecting its resistance to deformation; the cement should be used only in restorations with good inherent retention form where emphasis is on biocompatibility and pulpal protection. The EBA cement has a relatively short working time, and excess material is difficult to remove.

Resin-modified Glass ionomer Luting Agents. Resin-modified glass ionomers* were introduced in the 1990s in an attempt to combine some of the desirable properties of glass ionomer (i.e., fluoride release and adhesion) with the higher strength and low solubility of resins. These materials are less susceptible to early moisture exposure[35] than glass-ionomer and are currently among the most popular materials in general practice. Resin-modified glass ionomers should be avoided with all-ceramic restorations because they have been associated with fracture,[36,37] which is probably due to their water absorption and expansion.[38]

Resin Luting Agents. Unfilled resins have been used for cementation since the 1950s. Because of their high polymerization shrinkage and poor bio-

---

*The terminology for some of the newer glass-ionomer/resin combinations is rather confusing. In this textbook, the term *resin-modified glass ionomer* has been used. Other terms used for luting agents and restorative materials with a combination of glass ionomer and resin chemistries include *compomer* (mostly composite with some glass ionomer chemistry), *hybrid ionomer* (now considered obsolete), and *resin-reinforced glass ionomer.*

compatibility, these early products were unsuccessful, although they had very low solubility. Composite resin cements with greatly improved properties were developed for resin-retained prostheses (see Chapter 26) and are extensively used for the bonded ceramic technique (see Chapter 25). Resin cements are available with adhesive properties (i.e., they are capable of bonding chemically to dentin). Bonding is usually achieved with organophosphonates, HEMA (hydroxyethyl methacrylate), or 4-META (4 methacrylethyl trimellitic anhydride).[39] These developments, and their lack of solubility, have rekindled an interest in the use of resin cements for crowns and conventional fixed prostheses (Fig. 31-7). Resin luting agents are less biocompatible than cements such as glass ionomer, especially if they are not fully polymerized. They also tend to have greater film thickness.[40]

CHOICE OF LUTING AGENT
An ideal luting agent has a long working time, adheres well to both tooth structure and cast alloys, provides a good seal, is nontoxic to the pulp, has adequate strength properties, is compressible into thin layers, has a low viscosity and solubility, and exhibits good working and setting characteristics. In addition, any excess can be easily removed. Unfortunately, no such product exists (Tables 31-1 and 31-2).

Zinc Phosphate Cement. Despite its limited biocompatibility in terms of pulp irritation, zinc phosphate has a long history, and its limitations are well documented. This factor is important for cast restorations, which should be designed for long-term service. Zinc phosphate cement is probably still the luting agent of choice for otherwise normal, conservatively prepared teeth. Cavity varnish can be used to protect against pulp irritation from phosphoric acid and appears to have little effect on the amount of retention of the cemented restorations.[41]

Zinc Polycarboxylate Cement. This agent is recommended on retentive preparations when minimal pulp irritation is important (e.g., in children with large pulp chambers).

Glass Ionomer Cement. This has become a popular cement for luting cast restorations. It has good working properties, and because of its fluoride content, it may prevent recurrent caries.

Resin-modified Glass ionomer Luting Agents. Currently among the most popular luting agents, resin-modified glass ionomer luting agents have

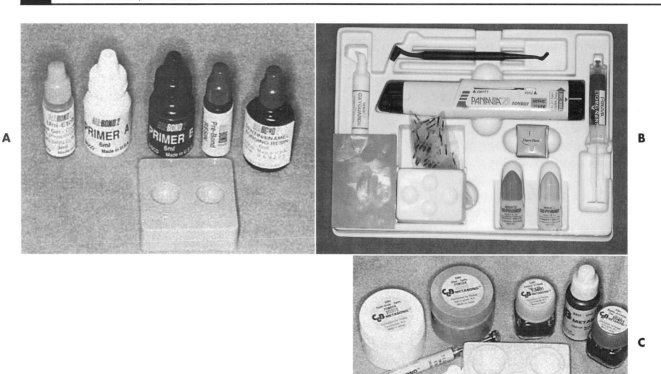

Fig. 31-7. Representative resin luting agents. **A,** All-Bond. **B,** Panavia. **C,** C & B Metabond.

Comparison of Available Luting Agents							TABLE 31-1
Property	Ideal Material	Zinc Phosphate	Poly-carboxylate	Glass Ionomer	Resin Ionomer	Composite Resin	Adhesive Resin
Film thickness (μm)*	Low	≤25	<25	<25	>25	>25	>25
Working time (min)	Long	1.5-5	1.75-2.5	2-3.5	2-4	3-10	0.5-5
Setting time (min)	Short	5-14	6-9	6-9	2	3-7	1-15
Compressive strength (MPa)†	High	62-101	67-91	122-162	40-141	194-200	179-255
Elastic modulus (GPa)‡	Dentin = 13.7 Enamel = 84-130§	13.2	nt‖	11.2	nt‖	17	4.5-9.8
Pulp irritation	Low	Moderate	Low	High	High	High	High
Solubility	Very low	High	High	Low	Very low	Very low	Very low
Microleakage¶	Very low	High	High to very high	Low to very high	Very low	High to very high	Very low to low
Removal of excess	Easy	Easy	Medium	Medium	Medium	Medium	Difficult
Retention#	High	Moderate	Low/ moderate	Moderate to high	nt‖	Moderate	High

*White SN, Yu Z: *J Prosthet Dent* 67:782, 1992; see also Fig. 31-2.
†See Fig. 31-4.
‡From Rosenstiel et al: *J Dent Res* 71:320, 1992.
§From O'Brien WJ: *Dental materials and their selection,* ed 2, Chicago, 1997, Quintessence, p. 351.
‖nt = not tested.
¶See Fig. 31-8.
#See Fig. 31-3.

Indications and Contraindications for Luting Agent Types   TABLE 31-2

Restoration	Indicated	Contraindicated
Cast crown, metal-ceramic crown, fixed partial denture	1,2,3,4,5,6,7	—
Crown or FPD with poor retention	1	2,3,4,5,6,7
MCC with porcelain margin	1,2,3,4,5,6,7	—
Casting on patient with history of post-treatment sensitivity	Consider 4 or 7	2
Pressed, high-leucite, ceramic crown	1,2	3,4,5,6,7
Slip-cast alumina crown	1,2,3,4,6,7	5
Ceramic inlay	1,2	3,4,5,6,7
Ceramic veneer	1,2	3,4,5,6,7
Resin-retained FPD	1,2	3,4,5,6,7
Cast post-and-core	1,2,3,5,6	4,7

Key:

Luting Agent Type	Chief Advantages	Chief Concerns	Precautions
1. Adhesive resin	Adhesive, low solubility	Film thickness, history of use	Moisture control
2. Composite resin	Low solubility	Film thickness, irritation	Use bonding resin, moisture control
3. Glass ionomer	Fluoride release	Solubility, leakage	Avoid early moisture exposure
4. Reinforced ZOE	Biocompatible	Low strength	Only for very retentive restorations
5. Resin ionomer	Low solubility, fluoride	Water sorption, history of use	Avoid with ceramic restorations
6. Zinc phosphate	History of use	Solubility, leakage	Use for "traditional" cast restorations
7. Zinc polycarboxylate	Biocompatible	Low strength, solubility	Do not reduce powder/liquid ratio

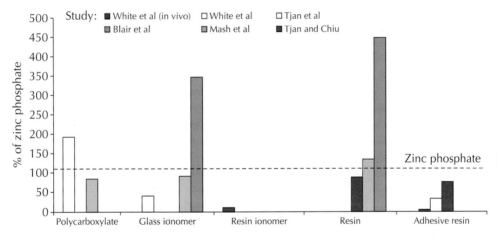

Fig. 31-8. Microleakage of luting agent. A comparison of data from one clinical and five laboratory studies expressed as a percentage of the value obtained for zinc phosphate cement. Considerable variation was reported, with adhesive resins and resin-modified glass ionomer exhibiting low microleakage values.
(From Rosenstiel SF et al: J Prosthet Dent 80:280, 1998.)

low solubility, adhesion, and low **microleakage** (Fig. 31-8). The popularity of these materials is mainly due to the perceived benefit of reduced post-cementation sensitivity.

Adhesive Resin. Long-term evaluations of these materials are not yet available, so they cannot be recommended for routine use. Laboratory testing yields high retention strength values,[42] but there is concern that stresses caused by polymerization shrinkage, magnified in thin films,[43] lead to marginal leakage.

Adhesive resin may be indicated when a casting has become displaced through lack of retention.

PREPARATION OF THE RESTORATION AND TOOTH SURFACE FOR CEMENTATION (Fig. 31-9)

The performance of all luting agents is degraded if the material is contaminated with water, blood, or saliva. Therefore the restoration and tooth must be carefully cleaned and dried after the try-in procedure, although excessive drying of the tooth must be avoided to prevent damage to the odontoblasts. The

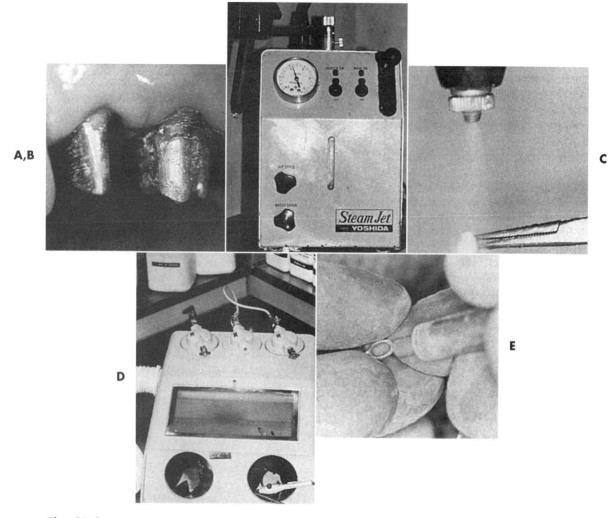

Fig. 31-9.   Tooth preparations and restorations must be carefully prepared immediately before cementation. **A,** Clean and dry preparations. **B** and **C,** Steam cleaner is convenient for removing traces of polishing compound from the restorations. **D** and **E,** Air abrasion of internal restoration surface.

casting is best prepared by air-abrading the fitting surface with 50-μm alumina. This should be done carefully to avoid abrading the polished surfaces or margins. Air abrasion has increased the in vitro retention of castings by 64%.[44] Alternative cleaning methods include steam cleaning, ultrasonics, and organic solvents.

Before the initiation of cement mixing, isolating the area of cementation and cleaning and drying the tooth is mandatory. However, the tooth should never be excessively desiccated. Overdrying the prepared tooth will lead to postoperative sensitivity. (The techniques for moisture control, essential to proper cementation, are described in Chapter 14.) If a nonadhesive cement (zinc phosphate) is to be used, the tooth should be cleaned,* gently dried, and coated with cavity varnish or dentin bonding resin.

Armamentarium (Fig. 31-10)
- Mirror
- Explorer
- Dental floss
- Cotton rolls
- Prophylaxis cup
- Flour of pumice
- Cement (powder and liquid)
- White stones
- Cuttle disks
- Local anesthetic (if needed)
- Saliva evacuator
- Forceps
- Thick glass slab (chilled)
- Cement spatula
- Gauze squares
- Adhesive foil
- Plastic instrument

*Pumice and/or a chlorohexadine preparation such as Consepsis (Ultradent) is recommended.

Step-by-step Procedure (Fig. 31-11). Zinc phosphate cement is used to illustrate a typical proce-

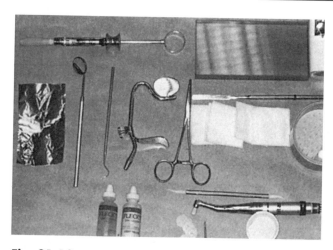

Fig. 31-10. Armamentarium for permanent cementation.

dure, but the steps may vary slightly, depending on the cement chosen. The differences with glass-ionomer are pointed out in the description.

1. Immediately before cementation, inspect all preparation surfaces for cleanliness. Remove any provisional luting agent with a pumice wash or hydrogen peroxide (see Fig. 31-9, A). Since the casting-cement interface is where failure occurs when a crown is displaced, the casting should be air-abraded, steam cleaned, or cleaned ultrasonically and washed with alcohol to remove any remaining rouge or Tripoli that might interfere with retention of the finished restoration (see Fig. 31-9 B, E).

2. Isolate the area with cotton rolls and place the saliva evacuator. On occasion, a rubber dam can be used but only rarely for extracoronal restorations. Avoid using cavity cleaners to aid in drying the preparation because they may adversely affect pulpal health.

3. Apply cavity varnish to reduce pulp irritation from the zinc phosphate cement. Obviously, a varnish should not be applied with polycarboxylate or glass ionomer cements, since it would prevent their adhesion to dentin.

4. Cool the glass slab under running water, dry it, and dispense the proper amount of powder and liquid. The cooled slab retards setting and allows additional powder to be incorporated in the liquid. This results in higher compressive strength and reduced solubility of the set cement. A paper mixing pad is generally used with glass ionomer or polycarboxylate cements.

Frozen Slab Technique. This technique presents a practical way to increase the working time and reduce the setting time of zinc phosphate cement.[45,46] The technique uses a 50% increased powder/liquid ratio, and mixing is performed on a frozen glass slab. There is no adverse effect on compressive strength, solubility, or retention,[47,48] and the pH rise in the cement may be accelerated.[49] The frozen slab technique is reliable and is particularly effective when multiple castings are to be cemented. An incidental advantage of this technique is that the condensation that forms on the glass slab facilitates cleanup of excess cement. Reduced temperature mixing has also been applied to glass ionomer cements as a way of increasing working time and increasing powder/liquid ratio. Film thickness measurements suggest that the procedure is beneficial.[50]

5. Divide the powder into small quantities (each about one sixth of the total mix) and add them one at a time to the liquid (Fig. 31-11, B). After the first increment of powder has been incorporated for 15 to 20 seconds, a second is added, and so on. During mixing, a large surface area (e.g., 60% of the slab) should be used so that the heat of the exothermic setting reaction will be dissipated. The mixing continues until all powder has been incorporated (about 90 seconds). For glass ionomer cement, the measured powder is divided into two equal parts and mixed with a plastic spatula. The first increment is rapidly incorporated in 10 seconds, and the second increment is incorporated and mixed for an additional 10 seconds.

6. When the mixing procedure is completed, check the consistency by lifting some cement off the slab with the spatula (Fig. 31-11, C). The cement is of proper consistency if it pulls into a thread of about 20 mm in length before "snapping" back onto the slab. The consistency of properly mixed glass ionomer is noticeably more viscous than zinc phosphate, but the material thins out with seating pressure.

7. Apply a thin coat of cement to the clean internal surface of the restoration (Fig. 31-11, D). To extend working time, the cement should be applied to a cool restoration rather than to a warm tooth.

8. Dry the tooth again with a light blast of air and push the restoration into place (Fig. 31-11, E). Final seating is achieved by rocking with an orangewood stick until all excess cement has escaped (Fig. 31-11, F). Seating the restoration firmly with a rocking, dynamic seating force is important (Fig. 31-11, G). Using a static load may cause binding of the restoration and lead to incomplete seating. Without rocking the casting, increasing the load only seems to increase the binding reaction.[51] Excessive force during seating should be avoided, especially with metal-ceramic or all-ceramic restorations, which may fracture.

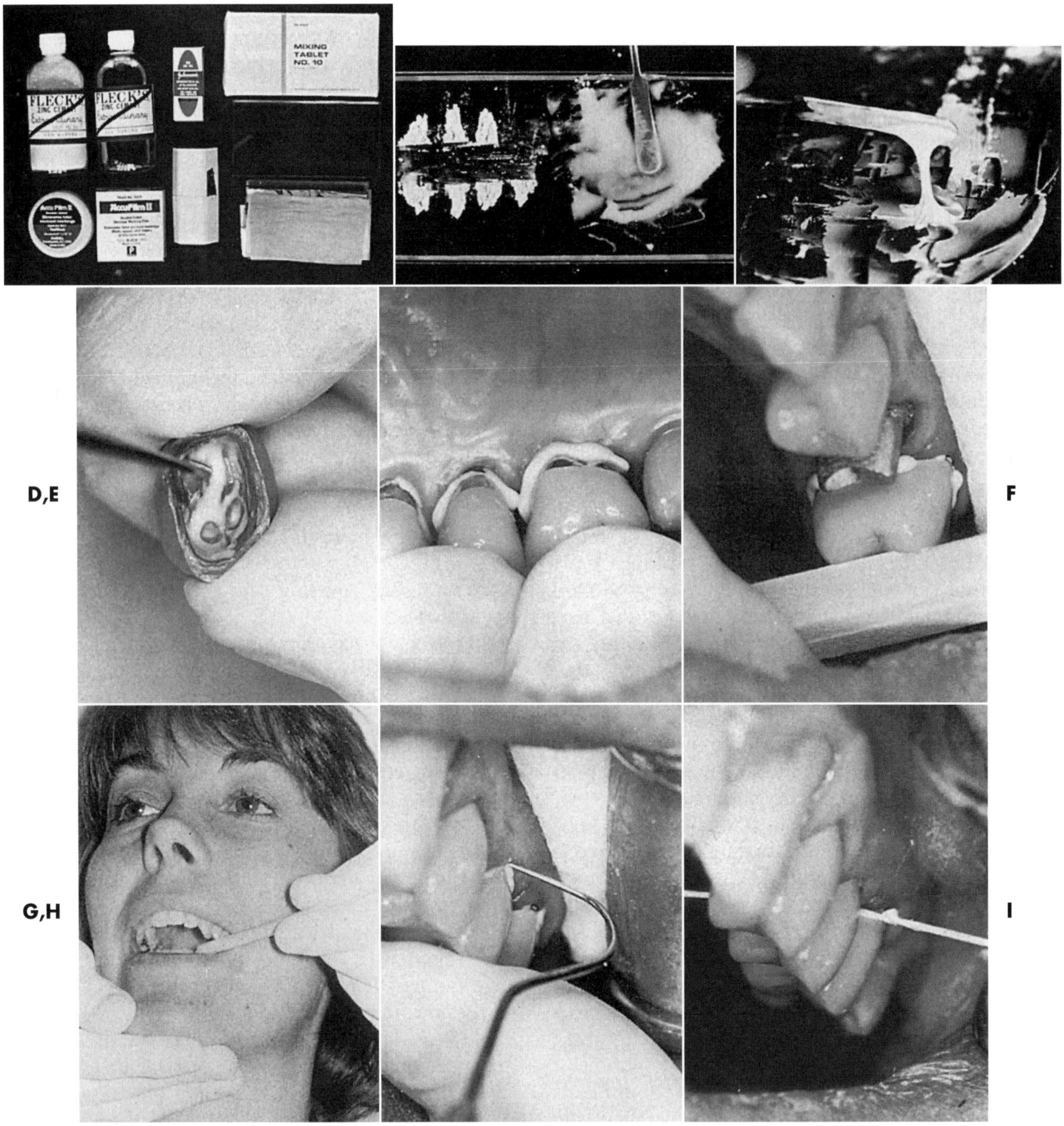

Fig. 31-11. Cementation technique with zinc phosphate. **A,** Armamentarium. **B,** The powder is divided into small increments and mixed with liquid on a cool slab over a large surface area. **C,** The consistency of the mix is evaluated by pulling out a "thread" of cement. The thread should break at about 20 mm. **D,** The internal surface of the restoration is coated. **E,** The restoration is seated. **F** and **G,** An orangewood stick applied with a rocking motion against the restoration will ensure that all excess cement is expressed. **H,** Complete seating is immediately verified with an explorer. **I,** When set, the excess cement is removed from around the margins. A length of dental floss with a knot tied in it is useful for removing excess interproximally. (*A to C courtesy Dr. J.H. Bailey; G rephotographed from Campagni WV:* Calif Dent Assoc J *12:21, 1984.*)

9. After the casting is seated, check the margins to verify that the restoration is fully in place (Fig. 31-11, *H*). Protect the setting cement from moisture by covering it with an adhesive foil (e.g., Dri-Foil*).

10. When it is fully set, remove excess cement with an explorer. Early cement removal may lead to early moisture exposure at the

Jelenko International: Armonk, N.Y.

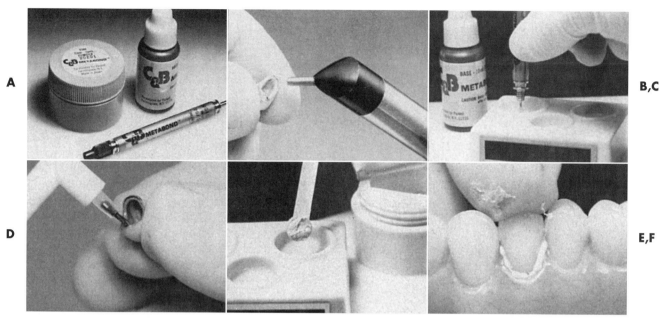

Fig. 31-12. **A,** C & B Metabond resin cement. **B,** The internal surface of the casting is cleaned in the laboratory with air-abrasion after clinical evaluation. The tooth surface is cleaned with pumice and water. The recommended dentin conditioner is applied for 10 seconds, rinsed off, and the tooth is dried. The refrigerated base liquid is dispensed into one well of the supplied ceramic mixing dish. The dish has a thermometer incorporated that should indicate between 16° and 22° C. **C,** One drop of catalyst is added to the base and stirred for 5 seconds. **D,** Both the tooth and the casting are painted with the mixed liquid. **E,** In a second well, another base/catalyst mixture is made, to which two scoops of powder are added and stirred. **F,** If the tooth or casting has dried, it is rapidly rewetted from the first well, the casting is filled with the resin, and the restoration is seated into place. Excess resin is removed after it has completely set (approximately 10 minutes). It is important not to remove resin before it has fully set because the rubbery material will pull away from the margins. *(Courtesy Parkell Products.)*

margins with increased solubility. Some cements, such as polycarboxylate or resin, tend to pull away from the margins if excess removal is performed too early. Dental floss with a small knot in it can be used to remove any irritating residual cement interproximally and from the gingival sulcus (Fig. 31-11, *I*). The sulcus should contain no cement. After the excess has been removed, the occlusion can be checked once more with Mylar shim stock.

11. Cements take at least 24 hours to develop their final strength. Therefore, the patient should be cautioned to chew carefully for a day or two.

Resin Luting Agents. Resin luting agents are available in a wide range of formulations. These can be categorized on the basis of polymerization method (chemical-cure, light-cure, or dual-cure) and the presence of dentin bonding mechanisms. Metal restorations require a chemically cured system, whereas a light- or dual-cure is appropriate with ceramics. Resins formulated for cementing conventional castings must have lower film thickness than materials

designed for ceramics or orthodontic brackets. However, this may be achieved at the expense of filler particle content and will adversely affect other properties such as polymerization shrinkage.

Manipulative techniques vary widely, depending on the brand of resin cement. For example, Panavia Ex* sets very rapidly when air is excluded. The directions call for the material to be spatulated in a thin film. It will set rapidly if piled up on the mixing pad. Another material, C & B Metabond† is mixed in a ceramic well that must be chilled to prevent premature setting. Mixing techniques for these materials are illustrated in Figs. 31-12 and 31-13.

■ CEMENTATION PROCEDURES FOR CERAMIC VENEERS AND INLAYS

These restorations rely on resin bonding for retention and strength. The cementation steps are critical to the restoration's success; careless handling of the resin lut-

---

*J. Morita USA, Inc.: Irvine, Calif.
†Parkell Products: Farmingdale, N.Y.

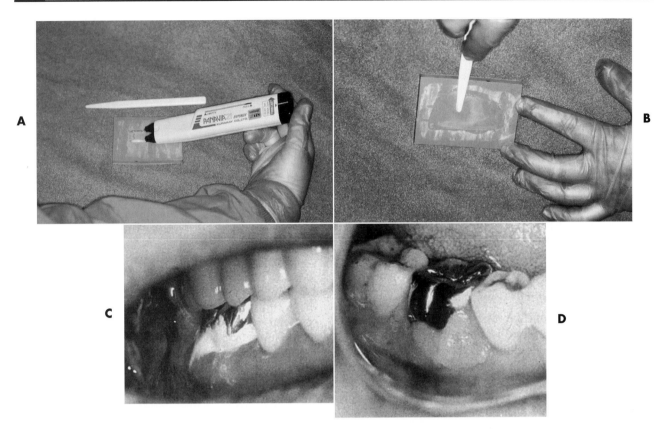

Fig. 31-13. **A,** Panavia resin cement. **B,** Measured powder and liquid spatulated for 60 to 90 seconds. The mix becomes more creamy as it is mixed. The cement sets if oxygen is excluded, so it should not be piled up. Instead, it should be spread out over a large surface area. **C,** Apply a thin coat of the cement, seat the restoration, and remove excess cement. **D,** The cement is coated with oxygen-inhibiting gel to promote polymerization.
(Courtesy J. Morita USA, Inc.)

ing agent may be a key factor in their prognosis. Bonding is achieved by performing the following steps:
1. Etching the fitting surface of the ceramic with hydrofluoric acid
2. Applying a silane coupling agent to the ceramic
3. Etching the enamel with phosphoric acid
4. Applying a resin bonding agent to etched enamel and silane
5. Seating the restoration with a composite resin luting agent (Fig. 31-14)

The etching and silanating steps are presented in Chapter 25.

SELECTION OF RESIN LUTING AGENT

Composite resin luting agents are available in a range of formulations. For veneers, a light-cured material can be used. For inlays, a chemical- or dual-cure material is preferred to ensure maximum polymerization of the resin in the less accessible proximal areas. Dual-cured resin provides better marginal adaptation at the critical gingival margin area,[52] because voids incorporated during mixing may reduce the harmful contraction stresses of the resin.[53]

The shade of veneers can be modified by the shade of the luting agent. To facilitate shade selection, color-matched try-in pastes are available from some manufacturers (e.g., Nexus*).

BONDING THE RESTORATION
Armamentarium (Fig. 31-15)
- Mirror
- Explorer
- Rubber dam kit
- Local anesthetic
- Saliva evacuator
- Forceps
- Scalpel
- Curette
- Plastic instrument
- Dental tape
- Mylar strips
- Cotton rolls

*SDS Kerr: Orange, Calif.

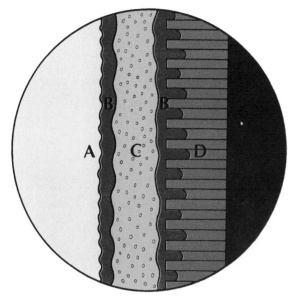

Fig. 31-14. Schematic of resin bonding technique. **A,** Ceramic surface (etched and silanated). **B,** Unfilled resin. **C,** Resin luting agent. **D,** Etched enamel.

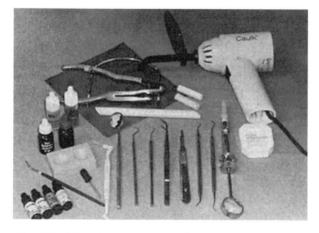

Fig. 31-15. Armamentarium for bonding procedure.

- Prophylaxis cup
- Flour of pumice
- Acid etchant
- Porcelain etchant
- Silane coupling agent
- Acetone
- Glycerin or try-in paste
- Bonding agent
- Brush
- Resin luting agent
- Curing light
- Fine grit diamonds
- Porcelain polishing kit

Step-by-step Procedure (Fig. 31-16)

1. Clean the teeth with pumice and water (or a chlorhexadine preparation). Isolate them with the rubber dam or displacement cord. A luting agent that contains zinc oxide-eugenol should be avoided for cementing provisional restorations before resin bonding. Eugenol inhibits the polymerization of the resin. Cleansing with pumice will leave a ZOE residue mixed with pumice, which can inhibit bonding.[54] Etching with 37% phosphoric acid after cleaning with pumice may be the best way to remove ZOE.[55]
2. Try in restorations with glycerin or a try-in paste (Fig. 31-16, *A*). Verify fit, shade, and insertion sequence.
3. Clean the restorations thoroughly in water with ultrasonic agitation. Use acetone if luting resin was used to verify the shade at try-in.* Dry the restorations.
4. Etch and silanate the restorations as described in Chapter 25 (Fig. 31-16, *B*).
5. Acid etch the enamel; 37% phosphoric acid is generally used and is applied for 20 seconds. Rinse thoroughly and dry.
6. Apply a thin layer of bonding resin to the preparation. Brush, rather than air-thin, the bonding resin, because air-thinning might inhibit polymerization. Do not polymerize this layer, because it might interfere with complete seating.
7. For veneers, place a Mylar matrix strip at the mesial and distal surfaces of the prepared tooth (Fig. 31-16, *C*).
8. Apply composite resin luting agent to the restoration; be especially careful to avoid trapping air. (Dual-cure is recommended for inlay and onlays; light cure is recommended for veneers) (Fig. 31-16, *D*).
9. Position the restoration gently, removing excess luting agent with an instrument (Fig. 31-16, *E*).
10. Hold the restoration in place while light-curing the resin. Do not press on the center of veneers; they may flex and break (Fig. 31-16, *F*).
11. Use dental tape to remove resin flash from the interproximal margins of inlays and onlays before curing these areas.

---

*This technique requires care. The restoration should not be exposed to the unit light; otherwise, the resin will polymerize prematurely.

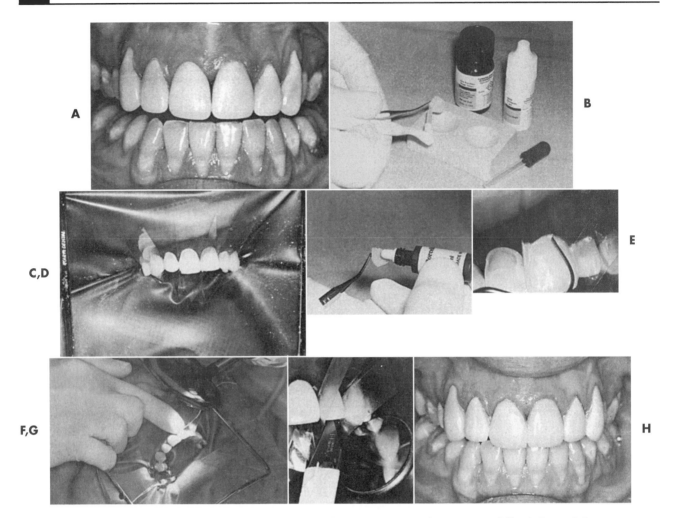

Fig. 31-16. Try-in and bonding procedure. **A,** The veneers are tried in very carefully. A drop of glycerin on the fitting surface aids in shade assessment and provides retention. If necessary, the shade can be modified slightly with colored luting agents. The luting agent must not polymerize during try-in; in particular, the unit light must not shine directly on the restoration. **B,** The veneers are thoroughly cleaned in acetone and are silanated according to manufacturer recommendations. **C,** The teeth are isolated, pumiced, and etched. Mylar strips are placed between adjacent teeth. **D,** The veneers are filled with resin luting agent and gently seated. **E,** Excess resin is removed with an explorer. **F,** The resin is polymerized. **G,** Gross excess resin is trimmed with a scalpel, and the margins are finished with fine-grit diamonds and diamond polishing paste. **H,** The completed restorations.

12. Do not undercure the resin cement. Allow at least 40 seconds for each area.
13. Remove resin flash with a scalpel or sharp curette (Fig. 31-16, *G*).
14. Finish accessible margins and occlusion with fine diamonds, using water spray. Use finishing strips for the interproximal margins.
15. Polish adjusted areas with rubber wheels or points and then with diamond polishing paste.

◼ REVIEW OF TECHNIQUE

Fig. 31-17 illustrates the cementation of six maxillary anterior metal-ceramic crowns.

1. The preparations are thoroughly cleaned, making sure all provisional luting agent is removed (Fig. 31-17, *A*).
2. The restorations are seated, and a readily accessible area of the margin is examined with an explorer (Fig. 31-17, *B*); this evaluation will provide a reference for complete seating during cementation.
3. The restorations are thoroughly cleaned with air abrasion, steam cleaning, or ultrasonics (Fig. 31-17, *C*).
4. The cement is mixed according to the manufacturer's recommendations (Fig. 31-17, *D*).
5. The restorations are seated to place with a firm rocking pressure (Fig. 31-17, *E*).

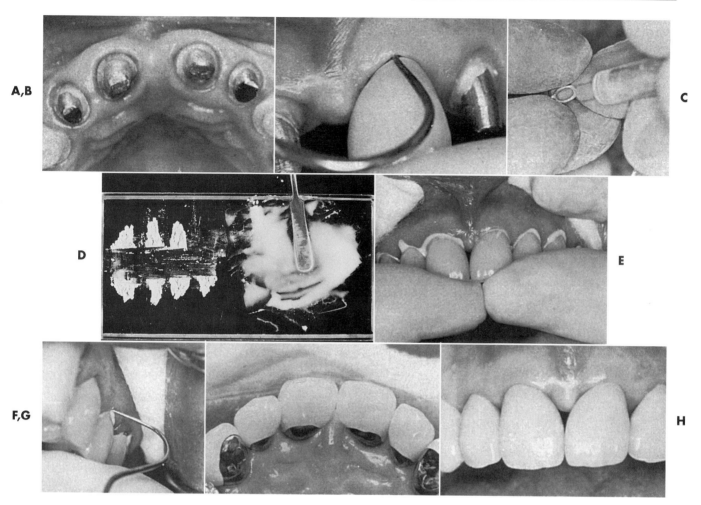

A,B

C

D

E

F,G

H

Fig. 31-17. Technique review.

6. The accessible margin area is quickly reexamined to ensure complete seating (Fig. 31-17, *F*).
7. Once the cement has completely set, all excess is removed (Fig. 31-17, *G* and *H*).

SUMMARY

Proper moisture control is essential for the cementation step. The restoration must be carefully prepared for cementation, including the removal of all polishing compounds. Air-abrading the fitting surface is recommended. The luting agent of choice is mixed according to manufacturer recommendations, and the restoration is seated, using a rocking action. The cement must be protected from moisture during its initial set. Removal of excess cement from the gingival sulcus is critical for continued periodontal health.

Additional steps are necessary for adhesively bonded restorations. These steps must be carefully sequenced according to manufacturer directions.

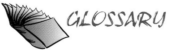

GLOSSARY

cement: *n 1:* a binding element or agency used as a substance to make objects adhere to each other, or something serving to firmly unite. *2:* a material that, on hardening, will fill a space or bind adjacent objects.

cementation: *obs 1:* the process of attaching parts with a cement. *2:* attaching a restoration to natural teeth with a cement.

placement: *v:* the process of directing a prosthesis to a desired location; the introduction of prosthesis into a patient's mouth—also called denture placement, prosthesis placement.

Study Questions

1. Discuss the principal differences in chemistry, physical properties, and manipulative variables for three different types of luting agents. How do the differences affect their clinically indicated use?
2. What are properties of the "ideal" luting agent?
3. Compare the recommended techniques for mixing zinc phosphate cement and Panavia Ex.
4. Describe how the tooth and the restoration are prepared before cementing a metal-ceramic crown with glass ionomer cement. How does this change when a different luting agent is selected?
5. Discuss the steps involved in cementation of two laminate veneers on teeth # 8 and # 9.

REFERENCES

1. Swartz ML et al: In vitro degradation of cements: a comparison of three test methods, *J Prosthet Dent* 62:17, 1989.
2. Stannard JG, Sornkul E: Demineralization resistance and tensile bond strength of four luting agents after acid attack, *Int J Prosthod* 2:467, 1989.
3. Dewald JP, Arcoria CJ, Marker VA: Evaluation of the interactions between amalgam, cement and gold castings, *J Dent* 20:121, 1992.
4. Knibbs PJ, Walls AW: A laboratory and clinical evaluation of three dental luting cements, *J Oral Rehabil* 16:467, 1989.
5. Jacobs MS, Windeler AS: An investigation of dental luting cement solubility as a function of the marginal gap, *J Prosthet Dent* 65:436, 1991.
6. Dupuis V et al: Solubility and disintegration of zinc phosphate cement, *Biomaterials* 13:467, 1992.
7. Dedmon HW: Ability to evaluate nonvisible margins with an explorer, *Oper Dent* 10:6, 1985.
8. Phillips RW: *Skinner's science of dental materials*, ed 9, Philadelphia, 1991, WB Saunders, p. 491.
9. Langeland K, Langeland LK: Pulp reactions to crown preparation, impression, temporary crown fixation, and permanent cementation, *J Prosthet Dent* 15:129, 1965.
10. Going RE, Mitchem JC: Cements for permanent luting: a summarizing review, *J Am Dent Assoc* 91:107, 1975.
11. Dahl BL et al: Clinical study of two luting cements used on student-treated patients: final report, *Dent Mater* 2:269, 1986.
12. Black SM, Charlton G: Survival of crowns and bridges related to luting cements, *Restor Dent* 6:26, 1990.
13. Phillips RW: *Skinner's science of dental materials*, ed 9, Philadelphia, 1991, WB Saunders, p. 490.
14. Osborne JW, Wolff MS: The effect of powder/liquid ratio on the in vivo solubility of polycarboxylate cement, *J Prosthet Dent* 66:49, 1991.
15. Øilo G, Jørgensen KD: The influence of surface roughness on the retentive ability of two dental luting cements, *J Oral Rehabil* 5:377, 1978.

16. Mausner IK, Goldstein GR, Georgescu M: Effect of two dentinal desensitizing agents on retention of complete cast coping using four cements, *J Prosthet Dent* 75:129, 1996.
17. Swartz ML et al: Long term F release from glass ionomer cements, *J Dent Res* 63:158, 1984.
18. Muzynski BL et al: Fluoride release from glass ionomers used as luting agents, *J Prosthet Dent* 60:41, 1988.
19. Rosenstiel SF et al: Dental luting agents: a review of the current literature, *J Prosthet Dent* 80:280, 1998.
20. Um CM, Øilo G: The effect of early water contact on glass-ionomer cements, *Quintessence Int* 23:209, 1992.
21. Curtis SR, Richards MW, Meiers JC: Early erosion of glass-ionomer cement at crown margins, *Int J Prosthodont* 6:553, 1993.
22. McLean JW: Glass-ionomer cements, *Br Dent J* 164:293, 1988.
23. Cho E, Kopel H, White SN: Moisture susceptibility of resin-modified glass-ionomer materials, *Quintessence Int* 26:351, 1995.
24. Council on Dental Materials, Instruments, and Equipment, American Dental Association: Reported sensitivity to glass ionomer luting cements, *J Am Dent Assoc* 109:476, 1984.
25. Heys RJ et al: An evaluation of a glass ionomer luting agent: pulpal histological response, *J Am Dent Assoc* 114:607, 1987.
26. Pameijer CH, Stanley HR, Ecker G: Biocompatibility of a glass ionomer luting agent. II. Crown cementation, *Am J Dent* 4:134, 1991.
27. Torstenson B: Pulpal reaction to a dental adhesive in deep human cavities, *Endod Dent Traumatol* 11:172, 1995.
28. Johnson GH, Powell LV, DeRouen TA: Evaluation and control of post-cementation pulpal sensitivity: zinc phosphate and glass ionomer luting cements, *J Am Dent Assoc* 124:38, 1993.
29. Bebermeyer RD, Berg JH: Comparison of patient-perceived postcementation sensitivity with glass-ionomer and zinc phosphate cements, *Quintessence Int* 25:209, 1994.

30. Kern M et al: Clinical comparison of postoperative sensitivity for a glass ionomer and a zinc phosphate luting cement, *J Prosthet Dent* 75:159, 1996.

31. Pameijer CH et al: Influence of low-viscosity liners on the retention of three luting materials, *Int J Periodont Restor Dent* 12:195, 1992.

32. Goshima T, Goshima Y: Radiographic detection of recurrent carious lesions associated with composite restorations, *Oral Surg* 70:236, 1990.

33. Brackett WW, Metz JE: Performance of a glass ionomer luting cement over 5 years in a general practice, *J Prosthet Dent* 67:59, 1992.

34. Silvey RG, Myers GE: Clinical study of dental cements. VI. A study of zinc phosphate, EBA-reinforced zinc oxide eugenol and polyacrylic acid cements as luting agents in fixed prostheses, *J Dent Res* 56:1215, 1977.

35. Cho E, Kopel H, White SN: Moisture susceptibility of resin-modified glass-ionomer materials, *Quintessence Int* 26:351, 1995.

36. Letters to the editor: *Quintessence Int* 27:655, 1996.

37. Leevailoj C et al: In vitro study of fracture incidence and compressive fracture load of all-ceramic crowns cemented with resin-modified glass ionomer and other luting agents, *J Prosthet Dent* 80:699, 1998.

38. Knobloch L, Kerby RE, McMillen K: Solubility and sorption of resin-based luting cements, *J Dent Res* 75:372, 1996 (abstract no. 2840).

39. Phillips RW: *Skinner's science of dental materials*, ed 9, Philadelphia, 1991, WB Saunders, p. 497.

40. Caughman WF et al: Glass ionomer and composite resin cements: effects on oral cells, *J Prosthet Dent* 63:513, 1990.

41. Felton DA et al: Effect of cavity varnish on retention of cemented cast crowns, *J Prosthet Dent* 57:411, 1987.

42. Tjan AHL, Tao L: Seating and retention of complete crowns with a new adhesive resin cement, *J Prosthet Dent* 67:478, 1992.

43. Feilzer AJ et al: Setting stress in composite resin in relation to configuration of the restoration, *J Dent Res* 66:636, 1987.

44. O'Connor RP et al: Effect of internal microblasting on retention of cemented cast crowns, *J Prosthet Dent* 64:557, 1990.

45. Henschel CJ: The effect of mixing surface temperatures upon dental cementation, *J Am Dent Assoc* 30:1583, 1943.

46. Kendzior GM, Leinfelder KF: Characteristics of zinc phosphate cements mixed at sub-zero temperatures, *J Dent Res* 55(special issue B):B95, 1976 (abstract no. 134).

47. Myers CL et al: A comparison of properties for zinc phosphate cements mixed on room temperature and frozen slabs, *J Prosthet Dent* 40:409, 1978.

48. Rosenstiel SF, Gegauff AG: Mixing variables of zinc phosphate cement and their influence on the seating and retention of complete crowns, *Int J Prosthodont* 2:138, 1989.

49. Fakiha ZA et al: Rapid mixing of zinc phosphate cement for fixed prosthodontic procedures, *J Prosthet Dent* 67:52, 1992.

50. Brackett WW, Vickery JM: Reduced temperature mixing of glass-ionomer luting agents (in press).

51. Rosenstiel SF, Gegauff AG: Improving the cementation of complete cast crowns: a comparison of static and dynamic seating methods, *J Am Dent Assoc* 117:845, 1988.

52. Noack MJ et al: Marginal adaptation of porcelain inlays luted with different composite materials, *J Dent Res* 69:161, 1990 (abstract).

53. Alster D et al: The dependence of shrinkage stress reduction on porosity concentration in thin resin layers, *J Dent Res* 71:1619, 1992.

54. Mojon P, Hawbolt EB, MacEntee MI: A comparison of two methods for removing zinc oxide-eugenol provisional cement, *Int J Prosthodont* 5:78, 1992.

55. Schwartz R, Davis R, Mayhew R: Effect of a ZOE temporary cement on the bond strength of a resin luting cement, *Am J Dent* 3:28, 1990.

56. White SN, Yu Z: Physical properties of fixed prosthodontic, resin composite luting agents, *Int J Prosthodont* 6:384, 1993.

POSTOPERATIVE CARE

After placement and cementation of a fixed partial denture (FPD), patient treatment continues with a carefully structured sequence of postoperative appointments designed to monitor the patient's dental health (Fig. 32-1), stimulate meticulous **plaque-control** habits, identify any incipient disease, and introduce whatever corrective treatment may be needed before irreversible damage occurs.

Patients should be instructed in special plaque-control measures, especially around pontics and connectors, and the use of special oral hygiene aids such as floss threaders (Fig. 32-2). If pontics are appropriate in design (see Chapter 20), floss can be looped through the embrasure spaces on each side; the loop can be pulled tightly against the convex pontic tissue surface. A sliding motion is then used to remove dental plaque (Fig. 32-3). Flossing under pontics is essential to improve prosthesis longevity. When dental floss is used, the mucosa beneath pontics remains healthy; without it, mild or moderate inflammation results.[1] Furthermore, tissue response is independent of the pontic material.[2]

Recall examinations are especially important for patients with extensive restorations and should be carried out by the dentist. Responsibility for follow-up care should not be delegated to auxiliary personnel (although good cooperation with a dental hygienist can be beneficial for success).

Detecting disease around an FPD can be extremely difficult at a stage when corrective treatment is still relatively simple. For instance, partial dissolution of the luting agent may be difficult to diagnose next to a subgingival margin. Caries is often

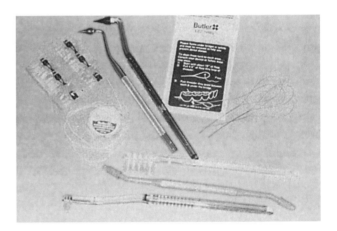

Fig. 32-2. Oral hygiene aids designed to maintain FPDs.

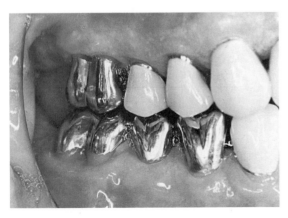

Fig. 32-1. Treatment after placement of multiple restorations. To ensure tissue health and long-term success, proper oral hygiene is mandatory.

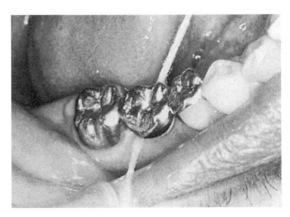

Fig. 32-3. The patient should be instructed in the use of floss to clean FPDs.

detected only after irreversible pulp involvement has resulted. Caries under a crown is more difficult to detect radiographically, although bitewings provide some information interproximally. Follow-up studies on patients with FPDs reveal that identifying risk factors and predicting the development of caries in any particular patient is complicated. However, there is no indication that caries is more likely in association with prostheses than on unrestored teeth.[3]

If caries is overlooked, disease may rapidly progress to the point where the fabrication of a new prosthesis becomes inevitable, or even worse, where tooth loss results.

POSTCEMENTATION APPOINTMENTS

To enable the dentist to monitor the function and comfort of the prosthesis and to verify that proper plaque control has been mastered by the patient (Fig. 32-4), an appointment is generally scheduled within a week to 10 days after the cementation of an FPD. The dentist should check carefully that the gingival sulcus remains clear of any residual cement that may have been overlooked previously and that all aspects of the occlusion remain satisfactory.

Radiolucent cements should be avoided because detecting excess luting agent radiographically is impossible if that material is effectively radiolucent. As the radiopacity of the luting agent increases, the detection threshold for marginal overhangs decreases; therefore, a luting agent should be chosen that is as radiopaque as possible. In practice, available luting agents come in a wide range of radiopacities.[4-6] Fig. 32-5 summarizes data from these studies.

The presence of "polished" facets on the contacting surfaces of cast restorations at the postcementation appointment should lead to a careful reassessment and correction of the occlusion. If any minor shift in tooth position has occurred, some **occlusal**

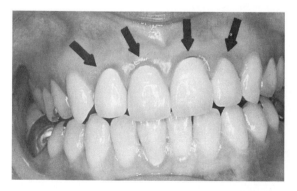

Fig. 32-4. Postcementation monitoring of plaque control is necessary around recently cemented restorations. Poor oral hygiene has led to gingival inflammation *(arrows)*.

adjustment may be necessary. If so, the patient is rescheduled for the following week to ensure that no further correction is needed.

PERIODIC RECALL

Patients with cast restorations should be recalled at least every 6 months. Less frequent recall may lead to oversight of recurrent caries or the development of periodontal disease. Patients who have been provided with extensive fixed prostheses (Fig. 32-6) will need more frequent recall appointments, particularly when advanced periodontal disease was present. The appointments can be coordinated by the restorative dentist or the periodontist. To ensure treatment continuity, establishing in advance who will assume primary responsibility for coordinating recall appointments is imperative.

HISTORY AND GENERAL EXAMINATION

The patient's medical history should be reviewed and updated at least annually. The patient should be examined using the principles introduced in Chapter 1. Particular attention is paid to the soft tissues, because early signs of oral cancer may be detected at a recall appointment.

ORAL HYGIENE, DIET, AND SALIVA

Patients tend to become somewhat less diligent in their plaque-control efforts when the active phase of their treatment is completed. The dentist should look carefully for any signs of deterioration in oral hygiene and assess the general effectiveness of plaque control at every recall with an objective index (Fig. 32-7). Deficiencies must be identified early, and corrective therapy should be initiated. The dentist should ask about changes in diet, particularly increased sugar consumption or "fad" diets. Excessive weight loss or gain should also be investigated. For instance, a patient who has recently stopped smoking may start ingesting large amounts of candy, with a resulting increase in carious damage.

Saliva plays an important role in dental caries. Patients with xerostomia can rapidly develop extensive carious lesions.[7] Diagnosing the cause of reduced saliva is imperative and is often due to drug side effects.

DENTAL CARIES

Dental caries (Fig. 32-8) is the most common cause of failure of a cast restoration.[8-11] Detection can be very difficult,[12] particularly where complete coverage is used. At each appointment, the teeth should be thoroughly dried and visually inspected (Fig. 32-9). The explorer must be used very carefully

Radiopacity
Luting Agents

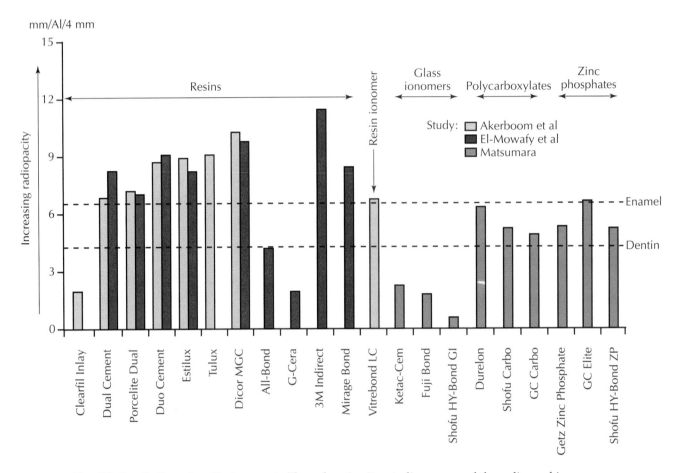

Fig. 32-5. Radiopacity of luting agents. These three in vitro studies compared the radiographic appearance of various luting agents to aluminum. The data were normalized to account for different specimen thicknesses used by the investigators. Excess luting agent will be more difficult to detect if materials with lower values are chosen. In addition, margin gaps and recurrent caries will be more difficult to diagnose.

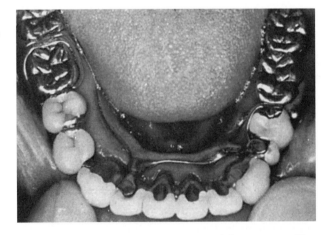

Fig. 32-6. Patients who have received extensive treatment of this nature will require more frequent follow-up care.

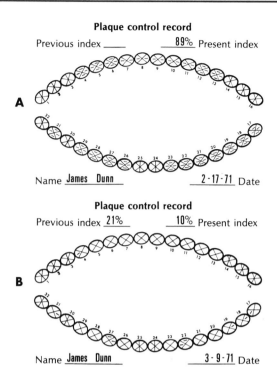

Plaque control record

Previous index _____   89% Present index

A

Name James Dunn   2-17-71 Date

Plaque control record

Previous index 21%   10% Present index

B

Name James Dunn   3-9-71 Date

Fig. 32-7. **A,** Plaque control record filled out at the first appointment for teaching proper oral hygiene measures. **B,** Plaque control record after four sessions of instruction. This patient's plaque level is such that definitive treatment can begin. This level of plaque control needs to be maintained during the follow-up phase of treatment. *(From Goldman HM, Cohen DW:* Periodontal therapy, *ed 5, St. Louis, 1973, Mosby.)*

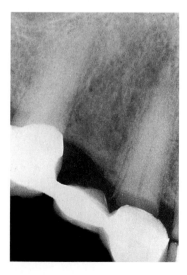

Fig. 32-8. Undetected caries beneath this FPD resulted in serious complications.

when assessing early enamel lesions because a "heavy-handed" examination may damage the fragile demineralized enamel matrix. An intact enamel matrix is essential for procedures that induce remineralization[13] (e.g., improved plaque control, dietary changes, topical fluoride applications).

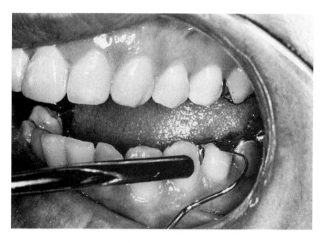

Fig. 32-9. Drying the teeth facilitates assessment of the margin integrity of a cemented prosthesis.

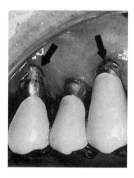

Fig. 32-10. Occasionally, cervical amalgam restorations *(arrows)* can extend the useful life of a previously placed cast restoration and will prevent unnecessary and complicated replacement of the prosthesis.

Conservative treatment of caries at the cavosurface margin is especially problematic. The lesion can spread rapidly, particularly if the restoration has a less than optimal marginal fit. Correcting the problem with a small amalgam, composite resin, or gold foil restoration is sometimes possible (Fig. 32-10). If the cast restoration is supported by an amalgam or composite resin core, the extent of the caries may be difficult to determine. When there is doubt that all carious dentin has been removed, replacing the entire restoration is recommended.

Root Caries. Caries of exposed root surfaces (Fig. 32-11) can be a severe problem in the age group commonly seeking fixed prosthodontic care.[14-16] In the classic Vipeholm study,[17] **root caries** accounted for more than 50% of new lesions in patients in the 50-year-old age group. Root caries incidence increased considerably with age.[18] In the caries examination from Phase 1 of the Third National Health and Nutrition Examination Survey, root caries affected

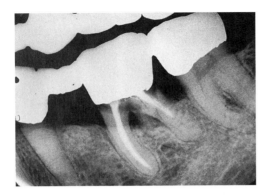

Fig. 32-11. Extensive root caries beneath a cemented FPD.
(Courtesy Dr. J. Keene.)

22.5% of the dentate population.[19] Root surface caries seems to be associated with individual dental plaque scores and high counts of salivary mutans streptococci.[20] Age-related xerostomia or that caused by medication or radiation treatment has been implicated in the etiology of rampant caries.[21-23] Other factors include the patient's economic status, diet, oral hygiene, and ethnic background.[24] Only a most vigorous effort on the part of the dentist and patient will lead to resolution of the problem. Prevention is focused on diet counseling and fluoride treatment. Treatment often requires the placement of large cervical amalgam or glass ionomer restorations that wrap around the periphery of previously placed cast restorations. Such restorations are difficult to place. However, in view of the constraints, they are a preferred alternative to comprehensive retreatment with elaborate fixed prostheses.

PERIODONTAL DISEASE

Unfortunately, periodontal disease often occurs following placement of fixed prostheses,[25] especially where the cavosurface margin is placed subgingivally[26-28] or the prosthesis is overcontoured.[29] Inflammation is more severe with poorly fitting restorations[30] (Fig. 32-12), but even "perfect" margins have been associated with periodontitis.[31] At recall appointments, particular attention is given to sulcular hemorrhage, furcation involvement, and calculus formation as early signs of periodontal disease. Improperly contoured restorations should be recontoured or replaced.

OCCLUSAL DYSFUNCTION

The patient is examined for signs of occlusal dysfunction at each recall appointment (Fig. 32-13). The patient should be asked about any noxious habits such as bruxism. An examination of the occlusal surfaces may reveal abnormal wear facets. In particular, the canines should be inspected because wear in this area will soon lead to excursive interfering contacts on the posterior teeth. Abnormal tooth mobility is investigated, as is muscle and joint pain. A standardized muscle-and-joint palpation technique (see Chapter 1) is helpful. Articulated diagnostic casts should be periodically remade (Fig. 32-14) and compared with previous records so that any occlusal changes can be monitored and corrective treatment initiated.

A small number of patients may not have responded well to previous occlusal treatment or may resume parafunctional activity some time after completion of the active phase of treatment. Although resolving the underlying etiology is preferable, a nightguard can occasionally be prescribed. Its design is identical to the occlusal device described in Chapter 4 for treating neuromuscular symptoms resulting from malocclusion. However, the device is only worn at night. If the patient primarily clenches, the dentist should consider a slightly flatter anterior ramp than is ordinarily incorporated in the conventional device.

PULP AND PERIAPICAL HEALTH

At the recall appointment, the patient may describe one or more episodes of pain during the previous months. This could indicate the loss of vitality of an abutment tooth and should be investigated. Appropriate corrective measures can then be taken.

One advantage of partial-coverage restorations is that pulp health can be monitored with an electric pulp tester (Fig. 32-15), although the vitality of any tooth with a complete crown can still be assessed by thermal means. Correlating the histologic condition of a pulp directly with the patient's response to pulp testing is difficult.[32] Therefore, such results should be combined with other clinical data that result from careful patient history information and examination. Seeking the opinion of an endodontist is often a good idea (Fig. 32-16). Radiographs provide useful information about the presence of periapical pathosis. Teeth with fixed restorations should be reviewed radiographically every few years. The use of a standardized technique enables the dentist to make an objective comparison with previous films. Although some studies have shown a high incidence of periapical disease associated with fixed prostheses,[33,34] other studies have shown a low incidence of this complication.[28,35,36]

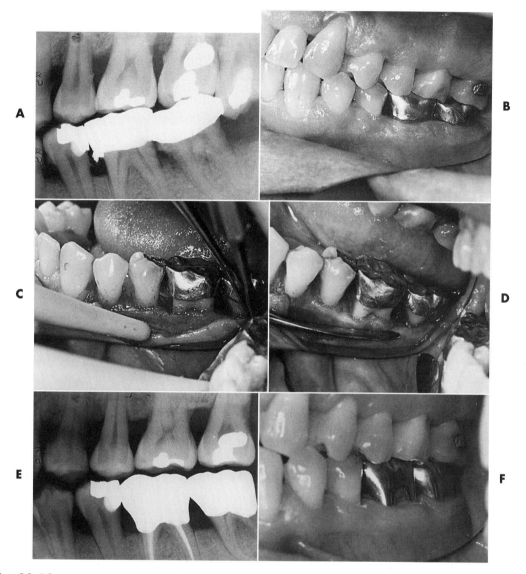

Fig. 32-12. Periodontal failure resulting from defective fixed prostheses. **A,** Inadequate margins and contour. **B,** Before surgery. **C,** Flap reflected. **D,** After surgical recontouring. **E,** Radiograph of new cast restorations. **F,** Replacement restorations.
(Courtesy Dr. D. Politis.)

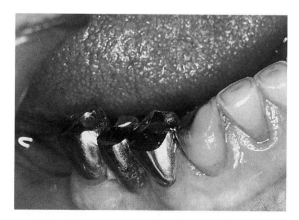

Fig. 32-13. If a cast restoration is not designed according to neuromuscular and temporomandibular controls, extensive wear can result after a relatively short time.

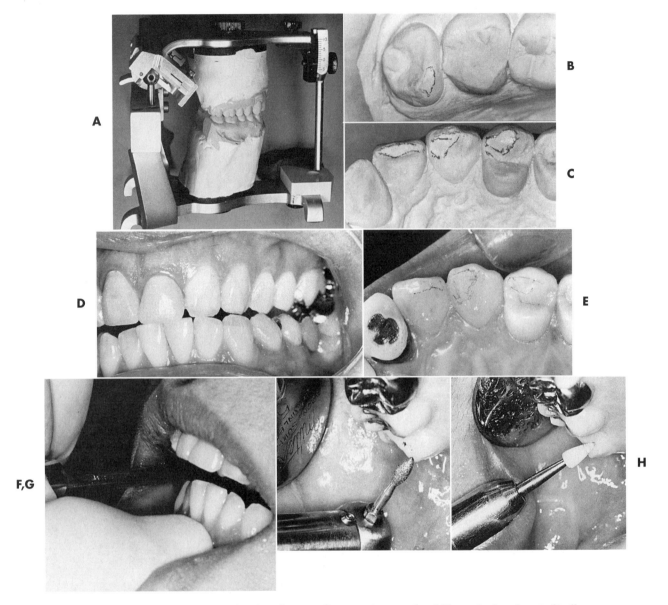

Fig. 32-14. Posttreatment occlusal analysis. **A,** Diagnostic casts should be articulated periodically. **B** and **C,** Wear facets on the maxillary molar correspond to faceting on the premolar, canine, and lateral incisor. **D** and **E,** Mandibular excursion corresponding to the observed wear patterns. **F** to **H,** After marking, the newly detected interferences can be easily removed.

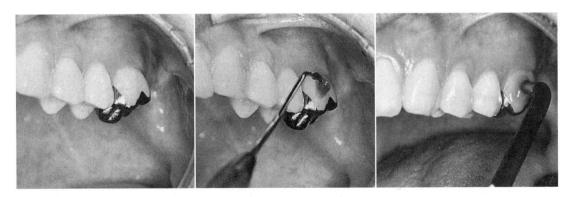

Fig. 32-15. Partial-coverage restorations offer the advantage of convenient vitality assessment with an electric pulp tester.

A   **B**   **C**

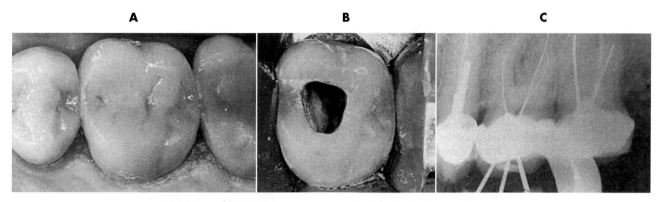

Fig. 32-16. Endodontic treatment after crown cementation. **A,** Symptomatic maxillary molar with a metal-ceramic crown. **B,** Access cavity prepared through the crown. **C,** Endodontic therapy in progress. *(Courtesy Dr. D. A. Miller.)*

EMERGENCY APPOINTMENTS

Occasionally patients have an emergency between routine recall visits. With carefully planned and executed treatment, however, these should be rare (although problems can still develop even with the best treatment). Patients should be taught to notice small changes in their oral health and to report them without delay. For instance, the porcelain veneer of a metal-ceramic restoration may be shielded from further fracture when a small chip is promptly rounded off and the occlusion adjusted immediately after it is first noticed. Postponement of corrective treatment can be especially costly, requiring a remake of a complex prosthesis that could have been saved with prompt attention.

PAIN

A patient presenting with pain should be asked about its location, character, severity, timing, and onset. Factors that precipitate, relieve, or change the pain should be investigated, and appropriate treatment measures should be initiated (see Chapter 3).

Although most oral pain is of pulpal origin, this should never be assumed. A detailed investigation is always recommended. In difficult or questionable situations, the diagnosis should be confirmed by an appropriate specialist.

If the patient has several endodontically treated teeth that have been restored with posts-and-cores and fixed prostheses, the possibility of root fracture should be considered, especially for teeth that were internally weakened as a result of endodontic treatment in conjunction with oversized posts of less than optimal length. If a fracture has occurred, the tooth is almost invariably lost, which can significantly complicate follow-up treatment, especially if it involves an abutment tooth for an FPD (Fig. 32-17).

LOOSE ABUTMENT RETAINER

A **loose retainer** (Fig. 32-18) may not be easily perceived by the patient, especially if it is part of a fixed prosthesis supported by several abutment teeth. The patient may have noticed a bad taste or smell rather than detecting movement.

Unless appropriate instrumentation is available, removing the prosthesis intact for recementation is often difficult or impossible. The more recently developed devices shown in Figs. 32-19 to 32-21 have been successful, but they are expensive. The devices shown in Fig. 32-22 are less reliable and can be quite intimidating and uncomfortable for the patient. On occasion, a direct pull with hemostat forceps succeeds. (Metal-ceramic crowns should first be coated with autopolymerizing acrylic resin to prevent chipping or cracking.) Applying the tip of an ultrasonic scaler to the restoration is recommended because prolonged ultrasonic vibration can decrease crown retention.[37] A procedure for removing crowns and FPDs with a strongly adhesive resin[38] has been used successfully in certain cases[39] (Fig. 32-23). When trying to remove a permanently cemented prosthesis, the dentist must use great caution. Unless force is applied in the path of withdrawal, an abutment tooth may fracture.

A loose retainer usually indicates inadequate tooth preparation, poor cementation technique, or caries. In this case, the tooth requires repreparation and a new prosthesis. Sectioning the prosthesis rather than attempting to remove it intact is often the best policy (Fig. 32-24).

FRACTURED CONNECTOR

An improperly fabricated connector may fracture under functional loading (Fig. 32-25). Depending on the design and location of the FPD, the patient may

Text continued on p. 795

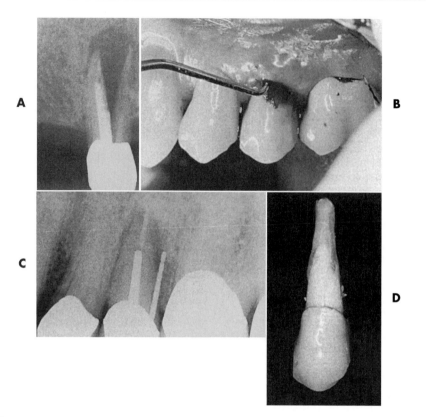

Fig. 32-17. **A,** Longitudinal root fracture of RPD abutment necessitated extraction. **B** and **C,** Longitudinal fracture with resulting periodontal defect. **D,** Fracture is clearly visible after extraction. *(Courtesy Dr. D.A. Miller.)*

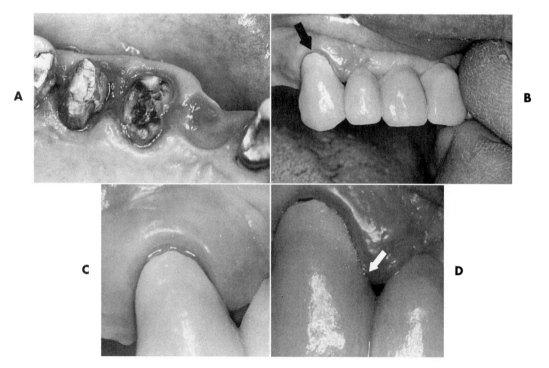

Fig. 32-18. **A,** Severe tooth destruction may result when a loose retainer goes undetected. **B,** Looseness of one retainer can occasionally be observed directly *(arrow)* when force is exerted in an occlusal direction. **C,** Water is then applied to the cervical area, and the diagnosis is confirmed if bubbles appear when pressure is exerted **(D).**

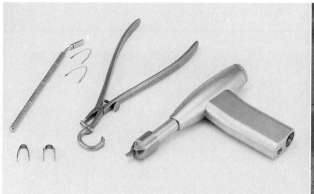

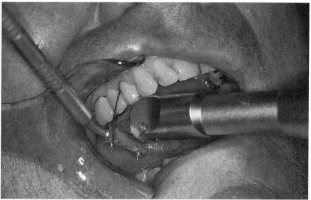

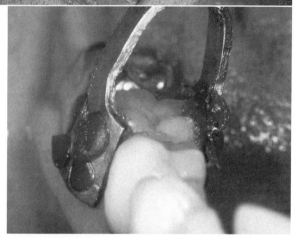

Fig 32-19. Coronaflex crown remover.* This is an air-driven device that connects to standard dental handpiece hoses via KaVo's Multiflex coupler. The crown remover delivers a controlled low amplitude impact at its tip. The device works well on FPDs and is well-tolerated by patients. **A,** The kit includes loops to thread under FPD connectors that attach to a holder, calipers, and an adhesive clamp to obtain a purchase on single crowns. The goal is to deliver the impact in the long axis of the abutment tooth. **B,** The loop is threaded under the connector. The tip of the crown remover is placed on the bar, and the impact is activated by releasing the index finger from the air valve. **C,** The adhesive clamp is attached with autopolymerizing resin used to remove a single crown. (*A courtesy Sullivan-Schein Dental; C courtesy KaVo America.*)

*KaVo America: Lake Zurich, Ill.

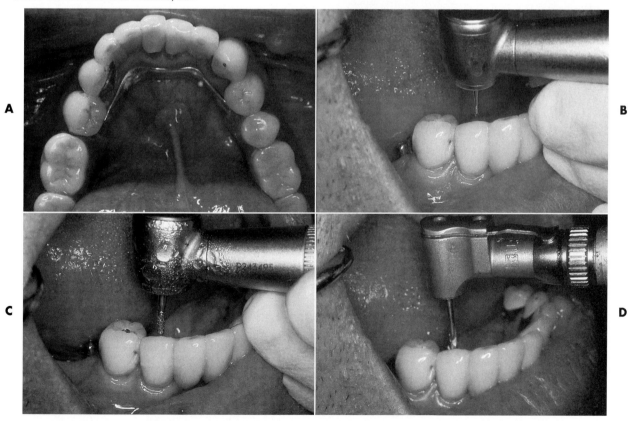

Fig. 32-20. The Metalift Crown and Bridge Removal System.† **A,** Five-unit FPD supporting an RPD. The anterior abutment (tooth # 25) is loose; the posterior abutments (tooth # 28 and # 29) are firmly cemented. **B,** Access to the metal on each abutment is provided by preparing through the porcelain with a diamond. **C,** The metal is penetrated with a no. 1 round bur to create a pilot channel in each abutment. **D,** The pilot hole is followed by the special drill. (*Courtesy Dr. R. D. Westerman.*)

Continued

†Classic Practice Resources: Baton Rouge, La.

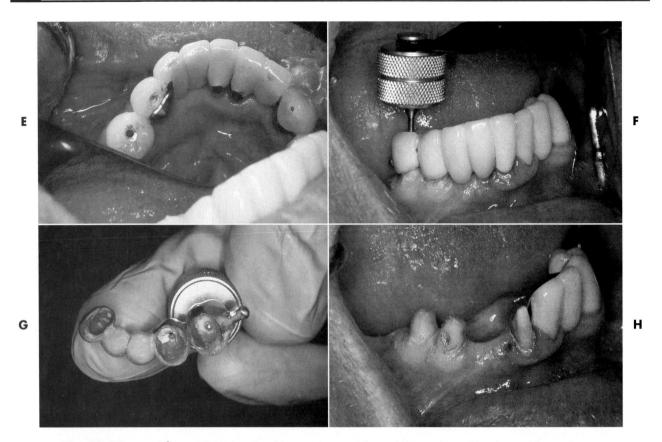

Fig. 32-20, cont'd.   E, The holes should just penetrate the metal as indicated by the visible cement. F, The Metalift instrument is threaded into both crowns, breaking the cement seal. **G,** The FPD is re-moved and, if the abutments are satisfactory as seen here **(H),** it can be recemented for further service. The manufacturer supplies threaded keys that can be used to seal the occlusal hole. To facilitate recovery, they can also be incorporated in crowns before cementation.

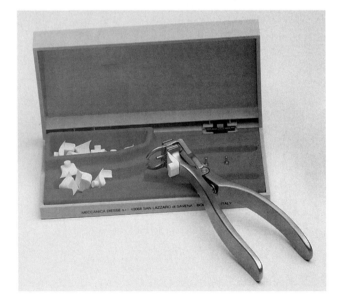

Fig. 32-21.   Roydent Bridge and Crown Remover.* This device is designed to grip a crown or FPD and to deliver a removal force along the long axis.
(Courtesy Sullivan-Schein Dental.)

*Roydent Dental Products: Rochester Hills, Mich.

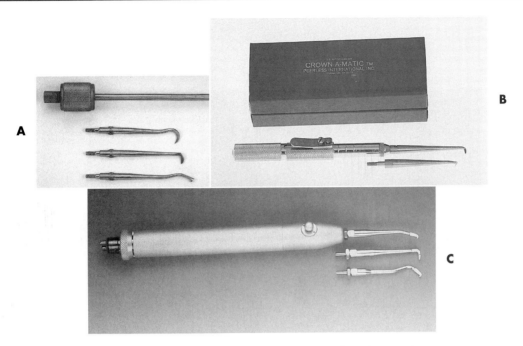

Fig. 32-22. Crown removers. **A,** Back-action. **B,** Spring-activated. **C,** Pneumatic. *(Courtesy Sullivan-Schein Dental.)*

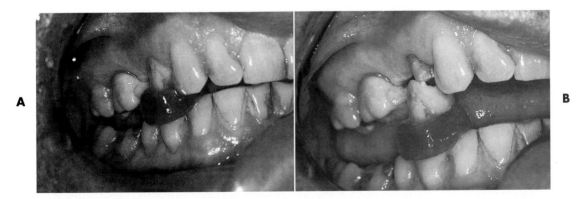

Fig. 32-23. Richwil Crown and Bridge Remover.* This adhesive resin tablet is softened in warm water for 1 to 2 minutes, and the patient is instructed to occlude into it **(A)** (the manufacturer recommends tying a length of floss to the tablet to prevent aspiration). The resin is cooled with water. A sharp opening action should remove the crown **(B).** Care is needed to avoid removing a restoration in the opposing jaw.

*Almore International, Inc: Portland, Ore.

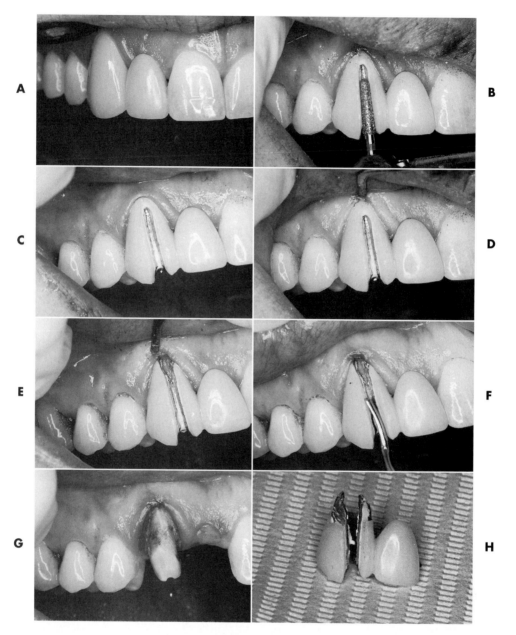

Fig. 32-24. Removal of an existing crown by sectioning. **A,** This cantilever FPD required replacement for esthetic and periodontal reasons. **B,** The restoration is carefully sectioned, initially cutting just through the ceramic to the metal. It is easiest to do this on the facial and incisal surfaces. **C,** The goal is to cut just through the metal to the cement and follow the cement toward the gingival margin. **D,** Displace the gingiva with an instrument and carefully section the crown to the gingival margin **(E).** **F,** Place a suitable instrument (e.g., a cement spatula or sterilized screwdriver) in the cut and gently rotate to force the halves of the crown apart. It may be necessary to section part of the lingual surface to facilitate this step. **G,** The abutment. Additional incisal reduction was necessary; the notch in the incisal edge is of no concern. **H,** Removed prosthesis.
(Courtesy Dr. D.H. Ward.)

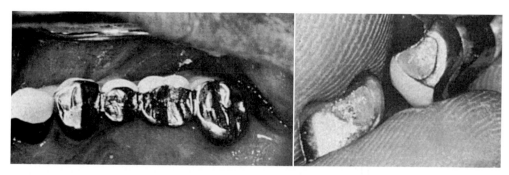

Fig. 32-25. The soldered connector of a four-unit FPD fractured during function. The patient's chief complaint was molar pain, although the fracture was between the premolars.

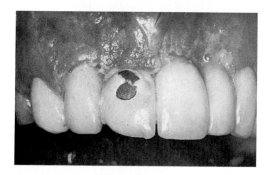

Fig. 32-26. Fractured metal-ceramic veneer.

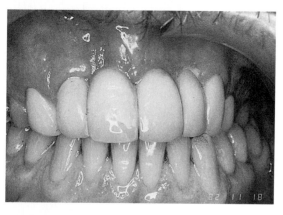

Fig. 32-27. On occasion, repairing a fractured metal-ceramic veneer rather than replacing the entire FPD is advantageous. In this example, the porcelain surface has been etched; a resin repair system has been used.

complain of varying degrees of pain. Extra force is typically transmitted to the abutment teeth, and discomfort from overloading the periodontal ligament may draw attention away from the location of the actual problem. If the abutment teeth have good bone support and minimal mobility, **fractured connectors** can be very difficult to detect clinically. Wedges can sometimes be positioned to separate the individual FPD components enough to confirm the correct diagnosis.

FRACTURED PORCELAIN VENEER

Mechanical failure of a metal-ceramic restoration (Fig. 32-26) is not uncommon. It is usually related to faults in framework design, improper laboratory procedures, excessive occlusal function, or trauma (e.g., an automobile or sports accident).

If the porcelain has fractured on an otherwise satisfactory multi-unit prosthesis, an attempt at repair rather than a remake may be justified to save the patient additional discomfort, time, and expense. When the fractured porcelain is not missing and there is little or no functional loading on the fracture site, it can sometimes be bonded in place with a **porcelain repair** system (Fig. 32-27) using silane coupling agents or 4-META to promote bonding

with acrylic or composite resin.[40-43] Unfortunately, the strength of joints made this way seems to diminish with changes in temperature[44] and with prolonged water storage.[45] Benefits from such repair are considered temporary, but it may be preferable to dismantling and remaking a complex FPD. In other circumstances, the fractured area may be repaired with composite resin retained by means of mechanical undercuts in the metal framework.[46] The use of a silane coupling agent is also recommended for these repairs.

A more permanent repair can sometimes be effected by making a metal-ceramic restoration to fit over the fractured original. This technique is appropriate when the pontic rather than an abutment retainer has fractured. A little ingenuity is needed to produce a suitable design.[47,48] The most common difficulty encountered when attempting such a repair is weakening of the connectors during the preparation, with the associated risk of subsequent prosthesis fracture (Fig. 32-28).

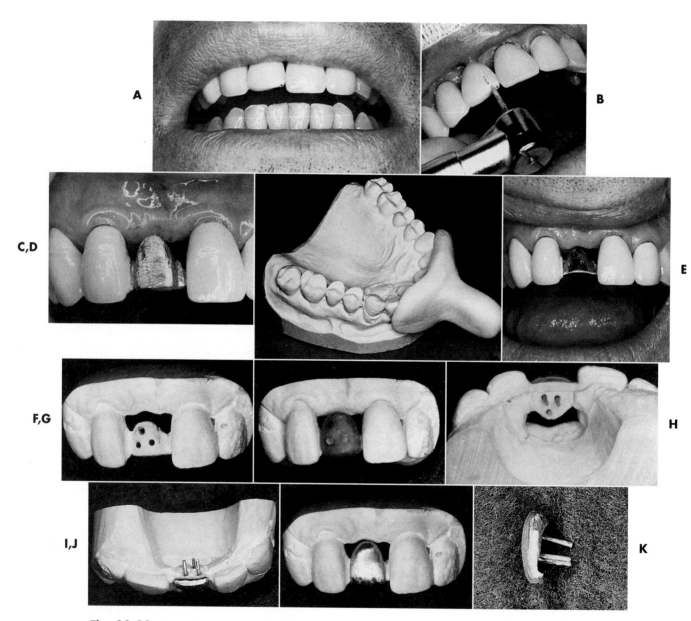

Fig. 32-28.   Repair of a fractured metal-ceramic pontic. **A,** Pretreatment appearance. **B,** The ceramic veneer is removed with diamond rotary instruments. **C,** After porcelain removal. **D,** Special impression tray. **E,** Pinholes are placed in the substructure. **F,** Cast of the substructure. **G,** Waxed overlay. **H,** Note the plastic pins used. **I,** Cast overlay. **J,** Facial aspect. **K,** Proximal aspect.
(Courtesy Dr. A. G. Gegauff.)

Continued

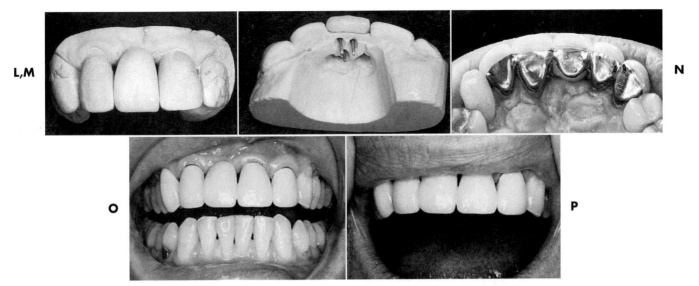

Fig. 32-28, cont'd.   L, Facial aspect after the porcelain application. **M,** Lingual aspect after firing (cast relieved). **N,** Following cementation. **O** and **P,** The finished repair.

RETREATMENT

Although fixed prostheses do not last forever, with good plaque removal, patient motivation, and average or above-average resistance to disease, a well-designed and well-fabricated restoration can provide many years of service. With poor care and neglect, even the "perfect" prosthesis or restoration can fail rapidly (Fig. 32-29). Because of exceptional host resistance, long-term success is sometimes possible with obviously defective restorations (Fig. 32-30).

Nevertheless, at some stage the decision about retreatment will have to be made. Much will depend on whether the retreatment is part of an ongoing program of comprehensive care or whether the existing prosthesis has been subjected to years of neglect.

PLANNED RETREATMENT

At the original treatment-planning stage, retreatment should be considered. This consideration may need to be general rather than specific because of difficulties in accurately predicting the pattern of future dental disease. Occasionally, however, a prosthesis is designed to accommodate the eventual failure of a doubtful abutment (Fig. 32-31). With a little foresight, survey contours can already be incorporated in the retainers of an FPD to accommodate a future removable partial denture (RPD) in the event of a terminal abutment loss. Similarly, accommodations can be made for future occlusal rests by deliberately increasing occlusal reduction during

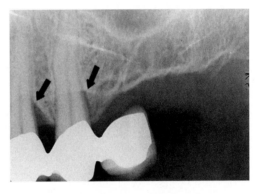

Fig. 32-29.   Osseous defects *(arrows)* within 2 years of the placement of this FPD.
(Courtesy Dr. J. Keene.)

tooth preparation and using metal occlusal surfaces. Furthermore, proximal boxes can be incorporated if it is anticipated that a nonrigid (dovetail) rest could simplify future retreatment (see Fig. 32-31).

When tooth preparations are conservative, margins are supragingival, and complicated FPD designs are avoided, replacement dentistry can be performed in an orderly manner, as long as plaque control and follow-up care are maintained.

The key to successful fixed prosthodontic treatment planning lies in anticipating potential areas of future failure. Ideally, the design of a prosthesis should incorporate an escape mechanism to allow simple and convenient alteration to accommodate future treatment needs.

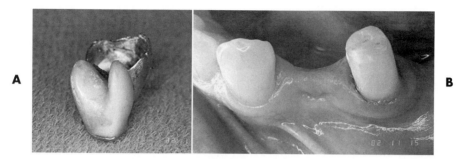

Fig. 32-30. A "saddle" pontic should not be fabricated, because it makes plaque control impossible. However, this particular FPD was replaced after 35 years of service. **B,** Despite poor pontic design, there are no significant signs of ulceration. This example illustrates the variability of tissue response due to differences in host resistance.

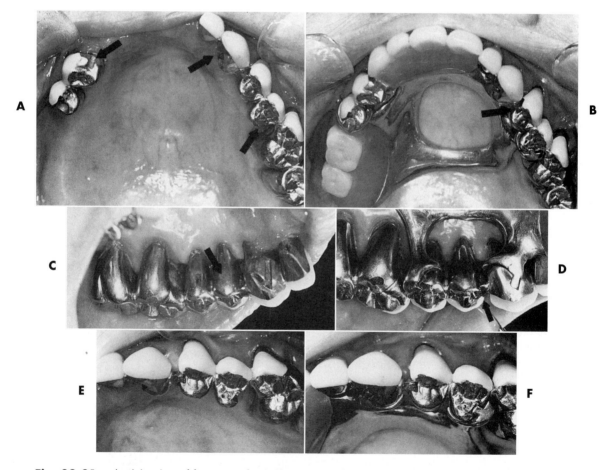

Fig. 32-31. Anticipation of future needs. **A,** Four years after the restoration of an arch with periodontally compromised teeth. Three intracoronal rests *(arrows)* were fabricated to support an RPD. **B,** An additional rest *(arrow)* was included as a nonrigid connector for splinting the prostheses in the maxillary left quadrant. This rest is parallel to the others, so it will be available (if needed) for future support of a modified or new RPD. **C,** The lingual of the premolar incorporates the appropriate survey contour *(arrow)* to accommodate such a prosthesis. **D,** The RPD in place. Note the third intracoronal rest *(arrow).* **E,** Occlusal aspect of the fixed prosthesis. **F,** The FPD with the RPD in place.

Continued

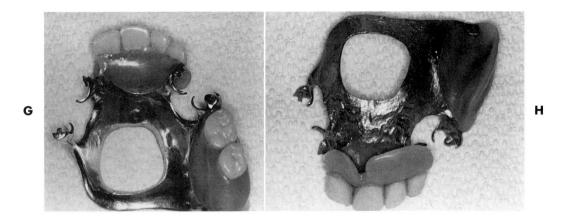

Fig. 32-31, cont'd.   G and H, External and internal aspects of the RPD. This was cast in Type IV gold, which allows the relatively easy addition of a new minor connector with conventional soldering techniques.

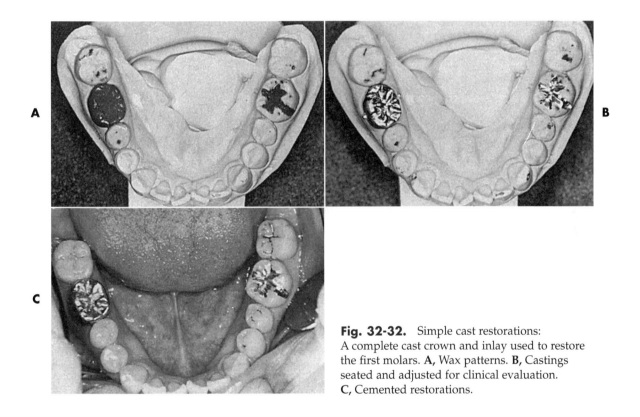

Fig. 32-32.   Simple cast restorations: A complete cast crown and inlay used to restore the first molars. **A,** Wax patterns. **B,** Castings seated and adjusted for clinical evaluation. **C,** Cemented restorations.

NEGLECT

The patient with an extensive fixed prosthesis that has been neglected is much more difficult to treat. Considerable expertise is needed to successfully perform the lengthy and demanding procedures. Specialized treatment is almost always necessary and usually includes controlling mobility of the abutment teeth, improving support for removable appliances in the edentulous area, and creating a more favorable load distribution.

▉ TREATMENT PRESENTATIONS

Several selected treatment results are presented, including follow-up documentation as appropriate. The treatments demonstrate successful treatment approaches consistent with the principles discussed in this text.

Treatment I (Fig. 32-32): Simple cast restorations
Treatment II (Fig. 32-33): Single cast restorations
Treatment III (Fig. 32-34): Simple fixed partial
  dentures

Text continued on p. 815

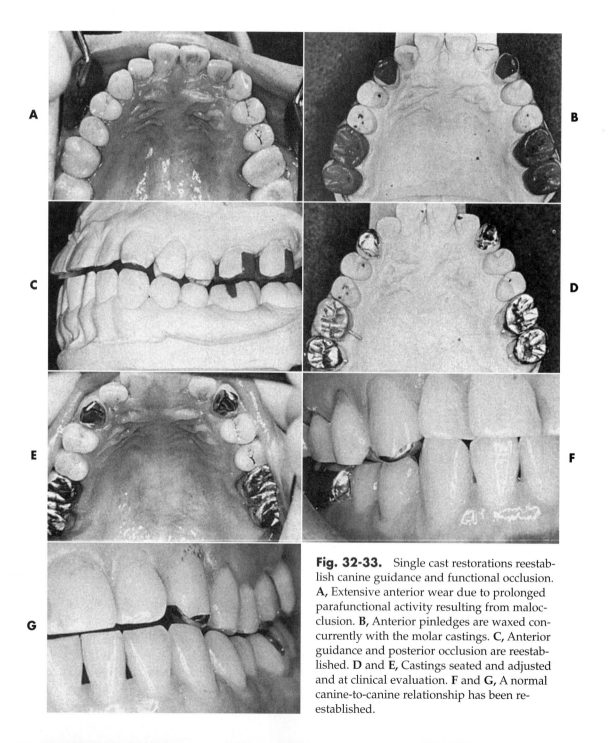

Fig. 32-33. Single cast restorations reestablish canine guidance and functional occlusion. **A,** Extensive anterior wear due to prolonged parafunctional activity resulting from malocclusion. **B,** Anterior pinledges are waxed concurrently with the molar castings. **C,** Anterior guidance and posterior occlusion are reestablished. **D** and **E,** Castings seated and adjusted and at clinical evaluation. **F** and **G,** A normal canine-to-canine relationship has been reestablished.

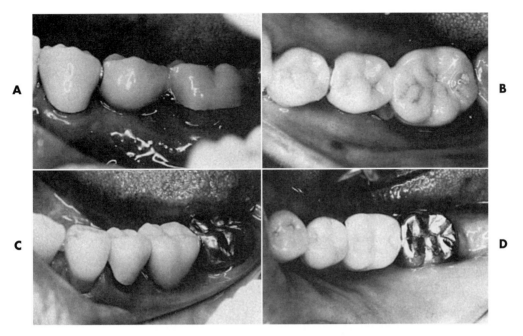

Fig. 32-34. Simple FPDs: Long-term follow-up: These small FPDs remain serviceable after 7 and 13 years, respectively. **A** and **B**, Seven-year follow-up. **C** and **D**, Thirteen-year follow-up.

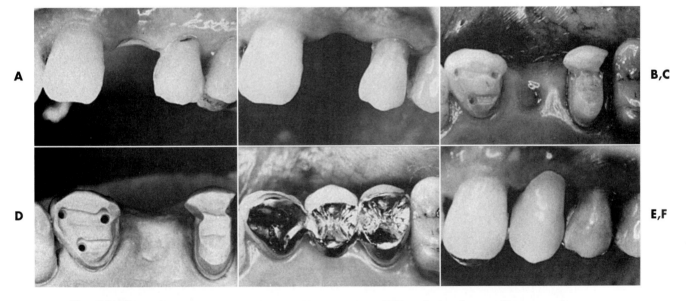

Fig. 32-35. Partial-coverage retainers used to support an FPD replacing the maxillary premolar. **A** and **B**, Abutment teeth before and after tooth preparation. **C** and **D**, Occlusal views of preparations. **E** and **F**, Occlusal and buccal views of cemented FPDs.

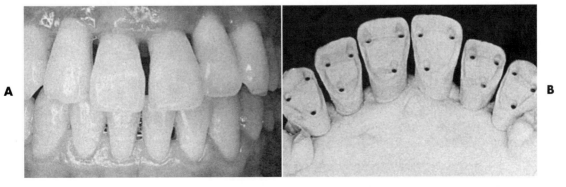

Fig. 32-36. Pinledge splint: **A** and **B**, Periodontally involved anterior teeth prepared for pinledges.

Continued

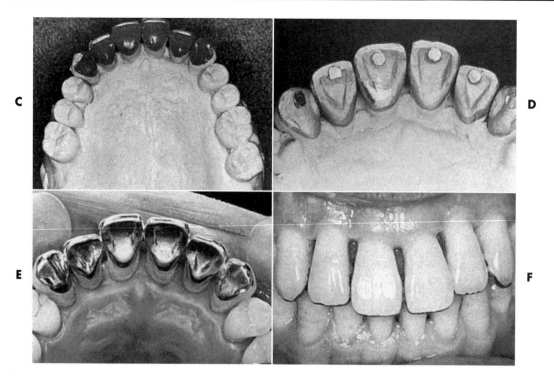

Fig. 32-36, cont'd. **C** and **D**, Pinledges waxed, cast, and seated on the working cast. **E** and **F**, Completed restorations. Some metal is displayed as a result of the long clinical crown length and opened embrasures resulting from periodontal surgery. However, this treatment approach is preferred because it is much more conservative of tooth structure than splinting with metal-ceramic crowns.

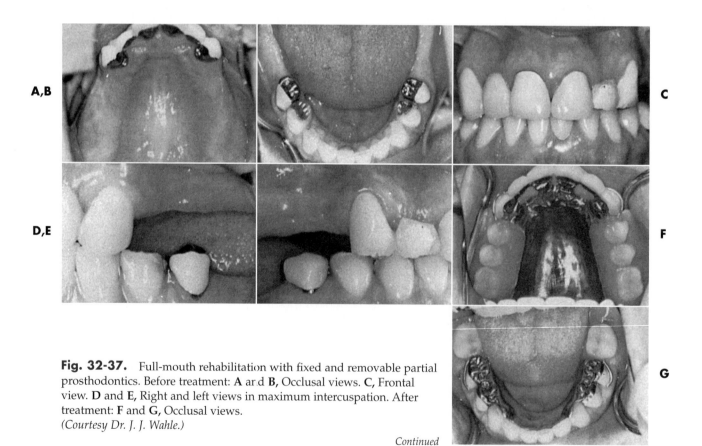

Fig. 32-37. Full-mouth rehabilitation with fixed and removable partial prosthodontics. Before treatment: **A** and **B**, Occlusal views. **C**, Frontal view. **D** and **E**, Right and left views in maximum intercuspation. After treatment: **F** and **G**, Occlusal views.
(Courtesy Dr. J. J. Wahle.)

Continued

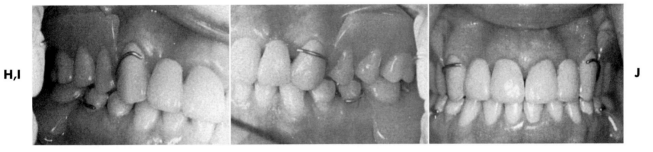

Fig. 32-37, cont'd. H and I, Right and left mirror views in maximum intercuspation. J, Frontal view.

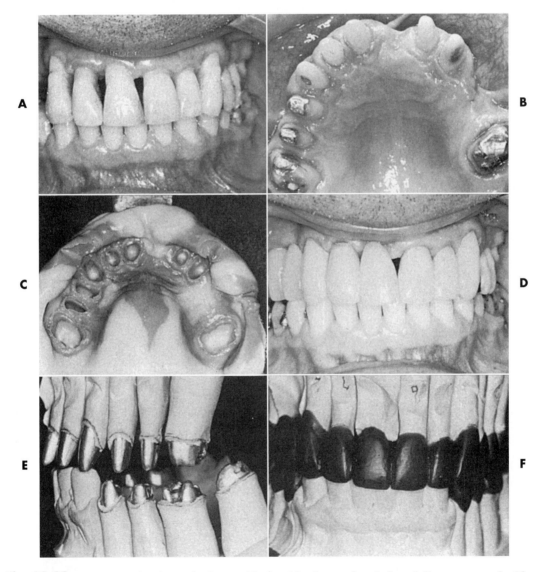

Fig. 32-38. Extensive fixed prosthodontics: Teeth with advanced periodontal disease restored with fixed prosthodontics. **A,** Initial presentation. The patient required extraction of the right maxillary incisor and surgical correction of the periodontal defects. **B,** Maxillary teeth prepared for metal-ceramic restorations. **C,** Reversible hydrocolloid impression. **D,** Provisional restorations. **E,** Working casts. **F,** Anatomic contour wax patterns.
(Courtesy Dr. M. T. Padilla.)

Continued

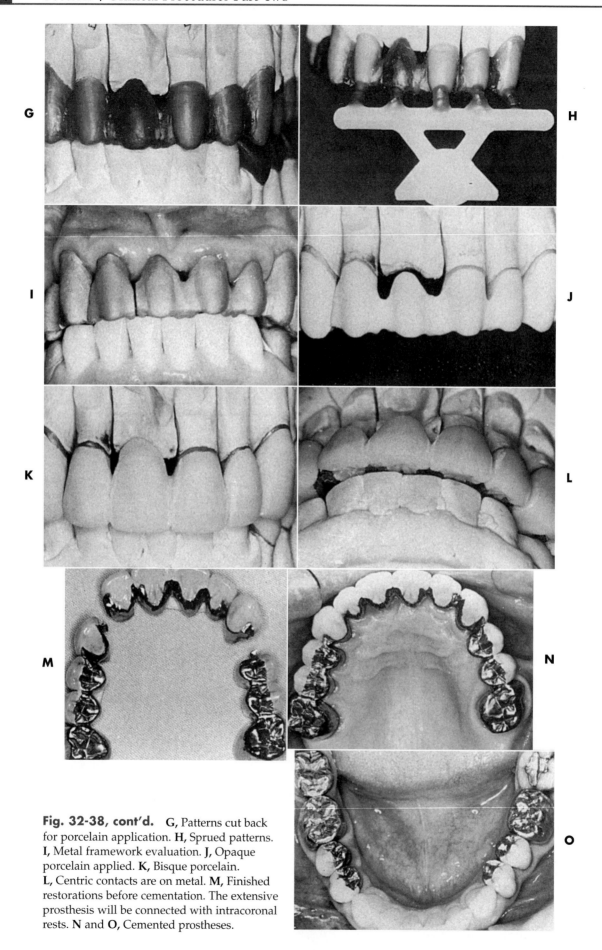

Fig. 32-38, cont'd.   G, Patterns cut back for porcelain application. **H,** Sprued patterns. **I,** Metal framework evaluation. **J,** Opaque porcelain applied. **K,** Bisque porcelain. **L,** Centric contacts are on metal. **M,** Finished restorations before cementation. The extensive prosthesis will be connected with intracoronal rests. **N** and **O,** Cemented prostheses.

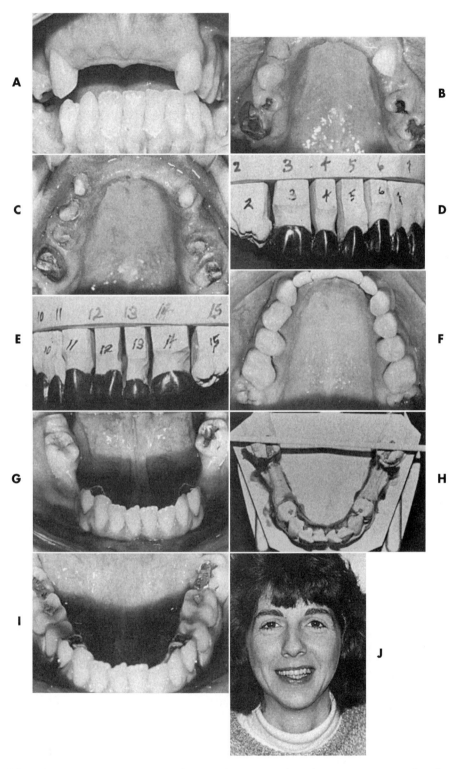

Fig. 32-39. Extensive fixed and removable prosthesis: **A** and **B,** The patient presented with missing maxillary anterior teeth and mandibular posteriors. There was a significant slide from centric relation to maximum intercuspation. The patient was treated with a combination of fixed and removable prostheses. **C,** Maxillary teeth prepared and foundation restorations placed. **D** and **E,** Maxillary teeth waxed to anatomic contour. **F** and **G,** Completed fixed restorations. **H,** Working cast for mandibular RPD framework before duplication. A rotational path of insertion was used to engage mesial undercuts in second molars. **I,** Completed mandibular RPD. Amalgam stops were placed in the first molars to prevent premature wear of the denture teeth. **J,** Completed treatment.
(Courtesy Dr. J. A. Holloway.)

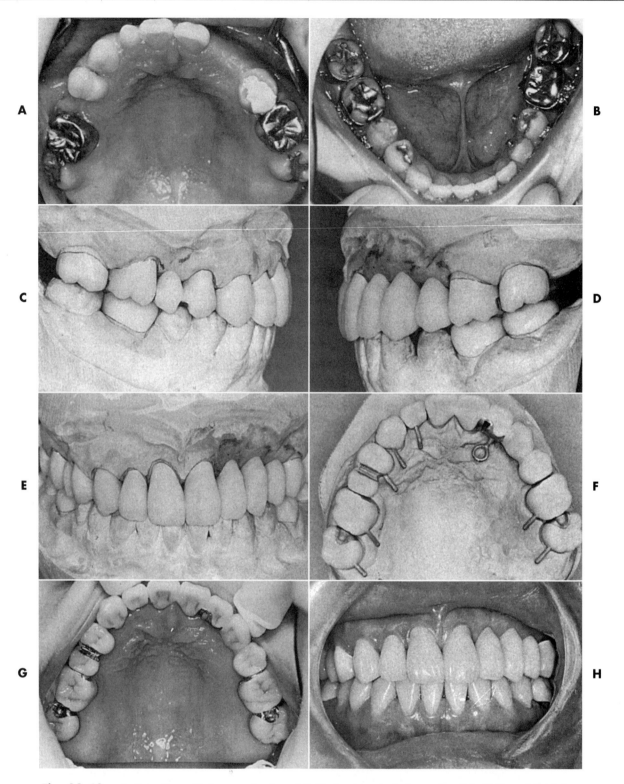

Fig. 32-40. Anticipation of future needs: **A** and **B**, Pretreatment photographs. **C** to **E**, Buccal/labial view of bisque bake. **F** and **G**, Occlusal view before and at clinical evaluation. Note the location of the occlusal rests to anticipate various future RPD designs. An intracoronal rest (dovetail) was incorporated in the left lateral incisor. It is filled with composite resin, which is easily removed if the need arises. **H**, Completed treatment.

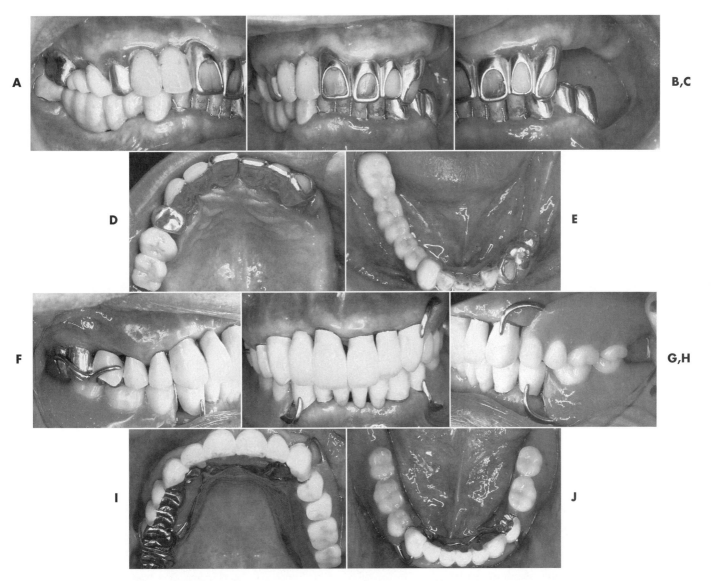

Fig. 32-41. This patient presented with multiple falling restorations and severely compromised function. **A** to **E,** Preoperative photographs. **F** to **J,** Post-treatment photographs. Where possible, I-bars were used to minimize clasp visibility. Also note the extensive use of metal occlusal surfaces. When designing prostheses for dentitions with compromised crown/root ratios, precise adjustment of the occlusion and anterior guidance components is critical.

Continued

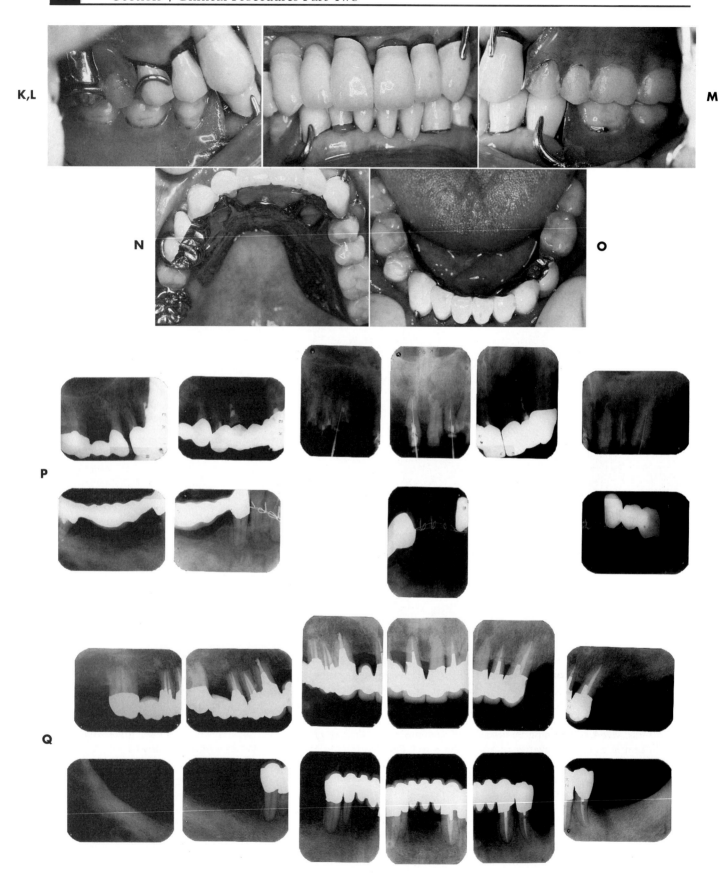

Fig. 32-41, cont'd. K to O, 17-year follow-up photographs. Note that the maxillary canine was lost and the existing retainer was modified into a pontic through the addition of composite resin. Additional endodontic treatment was needed as time passed. **P,** Preoperative radiographs. **Q,** Postoperative radiographs.

Continued

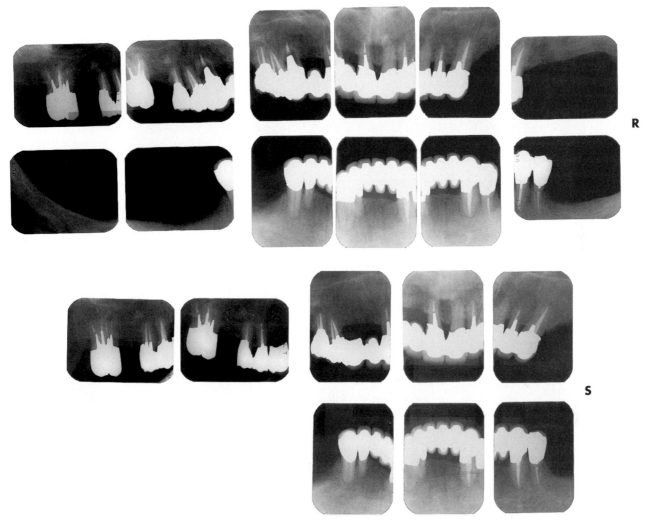

Fig. 32-41, cont'd. **R,** 8-year postoperative radiographs. **S,** 17-year postoperative radiographs. An FPD was fabricated, replacing the missing # 3 with teeth # 5, # 4, and # 2 as abutments. The teeth were prepared with minimal taper and the castings exhibited good retention. After 10 years, the FPD failed when # 2 became dislodged, possibly due to the additional loading by the RPD. # 2 and the pontic were removed, endodontic treatment was performed, a new crown was fabricated, and the # 3 pontic was incorporated in a new RPD. # 6 was lost due to internal resorption and caries. Initially, the tooth was discolored, but the lesion was inactive, and the attempt to save it failed after 8 years. Its guarded prognosis was discussed as a significant risk factor before treatment initiation. This suggests that teeth with a guarded prognosis can be maintained if attention is paid to the principles of casting adaptation and occlusion.

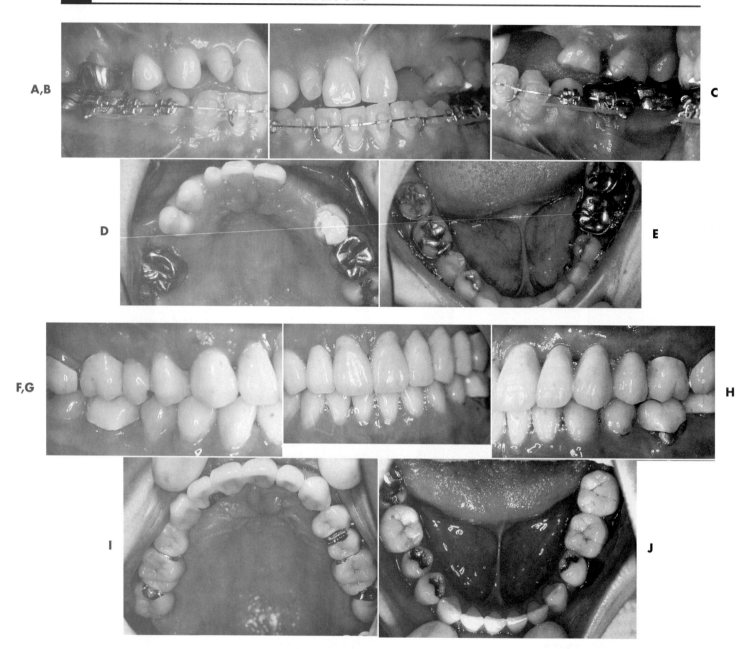

Fig. 32-42. Long-term follow-up after comprehensive treatment with fixed prostheses. **A** to **E**, Preoperative photographs. **F** to **J**, Postoperative photographs.

Continued

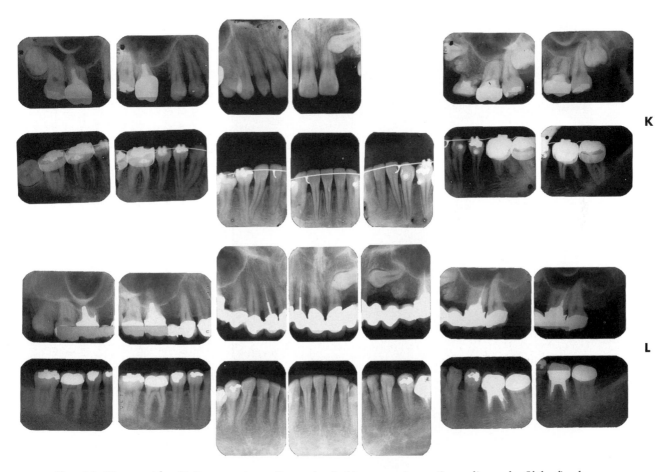

Fig. 32-42, cont'd. K, Preoperative radiographs. L, 14-year postoperative radiographs. If the fixed prostheses have been designed carefully and the patient is cooperative and maintains excellent plaque control, fixed partial dentures can withstand the test of time. Today, these prostheses continue to provide excellent esthetics and function after more than 16 years of service. Note that the impacted canine was ignored. Initially, this patient presented with only posterior guidance on the left and right first molars. A gingival graft was performed on the left side before the fixed prosthodontic treatment. Fourteen years later, all teeth are stable without any clinically significant mobility, and the anterior guidance components exhibit no visible facetting. No significant change has occurred in bone levels, whereas apparent radiographic bone densities appear slightly increased. Meticulous attention to precise adjustment of the occlusion, especially the anterior guidance component, contributed to the long-term success of this treatment. On the 14-year postoperative radiographs, no signs of occlusal trauma are seen. Also, note that three endodontically treated molars have very large access cavities. Such teeth have a guarded prognosis and are prone to fracture, but no fractures have occurred. Again, this suggests the importance of precise and optimal load distribution at the time of initial treatment and during periodic follow-up appointments. This patient was recalled every 6 months.

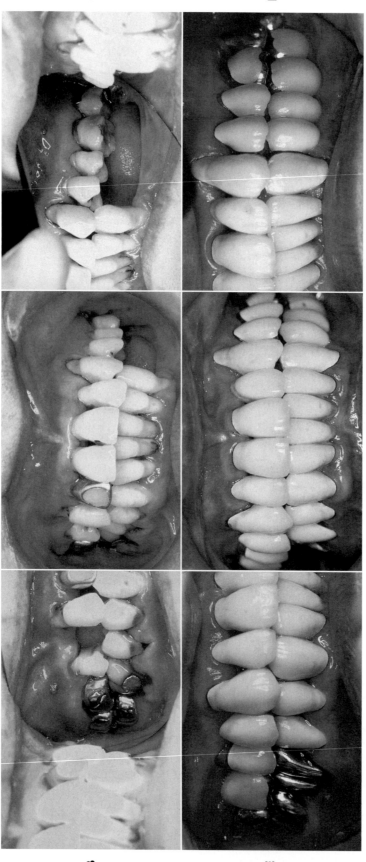

Fig. 32-43. Treatment of a severely periodontally compromised dentition. **A** to **C,** Preoperative photographs. **D** to **F,** 14-year postoperative photographs. When initially discussing an extensive treatment plan with a patient with a severely compromised dentition, a thorough understanding of the many risks and possibilities of failure must be fully understood by all parties. This extremely complex rehabilitation continues to serve well today. A meticulous design and frequent recall appointments, combined with outstanding home care, enables this patient to enjoy improved function 14 years later.

Throughout the follow-up, the patient was seen at 1-month and periodic 3-month recall appointments, depending on pocket charting and patient motivation. Today, tooth # 4 has no attached gingiva and little bone support, but *no pocket formation.* Initially, it was expected that this tooth would be the first to be lost. In conjunction with loss of # 1, this would have necessitated an RPD or implant-supported FPD. Occlusal rests, undercuts, and guide planes had been incorporated in the initial prosthesis to anticipate such failure.

After more than 14 years, the prostheses continue to serve satisfactorily. The anterior guidance component is starting to show some wear. Throughout the recall, wherever posterior tooth contact was observed in excursive movements, they were eliminated as part of ongoing occlusal adjustment. Meticulous management of load distribution has contributed to the long-term success of this very complex rehabilitation.

Continued

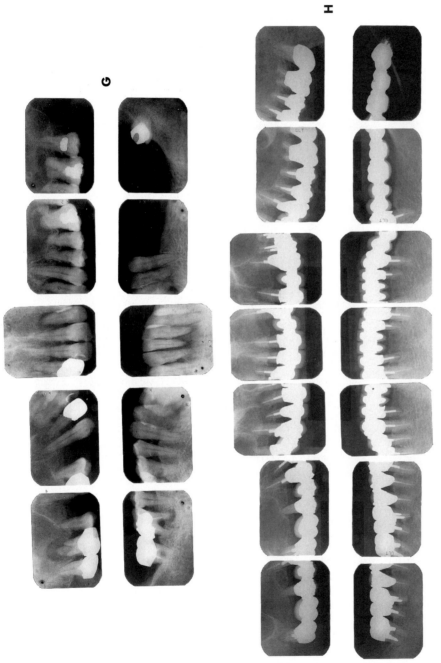

Fig. 32-43, cont'd. G, Preoperative radiographs. H, 14-year postoperative radiographs. This patient was referred initially for complete maxillary and mandibular denture fabrication. Implant-supported prostheses were rejected because of the necessity for a surgical sinus-lift procedure. Before prosthodontic treatment, the periodontal condition was treated. Treatment included a modified Widman flap, performed throughout both arches. A root resection was done for tooth # 14, and # 30 was hemisected, resulting in two premolar-like restorations. Use of the severely tilted # 17 as a single abutment to support a very long span posed a substantial risk to the long-term success of this treatment, and its future loss was anticipated in the design of the prostheses. Another risk was posed by the root morphology of tooth #1, with a small, fused root. This tooth was lost after 14 years due to a periodontal defect that progressed along a vertical groove in the fused root.

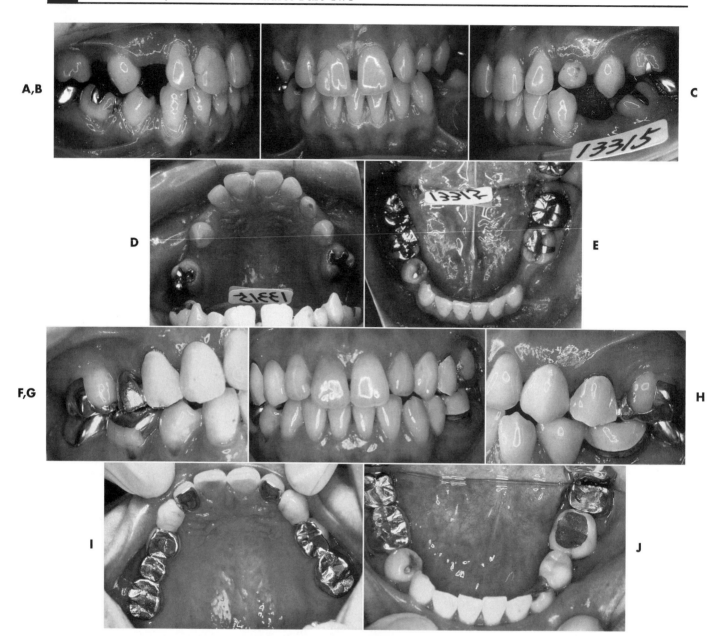

Fig. 32-44. Long-term evaluation: **A** to **E**, Preoperative photographs. **F** to **J**, 18-year post-treatment photographs. Three simple fixed partial dentures combining conventional and metal-ceramic prostheses with post-soldered connectors continue to serve 18 years after initial placement. Complications over the years included the reshaping of some restorations to correct occlusal discrepancies and the endodontic treatment of tooth # 19 through the prosthesis (the access cavity was restored with amalgam).
This patient presented with congenitally missing teeth # 4 and # 12. The maxillary canine was left in the premolar position for use as an abutment with posterior disocclusion resulting from guidance on the canine-shaped pontic. This is not ideal from the perspective of force distribution; however, the canine root successfully withstood the loading over time. Risk factors initially discussed with the patient included uncertainty regarding the impact of the crown/root ratios on the long-term prognosis. At the time of prosthetic treatment, more than 20 years ago, osseointegration was not the reliable treatment modality that it is today. This young female declined a removable prosthesis as an alternative to FPDs. A pinledge retainer was used on the small lateral incisor. Over time, not only was this esthetically effective, but it contributed to long-term maintenance of its periodontal health. Similarly, a pinledge was used on the left mandibular canine, a far more conservative option than a metal-ceramic restoration. If instead metal-ceramic retainers had been used, by now this likely would have resulted in additional treatment needs, and possibly the loss of the lateral incisor. Teeth # 18 , # 19, and # 3 were treated endodontically; cast post-and-cores were used. Also, note that tooth # 8 has served well over time. The conservative access cavity was restored, and the favorable position in the arch results in favorable loading. Recall appointments for this patient were scheduled at 6-month intervals throughout the evaluation period.

Continued

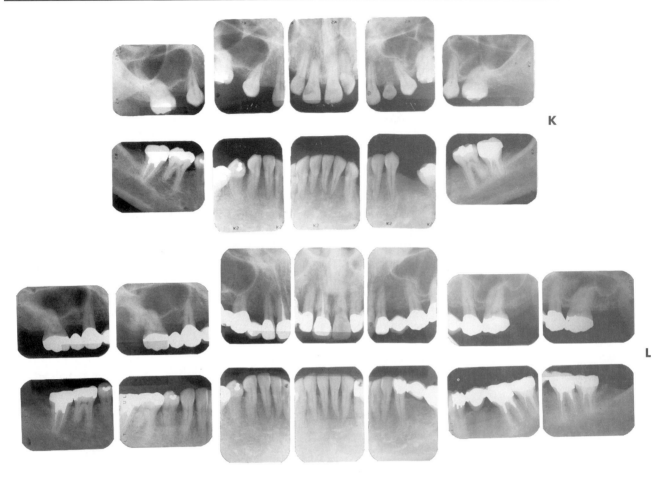

Fig. 32-44, cont'd.   K, Preoperative radiographs. L, Eighteen-year postoperative radiographs.

SUMMARY

Well-organized and efficient postoperative care is the chief mechanism for successful fixed prosthodontics. A restoration that is cemented, forgotten, and ignored is likely to fail, regardless of how skillfully it was designed and executed. Restored teeth require more assiduous plaque removal and maintenance than healthy unrestored teeth. An FPD requires additional care and attention.

Common complications after completion of the active phase of treatment include caries, periodontal failure, endodontic failure, loose retainers, porcelain fracture, and root fracture.

If possible, the dentist should anticipate the long-term prognosis and treatment needs of the patient and attempt to design the treatment plan accordingly. On occasion, FPDs can be designed so that future treatment can be simplified. However, it is not possible, even for the most experienced clinician, to anticipate every contingency and complication. The patient must understand the limitations of fixed prosthodontics before treatment begins.

Study Questions

1. What should be included in a typical post-treatment assessment once the previously rendered treatment has been completed? When and how often should the patient be reexamined? Provide examples of variables that influence this frequency.
2. What are typical complications for short-term post-cementation? How can they be avoided? Once they have been identified, how can they be resolved?
3. How can advanced root caries be satisfactorily resolved?
4. How is a loose retainer confirmed? Once this has been confirmed, how is the FPD removed?
5. Give three examples of treatment planning that takes future failure into consideration.

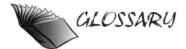

GLOSSARY

occlusal trauma: trauma to the periodontium from functional or parafunctional forces causing damage to the attachment apparatus of the periodontium by exceeding its adaptive and reparative capacities. It may be self-limiting or progressive.

overclosure: *n:* an occluding vertical dimension at a reduced interarch distance; an occluding vertical dimension that results in excessive interocclusal distance when the mandible is in the rest position; it results in a reduced interridge distance when the teeth are in contact.

overdenture: *n:* a removable partial or complete denture that covers and rests on one or more remaining natural teeth, roots, and/or dental implants; a prosthesis that covers and is partially supported by natural teeth, natural tooth roots, and/or dental implants—also called *overlay denture, overlay prosthesis, superimposed prosthesis.*

overhang: *n (1864):* excess restorative material projecting beyond a cavity or preparation margin.

REFERENCES

1. Tolboe H et al: Influence of oral hygiene on the mucosal conditions beneath bridge pontics, *Scand J Dent Res* 95:475, 1987.
2. Tolboe H et al: Influence of pontic material on alveolar mucosal conditions, *Scand J Dent Res* 96:442, 1988.
3. Ericson G et al: Cross-sectional study of patients fitted with fixed partial dentures with special reference to the caries situation, *Scand J Dent Res* 98:8, 1990.
4. Akerboom HB et al: Radiopacity of posterior composite resins, composite resin luting cements, and glass ionomer lining cements, *J Prosthet Dent* 70:351, 1993.
5. Matsumura H et al: Radiopacity of dental cements, *Am J Dent* 6:43, 1993.
6. el-Mowafy OM, Benmergui C: Radiopacity of resin-based inlay luting cements, *Oper Dent* 19:11, 1994.
7. Gibson G: Identifying and treating xerostomia in restorative patients, *J Esthet Dent* 10:253, 1998.
8. Walton JN et al: A survey of crown and fixed partial denture failures: length of service and reasons for replacement, *J Prosthet Dent* 56:416, 1986.
9. Libby G et al: Longevity of fixed partial dentures, *J Prosthet Dent* 78:127, 1997.
10. Sundh B, Odman P: A study of fixed prosthodontics performed at a university clinic 18 years after insertion, *Int J Prosthod* 10:513, 1997.
11. Priest GF: Failure rates of restorations for single-tooth replacement, *Int J Prosthod* 9:38, 1996.
12. Bauer JG et al: The reliability of diagnosing root caries using oral examinations, *J Dent Educ* 52:622, 1988.
13. Silverstone LM: Remineralization phenomena, *Caries Res* 11 (suppl 1):59, 1977.
14. Gordon SR: Older adults: demographics and need for quality care, *J Prosthet Dent* 61:737, 1989.
15. Hellyer PH et al: Root caries in older people attending a general dental practice in East Sussex, *Br Dent J* 169:201, 1990.
16. Guivante-Nabet C et al: Active and inactive caries lesions in a selected elderly institutionalised French population, *Int Dent J* 48:111, 1998.
17. Gustafsson BE et al: The Vipeholm dental caries study: the effect of different levels of carbohydrate intake on caries activity in 436 individuals observed for 5 years, *Acta Odontol Scand* 11:232, 1954.
18. Fure S: Five-year incidence of caries, salivary and microbial conditions in 60-, 70- and 80-year-old Swedish individuals, *Caries Res* 32:166, 1998.
19. Winn DM et al: Coronal and root caries in the dentition of adults in the United States, 1988-1991, *J Dent Res* 75(spec. no.):642, 1996.
20. Reiker J et al: A cross-sectional study into the prevalence of root caries in periodontal maintenance patients, *J Clin Periodont* 26:26, 1999.
21. Younger H et al: Relationship among stimulated whole, glandular salivary flow rates, and root caries prevalence in an elderly population: a preliminary study, *Spec Care Dentist* 18:156, 1998.
22. Powell LV et al: Factors associated with caries incidence in an elderly population, *Community Dent Oral Epidemiol* 26:170, 1998.
23. Sorensen JA: A rationale for comparison of plaque-retaining properties of crown systems, *J Prosthet Dent* 62:264, 1989.
24. Alexander AG: Periodontal aspects of conservative dentistry, *Br Dent J* 125:111, 1968.
25. Valderhaug J: Gingival reaction to fixed prostheses, *J Dent Res* 50:74, 1971.
26. Reichen-Graden S, Lang NP: Periodontal and pulpal conditions of abutment teeth. Status after four to eight years following the incorporation of fixed reconstructions, *Schweiz Monatsschr Zahnmed* 99:1381, 1989.
27. Wagman SS: The role of coronal contour in gingival health, *J Prosthet Dent* 37:280, 1977.
28. Mojon P et al: Relationship between prosthodontic status, caries, and periodontal disease in a geriatric population, *Int J Prosthodont* 8:564, 1995.

29. Rantanen T: A control study of crowns and bridges on root canal filled teeth, *Suom Hammaslaak Toim* 66:275, 1970.

30. Abou-Rass M: The stressed pulp condition: an endodontic-restorative diagnostic concept, *J Prosthet Dent* 48:264, 1982.

31. Saunders WP, Saunders EM: Prevalence of periradicular periodontitis associated with crowned teeth in an adult Scottish subpopulation, *Br Dent J* 185:137, 1998.

32. Karlsson S: A clinical evaluation of fixed bridges, 10 years following insertion, *J Oral Rehabil* 13:423, 1986.

33. Eckerbom M et al: Prevalence of apical periodontitis, crowned teeth and teeth with posts in a Swedish population, *Endod Dent Traumatol* 7:214, 1991.

34. Valderhaug J et al: Assessment of the periapical and clinical status of crowned teeth over 25 years, *J Dent* 25:97, 1997.

35. Olin PS: Effect of prolonged ultrasonic instrumentation on the retention of cemented cast crowns, *J Prosthet Dent* 64:563, 1990.

36. Oliva RA: Clinical evaluation of a new crown and fixed partial denture remover, *J Prosthet Dent* 44:267, 1980.

37. Parreira FR et al: Cast prosthesis removal using ultrasonics and a thermoplastic resin adhesive, *J Endod* 20:141, 1994.

38. Robbins JW: Intraoral repair of the fractured porcelain restoration, *Oper Dent* 23:203, 1998.

39. Chung KH, Hwang YC: Bonding strengths of porcelain repair systems with various surface treatments, *J Prosthet Dent* 78:267, 1997.

40. Kupiec KA et al: Evaluation of porcelain surface treatments and agents for composite-to-porcelain repair, *J Prosthet Dent* 76:119, 1996.

41. Pameijer CH et al: Repairing fractured porcelain: how surface preparation affects shear force resistance, *J Am Dent Assoc* 127:203, 1996.

42. Nowlin TP et al: Evaluation of the bonding of three porcelain repair systems, *J Prosthet Dent* 46:516, 1981.

43. Gregory WA et al: Composite resin repair of porcelain using different bonding materials, *Oper Dent* 13:114, 1988.

44. Barreto MT, Bottaro BF: A practical approach to porcelain repair, *J Prosthet Dent* 48:349, 1982.

45. Welsh SL, Schwab JT: Repair technique for porcelain-fused-to-metal restorations, *J Prosthet Dent* 38:61, 1977.

46. Miller TH, Thayer KE: Intraoral repair of fixed partial dentures, *J Prosthet Dent* 25:382, 1971.

47. Cardoso AC, Spinelli Filho P: Clinical and laboratory techniques for repair of fractured porcelain in fixed prostheses: a case report, *Quintessence Int* 25:835, 1994.

48. Westerman RD: A new paradigm for the construction and service of fixed prosthodontics, *Dent Today* 18:62, 1999.

DENTAL MATERIALS AND EQUIPMENT INDEX

■ AIR ABRASIVE UNITS
RECOMMENDED USE
> Metal preparation before porcelain (Chapter 24)
> Identification of unwanted metal contact (Chapters 22 and 30)
> Preparation of casting before cementation (Chapter 31)

SELECTED SUPPLIERS
> Belle de St. Claire
> Jelenko International
> Paasche Airbrush Co.
> APM-Sterngold
> Buffalo Dental Mfg. Co., Inc.
> Hydro-Cast Dental Products
> Denerica Dental Corporation
> Danville Engineering, Inc.

■ ARTICULATORS
Fully adjustable
RECOMMENDED USE
> Complex prosthodontics
> selected products
> Denar D5A (Teledyne Water Pik)
> Stuart Articulator (CE Stuart)

Semiadjustable
RECOMMENDED USE
> Most prosthodontic diagnosis and treatment

SELECTED PRODUCTS
> Denar Mark II, Advantage (Teledyne Water Pik)
> Panadent (Panadent Corporation)
> Hanau 183-2 (Teledyne Water Pik)
> Model 2240, Model 2340 (Whip Mix Corp.)

■ ASH'S METAL; see SOFT METAL SHEET

■ ATTACHMENTS
Bar attachments
RECOMMENDED USE
> RPD and overdenture support and retention

SELECTED PRODUCTS
> ABS Bar, CBS Bar, Dolder Bar, Hader Bar (Attachments International)
> CM 342 (APM-Sterngold)

Intracoronal rests
RECOMMENDED USE
> RPD support (Chapter 21)
> FPD connectors (Chapter 28)

SELECTED PRODUCTS
> PRP Mandrels (Ticonium Co.)
> PD Attachments (Austenal, Inc.)
> P/S Splint (Bell International)
> Interlock, Omega-M, PDC, Swiss Taper (Attachments International)

Intracoronal slider attachments
RECOMMENDED USE
> RPD retention and support (Chapter 21)

SELECTED PRODUCTS
> Chanes No. 9 (Degussa-Ney Dental, Inc.)
> Sterngold G/A (APM-Sterngold)
> Crismani, McCollum (Attachments International)

Stud attachments
RECOMMENDED USE
> Overdenture retention (Chapter 21)

SELECTED PRODUCTS
> Gijin (Bell International)
> ERA Attachment (Sterngold)
> ORS-OD, Rothermann (Attachments International)
> ZAAG, Zest (Zest Anchors, Inc.)
> Flexi-Post (Essential Dental Systems)

■ BURS, DIAMONDS, AND STONES
High-speed diamonds
RECOMMENDED USE
> Extracoronal tooth preparation (Chapters 8 to 11)

SELECTED PRODUCTS
> Two Striper (Premier Dental Products Co.)
> Brasseler Diamonds (Brasseler USA)
> BluWhite Diamonds (SDS Kerr)

Tungsten-carbide burs
RECOMMENDED USE
> Intracoronal tooth preparation
> Retention features (Chapters 8 to 11)
> Finishing preparations

SELECTED PRODUCTS
> Midwest American Burs (Midwest Dental Products Corporation)
> Brasseler Burs (Brasseler USA)
> Busch Burs (Pfingst & Co., Inc.)
> Carbide Burs (SS White Burs, Inc.)

Laboratory stones (for metal)
RECOMMENDED USE
> Grinding castings (Chapter 29)

SELECTED SUPPLIERS
> Degussa-Ney Dental, Inc.
> Brasseler USA
> Shofu Dental Corp.

Jelenko International
Laboratory stones (for porcelain)

RECOMMENDED USE
Grinding porcelain (Chapters 24 and 25)

SELECTED PRODUCTS
Ceramiste Mounted Points (Shofu Dental Corp.)
Busch Silent, Horico Diamond (Pfingst & Co., Inc.)
Unitek Green Stones (3M-Unitek Corp.)
Green Mounted Points (Jelenko International)

■ CASTING ALLOYS

ADA Type III gold casting alloys

RECOMMENDED USE
Extracoronal and intracoronal restorations (Chapter 22)

SELECTED PRODUCTS
Firmilay (Jelenko International)
Degulor C (Degussa-Ney Dental, Inc.)
Ney-Oro B-2 (Degussa-Ney Dental, Inc.)
Williams Harmony Line Hard (Ivoclar North America)

ADA Type IV gold casting alloys

RECOMMENDED USE
Extracoronal restorations (high stress)

SELECTED PRODUCTS
Jelenko No. 7 (Jelenko International)
Primallor G (Degussa-Ney Dental, Inc.)
Ney-Oro G3 (Degussa-Ney Dental, Inc.)

Lower gold casting alloys

RECOMMENDED USE
Extracoronal and intracoronal restorations

SELECTED PRODUCTS
Midas (Jelenko International)
Midigold (Ivoclar North America)
Miracast (Degussa-Ney Dental, Inc.)
Rx Midacast (Jeneric/Pentron)

Metal-ceramic alloys (base metal)

RECOMMENDED USE
Substructure for metal-ceramic restorations

SELECTED PRODUCTS* (SEE TABLE 19-1)
Rexillium III (Jeneric/Pentron Inc.)
Neobond II (Neoloy Products, Inc.)

Metal-ceramic alloys (high noble metal)

RECOMMENDED USE
Substructure for metal-ceramic restorations (Chapter 19)

SELECTED PRODUCTS*
(see Table 19-1)

■ CEMENTS/LUTING AGENTS

Glass ionomer

RECOMMENDED USE
Permanent cementation (especially with esthetic considerations)

SELECTED PRODUCTS
Ketac-Cem, Ketac-Cem Aplicap (ESPE)
Fuji I (GC America Inc.)
Vivaglass Cem (Ivoclar/Vivadent)

Provisional

RECOMMENDED USE
Luting provisional restorations (Chapter 15)

SELECTED PRODUCTS
Temp-Bond (SDS Kerr)

*Choice may depend on porcelain used

Zone (Cadco)
Resin (adhesive)

RECOMMENDED USE
Permanent cementation (Chapter 31)

SELECTED PRODUCTS
Panavia (J. Morita USA Inc)
C&B Metabond (Parkell Products)

Resin (autopolymerizing)

RECOMMENDED USE
Luting ceramic inlays and veneers (Chapter 25)

SELECTED PRODUCTS
Comspan (Caulk/Dentsply)
Conclude (3M-Dental Products Division)
C&B Luting Composite (Bisco)
Cement-It! (Jeneric/Pentron)

Resin (photopolymerizing)

RECOMMENDED USE
Luting ceramic inlays and veneers (Chapter 25)

SELECTED PRODUCTS
Nexus (SDS Kerr)
Dual Cement (Ivoclar-Vivadent)
Duo-Link (Bisco)
EnForce (Dentsply/Caulk)
Lute-It! (Jeneric/Pentron Inc.)
Ultra-Bond (Den-Mat Corporation)
Variolink II (Ivoclar-Vivadent)

Resin-modified glass ionomer

RECOMMENDED USE
Permanent cementation (Chapter 31)

SELECTED PRODUCTS
Fuji Plus (GC America)
Vitremer (3M Dental)
Principle (Dentsply/Caulk)
ProTec CEM (Ivoclar-Vivadent)

Zinc phosphate

RECOMMENDED USE
Permanent cementation (Chapter 31)
Bases (Chapter 6)

SELECTED PRODUCTS
Fleck's Extraordinary (Keystone Industries)
Tenacin (Caulk)
Smith's Zinc (Teledyne Water Pik)

Zinc polycarboxylate

RECOMMENDED USE
Permanent cementation (Chapter 31; especially with pulpal considerations)

SELECTED PRODUCTS
Durelon, Durelon Aplicap (ESPE)
Hy-Bond (Shofu Dental Corp.)
Liv Carbo (GC America, Inc.)
PCA (Mission Dental, Inc.)

■ CROWN AND FPD REMOVERS

RECOMMENDED USE
See Chapter 32

SELECTED PRODUCTS
Coronaflex crown remover (KaVo America)
Metalift Crown and Bridge Removal System (Classic Practice Resources)
Roydent Bridge and Crown Remover (Roydent Dental Products)

Richwell Crown and Bridge Remover (Almore International, Inc.)

Atwood Crown and Bridge Remover (Atwood Industries)

Crown and Bridge Removers (Parkell Products)

■ CYANOACRYLATE RESIN

RECOMMENDED USE

Impregnating stone dies (Chapters 17, 18, 19, and 24)
Cementing Pindex dowel pins (Chapter 17)

SELECTED PRODUCTS

Hot Stuff (Satellite City, Inc.) (hardware stores)
Permabond 910 (George Taub Products & Fusion Co.)
Krazy Glue (hardware stores)
DVA Rocket (Dental Ventures of America, Inc.)

■ DENTURE TEETH

SELECTED PRODUCTS

Trubyte (Dentsply/York Division)
Justi (American Tooth Industries)
Ivoclar (Ivoclar North America)
Vitapan (Vident)

■ DIAMONDS; see BURS, DIAMONDS, AND STONES

■ DIE LUBRICANT

RECOMMENDED USE

Lubricating dies before waxing (Chapter 17)

SELECTED PRODUCTS

Slikdie Lubricant (Slaycris Products, Inc.)
Gator Die Lube (Whip Mix Corp.)
Die Lube (Degussa-Ney Dental, Inc.)
Isolit (Degussa-Ney Dental, Inc.)

■ DIE MATERIALS (ALTERNATIVES TO GYPSUM)

RECOMMENDED USE

Dies for complete ceramic crowns (Chapter 25)

Electroplating materials

SELECTED SUPPLIERS

Engelhard/Baker Dental

Epoxy resins

SELECTED PRODUCTS

Epoxy-Die (Ivoclar North America, Inc.)
Poly-Roqq (Dental Ventures of America, Inc.)

■ DIE SAWS

RECOMMENDED USE

Sectioning working casts (Chapter 17)

SELECTED PRODUCTS

Ney Die Saw (Degussa-Ney Dental, Inc.)
Pindex Hand Saw (Coltène/Whaledent, Inc.)

DIE SPACERS

RECOMMENDED USE

To increase space for luting agent (Chapter 17)

SELECTED PRODUCTS

Pactra Aerogloss (hobby stores)
Die Spacer (SDS Kerr)
Tru-Fit (George Taub Products & Fusion Co.)

■ DIE SYSTEMS

RECOMMENDED USE

Fabricating removable dies (Chapter 17)

SELECTED PRODUCTS

(See Table 17-2)
Pindex (Coltène/Whaledent, Inc.)
Dilok (Di-Equi Dental Products)
DVA Model System (DVA, Inc.)
Zeiser model system (Girrbach Dental GmbH)
Dowel pins (Buffalo Dental Mfg. Co., Inc.; Degussa-Ney Dental, Inc.)

■ ELECTROPLATING MATERIALS; see DIE MATERIALS

■ ELECTROSURGICAL EQUIPMENT

RECOMMENDED USE

Removal of hyperplastic tissue before impression making (Chapter 14)

SELECTED PRODUCTS

Electrosurgical Unit (Macan Engineering & Mfg. Co.)
Dento-Surg 90 (Ellman International Manufacturing Co.)
PerFect TCS (Coltène/Whaledent, Inc)
Sensimatic (Parkell Products)
Macan MC-6 (Macan Engineering & Mfg. Co.)

■ EPOXY RESIN DIE MATERIALS; see DIE MATERIALS

■ FACEBOWS

RECOMMENDED USE

Articulator mounting casts (Chapters 2 and 17)

SELECTED PRODUCTS

Slidematic (Teledyne Water Pik)
Quick Mount (Whip Mix Corp.)
Earpiece Facebow (Teledyne Water Pik)
Hinge Axis Locator (Almore International, Inc.)

■ FIBER-REINFORCED COMPOSITES

RECOMMENDED USE

Alternative to metal ceramic restorations (Chapter 27)

SELECTED PRODUCTS

Ribbond/BelleGlass (SDS Kerr)
Connect (GlasSpan, Inc.)
Vectris/Targis (Ivoclar North America)
Fiberkor/Sculpture, Splint-It (Jeneric/Pentron Inc)

■ GINGIVAL DISPLACEMENT

Astringent solutions

RECOMMENDED USE

Gingival displacement before impression making (Chapter 14)

SELECTED PRODUCTS

Hemodent (Premier Dental Products Co.)
Gingi-Aid (Belport Corp./Gingi-Pak)
Astringedent (Ultradent Products Inc.)
Visine Eye Drops (Pfizer)
Afrin (oxymetazoline) Nose Spray (Schering-Plough HealthCare Products, Inc.)

Displacement cord

RECOMMENDED USE

Gingival displacement before impression making (Chapter 14)

SELECTED PRODUCTS

Gingi-Pak (Belport Corp./Gingi-Pak)

Gingibraid, Gingigel (Van R Dental Products)

Sil-Trax (Pascal Company, Inc.)

Ultrapak (Ultradent Products, Inc.)

■ GYPSUM PRODUCTS

ADA Types IV and V die stones

RECOMMENDED USE

Casts and dies (Chapters 2 and 17)

SELECTED PRODUCTS

Silky-Rock, Prima-Rock, Jade Stone Super-Die, Resin-Rock, Hard Rock (Whip Mix Corp.)

Vel-Mix Stone, Supra Stone (SDS Kerr)

Glastone, Glastone 2000 (Dentsply/Trubyte)

Die-Keen, Milestone, Die-Stone, Tru-Stone (Modern Materials, Heraeus Kulzer, Inc.)

Synthetic Die Stone (Microstar Corporation)

Impression plaster

RECOMMENDED USE

Soldering index (Chapter 28)

Occlusal registration (Chapter 17)

SELECTED PRODUCTS

Snow White No 2 (SDS Kerr)

Mounting stone

RECOMMENDED USE

Articulator mounting casts (Chapters 2 and 17)

SELECTED PRODUCTS

Mounting Stone (Whip Mix Corp.)

Castone Dental Stone (Dentsply/Trubyte)

■ IMPLANT MATERIALS

SELECTED SUPPLIERS

Nobelbiocare

Sulzer Calcitek

Astratech

3i (Implant Innovations)

Strauman (I.T.I.)

Paragon (Core-Vent)

Implant Support Systems, Inc.

Lifecore Biomedical

Friadent

■ IMPRESSION MATERIALS

Addition silicone

RECOMMENDED USE

Impressions of preparations (Chapter 14)

SELECTED PRODUCTS

Extrude, Take 1 (SDS Kerr)

Reprosil, Aquasil (Caulk/Dentsply)

Exaflex, Examix (GC America Inc.)

Imprint, Express (3M-Dental Products Division)

President (Coltène/Whaledent, Inc.)

Irreversible hydrocolloid (alginate)

RECOMMENDED USE

Impressions for diagnostic casts (Chapter 2)

Duplicating diagnostic waxing

SELECTED PRODUCTS

Jeltrate (Caulk/Dentsply)

Coe Alginate (GC America, Inc.)

Supergel (Harry J. Bosworth Co.)

Polyether

RECOMMENDED USE

Impressions of preparations (Chapter 14)

SELECTED PRODUCTS

Impregum, Permadyne (ESPE America)

Polygel (Caulk/Dentsply)

Polysulfide polymer

RECOMMENDED USE

Impressions of preparations (Chapter 14)

SELECTED PRODUCTS

Permlastic (SDS Kerr)

Coe-Flex (GC America, Inc.)

Reversible hydrocolloid (agar)

RECOMMENDED USE

Impressions of preparations (Chapter 14)

SELECTED PRODUCTS

Rubberloid, Acculoid (Van R Dental Products)

GingiPak (Belport Corp./Gingi-Pak)

Silicone putty

RECOMMENDED USE

External mold for provisionals (Chapter 15)

Preparation reduction guide (Chapters 8 to 11)

SELECTED PRODUCTS

Citricon (putty) (SDS Kerr)

Accoe Silicone Tray Impression Material (GC America, Inc.)

Zinc oxide-eugenol occlusal registration (impression) pastes

RECOMMENDED USE

Occlusal records (Chapters 2 and 17)

Soldering records (Chapter 28)

Remount procedure (Chapter 30)

SELECTED PRODUCTS

Superpaste (Harry J. Bosworth Co.)

Luralite (SDS Kerr)

■ IMPRESSION SYRINGES

RECOMMENDED USE

Making elastomeric impressions (Chapter 14)

SELECTED PRODUCTS

Coe Syringe, Plastic Syringe (GC America, Inc)

Free-Flo Syringe (SDS Kerr)

Impregum Syringe (ESPE America)

■ INTERNAL FITTING AGENTS

RECOMMENDED USE

Evaluating and refining internal fit of restoration (Chapter 30)

SELECTED PRODUCTS

Fit Checker (GC America, Inc.)

Disclosing Wax (SDS Kerr)

PIP Pressure Indicator Paste (Mizzy, Inc.)

■ INVESTING EQUIPMENT

Casting rings, liners, and crucible formers

SELECTED SUPPLIERS

Whip Mix Corp.

Degussa-Ney Dental, Inc.
SDS KerrBelle de St. Claire
Buffalo Dental Mfg. Co., Inc.

■ INVESTMENT MATERIALS
Gypsum bonded
RECOMMENDED USE
Conventional (low-heat) casting (Chapter 22)
SELECTED PRODUCTS
Beauty Cast (Whip Mix Corp.)
Luster Cast (SDS Kerr)
Investments for porcelain
RECOMMENDED USE
Ceramic inlays and veneers (Chapter 25)
selected products (*Note*: some ceramic systems require manufacturer's specified material)
V.H.T., Polyvest (Whip Mix Corp.)
Neo-Brillat (Vident)
Phosphate bonded
RECOMMENDED USE
Casting metal-ceramic alloys (Chapter 19)
Pre-ceramic application soldering (Chapter 28)
SELECTED PRODUCTS
Cerafina, Ceramigold, Hi-Temp, FastFire 15, Power-Cast (Whip Mix Corp.)
Complete, High-Span II, JelVest (Jelenko International)
Deguvest F (Degussa-Ney Dental, Inc.)
Soldering investment
RECOMMENDED USE
Soldering (Chapter 28)
SELECTED PRODUCTS
Hi-Heat, Speed-E, Soldering Investment (Whip Mix Corp.)
Quick Set Soldering Investment (SDS Kerr/Belle de St. Claire)

■ MAGNIFICATION EQUIPMENT
Laboratory microscope
SELECTED SUPPLIERS
Nikon, Inc. Instrument Group
Olympus America, Inc.
Austenal, Inc.
Carl Zeiss, Inc.
Loupes
SELECTED SUPPLIERS
Almore International, Inc.
Lactona/Universal
Designs for Vision, Inc.
American Optical
Orascoptic Research, Inc.
General Scientific Corporation

■ MARKING AGENTS
RECOMMENDED USE
Identifying unwanted contacts on the fitting surface of castings (Chapters 20 and 26)
SELECTED PRODUCTS
Occlude (Pascal Company, Inc.)
Accufilm IV (Parkell Products)
Liqua-Mark (The Wilkinson Company)

■ MODELING COMPOUND
RECOMMENDED USE
Modifying impression trays (Chapter 2)
Supporting rubber dam clamps, matrix bands (Chapter 6)
Transfer fork registration (Chapter 2)
SELECTED PRODUCTS
Mizzy Impression Compound (Mizzy, Inc.)
Impression Compound (SDS Kerr)

■ MOISTURE-CONTROL PRODUCTS
Adhesive foil
RECOMMENDED USE
Moisture control during cementation (Chapter 31)
SELECTED PRODUCT
Burlew Dryfoil (Jelenko International)
Saliva ejectors
RECOMMENDED USE
Moisture and tongue control (Chapters 8 to 11 and 14)
SELECTED PRODUCTS
Svedopta (E.C. Moore Co.)
Speejector (Pulpdent Corp.)

■ OCCLUSAL CONTACT INDICATORS
Articulating film
RECOMMENDED USE
Identifying the location of occlusal contacts (Chapters 4, 6, and 30)
SELECTED PRODUCTS
Accu-Film II (Parkell Products)
Articulating Silk-Mark Ribbon (J.R. Rand Corp.)
ArtTape, GHM Articulating film, Madam Butterfly Silk (Almore International, Inc.)
Powdered wax
RECOMMENDED USE
As an alternative to zinc stearate to identify wax contacts (Chapter 18)
SELECTED PRODUCTS
Powdered Dusting Wax (Almore International, Inc.)
Powdered Dusting Wax (DeLar Corporation)
Thin Mylar film
RECOMMENDED USE
Identifying the presence of occlusal contact (Chapters 4, 6, and 30)
SELECTED PRODUCTS
Plastic Shim Stock (.0005") (Artus Corporation)
Shimstock Occlusion Foil (Almore International, Inc.)

■ PICKLING SOLUTION
RECOMMENDED USE
Removing oxides from castings (Chapter 22)
SELECTED PRODUCT
Pickle-It (American Dental Supply, Inc.)
Prevox (Ivoclar North America)

■ POLISHING MATERIALS
Acrylic resins (Chapters 4 and 14)
SELECTED PRODUCTS
Pumice (Whip Mix Corp.)
Finalustre (Buffalo Dental Mfg. Co., Inc.)

Fabulustre (William Dixon Co.)

Castings (Chapter 29)
SELECTED PRODUCTS
Moore's Disks (E.C. Moore Co.)
White Flexies (Dedeco International, Inc.)
Tripoli, Rouge (Buffalo Dental Mfg. Co., Inc.)
BBC (Jelenko International)

Porcelain (Chapter 30)
SELECTED PRODUCTS
Porcelain Polishers (Brasseler USA, Inc.)
Two-Striper (Premier Dental Products Co.)
Porcelain Adjustment Kit (Shofu Dental Corp.)
Diamond Polishing Paste (Vident)

■ PORCELAIN
Complete ceramic
RECOMMENDED USE
Crowns, inlays, and veneers with high esthetic need (Chapter 25)
SELECTED PRODUCTS
Empress, Empress 2 (Ivoclar North America)
In-Ceram, Vitadur Alpha (Vident)
Optimal (Jeneric/Pentron, Inc.)

Metal-ceramic
RECOMMENDED USE
Esthetic crowns and FPDs (Chapter 24)
SELECTED PRODUCTS
IPS Classic (Ivoclar North America)
Vita VMK-95, Omega 900 (Vident)

■ PORCELAIN INSTRUMENTS
SELECTED SUPPLIERS
Vident
SDS Kerr/Belle de St. Claire
Jelenko International

■ PORCELAIN STAINS
RECOMMENDED USE
Staining ceramic restorations (Chapter 30)
SELECTED PRODUCTS
Vita-Chrom (Vident)
DTC Color System Kit (Jelenko International)
IPS Classic Stains-P (Ivoclar North America)

■ POST REMOVERS
SELECTED PRODUCTS
Masserann Kit (Medidenta International, Inc)
Post Puller (Star Dental/Den-tal-ez, Inc.)
Peerless Crown Remover (Peerless International, Inc)
Gonon (Thomas Extracteur De Pivots)

■ POST SYSTEMS
Post preparation drills
RECOMMENDED USE
Restoration of endodontically treated teeth (Chapter 12)
SELECTED PRODUCTS
Gates-Glidden drills (Pulpdent Corp.)

Posts
RECOMMENDED USE
Restoration of endodontically treated teeth (Chapter 12)

SELECTED PRODUCTS (*see also* TABLE 12-5)
EZ Cast Post (Merritt EZ Cast Post, Inc)
Endowel (Star Dental/Syntex Dental Products Inc)
ParaPost (Coltène/Whaledent, Inc.)
PGP Wire (Degussa-Ney Dental, Inc.)

■ PREFABRICATED CROWN FORMS
RECOMMENDED USE
Provisional restorations (Chapter 15)
Metal (posterior teeth)
SELECTED PRODUCTS
Aluminum Crowns (3M-Unitek Corp.)
Iso-Form Ion Crowns (3M-Dental Products Division)
Resin (anterior teeth)
SELECTED PRODUCTS
Ion Polycarbonate Crowns (3M-Dental Products Division)
B-Crowns (Harry J. Bosworth Co.)

■ RESINS
Autopolymerizing acrylic resin pattern material
RECOMMENDED USE
Direct patterns for post and cores (Chapter 12)
Soldering index (Chapter 28)
Recording occlusal relationship (Chapter 17)
SELECTED PRODUCTS
Duralay (Reliance Dental Mfg. Co.)
Pattern Resin (GC America, Inc.)
Relate (Parkell Products)
Palavit G (Heraeus Kulzer, Inc.)
Autopolymerizing clear acrylic resin
RECOMMENDED USE
Fabricating occlusal appliances (Chapter 4)
SELECTED PRODUCTS
Caulk Orthodontic Resin (Caulk/Dentsply)
COE Ortho-Resin II (GC America, Inc.)
Custom tray resin
RECOMMENDED USE
Impression trays (Chapter 14)
Anterior guide table (Chapter 2)
Remount procedure (Chapter 30)
SELECTED PRODUCTS
Formatray (SDS Kerr)
Tray Resin (Caulk/Dentsply)
TMJ Resin (TMJ Instrument Co., Inc.)
Hygon Tray Resin (Hygenic Corporation)
COE Tray Plastic (GC America, Inc.)
Heat-polymerized clear acrylic resin
RECOMMENDED USE
Fabricating occlusal appliances (Chapter 4)
SELECTED PRODUCTS
Perma-Cryl Clear (GC America, Inc.)
Lucitone Clear (Caulk/Dentsply)
Light-cured pattern resin
RECOMMENDED USE
Direct patterns for cores (Chapter 12)
Soldering index (Chapter 28)
Recording occlusal relationship (Chapter 17)
SELECTED PRODUCTS
Palavit G LC (Heraeus Kulzer, Inc.)
Luminex (Dentatus USA Ltd.)

Provisional resin

RECOMMENDED USE

Fabricating provisional restorations (Chapter 15)

SELECTED PRODUCTS

Jet (Lang Dental Mfg. Co., Inc.)

Temporary Bridge Resin (Caulk/Dentsply)

Alike (GC America, Inc)

Snap (Parkell Products)

Temporary Bridge Resin (Caulk/Dentsply)

Trim (Harry J. Bosworth Co.)

Temporary Bridge Resin (Caulk/Dentsply)

Protemp Garant (ESPE America.)

Integrity (Caulk/Dentsply)

Temphase (SDS Kerr)

Luxatemp (Zenith)

■ RESIN STAINS

RECOMMENDED USE

Staining provisional restorations (Chapter 15)

SELECTED PRODUCTS

Jet adjusters (Lang Dental Mfg. Co., Inc.)

Minute Stains (George Taub Products & Fusion Co.)

■ SEATING STICKS

RECOMMENDED USE

Seating cast restorations (Chapter 31)

SELECTED PRODUCTS

Aidaco Bite Sticks (Temrex Corporation)

■ SEPARATING FLUIDS; see also DIE LUBRICANT

RECOMMENDED USE

Fabricating provisional restorations (Chapter 15)

Fabricating occlusal appliances (Chapter 4)

SELECTED PRODUCTS

Al-Cote (Caulk/Dentsply)

Modern Foil (Jelenko International)

Foil Cote (Buffalo Dental Mfg. Co., Inc.)

■ SOFT METAL SHEET (ASH'S METAL)

RECOMMENDED USE

Reinforcing centric record (Chapter 2)

SELECTED PRODUCT

Relief Metal (William Dixon Co.)

■ SOLDERING FLUX

RECOMMENDED USE

Preventing oxidation during soldering (Chapter 28)

SELECTED PRODUCTS

DS 1 Soldering Flux (Degussa Corporation)

Soldering Flux (Degussa-Ney Dental, Inc.)

■ SOLDERS

High-heat

RECOMMENDED USE

Pre-ceramic soldering (Chapter 28)

SELECTED PRODUCTS

(Use material recommended by alloy manufacturer.)

Low-heat

RECOMMENDED USE

Soldered connectors for conventional gold restorations (Chapter 28)

Post-ceramic soldered connectors (Chapter 28)

SELECTED PRODUCTS

Slim strip 650 solder (Jelenko International)

Ney Balanced Line Regular Solder (Degussa-Ney Dental, Inc.)

Engelhard Dental Solders (Engelhard/Baker Dental)

■ STONES; SEE BURS, DIAMONDS, AND STONES

■ SURFACTANTS

RECOMMENDED USE

Painting patterns before investing (Chapter 22)

SELECTED PRODUCTS

Smoothex (Whip Mix Corp.)

DeBubblizer (SDS Kerr)

DeLar Surfactant (DeLar Corporation)

■ THERMOPLASTIC RESIN SHEETS

RECOMMENDED USE

External mold for provisionals (Chapter 15)

Matrix for occlusal appliance (Chapter 4)

Tooth-preparation reduction guides (Chapters 8 to 11)

SELECTED PRODUCTS

Sta-Vac (Buffalo Dental Mfg. Co., Inc.)

Temporary Splint (Dentiform, Inc.)

■ THICKNESS GAUGES

RECOMMENDED USE

Measuring thickness of patterns and restorations

SELECTED PRODUCTS

Dial Caliper (Almore International, Inc.)

Crown gauge (Miltex Instrument Co.)

Iwanson Spring Caliper (Hu-Friedy Mfr. Co.)

Calipers (Buffalo Dental Mfg. Co., Inc.)

■ ULTRASONIC CLEANERS AND SOLUTIONS

RECOMMENDED USE

Cleaning restorations and provisionals

SELECTED SUPPLIERS

Jelenko International

L & R Mfg. Co.

Hu-Friedy Mfr. Co.

Coltène/Whaledent, Inc.

■ VACUUM FORMERS

RECOMMENDED USE

External molds for provisional restorations (Chapter 15)

Tooth preparation reduction guides (Chapters 8 to11)

SELECTED SUPPLIERS

Buffalo Dental Mfg. Co., Inc.

Ultradent Products, Inc.

■ WAXES

Boxing wax

RECOMMENDED USE

Boxing impressions (Chapter 14)

Boxing soldering assembly (Chapter 28)

SELECTED PRODUCTS

Boxing Wax (Hygenic Corporation)

Pro-Craft Boxing Wax Strips (William Dixon Co.)

also Magnetic Boxing Strips:

Magnetic Vinyl Strips (Almore International, Inc.)
DeLar Magnetic Boxing Strip (DeLar Corporation)

Inlay casting wax

RECOMMENDED USE
Making wax patterns (Chapter 18)
SELECTED PRODUCTS
Inlay Casting Wax (SDS Kerr)
Plastodent (Degussa Corporation)
Red Casting Wax (Jelenko International)
Flex 200 (MDL Dental Products)

Occlusal registration wax

RECOMMENDED USE
Centric recording for diagnostic casts (Chapter 2)
SELECTED PRODUCTS
Aluwax (Aluwax Dental Products Co.)
Delar Wax (Almore International, Inc.)

Sprue wax

RECOMMENDED USE
Sprue former (Chapter 22)
SELECTED PRODUCTS
Sprue Wax (SDS Kerr)
Sprue Wax (Jelenko International)
Stalite Round Wire Wax (Buffalo Dental Mfg. Co., Inc.)
Pro-Craft Sprue Rod Wax (William Dixon Co.)

■ WAXING INSTRUMENTS

SELECTED SUPPLIERS
American Dental Mfg.
Hu-Friedy Mfr. Co.
Premier Dental Products Co.
ELECTRIC INSTRUMENTS
Almore International, Inc.
Ultra-Waxer (SDS Kerr/Belle de St. Claire)

MANUFACTURERS' INDEX

ABRASIVE TECHNOLOGY, INC
8400 Green Meadows Drive
P.O. Box 6127
Westerville, OH 43081
(800) 964-8324
Fax: (740) 548-7617
www.abrasive-tech.com

ALMORE INTERNATIONAL, INC.
P.O. Box 25214
Portland, OR 97225
(800) 547-1511
Fax: (503) 643-9748
www.almore.com

ALUWAX DENTAL PRODUCTS CO.
4180 44th Street, SE
Grand Rapids, MI 49512
(616) 895-4385
Fax: (616) 895-5060

AMERADENT INC OF NEVADA
2533 North Carson Street
Carson City, NV 89706
(800) 959-8517
(916) 858-1250

AMERICAN DENTAL MFG. (*see* GC AMERICA INC)

AMERICAN DENTAL SUPPLY, INC.
2600 William Penn Highway
Easton, PA 18042
(800) 558-5925
Fax: (610) 252-2822

AMERICAN TOOTH INDUSTRIES
1200 Stellar Drive
Oxnard, CA 93033
(800) 235-4639
Fax: (805) 483-8482
www.americantooth.com

APM-STERNGOLD (*see* STERNGOLD)

ARTUS CORPORATION
P.O. Box 511
201 South Dean Street
Englewood, NJ 07631
(201) 568-1000
Fax: (201) 568-8865
www.artusshim.com

ASEPTICO INTERNATIONAL
P.O. Box 1548
Woodinville, WA 98072
(800) 426-5913
Fax: (360) 668-8722
www.aseptico.com

ASTRA TECH, INC.
430 Bedford Street, Suite 100,
Lexington, MA 02173.
(781) 861-7707
Fax: (781) 861-7787
www.astratech.com

ATTACHMENTS INTERNATIONAL
600 S. Amphlett Blvd
San Mateo, CA 94402
(800) 999-3003
Fax: (650) 340-8423
www.attachments.com

ATWOOD INDUSTRIES
1708 Rubenstein Drive
Cardiff-by-the-Sea, CA 92007
(619) 944-9884
Fax: (619) 944-0112

AURIUM RESEARCH, U.S.A.
5855 Oberlin Drive
San Diego, CA 92121
(800) 645-6110
Fax: (516) 763-6710

AUSTENAL, INC.
4101 W. 51st Street
Chicago, IL 60632
(800) 621-0381
Fax: (312) 735-3940

BAUSCH ARTICULATING PAPERS, INC.
11 Lacy Lane
Nashua, NH 03062
(800) 622-8724
Fax: (603) 595-9988
www.bauschdental.com

BAYER INC (*see* HERAEUS KULZER, INC.)

BELL INTERNATIONAL
31 Edwards Court
Burlingame, CA 94010
(800) 523-6640
Fax: (415) 348-3937

BELLE DE ST. CLAIRE A DIVISION OF SDS KERR
1717 West Collins Avenue
Orange, CA 92867
(800) 322-6666
Fax: (818) 341-1142
www.sybrondental.com

BELPORT CORP./GINGI-PAK
P.O. Box 240
4825 Calle Alto
Camarillo, CA 93011-0240

(800) 437-1514
Fax: (805) 484-5076

BENCO DENTAL
11 Bear Creek Boulevard
Wilkes-Barre, PA 18702
(800) 462-3626
(570) 823-9947
www.benco.com

BISCO DENTAL PRODUCTS
1100 W. Irving Park Road
Schaumburg, IL 60193
(800) 247-3368
Fax: (800) 959-9550
www.bisco.com

HARRY J. BOSWORTH CO.
7227 N. Hamlin Avenue
Skokie, IL 60076
(800) 323-4352
Fax: (708) 679-2080
www.bosworth.com

BRASSELER USA
800 King George Blvd.
Savannah, GA 31419
(800) 841-4522
Fax: (912) 927-8671
www.brasseler.com

BUFFALO DENTAL MFG. CO., INC.
99 Lafayette Drive
Syosset, NY 11791
(800) 828-0203
Fax: (516) 496-7751
www.buffalodental.com

JOHN O. BUTLER COMPANY
4635 West Foster Avenue
Chicago, IL 60630
(800) 528-8537
Fax: (312) 777-5101
www.jbutler.com

CADCO DENTAL PRODUCTS, INC.
600 East Hueneme Road
Oxnard, CA 93033
(800) 833-8267
Fax: (805) 488-2266
www.cadcodental.com

CALCITEK (*see* SULZER CALCITEK, INC.)

CAPTEK PRECIOUS CHEMICALS
2957 State Road 434, Suite 100
Longwood, FL 32750
(800) 921-2227
Fax: (407) 889-8893
www.captek.com

CARL ZEISS, INC.
One Zeiss Drive
Thornwood, NY 10594
(800) 442-4020
Fax: (914) 681-7446
www.zeiss.com

CAULK/DENTSPLY
38 West Clarke Avenue
Milford, DE 19963
(800) 532-2855
Fax: (800) 788-4110
www.caulk.com

CERAMCO, INC.
Six Terri Lane
Burlington, NJ 08016
(800) 487-0100
Fax: (609) 386-8282
www.ceramco.com

CHAMELEON DENTAL PRODUCTS
200 N 6th Street
Kansas City, KS 66101
(800) 366-0001
Fax: (913) 621-7012
www.miragecdp.com

R. CHIGE, INC.
4531 N. Dixie Highway
Boca Raton, FL 33431
(800) 645-2628
Fax: (561) 338-5668

CLASSIC PRACTICE RESOURCES
Div. Westerman Enterprises, Inc.
7855 Jefferson Highway
Baton Rouge LA 70809
(800) 928-9289
Fax: (504) 923-2499

COE LABORATORIES, INC. (*see* GC AMERICA, INC.)

COLGATE ORAL PHARMACEUTICALS
1 Colgate Way
Canton, MA 02021
(800) 527-0222
Fax: (617) 821-2187
www.colgate.com

COLTÈNE/WHALEDENT, INC.
750 Corporate Drive
Mahwah, NJ 07430
(201) 512-8000
Fax: (201) 539-2103
www.coltenewhaledent.com

COLUMBIA DENTOFORM
22-19 41 Avenue
Long Island City, NY 11101
(718) 482-1569
Fax: (718) 482-1585
www.columbiadentoform.com

COLUMBUS DENTAL *see* HERAEUS KULZER, INC.)

COPALITE/COOLEY & COOLEY, LTD.
8550 Westland West Blvd.
Houston, TX 77041

(800) 215-4487
Fax: (800) 215-4489
www.copalite.com

CORE-VENT CORP. (*see* PARAGON IMPLANT COMPANY)

COTTRELL LTD.
7399 S. Tucson Way
Englewood, CO 80112
(800) 843-3343
Fax: (303) 799-9408

CLIVE CRAIG
600 East Hueneme Road
Oxnard, CA 93033
(800) 833-8267
Fax: (805) 488-2266
www.clivecraig.com

CRESCENT DENTAL MFG. CO
7750 West 47th Street
Lyons, IL 60534
(800) 323-8952
Fax: (708) 447-8190
www.cresentproducts.com

CTH
393 Sunrise Highway
West Babylon, NY 11704
(800) 458-6152
Fax: (516) 661-8792

DANVILLE ENGINEERING, INC
1901 San Ramon Valley Blvd.
San Ramon, CA 94583
(800) 827-7940
Fax: (510) 838-0944
www.ddsnet.com/danville

DEDECO INTERNATIONAL, INC.
Route 97
Long Eddy, NY 12760
(888) 433-3326
Fax: (914) 887-5281
www.dedeco.com

DEGUSSA-NEY DENTAL, INC.
65 West Dudley Town Road,
Bloomfield, CT 06002
(860) 242-6188
Fax: (860) 769-5050
www.neydental.com

DeLAR CORPORATION
P.O. Box 226
Lake Oswego, OR 97034
(800) 669-7499
Fax: (503) 635-2978
www.delar.com

DENAR CORP. (*see* TELEDYNE WATER PIK)

DENERICA DENTAL CORPORATION
313 Oswalt Avenue
Batavia, Illinois 60510
(800) 336-7422
Fax: (630) 761-9663
www.denerica.com

DEN-MAT CORPORATION
P.O. Box 1729

Santa Maria, CA 93456
(800) 433-6628
Fax: (805) 922-6933
www.denmat.com

DENOVO
5130 Commerce Dr.
Baldwin Park, CA 91706
(800) 854-7949
Fax: (800) 847-8599
www.denovodental.com

DEN-TAL-EZ/STAR DENTAL
1816 Colonial Village Lane
Lancaster, PA 17601
(800) 275-3320
Fax: (717) 291-5699
www.dentalez.com

DENTAL POWER (*see* WESTERN DENTAL SPECIALTIES/DENTAL POWER)

DENTAL VENTURES OF AMERICA, INC.
217 Lewis Court
Corona, CA 91720
(800) 228-6696
Fax: (909) 270-0636
www.dentalventures.com

DENTATUS USA LTD.
192 Lexington Avenue
New York, NY 10016
(800) 323-3136
Fax: (212) 532-9026
www.dentatus.com

DENTIFORM, INC.
210 Division Street
Kingston, PA 18704
(800) 441-5421
Fax: (717) 283-9094

DENTIFAX/DI-EQUI
17 Old Route Nine
Wappingers Falls, NY 12590
(800) 643-1603
Fax: (914) 297-1626
www.dentifax.com

DENTSPLY INTERNATIONAL
570 W. College Ave
P.O. Box 872
York, PA 17405
(800) 877-0020
Fax: (717) 854-1599
www.dentsply.com

DESIGNS FOR VISION, INC
760 Koehler Avenue
Ronkonkoma, NY 11779
(800) 727-6407
Fax: (516) 585-3404
www.designsforvision.com

DI-EQUI (*see* DENTIFAX/DI-EQUI)

LESTER A. DINE, INC.
PGA Commerce Park
351 Hiatt Drive
Palm Beach Gardens, FL 33418
(800) 237-7226

Fax: (407) 624-9103
www.lesterdine.com

WILLIAM DIXON CO.
750 Washington Avenue
Carlstadt, NJ 07072
(800) 847-4188
Fax: (800) 243-2432
www.grobetusa.com

DMG-HAMBURG (*see* ZENITH)

ELLMAN INTERNATIONAL, INC.
1135 Railroad Avenue
Hewlett, NY 11557
(800) 835-5355
Fax: (516) 569-0054
www.ellman.com

ESPE NORTH AMERICA
1710 Romano Dr.
P.O. Box 111
Norristown, PA 19404
(800) 344-8235
Fax: (800) 458-3987
www.espeusa.com

ESSENTIAL DENTAL SYSTEMS
89 Leuning Street
South Hackensack, NJ 07606
(800) 223-5394
Fax: (201) 487-5120
www.edsdental.com

FILHOL DENTAL USA
1219B Greenwood Road,
Baltimore, MD 21208
(800) 910-2050
Fax: (410) 484-6354
www.filhol.com

FLORIDA PROBE CORPORATION
3700 NW 91st Street
Suite C-100
Gainesville, FL 32606
(352) 372-1142
Fax: (352) 372-0257
www.floridaprobe.com

GC AMERICA, INC.
3737 West 127th Street,
Alsip, IL 60803
(800) 323-7063
Fax: (800) 423-2963
www.gcamerica.com

GEL-KAM (*see* COLGATE ORAL PHARMACEUTICALS)

GENERAL SCIENTIFIC CORPORATION
77 Enterprise Drive
Ann Arbor, MI 48103
(800) 959-0153
Fax: (734) 662-0520
www.surgitel.com

GINGI-PAK (*see* BELPORT CORP./GINGI-PAK)

GIRRBACH DENTAL GmbH
PO Box 14 01 20
75138 Pforzheim

Germany
+49-(0)72 31-957-160
Fax: +49-(0)72 31-957-169
www.Girrbach.com

GLASSPAN, INC.
101 J.R. Thomas Drive
Exton, PA 19341
800-280-7726
Fax: 610-363-6391
www.dentalxchange.com/glasspan/

GRESCO PRODUCTS, INC.
12603 Executive Drive, 814
P.O. Box 865
Stafford, TX 77477
(800) 527-3250
Fax: (713) 240-2371

HANDLER MFR. COMPANY, INC.
P.O. Box 520
Westfield, NJ 07091-0520
(800) 274-2635
Fax: (908) 233-7340

HERAEUS KULZER, INC.
4315 S. Lafayette Blvd.
South Bend, IN 46614
(800) 343-5336
Fax: (219) 291-7248
www.kulzer.com

HU-FRIEDY MFR. CO., INC.
3232 N. Rockwell Street
Chicago, IL 60618
(800) 729-3743
Fax:(773) 975-1683
www.hufriedy.com

HYGENIC CORPORATION, THE
1245 Home Avenue
Akron, OH 44310
(800) 321-2135
Fax: (330) 633-9359
www.hygenic.com

HYDRO-CAST DENTAL PRODUCTS
A Division of Kay-See Dental Manufacturing Company
124 East Missouri Avenue
Kansas City, MO 64106
(800) 842-8844
Fax: (816) 842-3402
www.hydrocast.com

IMPLANT INNOVATIONS *see* 3I CORPORATION)

INTERPORE INTERNATIONAL
181 Technololgy Drive
Irvine, CA 92718
(800) 722-4489
Fax: (714) 727-7084
www.interpore.com

INTRATECH DENTAL PRODUCTS
3301 Conflans Rd. Suite 101
Irving,TX 75061
(800) 443-3536
Fax: (972) 790-9480

www.intratechdental.com

IVOCLAR NORTH AMERICA, INC.
175 Pineview Drive
Amherst, NY 14228
(800) 533-6825
Fax: (716) 691-2285
www.ivoclarna.com

JELENKO INTERNATIONAL
99 Business Park Dr.
Armonk, NY 10504
(800) 431-1785
Fax: (914) 273-9379
www.jelenko.com

JENERIC/PENTRON, INC.
53 North Plains Industrial Rd.
P.O. Box 724
Wallingford, CT 06492
(800) 551-0283
Fax: (203) 284-3310
www.jeneric.com

JENSEN INDUSTRIES
50 Stillman Road
North Haven, CT 06473
(800) 243-2000
Fax: (203) 239-7630
www.jensenindustries.com

KAVO AMERICA CORPORATION
340 East Main Street
Lake Zurich, IL 60047
(800) 323-8029
Fax: (847) 550-6434
www.kavousa.com

KERR DENTAL (*see* SDS KERR)

KEYSTONE INDUSTRIES
616 Hollywood Avenue
Cherry Hill, NJ 08002
(800) 333-3131
Fax: (609) 663-0381
www.keystoneind.com

KILGORE INTERNATIONAL, INC.
36 West Pearl Street
Coldwater, MI 49036 USA
(800) 892-9999
Fax: (517) 278-2956
www.dentalstudymodels.com

L & R MFG. CO.
577 Elm Street
Kearny, NJ 07032
(800) 572-5326
Fax: (201) 991-5870
www.dentalxchange.com/frames/frame184.htm

LACTONA/UNIVERSAL
201 Commerce Drive
Montgomeryville, PA 18936
(800) 523-2559
Fax: (215) 368-1659

LANG DENTAL MFG. CO., INC.
P.O. Box 969
175 Messner Drive

Wheeling, IL 60090
(800) 222-5264
Fax: (708) 215-6678
www.langdental.com

LARES RESEARCH
295 Lockheed Avenue
Chico, CA 95973
800-347-3289
Fax: (916) 345-1870
www.laresdental.com

LEACH & DILLON DENTAL PRODUCTS
5855 Oberlin
San Diego, CA 92121
(800) 375-9177
Fax: (619) 626-8686
www.argen.com

LEE PHARMACEUTICALS
1434 Santa Anita Avenue
South El Monte, CA 91733
(800) 950-5337
Fax: (818) 443-1561
www.leepharmaceuticals.com

MACAN ENGINEERING & MFG. CO.
1564 N. Damen
Chicago, IL 60622
(312) 772-2000
Fax: (312) 772-2003
www.macanengineering.com

MAILLEFER (*see* DENTSPLY INTERNATIONAL)

MEDIDENTA INTERNATIONAL, INC.
39-23 62nd Street
Woodside, NY 11377
(800) 221-0750
Fax: (718) 565-6208
www.medidenta.com

MEDESCO
23461 South Point Dr.
Laguna Hills, CA 92652
(800) 633-3726
Fax: (714) 588-9844
www.mtcnet.com/medesco.htm

MERRITT EZ CAST POST, INC.
609 Fleming St
Hendersonville, NC 28791
(828) 692-6226
Fax: (828) 692-6227
www.merrittezcastpost.com

METALOR DENTAL USA CORP.
255 John L. Dietsch Boulevard
P.O. Box 255
North Attleborough, MA 02761
(800) 554-5504
Fax: (508) 695-3447
www.metalor.com

MICROSTAR CORPORATION
4220 Steve Reynolds Blvd., Suite 19
Norcross GA 30093
(800) 313-6427
Fax: (770) 935-4460
www.microstarcorp.com

MIDWEST DENTAL PRODUCTS CORPORATION A DIVISION OF DENTSPLY INTERNATIONAL INC.
901 West Oakton St.
Des Plaines, IL 60018
(800) 800-2888
Fax: (800) 596-9190
www.midwestdental.com

MILES INC. (*see* HERAEUS KULZER, INC.)

MILTEX INSTRUMENT CO., INC.
700 Hicksville Road
Bethpage, NY 11714
(800) 645-8000
Fax: (516) 775-7185

MIRAGE DENTAL SYSTEMS (*see* CHAMELEON DENTAL PRODUCTS)

MISSION DENTAL, INC. (*see* KEYSTONE INDUSTRIES)

MIZZY, INC. (*see* KEYSTONE INDUSTRIES)

MODERN MATERIALS (*see* HERAEUS KULZER, INC.)

E.C. MOORE CO.
P.O. Box 353
Dearborn, MI 48121
(800) 331-3548
Fax: (313) 581-8348

J. MORITA USA, INC.
9 Mason
Irvine, CA 92618
(800) 752-9729
Fax: (949) 465-1095
www.jmoritausa.com

MOYCO TECHNOLOGIES, INC.
200 Commerce Drive
P.O. Box 505
Montgomeryville, PA 18936
(800) 331-8837
Fax: (215) 362-3809
www.pond.com/moyco/

MYRON INTERNATIONAL (*see* CHAMELEON DENTAL PRODUCTS)

NEOLOY PRODUCTS CO.
14807 S. McKinley Avenue
Posen, IL 60469
(800) 628-7336
Fax: (708) 371-8217

NEY DENTAL (*see* DEGUSSA-NEY DENTAL, INC.)

NIKON, INC., INSTRUMENT GROUP
1300 Walt Whitman Road
Melville, NY 11747
(516) 547-4200
Fax: (516) 547-0306
www.nikonusa.com

NOBEL BIOCARE USA, INC.
22895 Eastpark Drive,
Yorba Linda, CA 92887
(800) 993-8100
Fax: (714) 998-9236
www.nobelbiocare.se

OLYMPUS AMERICA, INC.
Precision Instrument Division
4 Nevada Drive
Lake Success, NY 11042
(800) 446-5967
Fax: (516) 328-9503
www.olympusamerica.com

ORASCOPTIC RESEARCH, INC.
5225-3 Verona Road
Madison, WI 53711
(800) 369-3698
Fax: (608) 278-0101
www.orascoptic.com

PAASCHE AIRBRUSH CO.
7440 W. Laurence Ave.
Harwood Heights, IL 60656
(800) 621-1907
Fax: (708) 867-9198
www.paascheairbrush.com

PANADENT CORPORATION
22573 Barton Road
Grand Terrace, CA 92324
(800) 368-9777
Fax: (909) 783-1896
www.panadent.com

PARAGON IMPLANT COMPANY
15821 Ventura Blvd, Suite 420
Encino, CA 91436
(800) 877-9991
Fax: (818) 789-3928
www.paragon-implant.com

PARKELL PRODUCTS
155 Schmitt Blvd.
Box 376
Farmingdale, NY 11735
(800) 243-7446
Fax: (516) 249-1242
www.parkell.com

PASCAL COMPANY, INC.
P.O. Box 1478
Bellevue, WA 98009
(800) 426-8051
Fax: (206) 827-6893
www.pascaldental.com

PATTERSON DENTAL COMPANY
1031 Mendota Heights Road
St. Paul, MN 55120
(800) 328-5536
www.pdental.com

PEERLESS INTERNATIONAL, INC.
438 Depot Street
South Easton, MA 02375
(800) 527-2025
Fax: (508) 230-2177
www.peerlessonline.com

PFINGST & CO., INC.
105 Snyder Road
P.O. Box 377
S. Plainfield, NJ 07080
(800) 221-1268
Fax: (908) 561-3213

PRECISION ROTARY INSTRUMENTS (*see* SDS KERR)

PREMIER DENTAL PRODUCTS CO.
3600 Horizon Avenue, Box 61574
King of Prussia, PA 19406
(888) 773-6872
Fax: (610) 239-6171
www.premusa.com

PRODONTA S.A. MICRO-MEGA *see* **MEDIDENTA INTERNATIONAL, INC.)**

PULPDENT CORP.
80 Oakland Street
P.O. Box 780
Watertown, MA 02272
(800) 343-4342
Fax: (617) 926-6262
www.pulpdent.com

J.R. RAND CORP.
100 S. East Jetryn Blvd.
Deer Park, NY 11729
(800) 526-7111
Fax: (516) 253-0505

RELIANCE DENTAL MFG. CO.
5805 W. 117th Place
Worth, IL 60482
(708) 597-6694
Fax: (708) 597-7560

ROYDENT DENTAL PRODUCTS, INC.
1010 West Hamlin Road
Rochester Hills, MI 48309
(800) 992-7767
Fax: (888) 769-3368
www.roydent.com

SATELLITE CITY, INC.
P.O. Box 836
Simi Valley, CA 93062
(805) 583-0994
Fax: (805) 527-9114

SDS KERR
1717 West Collins
Orange, CA 92867
(800) 537-7123
Fax: (800) 537-7345
www.kerrdental.com

HENRY SCHEIN, INC.
5 Harbor Park Drive
Port Washington, NY 11050
(800) 372-4346
Fax: (800) 732-7023
www.henryschein.com

SHOFU DENTAL CORP.
4025 Bohannon Dr.
Menlo Park, CA 94025
(415) 324-0085
Fax: (415) 323-3180
www.shofu.com

SIRONA USA
1200-A Westinghouse Blvd.
Charlotte, NC 28273

(704) 587-0453 ext.103
Fax: (704) 587-9394
www.sirona.com

SLAYCRIS PRODUCTS, INC.
1029 S.W. Washington Street
Portland, OR 97205
(503) 227-3583
Fax: (503) 227-6968

SOUTHERN DENTAL INDUSTRIES, INC.
246 First Street, Suite 204
San Francisco CA 94105
(800) 228-5166
(415) 975-8065
www.sdi.com.au

STAR DENTAL (*see* DEN-TAL-EZ/STAR DENTAL)

STERI-OSS INC. (*see* NOBEL BIOCARE USA, INC.)

STERNGOLD
23 Frank Mossberg Dr.
P.O. Box 2967
Attleboro, MA 02703
(800) 243-9942
Fax: (508) 226-5473
www.sterngold.com

STRAUMAN COMPANY
Reservoir Place 1601 Trapelo Road
Waltham, MA 02154
(800) 448-8168
Fax:(781) 890-6464
www.straumann.com

C.E. STUART
6663 W 120th Avenue
Suite 230
Broomfield, CO 80020
(800) 582-8190

SULZER CALCITEK, INC.
1900 Aston Avenue
Carlsbad, CA 92008
(760) 431-9515
Fax: (760) 431-7811
www.sulzercalcitek.com

SURGIDENT (*see* HERAEUS KULZER, INC.)

SURGITEL (*see* GENERAL SCIENTIFIC CORPORATION)

SUTER DENTAL MFG. CO., INC.
632 Cedar Street
Chico, CA 95928
(800) 368-8376
Fax: (916) 893-0473

GEORGE TAUB PRODUCTS & FUSION CO.
277 New York Avenue
Jersey City, NJ 07307
(800) 828-2634
Fax: (201) 659-7186

TELEDYNE WATER PIK
1730 E. Prospect Road
Fort Collins, CO 80553
(800) 525-2020

Fax: (800) 289-4389
www.waterpik.com

TEMREX CORPORATION
112 Albany Ave., P.O. Box 182,
Freeport, NY 11520
(800) 645-1226
Fax: (516) 868-5700
www.dentalxchange.com/temrex

THOMAS EXTRACTEUR DE PIVOTS
FFDM-Pneumat
Bourges
France
(33) 48246255

THOMPSON DENTAL MANUFACTURING COMPANY
1201 South 6th W.
Missoula, MT 59806
(800) 622-4222
Fax: (406) 728-4885
www.tdent.com

3I CORPORATION
20 William Street
Suite G90
Wellesley, MA 02481
(781) 235-9833
Fax: 781-235 9832
www.3i.com

3M-DENTAL PRODUCTS DIVISION
3M Center, 225-2SE-02
St. Paul, MN 55144
(800) 634-2249
Fax: (800) 888-3132
www.mmm.com/dental/

3M-UNITEK CORP.
2724 South Peck Rd.
Monrovia, CA 91016
(800) 423-4588
Fax: (818) 574-4793
www.mmm.com/market/dental/unitek

TICONIUM CO.
413 North Pearl St.
Albany, NY 12201
(800) 888-5868
Fax: (518) 434-1288

TRI HAWK
150 Highland Road
Massena NY 13662
(800) 874-4295
Fax: (315) 764-8128
www.trihawk.co

TMJ INSTRUMENT CO., INC.
1614 Industrial Avenue
Norco, CA 91760
(800) 225-5865
Fax: (909) 735-9979

TULSA DENTAL (*see* DENTSPLY INTERNATIONAL)

ULTRADENT PRODUCTS, INC.
505 W 10200 South
South Jordan, UT 84095
(800) 552-5512
Fax: (800) 842-9024
www.ultradent.com

UNION BROACH (*see* **MOYCO INDUSTRIES, INC.**)

VAN R DENTAL PRODUCTS
600 East Hueneme Road
Oxnard, CA 93033
(800) 833-8267
Fax: (800) 444-5170
www.vanr.com

VIDENT
3150 East Birch Street
Brea, California 92621
(800) 828-3839
Fax: (818) 962-4220
www.vident.com

VIVADENT USA, INC. (*see* **IVOCLAR NORTH AMERICA**)

WESTERN DENTAL SPECIALTIES/DENTAL POWER
3680 Charter Power Drive
San Jose, CA 95136
(800) 545-0727
Fax: (408) 266-0706

WHALEDENT INTERNATIONAL (*see* **COLTÈNE/WHALEDENT, INC.**)

WHIP MIX CORP.
361 Farmington Ave.
P.O. Box 17183
Louisville, KY 40217
(800) 626-5651
Fax: (502) 634-4512
www.whipmix.com

SS WHITE BURS, INC.
1145 Towbin Avenue
Lakewood, NJ 08701
(800) 535-2877
Fax: (908) 905-0987
www.sswhiteburs.com

THE WILKINSON COMPANY
590 Clearwater
Suite C, Selkirk Building
Post Falls, ID 83854

(208) 777-8332
(208) 777-8592

WILLIAMS DENTAL COMPANY, INC. (*see* **IVOCLAR NORTH AMERICA**)

WYKLE RESEARCH, INC.
2222 Hot Springs Road
Carson City, NV 89706
(800) 854-6641
Fax: (702) 882-7952

ZAHN DENTAL (**SEE HENRY SCHEIN, INC.**)

ZENITH
242 South Dean St.
Englewood, NJ 07631
(800) 662-6383
Fax: (201) 894-0213
www.dentalmaterial.com

ZEST ANCHORS, INC.
2061 Wineridge Place
Suite 100
Escondido, CA 92029
(800) 262-2310
Fax: (800) 487-1357
www.zestanchor.com

INDEX

A

Abfraction, 79
  clenching and, 94
Abrasion, 104, 730
  from bruxism, 94
  charting of, 13
  poor resistance of gypsum and, 433
Abrasive disk, 713
Abrasiveness of ceramic, 663
  polishing *versus* glazing and, 759
Abrasives for finishing-739, 738
Abscess, urgent treatment of, 76
Abutment, 79
Abutment analog, 335-336
Abutment driver, 328
Abutment healing cap, 328, 329
Abutment of implant, 330-333
Abutment post, 328, 336
Abutment teeth
  alignment during tooth preparation and, 196
  fiber-reinforced composite fixed prosthesis and, 701
  gingival preservation in residual ridge resorption and, 515-519
  indications for removable partial denture and, 74
  periodontal considerations, 108-134
    anatomy in, 108-109
    bone induction and, 119, 120
    classification of furcation involvements and, 121
    control of microbial plaque in, 113-115
    correction of defective restorations in, 115
    gingivectomy and, 116-117
    guided tissue regeneration and, 125-129, 130
    maintenance of periodontal status in, 129
    minor tooth movement and, 116
    mucosal repair and, 117-118
    odontoplasty-osteoplasty and, 122-123
    open debridement and, 117, 118
    osseous resection with apically positioned flaps and, 119-120
    periodontal disease and, 110-112
    prognosis in periodontal disease, 129-130
    provisionalization and, 124-125
    restoration of tooth with resected roots and, 125, 126, 127
    root amputation and, 123-124
    root anatomy and, 121-122
    root planing in, 115-116
    scaling and polishing in, 115
    stabilization of mobile teeth in, 116
    strategic tooth removal in, 116
    timing and sequence of treatment, 113
  replacement of single missing tooth and, 66-67

Abutment teeth—cont'd
  resin-retained fixed partial denture and, 683, 684-685
  retainer and, 62, 543-566
    attachments for, 557-562, 563
    bars, studs, and magnets for, 561-562, 563
    design of, 546-548
    extracoronal attachments for, 557, 558
    fabrication of crown for existing removable partial denture, 556-557
    finishing of, 555-556
    impression making for, 552
    intracoronal attachments for, 557-561, 562
    reciprocation and, 549
    retention and, 549
    tooth preparation for, 549-552
    try-in and cementation of, 556
    wax pattern fabrication for, 552-555
  selection of, 65-75
    indications for removable partial dentures, 74-75
    replacement of several missing teeth, 69-74
    replacement of single missing tooth, 65-69
Accelerated casting method, 582-583
Accelerator, 369, 377
AccessPost Overdenture, 291
Accufilm IV, 734
Achromatic, term, 605
Achromatic shade, 594
Achromatism, 598
Acid-etch technique, 265
Acid regurgitation
  abnormal tooth wear and, 97
  tooth damage caused by, 5
Acquired immunodeficiency syndrome, 6
Acquired pellicle, 110
Acrylic pontic, 526
Acrylic resin, 415
  in custom-made post, 297
  for custom tray fabrication, 364-365
  in fabrication of occlusal device, 100-103
  in provisionalization, 124-125
Acrylic resin record bases, 41
Acrylic resin veneer, 62
Acute necrotizing ulcerative gingivitis, 110
ADA type gypsum, 432, 435
  vacuum mixing of, 442-443
Adaptation, 484
  provision for adequate cement space and, 459
Add-on porcelain, 749
Addition silicone, 361, 363-364
Additive color mixture, 605
Adhesion bridge, 676-679
Adhesive failure of porcelain-metal interface, 619-620

Adhesive resin, 771
  for resin-retained fixed partial denture, 690, 691
Adjacent teeth, prevention of damage during tooth preparation, 166-167
Adjustable anterior guidance, 53
Advanced plaque-induced lesion, 112
Aestheti-Post, 290, 297
Agar, 49, 377
Agar hydrocolloid, 360, 361
Age
  chewing movements and, 92
  factor in prognosis of prosthodontic treatment, 19
Air cooling for heat generated during tooth preparation, 167
Air-firing, strength values and, 619
Airborne particle abrasion, 510, 693, 743
  with aluminum oxide, 618
  of cast alloy, 620
  before cementation, 772
  in finishing of cast restoration, 738
  to identify occlusal contacts, 752, 753
  for removal of investment, 611
  retention and, 185
  scanning micrograph of alumina and silicate particles, 679
  of slip-cast ceramic, 649, 652
  of veneering surface, 612, 613
Alcohol cleaning of metal framework, 613
Alginate, 26
Alignment
  evaluation of, 13, 15-16
  partial veneer crown and, 231
  tooth preparation and, 196
Alignment grooves for axial reduction, 208-209
All-Bond resin luting agent, 770
All-ceramic fixed partial dentures, 666
All-ceramic foundation restoration, 666-667
All-ceramic implant, 332
All-ceramic restoration, 262-271, 643-672
  aluminous core ceramics, 647, 648, 649, 650
  ceramic inlays and onlays, 265-267
  complete ceramic crown, 262-265
  esthetics and, 592-608
    balance in, 599, 600
    light and color in, 592-598
    midline and, 599-600
    proportion in, 598-599, 600
    shade selection and, 600-605
    smile anatomy in, 598, 599
  fixed partial dentures, 666
  foundation restoration, 666-667
  high-strength ceramics for, 644
  historical background of, 643-644
  hot-pressed ceramics, 653-656
  inlays and onlays, 665-666
  machined ceramics, 656-660
  metal-reinforced systems, 660-663